DENTAL LABORATORY PROCEDURES

FIXED PARTIAL DENTURES

VOLUME TWO

DENTAL LABORATORY PROCEDURES

FIXED PARTIAL DENTURES

JOHN E. RHOADS, B.S., D.D.S., F.A.C.D., F.I.C.D.
Formerly Associate Professor, Prosthetic Dentistry,
University of the Pacific, School of Dentistry,
San Francisco, California

KENNETH D. RUDD, D.D.S., F.A.C.D., F.I.C.D.
Associate Dean for Continuing Education,
Professor of Prosthodontics, Department of Prosthodontics,
The University of Texas Health Science Center
at San Antonio, Dental School,
San Antonio, Texas

ROBERT M. MORROW, D.D.S., F.A.C.D., F.I.C.D.
Associate Dean for Advanced Education,
Professor and Head, Postdoctoral Division, Department of Prosthodontics,
The University of Texas Health Science Center
at San Antonio, Dental School,
San Antonio, Texas

SECOND EDITION

with 1425 illustrations including 19 in full color

THE C. V. MOSBY COMPANY

ST. LOUIS · TORONTO · PRINCETON 1986

MOSBY

A TRADITION OF PUBLISHING EXCELLENCE

Editor: Darlene Warfel
Assistant Editor: Melba Steube
Manuscript Editor: Patricia J. Milstein
Designer: Jeanne Genz
Production: Barbara Merritt

SECOND EDITION

Printed in the United States of America

The C.V. Mosby Company
11830 Westline Industrial Drive, St. Louis, Missouri 63146

Library of Congress Cataloging in Publication Data
Main entry under title:

Dental laboratory procedures.

Contents: —v.1. Complete dentures—v.2. Fixed partial dentures—v.3. Removable partial dentures.
Includes bibliographies and index.
I. Dental technology—Laboratory manuals. I. Rhoads, John E. II. Rudd, Kenneth D. III. Morrow, Robert M., 1931– . [DNLM: I. Denture, Complete—laboratory manuals. 2. Technology, Dental—laboratory manuals. WU 500 D4135]
RK652,D47 1985 617.6 85-10599
ISBN 0-8016-4141-1 (v.2)

C/MV/MV 9 8 7 6 5 01/B 033

CONTRIBUTORS

WAYNE V. CAMPAGNI, B.S., D.M.D., F.A.C.D.

Associate Professor, Department of Restorative Dentistry, Ohio State University, College of Dentistry, Columbus, Ohio

C. WAYNE CASWELL, D.D.S., M.S.

Associate Professor, Director, Division of Occlusion and Fixed Prosthodontics, University of Florida, College of Dentistry, Gainesville, Florida

LEWIS A. CHAMBLESS, Jr., B.S., D.D.S.

Associate Professor, Fixed Prosthodontics, Baylor College of Dentistry, Dallas, Texas; Consultant, Post-graduate Prosthodontic Program, University of Missouri, Kansas City

RUSSELL T. DeVREUGD, C.D.T.

Dental Technologist, DeVreugd Dental Laboratory; Consultant and Lecturer, School of Dentistry, University of California, San Francisco, California

GORDON D. DOUGLASS, B.A., D.D.S., F.A.C.D.

Associate Clinical Professor, School of Dentistry, University of California, San Francisco; Consultant, Veterans Administration Hospital, Martinez, California

†HAROLD F. EISSMANN, D.D.S., F.A.C.D.

Formerly Clinical Professor, Department of Restorative Dentistry, School of Dentistry, University of California, San Francisco, California

NILES F. GUICHET, D.D.S

Diplomate, American Board of Prosthodontics; President, Society for Occlusal Studies, Anaheim, California

HAJIME HAMAGUCHI, D.D.S.

Clinical Professor, Department of Restorative Dentistry, School of Dentistry, University of California, San Francisco, California

MALCOLM D. JENDRESEN, D.D.S., Ph.D.

Professor and Chairman, Department of Restorative Dentistry, School of Dentistry, University of California, San Francisco, California

ALTON M. LACY, Ph.D., D.D.S.

Associate Professor, Department of Restorative Dentistry, School of Dentistry, University of California, San Francisco, California

CALVIN S. LAU, D.D.S.

Clinical Associate Professor, Department of Practice Dynamics, University of Southern California, School of Dentistry, Los Angeles, California

DOUGLAS B. LAW, B.S., D.D.S.

Lieutenant Colonel, U.S. Army Dental Corps, 98th Medical Detachment

BILL B. LEFLER, D.D.S.

Brigadier General, U.S. Army Dental Corps, Headquarters, 7th Medical Command

KENNETH A. MALAMENT, D.D.S., M.Sc.D.

Private Practice, Brookline, Massachusetts

CHARLES McNEILL III, D.D.S., F.A.C.D., F.I.C.D.

Associate Professor, Department of Restorative Dentistry; Director, Postgraduate Continuing Education Study Groups in Occlusion and Articulation, School of Dentistry, University of California, San Francisco

†Deceased.

ROBERT A. MELI, B.S., D.D.S.

Formerly Lecturer, Department of Restorative Dentistry, School of Dentistry, University of California, San Francisco, California

MERRILL C. MENSOR, B.A., D.D.S., F.I.C.D.

Formerly Assistant Clinical Professor, Department of Fixed Prosthodontics, University of the Pacific, School of Dentistry, San Francisco, California; Consultant, Veterans Administration Medical Centers

EVERITT V. PAYNE, D.D.S., F.A.C.D.

Professor, Department of Operative Dentistry, Baylor College of Dentistry, Dallas, Texas

RYLE A. RADKE, D.D.S., F.A.C.D.

Associate Professor, School of Dentistry, University of California, San Francisco, California

THOMAS G. REDDY, Jr., B.S., D.D.S.

Colonel, U.S. Army Dental Corps, San Francisco, California

JOHN E. RHOADS, B.S., D.D.S., F.A.C.D., F.I.C.D.

Formerly Associate Professor, Prosthetic Dentistry, University of the Pacific, School of Dentistry, San Francisco, California

ROBERT C. SPROULL, D.D.S., F.A.C.D.

Regional Consultant, Veterans Administration Hospital; Consultant, William Beaumont Medical Center, El Paso, Texas

ROBERT S. STAFFANOU, D.D.S., M.S., F.A.C.D.

Professor and Chairman, Department of Fixed Prosthodontics, Baylor College of Dentistry, Dallas, Texas

CLIFFORD L. STOCKS, D.D.S.

Formerly with Division of Biomaterials, School of Dentistry, University of California, San Francisco, California

G. ROGER TROENDLE, B.S., D.D.S., M.S.

Clinical Assistant Professor, Department of Prosthetic and Restorative Dentistry, University of Texas Health Science Center at San Antonio, Dental School, San Antonio, Texas

VERN M. TUELLER, D.D.S.

Clinical Professor and Chairperson, Division of Fixed Prosthodontics, School of Dentistry, University of California, San Francisco, California

HENRY N. YAMADA, D.D.S.

Clinical Associate Professor, Department of Biomaterials, University of Southern California, School of Dentistry, Los Angeles, California

It has been said that great men cast long shadows. Dentistry is deeply indebted to the great teachers of unusually high caliber who, through their knowledge, expertise, and generosity, have led the way toward enlightenment and improvement of our profession. To one of these giants, Dr. Harold F. Eissmann, this second edition is respectfully and humbly dedicated.

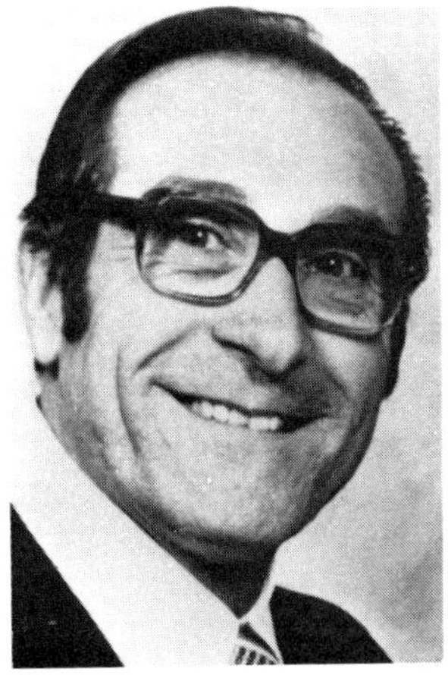

PREFACE

In undertaking the revision of this edition, we are working in the shadow of the late Harold F. Eissmann, whose great knowledge, talent, and expertise are rarely equalled. His loss has been felt by us personally and by the profession as well. His teachings have greatly influenced dentistry's understanding of esthetic concepts and the application of physiologic principles toward the improvement of cosmetic and hygienic restorations. The fundamental designs and concepts that he presented so beautifully have been retained without modification—first, in deference to his memory, and second, because it was felt that no improvement could be made. However, there has been a reorganization of the subject matter for better continuity, with updating of techniques, materials, and application of research findings.

We would be ungrateful if we did not express our gratitude to the many contributors without whose efforts this revision would have been impractical, if not impossible, to accomplish. Our sincere thanks is also extended to the many manufacturers who so graciously supplied photographs and descriptions of the equipment presented in the chapter on dental laboratory equipment. We are indebted to the teachers, practitioners, and students who have evaluated the current edition and offered suggestions for its improvement.

Much credit is due those individuals who, after discovery and development of techniques and processes, have presented them to the profession through publication in the scientific literature and through their own individual presentations. We are indebted to those whose contributions we have drawn upon for presentation in this revision.

We offer our heartfelt thanks to the clerical staff, primarily Mrs. Marjorie C. Rhoads, who has acted as secretary, typist, confidant, and "ear" in the development of this revision. Without her ever-present help the task would have been next to impossible.

It is hoped that this revision will satisfy the need for which it is intended in dental literature.

John E. Rhoads
Kenneth D. Rudd
Robert M. Morrow

CONTENTS

COLOR PLATES *following p. 256*

CHAPTER 1

IMPRESSIONS AND CASTS

inelastic impression materials Impression materials that cannot be removed intact from undercut areas, for example, impression compound, plaster, zinc oxide–eugenol pastes, and electrolytic waxes.

elastic impression materials Impression materials that can be removed intact from undercut areas if they are not too severe, for example, reversible hydrocolloids, irreversible hydrocolloids, polysulfides (mercaptans, Thiokols), silicones, polyethers, and polysiloxanes.

PART ONE

Impression materials and techniques

VERN M. TUELLER

SELECTION OF IMPRESSION MATERIAL

In addition to elasticity or lack of it, two major considerations in the selection of an impression material must be included: dimensional accuracy and stability, and the ability of the material to reproduce intricate detail. The material should be selected according to the intended use of the resultant cast and the severity of undercut areas that must be reproduced with accuracy. Irreversible hydrocolloid, for example, can be used in the production diagnostic casts or casts that will provide opposing occlusion. Although most irreversible hydrocolloid materials possess an acceptable dimensional stability, as a group they lack the ability to reproduce fine detail.

In those situations where greatest accuracy and the ability to reproduce finest detail are necessary (working dies for production of fine castings), either reversible hydrocolloid, polysulfide, silicone, or polysiloxane impression material would be appropriate. The clinical application of each of these products will be described, the extent and detail proportionate to the current popularity.

INELASTIC IMPRESSION MATERIALS

Impression compound

Impression waxes (compound) have been used effectively for making impressions of teeth prepared for complete crowns or simple inlays. These, being thermoplastic, require a confining tubular copper band or other rigid carrier for support when they are in the plastic state and to prevent deformation after chilling and removal from the prepared tooth or area being impressed (Fig. 1-1). Copper tube impressions can be used to advantage in those situations where the margins of the preparation are below the level of the gingival tissue. Care must be exercised that damage to the fibers of the periodontal ligament does not occur from the sharp edge of the confining band. If the impression material is heated to too high a temperature, damage to the dental pulp may occur during adaptation of the heated material to the prepared tooth surfaces.

Several different types of die materials may be employed in conjunction with impression compound–copper tube impressions. This material can be electroplated easily to produce copper or silver electroformed dies. Improved Hydrocal and epoxy die material can also be used effectively to produce working dies. After the die material has set, the impression compound is softened in hot water to facilitate removal from the die without damage.

There are several different types of impression waxes (compound) classed according to softening temperature (high, medium, low). They have also been classified according to the intended use and form in which they are

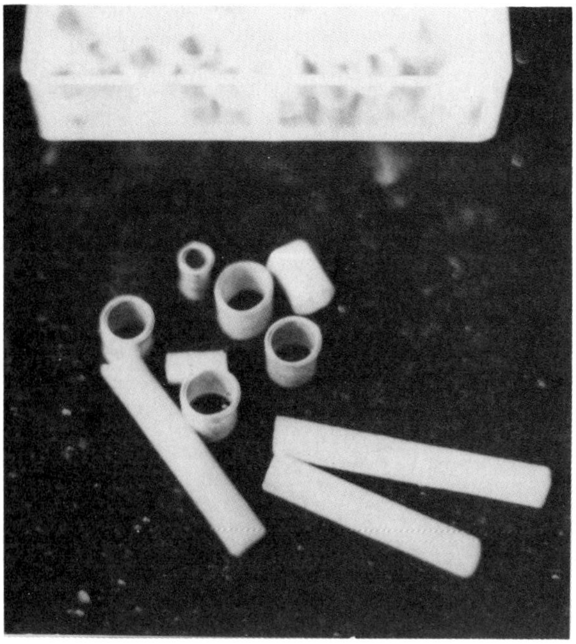

Fig. 1-1. Copper bands (assorted sizes) and stick compound.

supplied by the manufacturer. Type I or true *impression compound* is employed in those instances where the final surface characteristics, dimension, and detail are to be recorded in the impression material. Type II or *tray* compound is usually employed to make the preliminary border molded reproduction of edentulous areas. This procedure is followed by a secondary or "wash" impression, which employs the primary impression as a carrier, and which is used to record the fine detail and surface characteristics. This approach is of particular interest, since it probably was the precursor of our two-stage silicone impression, a method introduced in the 1960s and still enjoying great popularity. Polysulfides can also be used in this two-stage fashion, which will be described in detail.

Impression plaster

Impression plasters are plaster of Paris (calcium sulfate hemihydrate) to which modifiers have been added to regulate the setting time and to control setting expansion. Except for occasional use in the making of impressions of fully edentulous arches, these materials are now used primarily in producing indexes for soldering, remounting procedures, and interocclusal records. The rapid setting time is of great advantage when intraoral records are to be obtained. The rigidity and lack of distortion after setting are of particular advantage in indexing castings for soldering, transfer impressions, and accurate evaluation in refining the occlusion in rehabilitation procedures.

Zinc oxide–eugenol impression pastes

Zinc oxide–eugenol impression materials are extremely effective for the final impression when used in conjunction with a border molded impression of an edentulous ridge or arch. The reproduction of the fine detail of tissue surfaces makes them especially useful in obtaining impressions for mucostatic and altered cast techniques. Although several of these products are supplied in the traditional powder/liquid form, most are now supplied in easy-to-use paste form. One tube contains the formulated zinc oxide portion, and another contains the eugenol/rosin portion in paste form.

Accelerators, plasticizers, and fillers provide desirable properties to the basic zinc oxide–eugenol compound. The setting time and viscosity can be controlled by mixing conditions to provide the particular characteristics for a specific clinical procedure.

ELASTIC IMPRESSION MATERIALS

The accurate and detailed reproduction of the surfaces and contours of the teeth and associated soft tissues, including deeply undercut areas, requires an impression material that is sufficiently elastic to undergo deformation during the process of its removal from the subject and yet return to its original form and dimension without permanent deformation.

Impressions using elastic materials

Certain inaccuracies are inherent in all elastic impression materials. These inaccuracies center around the dimensional stability of the gelled or polymerized material and the elastic limit as evidenced by the ability of the material to reproduce severe undercut areas without permanent deformation.

The dimensional instability of the hydrocolloids and other water-based materials can be the result of loss of water volume and syneresis. Inaccuracy of elastomers can be the result of continued polymerization over an extended period of time.

It is well known that all elastomers that polymerize by a condensation reaction exhibit a certain degree of shrinkage that can continue for considerable time after the "clinical set" of the material.

All techniques that employ any of these elastic materials should be designed to minimize the inaccuracies inherent in them. General rules can be developed for the use of all elastic materials. Adherance to them will produce greater accuracy of the resultant casts.

GENERAL RULES

1. The tray or carrier must be rigid.
2. The impression material should be securely attached to the tray by adhesive, retentive holes, or locking rims.

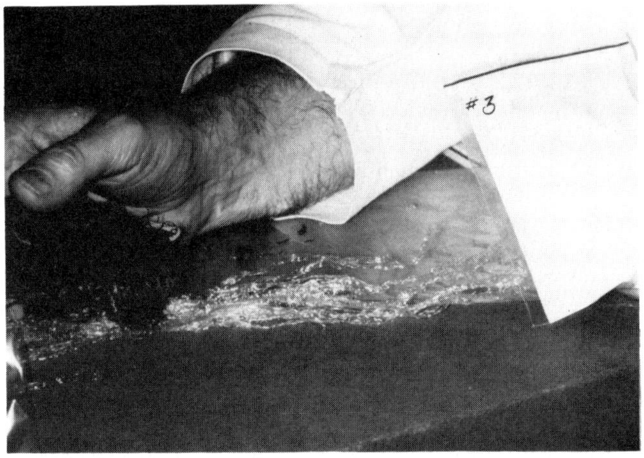

Fig. 1-2. Reversible hydrocolloid in various processing steps: *(left to right)* raw dried agar, processed agar in strands, and powdered agar containing some additives.

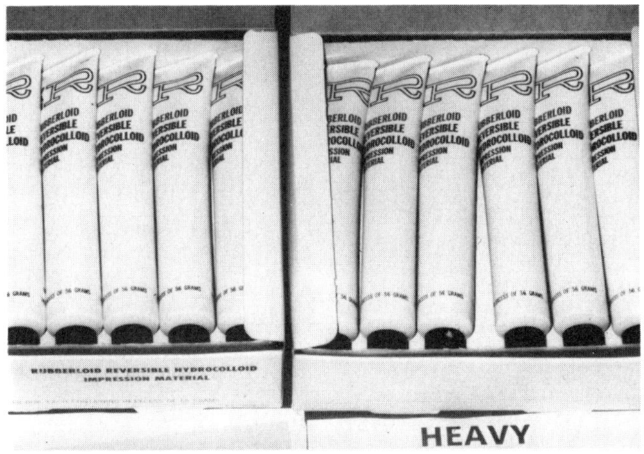

Fig. 1-3. Packaged reversible hydrocolloid in tubes (Poly tubes).

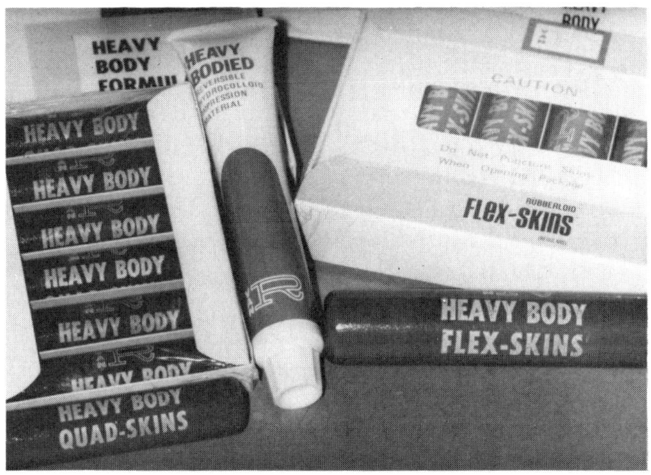

Fig. 1-4. Reversible hydrocolloid in plastic jackets.

3. The tray should be designed to allow a minimum thickness of impression material. Custom-made trays or stock trays modified with fillers are effective in controlling a uniform minimum amount of the impression material.

4. The cast material should be introduced into the impression as soon as practical after removal from the mouth. In the event that pouring of the impression must be delayed, care must be exercised to protect it from dehydration.

Inaccuracies that result from dimensional change of the impression material can be minimized by adherance to these rules. Inaccuracies that result from the limitation of the elasticity of the material can be controlled by eliminating or minimizing the undercut areas in preparation of the mouth so that the material is not overstressed.

The development of impression materials that could be applied to the area to be reproduced in a viscous condition and gel or "set" into a flexible elastic mass, which could return to its former dimensions, has been instrumental in the progress in much of fixed prosthodontics.

Water-based materials, colloidal in nature, have provided a basis for development of the elastic materials currently in use. More recently, the elastomeric materials, rubberlike in character, have given prosthetic and restorative dentistry the means to produce extremely accurate and finely detailed casts of the teeth.

Reversible hydrocolloid

Reversible hydrocolloid impression materials are essentially a suspension of agar particles in water with fillers and chemical agents that alter the physical properties of the material to best suit it to dentistry's use (Figs. 1-2 to 1-4). It is liquefied by heating to the boiling point of water and then cooled to a lower temperature (140 to 150° F, 61° to 65° C) for storage and manipulation. Immediately before insertion of the material into the oral cavity it is cooled or tempered to a point just above the gelling temperature (110° to 115° F, 44° to 46° C). At this temperature the material can be adapted to the teeth and tissues and then cooled to form a *gel* that provides the necessary body, elasticity, and ability to withstand permanent deformation during withdrawal. Technical aspects of the development and control of the physical properties of the material are described in textbooks dealing with dental biomaterials and will not be described here. The reader is referred to these publications for more technical information. Discussion will be limited to clinical application.

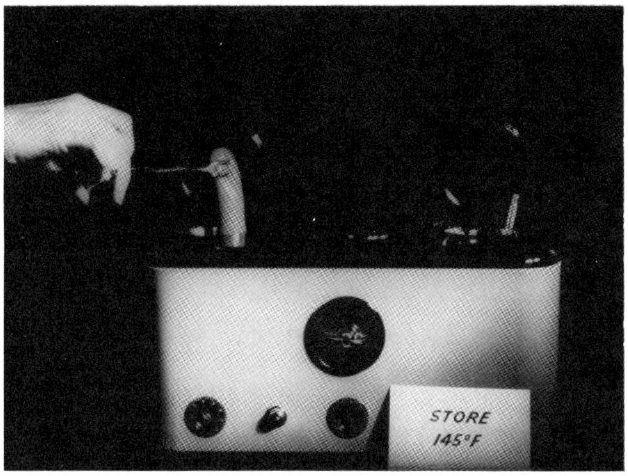

Fig. 1-5. Removing liquefied hydrocolloid from boiling bath.

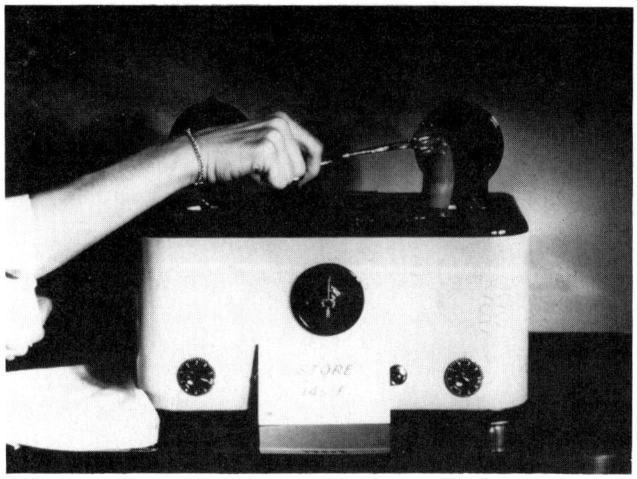

Fig. 1-6. Placing liquefied hydrocolloid in storage bath.

TYPICAL TECHNIQUE

For satisfactory use, hydrocolloid impression materials must be heated in a water bath to a temperature sufficiently high to change the material from the *gel* phase to the *sol* phase. This usually occurs at approximately the boiling point of water (212° F, 100° C). At high altitudes, where water boils at a lower temperature, liquefaction is usually accomplished under pressure in a closed vessel similar to an autoclave. Pressure-cooking pots have been used to advantage for attaining the desired liquefying temperature.

After liquefaction the impression material may be stored for as long as 8 to 10 hours in a water bath at approximately 145° to 150° F (63° to 65° C). It is not advisable to store the material in this bath for extended periods of time. Experience has shown that hydrocolloid materials tend to deteriorate if they are reliquefied repeatedly from the gelled state. An effort should be made to prepare (liquefy) only enough material for 1 day's anticipated use (Figs. 1-5 and 1-6).

Immediately before use (5 to 11 minutes), the impression material is placed into the prewarmed impression tray and tempered in a water bath. It is cooled to a temperature that can be tolerated by delicate oral tissues without injury (110° to 115° F, 44° to 46° C) (Fig. 1-7). Precaution should be taken to assure that the material is not so warm that the mouth tissues may be burned. Hydrocolloid materials have great potential for holding heat within the mass. Although surface temperatures may seem compatible, the temperature within the material may be sufficiently high to cause injury to the tissues.

The tempering of the impression material allows increased viscosity to develop. The increased firmness of the material in the tray will assure adequate adaptation of the material to the surfaces to be impressed.

Any retraction cord is removed from the tissue adjacent to the teeth and hydrocolloid material is injected from a suitable syringe into the critical areas.

Injection material is placed in small syringes developed for this purpose and processed in a manner similar to that just described. Because of the more rapid cooling of the impression material as it is extruded from the needle of the syringe, it is used directly from the storage bath without being immersed in the lower-temperature tempering bath.

The injected material should be placed with one continuous motion, into the more challenging areas first. Immediately after injection of the syringe material, the surface of the tray material is wiped with a 2 × 2 inch sponge on retrieval from the tempering bath, the water hose coupling is connected, and the tray is placed (Fig. 1-8).

Wiping the surface of the tray material ensures a bond between the injected hydrocolloid and the tray hydrocolloid. When the tray reaches the set position, which has been predetermined by try-ins and the use of stops, the waterflow is begun.

If the water temperature is between 68° and 74° F (20° to 24° C), an average size, full-arch impression will usually gel completely in 6 minutes. Quadrants require a little less time, and extremely large trays may require more. Cooling (gelling) water in the range indicated is ideal for this maturation process. Some believe that a radically cooler temperature can deform the negative. Certainly, on the other end of the scale, if the water is above 80° F (27° C), it will take longer for gelation or it will be necessary to add ice before running it through the system.

Packaging of the material varies: tubes (Poly tubes),

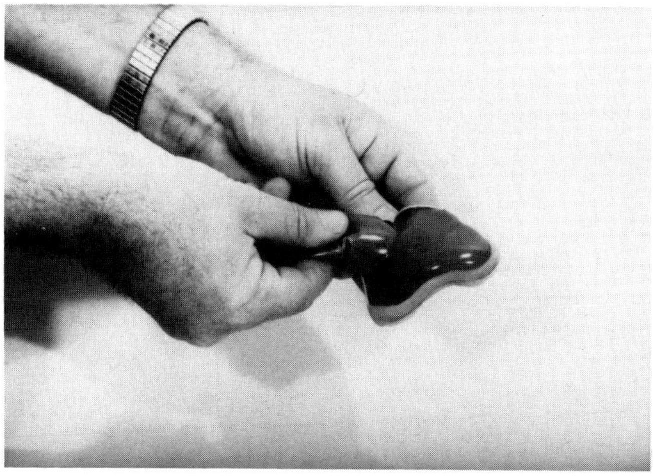

Fig. 1-7. Loading tray just before placement in tempering bath.

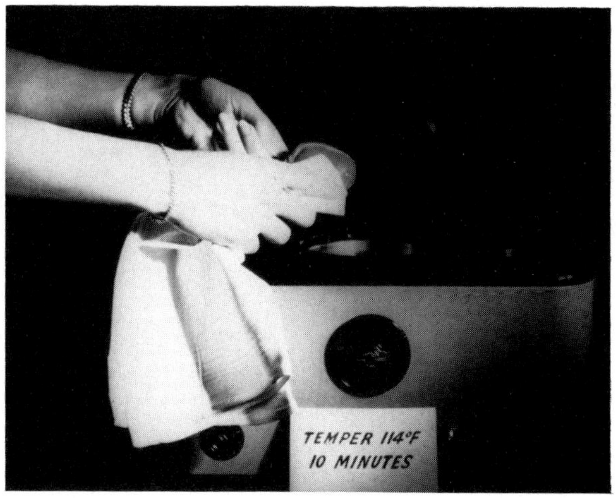

Fig. 1-8. "Freshening" surface of tray material just before placement in mouth.

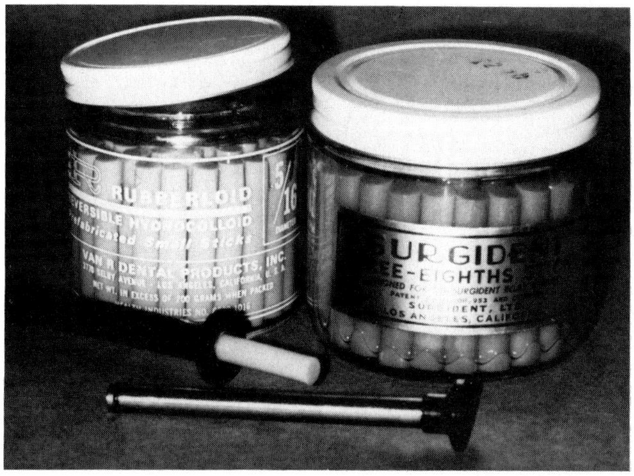

Fig. 1-9. Reversible hydrocolloid in sticks to place in syringes.

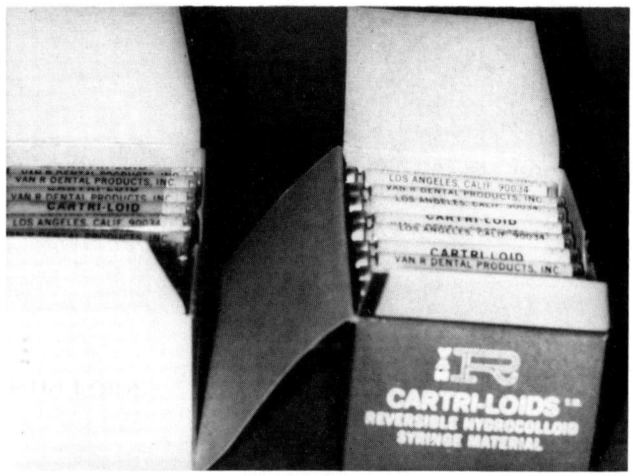

Fig. 1-10. Reversible hydrocolloid packaged in glass cartridges (Carpules).

plastic jackets, sticks in jars, and even glass, rubber-stoppered cartridges (Carpules). These different methods are intended to provide the operator with a means of injecting the liquefied material into the field and then following with a tray of much more viscous material. Different means of packaging are shown in Figs. 1-9 to 1-10.

There are at least three ways of handling the syringe material: (1) loading the sticks of material into Teflon syringes, boiling, and storing them with the tray material, (2) using material packaged in injection cartridges (Carpules) and then using the anesthetic syringe for injecting, or (3) using a backloading Poly tube that fits precisely into the cylinder of the Teflon syringe; these can be used to replenish syringe material coming directly from the storage bath (Figs. 1-11 to 1-15).

When complete gelation is reached, the tray is removed with a positive controlled thrust. Walking the hydrocolloid tray out of the mouth in a laborious fashion invites the possibility of tearing fragile extensions. Hydrocolloid has little tensile strength but is retrievable from even small precarious areas if done with one quick movement. This property can be portrayed by holding a stick of hydrocolloid and bending it on itself 180 degrees and then quickly letting it return to the original position. If this is done quickly, the material can tolerate this tension many times, but if done slowly, even the first bend will result in fissuring and then complete separation of the halves (Figs. 1-16 to 1-18).

After retrieval from the mouth, the impression should be trimmed of excess peripheral material and placed in a 2% potassium sulfate bath or in 100% hu-

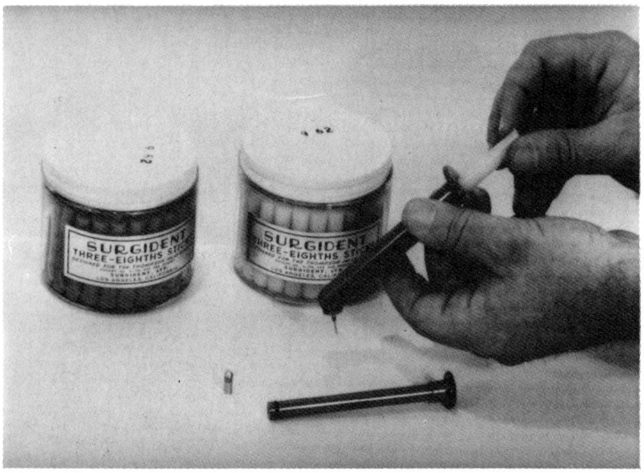

Fig. 1-11. Loading reversible hydrocolloid sticks into syringe.

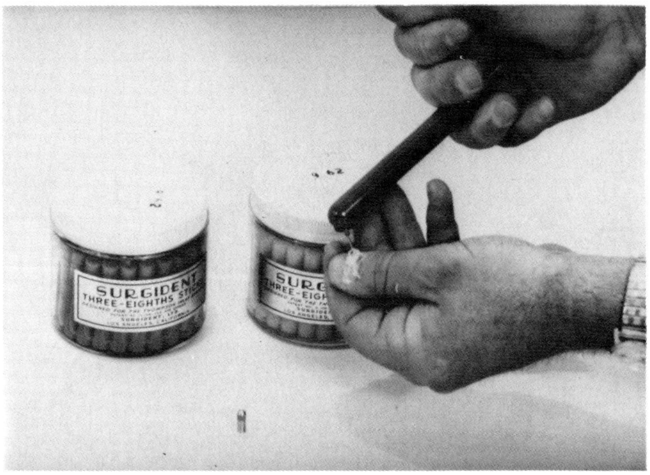

Fig. 1-12. Clearing syringe tip by extruding some of gelled material.

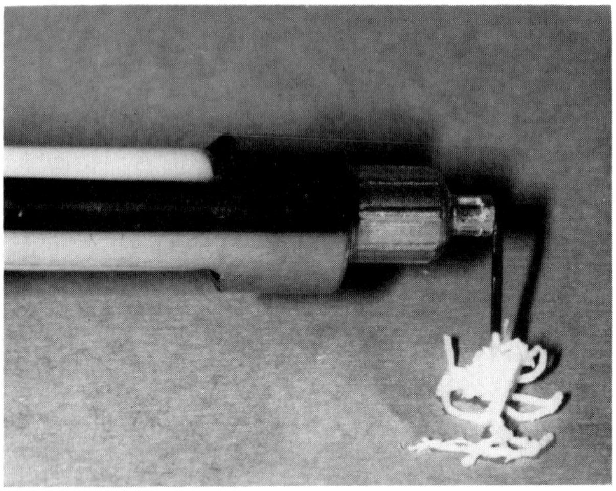

Fig. 1-13. Example of packaging injectable material in Carpule.

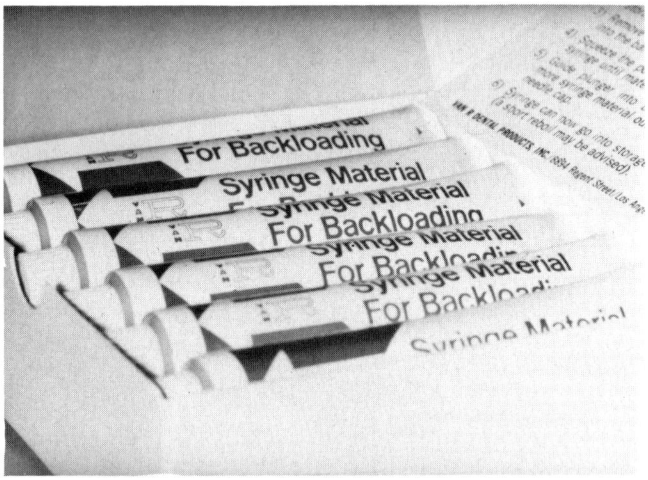

Fig. 1-14. Material used for "back-loading" method of filling syringe.

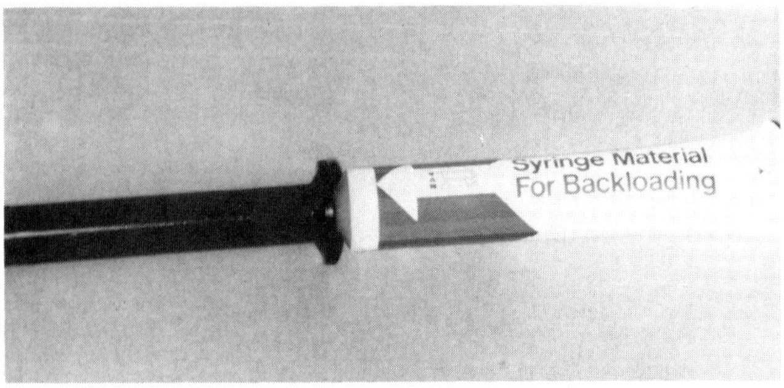

Fig. 1-15. Filling syringe by back-loading procedure.

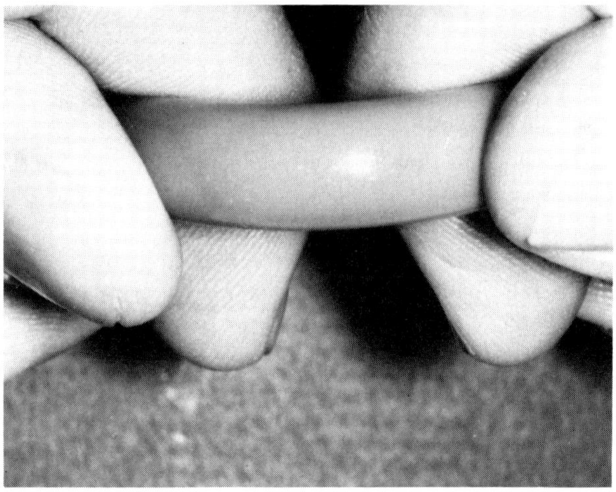

Fig. 1-16. No tearing where stick of reversible hydrocolloid is bent quickly.

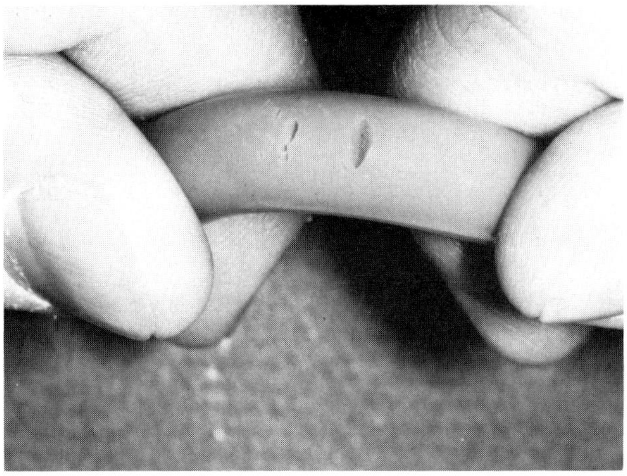

Fig. 1-17. When held in stressed position for just 1 or 2 seconds, hydrocolloid begins to fissure.

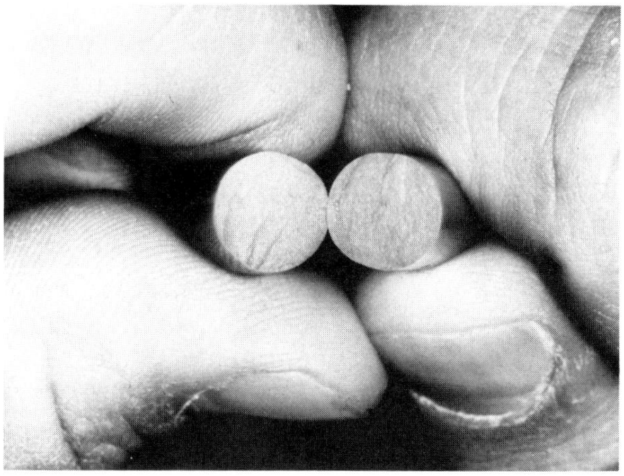

Fig. 1-18. Hydrocolloid under maintained tension severs completely.

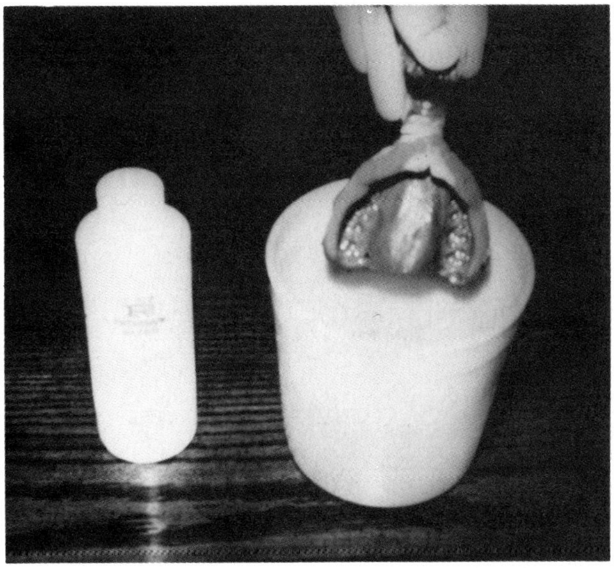

Fig. 1-19. Placing retrieved impression in 2% potassium sulfate bath.

midity (Fig. 1-19). Placing the impression in tap water, even for cleaning, is not recommended, since control of water volume is critical at this time.

The potassium sulfate bath accomplishes two main objectives: (1) control of water volume and (2) better surface integrity in the stone pour. Since most modern hydrocolloid formulas have potassium sulfate in them, some believe the bath is redundant. If the chemical bath is not used, an enclosed 100% humidity environment should be used until the cast is poured.

The stone should be hard die stone and vacuum mixed. Excess moisture in the negative can be handled by "running" it on a vibrator ahead of the properly mixed stone, until it runs out of the distal aspect of the pour (Figs. 1-20 and 1-21).

The pour is not inverted because this can cause "sagging" in the cast. The maturing stone should also be kept in 100% humidity until separation—the recommended time is 40 to 60 minutes, depending on the stone used (Fig. 1-22).

Irreversible hydrocolloids

Irreversible hydrocolloid, commonly called *alginate*, was introduced during World War II when agar was difficult to obtain, Japan being one of the largest producers. The use of this material exceeds all other impression materials. Alginate is usually the impression material of choice for production of orthodontic casts, diagnostic casts for prosthodontics, and working casts to function as opposing occlusion.

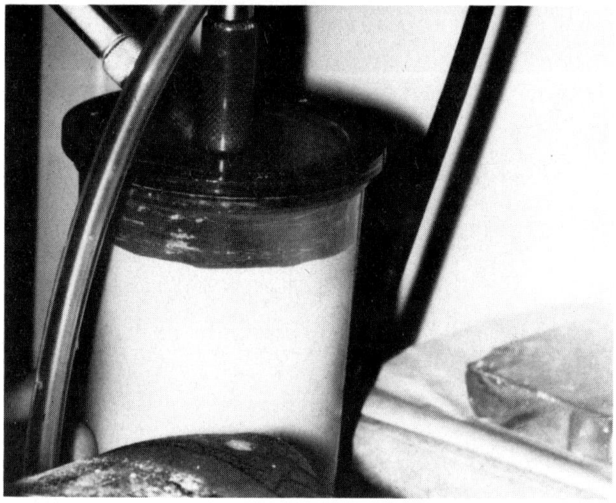

Fig. 1-20. Device for mechanical spatulation under vacuum.

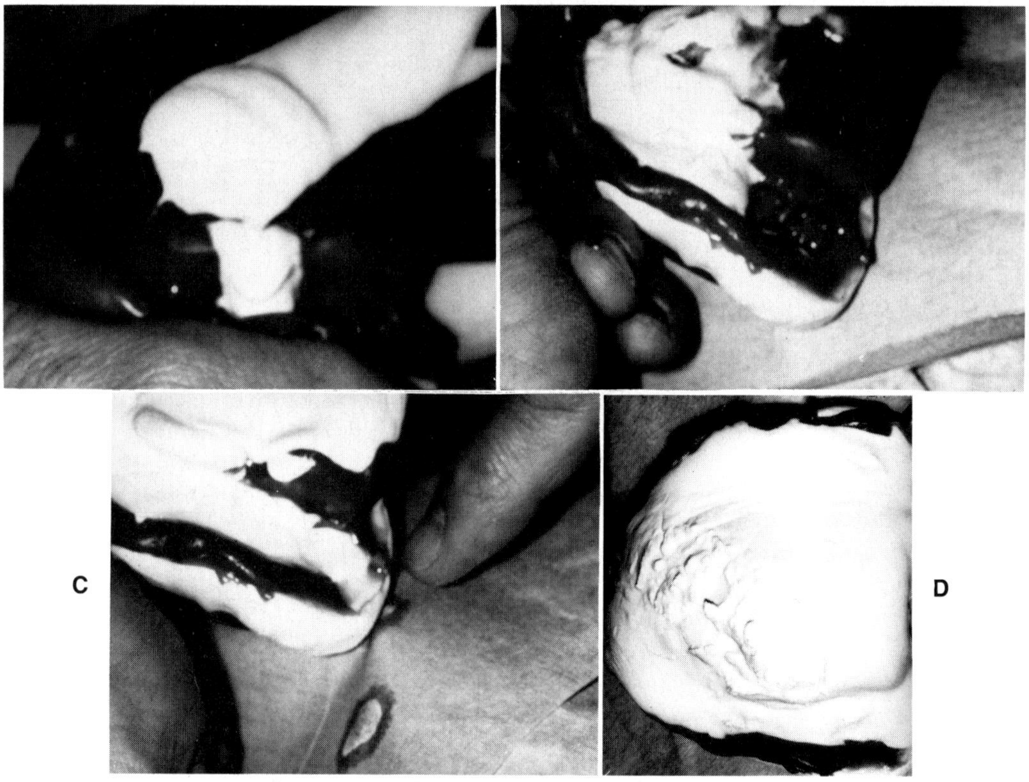

Fig. 1-21. Proper pouring of hydrocolloid impression **(A),** keeping excess moisture ahead of stone **(B),** carrying (pushing it out distal end of tray) **(C),** and impression completely poured **(D).**

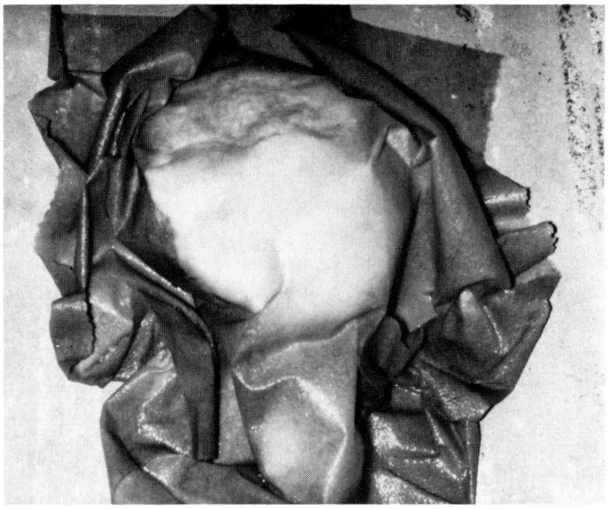

Fig. 1-22. If no enclosed humidifier is available, damp paper towel may be placed over pour for maturation period.

An irreversible chemical reaction is involved in setting the alginates. Actually two reactions occur: (1) calcium sulfate and trisodium phosphate give rise to calcium phosphate and sodium sulfate, then (2) when the supply of trisodium phosphate is exhausted, the calcium ions begin to react with the potassium alginate to produce calcium alginate. The two reactions occur as follows:

$$2Na_3PO_4 + 3CaSO_4 \rightarrow Ca_3(PO_4)_2 + 3Na_2SO_4 \quad (1)$$

$$K_nAlg + \frac{n}{2}CaSO_4 \rightarrow \frac{n}{2}K_2SO_4 + Ca_{\frac{n}{2}}Alg \quad (2)$$

A typical formulation of a current alginate by weight might be:

Diatomaceous earth	50%
Potassium alginate	20%
Calcium sulfate	16%
Zinc oxide	7%
Potassium titanium fluoride	6%
Sodium phosphate	1%

Potassium alginate and calcium sulfate are the main reactors. Diatomaceous earth is added as a filler; it increases strength and stiffness and produces a smooth texture and surface. Zinc oxide also acts as a filler and helps control the setting time. Potassium titanium fluoride assures a hard, dense stone surface in the cast, and sodium phosphate retards the setting time (Figs. 1-23 and 1-24).

When used properly the alginates have good dimensional stability, but have inherent difficulty in reproducing detail faithfully.

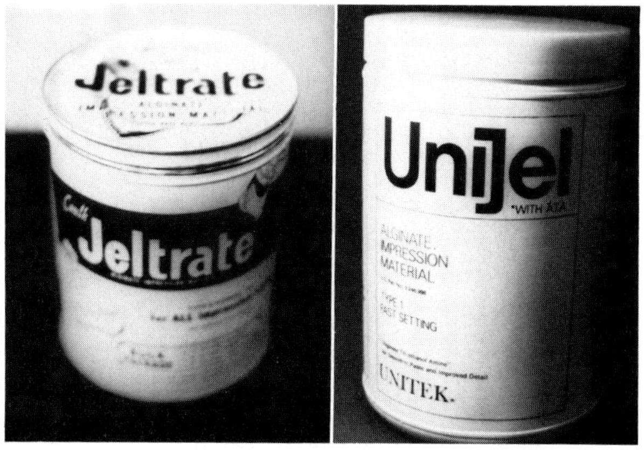

A **B**

Fig. 1-23. Two brands of alginates packaged in tins.

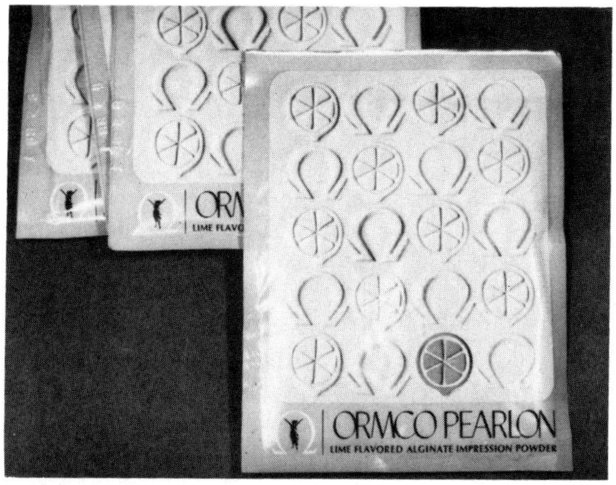

Fig. 1-24. Alginate packaged in individual envelopes.

TYPICAL TECHNIQUE

1. An appropriate tray or carrier is selected. A rigid tray with retentive elements in the form of a rim-lock or perforations that will allow the impression material to be firmly attached is recommended (Fig. 1-25). The alginate powder is agitated by rolling or shaking the container to ensure complete mixing of the contents. The powder (Fig. 1-26) and liquid are accurately measured.

2. In mixing, the rule of adding the powder to the liquid will tend to reduce entrapment of air. A wiping or spreading action of the broad spatula over the sides of the mixing bowel will aid in the production of a mix of impression material that is relatively bubble free.

3. The teeth should be clean and free of plaque and debris. The teeth and tissues should be moist but with any excess saliva removed by absorption from gauze sponges. The alginate material, at times, will adhere to

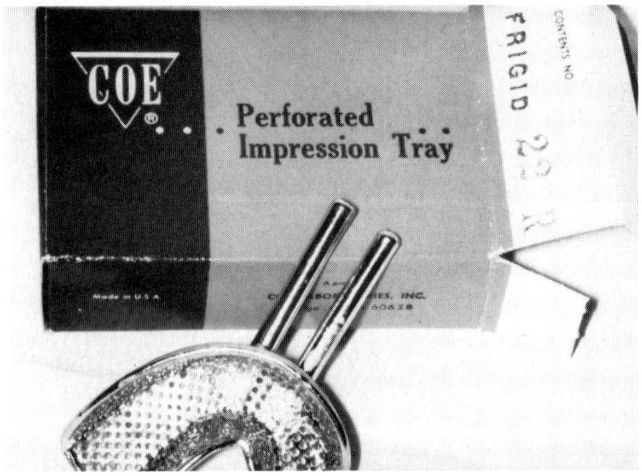

Fig. 1-25. Metal tray with rim lock and perforations for better retention of materials.

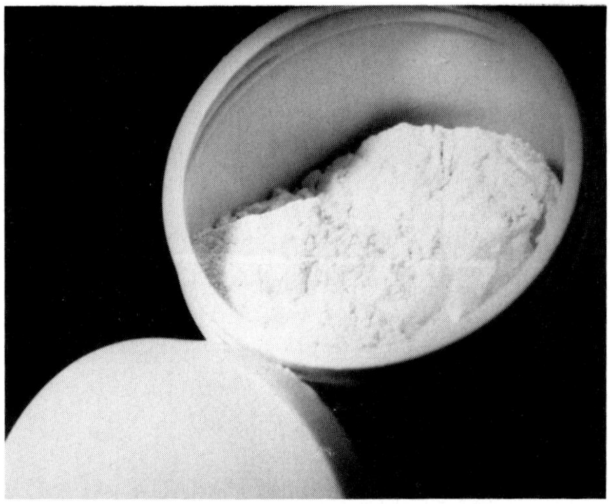

Fig. 1-26. Fluffed alginate ready for use.

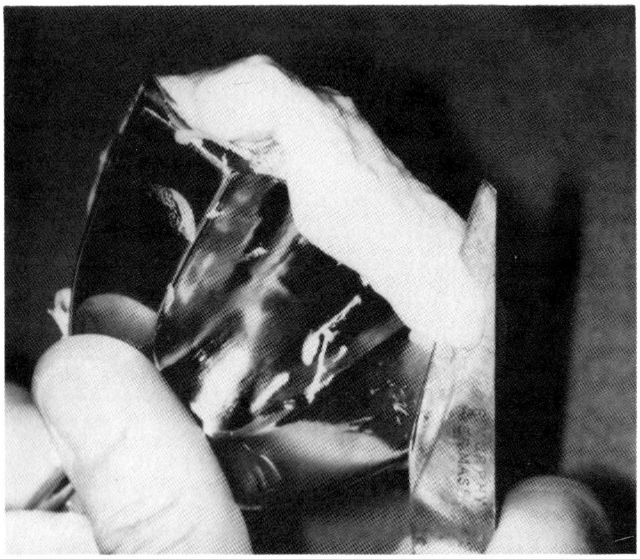

Fig. 1-27. Retrieved tray with excess material extending well beyond tray rim. (This material is trimmed away so that as tray is placed on bench following pour, no distortion will be relayed from redundant material to material inside tray.)

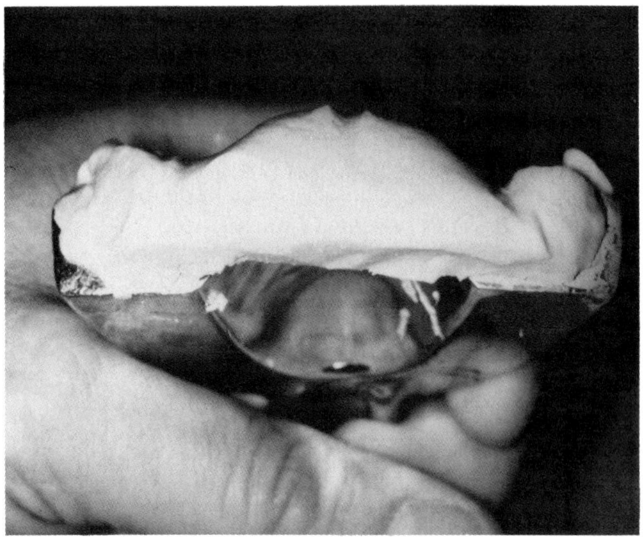

Fig. 1-28. Properly trimmed tray with no material extending beyond horizontal elevation of tray.

tooth structure that is absolutely dry. An excess of saliva around the teeth will cause bubbles in the interproximal areas and on the occlusal surfaces of the teeth. Air bubbles in the completed impression can be minimized by careful application of the impression material to the teeth and into the vestibular areas before placement of the filled tray.

4. The filled tray is joined to the preplaced material and seated. It should be held passively and motionless during the setting of the impression material.

5. Following setting (gelation) of the impression material the tray should be separated quickly from the teeth to avoid rocking and possible deformation of the fine areas of the impression. Excess material at the periphery of the impression should be trimmed (Figs. 1-27 and 1-28) and the impression stored in an environment of 100% humidity.

6. Cast material should be introduced into the impression as soon as practical and the poured impression returned to a humidor until setting is complete. The cast should be separated from the impression after 45 to 60 minutes.

GUIDELINES FOR MAKING ALGINATE IMPRESSIONS

1. A rigid tray that has positive retentive elements to prevent separation of the impression material from the tray is necessary. These trays either may be of perforated metal or may provide a rim lock.
2. The bulk of the impression material should be kept to a minimum. The use of beeswax adapted to the palatal area of upper trays and to edentulous areas will greatly reduce the thickness of impression material in these areas and will improve the accuracy of the resultant cast.
3. The teeth should be clean. Any excess debris or plaque should be removed. The interproximal areas should be cleaned with dental floss. The mouth should be rinsed and excess saliva absorbed with gauze sponges.
4. Impression material should be placed in critical and hard-to-reach areas, in the facial vestibules, and in deep palatal areas before the tray and main body of the impression material.
5. The impression material should be well mixed to produce a smooth uniform mix with minimum entrapment of air.
6. The impression should be poured with the cast material as soon as is practical after removal from the mouth. Storage of the impression should be in an atmosphere of 100% humidity before and after pouring.
7. The impression should be separated from the cast after approximately 60 minutes.
8. Impressions should not be "inverted" after pouring but should remain upright so that the cast material will not separate from the impression material. The cast material can be confined by judicious use of wax or metal boxing material placed so as not to distort peripheral areas of the impression.
9. Alginate impression materials properly manipulated will provide acceptable accuracy but do not provide fine detail necessary for master dies.

Alginate substitute-silicone impression system

A recently developed impression system has been introduced that combines the use of two different types of impression materials to produce a single completed impression. In this combination of seemingly incompatible materials, the manufacturer* claims to have combined the hydrophylic properties of hydrocolloid with the superior physical properties of the silicone impression materials.

Limited clinical trials have produced mixed reports from practitioners who have used the impression system. Some have reported favorably as to its accuracy while others have been disappointed with its ability to rebound completely after the distortion of retrieval from pronounced undercut areas.

The technique involves the concurrent but separate mixing of the silicone impression material (injection viscosity) and an alginate impression material to fill a tray or carrier. The silicone material is carefully introduced into the critical areas to be impressed and then immediately joined to the alginate material as the tray is placed in position—the entire procedure occurring before either material has polymerized or gelled.

After setting, the completed impression is retrieved from the mouth and poured with cast material as soon as is practical. If pouring of the cast must be delayed, the impression should be stored in a humidor at 100% humidity.

The impression system appears to be compatible with most die stones. After pouring of the cast material, the impression should be kept in an atmosphere of 100% humidity until the cast is separated from the impression. The care and handling of the completed impression should be similar to that of any reversible or irreversible hydrocolloid impression (Figs. 1-29 to 1-32).

Combination hydrocolloid impression techniques

A technique for production of impressions for master casts has been developed that combines the use of both reversible and irreversible hydrocolloid.

The procedure uses a specially formulated reversible hydrocolloid for injection into the critical areas (Fig. 1-33), joined with an irreversible (alginate) material in the carrier or tray that makes up the bulk of the impression. Formulation of the two materials has been adjusted so that a true bond results when they are combined in the impression. The greatest change in formulation appears to be in the reversible material. The manufacturers claim that the reversible injection material will bond with nearly all leading alginate products (Fig. 1-34).

The advantages of such a technique are obvious: (1) lower cost per impression, (2) liquefaction and storage of a smaller amount of the reversible material, (3) elimination of water cooled trays, and (4) reduced setting time of the impression.

After retrieval of the impression from the mouth, it is handled in a manner similar to that when other hydrocolloid materials are used. It is recommended that the impression be poured with the cast material as soon as is practical. Impressions that cannot be poured immediately should be stored in an atmosphere of 100% humidity to minimize loss of water volume and associated distortion.

After pouring, the impression should not be inverted but rather the cast material should be allowed to settle into the impression during setting. The impression

*Ultrafine—Buffalo Dental Corp., Brooklyn, N.Y.

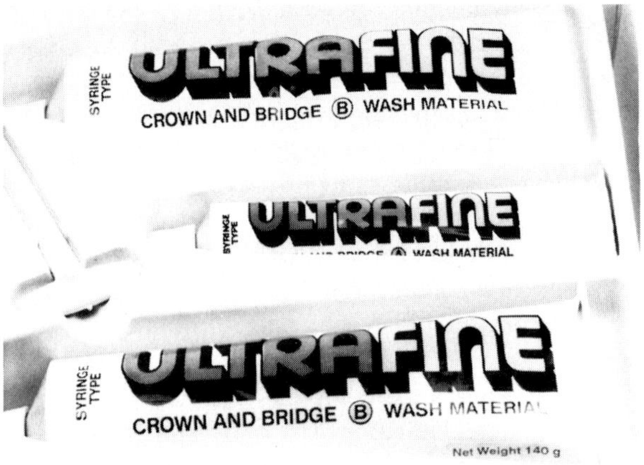

Fig. 1-29. Silicone portion of Ultrafine impression technique. Large tubes are base syringe material and single small tube accelerator portion of syringe material.

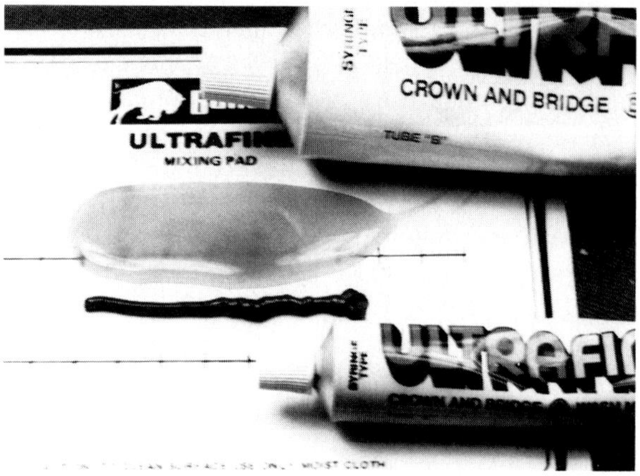

Fig. 1-30. Constituents of syringe material ready for mix. Syringe material is mixed concurrently with tray material.

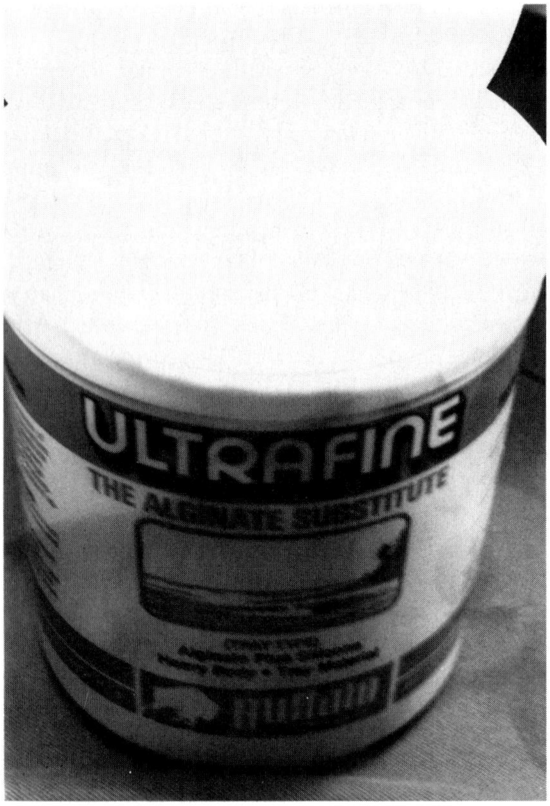

Fig. 1-31. Tray material for Ultrafine impression technique. It is said to be an alginate substitute.

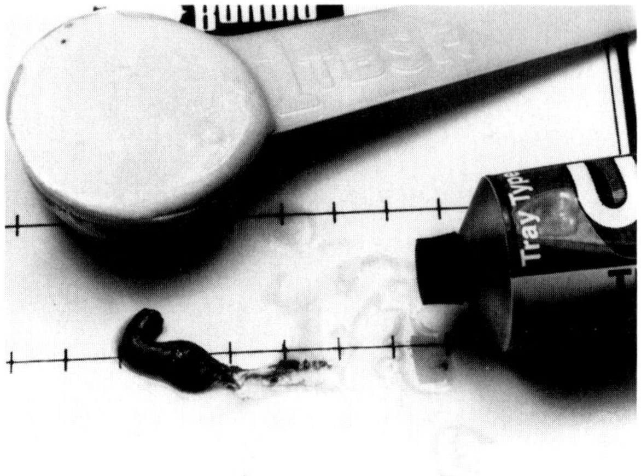

Fig. 1-32. Scoop of alginate substitute on pad ready to mix. Note that as accelerator was ejected, it lacked consistency (see puddles of uncolored material to right). This points up need for ambitious massage of tube before ejection. This holds for many materials packaged in this manner and that have the potential of separating component parts.

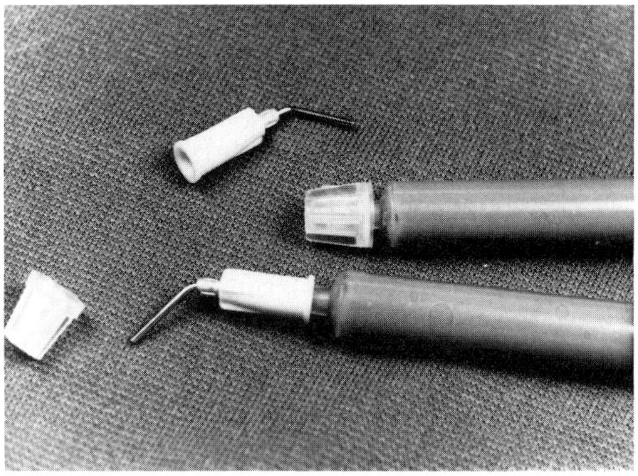

Fig. 1-33. Sample of reversible hydrocolloid packaged in disposable syringes. This material will bond with all alginates tested. Cap is kept on during boiling and into storage bath, but injecting tip should be placed on a few moments before ejecting and kept in the storage bath so that a cool needle tip will not tend to lessen working time with syringe.

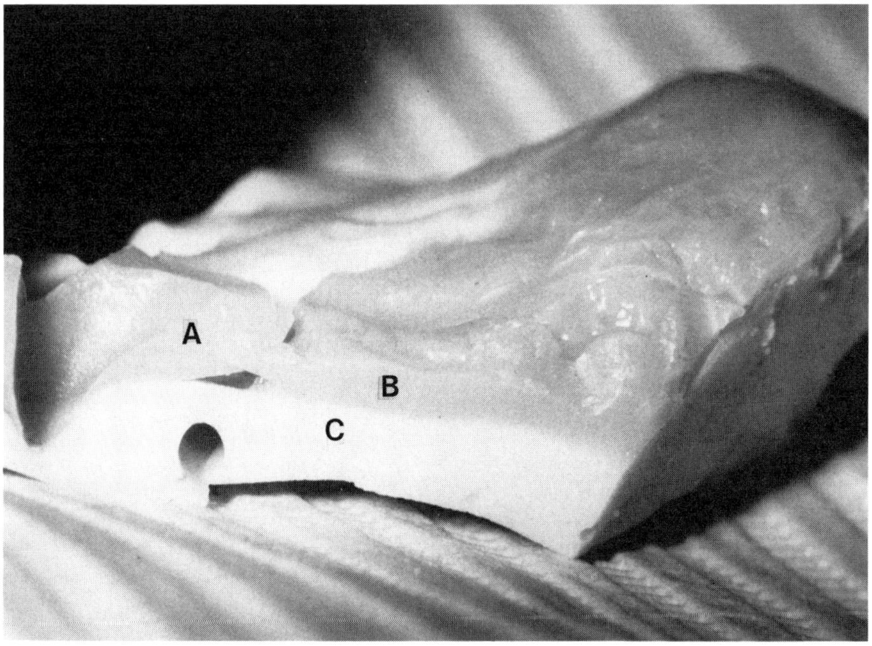

Fig. 1-34. Testing bonding potential of reversible and irreversible hydrocolloids. Two reversible hydrocolloids, *A* and *B,* and an irreversible hydrocolloid (alginate), *C,* are shown in cross section. *A* is clearly separating from *C,* while *B* shows a profound bond to *C.* *A* was orange and *B* was green so that delineation of materials was definite.

should be placed in a suitable humidor and the humidity maintained at 100% during the 45- to 60-minute setting period of the cast material.

It is claimed that a first pour can be made involving only the prepared teeth and removed for use as individual dies, followed by a second pour for the working cast. Individual experience will determine the practicality of the procedure.

Polysulfides

Polysulfides were one of the first of a large family of elastomeric compounds introduced to dentistry as impression materials. The polysulfides are also known as mercaptan and Thiokol rubbers. In two component systems polymerization occurs by a condensation reaction when activated by certain catalytic agents. The soft rubberlike materials possess great accuracy and remark-

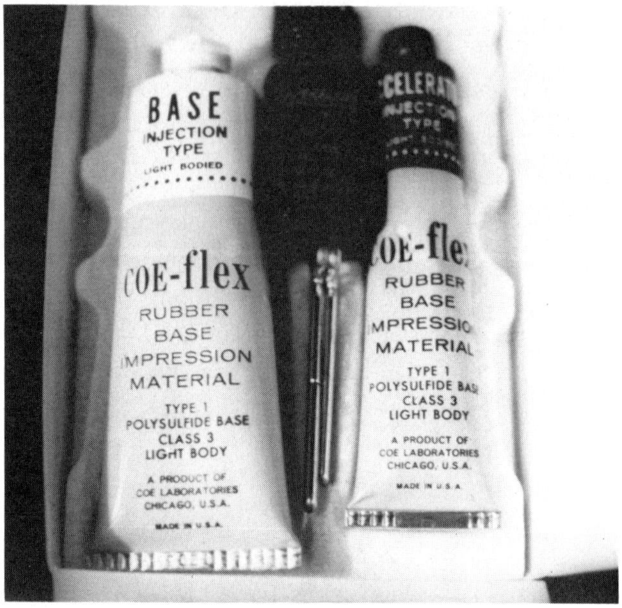

Fig. 1-35. One of the first polysulfides on market and still in widespread use.

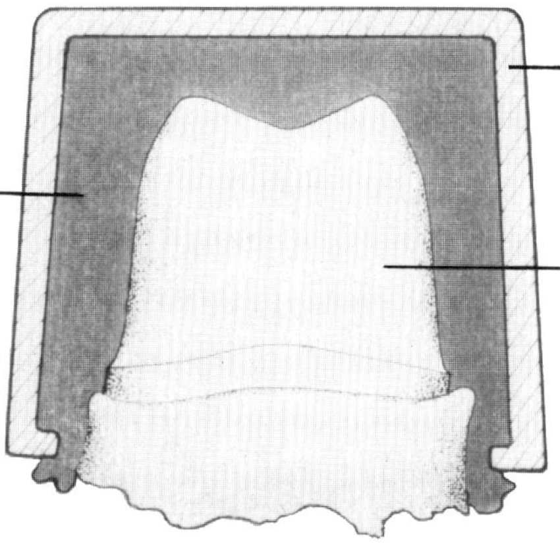

Fig. 1-36. Inconsistent abundance of reversible hydrocolloid within tray.

able elastic limit, which allows polymerized material to be removed from marked undercut areas with a minimum of permanent deformation.

The least dimensional error is obtained when the material is used in thin cross sections. Polymerization shrinkage is minimized by the use of custom-made trays, which allow a uniformly thin bulk and thickness of impression material (1 to 2 mm) in all areas of the impression. Comparison of thickness control is illustrated in Figs. 1-35 to 1-38.

TWO-STAGE (PUTTY-WASH) TECHNIQUE

Not long after the great acceptance of the two-stage silicone materials, a similar technique employing the polysulfide materials was developed. The method consisted of a first-stage customizing of a stock impression tray with polysulfide material of firm "puttylike" consistency either directly in the mouth or on a diagnostic cast. The second stage employed a relatively thin corrective layer of lower viscosity polysulfide material that could be introduced into the critical areas about the teeth and joined with similar "wash" material, which served as a reline impression (Figs. 1-39 to 1-41).

CUSTOM TRAY IMPRESSION TECHNIQUE

The fabrication of an impression tray specifically tailored to the contours of the patient's teeth or arch offers a distinct advantage in limiting and equalizing the amount of impression material necessary for the body of the impression. As described earlier, the use of uniform minimum thickness of material can materially improve dimensional accuracy in the impression.

The tray is constructed of autopolymerizing tray resin

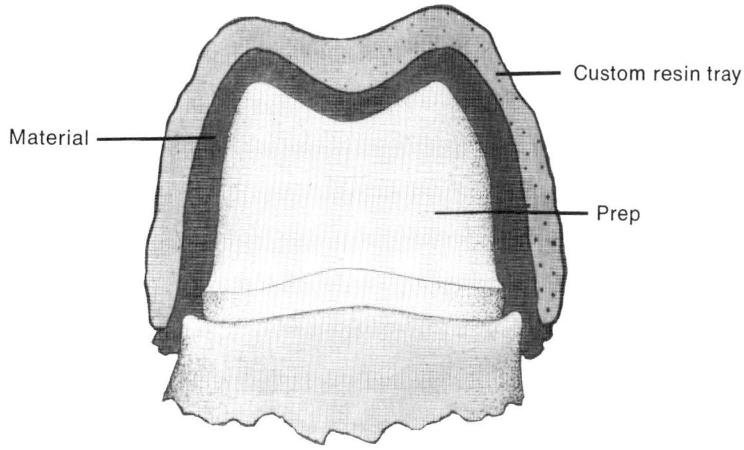

Fig. 1-37. Consistent small amount of polysulfide material is needed surrounding object. Because of polymerization shrinkage, this approach is needed to attain greatest accuracy.

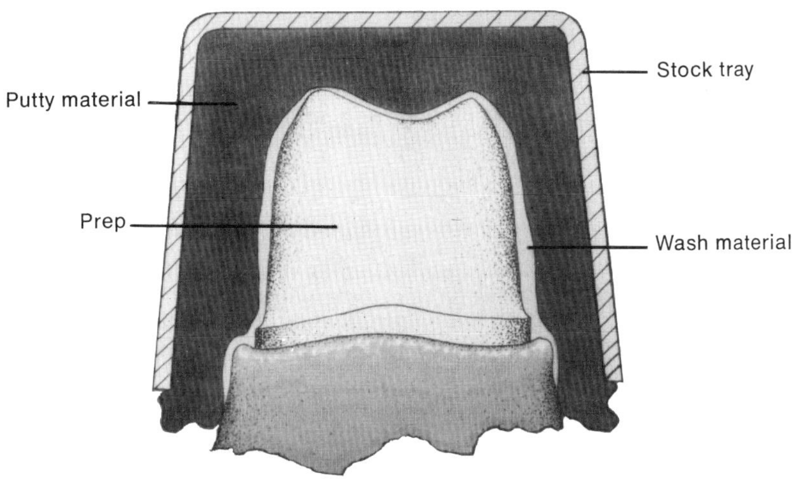

Fig. 1-38. Small consistent liner of material needed during final wash with silicones, as with polysulfides.

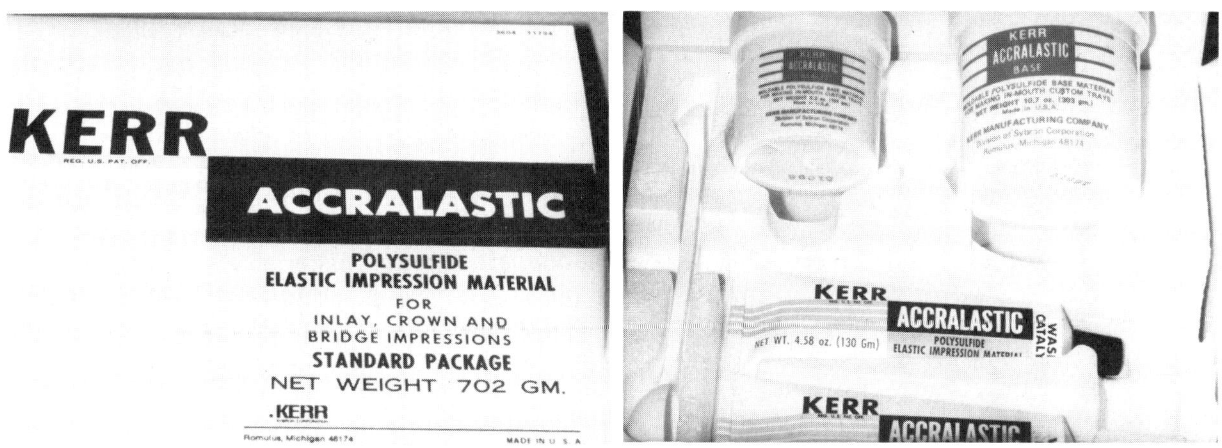

Fig. 1-39. Two-stage polysulfide that can be used with stock commercial tray.

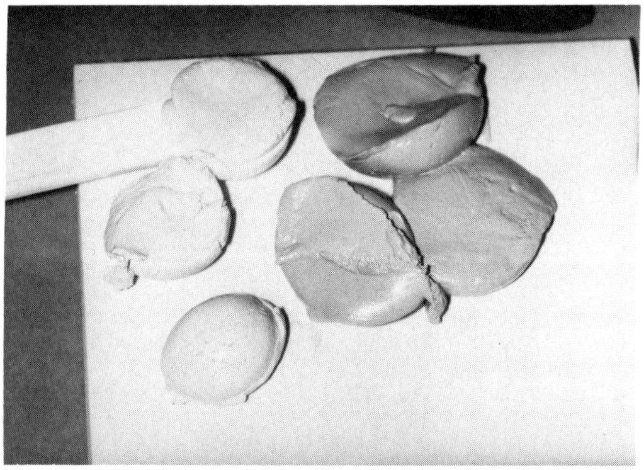

Fig. 1-40. Proportioned putty material, which is mixed, placed in tray, and then into mouth or over study model with proper relief.

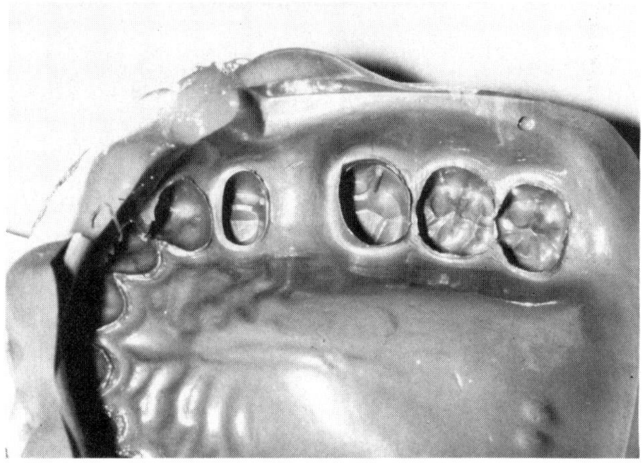

Fig. 1-41. Completed impression showing darker wash material over lighter putty.

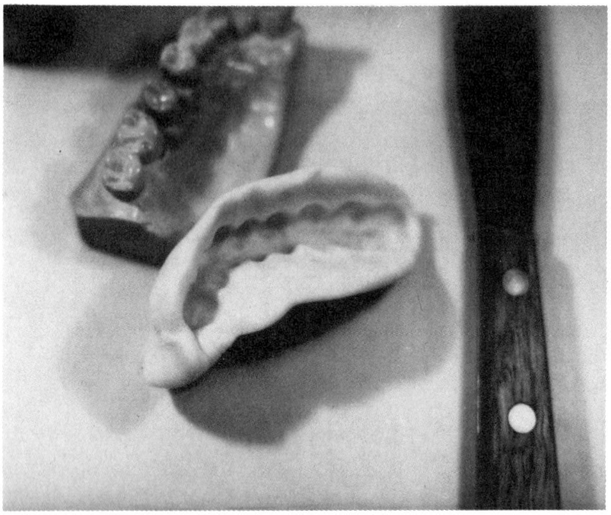

Fig. 1-42. Completed custom tray with relief over preparation area.

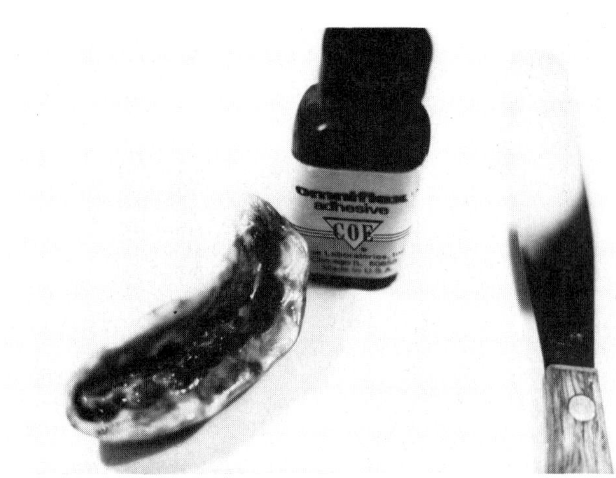

Fig. 1-43. Adhesive placed on tray and extended over borders.

adapted to a cast of the patient's teeth. A spacer of two sheets of base plate wax (2 mm) is first adapted to the cast. The wax spacer provides the necessary space within the tray being formed to allow the optimum thickness of impression material during the subsequent impression procedure (Fig. 1-42).

To assure bonding of the impression mixture to the tray, the inner surface and periphery of the tray are coated with a suitable adhesive. Proper proportions of the impression material are placed upon a mixing pad and mixed to a uniform consistency which exhibits no streaking of the different colored constituents (Figs. 1-43 to 1-47).

The mixed material is carefully inserted into the tray, avoiding entrapment of air masses within the viscous material (Fig. 1-48). The remaining material is carefully loaded into the injection syringe. Impression material is carefully placed into the critical areas to avoid entrapment of air or other innacuracy associated with the application of the material. The tray is placed over the teeth and seated with light uniform pressure to assure proper orientation. The tray should be maintained in its position with light finger pressure until polymerization has occurred. Care should be exercised that movement of the tray does not occur during the setting period.

After removal of the impression from the mouth (Fig. 1-49), the cast material should be introduced as described earlier.

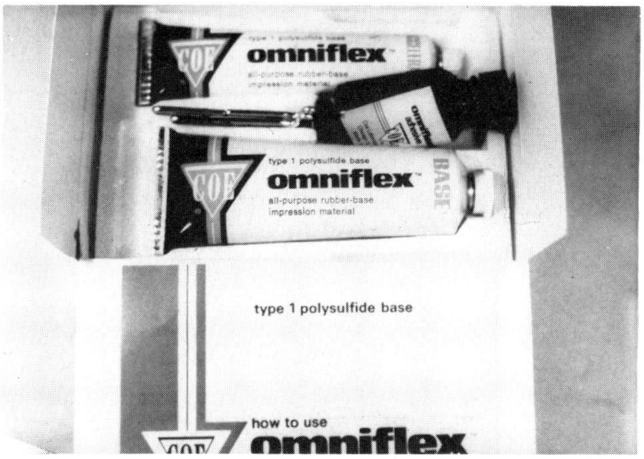

Fig. 1-44. Example of modern polysulfide.

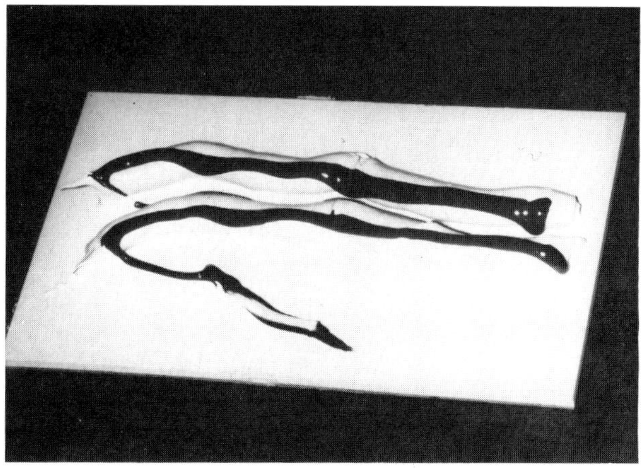

Fig. 1-45. Proportions measured out on pad.

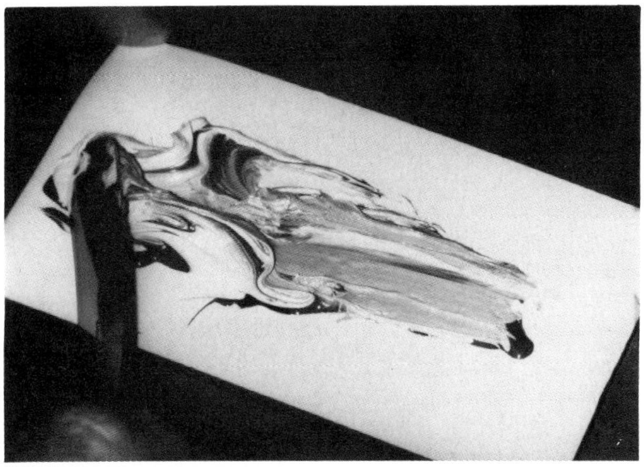

Fig. 1-46. Mix begun with spreading motion, not whipping.

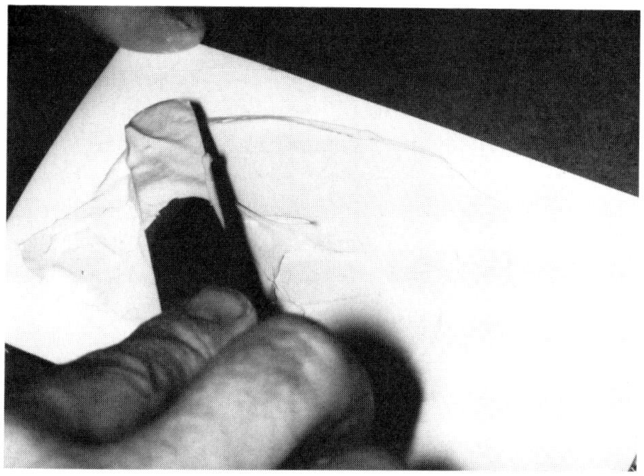

Fig. 1-47. Completed mix.

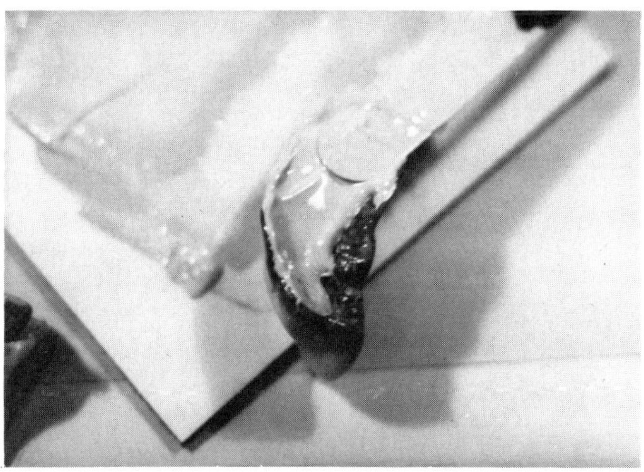

Fig. 1-48. Loading tray without incorporating or trapping air.

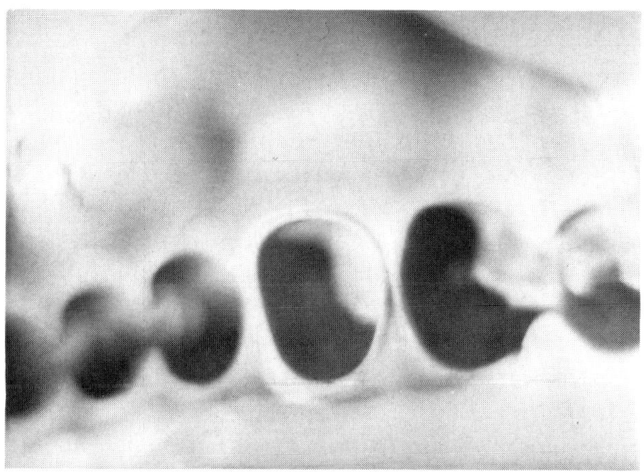

Fig. 1-49. Completed impression.

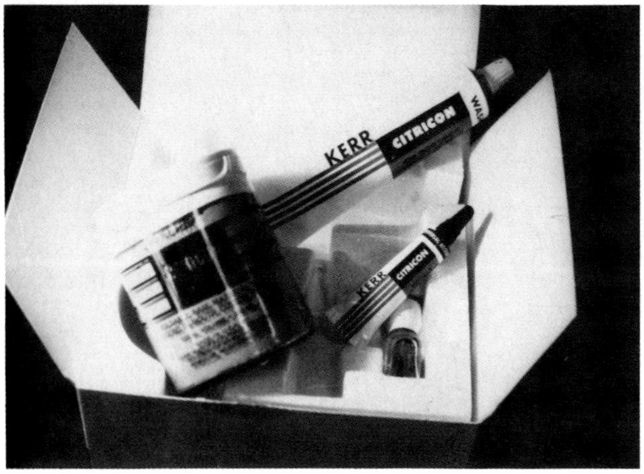

Fig. 1-50. Representative two-stage silicone.

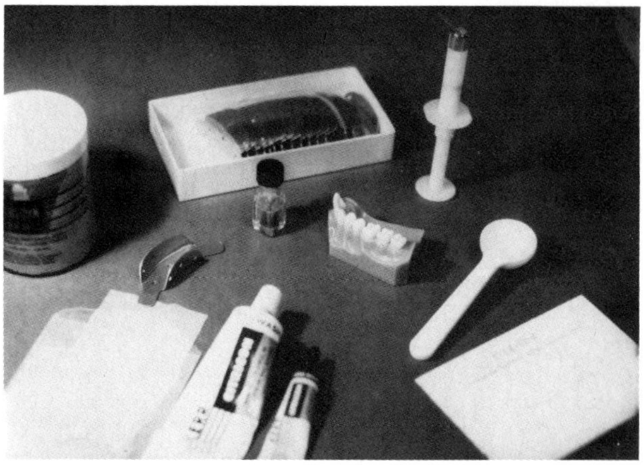

Fig. 1-51. Materials prepared for taking impression with two-stage silicone.

Silicones

Since their introduction to the dental profession about 1955, the silicone impression materials have undergone continual improvement in working properties, accuracy, and product reliability. The products currently available present a prolonged shelf life and a variety of forms or consistencies in which supplied. The different consistencies, being compatible with each other, allow considerable variation in technique of use depending upon the clinical conditions and the intended use.

Experience has shown that, like other elastomers that exhibit a condensation polymerization, increased accuracy can be attained by reducing the thickness and bulk of the material in the impression. This is accomplished through the use of custom-made trays that limit the amount of material or by the widely used two-stage or "putty-wash" technique.

TWO-STAGE (PUTTY-WASH) TECHNIQUE

The two-stage impression technique essentially makes a custom tray from a stock tray through the use of a heavy bodied silicone material that is formed directly over the teeth or upon a cast of the patient's dental arch. It is formed over an interspersed layer of relief material, which preforms the desired spacing. This space, approximately 2 mm in width, will be filled by the thinner viscosity material when the final impression is made (Figs. 1-50 and 1-51). The technique of developing the first-stage impression is described in Figs. 1-52 through 1-61.

The tray used for the first stage impression may be fabricated before the patient's appointment. It will be relined with the lower viscosity "wash" material after

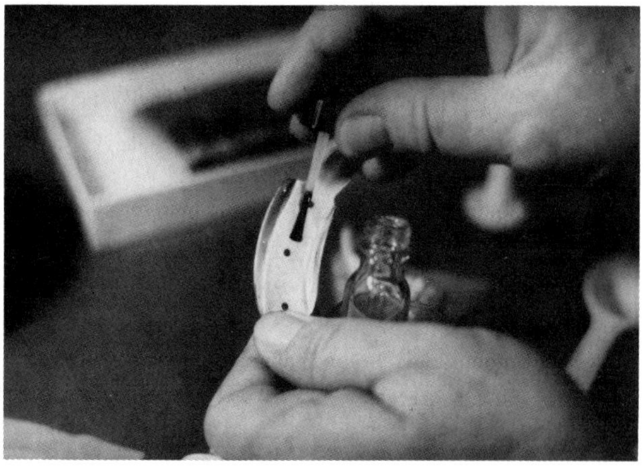

Fig. 1-52. Placing adhesive on stock commercial tray.

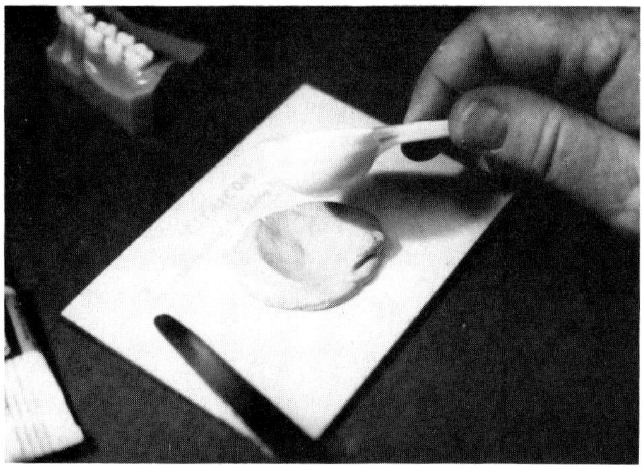

Fig. 1-53. Preparing putty base.

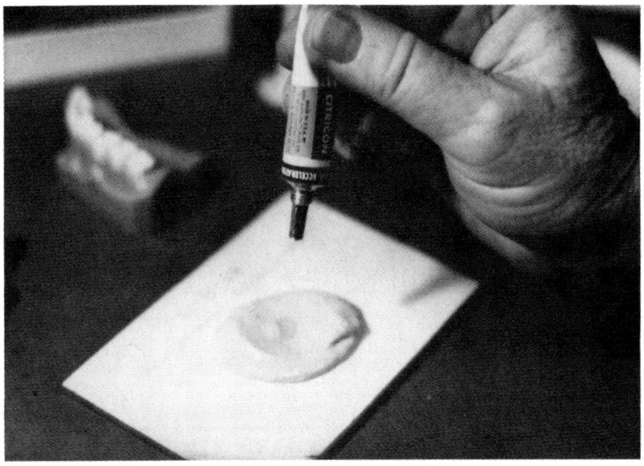

Fig. 1-54. Adding accelerator to putty material.

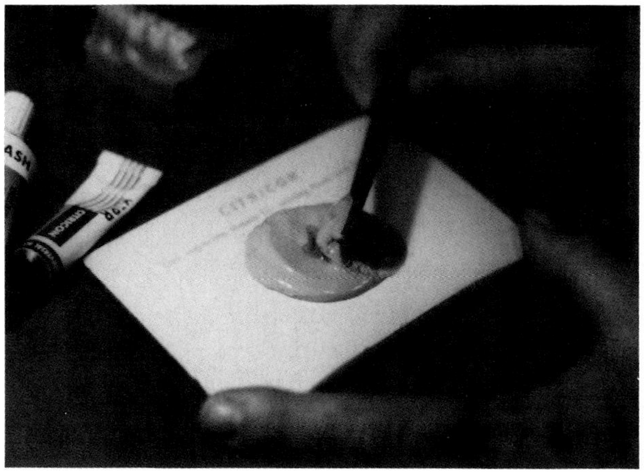

Fig. 1-55. Incorporating parts.

A 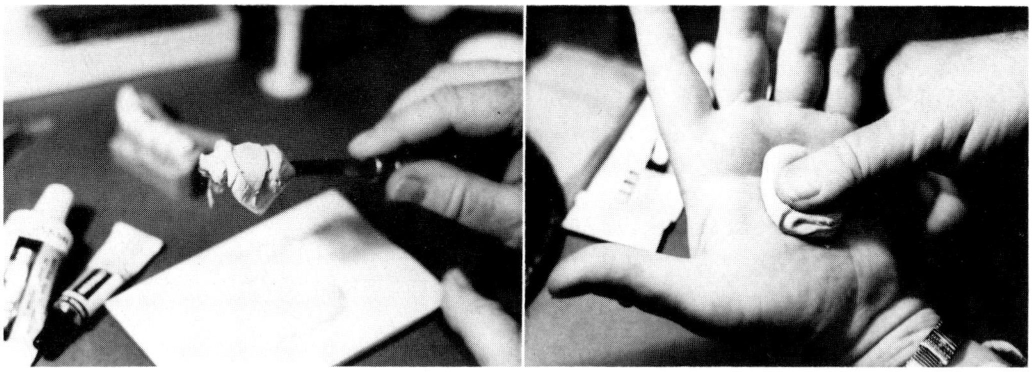 B

Fig. 1-56. Putty may be mixed with spatula, **A,** or kneaded with hands, **B.**

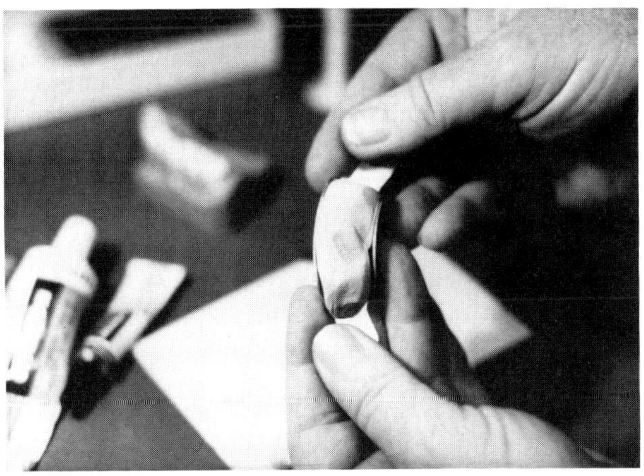

Fig. 1-57. Loading putty in tray.

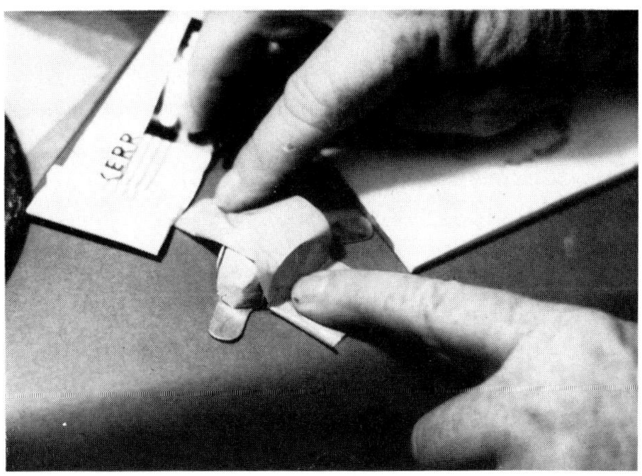

Fig. 1-58. Placing relief material over putty.

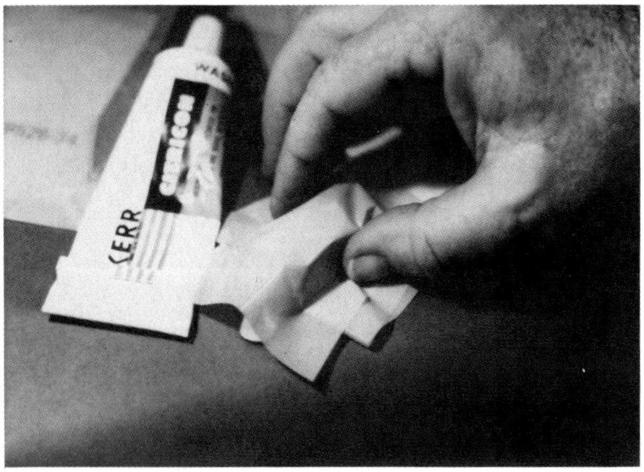

Fig. 1-59. Relief material in place.

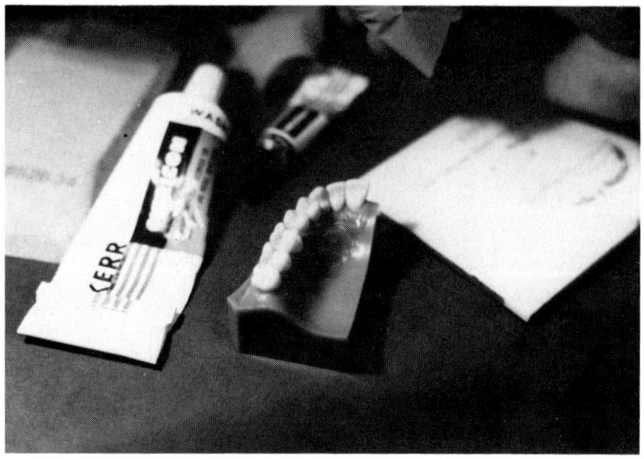

Fig. 1-60. Model to be impressioned.

the teeth have been prepared for the necessary restorative treatment. The second stage of the "wash" impression is described in Figs. 1-62 through 1-68.

Casts should be made from silicone impressions as soon as practical after removal from the mouth. It is possible, because of the strength and toughness of these materials, to obtain two or more casts from a single impression (multiple pours). The first cast should be removed from the impression after it has set for about an hour. Individual dies can be made from this cast for waxing and other fine work. The second cast, which should be poured as soon as the first is removed, can be used for relationships, working casts, and other duties that do not require the degree of accuracy required of individual dies upon which fine margins are developed.

Silicones also should be poured as soon as possible. Because of the tensile strength and stability of these materials, as well as the polysulfides, two models can generally be poured from one impression—the first for dies and the second for relationship.

The wettability of the stone mix on this material is no better and perhaps is a little more challenging than with the polysulfides. Thus until a satisfactory surfactant is found, the same slurry or thin mix of stone technique described for polysulfides is applicable with this family of impression materials.

Polyethers

Another group of elastomers, the polyethers (produced in Germany), came into general use in the early 1970's. These materials have been very accurate in dimensional stability and in reproducing detail. The polymerization shrinkage is not as great as with the polysulfides and silicones; however, for best results, a custom tray is recommended (Figs. 1-69 to 1-71).

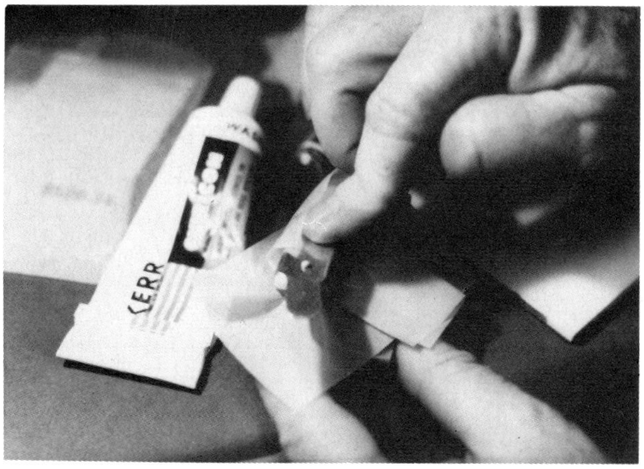

Fig. 1-61. Checking maturity of putty before placement.

Polyether impression materials are easily manipulated, even though they are stiffer in consistency and have a comparatively rapid clinical setting time. Because of the stiffness of the polymerized material, difficulty may be encountered in removing the impression from the mouth when significant undercut areas are present. Similarly, extreme care must be exercised in separation of the cast from the impression to avoid fracture of long and thin teeth or preparations. Some products supply modifiers or plasticizers that allow a certain degree of control of viscosity (stiffness) of the polymerized material (Fig. 1-72).

Polysiloxanes

Polysiloxane, one of the most recently introduced of the elastomeric impression materials, is of different chemical structure and composition than the other ma-

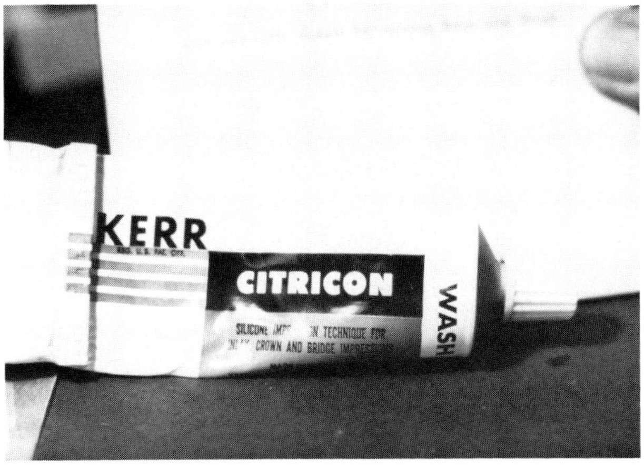

Fig. 1-62. Wash material.

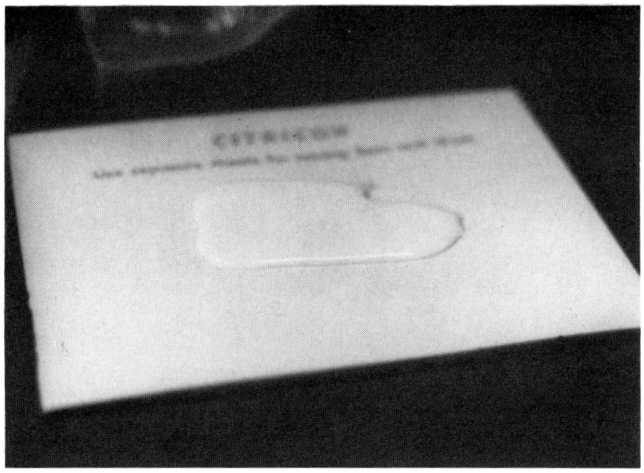

Fig. 1-63. Wash may be mixed on pad or in plastic cup.

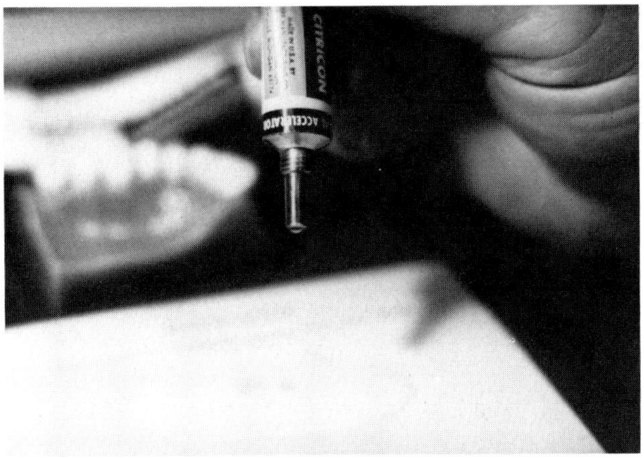

Fig. 1-64. Adding accelerator to wash.

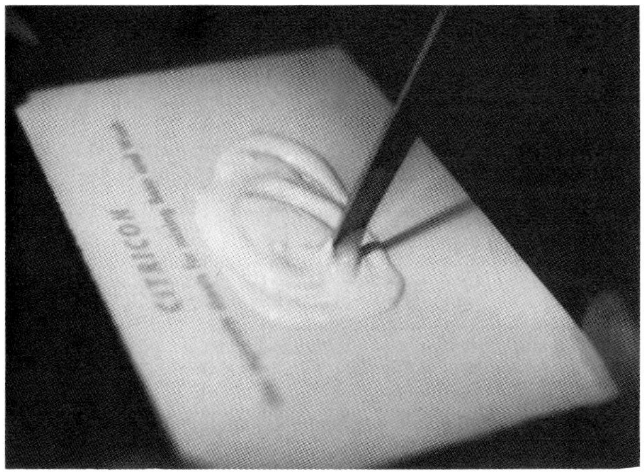

Fig. 1-65. Mixing parts of wash.

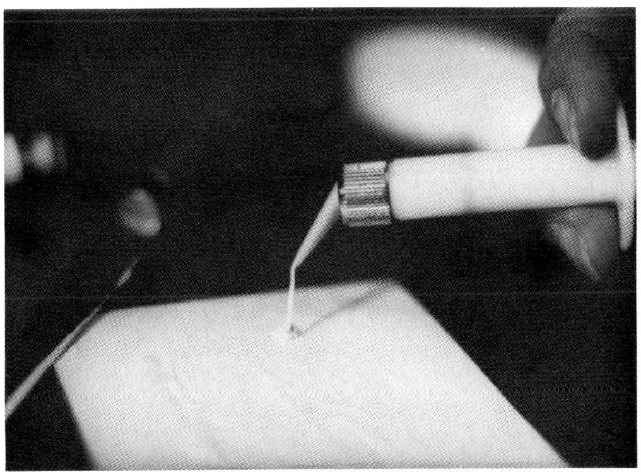

Fig. 1-66. Starting flow of wash from syringe.

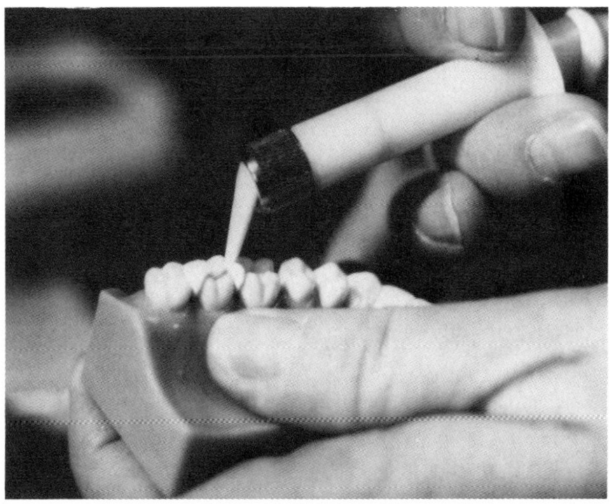

Fig. 1-67. Injecting wash into preparation area.

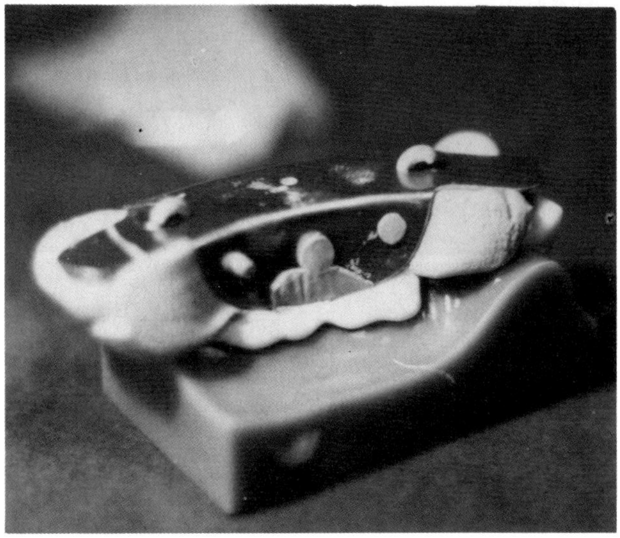

Fig. 1-68. After remaining wash is placed into putty, impression tray is carried to arch and seated according to previously designed stops.

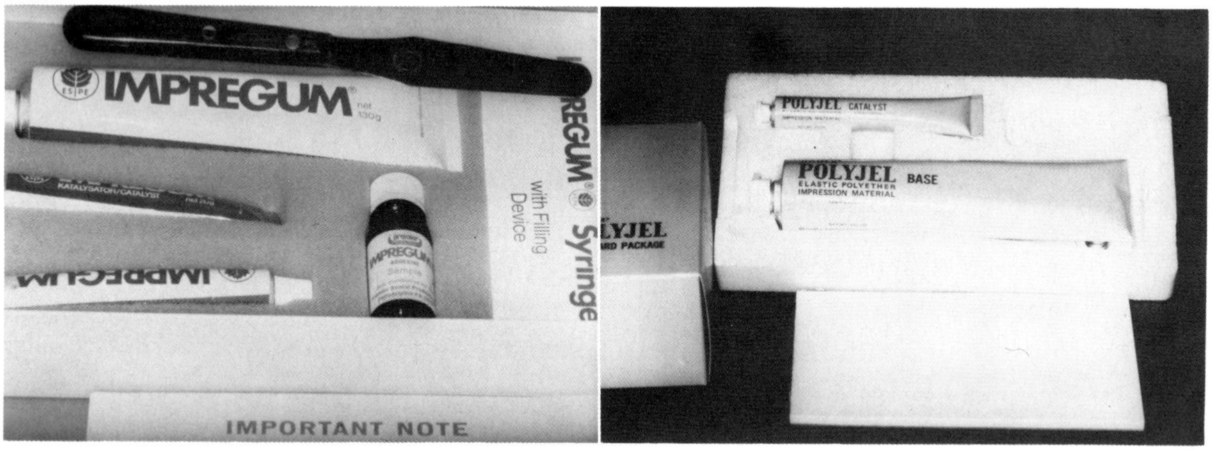

Fig. 1-69. Two representative brands of polyethers.

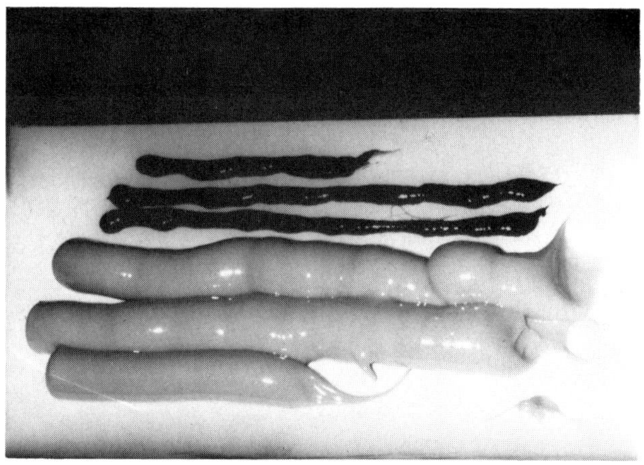

Fig. 1-70. Components of polyether before mixing.

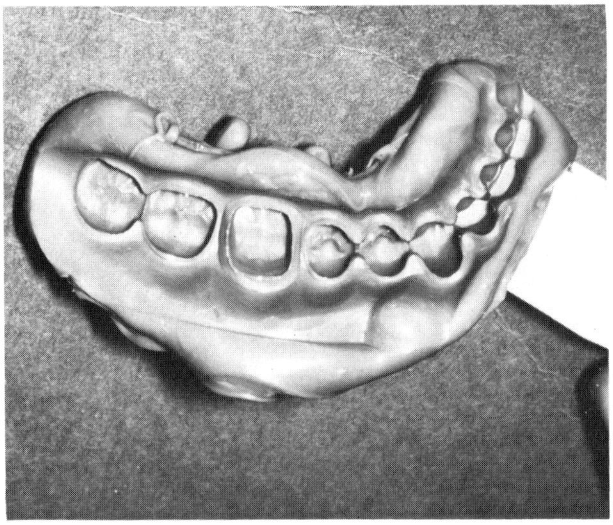

Fig. 1-71. Retrieved polyether impression.

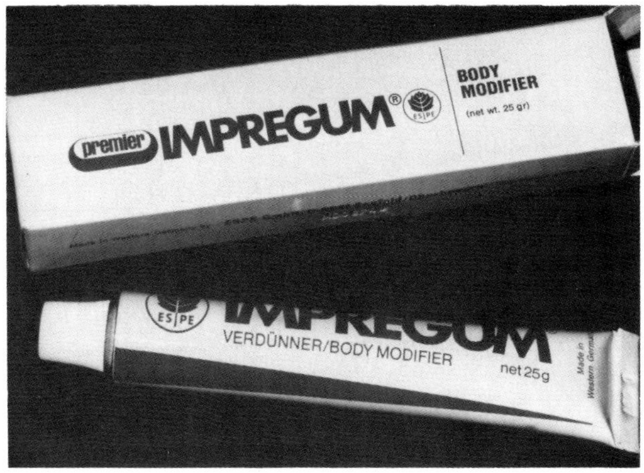

Fig. 1-72. Body modifier used to give mature impression material more elasticity.

terials and achieves its set by an addition-type polymerization. The dimensional change (shrinkage), which occurs in the setting of the other elastomeric compounds, is well controlled in the formulation of polysiloxanes so that casts of great accuracy can be produced from impressions made with this material (Figs. 1-73 to 1-76).

Polysiloxane impression materials are supplied in different forms and viscosities and can be employed successfully in several different clinical techniques. They are supplied in a stiff "putty-like" material suitable for two-stage impressions, previously described, in a viscosity developed for use with techniques that employ individual copper tube impressions, and in the other regular injection and tray viscosities.

Nearly all of the elastic impression materials currently available are capable of producing satisfactory results, provided they are employed within their capabilities. All have advantages and shortcomings. None is all things to all techniques. The techniques employed in their use must be designed to utilize favorable characteristics to the fullest while minimizing the unfavorable ones. Unsatisfactory results frequently are faults of technique and not necessarily of the impression material employed.

Tray carriers for elastic impression materials

Certain basic guidelines should be employed in the use of elastic impression materials. Knowledge of the physical properties and capabilities of the materials to be employed is one of the most important ones. Proper mixing and replacement of the material, proper and intelligent treatment of the impression after removal from the mouth, and proper introduction of a compatible cast

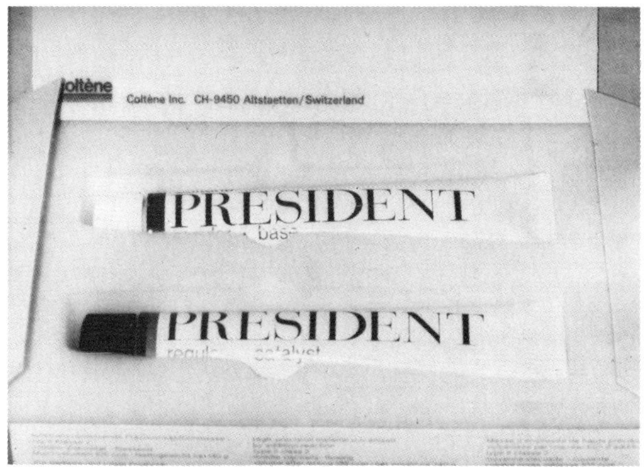

Fig. 1-73. Polysiloxane impression material.

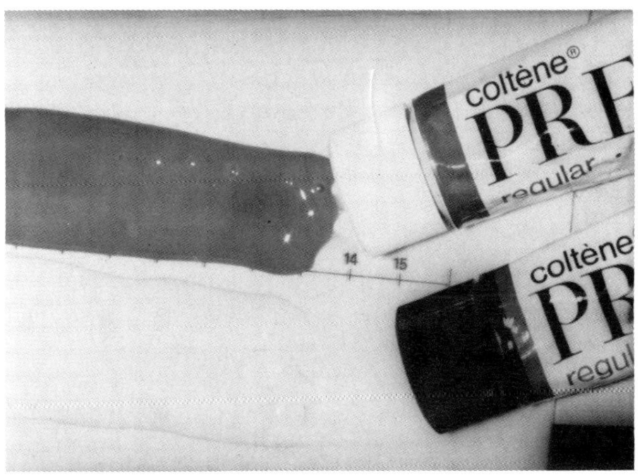

Fig. 1-74. Component parts of polysiloxane before mixing.

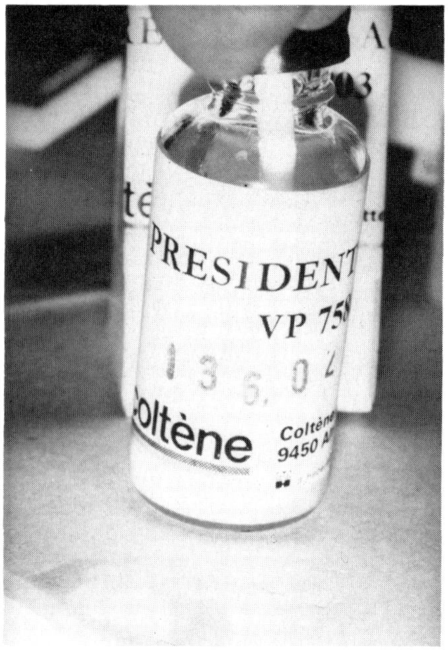

Fig. 1-75. Adhesive to be used with polysiloxane.

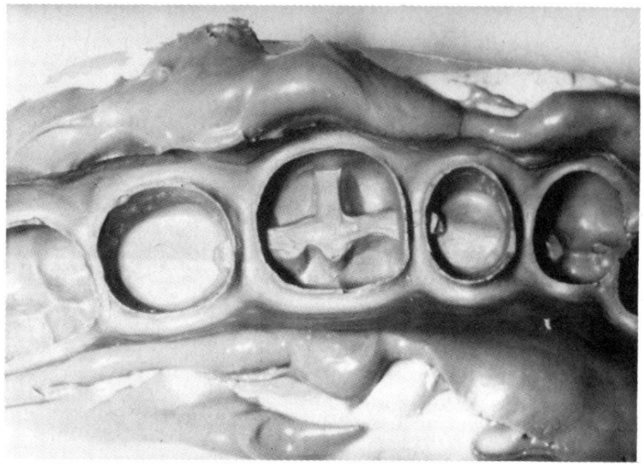

Fig. 1-76. Retrieved polysiloxane impression.

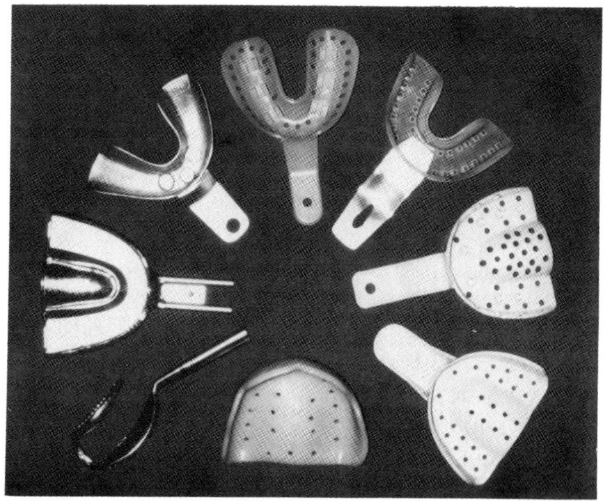

Fig. 1-77. Trays available on market today.

material are other factors that must receive care and attention.

A crucial consideration in any impression technique is the selection of a tray or carrier that will confine and support the impression material. Many different types, styles, and sizes of manufactured trays are available (Fig. 1-77). In addition, tray carriers can be fabricated in the laboratory from autopolymerizing tray resin, from thermoplastic resin sheets adapted by pressure of vacuum forming, and from perforated metal sheets of brass or aluminum.

The following suggestions are offered for tray selection for different types of impression materials:

1. Reversible hydrocolloid—positive mechanical retention must be provided by the design of the tray. Perforated metal appears to produce the most positive and uniform retentive capability. The rim-lock concept also retains the impression material in place in the tray, but this design can allow a separation between impression material and tray to occur over internal areas that are smooth and flat and afford no positive retentive elements (Figs. 1-78 and 1-79). Trays for reversible hydrocolloid must provide the capability for chilling the impression material. This is accomplished through incorporation of metal tubes or chambers through which cooling water can be circulated.

2. Irreversible hydrocolloid (alginate)—perforated metal or rim-lock trays can be used effectively and are the trays of choice for use with the alginate materials. Heavy-walled manufactured plastic trays that are rigid may also be used, provided an adequate number of retentive holes is present (Fig. 1-80). Alginate does not adhere to plastic tray material and positive mechanical retention must be supplied to prevent partial dislodgment of the impression mass upon its removal from the mouth.

3. Elastomeric impression materials—all elastomeric impression materials (polysulfides, silicones, polyethers, polysiloxanes) have similar characteristics and should receive similar evaluation so far as tray selection is concerned. All of these materials should employ a suitable adhesive, usually supplied by the manufacturer, to bind the material securely to the impression tray or carrier. Trays made of disposable plastic or custom-made carriers of autopolymerizing tray acrylic seem to be well suited for techniques using elastomeric materials. Most manufactured metal trays, although

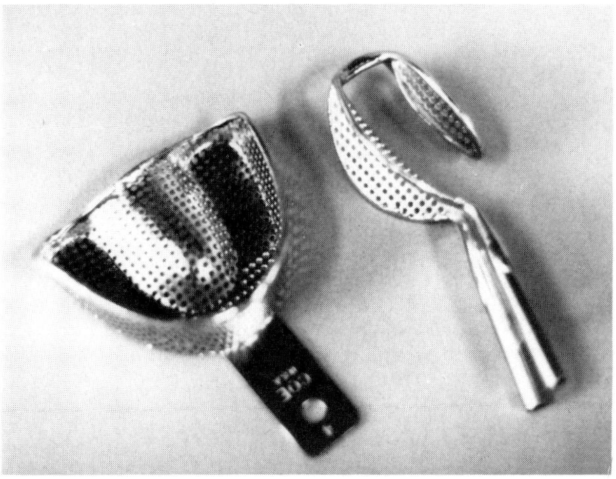

Fig. 1-78. Full-arch perforated metal tray and quadrant water-cooled tray for checkbite technique.

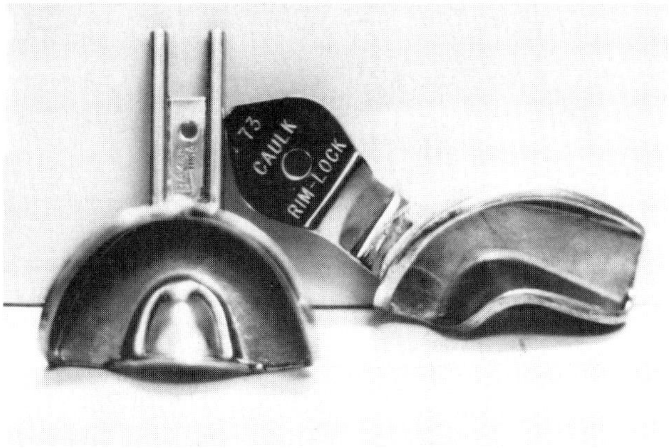

Fig. 1-79. Metal rim-lock water-cooled trays for both types of hydrocolloids.

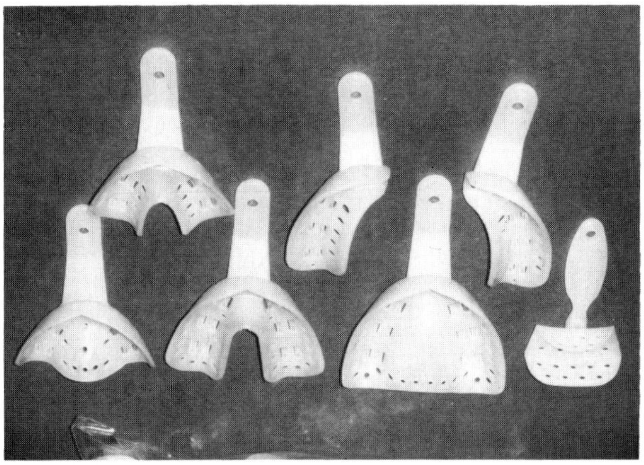

Fig. 1-80. Heavy plastic trays that can be customized with putty and then washed, using either polysulfide or silicone materials.

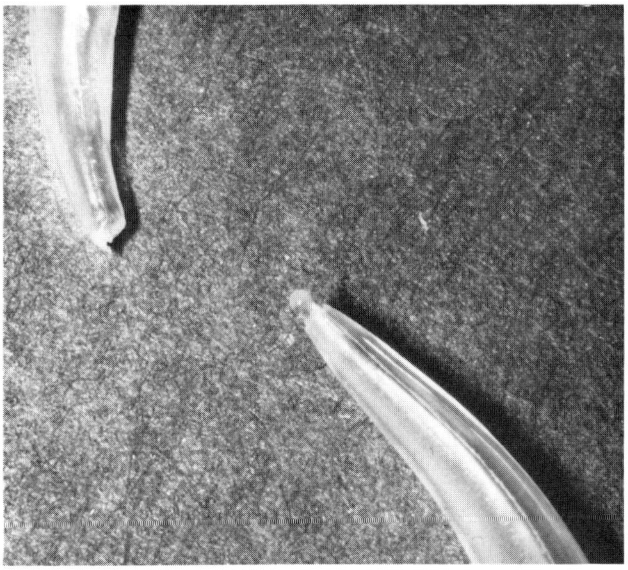

Fig. 1-81. Large, ragged tips of most disposable syringes.

they can be used, are less suitable because of the increased amount of expensive impression material that must be used. It is difficult to remove these materials from metal trays after use. The impression material is very adherent to the metal and is especially tenacious in the retentive holes and locks. Because of this factor, the use of expensive manufactured trays that must be reclaimed and reused is not advised for use with elastomeric impression materials.

Syringes

Several manufacturers have developed syringes, some disposable and some reusable, for injection of elastic impression materials into critical areas before the main mass of material is placed in position. Most are well suited for the intended purpose, but a few, especially the injection tips, must be carefully inspected and modified for most effective use. In the manufacturing process small tags of molding material may be left on the tips, or the small orifice through which the impression material must pass may be imperfectly cast. Close inspection and modification of any defect should be made before use (Fig. 1-81).

A suitable syringe should be easy to load, be easy to clean after use, allow a free effortless discharge of material, and have a well-formed tip that can deliver the impression material into the critical areas. Careful examination of the various products available should be

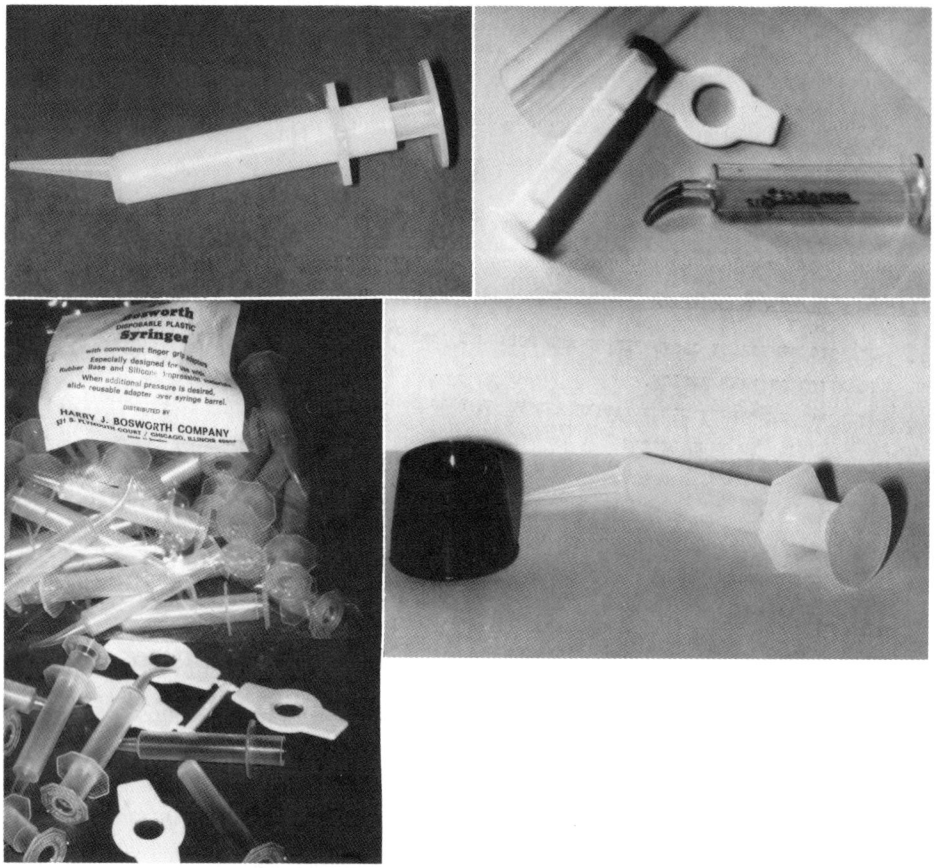

Fig. 1-82. Commercially available disposable syringes.

made so that a selection can be made that is most suitable for the intended use (Figs. 1-82 to 1-84).

Syringes for use with reversible hydrocolloid are usually made of metal (brass) with a covering of rubber or plastic insulating material to protect hands and lips from heat transfer. Such syringes should provide a seal for the needle while it is in the storage bath. Different gauge needles are available for most products, which enables careful injection of the impression material into critical areas (Figs. 1-85 and 1-86).

Syringes designed for use with the elastomeric impression materials have been made of aluminum and with Teflon. Both types are designed for complete disassembly for cleaning after use. Nearly all, except for the disposable types, incorporate a replaceable plastic tip that can be modified for the user's specific purpose.

A metal syringe developed for use with a polyether material (Impregel) has been well designed and is effective (Figs. 1-87 to 1-92). A removable filling reservoir and plunger assembly is particularly effective for loading the mixed impression material into the barrel of the syringe. The replaceable plastic injection tip has a fine orifice, which facilitates placement of the material into critical areas of the prepared teeth.

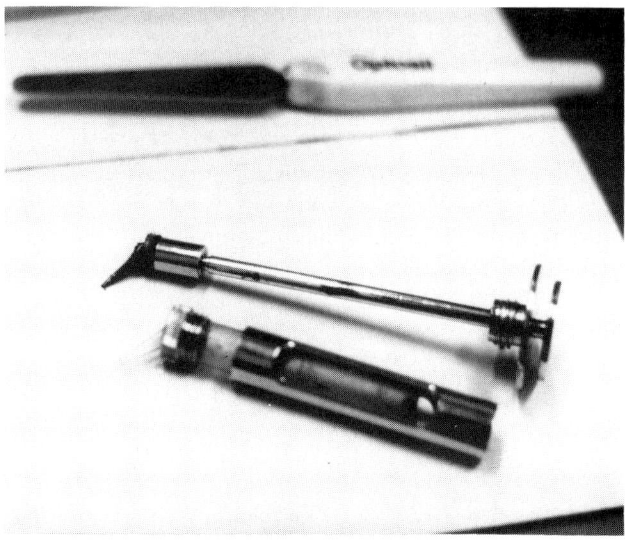

Fig. 1-83. Older model reusable syringe.

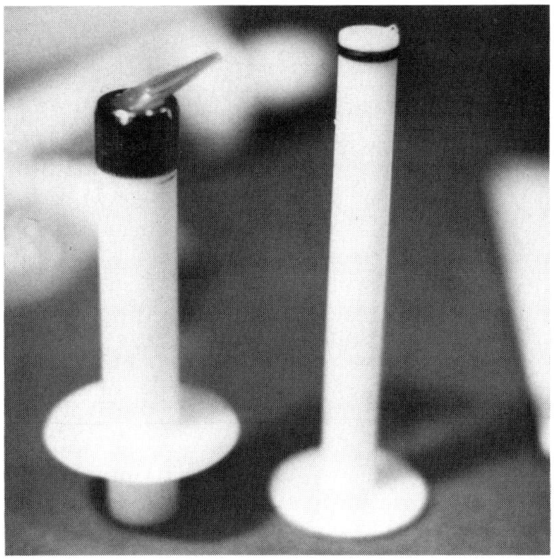

Fig. 1-84. Newer Teflon reusable syringe.

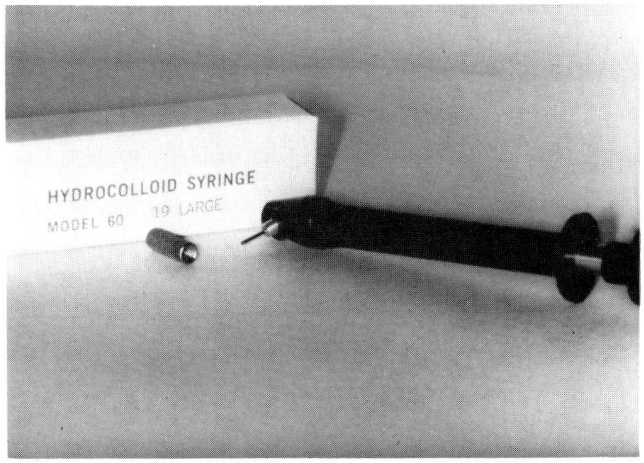

Fig. 1-85. A reversible hydrocolloid reusable syringe.

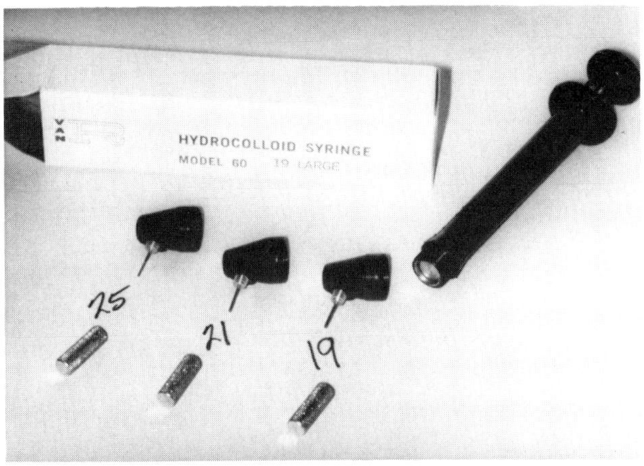

Fig. 1-86. Choice of three reversible hydrocolloid reusable tip sizes, gauges 25, 21, and 19, with syringe.

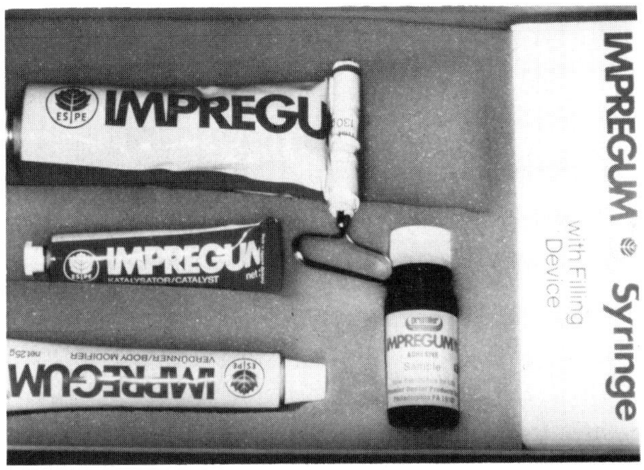

Fig. 1-87. Syringe called *filling device* packaged with polyether impression material (Impregum).

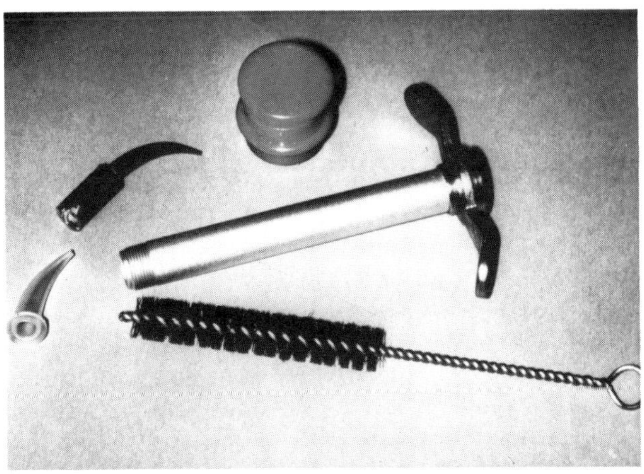

Fig. 1-88. Syringe parts.

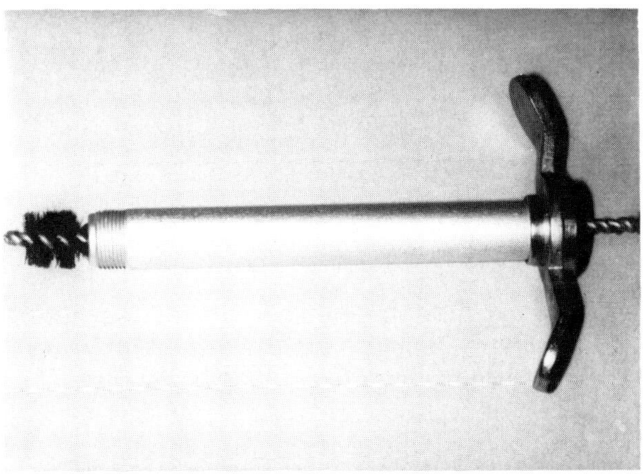

Fig. 1-89. Syringe barrel should be thoroughly cleaned with a brush.

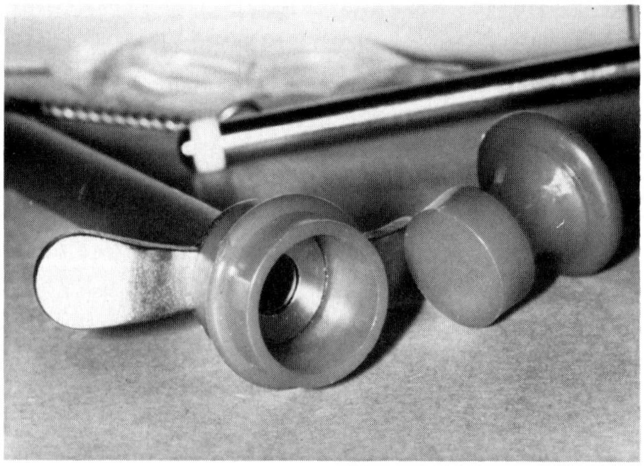

Fig. 1-90. Filling reservoir.

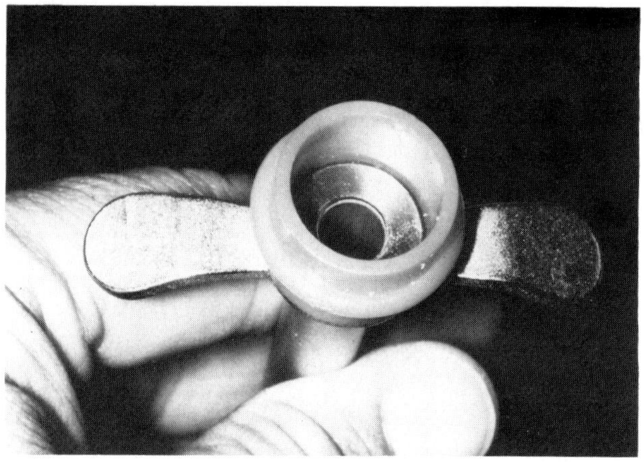

Fig. 1-91. Reservoir holds enough material to completely fill syringe barrel.

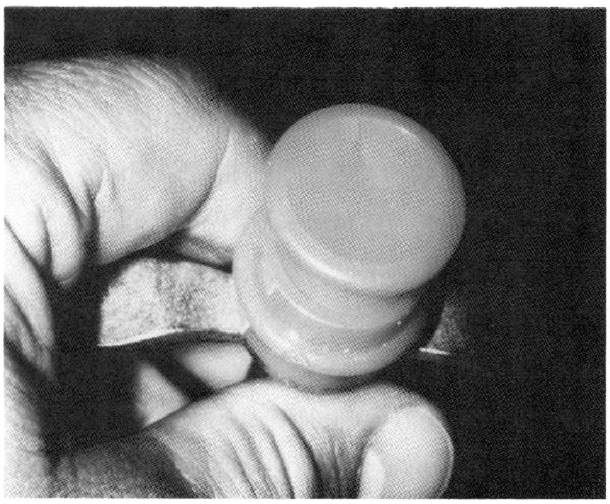

Fig. 1-92. Reservoir plunger pushes material into syringe barrel without air bubbles.

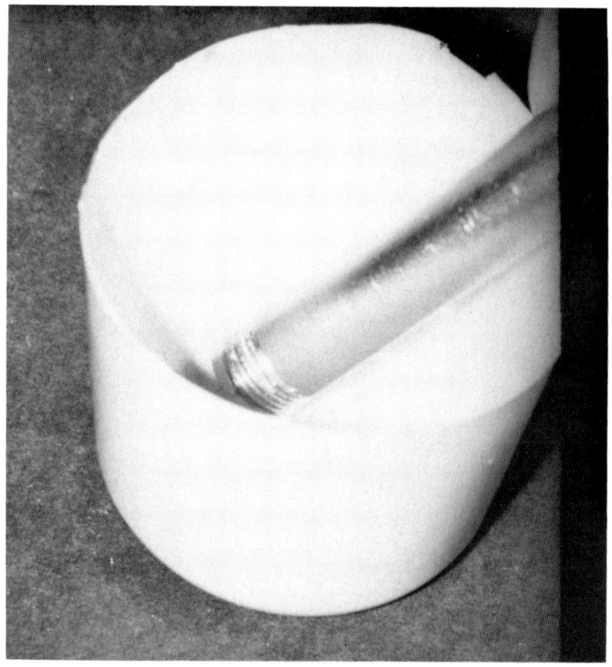

Fig. 1-93. Loading syringe by direct aspiration.

Other quick and efficient methods of loading the mixed impression material into the syringe barrel are: (1) direct aspiration from the mixing pad or from a container, (2) a paper cone formed from the mixing pad paper, and (3) quick passage of the end of the syringe over the mixed material on the pad in repeated strokes to force the material into the syringe barrel (Figs. 1-93 to 1-95). Care must be exercised that air bells or bubbles not be entrapped within the material as it is loaded into the syringe. Bubbles within the mass being injected can produce serious defects, usually on or adjacent to a critical margin, in the completed impression.

Mixing of elastomeric materials

In the mixing of the components of these materials, several basic considerations should be remembered. A spreading-gathering-spreading action of the spatula over the mixing pad should be employed to produce a uniform streak-free mix. Such action will tend to dispel any entrapped air bubbles from the material mass. A whipping action, on the contrary, may tend to incorporate air bubbles into the mix of impression material.

The components of the material should be kept separated until the actual mixing procedure is begun. The chemical polymerization of the elastomeric impression

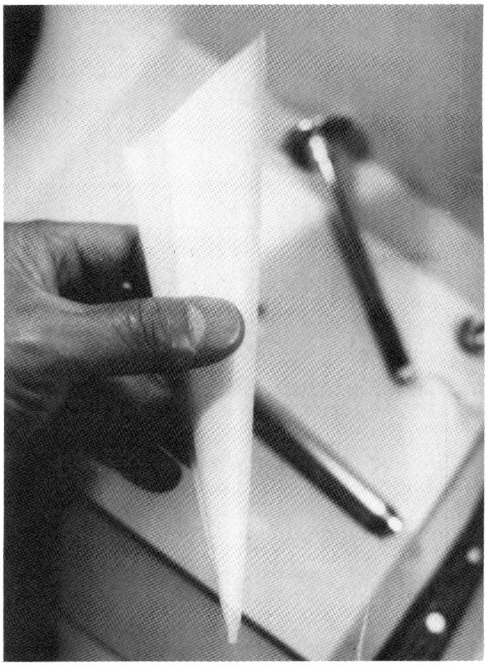

Fig. 1-94. Loading syringe by means of paper funnel.

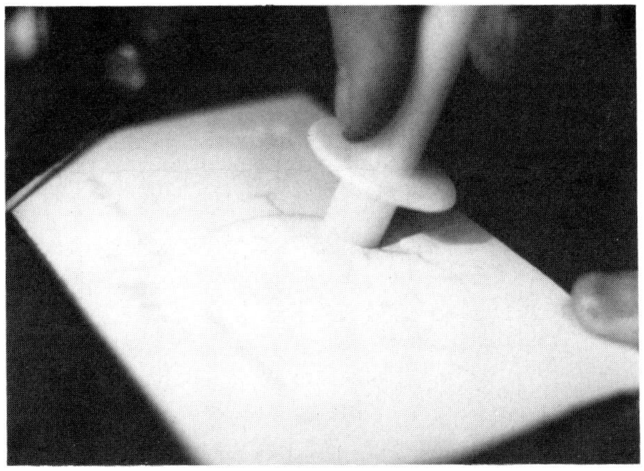

Fig. 1-95. Loading syringe by passing barrel quickly over mixing pad.

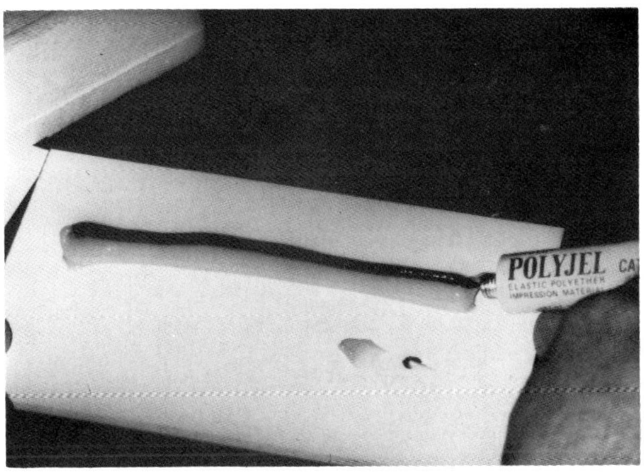

Fig. 1-96. Component parts of polyether impression material (Polyjel) placed in intimate contact on mixing pad few moments before mixing.

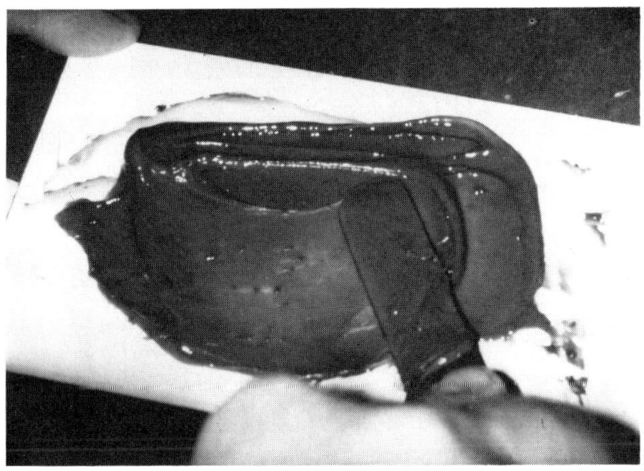

Fig. 1-97. Tiny globules that were impossible to eliminate because of procedure in Fig. 1-96.

materials begins as soon as the components contact one another. Accidental or preliminary contact before spatulation initiates this reaction and will result in particles of semipolymerized material becoming dispersed throughout the mix. In addition to the probability of obstructing the fine orifice of the injection tip, the presence of material in various stages of polymerization in the impression mass will produce an unknown result in the completed impression (Figs. 1-96 and 1-97).

PROBLEM AREAS

The major difficulties that can be encountered in the process of making impressions with elastic impression materials, the probable causes, and suggestions for solution are tabulated in Tables 1-1 to 1-3. The three basic types of impression materials—reversible hydrocolloid, irreversible hydrocolloid, and elastomer—are addressed.

Table 1-1. Reversible hydrocolloids

Problem	Probable cause	Solution
Nonunion of injected and tray material	Some contaminant at interface	Make sure injected material is not contaminated with saliva or other material in mouth Wipe surface of tray material with a 2 × 2-inch sponge prior to tray placement; in this process, remove some material
Syringe material too hot coming out of tip	Storage bath temperature too high or insufficient time in storage bath	Always monitor temperature of baths and be sure syringes are in storage bath at least 5 minutes
Syringe material exhibiting insufficient flow	Insufficient boiling period or storage bath temperature too low	Boil at least 8 to 10 minutes and constantly monitor temperature of baths; uninsulated syringes (Cartri-Loid) can cause loss of fluidity in injected material if time lapse is too long from bath retrieval to injection
Tearing of the material at or near marginal areas	Insufficient gingival retraction	Place sufficient bulk of material in sulcus (sometimes necessitating more ambitious cord retraction) or use electrosurgery
	Prolonged time and pressure in retrieving tray	Remove tray with one positive controlled thrust
	Incomplete set	Leave tray in mouth with water coolant at least 6 minutes.
Show of tray through material	"Floating" of tray, rather than positive seating	Use stops and other means to determine resting place of tray
Grainy texture in tray material	Insufficient liquefying	Boil material at least 10 to 15 minutes
	Storage or tempering bath temperatures too low	Constantly monitor temperature of baths
Rough or chalky stone casts	Contaminants in impression	Remove all contaminants (e.g., hemorrhage, saliva, water, potassium sulfate solution) before or during stone pour
	Removal of cast before complete maturation of stone	Remove cast from negative 45 to 60 minutes after pouring
	Poor stone mixing	Use proper water-powder ratio, pour powder into water, and use vacuum mixing device for specified time
	Maturation of stone in dry environment	Store for stone maturation in 100% humidity
Distortion in cast	Failure to control water volume in retrieved impression	Pour impression immediately after retrieval from mouth or store in potassium sulfate bath or 100% humidity environment
	Movement of tray during maturation	Stabilize during gelation
	Premature removal of tray from mouth	Keep tray in mouth 6 minutes with 60° to 72° F (16° to 22° C) water flowing through system
	Use of ice water during early stages of maturation	Maintain water at 60° to 72° F (16° to 22° C) is recommended; ice water during initial stages has shown potential of "shocking" and distorting material
	Maturation of stone in dry environment	Store maturing stone cast and negative in 100% humidity environment
	Inverting tray after pouring	Leave tray (negative) upright after pouring to avert "sagging" in wet stone
Bubbles	Incorporation of air during handling	Manipulate material more carefully during preparation in tray; syringe stick material more carefully

Table 1-2. Irreversible hydrocolloids

Problem	Probable cause	Solution
Distortion in stone cast	Impression not poured immediately	Pour immediately on retrieval from mouth
	Movement of tray during gelation	Hold tray stable during maturation; tray material must be sufficiently rigid to resist deformation from external forces
	Premature removal from mouth	Follow manufacturer's directions carefully
	Incomplete mix	Mix thoroughly without incorporating air
	"Settled" powder	"Fluff" powder before measuring
Poor stone surface	Contaminants in negative	Make sure impression is free of contaminants; if cleansing needed, use stone slurry
	Premature removal of stone casts	Leave casts in negative 45 to 60 minutes
	Leaving stone in impression too long	Leave casts in negative 45 to 60 minutes
	Poor stone mix	Thoroughly mix stone in vacuum mixer according to manufacturer's directions
Abnormal texture in mixed material	Mixing incomplete, too long, too short, or poor technique	Mix thoroughly, wetting every particle of powder for directed amount of time
	Incorrect water-powder ratio	Follow manufacturer's directions precisely
	"Settling" of material	"Fluff" material before measuring powder
Material sets too quickly	Elevated water temperature	Ideally, have water distilled and about 72° F (22° C)
	Powder-water ratio too high	Measure components exactly
Material sets too slowly	Low water temperature	Ideally, have water distilled and about 72° F (22° C)
	Powder-water ratio too low	Measure components exactly according to manufacturer's recommendations
Bubbles	Incorporation of air in mix and placement	Carefully mix and place material

Table 1-3. Elastomers

Problem	Probable cause	Probable solution
Distortion in stone cast	Incomplete polymerization	Make sure constituents are fresh and properly mixed
	Incomplete adhesion of material to tray	Make sure adhesion to tray is profound with adhesives and/or perforations
	Inconsistency of depth of material	For greatest accuracy, polysulfide or silicone must have consistently thin depth
	Lack of rigidity in tray	Use tray or combination tray and putty with unquestionable rigidity
	Impression not immediately poured	Pour all impressions as soon as possible
	Tray movement during polymerization	Place in predetermined spot to rest; hold it there with constant passive pressure
Bubbles	Poor mixing techniques in impression material and/or stone	Develop mixing technique for impression materials that completely incorporates components while not incorporating air; use vacuum mixer for stone

PART TWO

Working casts and dies

BILL B. LEFLER and THOMAS G. REDDY, Jr.

The final dental restoration can be only as accurate as the working cast on which it is fabricated. The working cast must be an accurate reproduction of the teeth and associated structures of the dental arch. An understanding of the materials used and an appreciation of the need to follow specific procedures in making the working cast and dies are essential to obtain an accurate working cast from an accurate final impression.

PHYSICAL AND CHEMICAL PROPERTIES OF DENTAL STONE

The gypsum used in dental stone is almost pure calcium sulfate dihydrate ($CaSO_42H_2O$). Grinding the gypsum and subjecting it to a temperature of 230° to 248° F (110° to 120° C) drives off part of the water of crystallization and produces calcium sulfate hemihydrate ($CaSO_4½H_2O$). Mixing the hemihydrate with water reverses the reaction and produces the dihydrate. The method of calcining gypsum determines whether the hemihydrate will be the beta or alpha form.

Calcining in an open kettle produces the beta form of the hemihydrate (i.e., plaster which has irregularly shaped and extremely porous crystals). A satisfactory mix requires 50 ml of water per 100 g of powder. The resultant plaster is relatively weak because of the high water content, porosity of the particles, and inability of these particles to fit together closely because of their irregular shape.

Calcining gypsum under steam pressure in an autoclave produces the alpha form of the hemihydrate (type I stone, Hydrocal). The crystals are dense, nonporous, regularly shaped, and cuboidal. Type I stone requires only 30 ml of water per 100 g of powder, and the resultant cast is approximately 2½ times as strong as plaster.

Calcining gypsum by boiling it in a 30% solution of calcium chloride ($CaCl_2$) produces another alpha form of the hemihydrate (type II stone, Densite). The crystals of this improved stone are even more dense and slightly larger than those of type I stone. Type II stone, which requires less water than type I stone (18 to 24 ml of water per 100 g of powder), results in a stronger cast with a harder surface.

Setting expansion

Linear expansion occurs during the change from a hemihydrate to dihydrate because of the outward thrust of needlelike crystals formed in the dihydrate. Although this expansion ranges from 0.06% to 0.5%, it is possible to control it to some extent to obtain the desired accuracy. Following are guidelines to controlling setting expansion:

1. The smaller the ratio of water to powder, the more the mix expands as a result of more nuclei of crystallization per unit volume and the outward thrust caused by growth interaction of the dihydrate crystals.
2. Longer mixing time results in the formation of more nuclei of crystallization and consequently more expansion.
3. Hygroscopic expansion follows the immersion of gypsum products in water during the setting process. Additional crystal growth takes place, and approximately twice the normal setting expansion occurs.
4. Accelerators and retarders, generally used to alter the setting time of gypsum products also usually reduce the setting expansion. The use of modifiers by the manufacturers generally limits the setting expansion of commercially available dental stones to between 0.06% and 0.12%, which is relatively insignificant in clinical use.

Setting time

Sometimes it is desirable to control the setting time of dental stone, and various methods are available to the manufacturer and operator.

Manufacturer

1. Accelerators, such as 2% potassium sulfate, decrease the setting time.
2. Retarders, such as 2% borax, increase the setting time.
3. Powdered calcium sulfate dihydrate mixed with hemihydrate powder acts as nuclei of crystallization and accelerates the setting time.
4. The finer the size particle of hemihydrate powder, the faster the set occurs.

Operator

1. Increasing the amount of water in the mix results in fewer nuclei of crystallization per unit volume and adds to the setting time.
2. The longer and faster the hemihydrate is mixed, the shorter the setting time is. The mixing spatula breaks up crystals that form, distributes them throughout the mixture, and results in the formation of more nuclei of crystallization.
3. The exposure of gypsum products to high humidity decreases the setting time, since an increase in the percentage of dihydrate provides more nuclei of crystallization. Therefore it is necessary to store powders in a moistureproof container.

The physical properties desired in a gypsum cast depend to a large extent on the correct water-powder ratio. Any attempt to influence the expansion or setting time by altering this ratio is questionable. Accurate measurement of powder and water is essential.

Compressive strength

Generally the strength of gypsum products is expressed in terms of compressive strength. This strength is inversely proportional to the water-powder ratio of the material, that is, the more water in the mix, the lower the compressive strength. Type II stone requires the least water and is the strongest, whereas plaster requires the most water and is the weakest. The 1-hour compressive strength values are as follows:

Dental plaster	1800 p.s.i.
Type I stone (Hydrocal)	4500 p.s.i.
Type II stone (Densite)	5500 p.s.i.

Two strengths of gypsum products are recognized: wet strength and dry strength. A gypsum product with wet strength has water in excess of the amount required for hydration of the hemihydrate left in the specimen. A gypsum product with dry strength has the excess water driven off. Dry strength, which is usually at least twice the wet strength, is of extreme importance.

Compressive strength is affected not only by the water-powder ratio, but also by accelerators and retarders, which decrease it. Increasing the spatulation time up to 1 minute increases the compressive strength. Surface hardness also depends on compressive strength, and soaking the gypsum cast in water, glycerin, or oils does not alter the hardness. The only advantage of soaking is to produce a smooth cast that resists abrasion.

POURING IMPRESSIONS

Clinical experience and the literature substantiate the value of some guidelines in pouring impressions for working casts. It is essential to pour them immediately after removal from the mouth regardless of the material used (Fig. 1-98). As much as 30 minutes can elapse by the time it is possible to clean and dry the impression, set the pins, and mix the stone. Additional time can lead to clinically significant changes in the impression.

PROCEDURE

1. Measure water and powder carefully according to the manufacturer's directions (Fig. 1-99). It is best to weigh prepackaged powder each time to make certain that the labeled amounts are consistently accurate. Variations in the water-powder ratio have a definite effect on the final compressive strength of the working cast. Use distilled water to eliminate the possibility of contamination of the mix with calcium and other minerals in tap water.
2. Vacuum mix the powder and liquid because it makes the mix more homogeneous than hand spatulation (Fig. 1-100). The resultant casts and dies are of higher density. Vacuum mix the base also to avoid the possibility of a void adjacent to the pin and resulting instability of the seated die.
3. Add the mixed stone to the impression in small increments, and vibrate it gently so that it flows over all surfaces to avoid air entrapment (Fig. 1-101). This is especially important when the preparations are long and thin. Allow the stone to flow down one side of the preparation to the incisal or occlusal portion, and fill the preparation gingivally. Make the first pour of stone approximately 5 mm above the margins of the preparations to avoid encroaching on these margins and weakening them. A larger amount of stone would be excessive and offer no advantage. While the stone is setting,

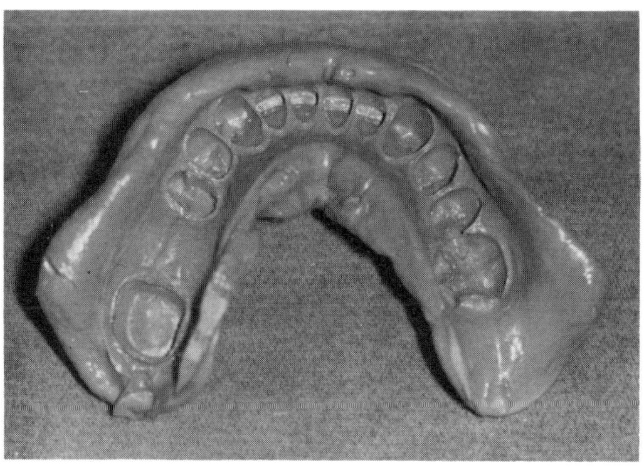

Fig. 1-98. Cleaned and dried mandibular impression.

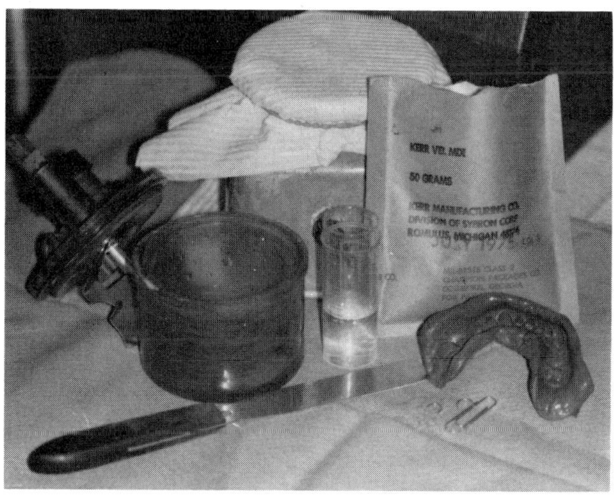

Fig. 1-99. Prepackaged powder, distilled water, final impression, vibrator, mixing bowl, spatula, and paper clips.

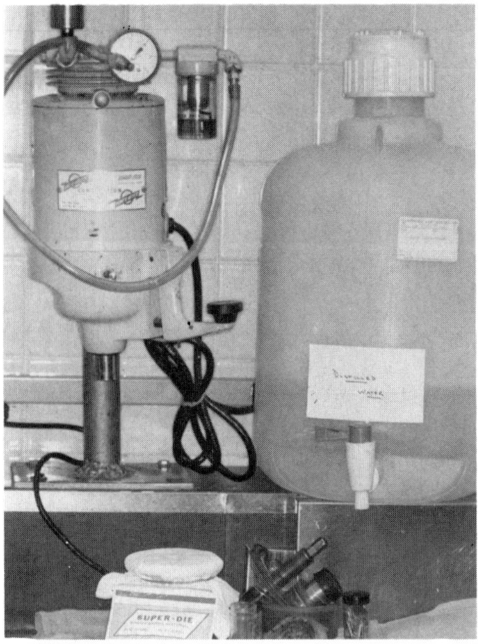

Fig. 1-100. Vacuum mixer and distilled water.

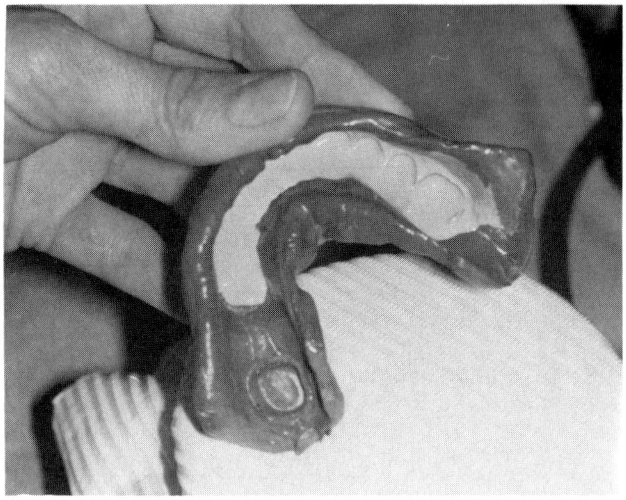

Fig. 1-101. Dental stone is vibrated gently to flow over surface of impression to avoid air entrapment.

place the poured impression in a humidor with 100% humidity (Fig. 1-102).

4. The base should be poured of a different color stone than the first pour to facilitate visualizing where to end the saw cuts when sawing out the dies.

5. Recover the working cast in not less than 45 minutes after pouring. With hydrocolloid materials recover the working cast in not more than 1 hour to prevent surface damage.

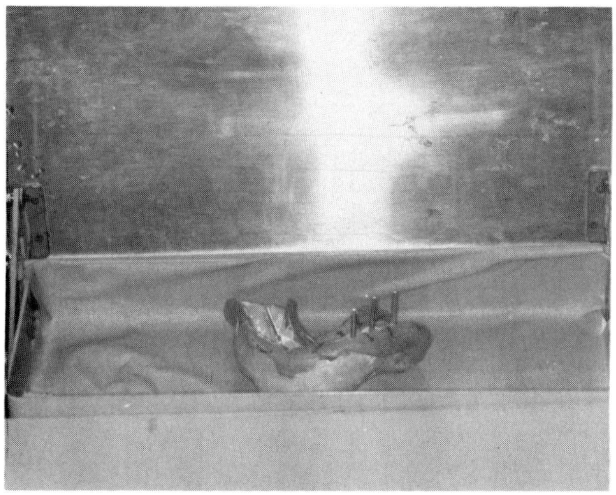

Fig. 1-102. Poured impression is placed in humidor.

PREPARATION OF WORKING CASTS WITH REMOVABLE DIES

The primary advantage of fabricating working casts with removable dies is to enable complete fabrication and insertion of fixed prosthodontic restorations in two appointments. This technique allows the restoration to be soldered in the laboratory without an extra appointment to obtain a solder index in the mouth of the patient. The resultant chair time and trauma are less for both the dentist and the patient. Many techniques and commercial products are available for fabricating working casts with removable dies. Following is a technique that is consistently successful, simple, and accurate.

PROCEDURE

1. Position the dowel pin used for producing removable dies before or after the initial stone pour. This preference depends on the skill of the dentist or technician. The experienced operator can mark the borders of the impression with an indelible pencil to guide in positioning the pins accurately in the soft stone after the initial pour (Figs. 1-103 and 1-104). However, an inexperienced operator can position these pins either too deep or too shallow in the preparation, too close to a proximal wall, or impinging on a margin of the preparation. It is easier to position the dowel pins in the impression prior to the initial pour to reduce the chances for error.

2. Position the dowel pins in the cleaned impression, and stabilize them by using paralleling instruments, needles, pins, paper clips, or bobby pins, whichever the operator prefers (Figs. 1-105 and 1-106).

3. Mix the stone properly, and pour it in the impres-

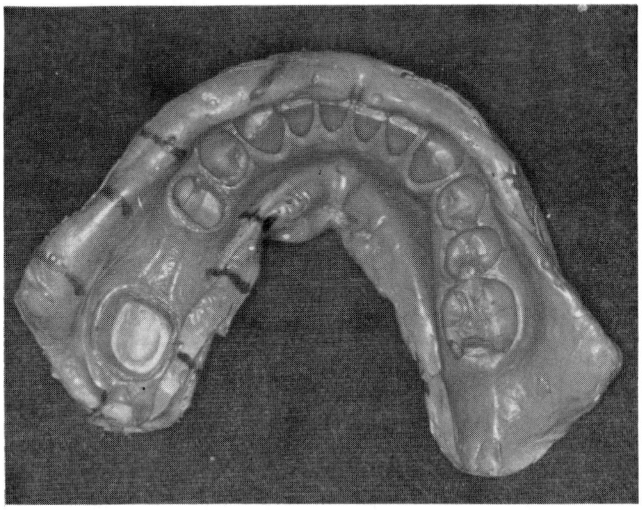

Fig. 1-103. Borders of final impression marked to indicate placement of pins after initial pour of dental stone.

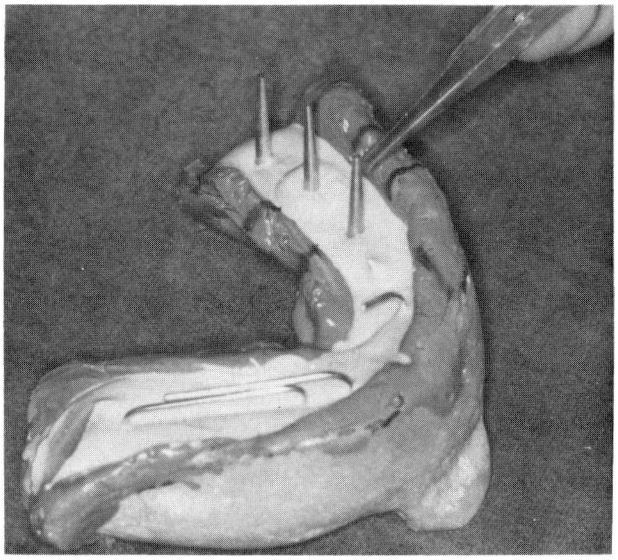

Fig. 1-104. Dowel pins are placed in impression according to marks on borders of impression.

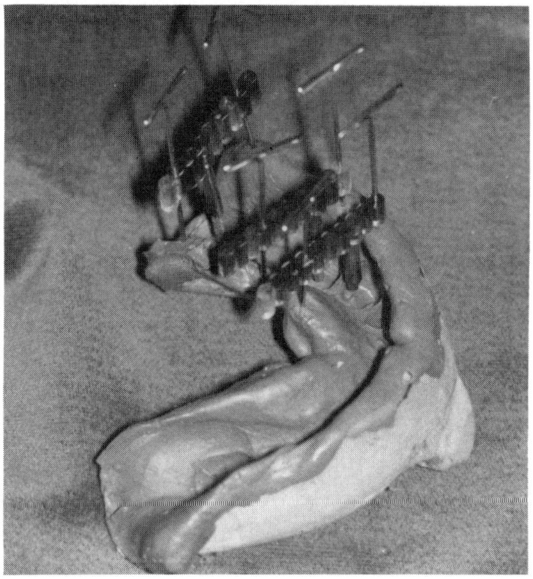

Fig. 1-105. One method of positioning pins before initial pour of stone.

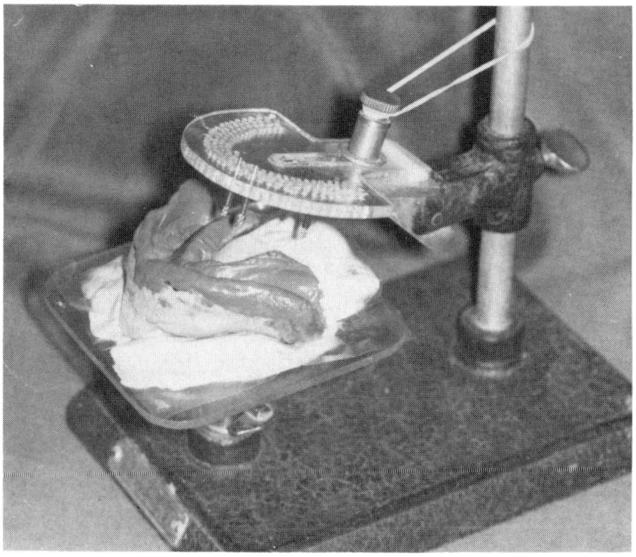

Fig. 1-106. Another method of positioning pins before initial pour of stone.

sion to a depth of not more than 5 mm over the margin of the preparation (Fig. 1-107). Make certain that the stone covers the gnarled retentive portion of the pin (Fig. 1-108).

4. Prior to the setting of the initial pour, add some form of mechanical retention to the areas of the impression that do not include the prepared teeth. Use paper clips, metal washers, or even stone (Fig. 1-107). When the stone has set, remove the dowel pin supports and any wax on the pins.

5. Incorporate a positive seat into the stone at this time so that the removable dies do not rotate when seated in the working cast (Fig. 1-109). Use either a V-shaped trench or a depression made with a No. 8 round bur. Apply a small ball of wax to the top of each dowel pin, and lubricate the area of the cast adjacent to the dowel pin with a thin film of separating medium (Figs. 1-110 and 1-111).

6. Place the cast in water briefly, and pour the base carefully with stone of a different color than the original stone pour. Recover the impression approximately 1 hour after the initial pour.

7. After recovering the cast, apply separating medium to the prepared and unprepared teeth immedi-

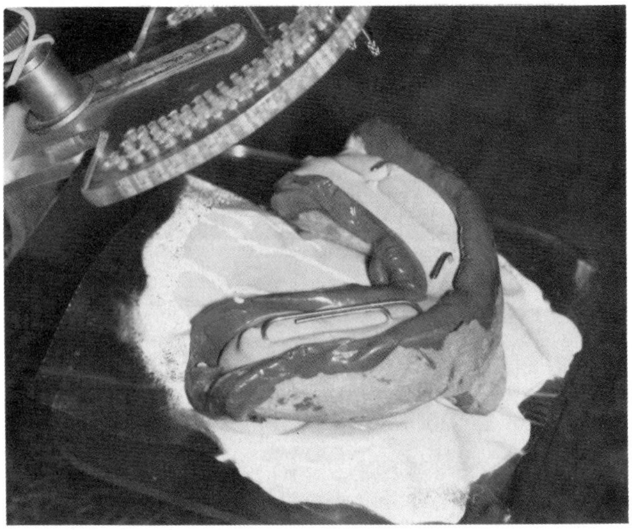

Fig. 1-107. Initial pour of stone with mechanical retention provided by paper clips.

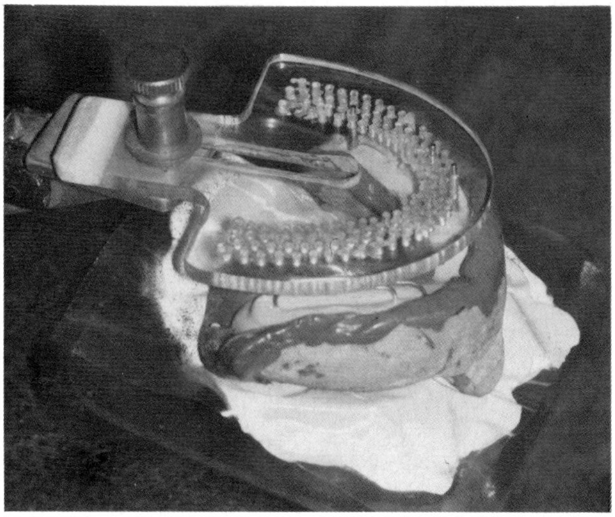

Fig. 1-108. Dowel pins are positioned in initial pour of stone in impression by pin setter.

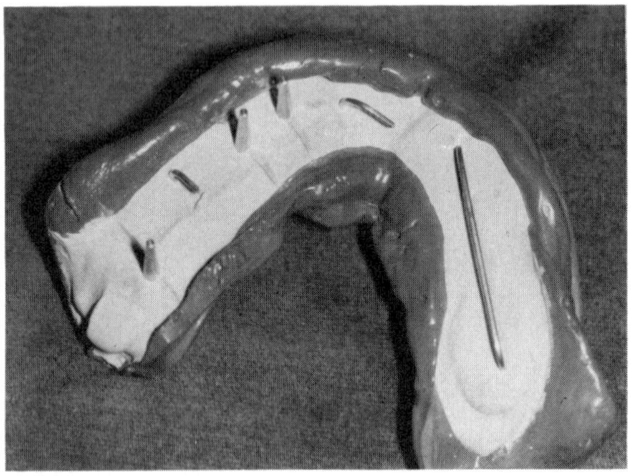

Fig. 1-109. Positive seat is provided in base of initial pour of set stone by V-shaped trenches.

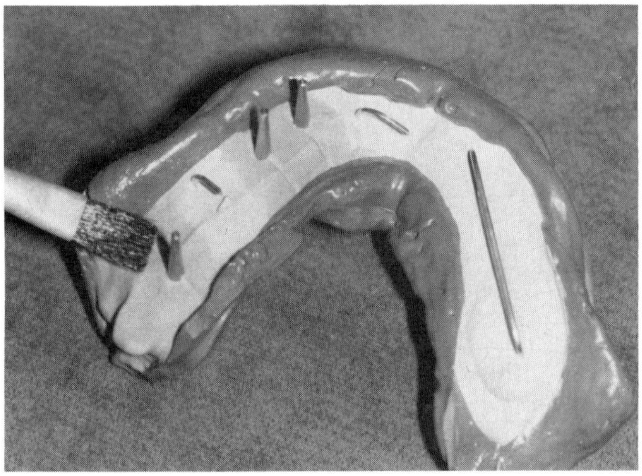

Fig. 1-110. Separating medium is painted on area of cast adjacent to each dowel pin.

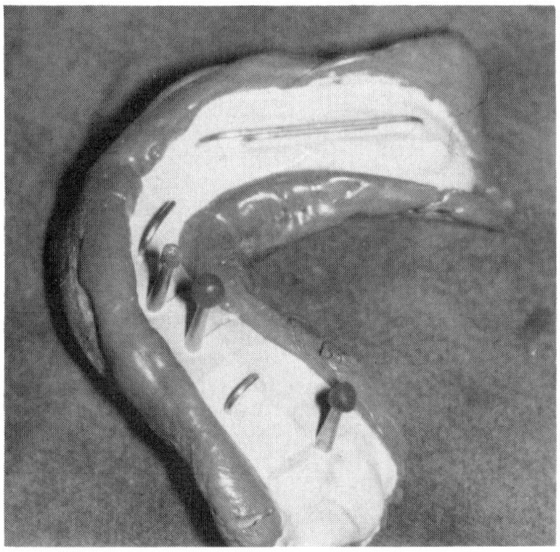

Fig. 1-111. Small balls of wax are placed on tips of dowel pins.

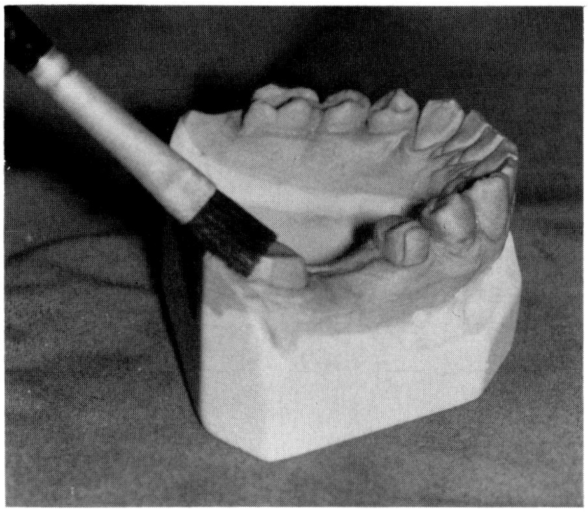

Fig. 1-112. Separating medium is applied to teeth after recovery of final cast from impression.

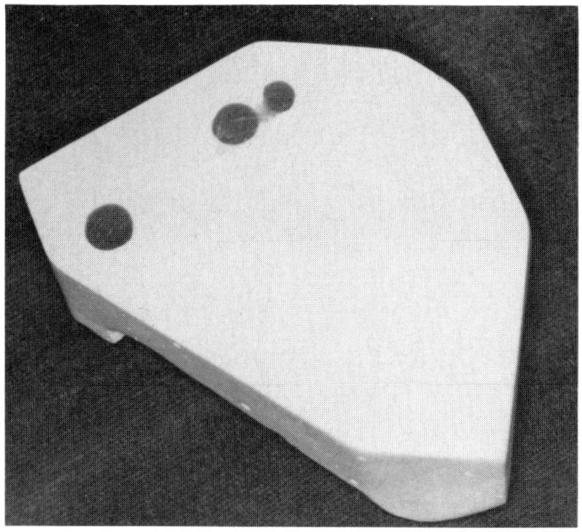

Fig. 1-113. Wax balls are located by trimming base of cast on model trimmer.

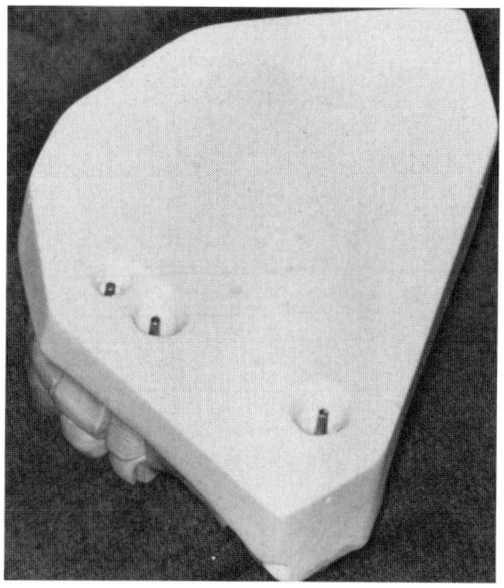

Fig. 1-114. Tips of dowel pins are exposed after removal of wax.

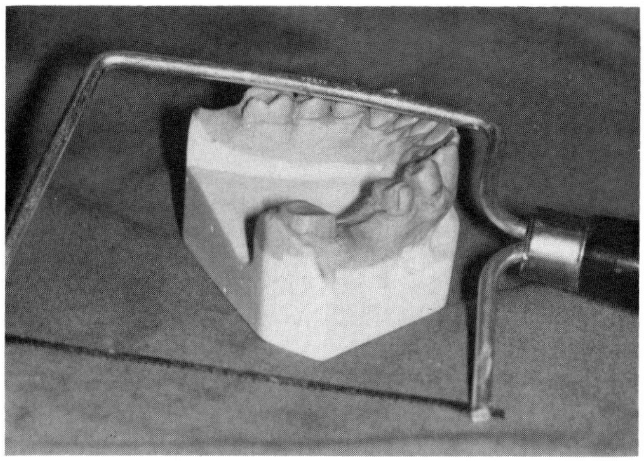

Fig. 1-115. Jeweler's saw used to cut through stone.

ately (Fig. 1-112) to prevent any possible etching of the stone surfaces by water left in contact with the cast.

8. Trim the cast properly, and locate the wax balls on the tips of the dowel pins by using the cast trimmer (Fig. 1-113). Remove the wax carefully, and clean the exposed tips of the dowel pins with chloroform (Fig. 1-114).

9. Make tapered cuts proximal to each preparation with a jeweler's saw (Fig. 1-115). These cuts should taper to prevent undercuts, but they should not impinge on the margins of the preparations or include too much of the edentulous ridge area needed for a proper ridge-pontic relationship. Make these saw cuts through the initial pour of stone (Fig. 1-116). Remove the dies by tapping lightly with a simple instrument and a mallet (Figs. 1-117 to 1-119).

10. Trim and ditch the dies, and mark the margins with a crayon pencil (Figs. 1-120 and 1-121). Do not use a lead pencil because it will result in rough and inaccurate margins. Check the dies for complete seating in the working cast with light pressure. If there is any interference, clean the pinhole with a pipe cleaner, and check to make certain that the dowel pin and the base of the removable die are free of debris before reseating the die in the pinhole (Fig. 1-122).

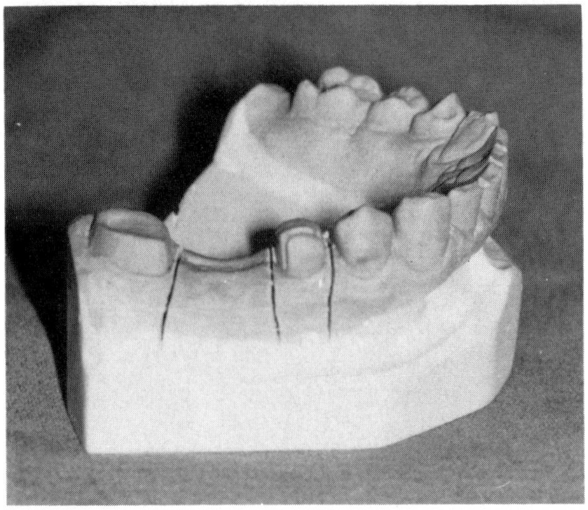

Fig. 1-116. Tapered saw cuts are made through initial pour of stone.

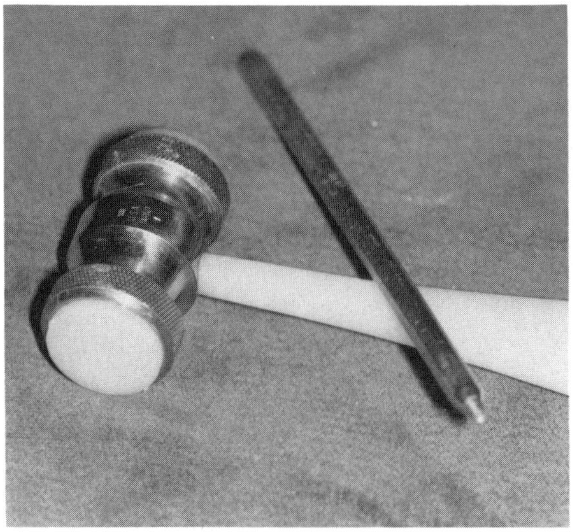

Fig. 1-117. Rubber mallet and instrument are used to tap out sawed dies.

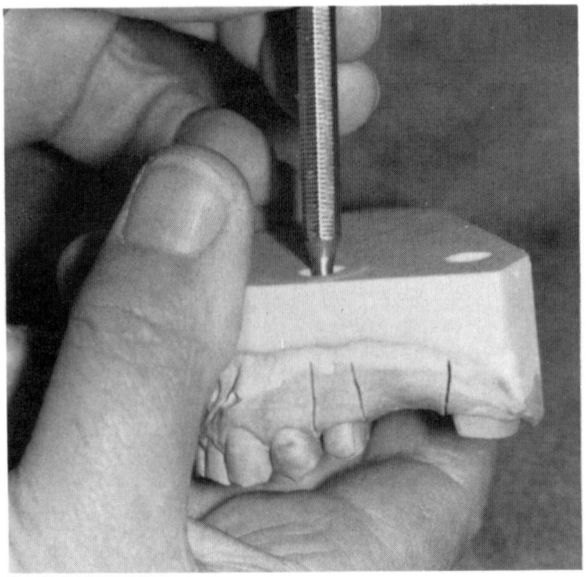

Fig. 1-118. Instrument is placed on tip of dowel pin.

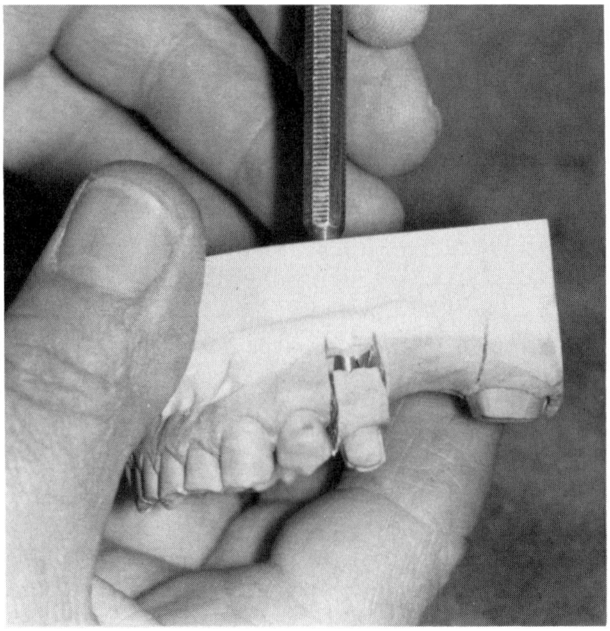

Fig. 1-119. Die is removed by tapping instrument with mallet.

Dry-pinning technique

Many different systems have been advocated and devised to enable working casts to be prepared that have dies that can be removed from the base. The precise placement of tapered die pins to allow the removal of individual dies presents a number of technical problems:

1. Optimum location of the pin to the removable die
2. Parallelism of the die shafts
3. Uniformity of length of the die pins in relation to the base of the cast
4. Smoothness of the die base at the interface with the cast base material
5. Guidance to prevent rotation and allow precise repositioning of the die
6. Stabilization of die pins during setting of the primary pour (during wet-pinning techniques)

Several different systems and accompanying appa-

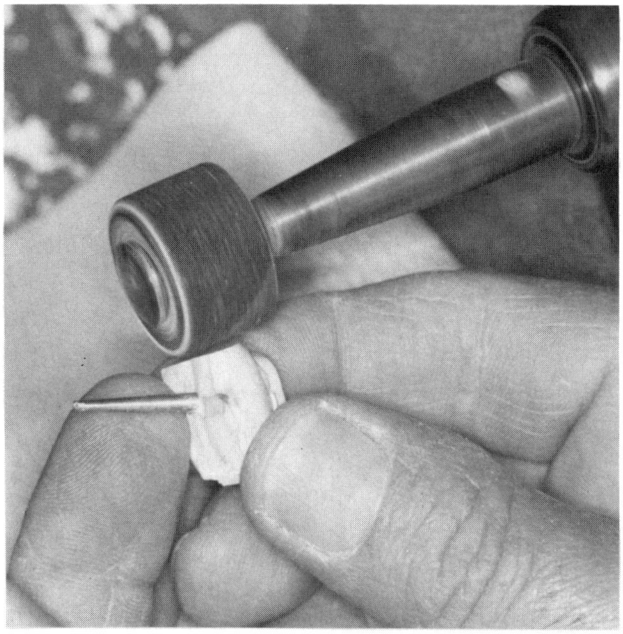

Fig. 1-120. Excess stone is removed from base of die by arbor band.

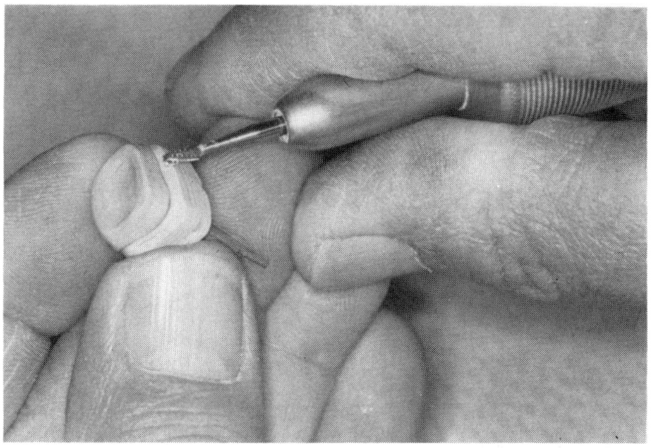

Fig. 1-121. Die is ditched with fissure bur.

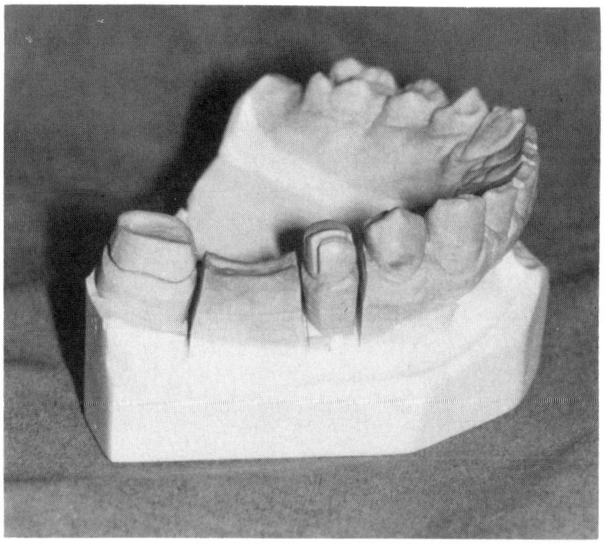

Fig. 1-122. Final working cast with trimmed, ditched removable dies.

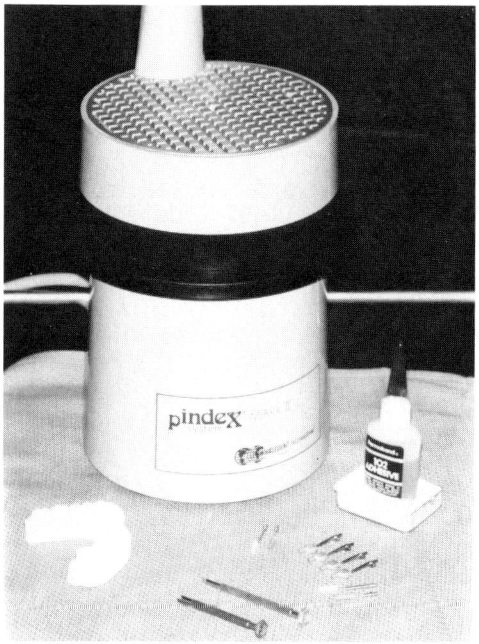

Fig. 1-123. "Pindex" drilling apparatus (developed by Whaledent, Inc.) for dry-pinning process. Prepared tooth on the cast is positioned beneath a pointer aligned with drill. As table is lowered, drill, which is positioned beneath, raises to form retentive hole in cast base. Die pin is later cemented into position.

ratus have been developed to allow the exact placement of die pins after the cast has been removed from the impression and inspected for completeness (Fig. 1-123). The dry-pinning approach allows the critical impression to be poured with die material immediately, thereby eliminating delay caused by adjustment apparatus for die pin orientation, which is necessary in a wet-pinning procedure.

PROCEDURE

1. Die stone is introduced into the impression, allowed to set, and separated from the impression. If second pour casts are desired for working, assembly, or back up casts they may be obtained by an immediate repouring of the impression.
2. The base of the separated cast is trimmed flat to about 15-mm thickness.
3. Exact position for the long index pin within the

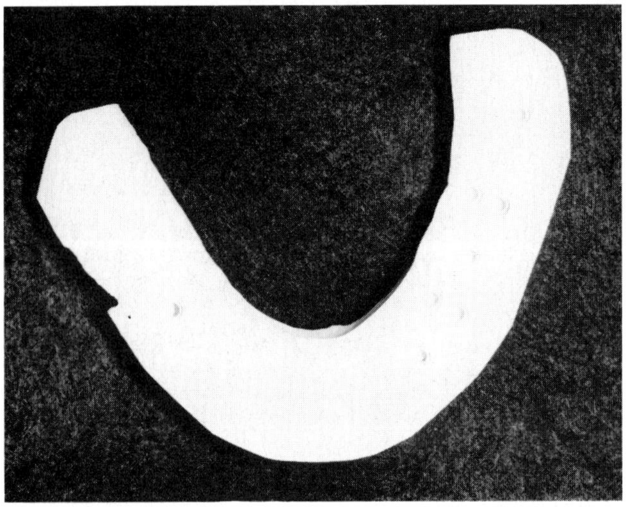

Fig. 1-124. Flattened side of cast showing retentive holes that have been precisely prepared to receive die pins. Flattened surface of die stone will permit a smooth interface and easy separation from base portion, which will be fabricated later.

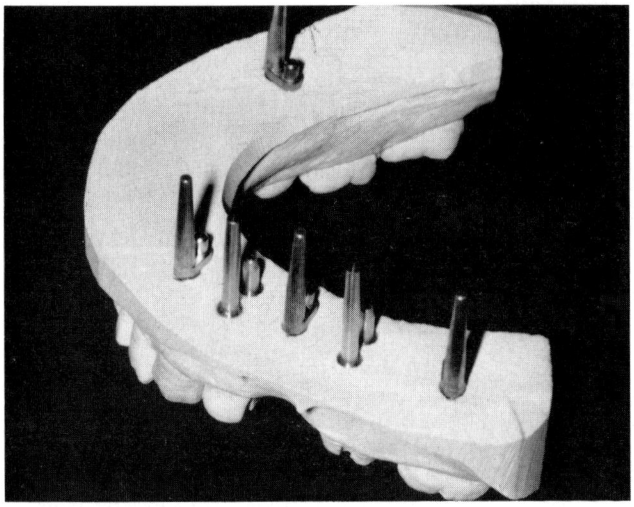

Fig. 1-125. Base side of cast showing die pins cemented into position. Note shorter secondary pins for orientation of die in base portion of cast.

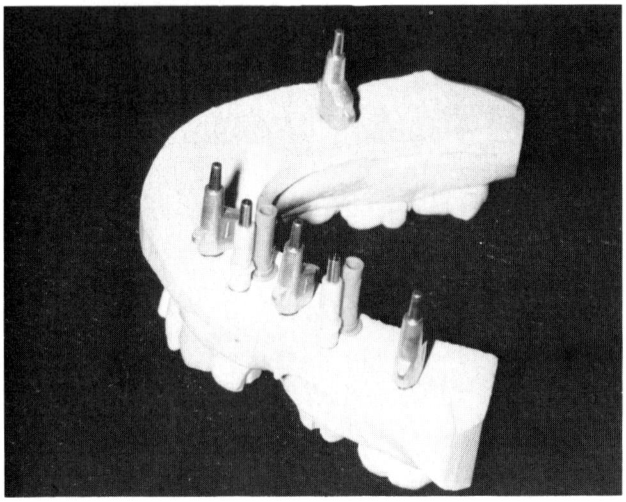

Fig. 1-126. Sleeves that fit die pins are positioned before base portion of cast is poured. Sleeves permit easy separation of pins and their precise replacement.

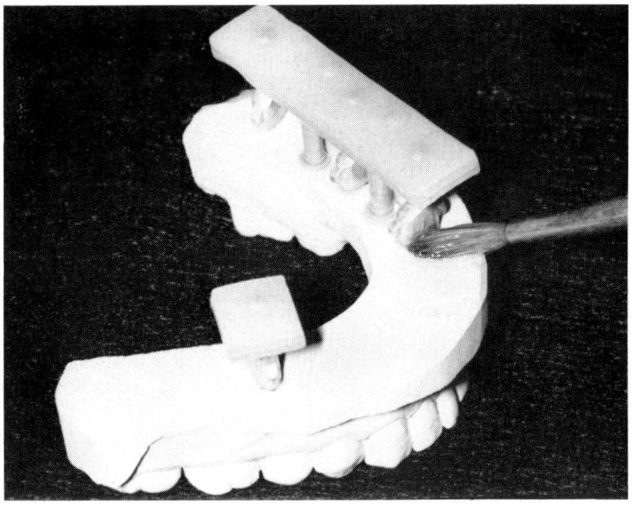

Fig. 1-127. Wax spacers placed over tips of die pins preform a channel in base portion of cast. When wax is removed from base portion of cast, pin tips are readily accessible. Separating medium is applied before base portion of cast is poured, to permit easy separation of die stone from base portion.

confines of the die crown is determined. A retentive hole is drilled in the base of the cast opposite this position to receive the retentive nib of the die pin. A similar hole is drilled adjacent to the first to receive a shorter auxiliary pin, which serves to orient the die assembly at any time it (the die) is returned to the cast (Fig. 1-124).

4. All pins are firmly cemented into the drilled holes with suitable cement (cyanoacrylate) (Fig. 1-125).

5. Plastic sleeves, manufactured to fit the pins precisely, are positioned over the dies (Fig. 1-126). The tips of the die pins are protected by a wax spacer. This spacer will allow the tips of the die pins to be located easily in the cast base (Figs. 1-126 and 1-127).

6. After placement of a suitable separating material (Fig. 1-127) and proper boxing of the cast, the base portion is poured with a different colored stone so that the division line can be identified (Fig. 1-128).

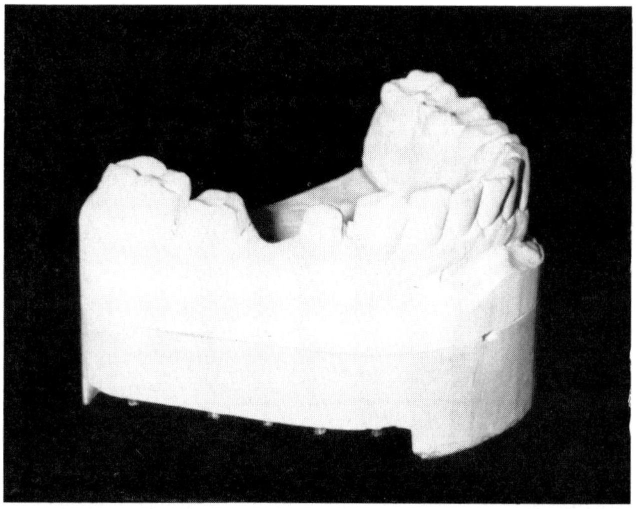

Fig. 1-128. Cast with base portion completed. Vertical saw cuts are made using a fine jeweller's saw, through interproximal areas of die stone to depth of cast base.

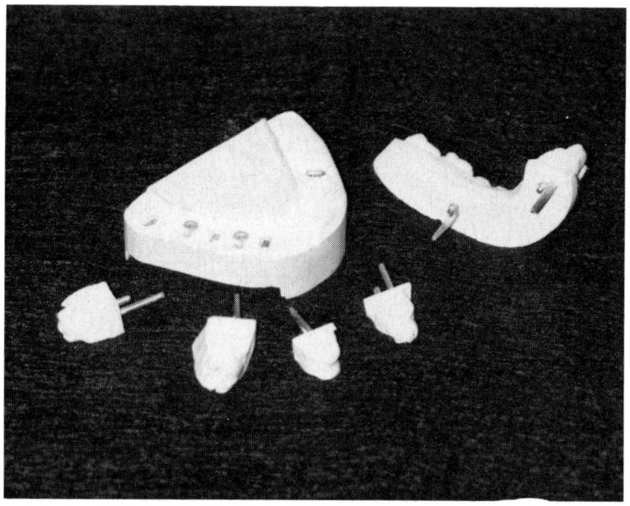

Fig. 1-129. Individual dies can be removed readily by tapping on tips of dies, which are exposed in channel of base. Pins will permit dies to be replaced in their exact positions.

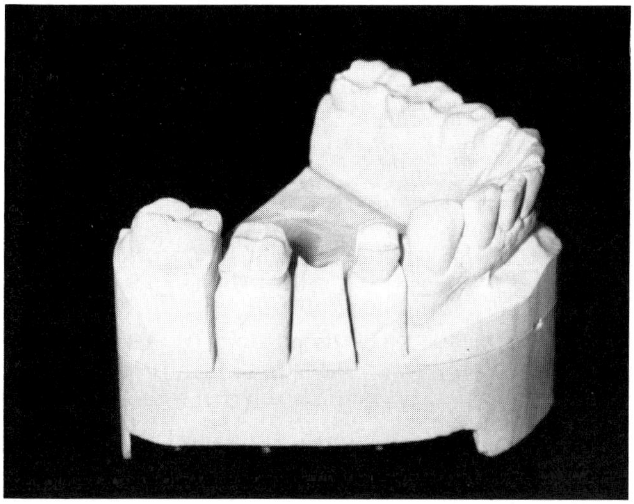

Fig. 1-130. Completed cast with removable dies after trimming and replacement. Saw cuts have been directed to allow removal and replacement of dies without impingement on adjacent surfaces of cast.

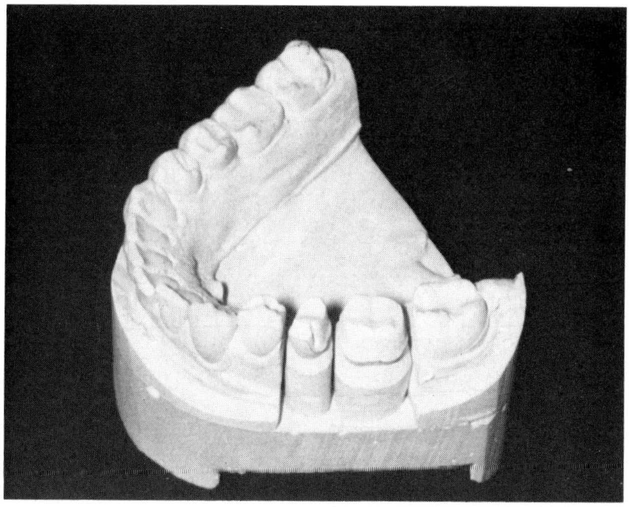

Fig. 1-131. Individual removable dies have been trimmed so that waxing procedures can be completed with access to margin areas.

7. With a fine jeweler's saw, the die stone portion of the cast is sectioned in the interproximal spaces to the depth of the base portion of the cast.
8. The dies can be removed by tapping lightly on the tips of the die pins that protrude into the channel previously formed by the wax spacer, which was in position at the time the cast base was poured.
9. Die margins can be trimmed in preparation for subsequent waxing procedures (Figs. 1-129 to 1-131).

Die spacing

Considerable attention has been focused on the role that internal relief of crown castings plays in margin adaptation. Internal relief of castings has been advocated for many years to provide space for the cementing medium and to allow a more complete seating of the casting on the prepared tooth. Recent investigations advocate the use of several layers of lacquer or other material to preform the relief layer in the wax pattern

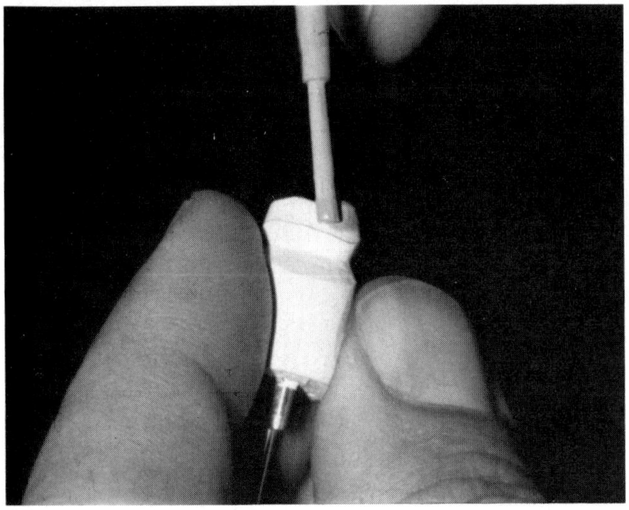

Fig. 1-132. Die spacing material is applied to the die over coronal and axial surfaces of preparation. Spacing material is carried no closer than 1 mm from cavosurface margin. Die spacing allows space for cementing medium between casting and prepared tooth surface and allows more complete seating of casting on tooth.

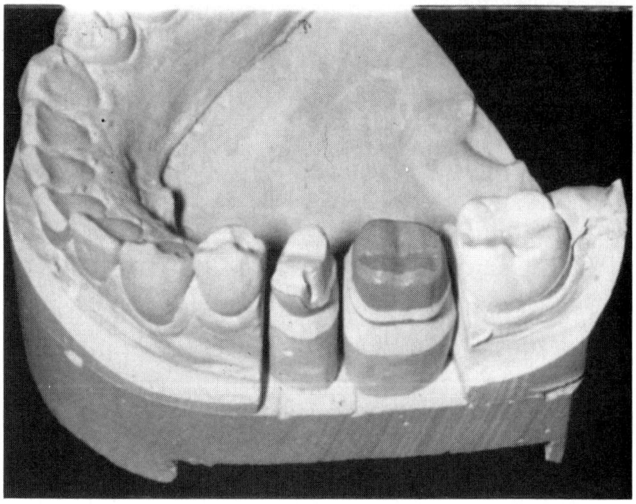

Fig. 1-133. Preparation after die-spacing lacquer is applied. Note complete coverage except for area immediately adjacent to margin. Die-spacing material should flow evenly, dry to a smooth surface, and be of contrasting color to both wax and die stone.

before it is invested and cast. It appears that the amount of internal relief can be more accurately controlled by the "die-spacing" method than by etching or milling processes that have been employed for so many years.

PROCEDURE

The technique of die spacing is relatively simple: successive layers of lacquer, fingernail paint, or model aircraft "dope"* are placed over the die surfaces (Fig. 1-132). The covering should stop approximately 1 mm from the margin of the preparation. Properly applied, the die spacing material should provide from 10 to 15 μm relief. The material should be of a color that is readily identifiable on the die (Fig. 1-133) and under the wax buildup so that wax thickness can be determined easily.

ALTERNATIVE DIE AND CAST MATERIALS

The materials used to construct dies and casts from dental impressions are dental stone, amalgam, resins, and electrodeposits of metal. Dental stone, which was discussed earlier in the chapter, is the most frequently used material; this chapter will present only a brief discussion on the alternative materials. The materials used for impressions often limit the types of casts or dies that it is possible to make. For example, hydrocolloid impressions are effective only with gypsum products. On the other hand, compound impressions are usable with dental stone, amalgam, and electrodeposits of metal. Polysulfide impressions are usable with dental stone, resin, or electrodeposits of metal. The type of impression material determines the choice of die or cast material.

The copper band–modeling plastic impressions used to make amalgam dies require wrapping in wax or tape and embedding in a rigid matrix, such as plaster, to resist the pressure necessary to condense the amalgam effectively. This technique is not only time consuming, but it also requires some degree of skill to condense the amalgam into the impression properly. Alloy takes at least 12 hours to harden before it is possible to recover the die. Improper manipulation of the amalgam can lead to clinically significant dimensional changes in the resulting die.

Other die materials are acrylic and epoxy resins. An acrylic resin is available as a powdered polymer with a liquid monomer, whereas an epoxy resin is available as a jar of resin with a syringe of hardener. These materials are for painting or pouring into the impression material (preferably polysulfide or polyether impression material). Resin materials are more viscous than dental stone and more prone to trap air in the preparations. Therefore a centrifuge technique is recommended to reduce the resulting air bubbles. Resin dies resist abrasion better and have higher compressive strength than dental stone. Resins shrink up to 0.02% on polymerization, whereas gypsum products expand on setting. The resin die can be smaller than the prepared tooth and,

*Aero Gloss, Hot Fuel Proof Dope, Pactra Industries, Inc., Upland, Calif. 91786.

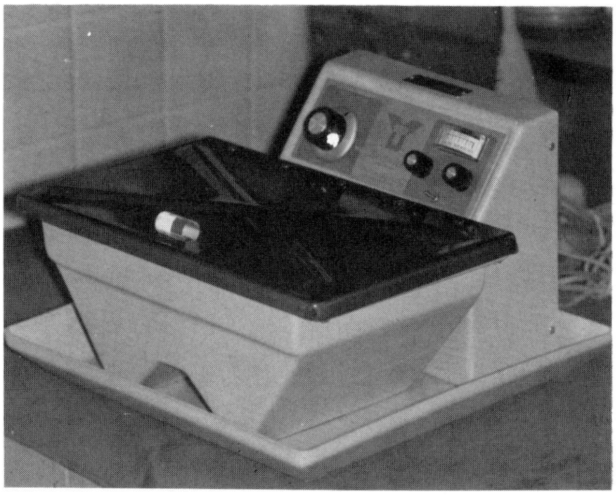

Fig. 1-134. Commercially available plating unit.

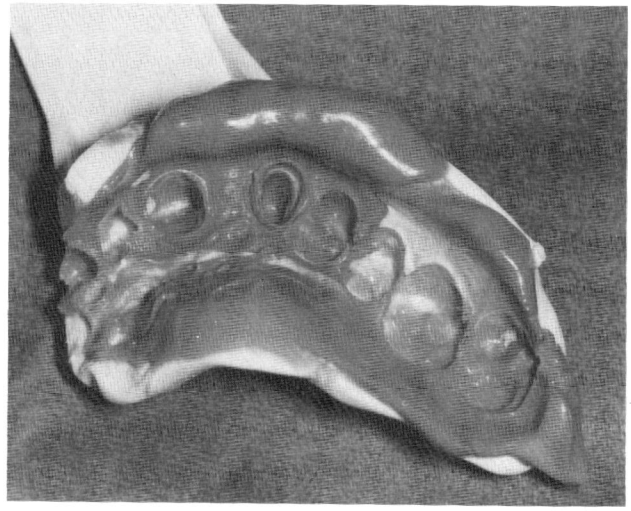

Fig. 1-135. Final impression after cleaning and drying.

unless the dentist makes some adjustment for this situation during the investing and casting procedure, it can be clinically significant.

Electrodeposition of metals or electroplating of impressions produces dies that have advantages over other materials discussed. An electroplated die has more surface hardness, better resistance to abrasions, and generally superior surface detail. Several commercially made plating units that produce these dies are available at moderate cost (Fig. 1-134).

The basic system consists of an electrolytic solution, such as copper sulfate or silver cyanide, and a source of direct current. The anode, which is either pure silver or pure copper, regenerates the solution during the migration of the copper from the cathode and to the surface of the impression. Generally, copperplating is used for wax or compound impressions and silver plating for polysulfide impressions. Although silver plating silicone impressions has been successful, distortion can be a problem.

PROCEDURE

The procedure for silver plating polysulfide and silicone impressions is the most commonly used method of electroplating removable dies.

1. After cleaning and drying the impression (Fig. 1-135), metalize the area to be plated with a fine silver powder by burnishing it with a sable brush (Fig. 1-136).
2. Insert the cathode wire in the border of the impression in the metalized area, but not too close to the preparations (Fig. 1-137).

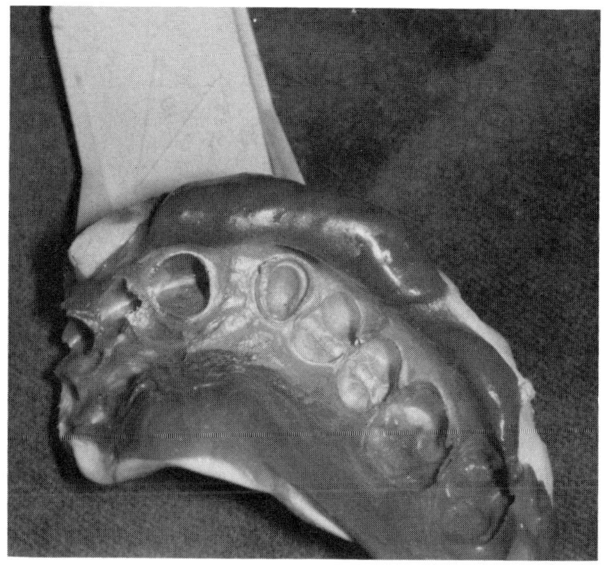

Fig. 1-136. Final impression is metalized with fine silver powder.

3. Fill the preparations and the teeth with the electrolytic solution by using an eyedropper to prevent air bubbles and resulting voids (Fig. 1-138).
4. Completely submerge the impression in the plating solution (Fig. 1-139). The silver anode immersed in the solution should be at least equal in size to the area of the surface to be plated.
5. Proceed with the plating initially at approximately 5 ma per tooth for 1 hour. Examine the impression after 1 hour to check for an even deposition of metal and to

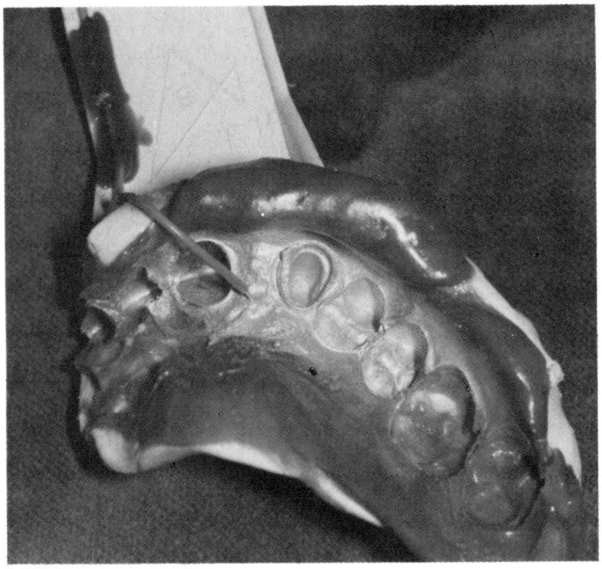

Fig. 1-137. Cathode wire is inserted in metalized area of impression.

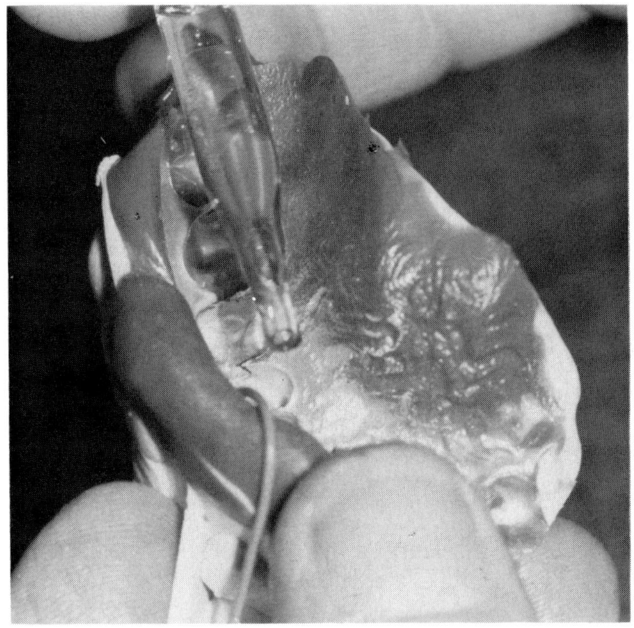

Fig. 1-138. Electrolytic solution is placed in preparation with eyedropper to prevent air bubbles.

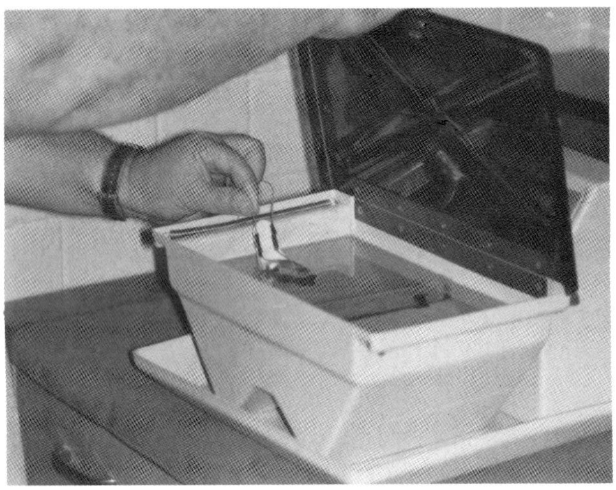

Fig. 1-139. Impression is connected to electrical source and submerged in plating solution. Note anode in middle of solution bath.

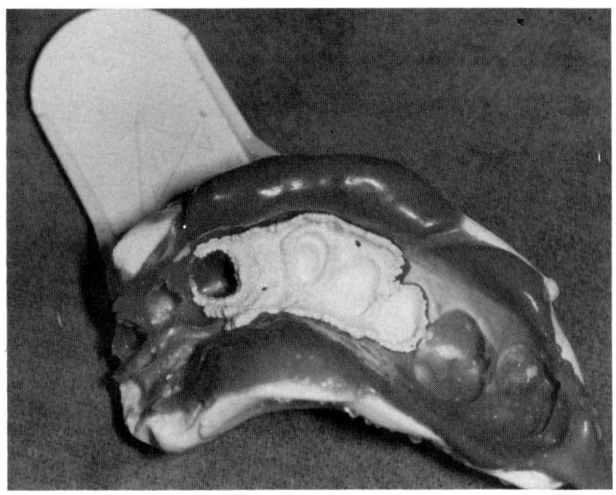

Fig. 1-140. Electroplated impression.

make certain that there are no voids. If any are present, remetalize them with silver powder. Resubmerge the impression in the plating solution, and plate it for approximately 12 hours at 10 ma per tooth.

6. After completion of the electroplating (Fig. 1-140), wash and dry the impression, and use dental stone to construct working casts with removable dies, as described previously (Figs. 1-141 and 1-142).

PROBLEM AREAS

The silver cyanide solution is extremely dangerous, because if it contacts acid, it produces fumes of extremely toxic hydrocyanic acid. Therefore place the bath in a well-ventilated area, and avoid all use of acids near the bath.

Silverplated dies are not significantly more or less accurate than stone dies. The possibility of continued po-

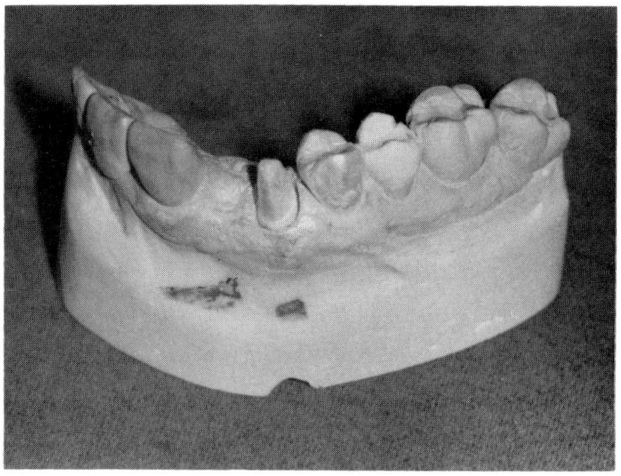

Fig. 1-141. Final working cast.

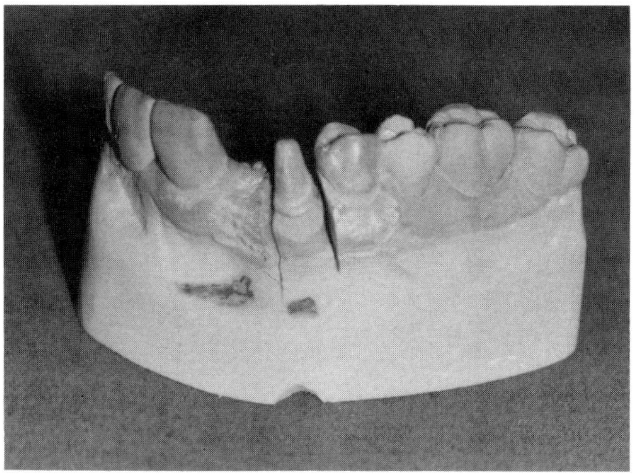

Fig. 1-142. Final working cast with trimmed and ditched removable die.

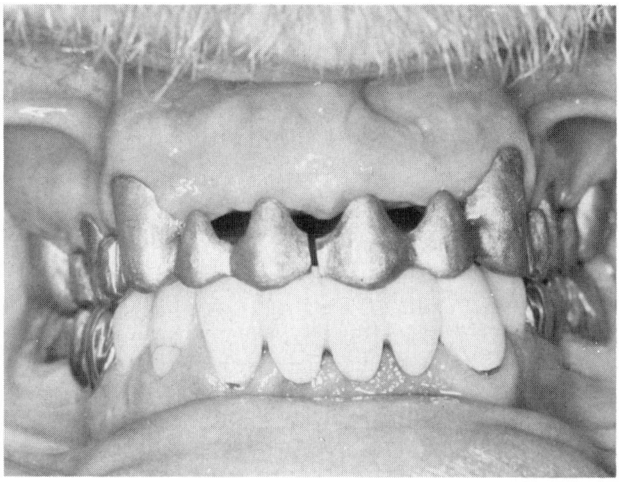

Fig. 1-143. Castings have been seated in mouth of patient. It was necessary to section anterior segment to seat it completely. It will be soldered from final remount cast by means of solder index.

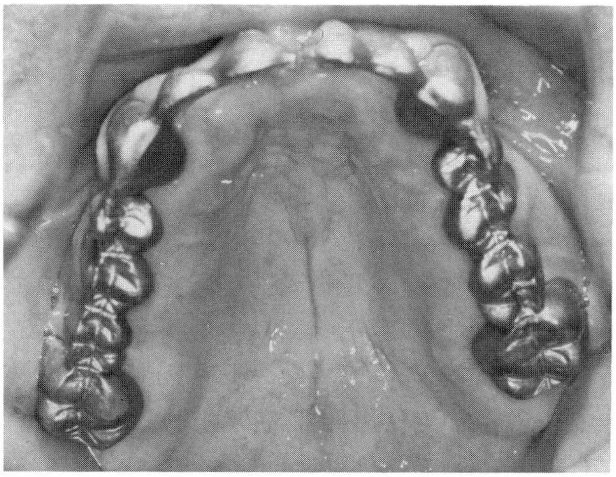

Fig. 1-144. Occlusal view of seated castings.

lymerization and distortion of the impression during electroplating may lead to a clinically significant dimensional change in the impression. This technique also precludes the possibility of returning the final working cast and dies in less than 12 hours, whereas other die materials can reduce the time dramatically.

FABRICATION OF REMOUNT CASTS

Remounting restorations on an articulator accurately in the same relationship as when they articulate in the mouth of the patient is exremely important in occlusal rehabilitation. It allows for the minute refinement of occlusal relationships and the observation of interocclusal relationships, which are extremely difficult to accomplish in the mouth. Of the several techniques commonly used to produce an accurate remount cast, the two described are precise and simple.

The dentist checks the restorations in the mouth of the patient for proper fit, contact, and contour (Figs. 1-143 and 1-144). The restorations can then be stabilized with a mixture of temporary cement and petroleum jelly. An accurate face-bow transfer and at least two centric records are made and set (Figs. 1-145 and 1-146). The second centric relation record is used to confirm the accuracy of the initial record, which was used to mount the mandibular cast to the face-bow–transferred maxillary cast.

To position the castings in the impression accurately, it is important to position the castings against a positive material. This requirement precludes the use of such

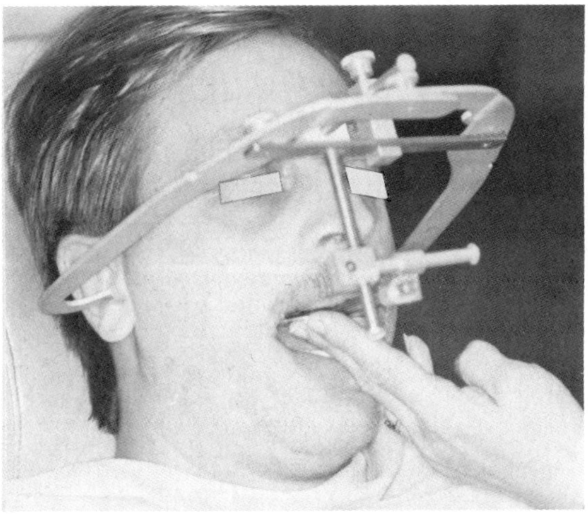

Fig. 1-145. Face-bow transfer record is made.

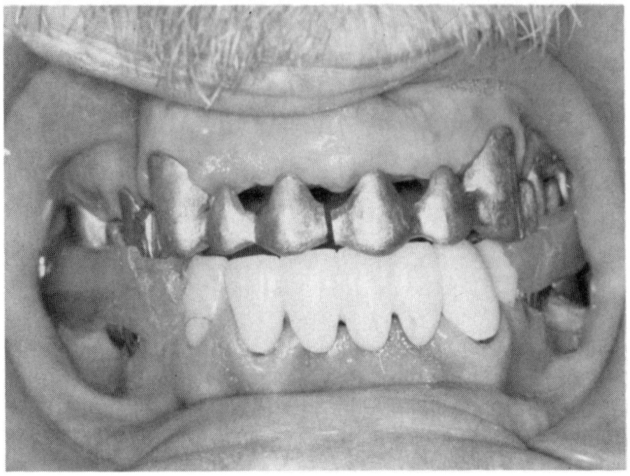

Fig. 1-146. Centric relation record is made.

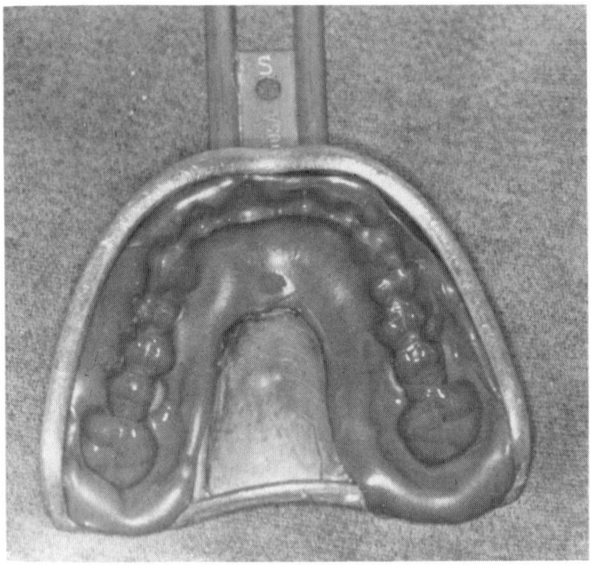

Fig. 1-147. Modeling plastic occlusal index of seated castings in water-cooled tray.

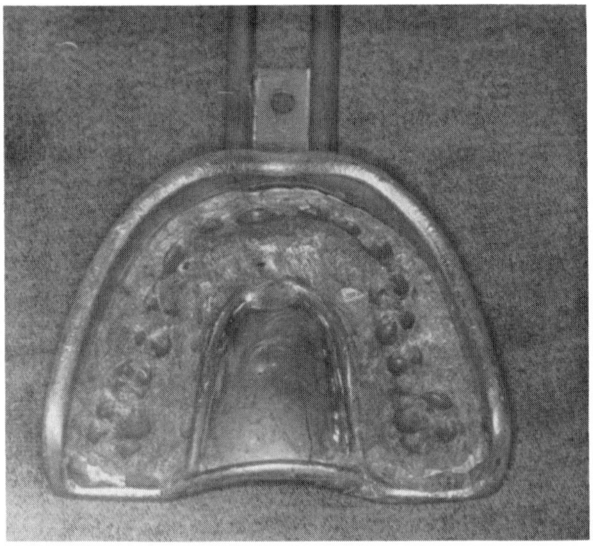

Fig. 1-148. Modeling plastic is trimmed back to imprints of tips of cusps.

materials as hydrocolloid, alginate, or polysulfide alone. For absolute accuracy it is necessary to combine them with plaster, acrylic, or compound.

Hydrocolloid compound technique

PROCEDURE

1. Soften modeling plastic in a water heater, and place it in a hydrocolloid water-cooled tray in the areas of the mouth containing the seated restorations; then remove it, and cool it (Fig. 1-147)

2. Remove any modeling plastic in contact with natural teeth, and trim it back where it is in contact with the restorations until only the tips of the cusps are present (Fig. 1-148).

3. Heat the modeling plastic with an alcohol torch (Fig. 1-149), and place softened hydrocolloid material in the tray to fill all areas.

4. Temper the tray in 100° F (38° C) water bath, place it firmly over the patient's teeth, and chill it for 5 minutes (Fig. 1-150).

5. On removal of the tray, place the restorations in the impression positively against its compound occlusal surfaces (Fig. 1-151). The compound produces a positive unyielding seat for the restorations.

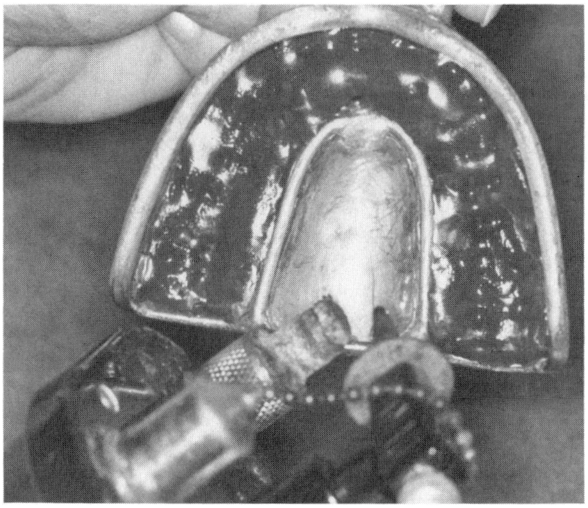

Fig. 1-149. Modeling plastic is heated with alchohol torch.

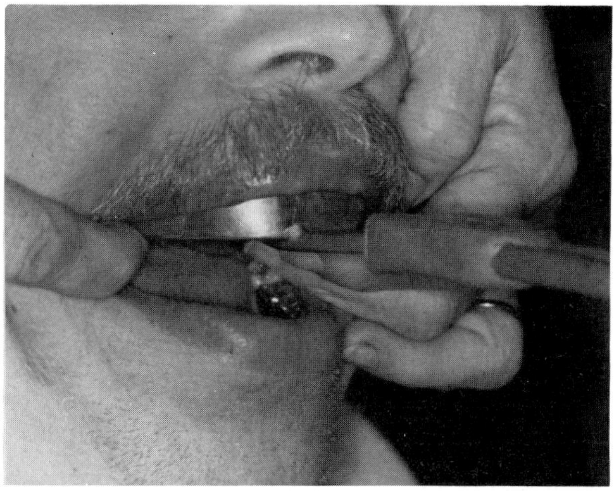

Fig. 1-150. Hydrocolloid–modeling plastic impression is made.

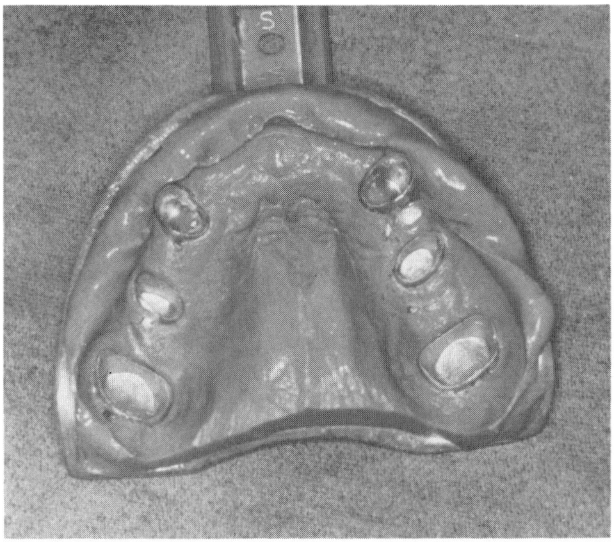

Fig. 1-151. Castings are positioned in impression.

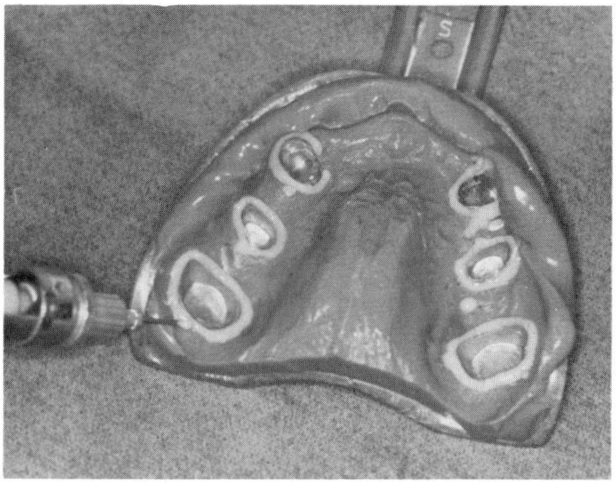

Fig. 1-152. Hydrocolloid is injected around exposed proximal surfaces of castings.

6. Apply a thin film of petroleum jelly to the internal portion of the restorations to facilitate removal from the cast at this time. Another method is to inject hydrocolloid around the exposed proximal surfaces of the restorations in the impression (Figs. 1-152 and 1-153). When using dental stone to pour the impression, do not vibrate it into the impression; paint it on to avoid dislodging the castings. A simpler method that also makes a stronger cast is to use low-fusing metal, such as Melotte's metal, for the first pour of this impression. Then it is easy to make the second pour of the impression with dental stone after providing adequate retention with paper clips in the metal (Figs. 1-154 to 1-156).

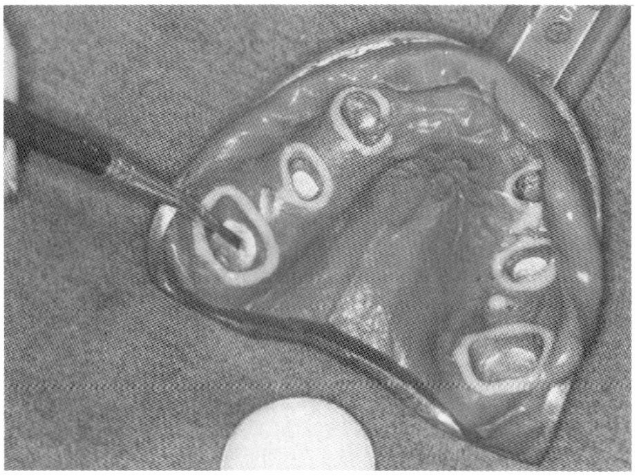

Fig. 1-153. Petroleum jelly is applied to internal surface of castings.

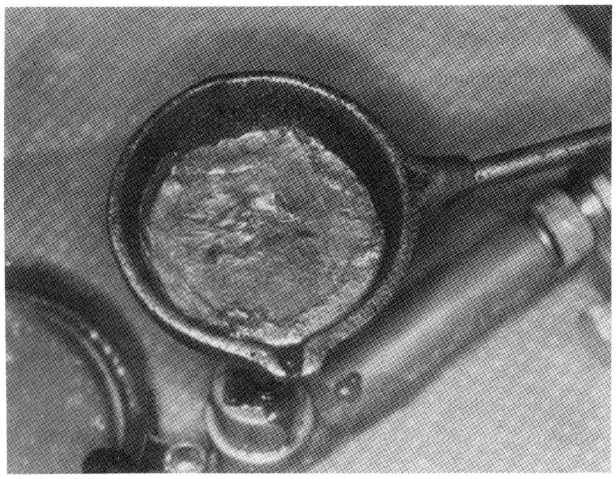

Fig. 1-154. Low-fusing metal is softened over Bunsen burner.

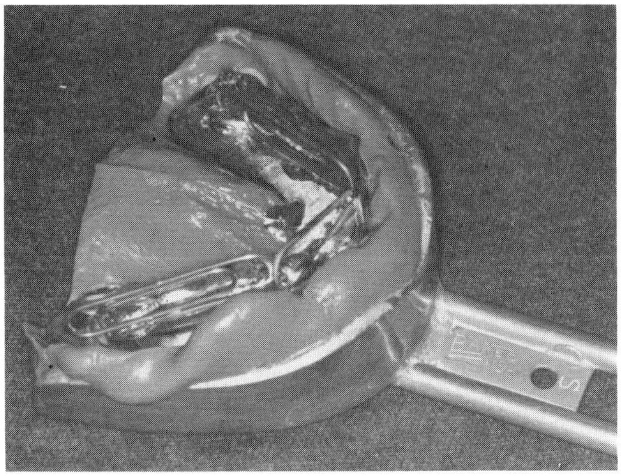

Fig. 1-155. Low-fusing metal is poured in impression, and retention is provided with paper clip.

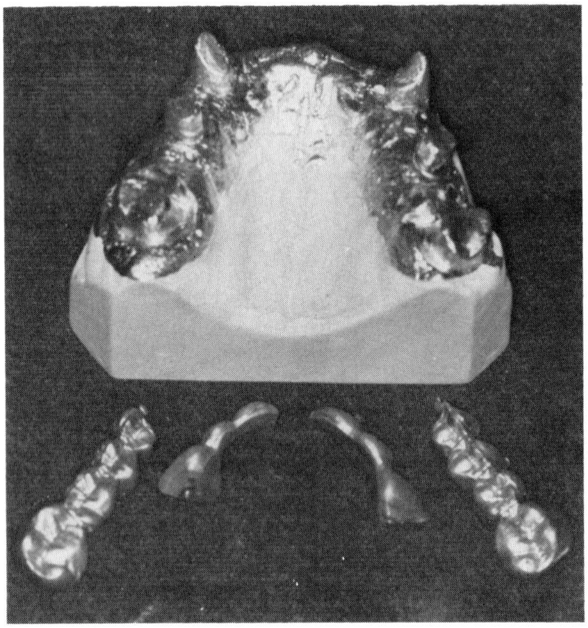

Fig. 1-156. Remount cast with castings removed.

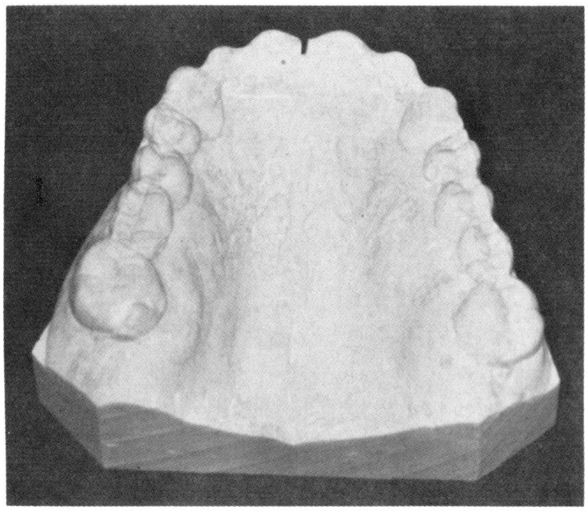

Fig. 1-157. Cast of castings in mouth of patient.

Plastic occlusal matrix

PROCEDURE

1. Make an alginate impression of the arch or arches containing the restorations to be remounted.

2. Pour the impression in dental stone mixed with slurry water to reduce the setting time (Fig. 1-157).

3. On the resultant cast, make an acrylic occlusal matrix. Contour heavy wire, such as a coat hanger, to fit the occlusal surfaces of the posterior teeth and the lingual surfaces of the anterior teeth. Paint a separating material on these surfaces, and use autopolymerizing acrylic resin to fabricate an index by sprinkling powder and liquid on these coated surfaces (Figs. 1-158 to 1-161). Incorporate the wire in this index for rigidity. The acrylic should bypass the natural teeth and not make contact with them. After the acrylic has hardened, remove the matrix, trim it, and try it in the mouth to assure accuracy.

4. Select a rim-lock tray to fit over the index. Roughen the index, and modify it to assure retention in the impression material.

5. Make a thin mix of zinc oxide–eugenol paste, ap-

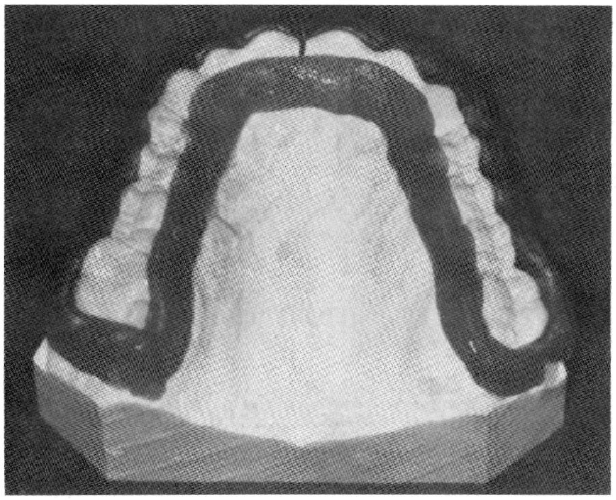

Fig. 1-158. Occlusal surfaces of cast are boxed with beading wax.

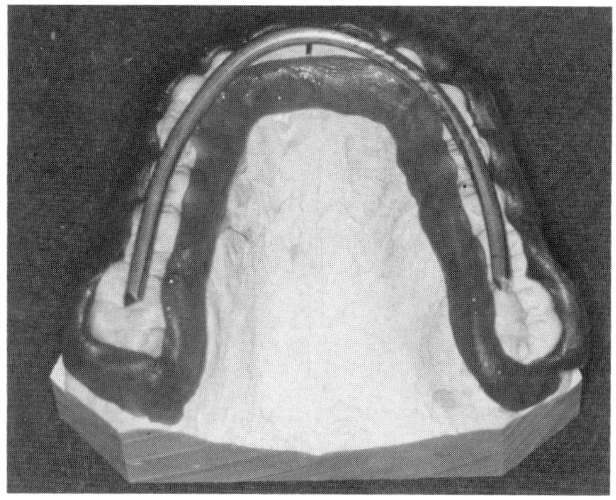

Fig. 1-159. Heavy-gauge wire is bent to conform to arch form.

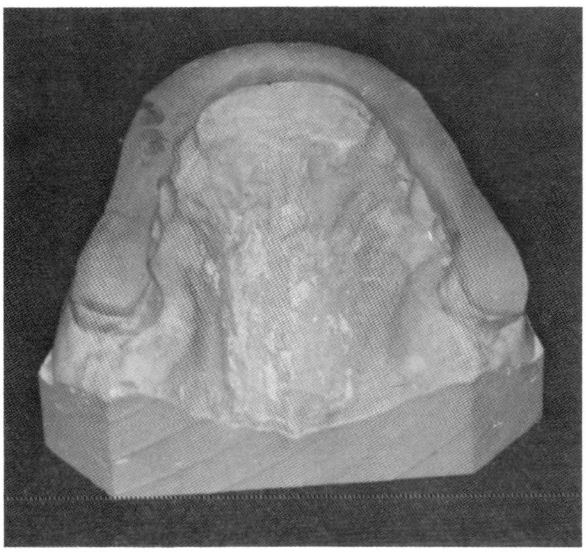

Fig. 1-160. Acrylic index is positioned on cast.

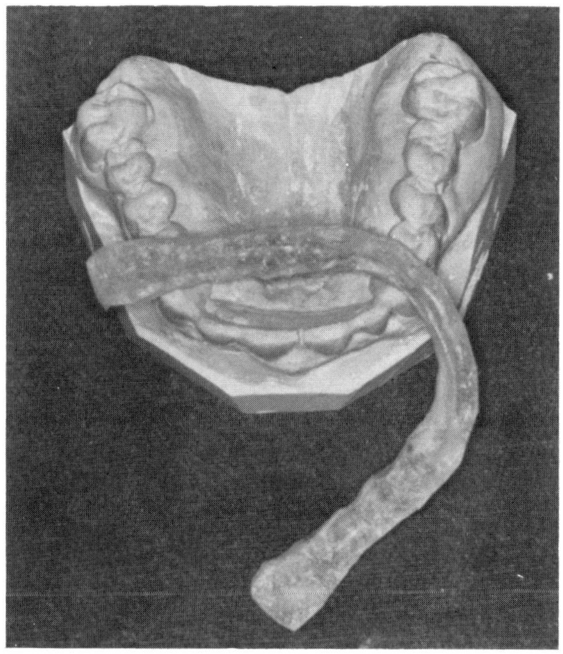

Fig. 1-161. Occlusal view of acrylic index.

ply it to the index, then lightly seat the index in the mouth of the patient, and hold it in place until set (Fig. 1-162).

6. After the paste has set, make an alginate impression of the castings and index in place. On removal of the impression, seat the castings in the impression against the positive stops provided by the zinc oxide–eugenol paste and acrylic index (Fig. 1-163). Apply a thin film of petroleum jelly to the casting, and block out the proximal surfaces with hydrocolloid or wax (Fig. 1-164).

7. Pour the remount cast in the manner described earlier with either stone or a combination of low-fusing metal and stone. This technique has the advantage of relating the castings under light pressure and not by means of seating the hydrocolloid and compound impressing firmly, as in the previous technique. It also allows registration of periodontally involved teeth in a relatively passive state.

8. Transfer the remount casts obtained by either technique to the articulator by using the previously made face-bow record and centric relation records, and

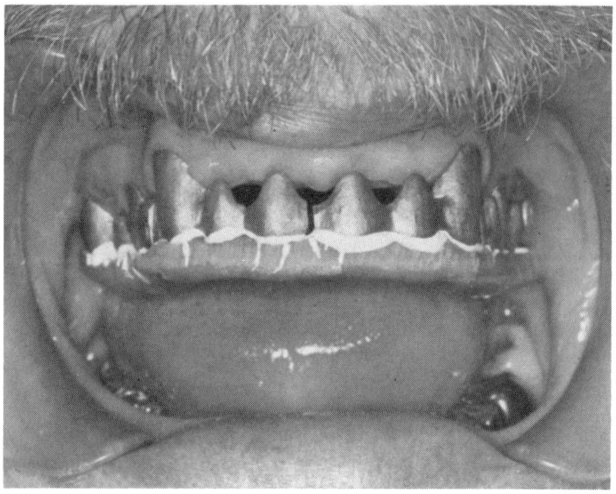

Fig. 1-162. Acrylic index is seated on casting with zinc oxide–eugenol paste.

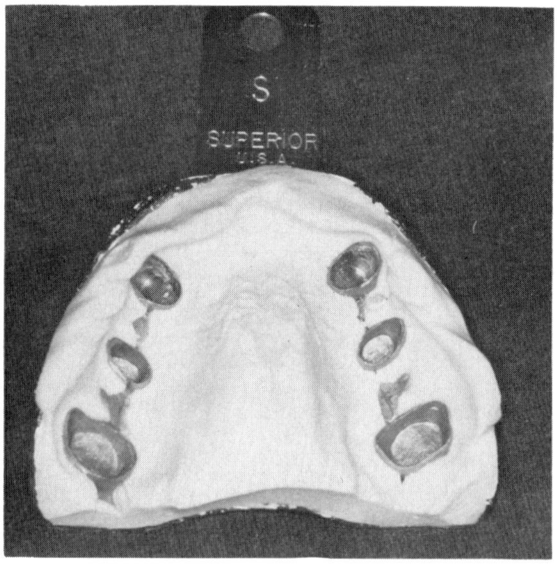

Fig. 1-163. Castings are positioned in impression.

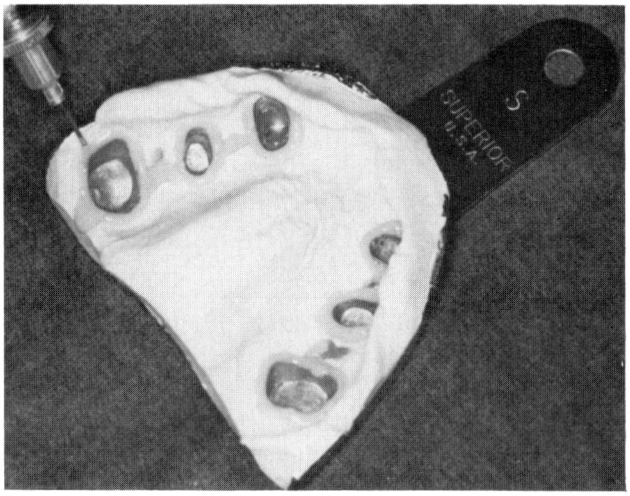

Fig. 1-164. Hydrocolloid is injected around exposed proximal margins of castings.

verify the mounting with the second centric relation. With an accurate representation of the relationships of these restorations in the mouth of the patient, refining the occlusion, contour, and interocclusal relationships is much easier and more accurate.

Acrylic resin also can serve as a substitute for stone or low-fusing metal when pouring the previously described remount casts. Exercise care, since shrinkage of this material can be significant clinically, and the resulting remount cast may not be as accurate. Little dimensional change occurs when using low-fusing alloys and dental stone.

For many techniques in restorative procedures, the use of transfer copings is essential. Precision attachment partial dentures fabricated with copings for the fixed restorations require the transfer of an accurate intraoral relationship. It is possible also to use copings to relate individually constructed dies within a full-arch impression to assure an accurate relation with each other, as well as with the edentulous area. Use of the remount procedures described makes it simple and practical to produce an accurate cast on which to finish the restorations.

PROBLEM AREAS

Problems that can arise during the fabrication of working casts and dies are outlined in Table 1-4.

1. Working casts should have a smooth hard surface that precisely reproduces every detail of the impres-

Table 1-4. Working casts and dies

Problem	Probable cause	Solution
Voids or air bubbles on working cast	Stone not vacuum mixed	Vacuum mix dental stone
	Stone added to impression too rapidly	Add stone in small increments at one border of impression; allow it to flow throughout impression; paint stone in narrow preparations with sable brush
Removable dies fracturing at neck	Dowel pin placed too deep in impression	Place gnarled portion of pin in middle of preparation; end at or slightly below gingival margin of preparation
	Die ditched too deeply	Ditch die to maximum depth of 0.5 mm to avoid weakening die in this area
Removable die rotating in working cast	Dowel pin too short in base of cast	Initially pour no more than 5 mm over margin of preparation and slightly over gnarled portion of dowel pin (Fig. 1-165)
	Base of die lacking positive seat	Augment base of die with grooves or depressions to give positive unyielding seat to resist rotation (Fig. 1-166)
Unable to remove dies after saw cuts made	Saw cuts not tapered	Taper cuts to make narrow portion adjacent to base of cast
	Adjacent natural teeth restricting removal of die	Place dowel pin in natural teeth adjacent to preparations to make teeth removable and allow for removal of preparation dies (Figs. 1-167 and 1-168)
Loosening of edentulous ridge on working cast	Insufficient retention placed in initial pour	Place dowel pin in edentulous area of impression; if ridge loosens, reseat it like removable die (Fig. 1-169)
Removable die unable to seat completely in die	Debris (stone and wax) in pinhole, on pin, on base of die, or on die seating area of cast	Examine all areas closely before using excessive pressure in attempt to seat die; clean them with air pressure, pipe cleaners, toothbrush, or pumping action of dowel pin in pinhold under flowing water (Fig. 1-170)
Surface of electroplated casts granular and porous	Current setting too high on plating unit	Decrease amount of current
Thin deposit of metal in deeper areas of depression	Current setting too high on plating unit	Decrease amount of current
	Impression too close to anode in bath	Move impression further away from anode (approximately 6 inches [15 cm]) to allow for more even deposition of metal
Inaccurate surface detail of remount cast poured in low-fusing metal	Metal either too cold or too hot when poured in impression	Have metal at correct temperature to pour and not too hot to touch

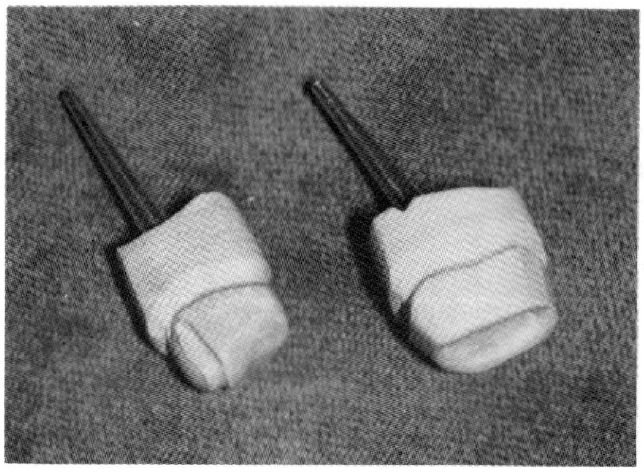

Fig. 1-165. Removable dies have been ditched to depth of approximately 0.5 mm. Length of exposed dowel pin is correct.

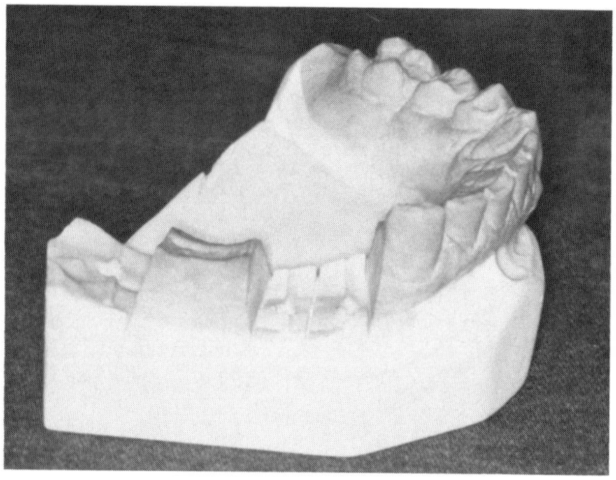

Fig. 1-166. Positive seat for removable dies is incorporated in base by means of V-shaped ridges to resist rotation.

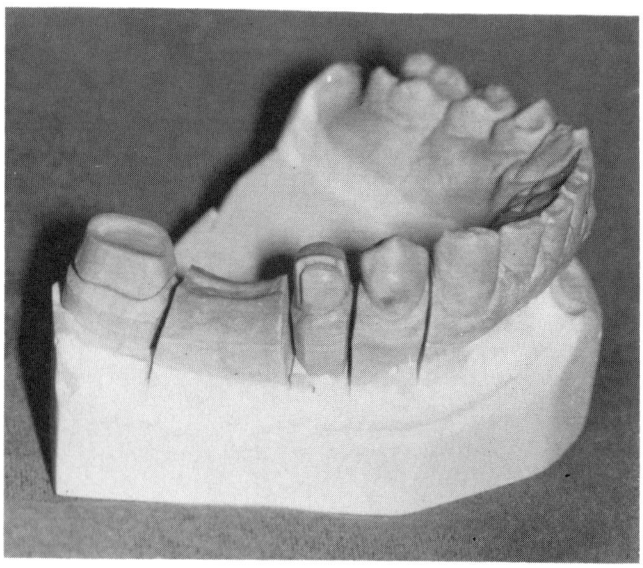

Fig. 1-167. Saw cuts are made through natural tooth adjacent to preparation to allow for removal of restricted die.

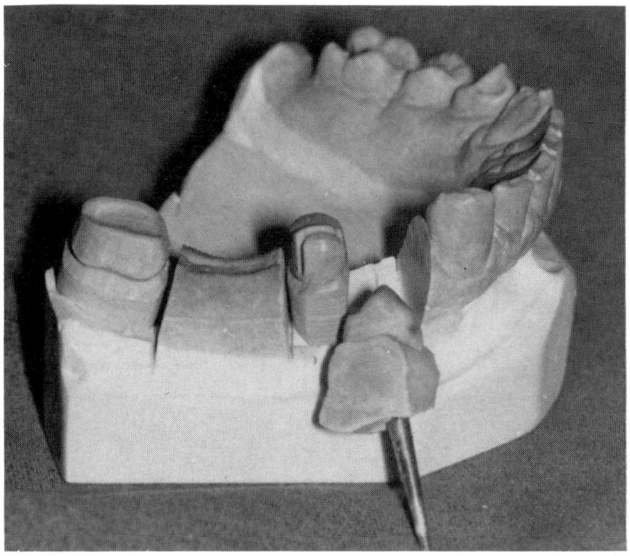

Fig. 1-168. Natural tooth is removed to allow for unimpeded removal of preparation die.

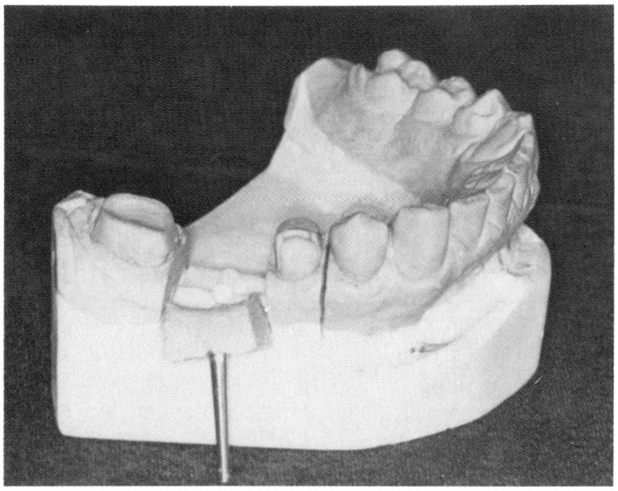

Fig. 1-169. Edentulous ridge is made removable with dowel pin to solve problem of possible ridge fracture.

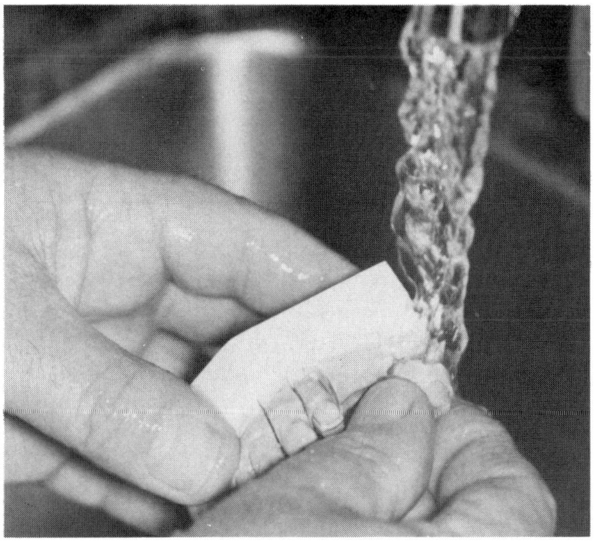

Fig. 1-170. Pumping action of dowel pin in pinhole under flowing water to remove debris.

sion. Voids, air bubbles, and chalky surface areas point to improper mixing and pouring technique. The water-powder ratio is critical for hardness of the cast. The manufacturer's recommendations should be followed. Vacuum spatulation for 1 minute will produce a smooth and dense mix of dental stone. The impression must be thoroughly rinsed under tap water to remove any saliva or debris. A gentle airstream is used to remove excess moisture prior to pouring the impression. Small increments of stone are added near the periphery of the impression and allowed to flow slowly into the deepest recess of the impression. Stone may be painted into narrow preparations with a sable brush.

2. The use of removable dies requires certain precautions to prevent some common problems, such as unstable dies, dies that are difficult to remove, and dies that will not reseat on the working cast. A positive reseating of the die is augmented by the use of a long dowel pin and by orientation grooves or depressions that will resist rotation of the die. Adjacent natural teeth may be sufficiently inclined to restrict removal of the die. This should be anticipated by placing a dowel pin in the teeth adjacent to the preparation to make them also removable. Debris, stone, or wax may attach to the base of the die or clog the pin channel and prevent proper reseating of the die. Examine these areas frequently, and keep them clean with air pressure.

3. The electroplated surface can be granular or porous, if the current setting is too high on the plating unit. A thin deposit of metal near the incisal or occlusal surface of the preparation may be due to a high current setting or placing the impression too close to the anode.

SUMMARY

In this section, the fabrication of working casts with removable dies has been presented. Dental stone is the most widely used cast and die material, therefore the physical and chemical properties and their effect on procedures and techniques using dental stone were discussed. The procedure of fabrication of remount casts was described, as well as alternate die materials, such as epoxy resin and electroplating of impressions. The final restoration can only be as accurate as the working cast and the dies on which it is constructed; therefore it is essential to gain a thorough understanding of the materials used and an appreciation of the need to follow specific procedures.

PART THREE

Mounting the master casts

LEWIS A. CHAMBLESS, Jr., and DOUGLAS B. LAW

Mounting the working casts on an articulator is the direct link between the patient and laboratory. The accuracy of this procedure is of primary importance because it represents the anatomic and functional relationships of the maxillomandibular articulation of the patient. Attention to detail as well as accuracy also will facilitate the laboratory phase of construction and reduce the amount of time required for adjusting the final prosthesis in order to retain the complicated anatomy developed especially for it.

The transfer and subsequent mounting of the working cast preserve the anatomic and functional relationships of the maxillomandibular relations of the patient and enable the laboratory to reproduce the basic spatial positions that the prosthesis will occupy (Fig. 1-171).

Mounting working casts can range from mounting quadrant models on a simple hinge apparatus to transferring complete arch casts and mounting them on a fully adjustable articulator or gnathologic instrument. Similarly, the relationships reproduced range from simple opening and closing to simulation of the full range of mandibular motion.

PREPARING CASTS FOR MOUNTING

In preparing casts for mounting on an articulator, it is necessary to perform several preliminary checks. Inspect the occlusal surfaces of the teeth in both the working and opposing casts. Carefully remove all blebs, nodules, or bubbles of stone with an instrument so that there is no interference with the tooth-to-tooth contact (Fig. 1-172). If there are broken or chipped working cusps on the buccal surface of the mandibular cast or the lingual surface of the maxillary cast, consider obtaining new casts. Inspect thoroughly the surfaces of the teeth or the land areas of the cast for any interference with occlusion (Fig. 1-173). Occasionally, the retromolar or tuberosity areas may require trimming because of their interference. If most of the teeth are present and in good condition and no interference remains, visual examination for facets and intercuspation will make it possible to articulate the casts by hand (Fig. 1-174).

Position the casts between the upper and lower members of the articulator, and determine whether the thickness of the bases will facilitate mounting. If a face-bow is available, make certain that the model will fit in the face-bow, without touching the mounting plate. Trim the casts unless they are the desired thickness. Notch the bottom of each base to create a positive index

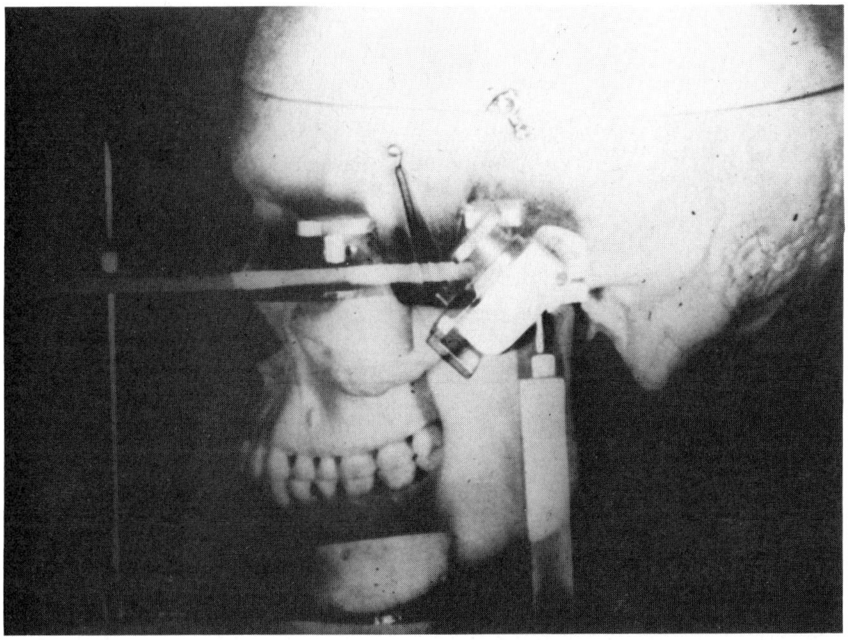

Fig. 1-171. Anatomic relationship of articulator to skull.

A 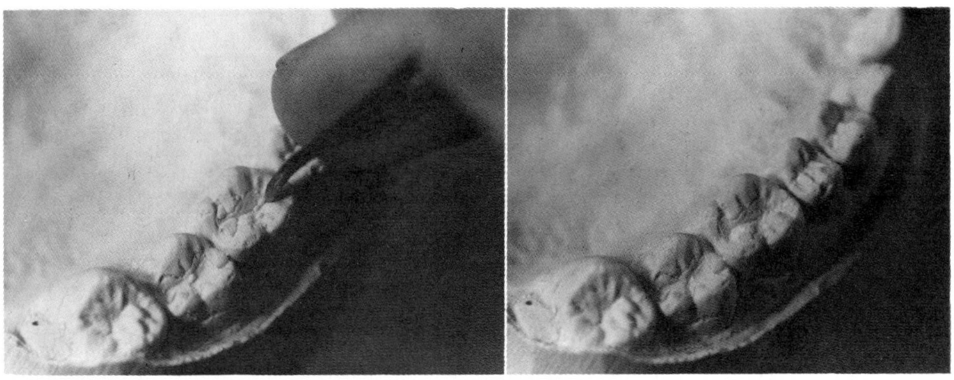 B

Fig. 1-172. A, Nodules that will interfere with intercuspation of casts are removed with sharp instrument. **B,** Interferences have been removed, and casts are occluded.

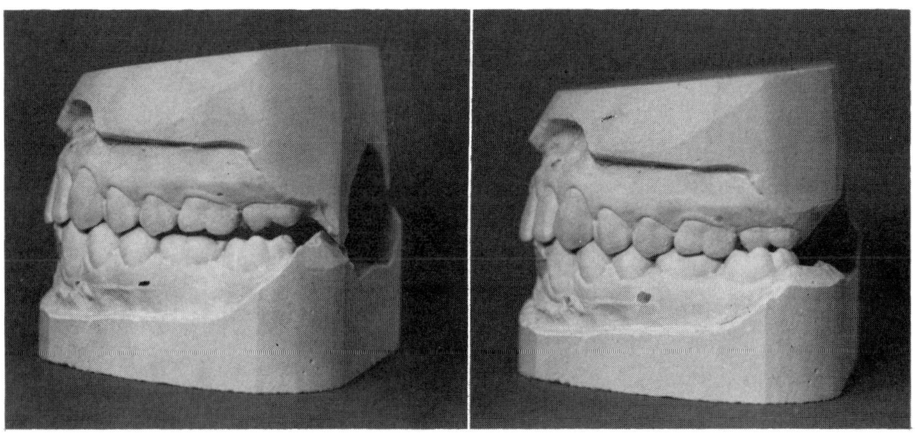

Fig. 1-173. Tuberosity and retromolar land area interferences.

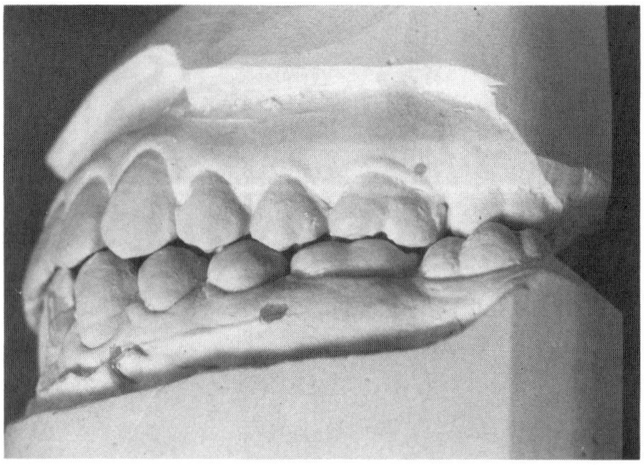

Fig. 1-174. Casts are articulated by hand, using intercuspation and visual examination for facets.

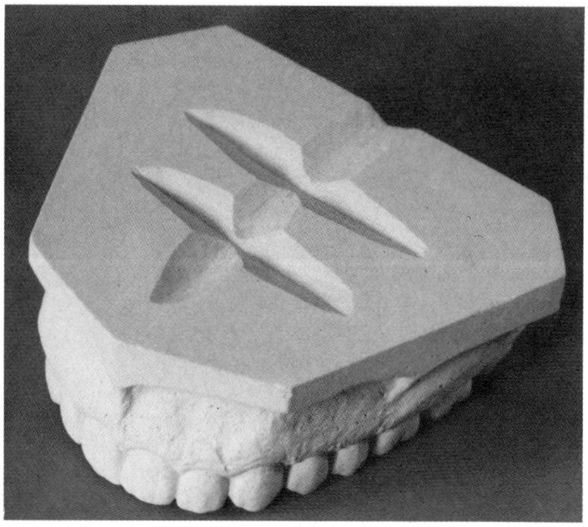

Fig. 1-175. Notches in base are made before mounting.

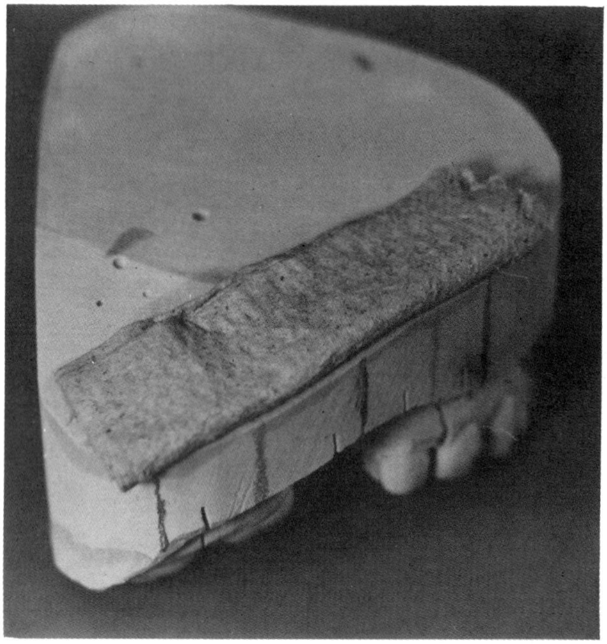

Fig. 1-176. Dowel-pin area is blocked out with wet asbestos to prevent stone from blocking access to ends of pins.

for accurate remounting of the casts (Fig. 1-175). Block out the dowel pin recesses with wet asbestos or soft wax to permit access to the pins after mounting and to prevent interference with accurate and positive seating of the dies and dowel pins in the model (Fig 1-176).

Mounting media

Dental plaster is a medium that will allow fast, accurate, and inexpensive attachment of a cast to the articulator or mounting ring. Although it is not as strong or as dimensionally stable as dental stone, it is adequate.

Dental stone and especially dental plaster expand to some extent while hardening. Normally, this is not a factor when mounting models unless using an especially large bulk of plaster. In that instance, it is advantageous to use two mixes of plaster. The first mix supplies most of the height necessary for mounting (Fig. 1-177, *A*). The second smaller mix attaches the cast to the larger and now stable, set portion of plaster (Fig. 1-177, *B*).

Whether using one or two mixes, allow adequate working time, and manipulate the plaster to a creamy mixture. Do not use a thick mix or an especially fast-setting plaster because the resistance of the material to flow can cause distortion of the mounting.

Orienting the maxillary cast

Determine the position of the maxillary cast in the articulator by one of several methods, depending on the complexity of the technique and the difficulty of the contemplated rehabilitation. It can range from the arbitrary positioning in a simple articulator to a hinge axis face-bow.

In the absence of a face-bow, position the cast in a simple hinge articulator arbitrarily. Exercise care to see that the casts fit between the members of the articulator, since there is no specific information on the location of the maxillary cast in relation to the hinge.

When a face-bow is available, orient the maxillary cast by the actual position of the maxilla of the patient with respect to fixed references. In mounting a maxillary cast on the articulator with a face-bow, make certain to satisfy several requirements. The cast must fit accurately into the indentations of the trimmed face-bow fork; otherwise, it is impossible to orient the cast

A 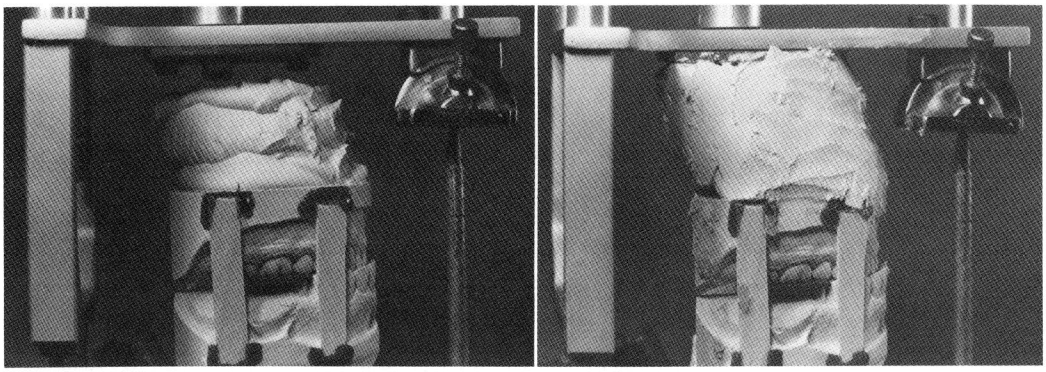 B

Fig. 1-177. A, Initial mix of plaster should provide most of height necessary for mounting. **B,** Second mix attaches cast to mounting.

A 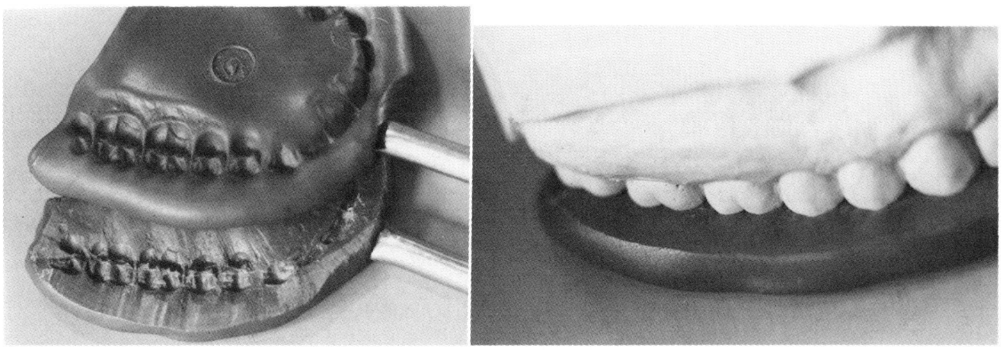 B

Fig. 1-178. A, Properly trimmed face-bow fork registration *(bottom)* shows registration material trimmed away until only indentations of tips of cusps are left. **B,** Cast seated in bite fork registration.

precisely (Fig. 1-178). There must be adequate room for the upper member of the articulator to close with the mounting plate in position (Fig. 1-179). Support of the face-bow fork, with the cast, is essential to prevent distortion of the face-bow during mounting. Use a vertical support, such as a T support or sliding blocks of wood to keep the weight of the cast on the fork or the placement of the plaster from distorting the face-bow record (Fig. 1-180). Exercise care to see that the upper member can close down to the terminal position with the plaster in place. Following these steps will make it possible to orient the maxillary cast in the articulator correctly.

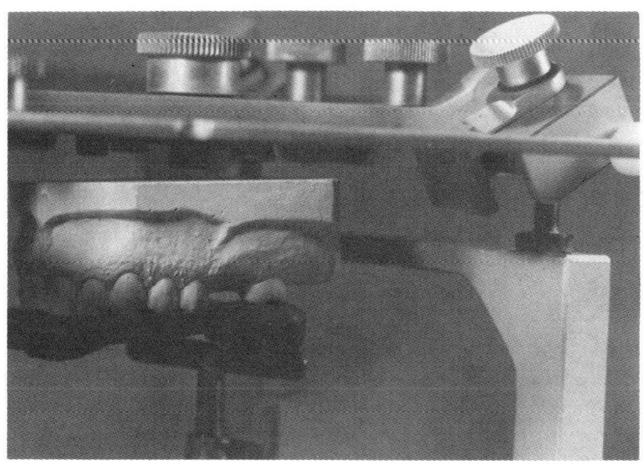

Fig. 1-179. Space between maxillary cast and mounting plate is adequate for plaster. Cast is supported from below with adjustable support.

Orienting the mandibular cast to the maxillary cast

When sending instructions about casts to the laboratory, the dentist can include one of several techniques for aligning the maxillary and mandibular casts. If the patient has an adequate number of teeth left, simple

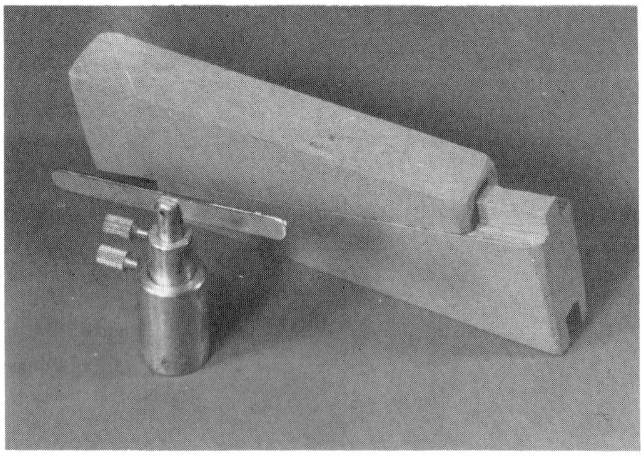

Fig. 1-180. Two types of adjustable supports that can be used during mounting to prevent movement of face-bow fork.

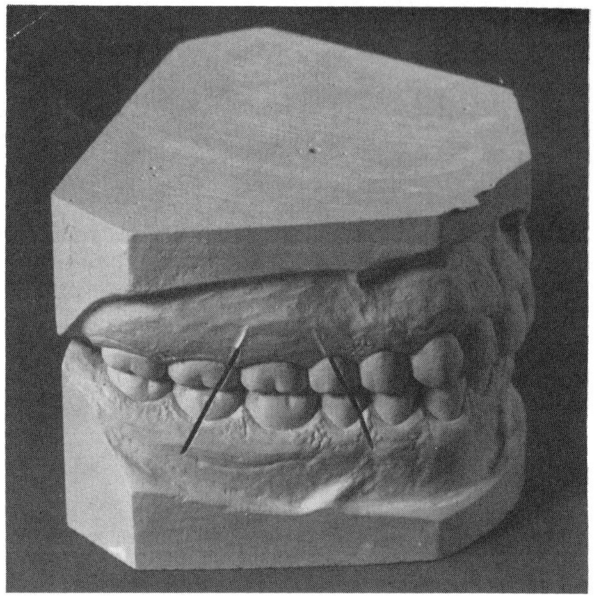

Fig. 1-181. Index cuts on cast are made in opposing directions to orient casts accurately.

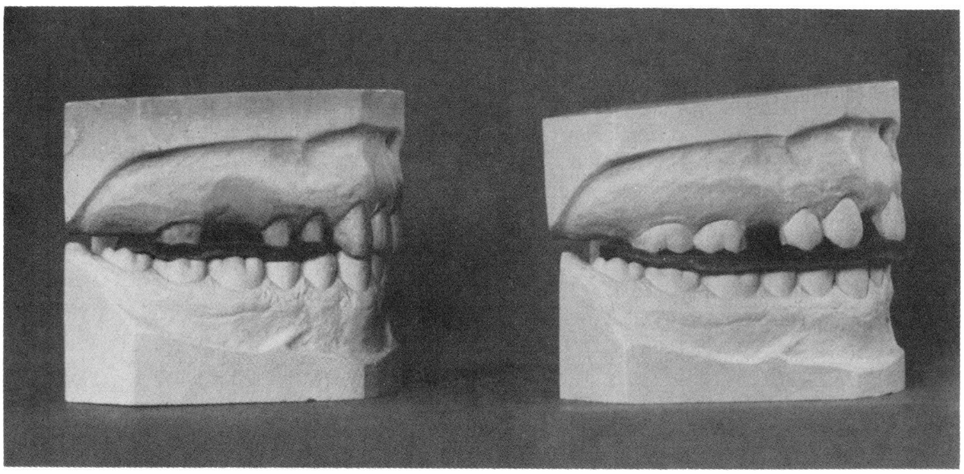

Fig. 1-182. Full-arch interocclusal record that separates casts *(right)*. Unilateral record is taken with unprepared teeth in contact.

tooth-to-tooth articulation of the casts may be adequate. However, when planning to articulate a model by hand using tooth-to-tooth contacts, place pencil marks or cuts on adjacent noncritical areas of the maxillary and mandibular casts to indicate to the laboratory the position of centric relation (Fig. 1-181).

When preparing several teeth or having no distal intact tooth to orient the casts, include a centric relation record for mounting the casts. Otherwise, it can result in a unilateral interocclusal record taken with the teeth slightly separated (Fig. 1-182). Either of these records will allow for precise alignment of the mandibular cast to the maxillary cast.

MOUNTING ANATOMIC MODELS

Nonadjustable articulators

PROCEDURE

1. Mount a quadrant cast in a tooth-to-tooth relationship without any interocclusal separation, since the opening and closing axis of the articulator can differ considerably from that of the patient. Tooth contact must be in proper intercuspation to assure correctness of the horizontal relationship and maintenance of the sagittal and frontal relationships (Fig. 1-183).

2. It is possible to mount full-arch casts on a plain-line articulator accurately, because it is easy to maintain the frontal and sagittal planes. Establish tooth-to-tooth

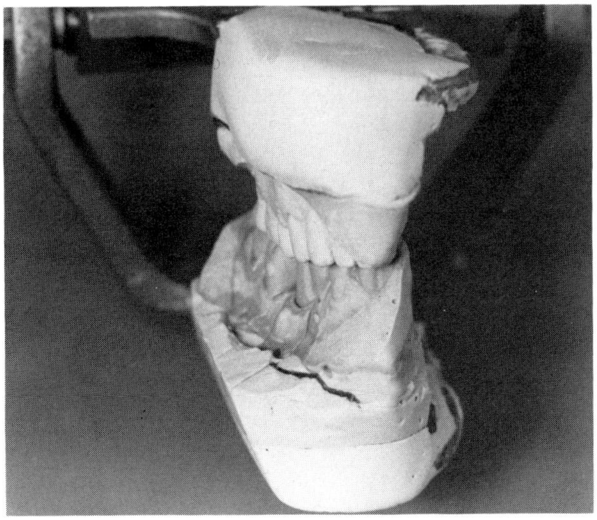

Fig. 1-183. Lack of cross-arch stability makes quadrant casts especially difficult to orient and mount. It is easy to disturb relationships of two casts in several directions.

A

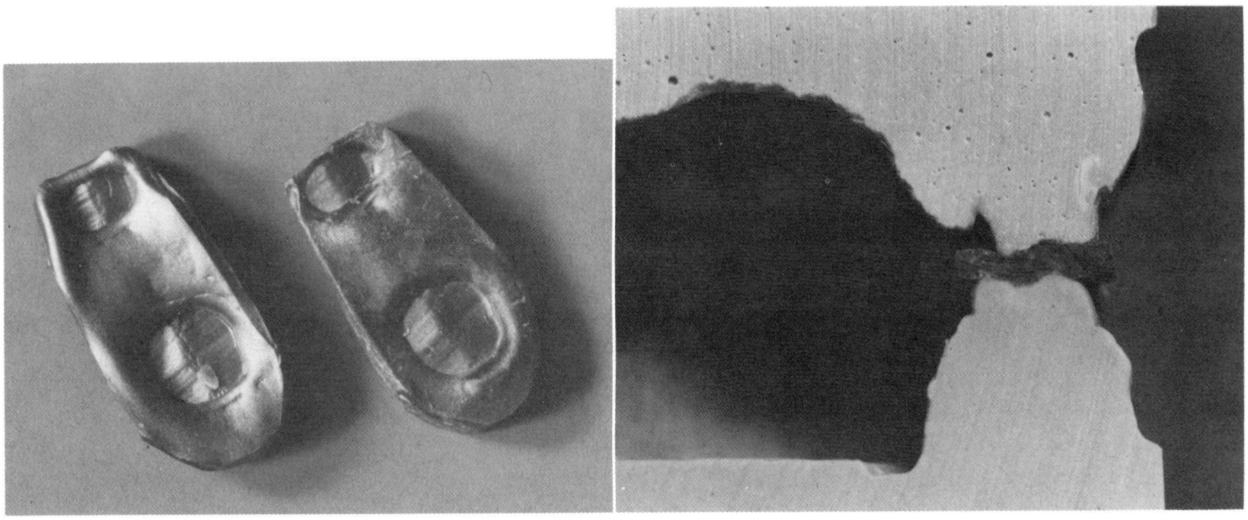

B

Fig. 1-184. A, Correctly trimmed unilateral record *(right).* Untrimmed record *(left).* **B,** Sagittal section through casts and record shows proper relationship with only tips of cusps in record.

contact, and avoid interocclusal separation. If the prepared tooth is a terminal abutment with no distal stop, include a simple interarch record to provide stability for the mounting. Although the material used for this record is unimportant, it is essential that the record fulfill criteria at the time of mounting. Include only the prepared distal abutment to give stability to the casts in centric relation. Trim the record to include only the tips of the cusps and make it possible to observe the relationships of the opposing cusps (Fig. 1-184). Include in the record no teeth anterior to the preparation to prevent improper separation and distortion of both vertical and frontal occlusal relationships.

3. After properly relating the casts in a tooth-to-tooth relationship with either intercuspation by hand or a unilateral record, maintain the relationship during the mounting procedure. One method uses sticky wax directly on the teeth, but it can present some hazards. The wax can distort the relationship and prevent observation of any change or slipping that may occur. After mounting, removal of the wax can result in fractures of the casts or modifications to their surface. A more reliable method is to lute the casts together by means of struts and sticky wax. Make the struts from segments of tongue blades, applicator sticks, or coat-hanger wire, and attach them to the bases of the casts with sticky wax or dental compound (Figs. 1-185 and 1-186). This method makes it possible to observe the intercuspation of the arches readily and to see and correct any change in the relationships.

4. A quick method of maintaining complete arch casts during mounting is to use rubber bands. Merely bind

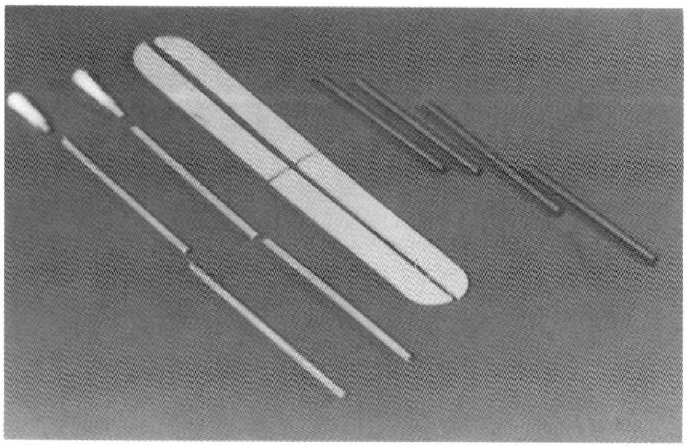

Fig. 1-185. Variety of materials can be used with sticky wax to stabilize casts.

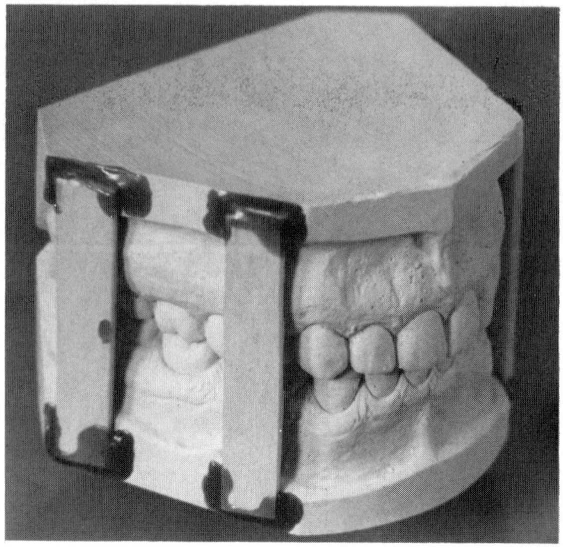

Fig. 1-186. Good method of stabilizing casts is to use sections of tongue blade and sticky wax.

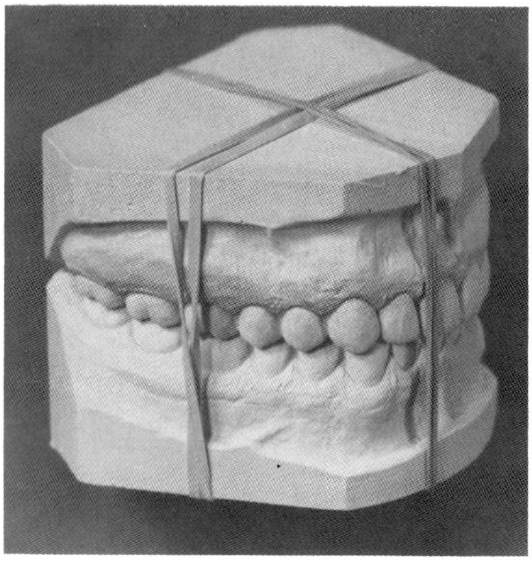

Fig. 1-187. Simple method of stabilizing casts is to use tightly wound opposing rubber bands.

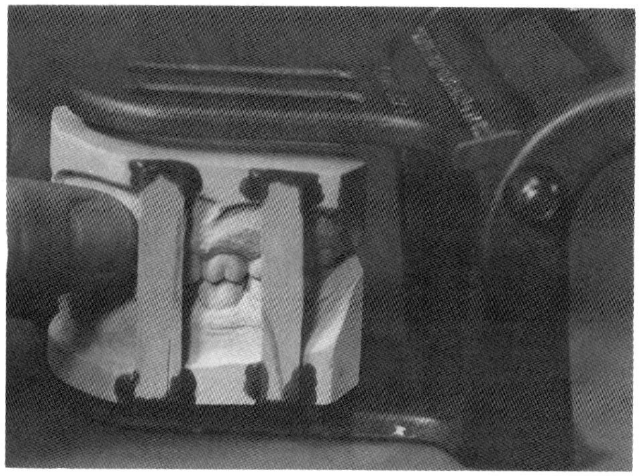

Fig. 1-188. Casts are held in hands between arms of articulator to make certain that there is adequate space for them and plaster.

the casts together with two rubber bands in opposing directions and mount them (Fig. 1-187). After completion of mounting, cut the rubber bands, and separate the casts.

5. To mount the articulated casts, place the nonanatomic articulator on a flat surface, and verify the adequacy of the space for the casts by holding them in position with the hands (Fig. 1-188). Mix the plaster, and place a portion on the lower mounting member. Position the articulated casts, and manipulate the plaster to secure the attachment (Fig. 1-189). When using mandibular removable dies, exercise care to prevent distortion of the blockout of the dowel pins.

6. Place another portion of plaster on the maxillary cast, and close the upper member until it engages the vertical stop on the articulator (Fig. 1-190). Manipulate the plaster to a smooth contour, and attach it securely (Fig. 1-191). After the plaster has set, remove the stabilizing struts, verify the mounting, and trim and smooth the excess bulk of plaster. Exercise care to prevent modification of the vertical stop (Fig. 1-192).

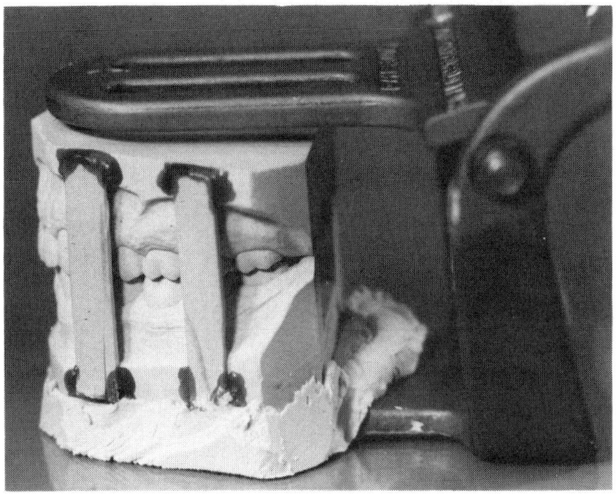

Fig. 1-189. Lower cast is attached to articulator with plaster.

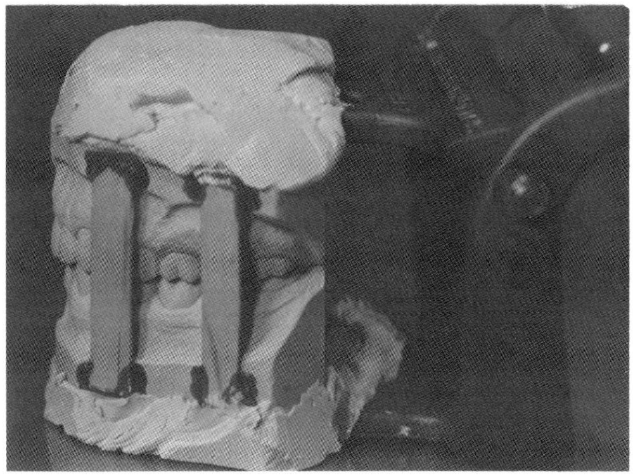

Fig. 1-190. Maxillary cast is attached to articulator with second mix of plaster.

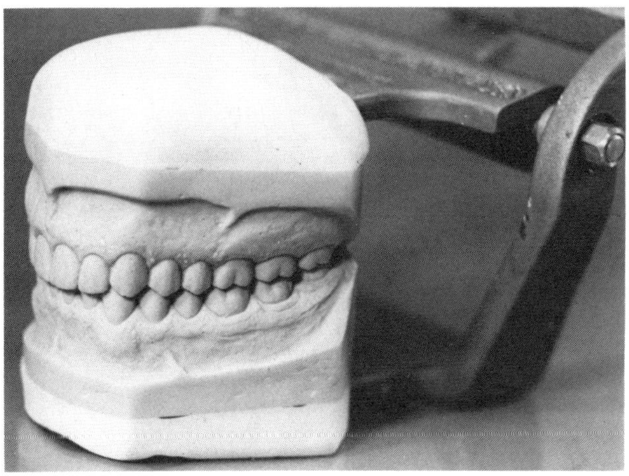

Fig. 1-191. Struts and sticky wax have been removed and plaster smoothed for finished mounting.

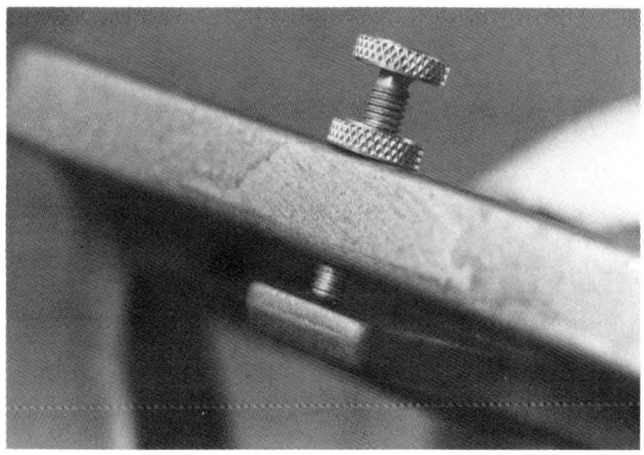

Fig. 1-192. When mounting is finished, vertical stop is checked to make certain that it is engaged.

Semiadjustable articulators

PROCEDURE

1. Before mounting the face-bow on a semiadjustable articulator, such as the Whip-Mix articulator,* several preparatory steps are necessary (Fig. 1-193). Make certain that the intercondylar width, determined by some face-bows, is correct for the patient, and then set it on the articulator (Fig. 1-194). Secure a mounting plate to the upper member, and if there is a lower mounting plate, remove it. Use some type of vertical support for the face-bow fork and cast, such as a T support or sliding blocks of wood (Fig. 1-180).

2. Examine the face-bow fork and its occlusal surface registration, and determine whether the maxillary cast will seat accurately in the indentations. If excess registration material prevents proper seating, trim it off carefully (Fig. 1-178). Proper face-bow fork registrations provide stable anterior and posterior seats and include only incisal edges and tips of cusps. Relate and attach the face-bow to the articulator according to the manu-

*Whip-Mix Corp., Louisville, Ky.

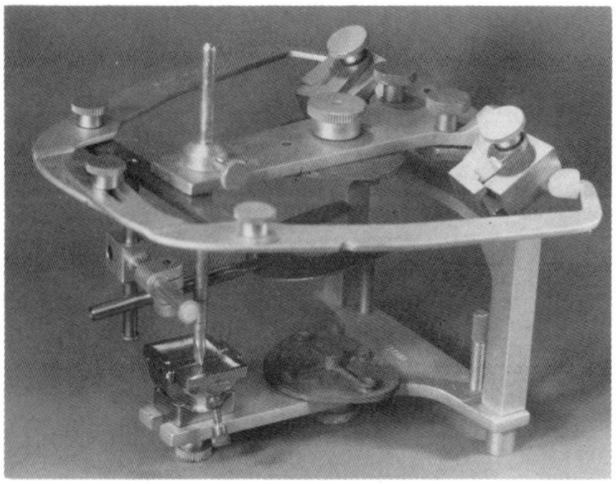

Fig. 1-193. Whip-Mix articulator with face-bow and face-bow fork.

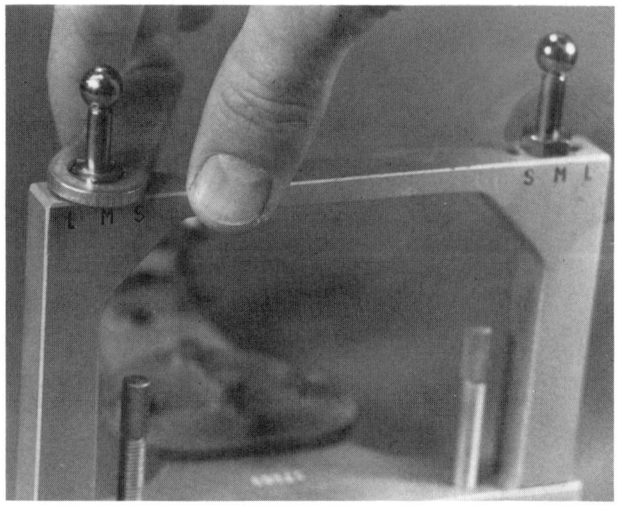

Fig. 1-194. Intercondylar width is set to match that of patient.

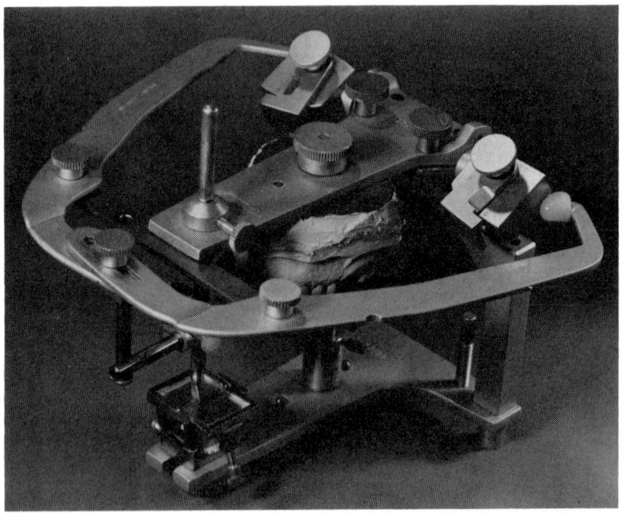

Fig. 1-195. Maxillary cast is supported from below to prevent distortion while it is attached to mounting ring with plaster.

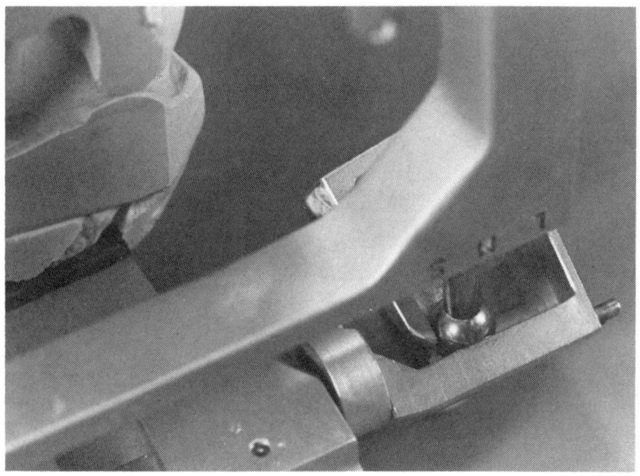

Fig. 1-196. Correct position of condyles in fossa assembly is maintained throughout procedure. Condyles must be in contact with metal walls of assembly.

facturer's instructions. Examine the clearance between the mounting plate and the cast to make certain that there is no contact to cause possible distortion of the face-bow relationships being transferred (Fig. 1-179).

3. Mix an appropriate portion of dental plaster, and apply it carefully to the top of the cast. Close the articulator firmly, but gently, to complete the attachment. Manipulate the plaster to engage the mounting plate and the cast, and allow the plaster to set (Fig. 1-195).

4. After attaching the upper cast to the articulator, turn the articulator upside down, orient the lower cast to the upper cast by means of the centric relation record, and hold them in place with struts and sticky wax. Put the lower member of the articulator in place, and make absolutely certain to seat the condylar heads in the upper member completely and to have the incisal pin contacting the incisal table (Fig. 1-196).

5. Attach the cast to the mounting plate on the lower member of the articulator with one or two creamy mixes of plaster (Fig. 1-177). The incisal pin will maintain the vertical separation of the casts. In addition, a full-arch centric relation record used to orient the casts will separate them. Raise the pin the same amount as the size of the opening created by the record. Although it is necessary to open the articulator somewhat arbitrarily, the upper and lower members will be nearly

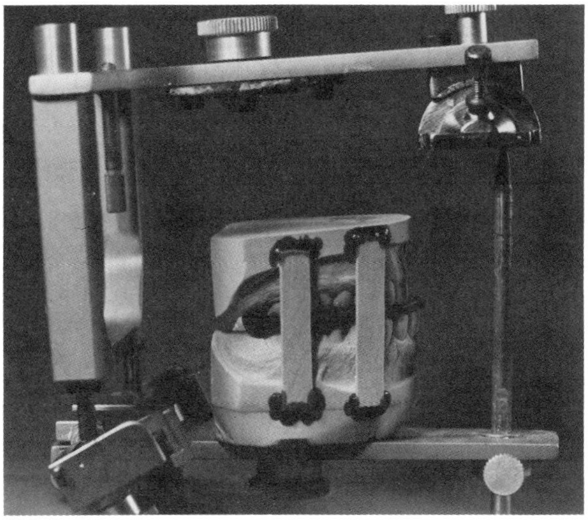

Fig. 1-197. Incisal pin is lengthened until members of articulator are parallel after full-arch centric relation record is removed from between casts.

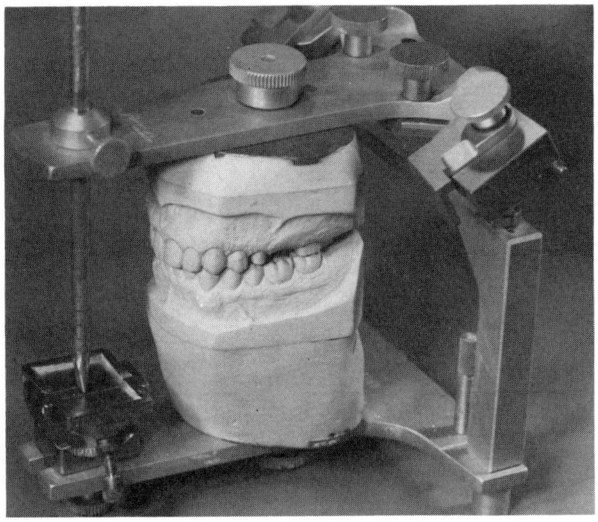

Fig. 1-198. Completed mounting on semiadjustable articulator.

parallel after removing the full-arch centric relation record (Fig. 1-197). When the plaster has set, remove the struts and centric relation record, and verify the accuracy of the mounting visually (Fig. 1-198).

Fully adjustable articulators

The clinical aspects of using and setting a fully adjustable articulator are much more complex than those of a semiadjustable articulator (Fig. 1-199). However, the laboratory phase of mounting the master casts is the same.

PROCEDURE

1. Place special mounting studs on the condylar heads of the (Denar*) to allow the face-bow to be attached to the articulator (Fig. 1-200). The hinge axis style of the face-bow will fit into these pins for mounting the face-bow record. Carefully place the master cast on the trimmed face-bow fork to check for proper seating in the record and for clearance beneath the mounting plate (Fig. 1-201).

2. Use a T support or wooden supports for the face-bow and cast, as seen previously (Fig. 1-180). Exercise even more care in manipulating this face-bow because the locking adjustments are lighter and more numerous, and any amount of pressure can distort the face-bow record. Now attach the maxillary cast to the mounting plate with a mix of dental plaster. Remove the face-bow and mounting studs carefully, and invert the articulator.

3. Use the centric relation record, sticky wax, and struts to lock the maxillary and mandibular casts together in centric relation prior to mounting the lower cast (Fig. 1-202). Carefully put the lower member of the articulator into position so that the condylar heads fit back completely into the condylar boxes (Figs. 1-196). This articulator also has a centric latch to help hold the upper and lower members in the proper position (Fig. 1-203). Open the incisal pin when using a full-arch centric relation record for mounting. Mount the mandibular cast with plaster, and, after it has set, remove the struts and centric relation record. Check the occluded casts to verify the accuracy of the mounting (Fig. 1-204).

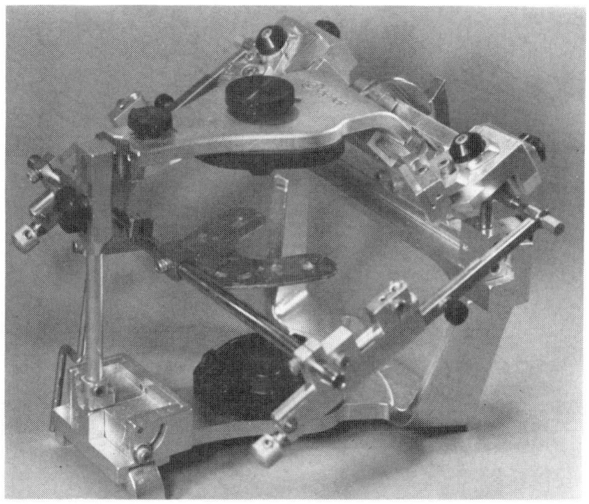

Fig. 1-199. Denar fully adjustable articulator with hinge axis face-bow assembly and face-bow fork.

*Denar Corp., Anaheim, Calif.

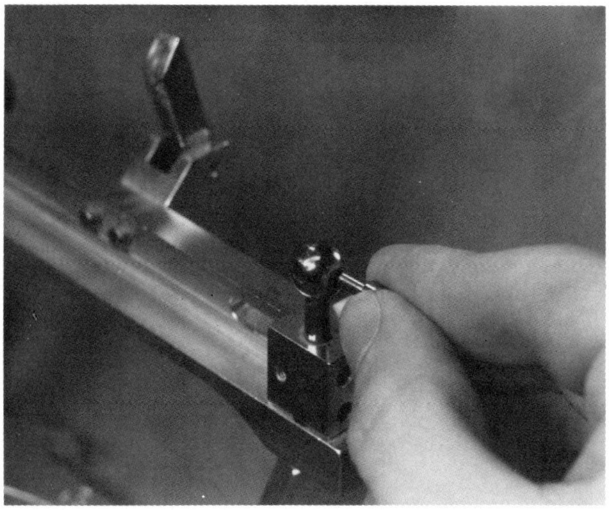

Fig. 1-200. Mounting stud is placed on metal condyle before placing face-bow.

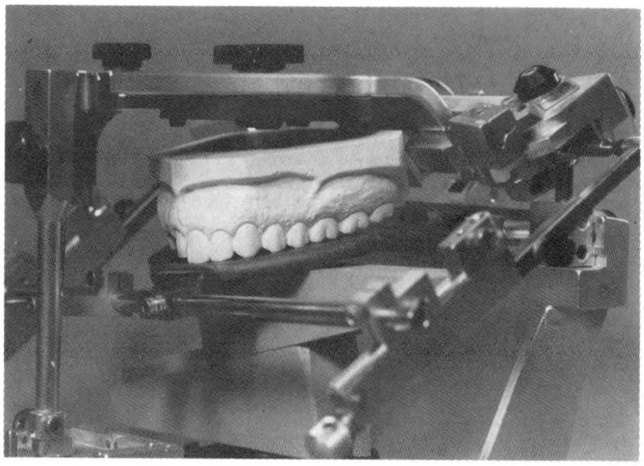

Fig. 1-201. Cast is shown on supported face-bow fork with adequate space for mounting with plaster.

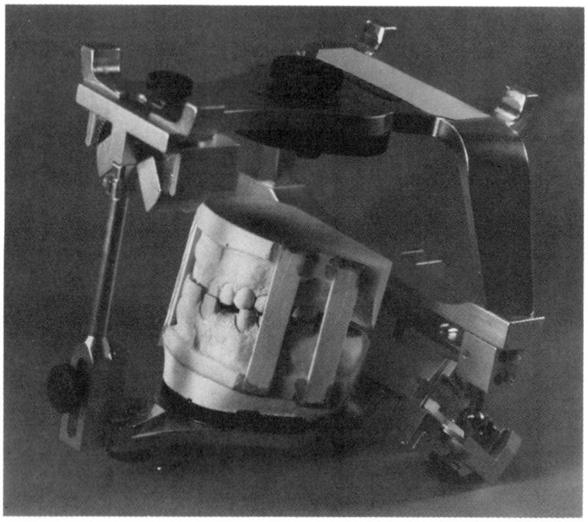

Fig. 1-202. After maxillary cast has been mounted, mandibular cast is stabilized to maxillary cast, and articulator is inverted.

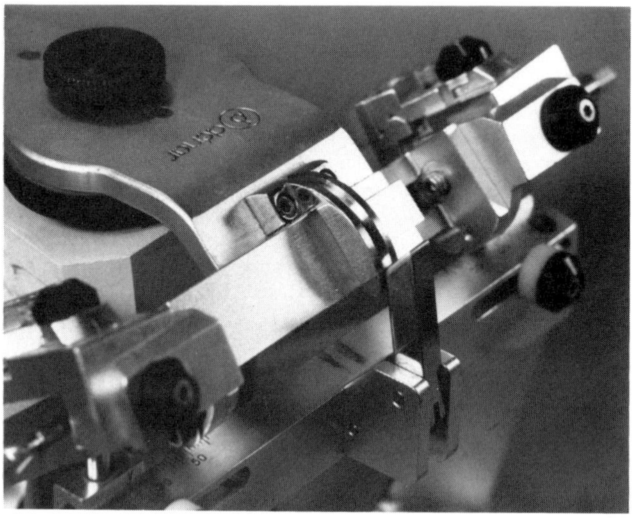

Fig. 1-203. Centric latch must be in place to help hold articulator in its proper position.

Fig. 1-204. Fully adjustable articulator with casts completely mounted.

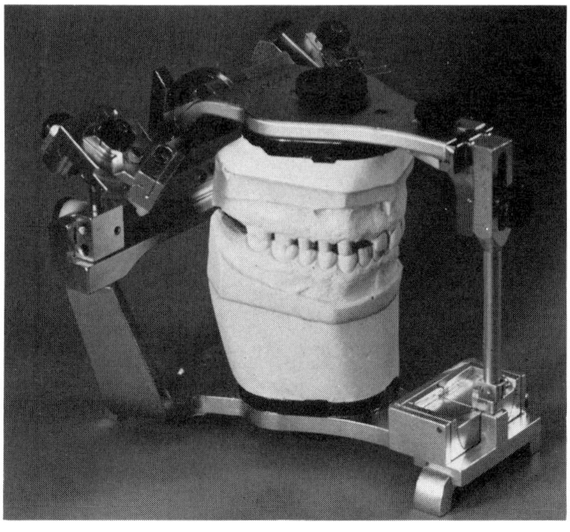

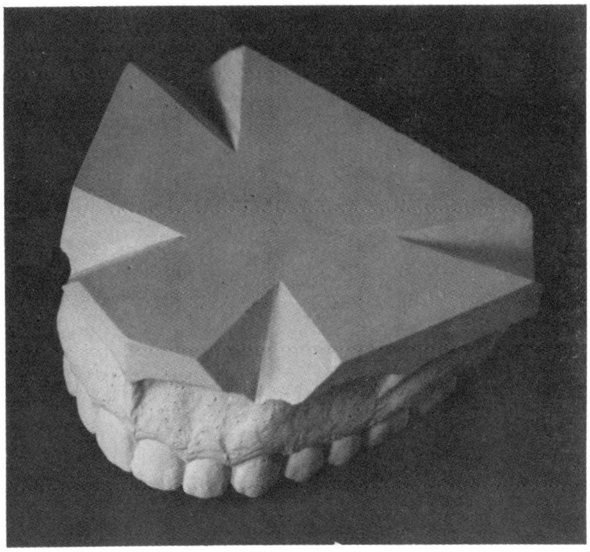

Fig. 1-205. Border of maxillary cast is notched in four or five places for split cast technique.

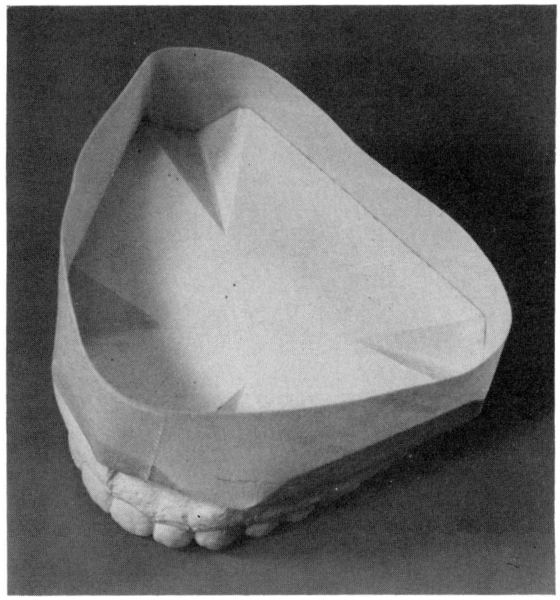

Fig. 1-206. Cast has been boxed with tape to receive stone, and separating medium has been applied to stone surfaces.

ALTERNATIVE MOUNTING TECHNIQUES

Split cast techniques

When the dentist requests verification of the centric relation by the split cast technique, it is necessary to use a variation of the typical mounting technique on the maxillary cast. It allows separation of the master cast and its base so that when placing a new centric record between the casts, it is possible to check the upper member with the mounted base as it closes into the maxillary cast. This procedure is much more definitive than trying to see whether the teeth on the casts intercuspate properly into a wax record.

PROCEDURE

1. Trim the maxillary cast flat, and make four notches in the outer border of the cast (Fig. 1-205). Put tape around the cast to box the cut portion of the cast, and extend it at least ¾ inch (1.8 cm) beyond the cast (Fig. 1-206). Paint a separating medium over the boxed portion of the maxillary cast, and pour enough dental stone into the boxing to fill the notches, making at least a ½ inch (1.3 cm) base. Leave retention mounds of stone on the stone base for mounting (Fig. 1-207).
2. After the stone has set, remove the boxing, and separate the base from the cast. If the base fits back on the cast properly, use sticky wax to put the two units together, and proceed with the usual mounting of the maxillary cast on an articulator.
3. Verify the centric relation by placing a new record between the maxillary and mandibular casts after separating the maxillary cast from its base. If the record is

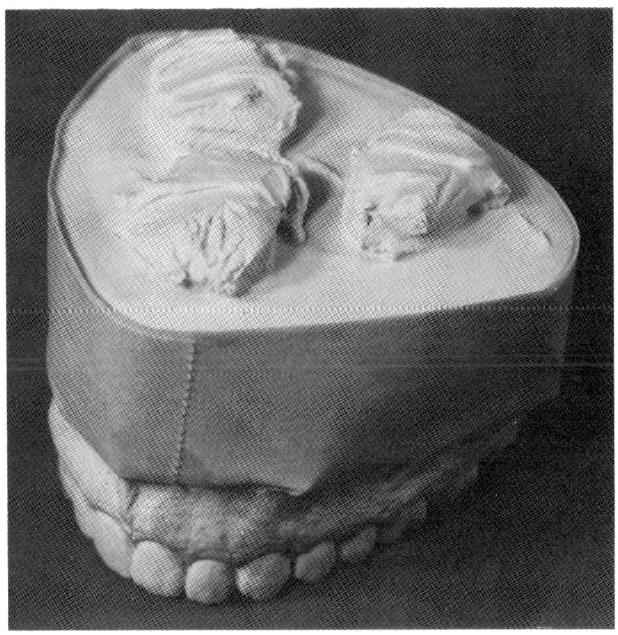

Fig. 1-207. Retentive nodules are left on stone to provide mechanical retention for mounting.

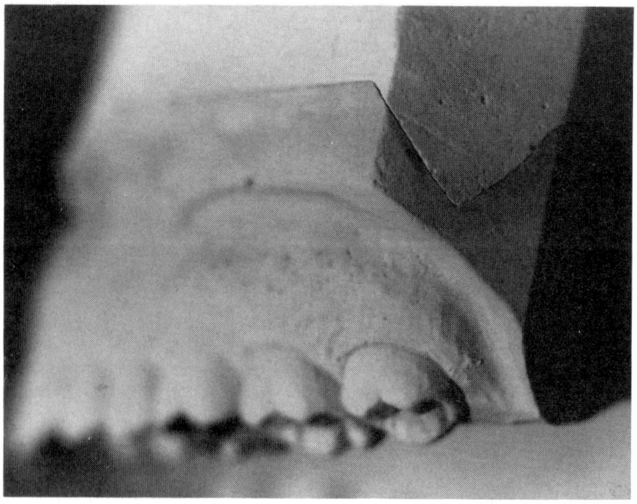

Fig. 1-208. Centric relation record is verified if base fits back perfectly in notched cast.

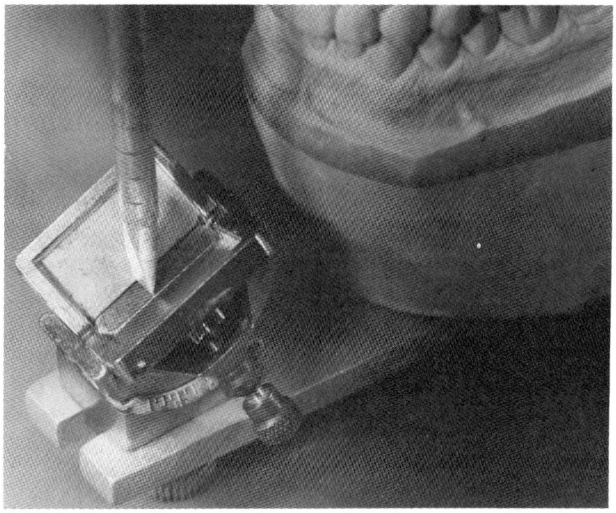

Fig. 1-209. Mechanical incisal guide table of manufacturer.

correct, the base and the cast will align perfectly with the articulator closed (Fig. 1-208). After verifying the centric relation, put the maxillary cast and base together with sticky wax, and continue with the routine procedures.

Custom incisal guide table

The last step in setting up mounted models may be fabrication of a custom incisal guide table. In most instances, it is necessary to restore only a few teeth, and the mechanical incisal guide table of the manufacturer is satisfactory (Fig. 1-209). The table will prevent undue wear on the stone teeth by guiding the movement of the articulator. When restoring the cuspid or working with a large number of prepared teeth, a custom incisal guide table may be advantageous because it duplicates more closely the incisal guidance of the patient (Fig. 1-210).

PROCEDURE

1. Remove the mechanical incisal guide table, and place an acrylic blank on the articulator (Fig. 1-211). Separate the upper and lower members of the articulator, and lubricate the tip of the incisal pin with petroleum jelly or a similar material. Mix a small batch of self-curing acrylic resin, and place it on the blank table where the incisal pin will make contact (Fig. 1-212). As the acrylic resin begins to attain some body and reaches the doughy stage, place the upper member back on the articulator. The incisal pin will sink into the soft acrylic resin on the blank. Now move the articulator into several right, left, and protrusive excursions. The incisal pin will push the acrylic resin into a perfect duplication of the incisal guidance of the patient (Fig. 1-213).

2. For canines or incisors prepared on the master cast, mount the diagnostic cast, and make the custom incisal guide table with them. Then replace the master cast, which will function with the custom incisal guide table that duplicated what the patient had prior to the preparations.

Mounting a functionally generated occlusal path record

Mounting a functionally generated occlusal path record requires mounting of the master cast with the dies, so that it can articulate with an opposing anatomic cast. Mount the master cast with the opposing anatomic cast in precisely the same manner and with the same precautions as the casts on the nonadjustable or plain-line articulator. The articulators used most frequently for this technique are the Hanau Twin-Stage Occluder* or the Ventriculator† (Fig. 1-214).

The Twin-Stage Occluder is a device that permits accurate articulation of one cast, the master cast, against two opposing casts, the anatomic cast and the functionally generated occlusal path record. The clinical technique followed when using a functionally generated occlusal path record often makes the prepared arch the maxillary arch. Since the single arm is on the lower portion of the articulator, it is necessary to put the prepared master cast there. At first it seems a little unnatural to have the two upper arms occlude with the one lower arm.

*Teledyne Dental Products Co., Hannau Division, Buffalo, N.Y.
†J.F. Jelenko & Co., New Rochelle, N.Y.

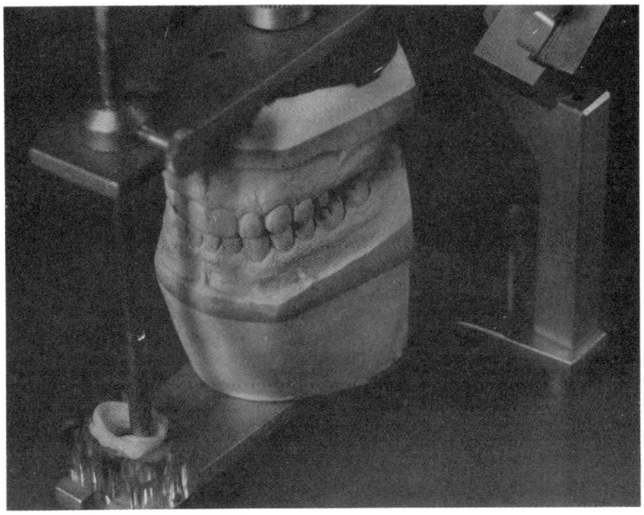

Fig. 1-210. Custom incisal guide table.

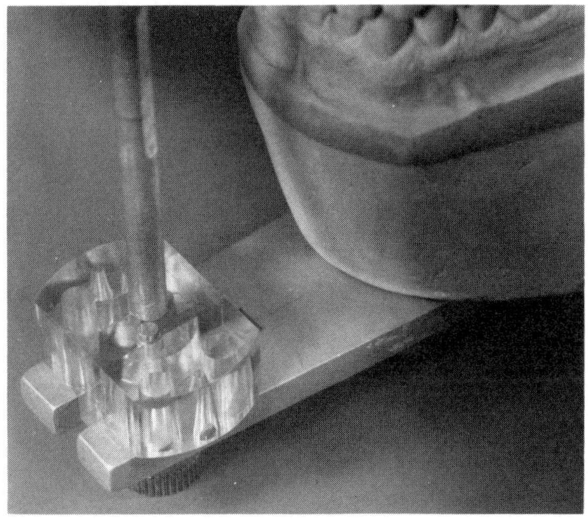

Fig. 1-211. Acrylic blank to be used in fabricating custom incisal guide table.

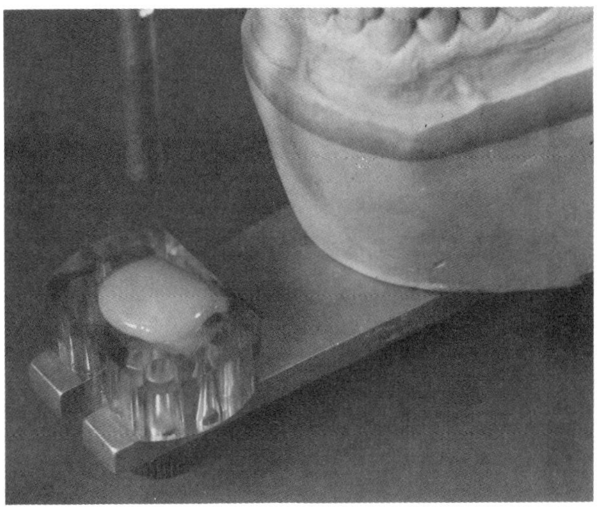

Fig. 1-212. Autopolymerizing acrylic resin is placed on acrylic blank where incisal pin will make contact.

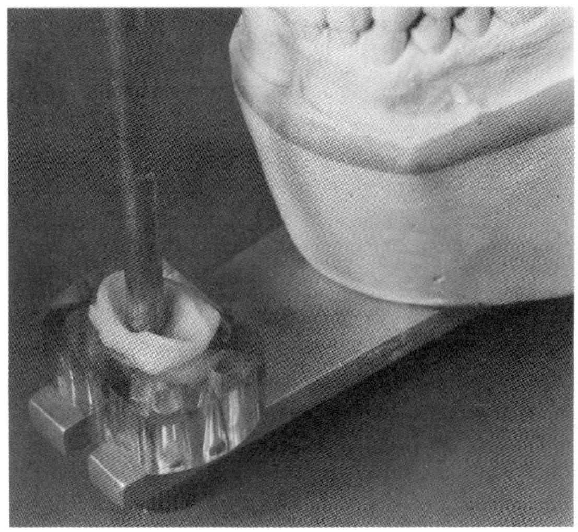

Fig. 1-213. Articulator is moved in various excursions to mold acrylic resin into duplicate of pathway.

A

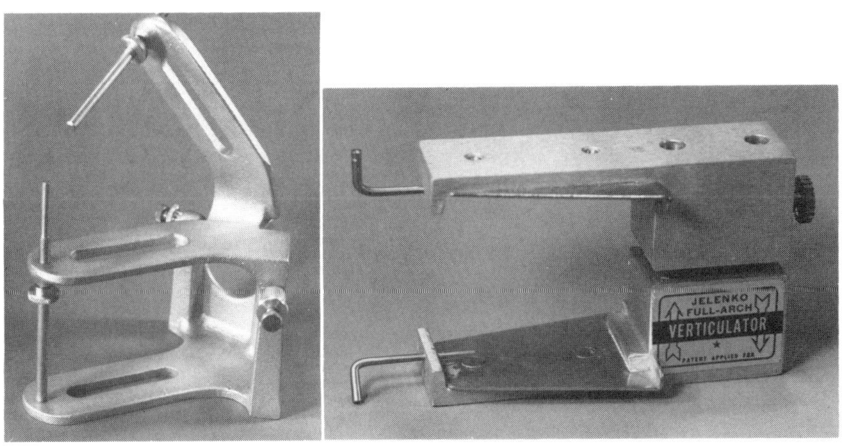

B

Fig. 1-214. A, Hanau Twin-Stage Occluder. **B,** Jelenko Verticulator.

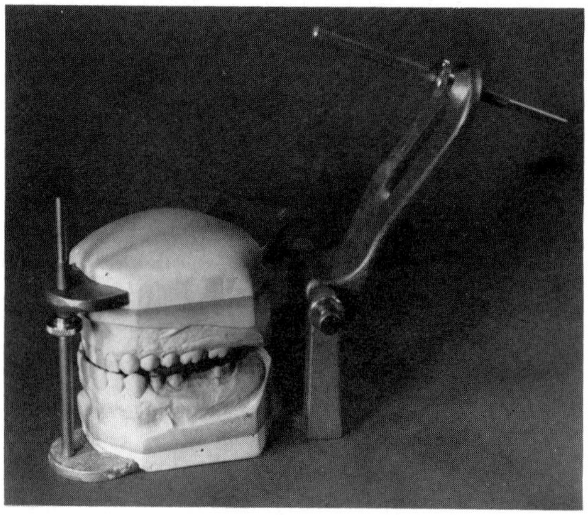

Fig. 1-215. Anatomic casts are mounted on articulator. Note that maxillary cast is on lower member in this instance.

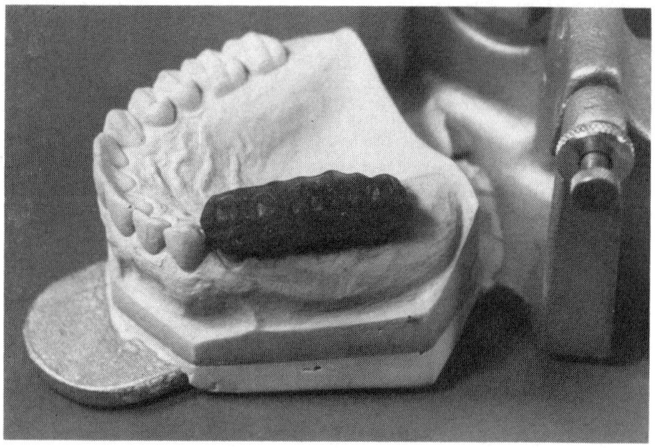

Fig. 1-216. Functionally generated occlusal path record is seated on dies completely and accurately.

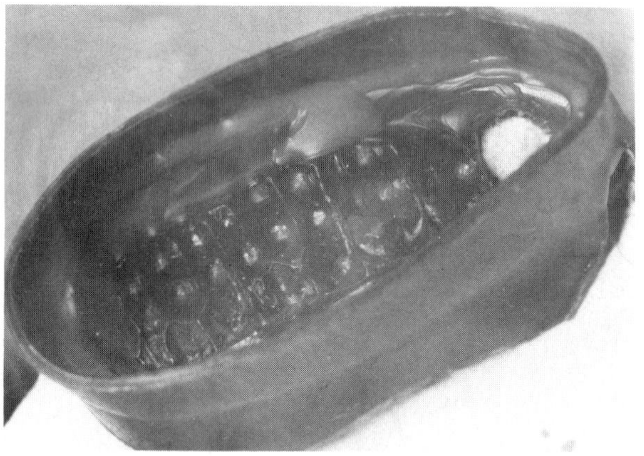

Fig. 1-217. Beading and boxing includes record and one tooth anterior to record. Separating medium is placed on any exposed stone.

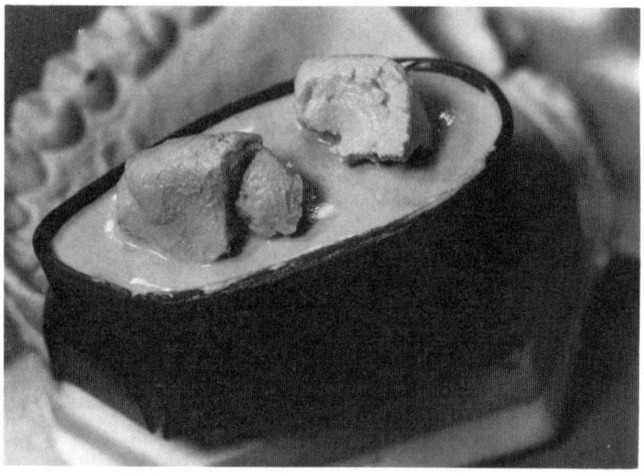

Fig. 1-218. Boxed record has been poured with stone and retention nodules left on surface for mounting.

PROCEDURE

1. After properly mounting the master cast and the anatomic cast, mount the functionally generated occlusal path record (Fig. 1-215). Place the occlusal path registration on the dies so that it is stable and completely seated (Fig. 1-216). Then bead the recording table, and box it with wax (Fig. 1-217). When boxing the table, make certain that the boxing includes one uncut tooth anterior to the preparations. It provides a positive vertical stop as well as a check on the accuracy of the closing of the record against the master cast. A good method of verifying the seal of the boxing is to pour some water into it and check for leaks. This is an important step because it is essential to fill the boxed record with stone. Any leak will permit stone to seep through and obliterate the underlying dies. Pour a mix of dental stone into the boxed record, and place retention nodules on the exposed portion (Fig. 1-218). After the initial set, attach the record to the other arm of the Twin-Stage Occluder with plaster (Fig. 1-219).

2. After the plaster has set, remove the boxing and beading, and open the device. Remove the table from the master cast, and observe the articulation. It is possible to articulate the master cast with the anatomic cast to accomplish the waxing and establish the proper intercuspation (Fig. 1-220, *A*). Then occlude the wax patterns with the functionally generated occlusal path record to detect and eliminate any interferences with occlusion (Figs. 1-220, *B* and 1-221).

Both the Twin-Stage Occluder and the Verticulator allow no lateral movement of the upper and lower members. Since the functionally generated occlusal

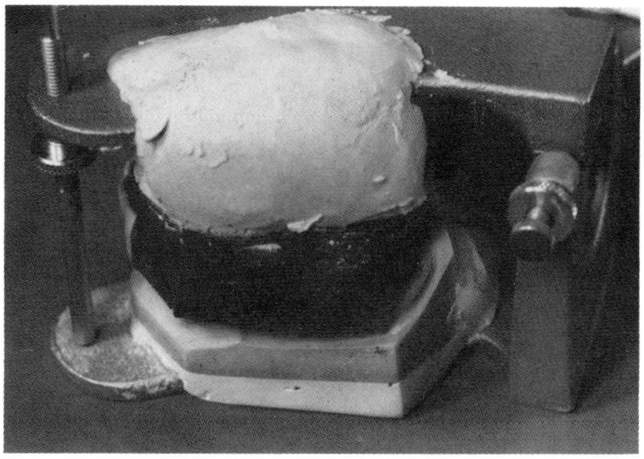

Fig. 1-219. Poured record is attached to articulator with plaster.

A

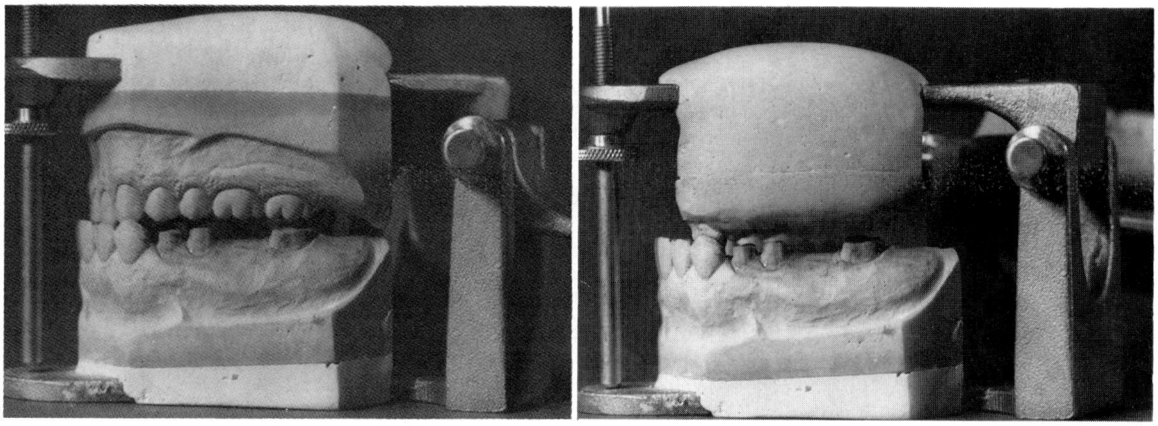

B

Fig. 1-220. A, Articulation of master cast with anatomic model. **B,** Articulation with functionally generated occlusal path record. Note positive stop anterior to record.

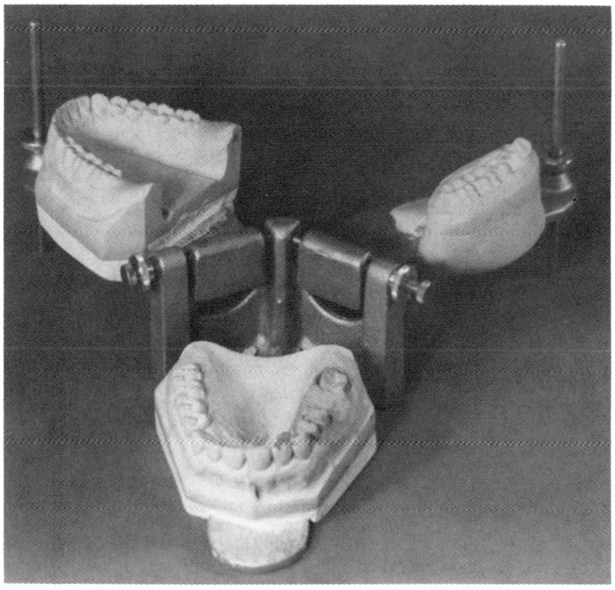

Fig. 1-221. Master cast can be occluded with anatomic record or functionally generated occlusal path record.

Table 1-5. Mounting the master cast

Problem	Possible cause	Solution
Condyles not fully seated in fossa assemblies	Condyles not held against metal walls of assembly during mounting	Remount Mandibular cast
Incisal pin not touching incisal guide table	Articulator not closed down to contact when mounting mandibular cast	Adjust incisal pin for small error, but remount mandibular cast for gross error
Upper and lower members of articulator not parallel	Incisal at incorrect position during mounting, or no allowance made for full-arch centric relation record	No change for small error, but remount lower cast for large error
Obvious error in centric relation	Cast not held together by cast stabilization, or articulator not in its proper relations during mounting	Remount mandibular cast
Obvious error in plane of occlusion	Face-bow not supported properly with face bow fork support	Obtain new face-bow and remount both casts
Cast broken loose from plaster mount	Plaster allowed to set too long before use or mixed too dry	Attach cast with sticky wax if able to be set back positively into remount grooves
Failure of split cast base to separate from cast	Failure to apply adequate amount of separating medium before pouring base	Break off base; clean up cast and notches Apply separating medium and pour new base
Failure of split cast base and cast to intercuspate with new centric relation record	Failure of original and second centric relation records to check	Try third record; on failure of third record to check, remount mandibular cast with another record; check it in same manner
Obvious improper articulation of functionally generated occlusal path record	Record probably not seated completely on dies	Reset record on dies and pour new cast
Stone from functionally generated occlusal path cast obilitering dies on master cast	Beading and boxing of record not watertight	Proceed if dies not damaged; if dies damaged, redo cast from new impressions
Vertical stop on cast not occluding with opposing cast	Incisal pin possibly in need of adjustment to allow cast to occlude or functionally generated occlusal path not mounted properly	Adjust incisal pin; if problem not corrected, remount functionally generated occlusal path record

path record represents the excursive movements of the opposing cusps, later movements of the articulating device are unnecessary. By interchanging the anatomic and functionally generated occlusal path records, it is possible to perform the same functions with the Verticular as with the Twin-Stage Occluder.

PROBLEM AREAS

Those problems which arise when mounting the master cast, their probable causes, and solutions are presented in Table 1-5.

1. When condyles are not fully seated within the fossa assembly, the proper interarch relationship is lost, and the mandibular cast has to be remounted. The condylar posts must be held firmly against the median and posterior walls of the fossa assembly until the mounting plaster has set. Similar discrepancies in the interarch relationship are found when the casts were not securely seated into the interocclusal record or when the casts were not securely fastened together with sticky wax or hand held during mounting.

2. Noticeable errors in the plane of occlusion can be traced to sagging of the bite fork, which has not been properly supported by a sliding block or T device. Also, when the articulator was not closed during the mounting of the maxillary cast, the occlusal plane will not be aligned anatomically correct with the condylar elements. Remounting the casts is usually indicated.

3. When the split cast mounting procedure is used, an adequate amount of separating medium applied will assure separation of the cast from its base. The split cast base and cast may not interdigitate with the second interocclusal record. A third record should be used as a double check. If the discrepancy persists, remounting of the mandibular cast with a new interocclusal record is indicated.

4. Problems that arise when functionally generated path records are used can be frequently traced to improper trimming and mounting of these records. Verify the complete and positive seating of the record on the working cast. Be certain that the record is trimmed smooth so it can be boxed watertight for pouring the opposing cast. Then excess stone or moisture cannot leak and compromise the master cast.

SUMMARY

This section has described mounting working casts on various articulating devices: nonadjustable, semiadjustable, and fully adjustable. Methods of orienting the maxillary cast on the articulator were detailed, as well as the orientation of the mandibular cast to the mounted maxillary cast. Here, the importance and proper handling of interocclusal records, fabrication of interocclusal records, fabrication of split cast mounting, and mounting of functionally generated path records were stressed.

Mounted working casts on an articulator are the direct link between the patient and laboratory. The accuracy with which this is accomplished will facilitate the construction of the prosthesis and minimize the time required for adjustment on the patient.

CHAPTER 2

DIAGNOSTIC PROCEDURES

GORDON D. DOUGLASS

MAKING DIAGNOSTIC CASTS

Diagnostic casts (study casts) are casts made of impressions taken prior to treatment and mounted anatomically in centric jaw relation. Impression materials used for diagnostic casts are most frequently those of the irreversible hydrocolloid varieties (alginates), primarily because of their fast setting times and ease of use. Recently, bonding hydrocolloids have been introduced to dentistry; these can be valuable for enhancing the surface characteristics of alginate impressions because reversible hydrocolloid is first injected over the tooth surface and then irreversible hydrocolloid is placed over it. The combination gives the surface accuracy of the reversible hydrocolloid with the economies of the irreversible. Some loss of detail results where the reversible hydrocolloid is completely displaced by the irreversible, as might occur on a cusp tip.

The preparation of diagnostic casts begins with careful handling of the impressions. As with all hydrocolloid impression materials, it is essential to prevent an exchange of water between the set alginate and its environment. It is preferable to pour casts immediately, although it is possible to store impressions in a humidor for a short time. Humidors are containers with moist atmosphere, and they vary in design. A simple humidor is a plastic container with moist towels on the bottom. A slot in the top of the humidor permits the handle to be secured outside and the tray to be suspended in the moist atmosphere (Fig. 2-1). Generally, this type of humidor is better than one that allows the impression to contact moist surfaces because of the risk of a change in the water content of the alginate. Do not store alginate impressions in water because they will absorb more water, causing the dimensions to change.

Before pouring casts, it is necessary to examine the impressions for apparent imperfections that will result in inaccurate casts. The following inaccuracies are found most frequently: (1) pulling away of the impression material from the periphery of the tray, (2) bubbles in the material, (3) perforation of the impression material by soft or hard tissues that also contact the metal of the tray, (4) extension of unsupported impression material beyond the tray, (5) apparent flowing of the alginate in areas during seating of the tray in the mouth, and (6) surface tearing usually associated with maxillary anterior teeth and interproximal areas. It is imperative for the dentist to correct inaccuracies in an impression prior to making the cast.

PROCEDURE

1. Trim any impression material extending beyond the tray with a sharp knife so that the impression rests on the metal tray when set on a flat surface (Figs. 2-2 and 2-3). Improper trimming will result in distorted casts.
2. Rinse the impression in running cold tap water to remove both saliva and blood, which increase the setting time of the stone. Occasionally, the consistency of saliva is heavy and mucinous. In this instance, sprinkle unmixed stone powder from a plastic squeeze bottle into the impression, and then immediately wash it out to aid in cleaning the surface of the impression (Fig. 2-4).
3. Shake the impression over a basin or blot the surface lightly with a paper towel to remove freestanding

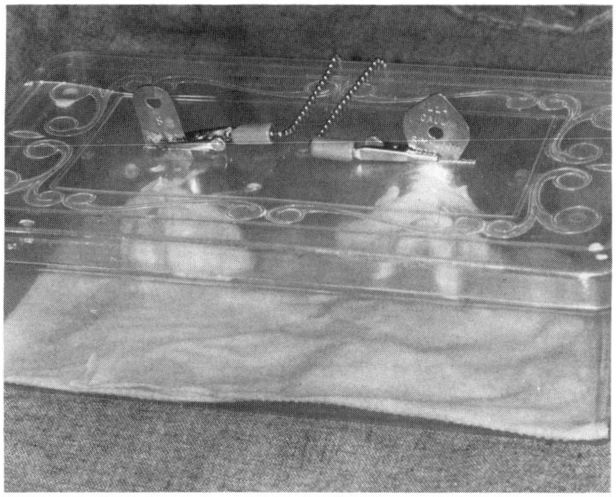

Fig. 2-1. Alginate impressions are rinsed and suspended in humidor until casts are made.

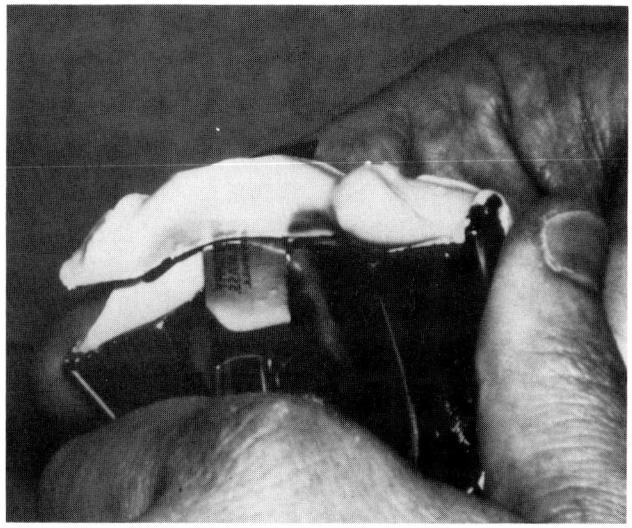

Fig. 2-2. Unsupported alginate is trimmed with sharp knife.

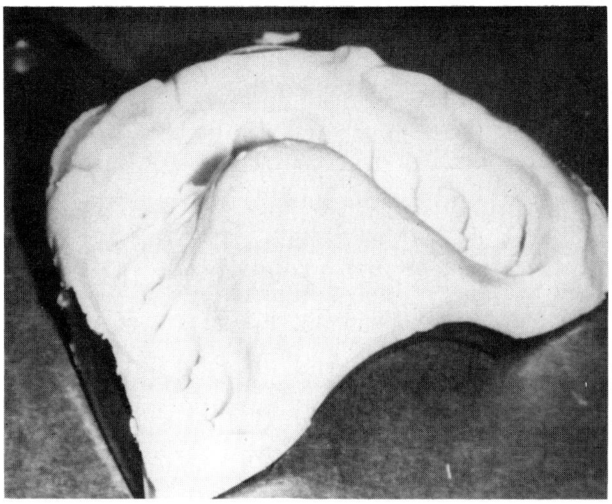

Fig. 2-3. Impression tray rests on flat surface and supports alginate to avoid displacement of unsupported alginate when making cast.

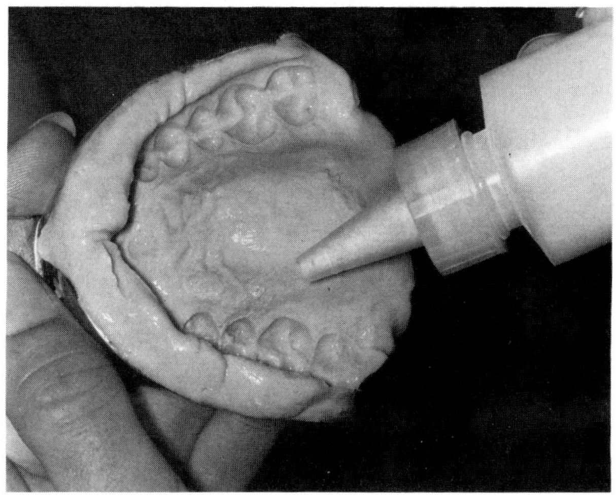

Fig. 2-4. Dry stone powder sprinkled in impression and washed out immediately acts as cleaning agent.

water. Do not dry alginate impression materials with compressed air because it can dehydrate the surface and cause distortion.

4. Make a proper mix of stone, place the tray handle on a vibrator, and begin the pour.

MAXILLARY CAST. Place a small amount of stone on the palate and allow a small stream to run toward the anterior teeth (Fig. 2-5). Continue to add small amounts of stone at the same point and allow the advancing stone to flow into the right and left sides of the mold until they are full (Fig. 2-6). Add the remaining bulk of stone to the palatal area, and shape it with a plaster spatula. Exercise care to prevent the stone from overflowing and locking onto the tray (Fig. 2-7). Add small amounts of stone to the surface of the freshly poured cast to facilitate mounting (Fig. 2-8).

MANDIBULAR CAST. Place a small amount of stone at the retromolar area on either the right or left side, and vibrate a small stream of stone into and along the arch on that side (Fig. 2-9). Continue adding small amounts of stone, and work the tray so that the advancing stone has a low angle of incidence with the surface (Fig. 2-10). As the stone fills the area of the anterior teeth take special care to avoid trapping air in the incisal corners. When full, add stone, and shape it carefully to avoid locking it over the edge of the tray. Add small amounts of stone to the surface of the freshly poured cast to facilitate mounting (Fig. 2-11).

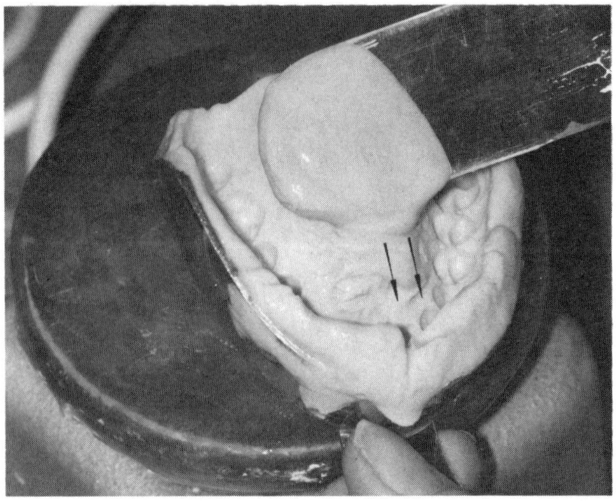

Fig. 2-5. Stone placed on palate is allowed to flow down lingual surfaces of maxillary teeth.

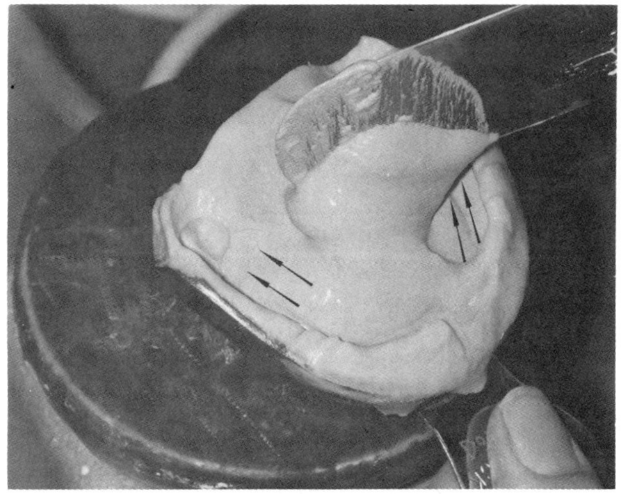

Fig. 2-6. Stone is added as pour advances posteriorly.

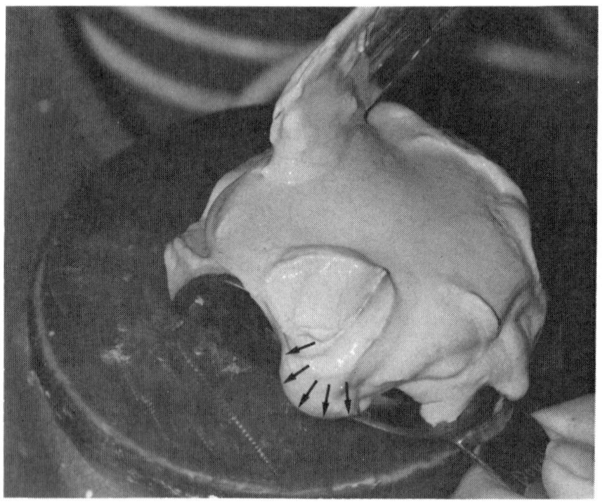

Fig. 2-7. Care must be exercised to prevent stone from flowing beyond periphery *(arrows).*

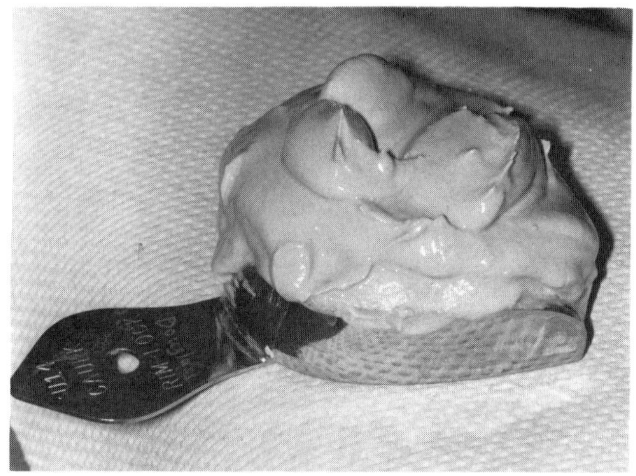

Fig. 2-8. Exposed surface of cast is made rough to facilitate mounting.

5. After making the cast set the tray upright in a humidor until the stone is set (Fig. 2-12). Do not invert a freshly poured cast because it causes "slumping" of the stone in the impression and distortion of the cast.

6. Do not allow stone to remain in the alginate after the final set. It is possible to store poured casts in a humidor for a short time. Excessive setting time prior to separation can result in loss of surface detail.

PROBLEM AREAS

Frequently found problems in making diagnostic casts, probable causes, and solutions are presented in Table 2-1.

1. Separating a cast from an impression is not always easy. It is especially difficult if stone has flowed beyond the impression material and locked under or around the tray. If this occurs, chip away the excess stone carefully until the cast is free from the tray. Extreme care in removing a cast is essential to avoid fracturing any portions. To loosen the cast and facilitate its removal, use a blast of compressed air at the periphery (Fig. 2-13). Then remove the cast with finger pressure alone. The use of instruments to pry a cast loose results in scarring and damaging the cast.

2. After removal, examine the cast thoroughly for apparent inaccuracies, such as broken teeth remaining in the alginate impression; bubbles of stone, usually in grooves of teeth and gingival borders; air bubbles, usu-

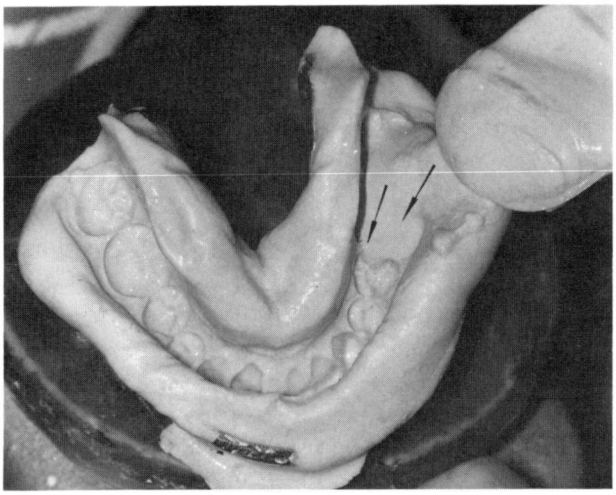

Fig. 2-9. Stone is started at distal aspect on one side of mandibular impression and allowed to flow anteriorly.

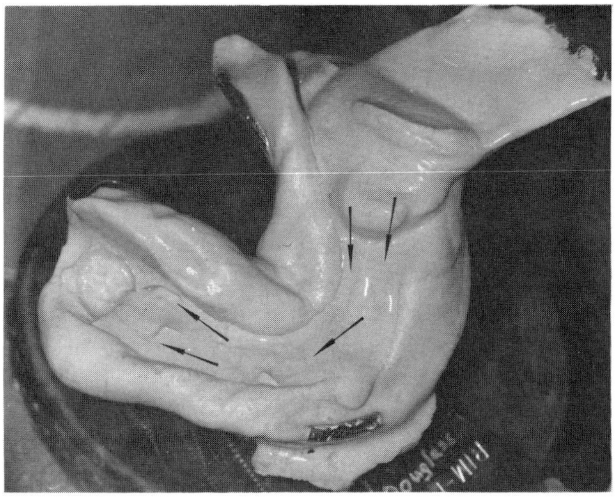

Fig. 2-10. Stone is added to mandibular impression until casting is complete.

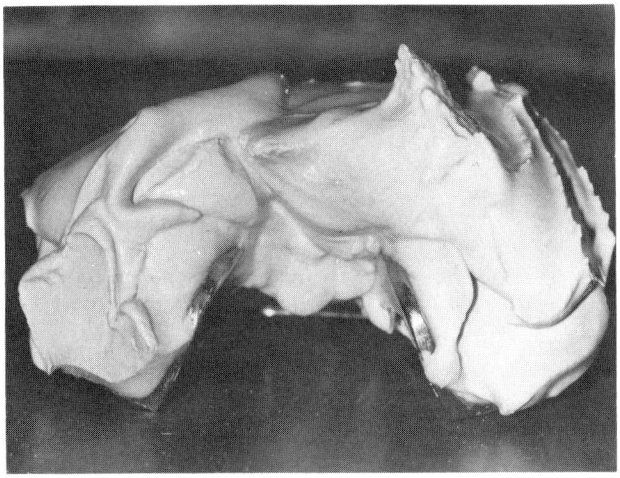

Fig. 2-11. Surface of mandibular cast is rough to facilitate mounting.

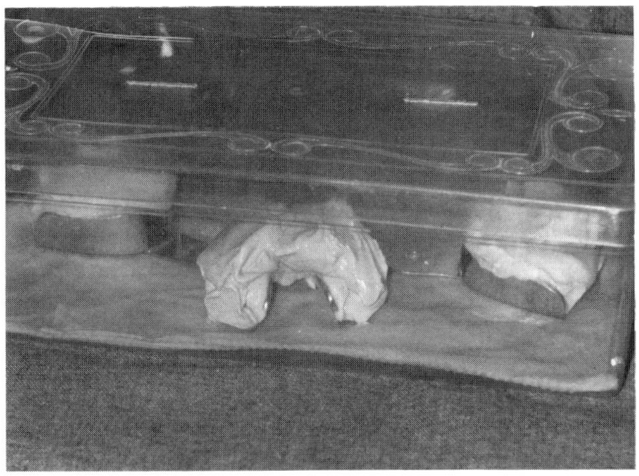

Fig. 2-12. Poured impressions are placed upright in humidor until final set.

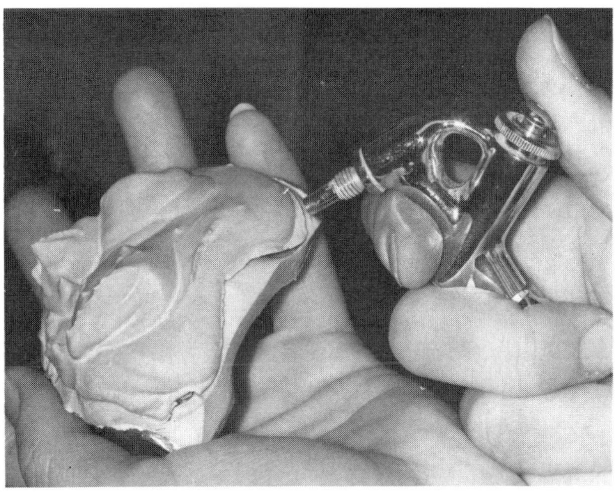

Fig. 2-13. Blast of compressed air at periphery of set cast will facilitate cast removal.

Table 2-1. Making diagnostic casts

Problem	Probable cause	Solution
Chalky occlusal surfaces on cast	Failure to remove free-standing water from impression adequately	Blot impression with small pieces of paper towel to facilitate removal of water
	Mucinous saliva remaining in impression after rinsing	Sprinkle dry stone powder into impression; immediately rinse before pouring
Cast unable to be removed from impression	Stone locked beyond periphery of tray	Shape stone away from periphery with spatula before setting
	Incompletely filled tray, allowing stone to flow under impression material	Add small amounts of freshly mixed impression material to areas destined to be undercuts
Alveolar ridge on cast appears narrower on one side than other	Impression material pulled away from periphery of tray during removal from mouth	Retake impression; reseat impression material against tray; note inherent inaccuracy
Air bubbles over entire surface of cast	Stone improperly mixed	Follow manufacturer's specifications; mix stone under vacuum on vibrator
Air bubbles at incisal edges and tips of cusps	Air trapped in corners of impression by stone flowing over surface	Rotate and tip tray while introducing stone into impression
Teeth broken off in impression	Carelessness in removing cast from impression	Trim and mount cast; allow it to dry; cement fractured teeth back in place with household cement
Failure of articulator to seat together firmly	Intercondylar distance not set for upper and lower members at same width	Reset intercondylar distances; completely remount
	Wrong lower member connected to articulator	Avoid intermixing of different articulators
Interocclusal record loose between casts after cast mounted	Lower cast disturbed when mounted to articulator	Have cast held in place during mounting or use sticky wax to hold it in place
	Instrument not in centric relation when lower cast mounted	Remount lower cast with condyle posts firmly seated in respective housings
Cast not centered in articulator	Slipping of face-bow on articulator during mounting of upper cast	Remount upper cast
	Patient asymmetrical	Recheck face-bow and maxillary record to verify asymmetry
Failure of cast to seat in interocclusal records	Inaccurate cast	Check for additional bubbles or soft tissue areas impinging on record; if there are none, retake impression
	Records distorted	Mount casts immediately or store records in contact with casts for only short time

ally on tips of cusps and incisal edges; chalky surfaces associated with inadequate drying of the impression; and distortions in size as a result of displaced alginate (Figs. 2-14 and 2-15). After the cast has dried thoroughly, cement any teeth that remained in the impression in place on the cast with a thin film of household cement.

3. Wet the cast to facilitate trimming and to preserve the trimming wheel. Trim casts soon after the final set of the stone. Soaking stone casts in tap water results in dissolution of the surface and loss of the detail (Fig. 2-16). Make slurry water by placing discarded stone in water for 48 hours. Use of the resulting water to soak casts prior to trimming will minimize the risk of damage to the surface.

4. The boundaries to which it is necessary to trim a cast depend on the area of interest. Usually, it is possible to trim casts to the base of the reflex surrounding the alveolar ridge. Trimming should be both esthetic and functional (Fig. 2-17). Excess stone left around the dental arch not only detracts from the esthetic result, but also can hamper either the mounting of casts or the visual access to the occluding surfaces after mounting. Do not trim the surface to be mounted to the articulator unless it becomes necessary during mounting.

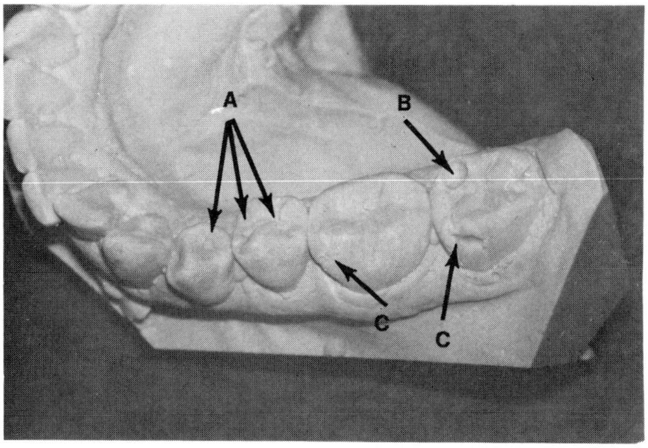

Fig. 2-14. Irregularities found on casts are bubbles of stone in grooves *(A)*, air bubbles on tips of cusps, *(B)*, and chalky areas *(C)*.

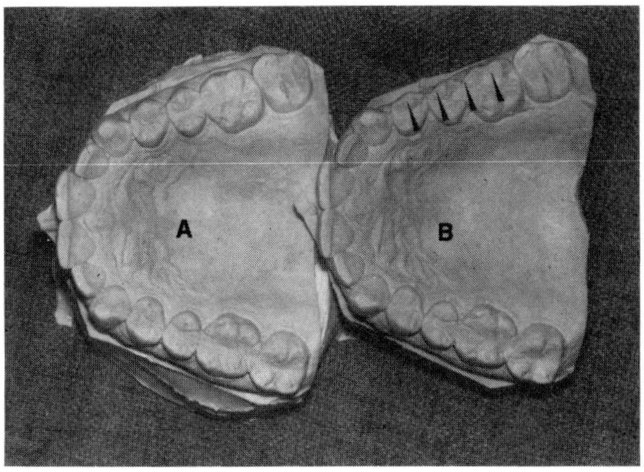

Fig. 2-15. Comparison of arch *A* with arch *B* of two casts for same patient shows distortion of *B* caused by alginate pulling loose from rim-lock tray.

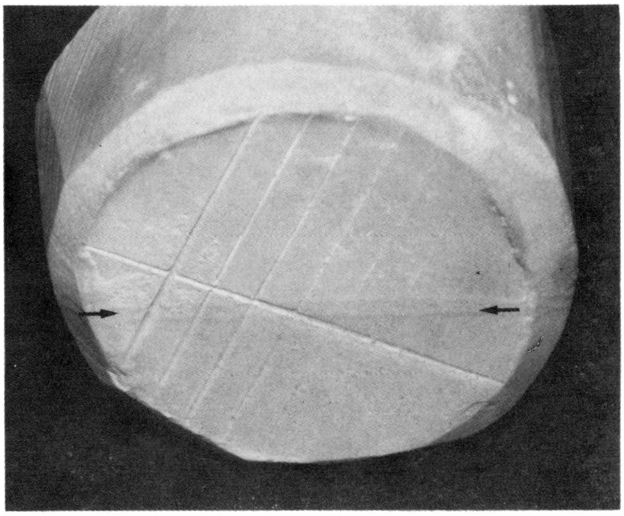

Fig. 2-16. Stone cast soaked in tap water for only 2 hours shows significant loss of detail below waterline *(arrows)*.

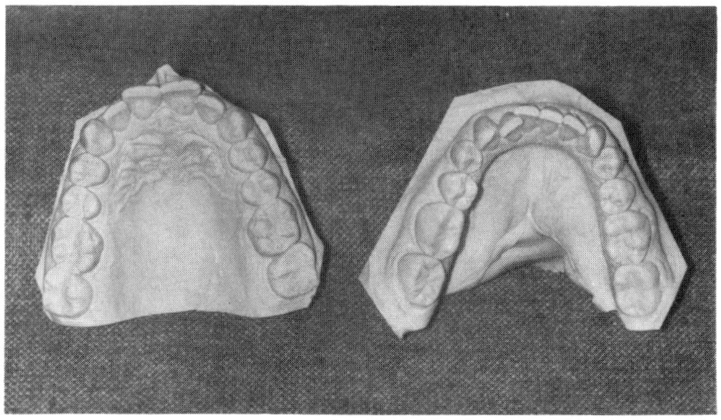

Fig. 2-17. Set of properly trimmed casts ready for mounting.

MOUNTING DIAGNOSTIC CASTS

The arbitrary mounting of casts usually is adequate for diagnostic purposes. In our opinion, the sophisticated hinge axis, split cast, and pantographic tracing techniques relate more properly to a procedure and treatment than to making a diagnosis. Therefore only the more commonly used arbitrary mounting procedure will be described here.

Two types of face-bow devices are in general use for mounting diagnostic casts to an arbitrary hinge axis. One type uses the ear meatus as an arbitrary point of reference to the hinge axis. A second type requires measuring an average distance anterior to each ear and using these points as arbitrary references. Since neither instrument results in an accurate determination of the hinge axis, the choice is a matter of personal preference.

The records necessary for the proper arbitrary mounting of diagnostic casts are a face-bow that has recorded the relationship of a maxillary index (bite fork) to an arbitrary plane, an interocclusal record, two trimmed casts, and an articulator capable of receiving the recorded information.

Although many instrument systems of each type are available, this section will discuss the use of only one of the more common instruments. However, the basic principles of all systems are similar. These principles relate the (1) maxillary cast to the opening axis of the articulator in a manner that is reasonably correct anatomically for that patient and (2) mandibular cast to the maxillary cast in centric jaw relation.

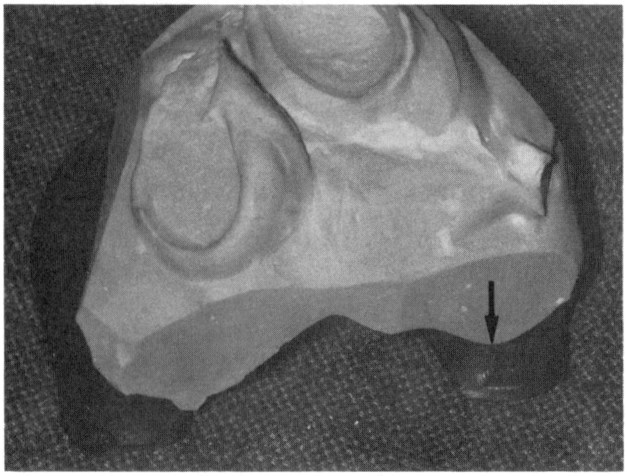

Fig. 2-18. Soft tissues recorded in cast sometimes contact wax records *(arrow).*

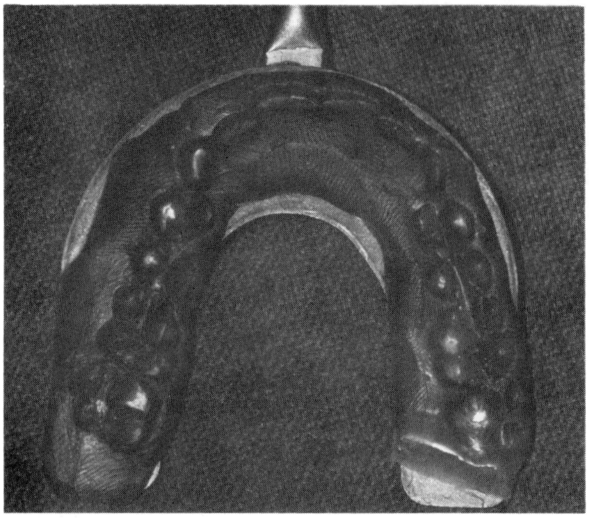

Fig. 2-19. Recorded area of soft tissue in wax record is cut away with sharp knife.

PROCEDURE USING QUICK-MOUNT WHIP-MIX* ARTICULATOR SYSTEM.

Before mounting the casts, verify the accuracy of the bite records by setting the maxillary cast carefully, first into the interocclusal record and then into the maxillary index (bite-fork record). If the cast seats completely without pressure, it is accurate. If the cast does not seat completely, recheck the cast for apparent inaccuracies as described for making diagnostic casts. Check also to make certain that the soft tissue areas recorded by the bite records are not in contact with the cast (Fig. 2-18). If they contact the cast, make appropriate adjustments of the offending bite record carefully with a sharp knife until the teeth on the cast provide the primary support for the records (Fig. 2-19).

1. Adjust the articulator to receive the face-bow by setting the intercondylar dimension to small, medium, or large by using the inserts supplied with the articulator. The intercondylar dimension can be determined from the registration on the hinge axis point of the face-bow (Figs. 2-20 and 2-21). Set the condylar inclination of the articulator at 30 degrees. This setting places the hinge axis point on the articulator at an average position with respect to the pin on the side of the condylar guide, and it serves as a standard position when mounting casts on the articulator (Fig. 2-22).

2. Attach a mounting plate to the upper member of the articulator, loosen the face-bow, and adjust it to place the earpieces over the pins on the side of the condyle guide of the articulator (Fig. 2-23). Rotate the upper member of the articulator forward until it rests on the cross-member of the face-bow (Fig. 2-24). NOTE: The face-bow S, M, and L indications are not accurate now because of the medial inset of the condyles from the face-bow attachment pins.

3. Place the maxillary cast in the maxillary bite record (bite fork), and check the available clearance between the cast and mounting plate. If the space does not allow the articulator to remain in contact with the cross-member of the face-bow as described in the preceding step, trim the cast until the space is sufficient for contact to be achieved (Fig. 2-25).

4. Using the lower member of the articulator as a mounting stand, place a fresh mix of plaster between the cast and mounting plate. Exercise care to avoid disturbing the position of the cast when placing the plaster, and make certain to have the upper member of the articulator in contact again with the cross-member of the face-bow (Fig. 2-26).

5. When the mounting plaster has set, remove the face-bow, and place the incisal guide pin in the articulator. In addition, position both side-shift plates (Bennett plates) at 0 (Fig. 2-27).

6. Reposition the lower condyle posts to correspond with the intercondylar distance setting of the upper member of the articulator. Put the two parts of the articulator together at this time to make certain that the intercondylar settings on the upper and lower members are identical. If they are not, the condyles will not seat firmly and positively in their respective housings (Fig. 2-28).

*Whip-Mix Corp., Louisville, Ky.

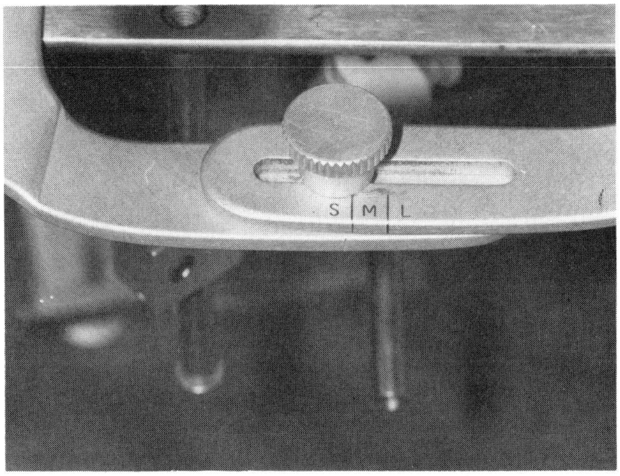

Fig. 2-20. Hinge point of Whip-Mix face-bow determines *S, M,* and *L* setting for use with articulator.

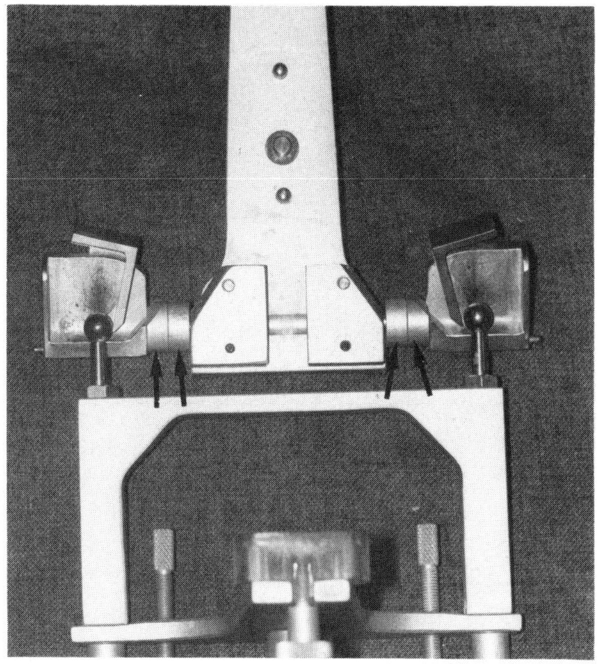

Fig. 2-21. Articulator with *L* setting of intercondylar width, as indicated by four inserts *(arrows).*

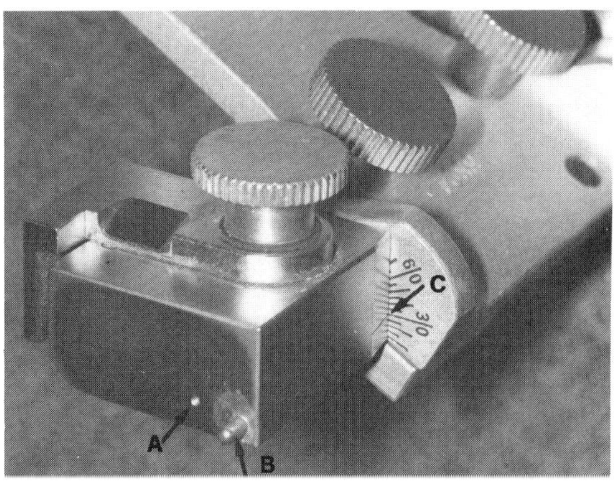

Fig. 2-22. Hinge axis point of articulator *(A)* is at average position with respect to mounting pin *(B)* when condylar inclination *(C)* is set at 30 degrees.

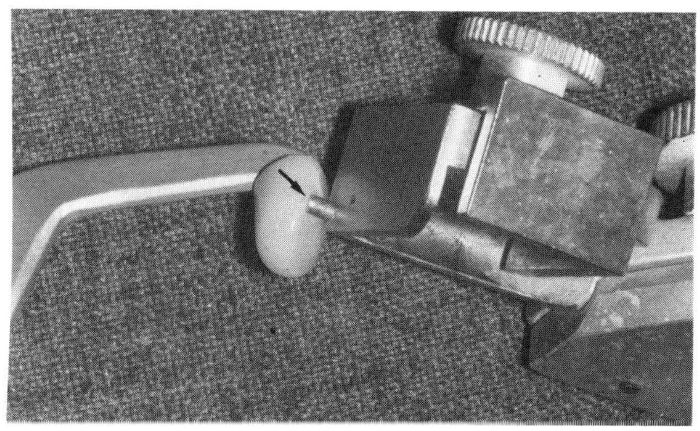

Fig. 2-23. Earpiece of face-bow is placed over mounting pin *(arrow)* in preparation for mounting maxillary cast.

7. Invert the upper member on a flat surface, place the interocclusal record in position on the maxillary cast, and place the mandibular cast in the record (Fig. 2-29).

8. Place the lower member of the articulator with a mounting plate attached on the upper member, and close the hinge. If the space is not adequate for the mounting plaster, trim the lower cast to provide space (Fig. 2-30).

9. Place a fresh mix of plaster between the lower cast and lower mounting plate. Exercise caution to avoid disturbing the position of the mandibular cast in the interocclusal record and make certain that the condyle posts seat firmly against the walls of their respective condylar housings (Fig. 2-31). This step completes the mounting of the upper and lower casts in an anatomically related position of centric jaw relation. Use this position as a basic reference when evaluating interarch relationships (Fig. 2-32).

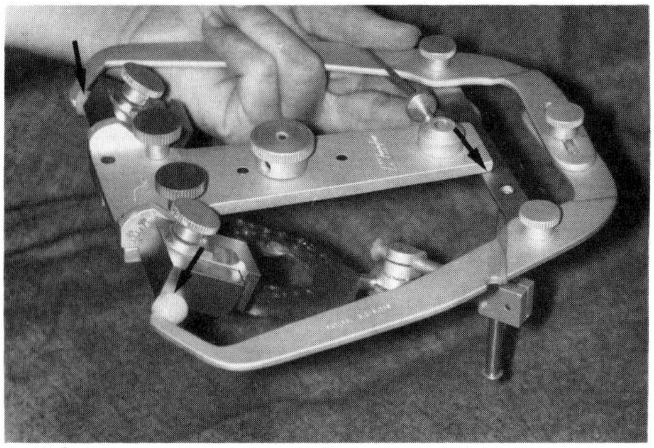

Fig. 2-24. Maxillary half of articulator is supported at three points of face-bow *(arrows).*

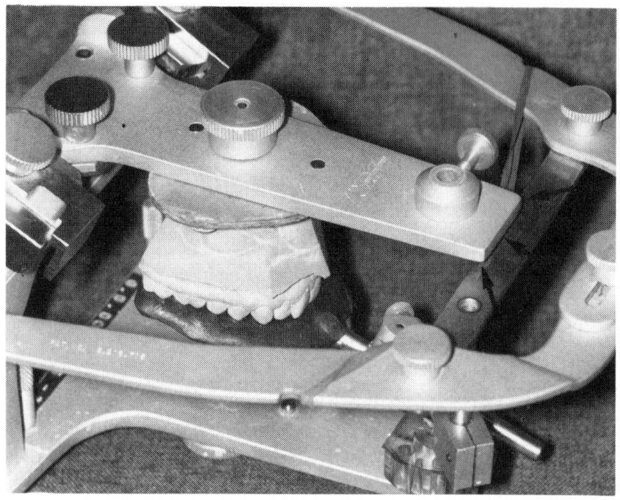

Fig. 2-25. This maxillary cast does not allow maxillary half of articulator to rest on face-bow *(arrow)* and requires trimming.

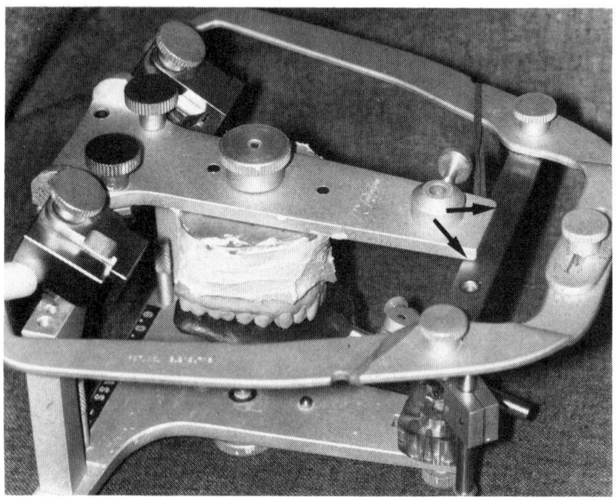

Fig. 2-26. Maxillary cast is mounted on articulator, which is checked to make certain that it contacts face-bow *(arrows).*

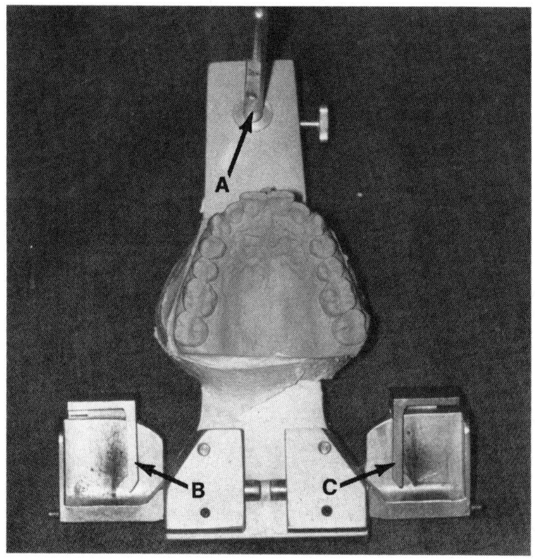

Fig. 2-27. Incisal guide pin *(A)* is placed, and two side-shift plates *(B)* and *(C)* are set at 0.

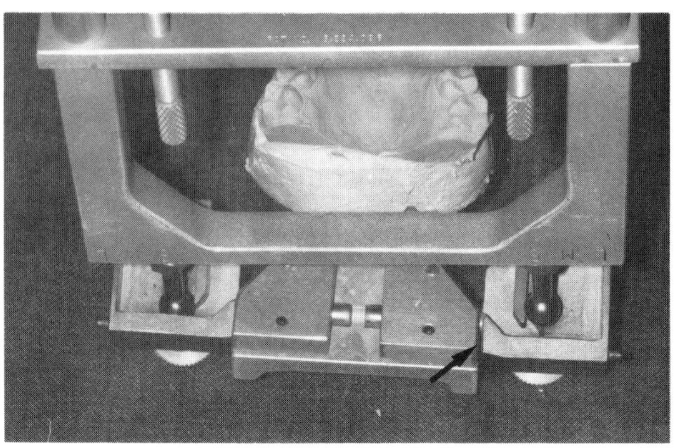

Fig. 2-28. Both condyles do not seat completely because condyle housing does not set tight against articulator *(arrow).*

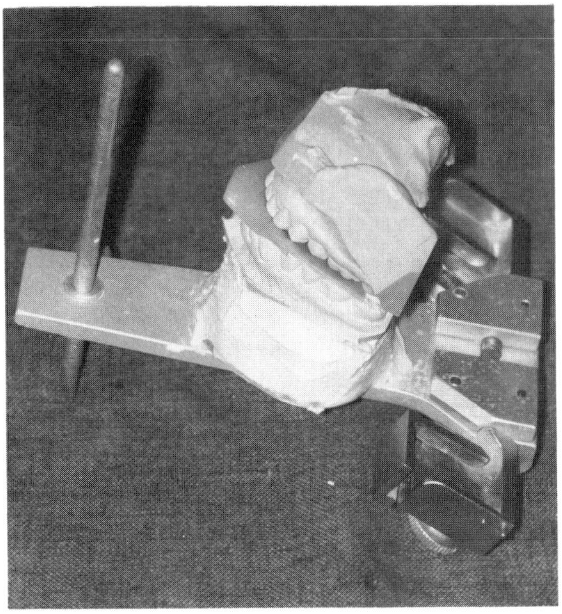

Fig. 2-29. Interocclusal record and mandibular cast in place.

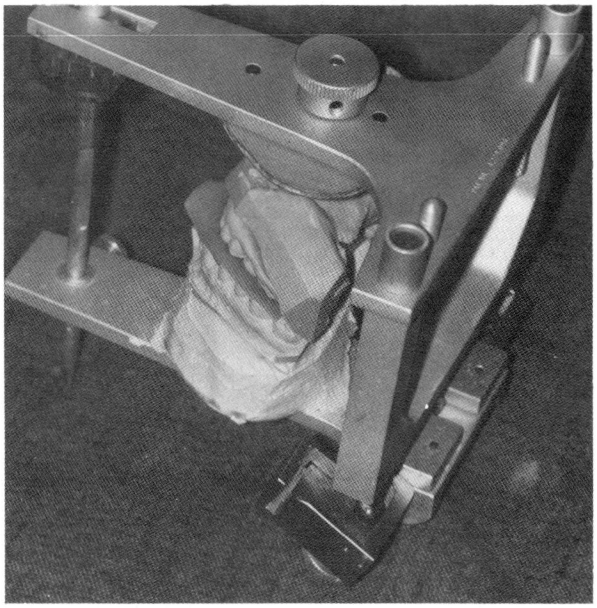

Fig. 2-30. Mandibular half of articulator is placed and checked for clearance between mounting plate and cast.

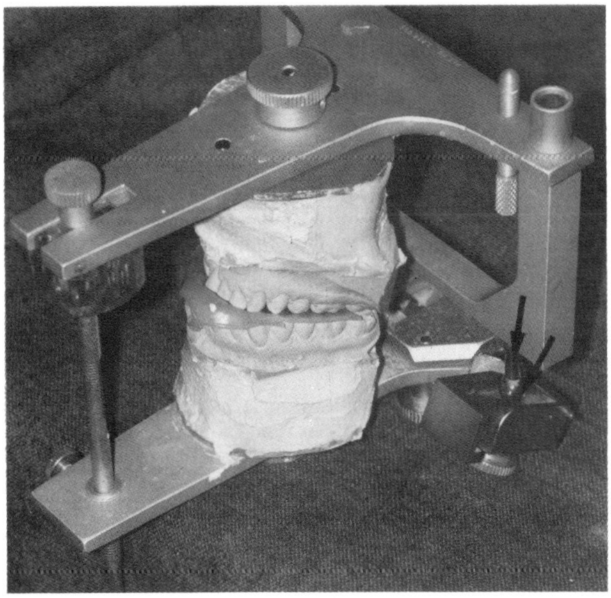

Fig. 2-31. Mounting stone is placed between mandibular cast and mounting plate, and condyle posts are checked to make certain that they seat against rear wall of condylar housing *(arrows).*

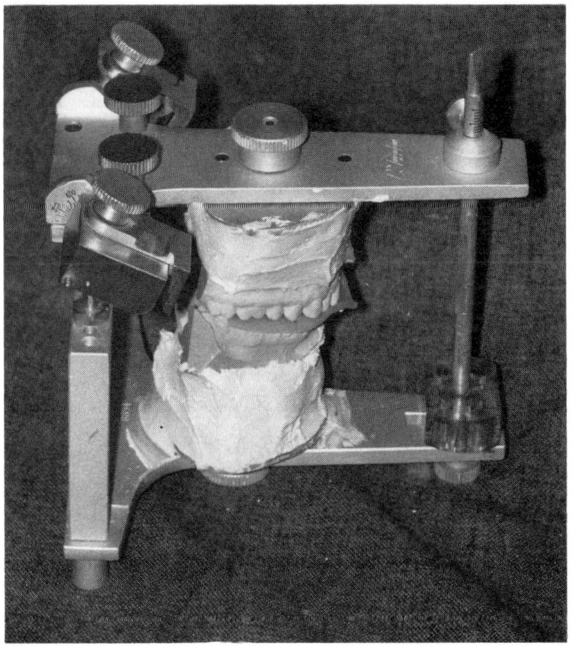

Fig. 2-32. Casts mounted in centric jaw relation.

USING DIAGNOSTIC CASTS

Dental care must begin with a thorough evaluation and an accurate diagnosis. The dentist is responsible for examining and recording all pertinent information to make the proper diagnosis. The history is of primary importance because it assists the dentist in making decisions that determine the type of objective information necessary for a proper diagnosis.

Objective information collected about an illness or a condition constitutes the signs. The dentist must look for signs from the moment a patient is first seen. Disfigured dentition, swelling, speech impairments, and facial expressions are objective signs. The dentist must also record other information, such as missing teeth, fillings, bacterial plaque retention, inflammation, periodontal pocket measurements, and tooth mobility. Frequently diagnostic mounted casts of the teeth and surrounding tissues must be added.

Diagnostic casts may be essential for formulating a diagnosis and treatment plan. If casts are to be of maximum value, they must meet specific criteria. First, they must be reasonably accurate; in most instances alginate materials are sufficient. Second, they must include the entire area of interest on inspection. Third, they must be related anatomically; usually casts mounted with arbitrary types of face-bows and simple interocclusal records are adequate.

The dentist uses diagnostic casts to evaluate intra-arch and interarch relationships of the teeth and surrounding tissues. In addition, mounted casts can serve as a guide in occlusal adjustments and for diagnostic waxing. The occluding surfaces of these casts must be free of defects before the dentist can make "trial" occlusal adjustment on the casts. A record of each adjustment should be made and used as a guide in adjusting the patient's teeth. For diagnostic waxing, the teeth are reduced and wax added to the surfaces. This procedure aids in deciding which teeth to prepare, how to prepare each tooth to allow adequate restoration, and how to contour the final restored result. Duplicate casts of the diagnostic wax-up can be invaluable aids in fabricating temporary restorations.

DIAGNOSTIC PREPARATION AND WAXING

Mounted diagnostic casts enable evaluation of the needs of the patient and formulation of a treatment plan. It is then possible to test procedures that could produce adverse results prior to their implementation. The objective of this discussion is to review some procedures proven valuable through usage.

diagnostic preparation The process of developing intra-arch and interarch relationships to establish crown contours and occlusal surfaces.

Intra-arch relationships

In restorative dentistry it is often necessary to involve other dental specialties in treating the patient. Diagnostic casts can be valuable for communication between the orthodontist and restorative dentist. The teeth are removed from the case and replaced in an appropriate relationship essential for restorations (Figs. 2-33 and 2-34). In this procedure cutting off only the incisal two thirds of the tooth and repositioning it allows the orthodontist to visualize both the direction and amount of movement desired by the restorative dentist. The therapists can then work together on decisions about the patient.

Perhaps the most common intra-arch relationship problem is the movement of teeth as a result of a loss of dental arch integrity. Frequently, drifting of the remaining teeth following tooth extraction presents the diagnostician with tipped teeth and open contacts (Fig. 2-35). Open contacts can be corrected in either of two ways: (1) orthodontic movement to close the contact or (2) increasing the mesiodistal width of the clinical crown with a restoration. The diagnostic cast with supplemental information acquired from the clinical examination is used to determine whether crown contours can be increased by restorations without adversely affecting the supporting structures. If contacts cannot be closed using restorations, orthodontic procedures may be instituted to accomplish the desired result.

Tipped teeth challenge the ingenuity of the restorative dentist. The tipped tooth that has achieved contact can be particularly difficult (Fig. 2-36). Frequently the mesiodistal width at the occlusal is less than the width at the proposed gingival margins. The diagnostician must determine from study casts and x-ray films the possibility of achieving a proper path of insertion. The case illustrated in Fig. 2-36 requires restoration of both molars or at least a serious recontouring of adjacent teeth.

When tipped teeth have not achieved contact, a fixed partial denture may be practical (Fig. 2-37). The casts indicate the severity of the problem of insertion. A path acceptable for the premolar may be unacceptable for the companion molar. In such an instance, a nonrigid connector might be considered were it not for the rotated premolar with a large pulp as indicated in the radiograph (Fig. 2-38). A common path of insertion even with a nonrigid connector at the distal of the premolar would be difficult to achieve. Several alternatives to the classic fixed partial denture design exist in this case. It is possible, for example, to right the molar by orthodontic treatment. If orthodontics were not feasible, a nonrigid connector could be placed in the pontic area. In this instance, however, such an approach would not

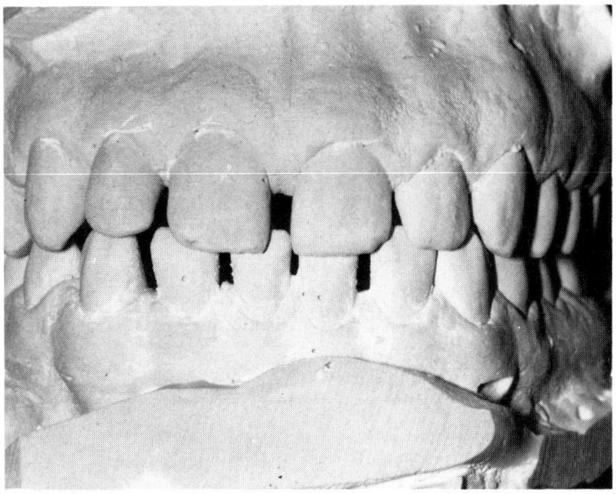

Fig. 2-33. Diagnostic casts with anterior spacing between teeth — to be repositioned diagnostically.

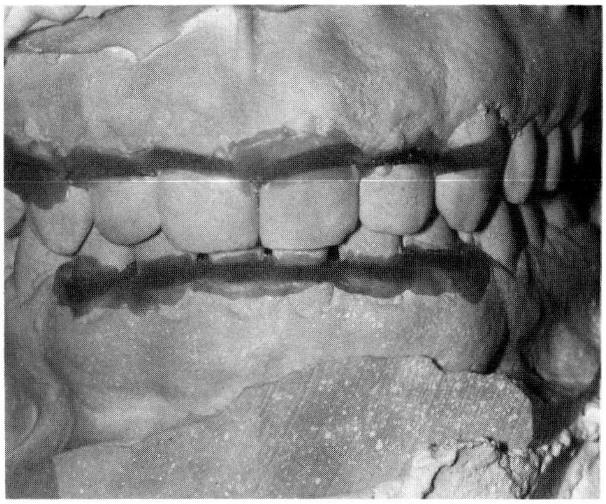

Fig. 2-34. Incisal two thirds has been cut off and repositioned for evaluation by orthodontist.

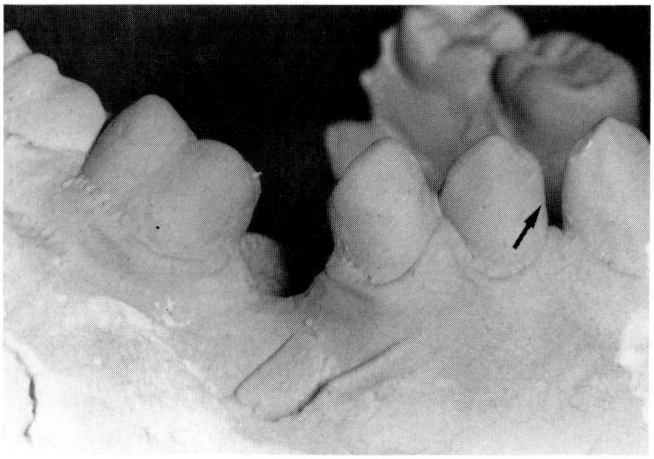

Fig. 2-35. Loss of a lower first molar has resulted in open contacts mesial to bicuspids *(arrow)* and mesial drifting of remaining lower molars.

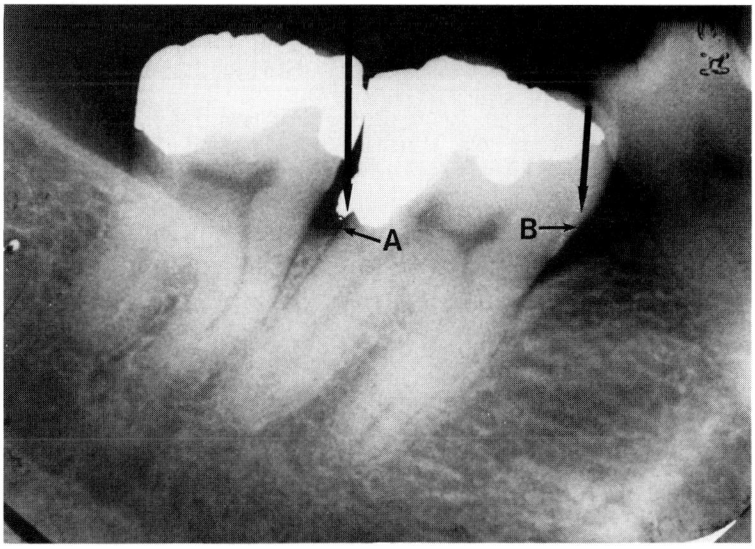

Fig. 2-36. Proposed placement of mesial and distal margins at *A* and *B* will result a path of insertion shown by arrows. In this case, without recontouring the adjacent teeth a path of insertion is not possible.

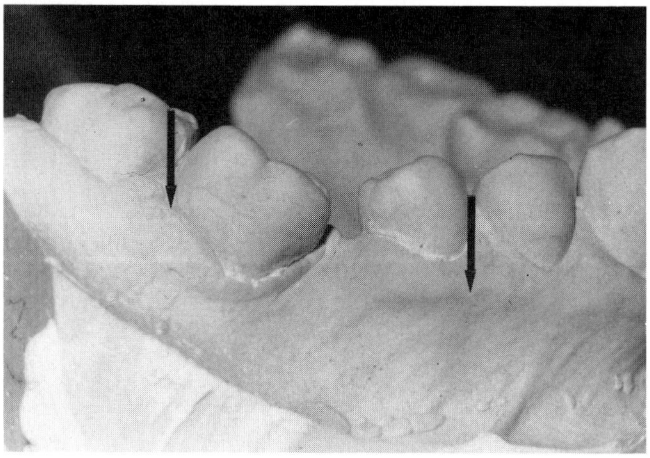

Fig. 2-37. Path of insertion *(arrows)* for bridge can be complicated by tipping of molars. In this case mesial of third molar interferes.

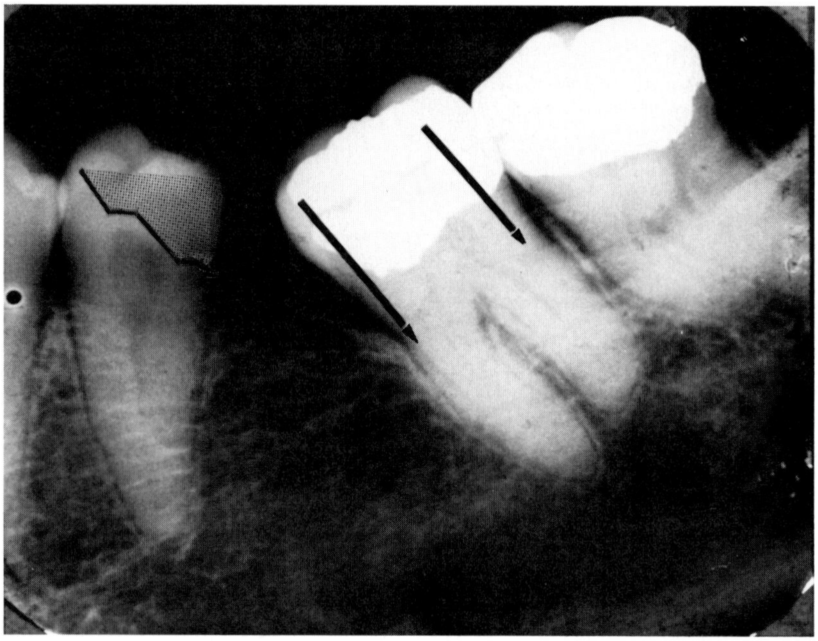

Fig. 2-38. Radiograph of case illustrated in Fig. 2-37 reveals a rotated premolar with a large pulp. Preparation of a "box" form in the premolar along the path of insertion dictated by the molar long axis would encroach on the pulp, as indicated by the outlined shaded area.

be acceptable because when such a connector is so positioned each retainer becomes a cantilever with its associated disadvantages. Finally, the placement of an inlay in the bicuspid and construction of a retainer and pontic for the molar with a shallow rest on the bicuspid might be considered.

Interarch relationships

In the least complex situation diagnostic casts are used to develop projected contours on deteriorated anterior teeth (Fig. 2-39). The illustration shows the teeth before and after the use of inlay wax on the mounted cast to replace the missing tooth structure. Not only does this procedure serve as a valuable guide to the

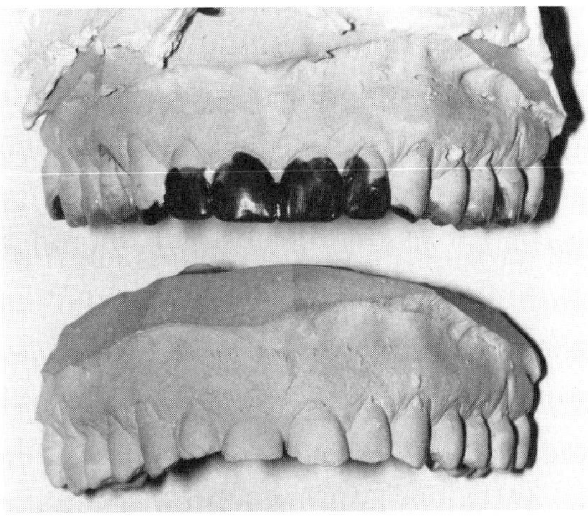

Fig. 2-39. Wax can be used to diagnostically replace lost tooth structure.

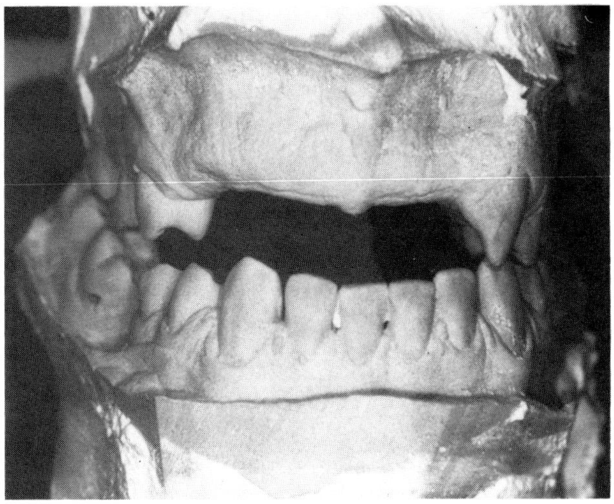

Fig. 2-40. Cast requiring multidisciplinary approach to treatment.

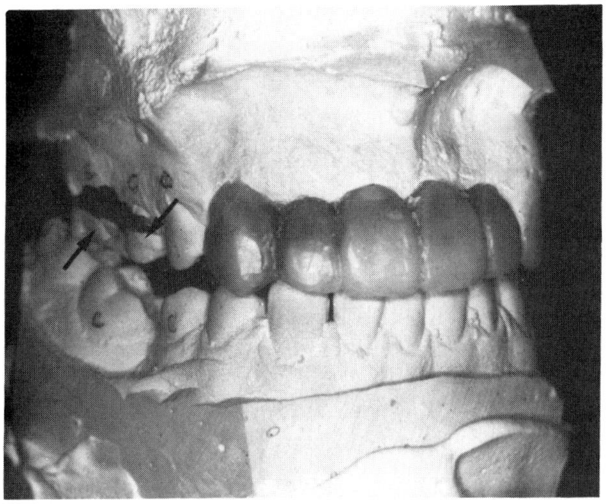

Fig. 2-41. Posterior teeth have been repositioned *(arrows),* and anterior teeth waxed to contour.

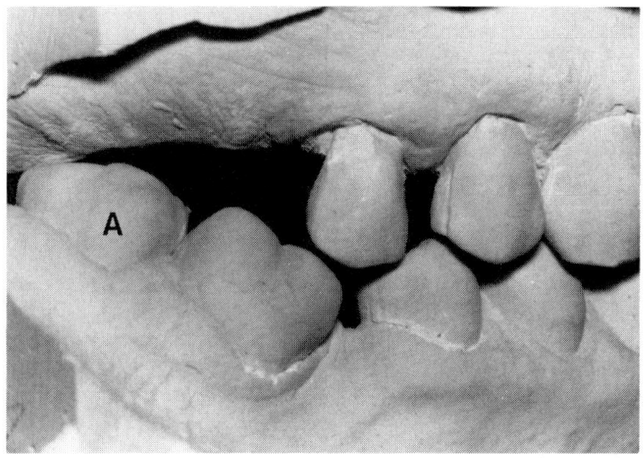

Fig. 2-42. Same case as Figs. 2-37 and 2-38 when placed in occlusion shows that third molar must be sacrificed to allow for upper partial restoration. Loss of third molar *(A)* would reduce dictating units affecting path of insertion of a fixed bridge between second bicuspid and molar.

final appearance, but it also becomes the model for constructing temporary restorations.

It is possible to use both repositioning of teeth and diagnostic waxing as communicative aids (Fig. 2-40). The mounted casts shown require a multidisciplinary approach. Repositioning the posterior teeth on the casts and waxing the anterior teeth diagnostically help determine the potential acceptability of a combined orthodontic-restorative approach without surgical intervention (Fig. 2-41).

Decisions that are based upon intra-arch conditions can or must be modified when interarch relationships are considered. The condition previously discussed and illustrated in Figs. 2-37 and 2-38 takes on a new perspective when maxillary and mandibular casts are placed in occlusion (Fig. 2-42). It becomes obvious that the second and third molars have extruded, with the third molar obliterating any space available for a removable partial denture. With this added information the diagnostician might consider the extraction of the third molar and construction of a fixed partial denture between premolar and first molar.

Potential problems of paths of insertion are greatly altered by the presence or absence of a "dictating unit," which can be described as a tooth or condition that affects the path of insertion of an intended restoration. In

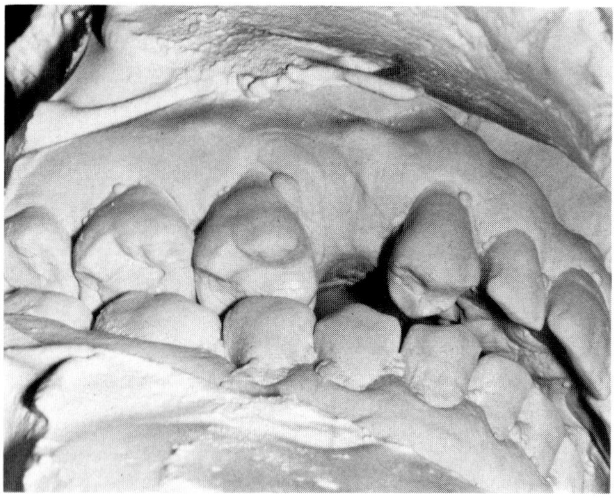

Fig. 2-43. Right side of unacceptable occlusal relationship before planned tooth reduction procedure on diagnostic casts.

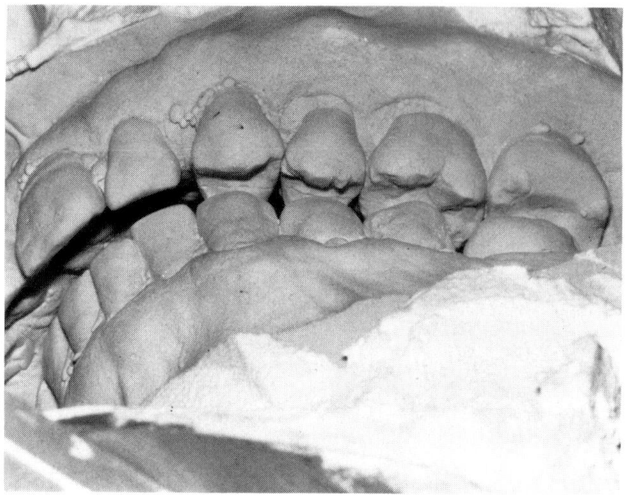

Fig. 2-44. Left side of same patient as in Fig. 2-43.

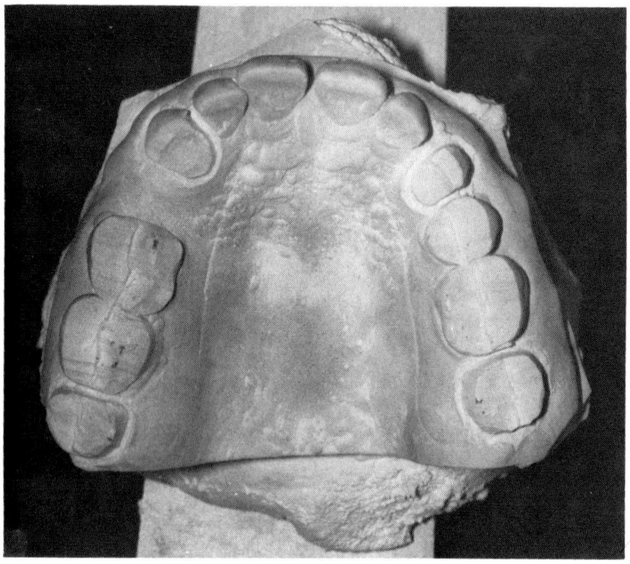

Fig. 2-45. Planned tooth reduction of 1.5 mm has been completed on maxillary cast.

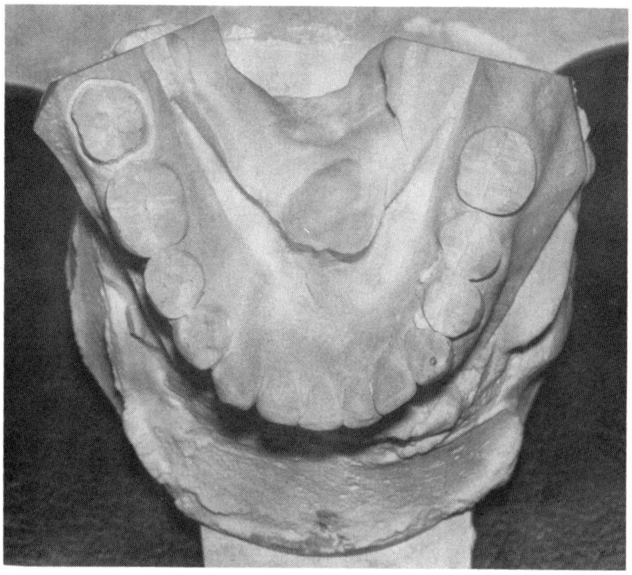

Fig. 2-46. Mandibular cast of patient in Fig. 2-45.

its simplest form a dictating unit could be a carious lesion on a facial surface requiring insertion of a restoration from the facial aspect. As the complexity of a restorative case increases (more complex restorations, tipped adjacent teeth, numerous abutments), so does the number of dictating units affecting the path of insertion of the restoration.

The problem discussed in Fig. 2-42 had four dictating units (two premolars and two molars) when only the intra-arch relationships were considered. As soon as the opposing arch was considered, one of the dictating units (the third molar) was found to be unacceptable because of extrusion. The removal of this molar would reduce the number of dictating units and make possible a greater number of alternative treatment designs.

Planned tooth reduction on the diagnostic casts is a useful aid. It may be necessary to remove a measured amount of tooth structure on the cast to predict the desired end result, as demonstrated by a postorthodontic patient with missing maxillary canines (Figs. 2-43 and 2-44). Interarch relationships in the patient shown in Fig. 2-43 are entirely unacceptable, since it is impossible to obtain anterior function by occlusal adjustment. Potentially, the best approach is restorative treatment.

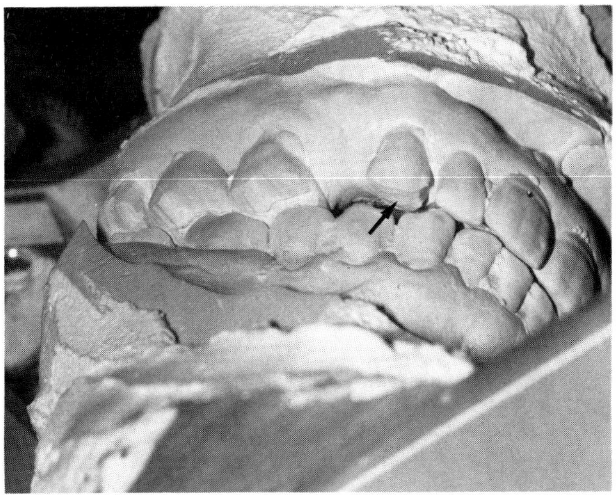

Fig. 2-47. Right-side articulation after planned reduction and recontouring of maxillary first premolar *(arrow).*

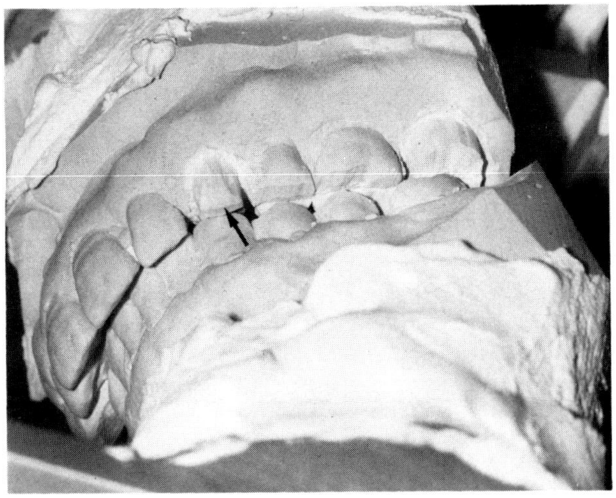

Fig. 2-48. Left side of patient in Fig. 2-47 showing similar treatment of left maxillary first premolar *(arrow).*

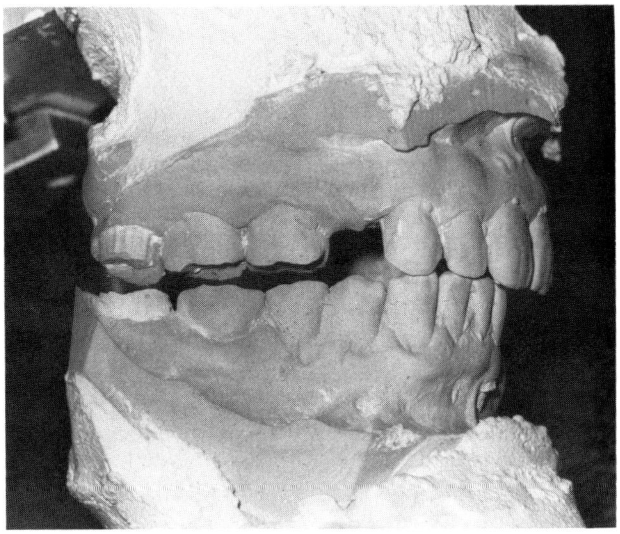

Fig. 2-49. Right side in right lateral (working) position. Clearance for posterior castings is adequate, and anterior function is acceptable.

To determine the feasibility of a restoration, it is necessary to reduce each occluding tooth exactly 1.5 mm, using a bur of measured diameter and following the occlusal contours of the teeth (Figs. 2-45 and 2-46). Even after this amount of reduction, interference of maxillary first premolars precluded development of a near-normal anterior relationship. Only removal of the lingual cusp of the premolars allowed the anterior function to occur (Figs. 2-47 to 2-50). A projected treatment plan for this patient would require intentional endodontic therapy for the maxillary first premolar teeth to allow a canine contour and function and to restore all opposing occlusal surfaces.

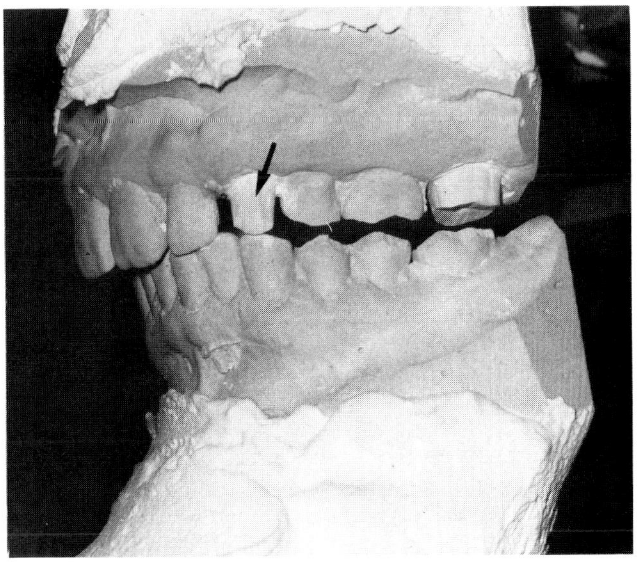

Fig. 2-50. Left side in left lateral (working) position. Although need of full veneer crown is anticipated for maxillary first premolar *(arrow),* anterior function is acceptable.

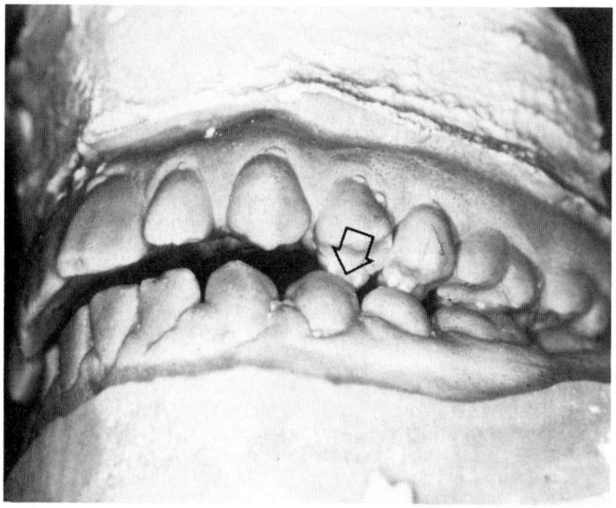

Fig. 2-51. Casts mounted in centric relation closure show lingual cusps directly over buccal cusps of lower teeth *(arrow)* on initial contact.

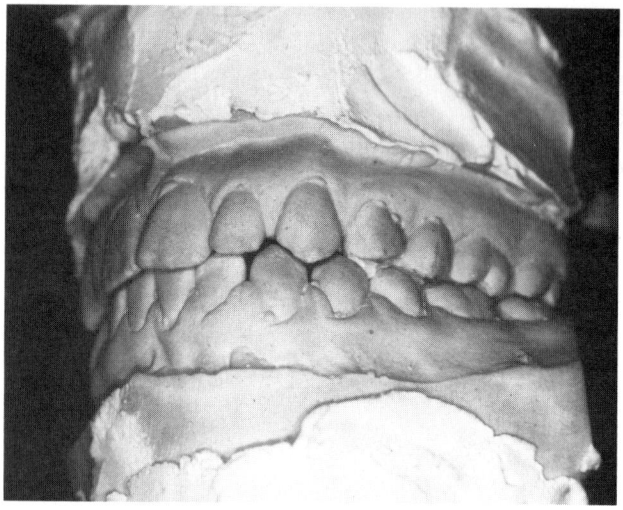

Fig. 2-52. Following adjustment of casts, closure in centric relation shows a near normal buccolingual relationship.

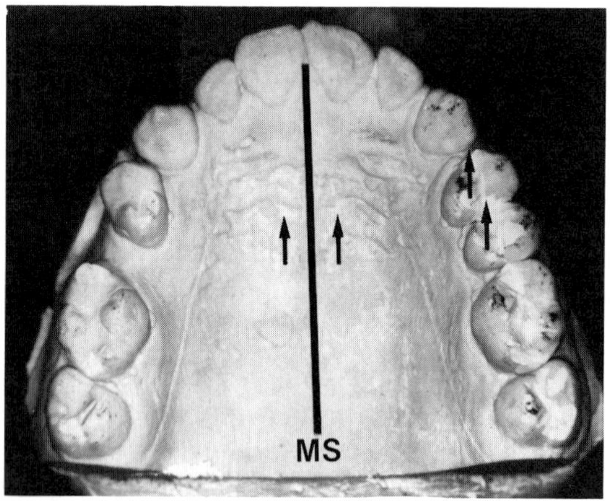

Fig. 2-53. Assuming a relatively symmetric arch form, closure around the midsagittal *(MS)* plane will result in lower cusps closing toward mesial, as indicated by arrows.

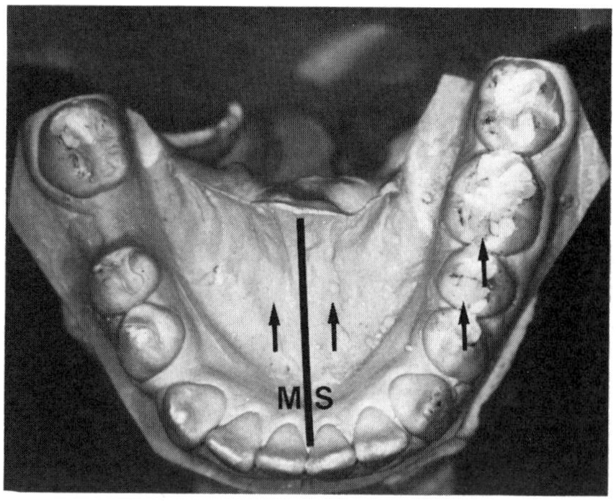

Fig. 2-54. Closure around midsagittal *(MS)* plane will result in upper cusps closing toward distal, as indicated by arrows.

OCCLUSAL ADJUSTMENT ON DIAGNOSTIC CASTS

Development of a harmonious relationship between centric jaw relation and centric occlusion with an acceptable anterior vertical and horizontal overlap is the primary goal of treatment planning occlusion. Occlusal adjustment can be performed on mounted diagnostic casts to determine the acceptability and potential for correction of occlusal disharmony.

A seemingly hopeless occlusal relationship (Fig. 2-51) can be modified on the mounted casts to determine the feasibility of adequate restorative results. Note the position of the premolars. The lingual premolar cusps appear to contact nearly end to end with the lower facial cusps. Careful adjustments of the casts allow the closure of the cast into an acceptable centric occlusion (Fig. 2-52). Notice the position of the premolar teeth after modification.

Analysis of the mechanics involved with the casts in Figs. 2-51 and 2-52 reveals that a closure around a hinge axis parallel with the midsagittal plane will allow the lower facial cusps to close into the fossae of the upper premolars (Figs. 2-53 and 2-54). Such a determination would not be possible without mounted casts.

These few patients illustrate the use of a diagnostic cast as a means for improved communication, preparation and waxing, and proper treatment planning. It is possible to develop many variations for any given situation. The diagnostician must consider every possibility; mounted diagnostic casts are a valuable aid.

SUMMARY

Diagnostic casts can be useful tools in communication and treatment planning. When unmounted, casts have a value limited to the evaluation of intra-arch tooth relationships. Frequently the relationships apparent within the same arch must be radically modified when evaluated using opposing casts.

The maximum value of diagnostic casts is achieved when casts are mounted in centric relation. Mounted casts can improve communication. Interarch relationships can be evaluated as they apply to the involved teeth and surrounding tissues. The added dimension provided by mounted casts allows their use as a guide in occlusal adjustment, tooth preparation, and diagnostic waxing. Every possible treatment approach for a given situation must be explored. Accurately fabricated *mounted* casts offer the opportunity for thorough case study and treatment planning.

CHAPTER 3

TOOTH MORPHOLOGY

HAJIME HAMAGUCHI

The study of tooth morphology is a visual experience. The use of text is to familiarize the student with descriptive terminology for anatomic landmarks and the morphologic nomenclature. To illustrate a composite of idealized tooth form, the entire dental arches, maxillary and mandibular, are shown from various views: occlusal, frontal, lingual, and lateral. These illustrations further demonstrate the relationship of adjacent and opposing teeth and also the alignment and integration of the individual tooth into the entire dental arch.

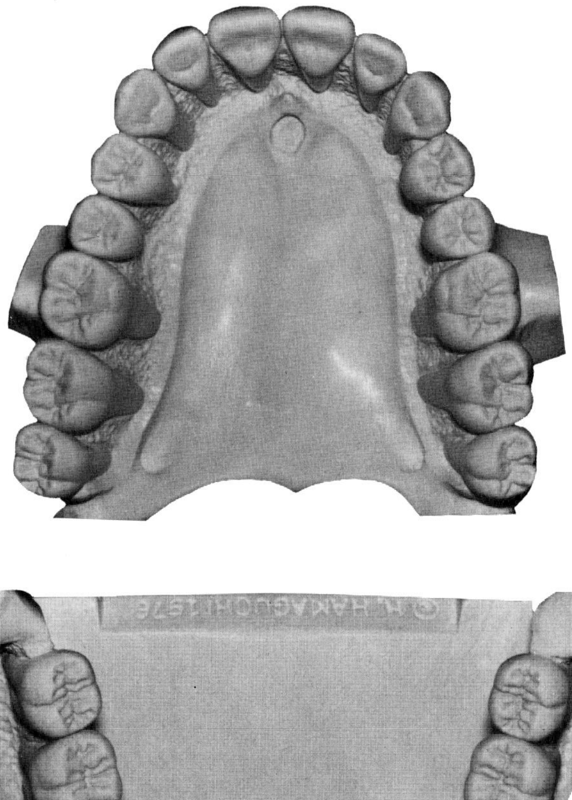

To study the morphologic features of the single tooth, the maxillary right side, central incisor to second molar, and the mandibular right side, central incisor to second molar, are illustrated and described. Each tooth is shown in five views. The views of the anterior teeth are facial, lingual, incisal, and proximal (mesial and distal). The views of the posterior teeth are facial, lingual, occlusal, and proximal (mesial and distal). Also, each tooth is shown in line drawings and in photographs of tooth models, which in form and proportion are representative of natural dentition.

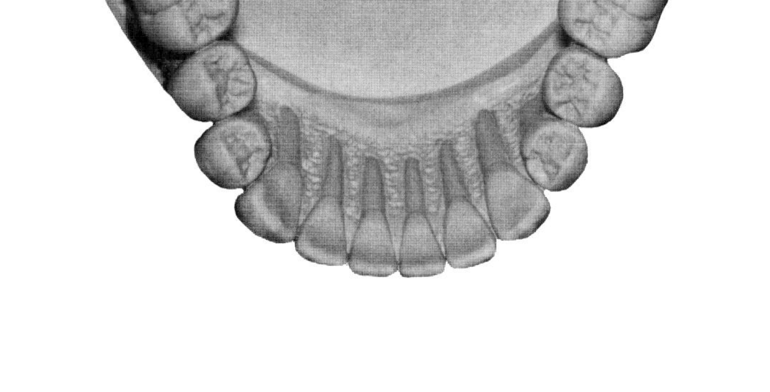

The complex curvature exhibited by the incisal and occlusal surfaces of the teeth can best be seen by observing casts of the mouth or dry specimens of human skulls from both the anterior and the posterior aspects. The intricate and geometric progression of these curves (curve of Spee, curve of Wilson) is illustrated in Fig. 3-1.

The maxillary and mandibular teeth, when viewed from the incisal or occlusal aspect, demonstrate the relationship of the facial and lingual embrasures in the formation of the contact areas of these teeth with their adjacent counterparts. The marked lingual convergence

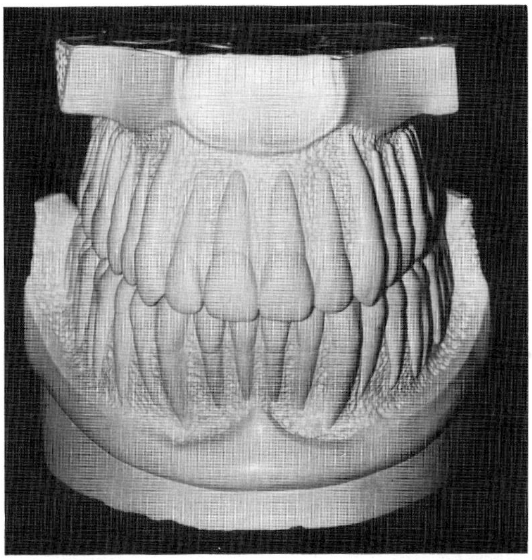

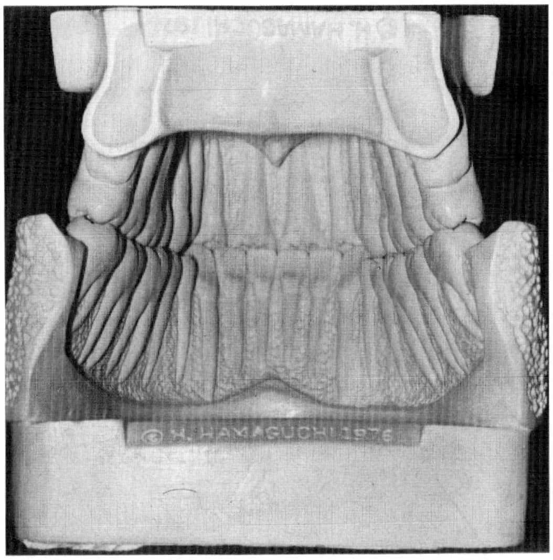
© H. HAMAGUCHI 1976

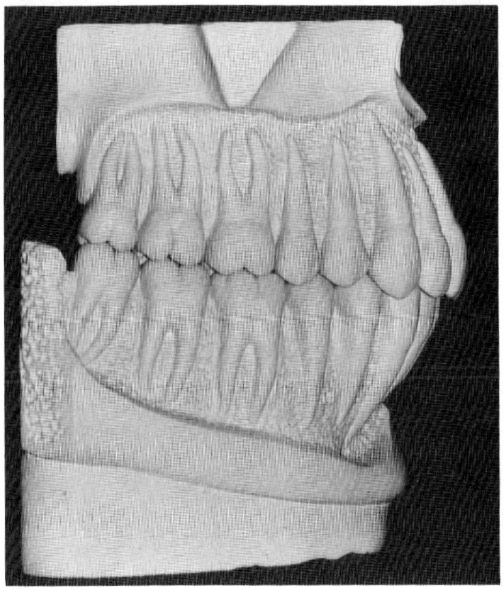

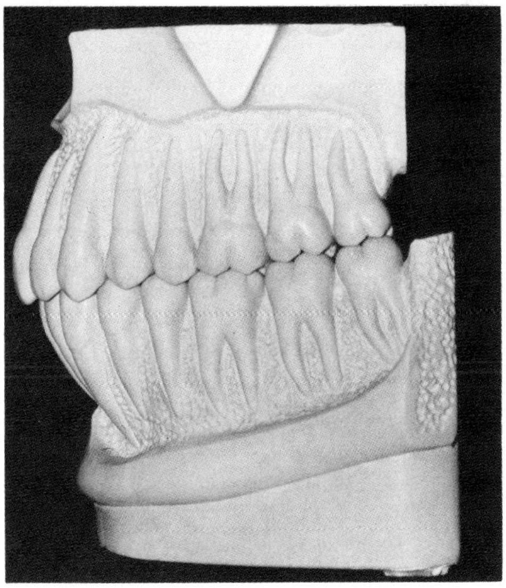

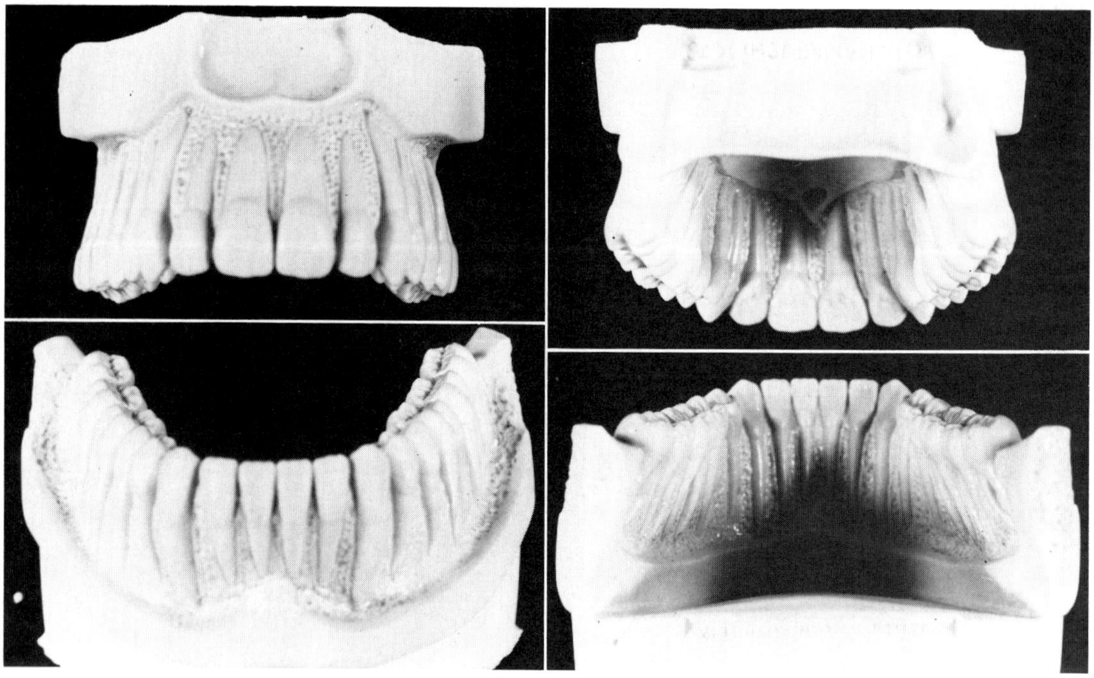

Fig. 3-1. Complex curvature of dental arches. Note interplay of cusp tips and incisal edges and alignment of crown-root axis.

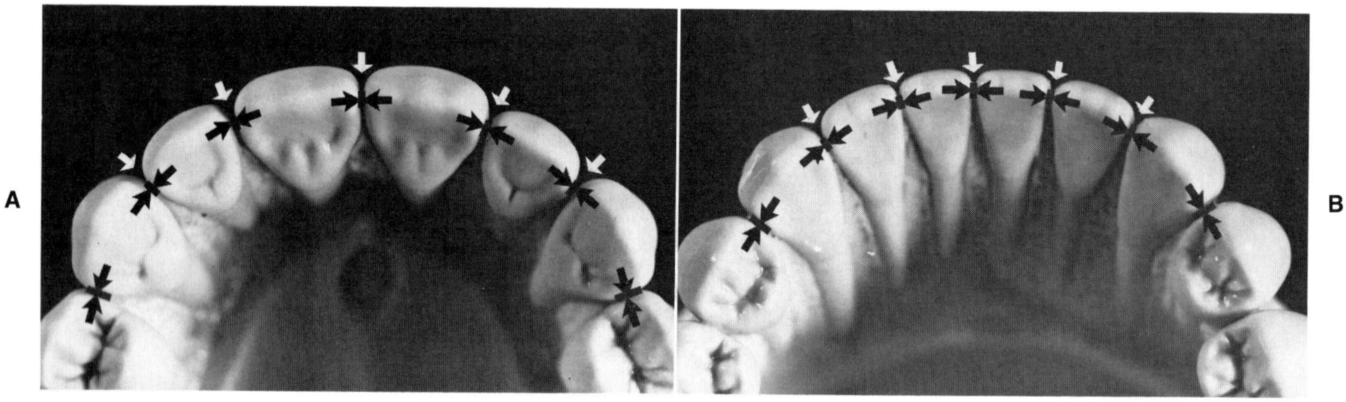

Fig. 3-2. Incisal view of **A,** maxillary and **B,** mandibular anterior teeth showing interrelationship of proximal contacts and embrasures. Note especially positions of facioproximal line angles of adjacent teeth and their formation of facial embrasures.

of the proximal surfaces of the anterior teeth, both maxillary and mandibular, allows contact of these teeth to be placed well toward the facial. This enables a symmetric and stable dental arch to be developed (Fig. 3-2).

The incisor teeth, being broad and bladelike and used for incision of food, must present interproximal contacts that are placed well toward the incising surfaces. The maxillary lateral incisors, being more rounded in the incisal third than the central incisors, present contact relationships that are farther from the incisal plane. The incisal embrasure deepens in relation to the incisocervical dimension of the crowns of the teeth as observation progresses distally (Fig. 3-3).

Proximal contact areas of the posterior teeth, both maxillary and mandibular, are normally placed in the facial half of the occlusal table. The maxillary molar teeth, an exception to this rule, have contact relationships approximately in the center of the faciolingual dimension. The facial embrasures are shallower and

A
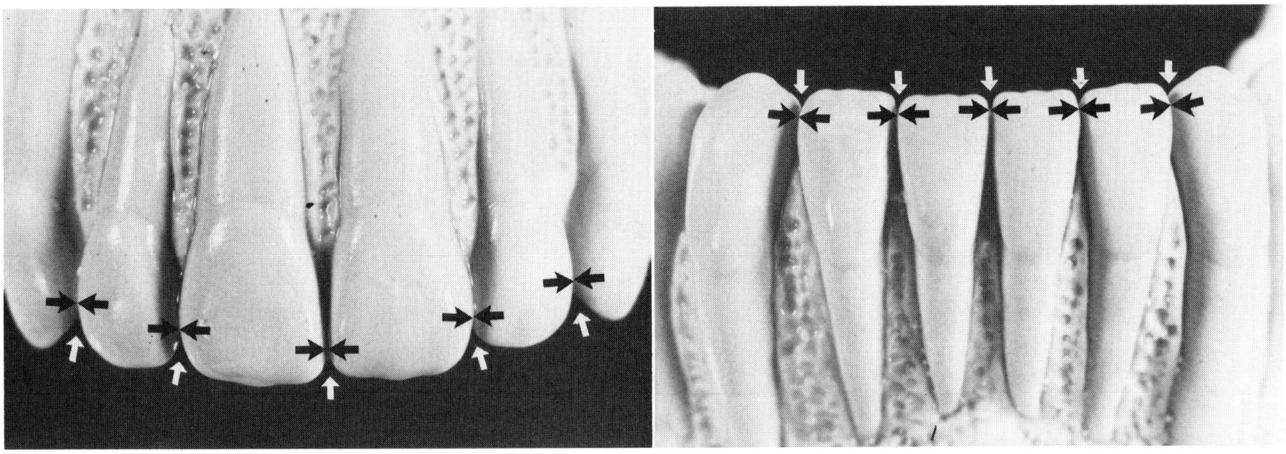
B

Fig. 3-3. Facial view of **A,** maxillary and **B,** mandibular anterior teeth showing incisogingival position of proximal contacts. Note forms of incisal embrasures.

A
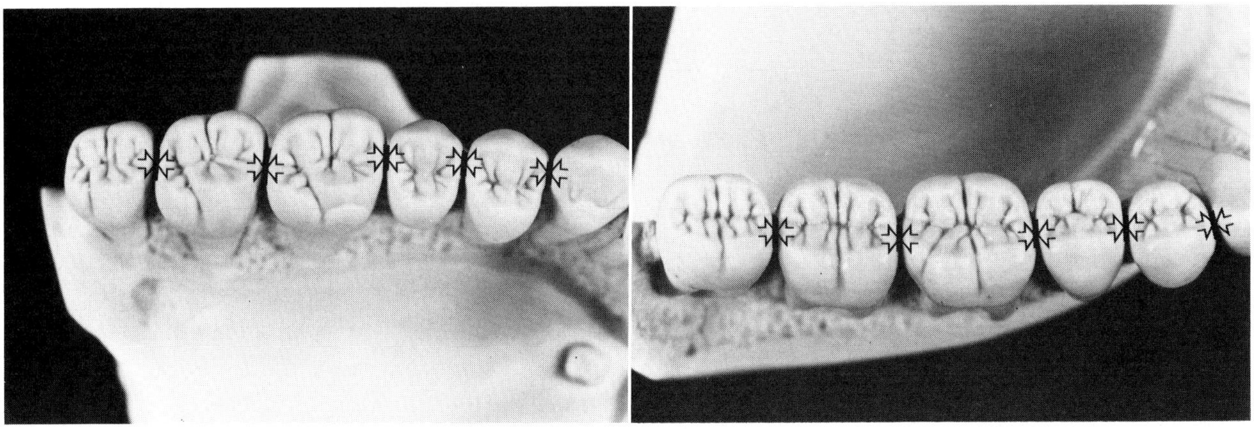
B

Fig. 3-4. Occlusal view of **A,** maxillary and **B,** mandibular posterior teeth showing position and form of proximal contacts and embrasures. Note that proximal contacts are in facial half of occlusal table (except between upper molars).

A
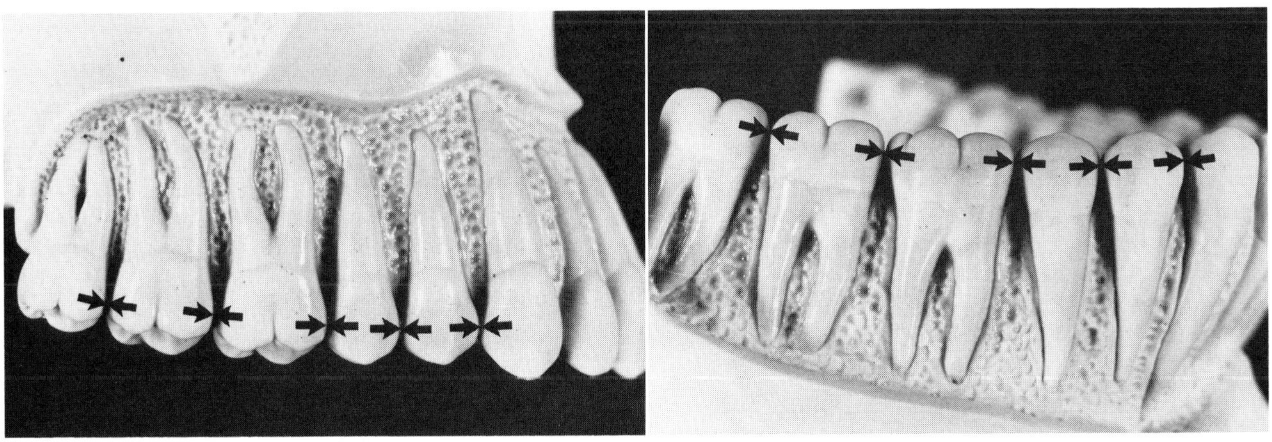
B

Fig. 3-5. Facial view of **A,** maxillary and **B,** mandibular teeth showing the position and form of proximal contacts and embrasures.

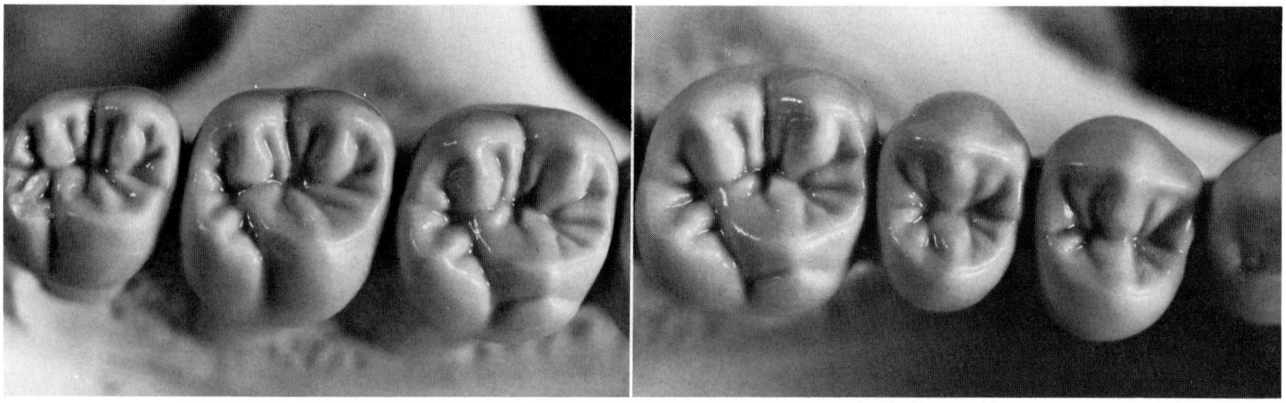

Fig. 3-6. Detailed occlusal view of the maxillary posterior teeth.

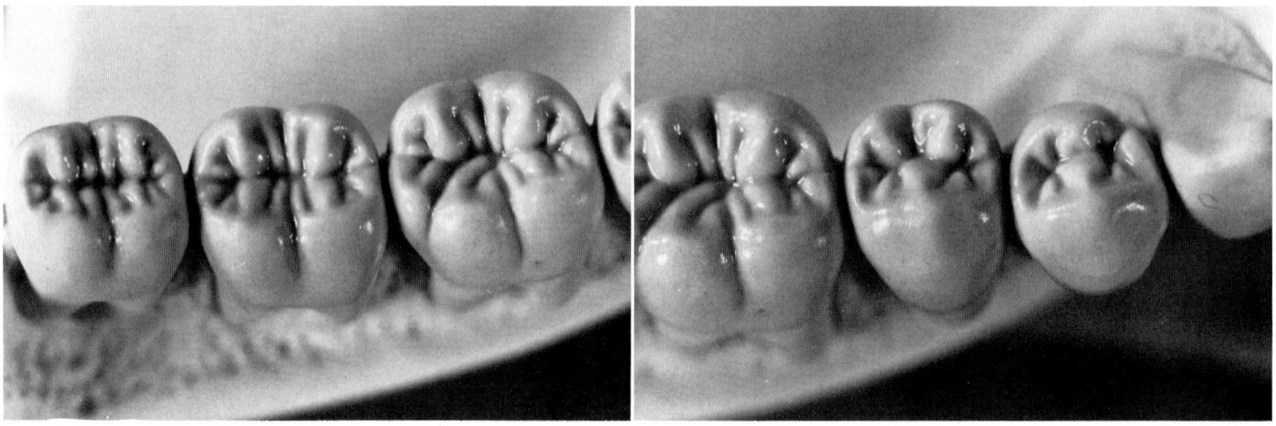

Fig. 3-7. Detailed occlusal view of mandibular posterior teeth.

broader when compared to the deeper and narrower lingual embrasures (Fig. 3-4).

The positions of the contact areas of the posterior teeth, when viewed from the facial aspect, depend on the height of the cusps and the steepness of the inclined planes in relation to the occlusocervical dimension of the crowns of the teeth. The proximal contours of the teeth determine the architecture of the gingival embrasures and the space available for the gingival papillae (Fig. 3-5).

The complex architecture of the occlusal surfaces of the posterior teeth, both maxillary and mandibular, is evident from observation of casts of the teeth and study of skulls presenting a complete dentition. The fossae and inclined planes are further embellished by supplementary grooves and sluiceways, which improve the efficiency of mastication and reduce the total contact area of the teeth in occlusion (Figs. 3-6 and 3-7).

MAXILLARY CENTRAL INCISOR

FACIAL VIEW

1. Crown longer incisocervically than mesiodistally.
2. Mesial outline slightly convex with proximal contact close to mesioincisal angle.
3. Distal outline more convex with proximal contact more cervical (in middle third).
4. Mesioincisal angle in outline forms 90-degree distoincisal angle more rounded in form.
5. Surface is smoothly convex but with labial lobe grooves.

LINGUAL VIEW

1. "Scooplike" form with concave lingual fossa bordered by mesial and distal marginal ridges.
2. Cingulum in cervical third with its prominence slightly distal of center.

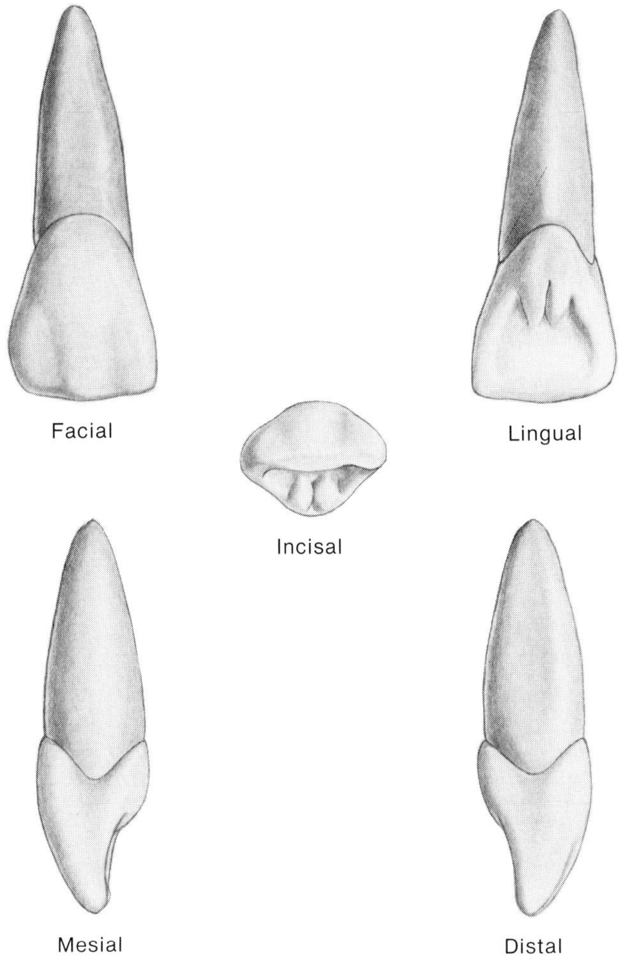

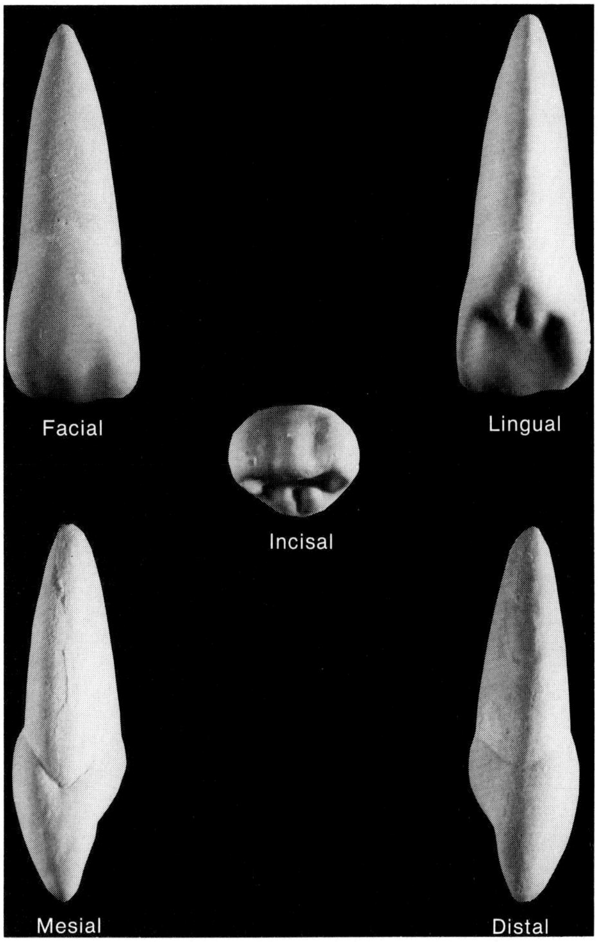

INCISAL VIEW

1. Crown wider mesiodistally than faciolingually.
2. Incisal edge in center faciolingually.
3. Facial outline convex to proximal contacts.
4. Proximal contacts approximately in center faciolingually.
5. Lingual outline tapers toward cingulum.
6. Prominence of cingulum slightly distal of center.

PROXIMAL (MESIAL AND DISTAL) VIEW

1. Crown longer incisocervically than faciolingually.
2. Both facial and lingual heights of contour relatively low (in cervical third).
3. Incisal edge centered in middle of crown.
4. Facial outline gently convex.
5. Lingual outline has flattened S shape with cingulum in cervical third.

MAXILLARY LATERAL INCISOR

FACIAL VIEW

1. Crown longer incisocervically than wide mesiodistally.
2. Mesial outline convex with proximal contact located approximately two thirds the cervicoincisal distance.
3. Distal outline even more convex with proximal contact located more cervically (in middle third).
4. Distoincisal angle more rounded in form than mesioincisal angle.
5. Surface smoothly convex except for facial lobe grooves.

LINGUAL VIEW

1. "Scoop-like" form with concave lingual fossa bordered by mesial and distal marginal ridges.
2. Cingulum in cervical third with its prominence slightly distal of center.
3. Fossa and marginal ridges are more prominent than in central incisor.

INCISAL VIEW

1. Crown wider mesiodistally than faciolingually.
2. Incisal edge in center faciolingually.
3. Facial outline convex to proximal contacts.
4. Proximal contacts approximately in center faciolingually.
5. Lingual outline tapers toward cingulum.
6. Prominence of cingulum slightly distal of center.

PROXIMAL (MESIAL AND DISTAL) VIEW

1. Crown longer incisocervically than wide faciolingually.
2. Both facial and lingual heights of contour relatively low (in cervical third).
3. Incisal edge centered in middle of crown.
4. Facial outline gently convex.
5. Lingual outline has flattened S shape with cingulum in cervical third.

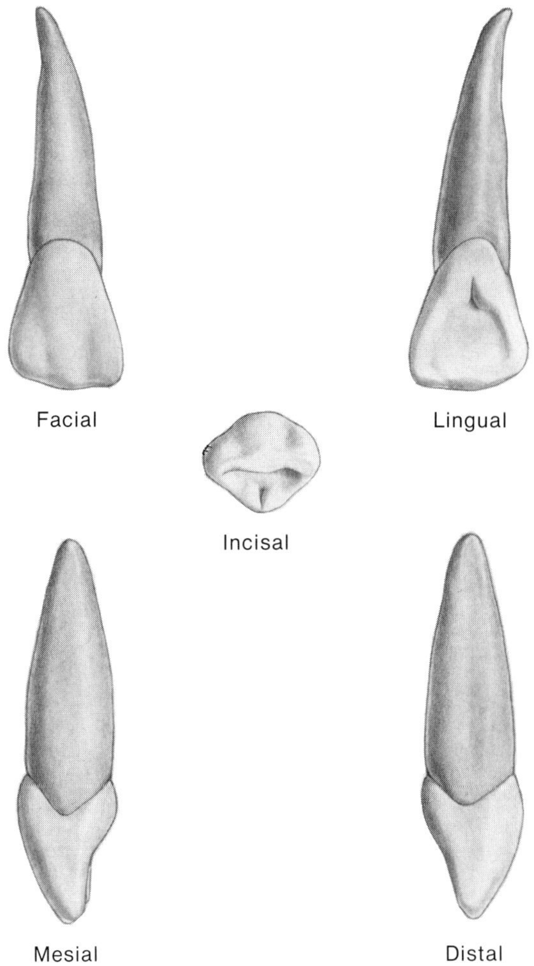
Facial
Lingual
Incisal
Mesial
Distal

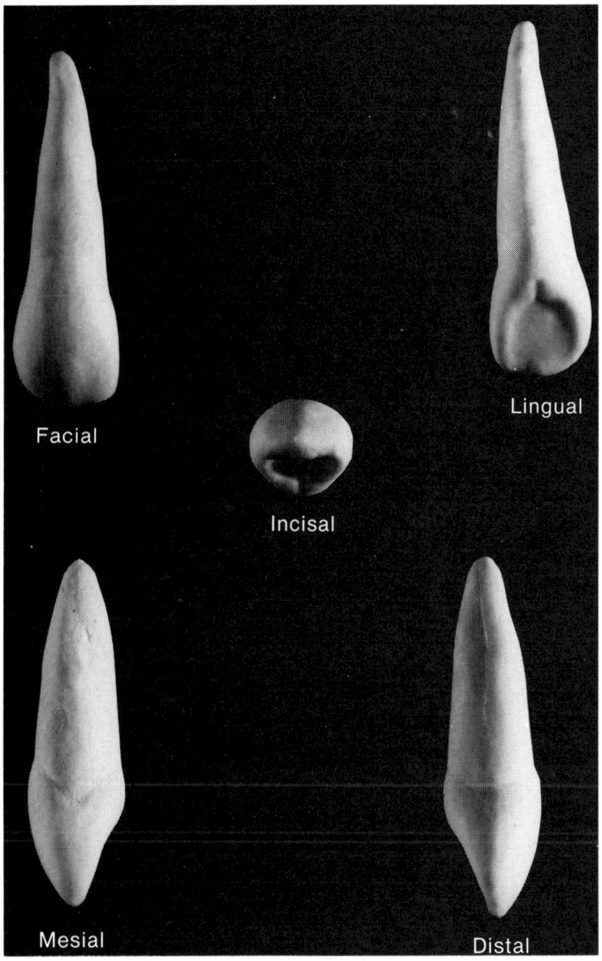
Facial
Lingual
Incisal
Mesial
Distal

MAXILLARY CANINE

FACIAL VIEW

1. Crown longer incisocervically than wide mesiodistally.
2. Mesial outline slightly convex cervically to proximal contact, which is approximately two thirds the cervicoincisal distance.
3. Distal outline concave between cervical line and proximal contact, which is in middle of crown.
4. Cusp tip approximately in center of crown.
5. Mesial slope of cusp shorter and at flatter angle than distal side.
6. Mesioincisal angle more incisal in position than distoincisal angle.
7. Surface is broken by prominent ridge in middle of crown.

LINGUAL VIEW

1. Mesial and distal marginal ridges with bulbous cingulum extending to middle of crown.
2. Lingual ridge extends from cusp tip to cingulum and is positioned in approximately center of crown mesiodistally.
3. Prominence of cingulum slightly distal of center.
4. Developmental grooves radiate from cingulum.

INCISAL VIEW

1. Crown wider faciolingually than mesiodistally.
2. Cusp tip facial to center of crown.
3. Mesial half of outline very convex and wider than distal half.
4. Distal half of outline also convex but interrupted by concavities both lingually and facially.
5. Lingual half is narrower than facial half.
6. Proximal contacts approximately in center of crown.

PROXIMAL (MESIAL AND DISTAL) VIEW

1. Longer incisocervically than wide faciolingually.
2. Both facial and lingual heights of contour relatively low (in cervical third).
3. Cusp tip slightly facial to middle of crown.
4. Facial outline convex but relatively flat.
5. Lingual outline relatively flat from height of contour (slightly concave near cusp tip).
6. Cingulum extends to half length of crown.

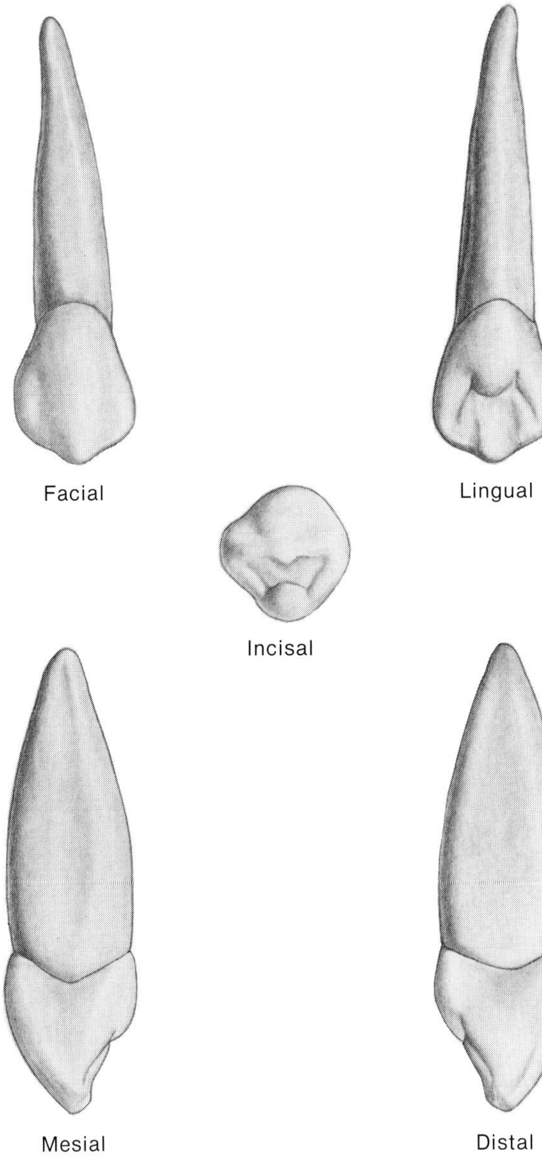
Facial
Lingual
Incisal
Mesial
Distal

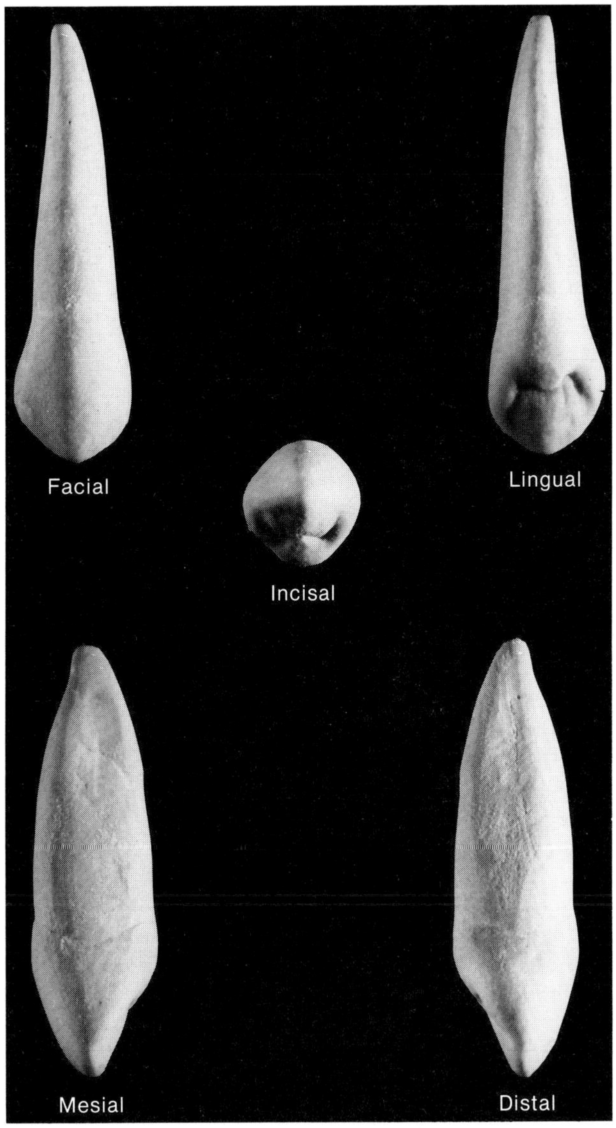
Facial
Lingual
Incisal
Mesial
Distal

MAXILLARY FIRST PREMOLAR

FACIAL VIEW

1. Crown longer occlusocervically than wide mesiodistally.
2. Mesial outline concave cervically to proximal contact, which is in middle third of crown.
3. Distal outline relatively straight to proximal contact, which is in middle third of crown.
4. Proximal contacts form a flattened convexity.
5. Cusp tip approximately in center of crown.
6. Cusp slopes at about 30-degree angle from tip.
7. Surface broken by prominent ridge in middle of crown.

LINGUAL VIEW

1. Cusp narrower and shorter than facial cusp.
2. Cusp tip slightly mesial of center.
3. Surface is smoothly convex.

OCCLUSAL VIEW

1. Crown wider faciolingually than mesiodistally.
2. Facial half of crown wider mesiodistally than lingual half.
3. Facial outline convex but interrupted by depressions marking facial ridge.
4. Lingual outline uniformly convex.
5. Occlusal table in middle of crown.
6. Facial cusp tip in center mesiodistally.
7. Lingual cusp tip slightly mesial of center.
8. Central groove in middle of occlusal table faciolingually.
9. Approximately half the mesiodistal width of crown separates mesial and distal pits.
10. Supplemental grooves and ridges radiate from pits.
11. Proximal contacts are facial to middle of crown.

PROXIMAL (MESIAL AND DISTAL) VIEW

1. Crown slightly wider faciolingually than occlusocervically.
2. Facial cusp longer than lingual cusp.
3. Both cusp tips positioned within cervical line.
4. Central groove in center of crown.
5. Facial outline relatively flat convexity with height of contour low in cervical third.
6. Lingual outline uniformly convex with height of contour more occlusal in position than facial.
7. Marginal ridges at approximately two thirds the occlusocervical distance.
8. Mesial concavity located at about one third the occlusocervical distance.

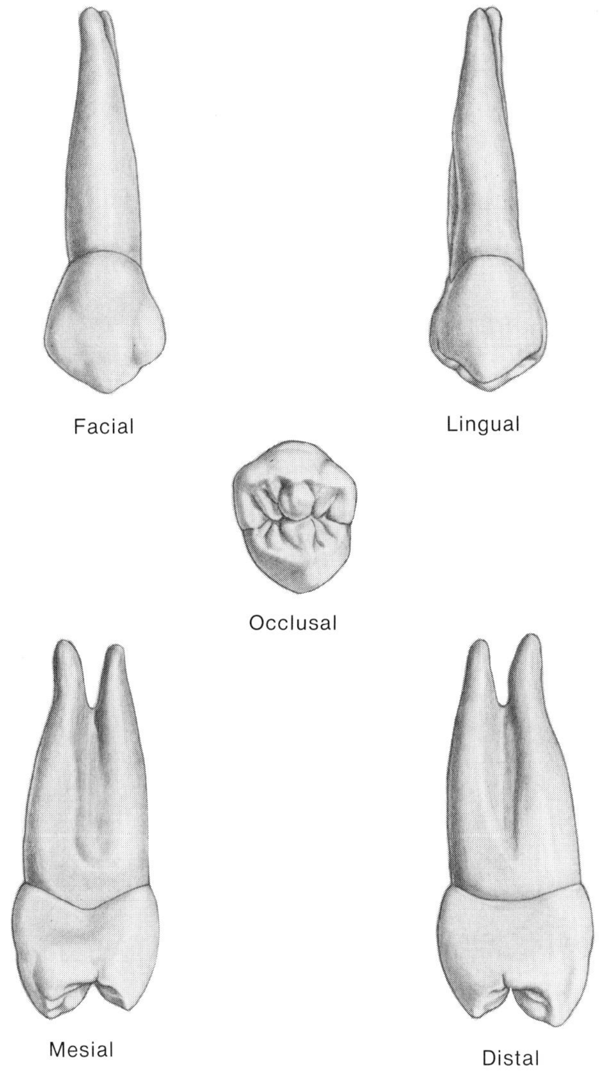
Facial
Lingual
Occlusal
Mesial
Distal

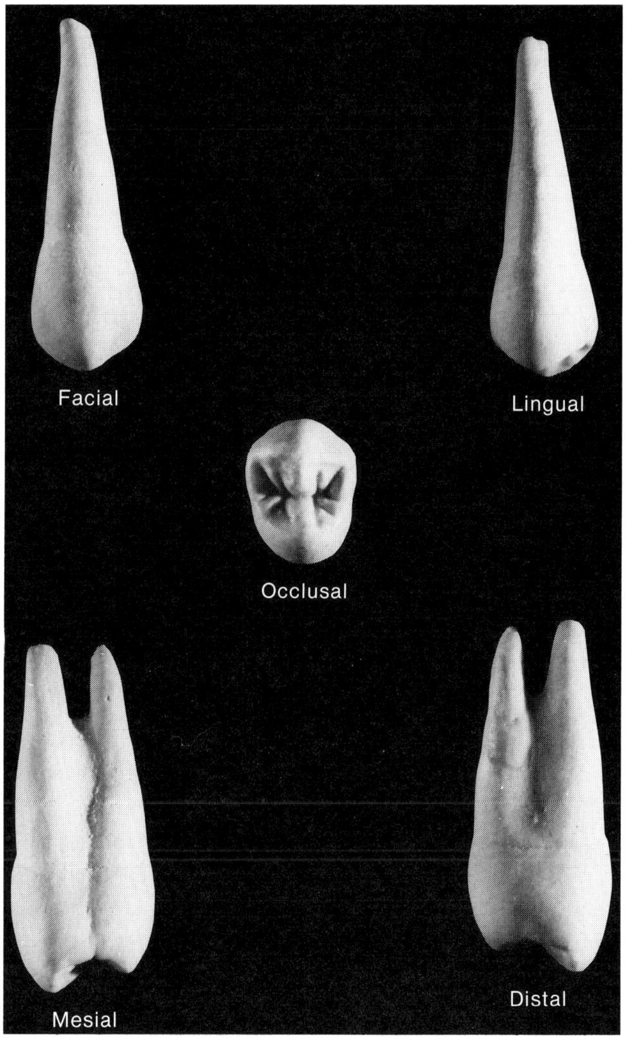
Facial
Lingual
Occlusal
Mesial
Distal

MAXILLARY SECOND PREMOLAR

FACIAL VIEW

1. Crown longer occlusocervically than wide mesiodistally.
2. Relatively symmetrical outline.
3. Mesial and distal outlines fairly straight and tapering cervically to proximal contacts, which are in middle third of crown.
4. Proximal contacts form a flattened convexity.
5. Cusp tip approximately in center of crown.
6. Cusp slopes at about 30-degree angle from tip.
7. Surface relatively smooth.

LINGUAL VIEW

1. Cusp slightly narrower and shorter than facial cusp.
2. Cusp tip slightly mesial of center.
3. Surface is smoothly convex.

OCCLUSAL VIEW

1. Crown wider faciolingually than mesiodistally.
2. Facial half of crown wider mesiodistally than lingual half.
3. Facial outline convex with only slight depression marking facial ridge.
4. Lingual outline uniformly convex.
5. Occlusal table in middle of crown.
6. Facial cusp tip in center mesiodistally.
7. Lingual cusp tip slightly mesial of center.
8. Central groove in middle of occlusal table faciolingually.
9. Approximately one third the mesiodistal width of crown separates mesial and distal pits.
10. Supplemental grooves and ridges radiate from pits.
11. Proximal contacts are facial to middle of crown.

PROXIMAL (MESIAL AND DISTAL) VIEW

1. Crown slightly wider faciolingually than long occlusocervically.
2. Facial cusp slightly longer than lingual cusp.
3. Both cusp tips positioned within cervical line.
4. Central groove in center of crown.
5. Facial outline relatively flat convexity with height of contour low in cervical third.
6. Lingual outline slightly more uniform in convexity with height of contour slightly more occlusal than facial.
7. Marginal ridges at approximately two thirds the occlusocervical distance.

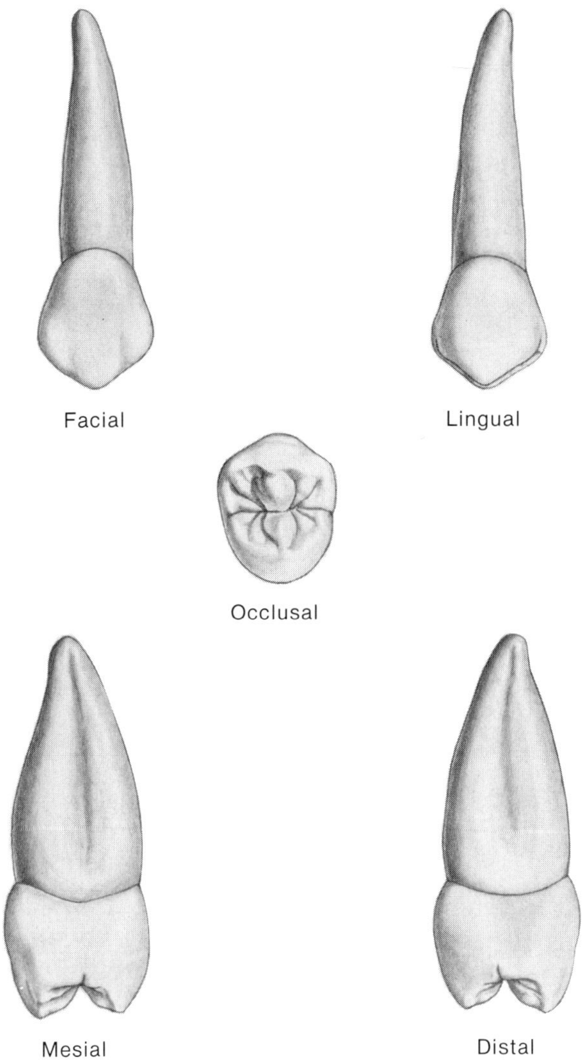
Facial
Lingual
Occlusal
Mesial
Distal

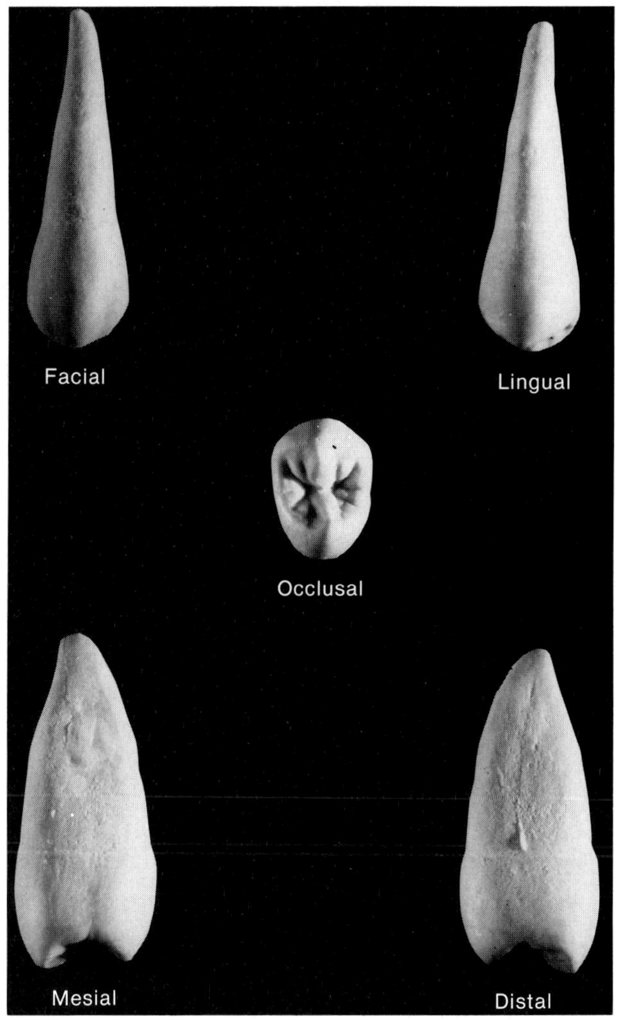
Facial
Lingual
Occlusal
Mesial
Distal

MAXILLARY FIRST MOLAR

FACIAL VIEW

1. Crown wider mesiodistally than long occlusogingivally.
2. Mesial outline relatively straight taper cervically to proximal contact, which is at about two thirds the occlusocervical length of crown.
3. Distal outline slightly more convex taper with proximal contact in middle third of crown.
4. Proximal contacts form flattened convexities.
5. Mesial and distal cusp tips and facial groove divide surface into approximately quarters.
6. Cusps slope at approximately 20-degree angle from tips.
7. Mesiolingual cusp tip visible distally to mesiofacial cusp tip.

LINGUAL VIEW

1. Lingual half slightly larger than facial half.
2. Mesiolingual cusp tip mesial of center and takes up three fifths the mesiodistal width of crown.
3. Distolingual cusp tip just mesial of cervical line and smaller than mesiolingual cusp.
4. Lingual groove in approximate center.
5. Fifth cusp attached to mesiolingual cusp and about level with distolingual cusp.

OCCLUSAL VIEW

1. Crown wider faciolingually than mesiodistally.
2. Mesial half of crown wider than distal half.
3. Lingual half of crown wider than facial half.
4. Facial outline convex but sloping lingually in distal half with height of contour mesial of center.

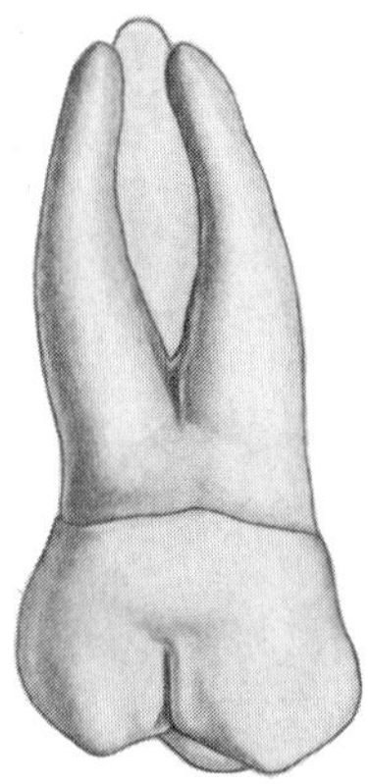

Facial

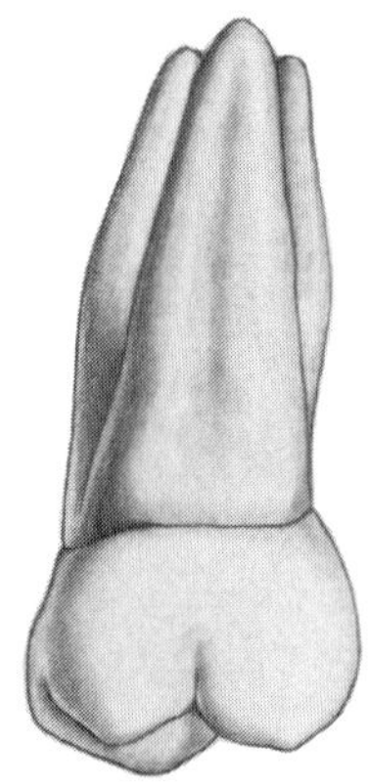

Lingual

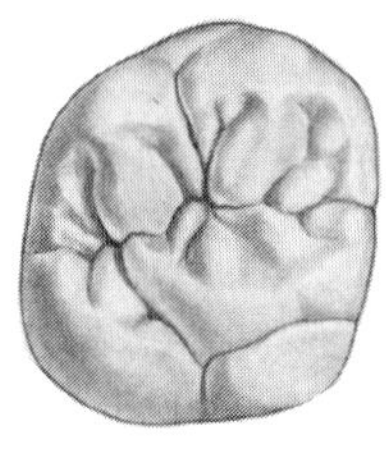

Occlusal

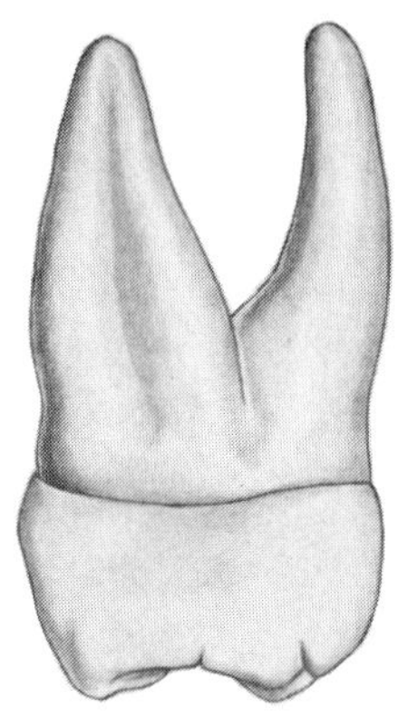

Mesial

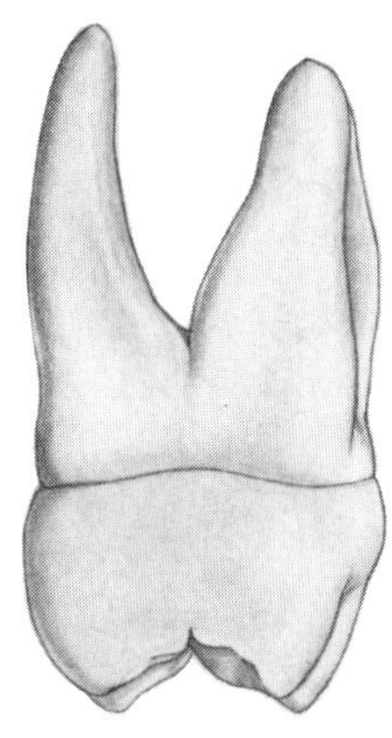

Distal

5. Lingual outline flattened convexity.
6. Mesial and distal outlines flattened convexities and approximately parallel to each other.
7. Mesioproximal contact facial to middle of crown.
8. Distoproximal contact lingual to middle of crown.
9. Straight lines connecting four major cusps form a rhomboid.
10. Occlusal table in middle of crown.
11. Central pit in approximate center of occlusal table.
12. Oblique ridge runs diagonally from distofacial to mesiolingual cusp tip.
13. Supplemental grooves and ridges radiate from pits.

PROXIMAL (MESIAL AND DISTAL) VIEW

1. Crown wider faciolingually than long occlusocervically.
2. Cusp tips about equal length except for distolingual cusp tip, which is shorter.
3. All cusp tips positioned inside cervical line.
4. Central groove slightly facial of center and equidistant between cusps.
5. Facial outline flattened convexity with height of contour in cervical third.
6. Lingual outline more uniformly convex with height of contour in cervical third.
7. Marginal ridges about level with middle of occlusal third.
8. From distal aspect the lingual slope on the facial surface should reveal mesiobuccal cusps as part of outline.

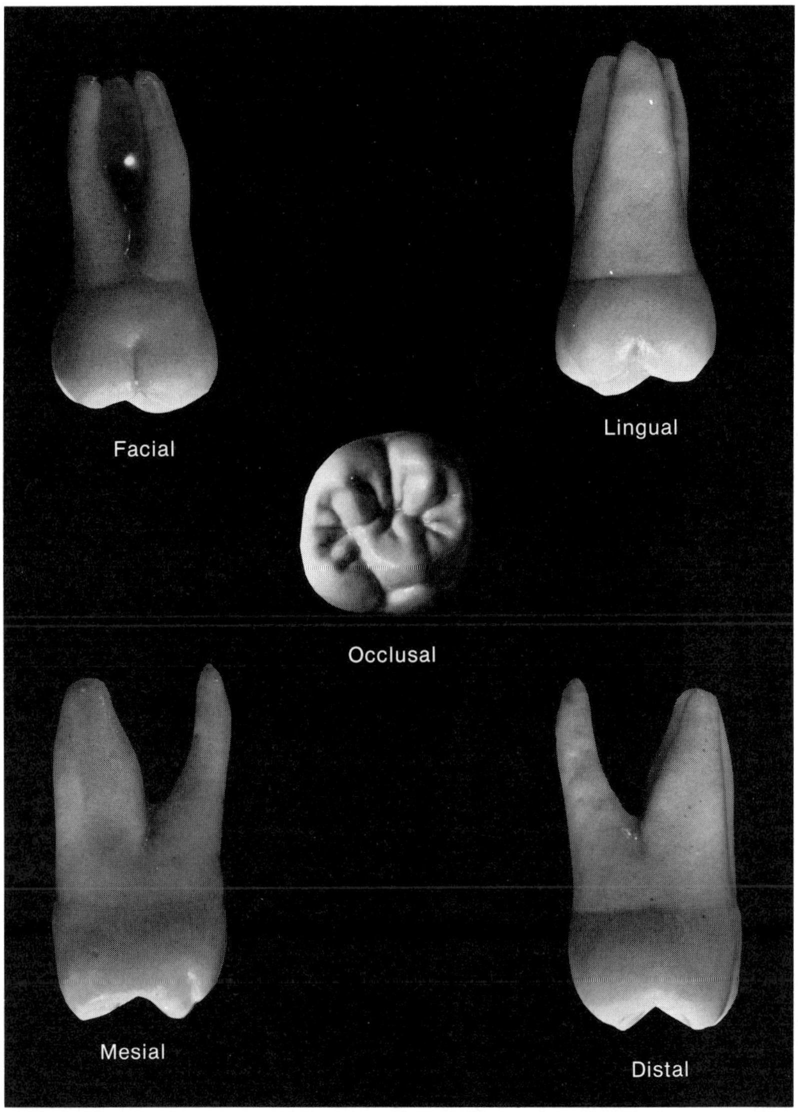

MAXILLARY SECOND MOLAR

FACIAL VIEW

1. Crown wider mesiodistally than long occlusocervically.
2. Mesial outline relatively straight taper cervically to proximal contact, which is at about two thirds the occlusocervical length of crown.
3. Distal outline more convex taper with proximal contact in middle third of crown.
4. Facial groove distal of crown center.
5. Mesiofacial cusp tip positioned well distal to cervical line.
6. Distofacial cusp tip positioned on line with cervical line.
7. Distal cusp smaller and shorter than mesial cusp.
8. Mesiolingual cusp tip visible distally to mesiofacial cusp.

LINGUAL VIEW

1. Lingual half approximately same size as facial half.
2. Mesiolingual cusp tip mesial of crown center.
3. Distolingual cusp shorter and narrower than mesiolingual cusp and positioned just mesially of cervical line.
4. Lingual groove distal of crown center.

OCCLUSAL VIEW

1. Crown wider faciolingually than mesiodistally.
2. Mesial half of crown wider than distal half.
3. Facial and lingual halves about same size.
4. Facial outline convex but sloping lingually in distal half with height of contour mesial of center.
5. Lingual outline flattened convexity.

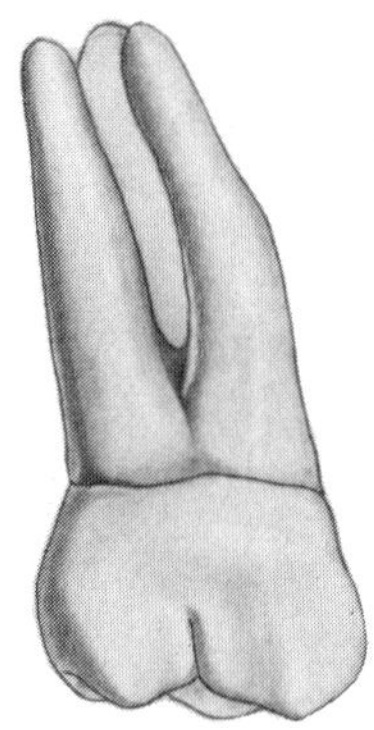

Facial

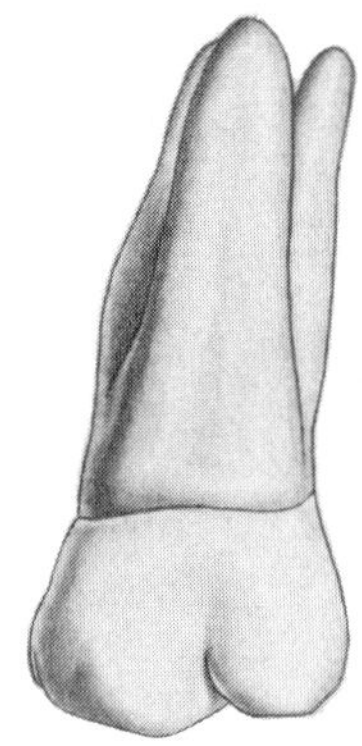

Lingual

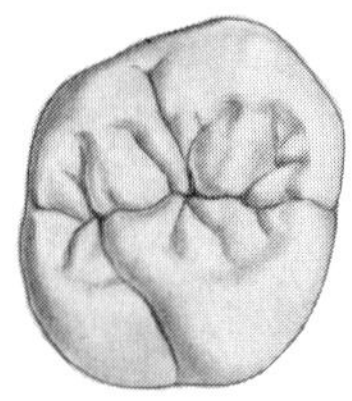

Occlusal

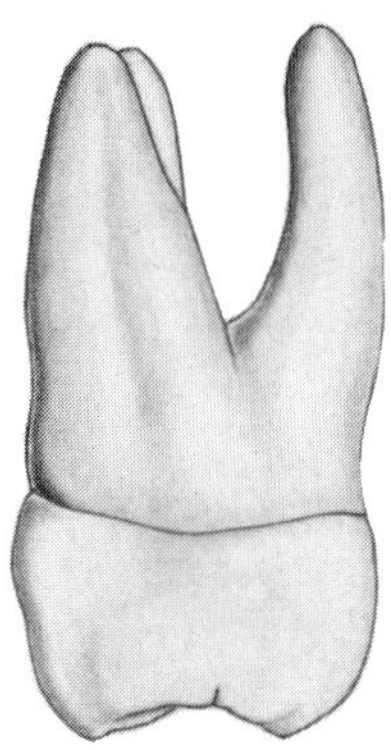

Mesial

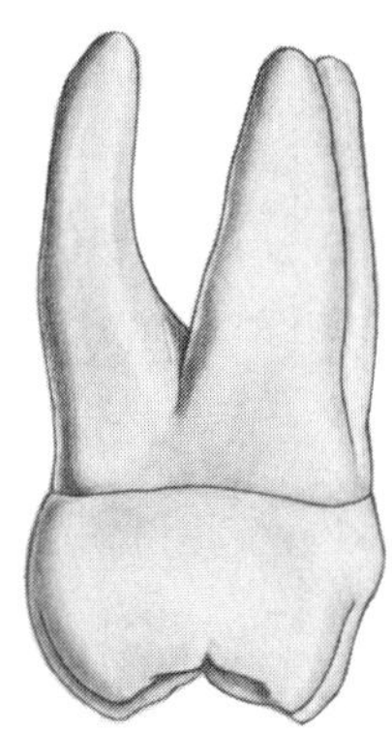

Distal

6. Mesial and distal outlines flattend convexity and parallel to each other.
7. Mesial contact facial to middle of crown.
8. Distal contact lingual to middle of crown.
9. Occlusal table in middle of crown.
10. Central pit in approximate center of occlusal table.
11. Oblique ridge runs diagonally from distofacial to mesiolingual cusp tip.
12. Supplemental grooves and ridges radiate from pits.

PROXIMAL (MESIAL AND DISTAL) VIEW

1. Crown wider faciolingually than long occlusocervically.
2. Mesiolingual and mesiofacial cusps about equal in length, whereas distal cusps are shorter.
3. All cusp tips positioned inside cervical line.
4. Central groove facial of center from mesial aspect and equidistant between cusps.
5. Facial outline flattened convexity with height of contour in cervical third.
6. Lingual outline more uniformly convex with height of contour in cervical third.
7. Marginal ridges about level with middle of occlusal third.
8. From distal aspect, lingual slope of facial surface and shortness of both distal cusps reveal both mesial cusps as part of outline.

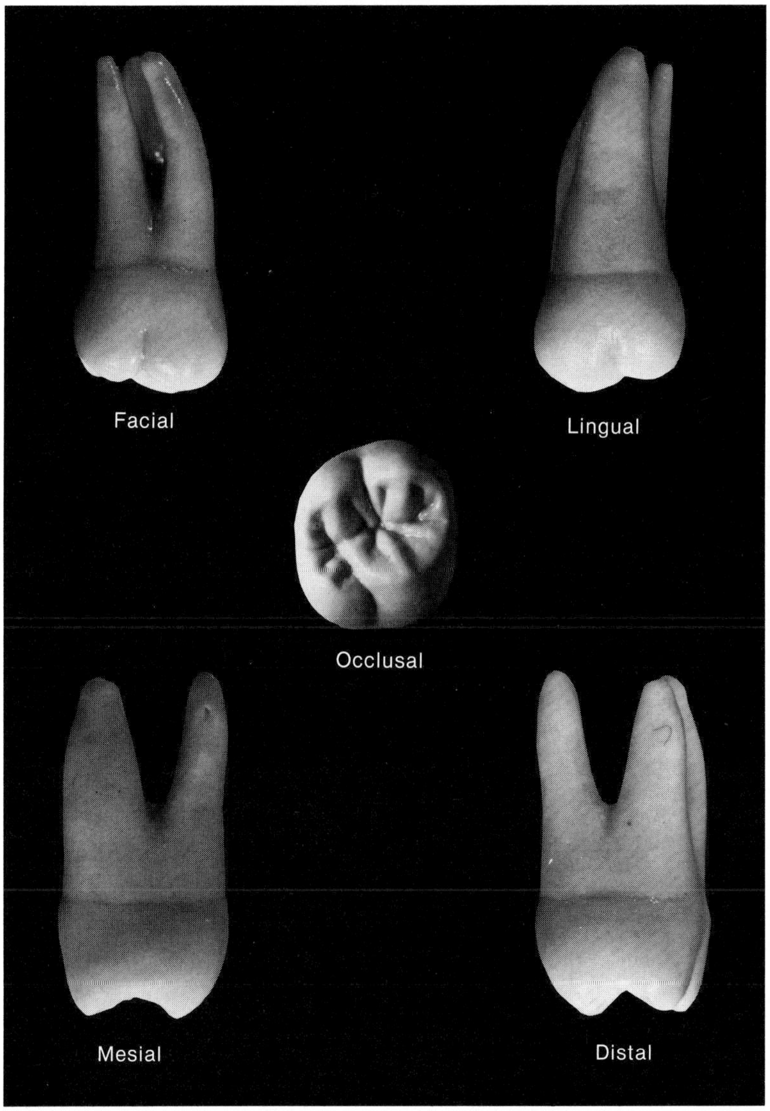

MANDIBULAR CENTRAL INCISOR

FACIAL VIEW

1. Crown longer incisocervically than wide mesiodistally.
2. Symmetrical outline.
3. Mesial and distal outlines taper evenly from incisal-edge proximal contacts in incisal third.
4. Both mesioincisal and distoincisal corners relatively square.
5. Incisal edge relatively straight and at right angles to long axis.

LINGUAL VIEW

1. Lingual fossa slightly concave with only slight marginal ridges.
2. Cingulum in cervical third with prominence in center.
3. Surface is smooth and symmetrical.

INCISAL VIEW

1. Crown wider faciolingually than mesiodistally.
2. Mesial and distal halves almost identical.
3. Incisal edge slightly lingual of center.
4. Facial outline highly convex to proximal contacts.
5. Proximal contacts approximately in center faciolingually or slightly lingual.
6. Lingual outline tapers toward cingulum.
7. Prominence of cingulum in center of crown.

PROXIMAL (MESIAL AND DISTAL) VIEW

1. Crown longer incisocervically than wide faciolingually.
2. Both facial and lingual heights of contour relatively low (in cervical quarter).
3. Incisal edge slightly lingual to middle of crown.
4. Facial outline almost straight from height of contour to incisal edge.
5. Lingual outline has flattened S shape with cingulum in cervical quarter.

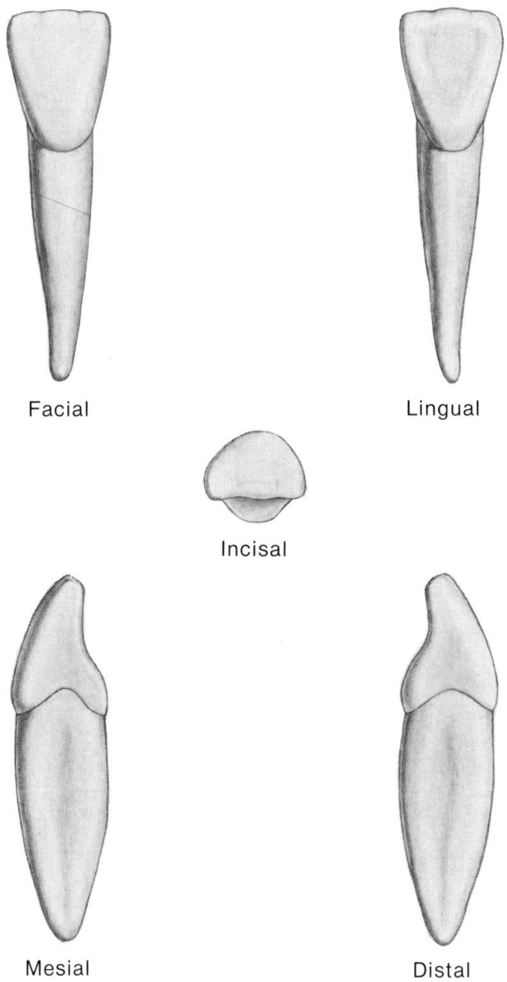
Facial
Lingual
Incisal
Mesial
Distal

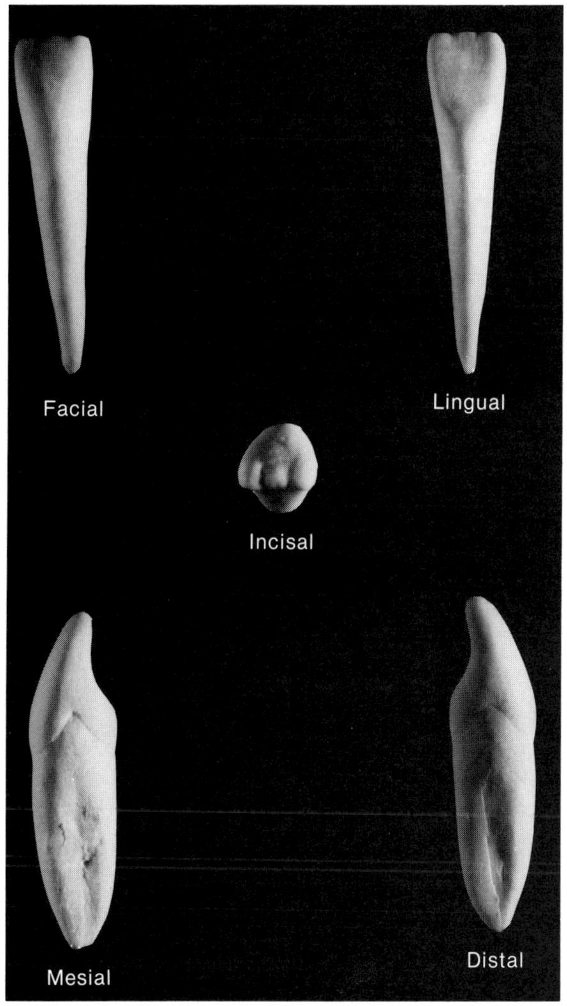
Facial
Lingual
Incisal
Mesial
Distal

MANDIBULAR LATERAL INCISOR

FACIAL VIEW

1. Crown longer incisocervically than wide mesiodistally.
2. Not symmetrical as with mandibular central.
3. Mesial outline tapers from proximal contact located close to incisal edge (incisal third).
4. Distal outline shorter than mesial outline and tapers from proximal contact located more cervically than mesially (in lower part of incisal third).
5. Incisal edge sloped cervically at distal angle.

LINGUAL VIEW

1. Lingual fossa slightly concave with only slight marginal ridges.
2. Cingulum in cervical third with prominence slightly distal of center.
3. Surface smooth.

INCISAL VIEW

1. Crown wider faciolingually than mesiodistally.
2. Incisal edge slightly lingual of center and sloping more lingually in distal half.
3. Facial outline highly convex to proximal contacts.
4. Proximal contacts approximately in center faciolingually with distal contact more lingual than mesial.
5. Lingual outline tapers toward cingulum.
6. Prominence of cingulum slightly distal of center.

PROXIMAL (MESIAL AND DISTAL) VIEW

1. Crown longer incisocervically than wide faciolingually.
2. Both facial and lingual heights of contour relatively low (in cervical quarter).
3. Incisal edge slightly lingual to middle of crown.
4. Facial outline almost straight from height of contour to incisal edge.
5. Lingual outline has flattened S shape with cingulum in cervical quarter.

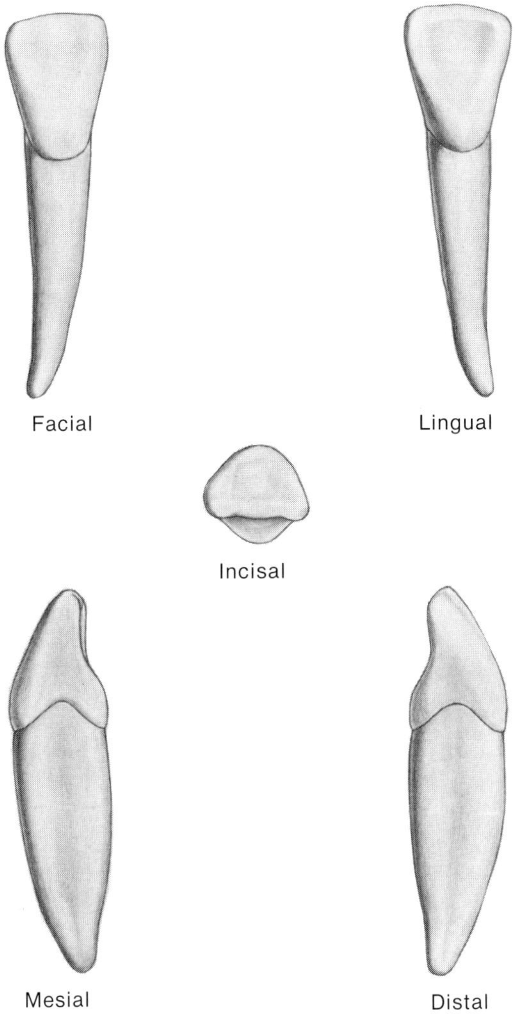
Facial
Lingual
Incisal
Mesial
Distal

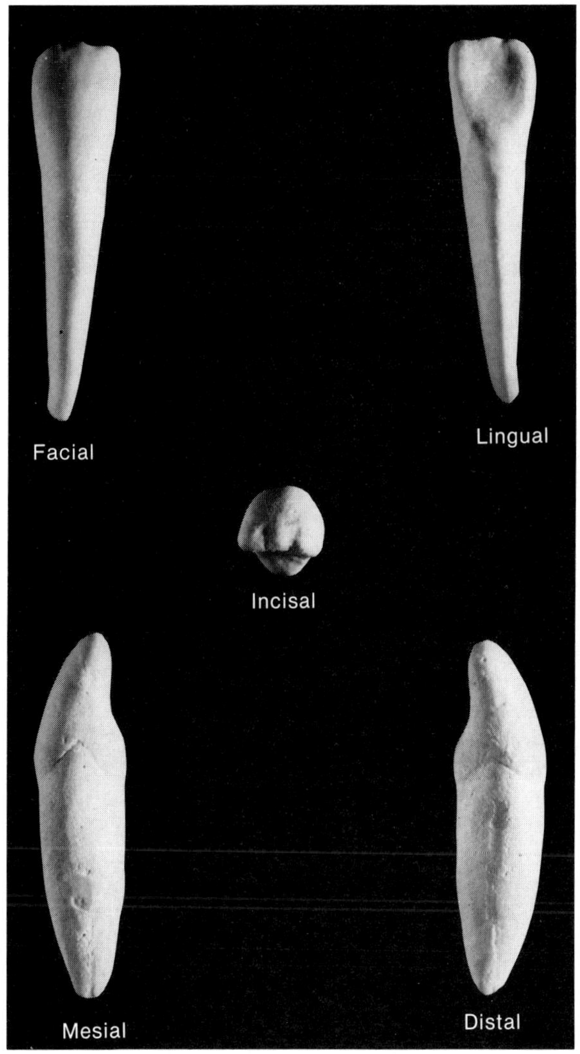
Facial
Lingual
Incisal
Mesial
Distal

MANDIBULAR CANINE

FACIAL VIEW

1. Crown longer incisocervically than wide mesiodistally.
2. Mesial outline nearly straight with proximal contact near mesioincisal angle.
3. Distal outline slightly concave cervically to proximal contact, which is at about two thirds the incisocervical distance.
4. Cusp tip in approximate center.
5. Mesial slope of cusp shorter and at flatter angle than distal slope.
6. Mesioincisal angle more incisal in position than distoincisal angle.
7. Surface is broken by prominent ridge in middle of crown.

LINGUAL VIEW

1. Slight mesial and distal marginal ridges with concave lingual fossa.
2. Narrow cingulum extends to about middle of crown.
3. Prominence of cingulum approximately in center of crown mesiodistally.
4. Surface relatively smooth.

INCISAL VIEW

1. Crown wider faciolingually than mesiodistally.
2. Cusp tip lingual to center of crown.
3. Mesial half of outline convex and wider than distal half.
4. Distal half of outline also convex but interrupted by concavities both lingually and facially.
5. Lingual half is narrower than facial half.
6. Proximal contacts approximately in center of crown.

PROXIMAL (MESIAL AND DISTAL) VIEW

1. Crown longer incisocervically than wide faciolingually.
2. Both facial and lingual heights of contour relatively low (cervical third), especially at facial height.
3. Cusp tip slightly lingual to middle of crown.
4. Facial outline convex.
5. Lingual outline has flattened S shape with cingulum extending to half the crown length.

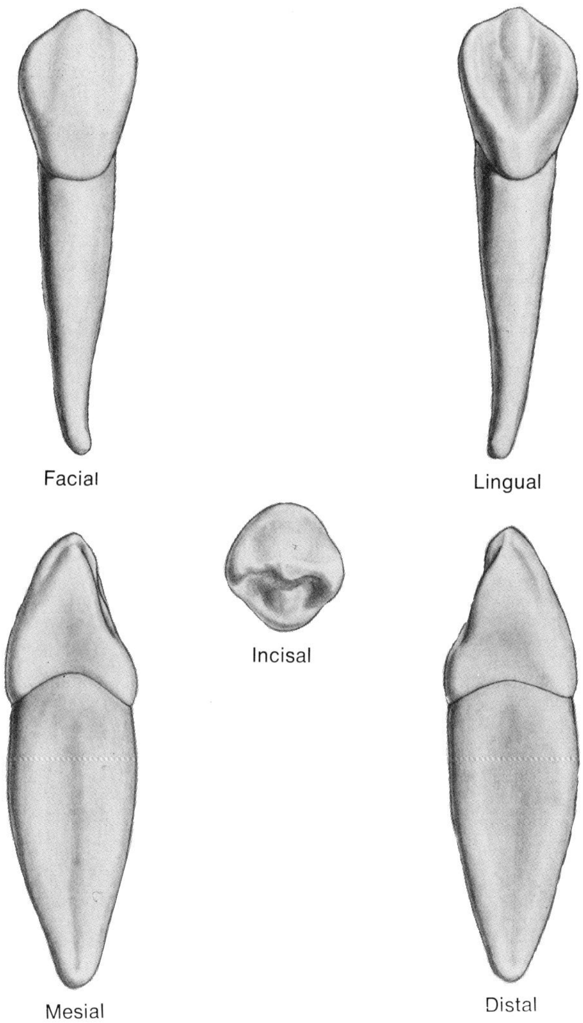
Facial
Lingual
Incisal
Mesial
Distal

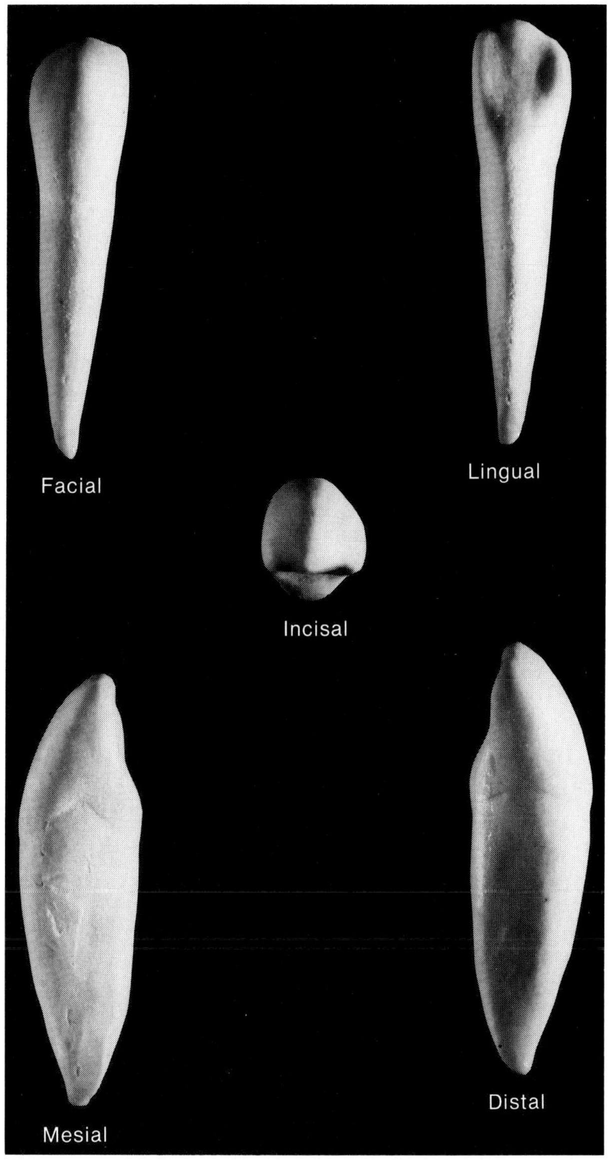
Facial
Lingual
Incisal
Mesial
Distal

MANDIBULAR FIRST PREMOLAR

FACIAL VIEW

1. Crown longer occlusocervically than wide mesiodistally.
2. Nearly symmetrical outline.
3. Mesial and distal outlines fairly straight taper cervically to proximal contacts, which are at about two thirds the occlusocervical length of crown.
4. Proximal contacts form a flattened convexity.
5. Cusp tip approximately in center of crown.
6. Cusp slopes at about 30-degree angle from tip.
7. Surface relatively smooth although facial ridge present in middle of crown.

LINGUAL VIEW

1. Lingual cusp tip slightly mesial of center and about two thirds the occlusocervical crown length in height.
2. Prominent triangular ridge extends from buccal cusp tip to central groove.
3. Marginal ridges incline cervically faciolingually.
4. Prominent mesiolingual groove at about one fourth the mesiodistal width of crown and half the occlusocervical length of crown.
5. Surface is uniformly tapered.

OCCLUSAL VIEW

1. Crown wider faciolingually than mesiodistally.
2. Facial outline very convex with buccal ridge in center.
3. Mesial and distal outlines convex and tapered lingually.
4. Proximal contacts in middle third of crown.
5. Lingual outline narrow and convex.
6. Occlusal table in lingual half of crown.
7. Central groove lingual to center of occlusal table.
8. Facial cusp tip in center of crown.
9. Lingual cusp tip slightly mesial of center and almost at edge of lingual surface.
10. Approximately one third the mesiodistal width of crown separates mesial and distal pits.
11. Supplemental grooves and ridges radiate from pits.

PROXIMAL (MESIAL AND DISTAL) VIEW

1. Crown longer occlusocervically than wide faciolingually.
2. Facial cusp tip in approximate center of crown.
3. Lingual cusp a little more than two thirds as long as facial cusp and approximately in line with cervical line.
4. Central groove just buccal to cervical line.
5. Facial outline very convex with height of contour at cervical third.
6. Lingual outline relatively flat with height of contour in occlusal half of crown.
7. Marginal ridges slightly more occlusal than two thirds the occlusocervical length of crown with cervical slope toward lingual surface.
8. Mesiolingual groove slightly lingual to central groove.

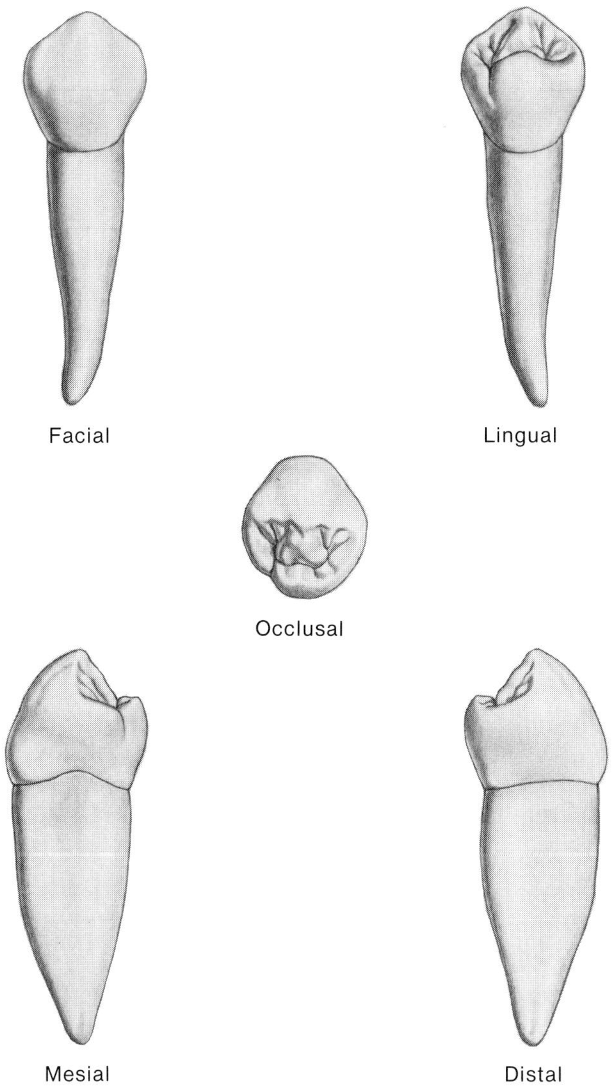
Facial
Lingual
Occlusal
Mesial
Distal

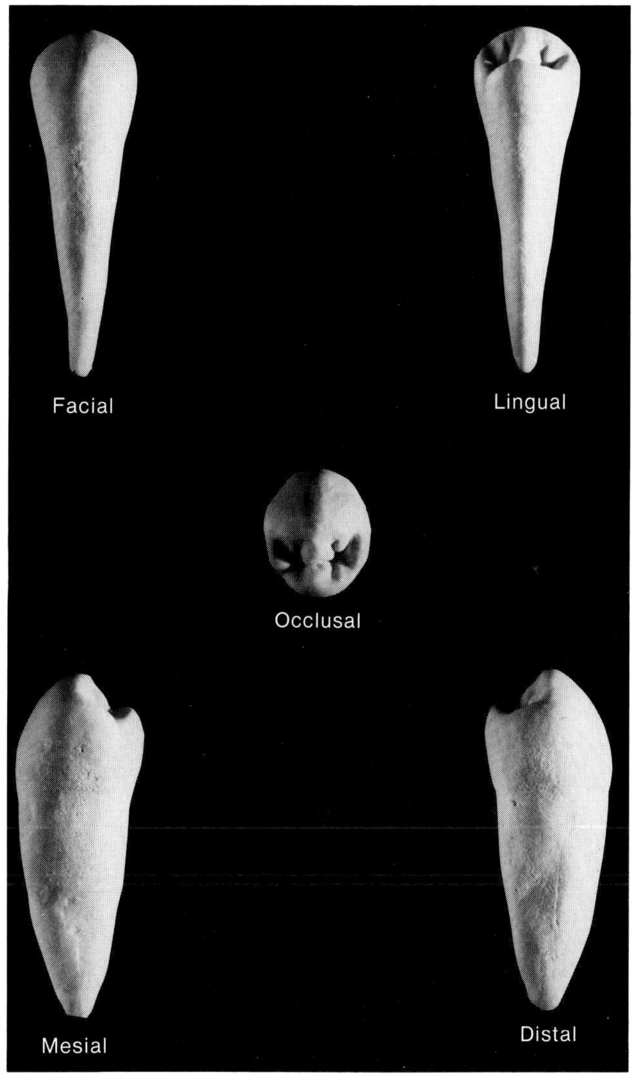
Facial
Lingual
Occlusal
Mesial
Distal

MANDIBULAR SECOND PREMOLAR

FACIAL VIEW

1. Crown longer occlusocervically than wide mesiodistally.
2. Nearly symmetrical outline.
3. Mesial and distal outlines fairly straight taper cervically to proximal contacts, which are at about two thirds the occlusocervical length of crown.
4. Proximal contacts form a flattened convexity.
5. Cusp tip approximately in center of crown.
6. Cusp slopes at about 20-degree angle from tip.
7. Surface relatively smooth although facial ridge present in middle of crown.

LINGUAL VIEW

1. Distolingual cusp tip just inside cervical line and about two thirds the occlusocervical crown length in height.
2. Mesiolingual cusp tip just inside cervical line and slightly longer than distolingual cusp.
3. Lingual groove slightly distal of center.
4. Triangular ridge extends from facial cusp tip to central groove.
5. Surface uniformly tapered.

OCCLUSAL VIEW

1. Crown wider faciolingually than mesiodistally.
2. Facial outline very convex with facial ridge in center.
3. Mesial and distal outlines relatively flattened convexity and approximately parallel to each other.
4. Proximal contacts in middle third of crown.
5. Lingual outline relatively flat and about as wide as facial outline.
6. Occlusal table in lingual two thirds of crown.
7. Y outline formed by mesial, lingual, and distal grooves.
8. Lingual groove just distal of center.
9. Buccal cusp tip approximately in center mesiodistally.
10. Lingual cusp tips almost at edge of mesiolingual and distolingual line angles.
11. Approximately half the mesiodistal width of crown separates mesial and distal pits.

PROXIMAL (MESIAL AND DISTAL) VIEW

1. Faciolingual width and occlusocervical length about equal.
2. Facial cusp tip slightly buccal of center of crown.
3. Distolingual cusp tip about two thirds as long as facial cusp and just slightly facial to cervical line.
4. Mesiolingual cusp tip slightly longer than distolingual cusp and just slightly facial of cervical line.
5. Central groove in lingual third of crown.
6. Facial outline broadly convex with height of contour at about cervical third of crown.
7. Lingual outline relatively flat with height of contour in occlusal third.
8. Mesial marginal ridge in occlusal third with distal marginal ridge at a slightly more cervical level.

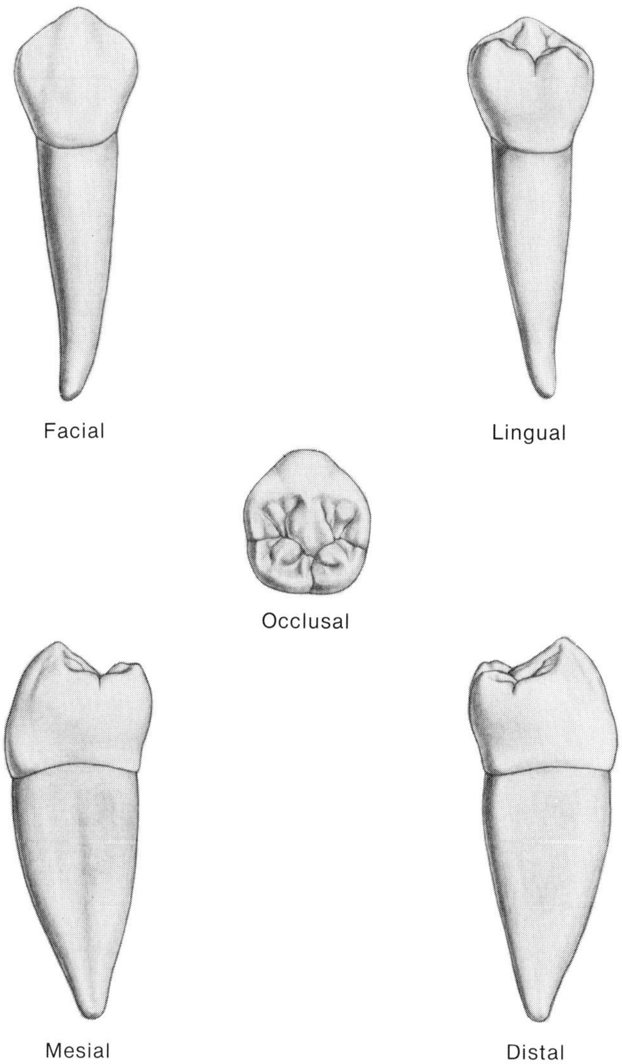
Facial
Lingual
Occlusal
Mesial
Distal

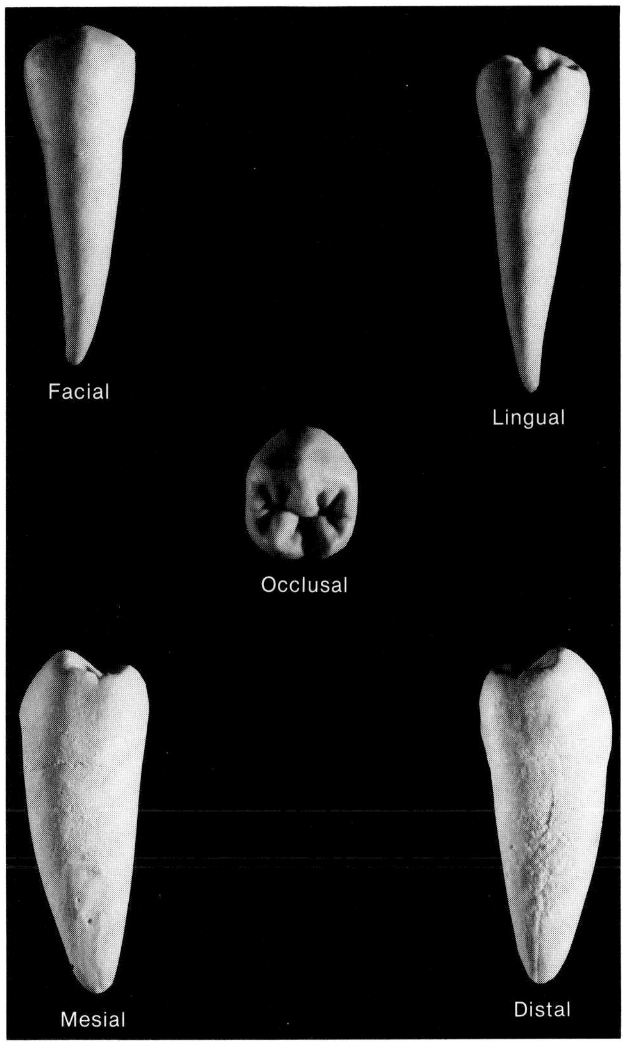
Facial
Lingual
Occlusal
Mesial
Distal

MANDIBULAR FIRST MOLAR

FACIAL VIEW

1. Crown wider mesiodistally than long occlusocervically.
2. Mesial and distal outline relatively straight taper cervically to proximal contacts, which are at about two thirds the occlusocervical length of crown.
3. Mesiofacial cusp is largest, and distal cusp is smallest.
4. Mesiofacial groove just mesial to bifurcation.
5. Distofacial groove mesial to cervical line.
6. Cusp outlines relatively flat.

LINGUAL VIEW

1. Lingual half narrower than facial half.
2. Both lingual cusps of approximate equal size.
3. Lingual groove about in line with bifurcation.
4. Mesial cusp tip in middle of mesial half, and distal cusp tip in middle of distal half.
5. Cusp slopes at steeper angle than facial cusps.

OCCLUSAL VIEW

1. Crown wider mesiodistally than faciolingually.
2. Mesial half of crown wider than distal half.
3. Lingual half narrower than facial half.
4. Facial outline convex but sloping lingually in distal half with height of contour mesial of center.
5. Lingual outline uniform flattened convexity with groove in middle of crown.
6. Mesial and distal outlines convex and tapering toward lingual surface with proximal contacts in middle of crown.
7. Occlusal table in lingual two thirds of crown.
8. Central groove equidistant between facial and lingual cusps.
9. Central pit in middle of occlusal table.
10. Lingual groove approximately in middle of crown.

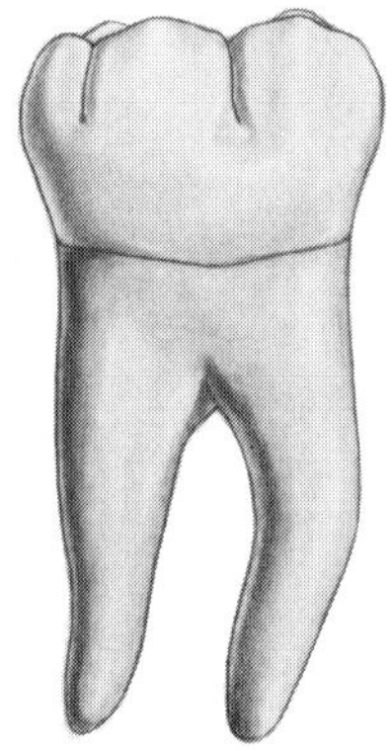

Facial

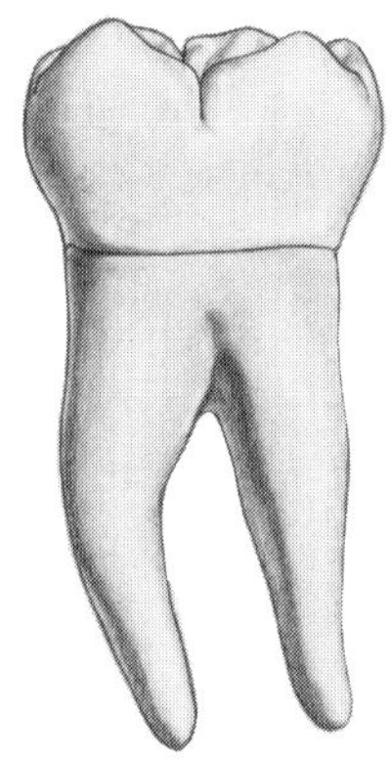

Lingual

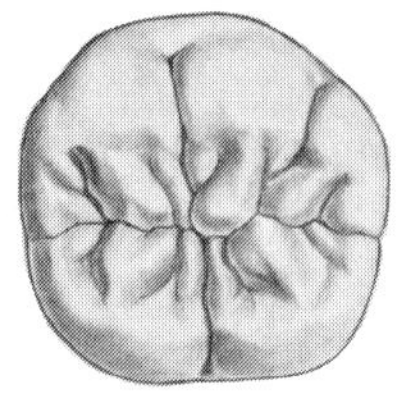

Occlusal

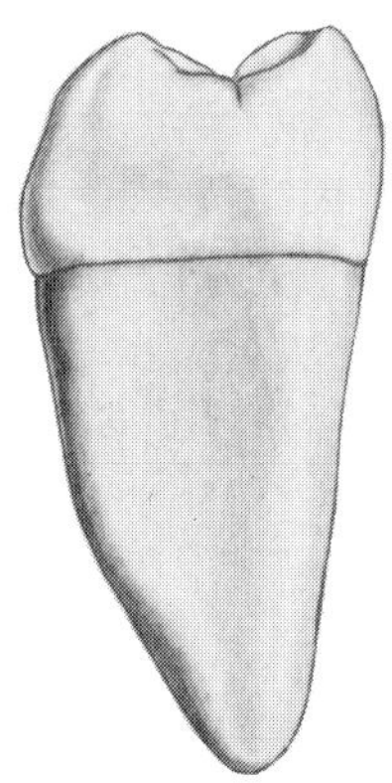

Mesial

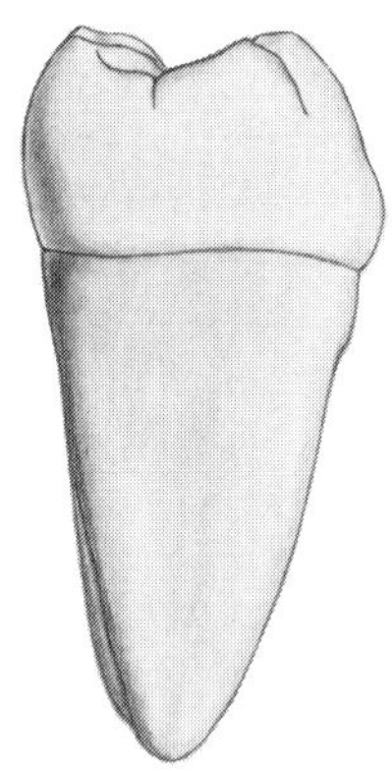

Distal

11. Distofacial groove angles diagonally from central pit.
12. Supplemental grooves and ridges radiate from pits.

PROXIMAL (MESIAL AND DISTAL) VIEW

1. Crown wider faciolingually than long occlusocervically.
2. Cusp tips approximately equal in length.
3. Facial cusp tips at about one third the buccolingual width of crown from facial height of contour.
4. Lingual cusp tips just buccal to the cervical line.
5. Central groove lingual to middle of crown.
6. Facial outline convex and leaning lingually with bulge in cervical third, denoting height of contour.
7. Lingual outline flattened convexity with height of contour in occlusal half.
8. Marginal ridges about level with middle of occlusal third.
9. Distal half narrower and shorter than mesial half.

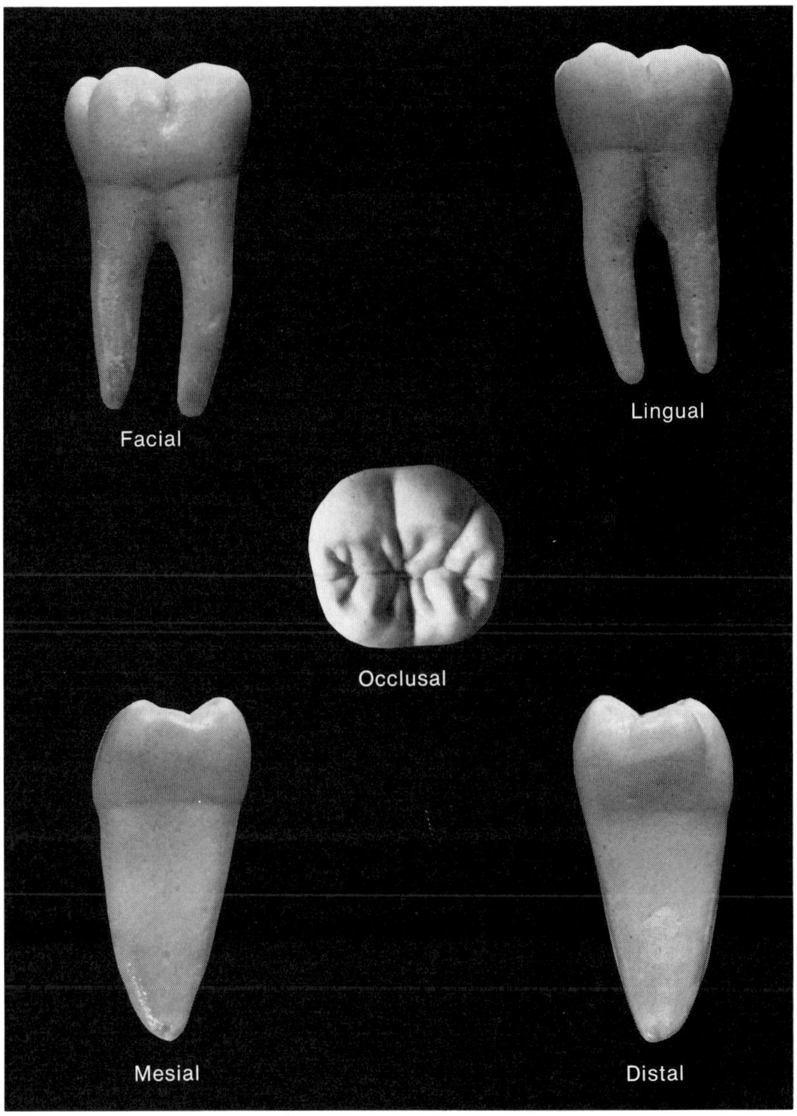

MANDIBULAR SECOND MOLAR

FACIAL VIEW

1. Crown wider mesiogingivally than occlusogingivally.
2. Mesial and distal outlines relatively straight taper cervically to proximal contacts, which are about two thirds the occlusocervical length of crown.
3. Both cusps approximately equal size.
4. Facial groove approximately in line with bifurcation.
5. Cusp tips and facial groove divide surface into approximately quarters.
6. Cusp outlines relatively flat.

LINGUAL VIEW

1. Lingual cusps about equal in size.
2. Lingual groove in line with bifurcation.
3. Mesial cusp in middle of mesial half, and distal cusp tip in middle of distal half.
4. Cusp slopes at steeper angle than facial cusps.

OCCLUSAL VIEW

1. Crown wider mesiodistally than faciolingually.
2. Mesial half wider than distal half.
3. Facial half and lingual half about equal in width.
4. Facial outline convex but sloping lingually in distal half with height of contour mesial of center.
5. Lingual outline uniform flattened convexity with lingual groove in middle of crown.
6. Mesial and distal outlines flattened convexity parallel to each other with proximal contact in middle of crown.
7. Occlusal table in lingual two thirds of crown.
8. Central groove equidistant between facial and lingual cusps.
9. Central pit in middle of occlusal table.
10. Occlusal table divided into quarters by central, facial, and lingual grooves.
11. Supplemental grooves and ridges radiate from pits.

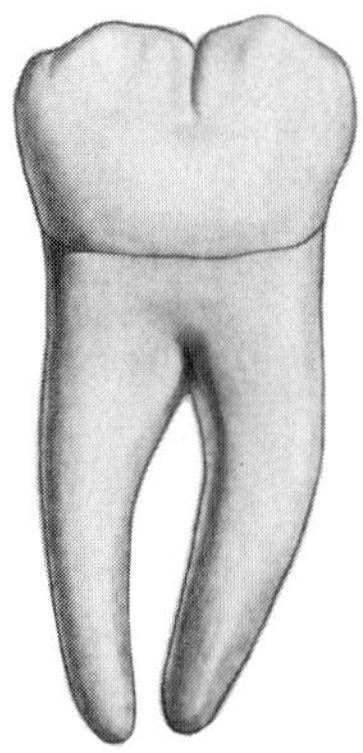

Facial

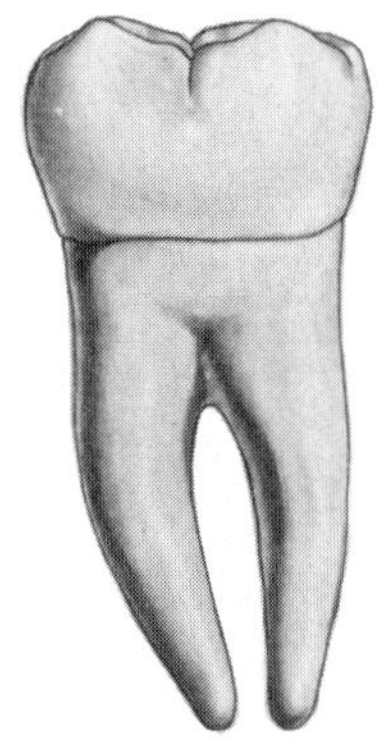

Lingual

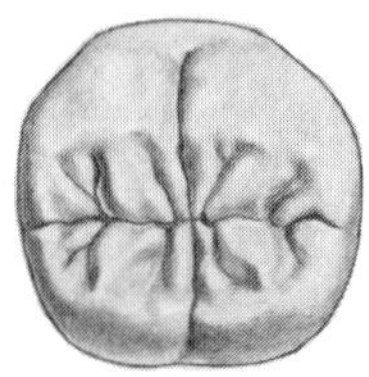

Occlusal

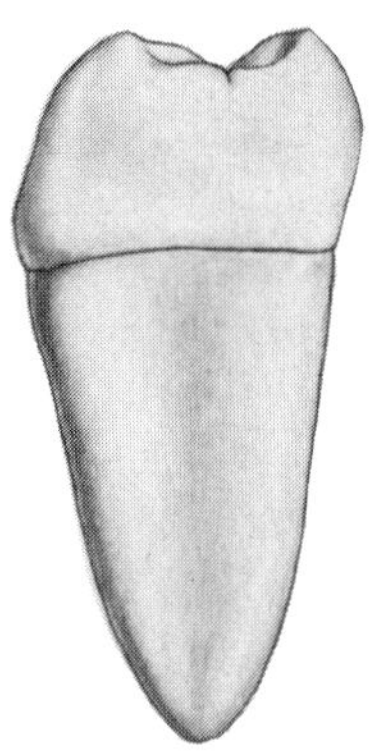

Mesial

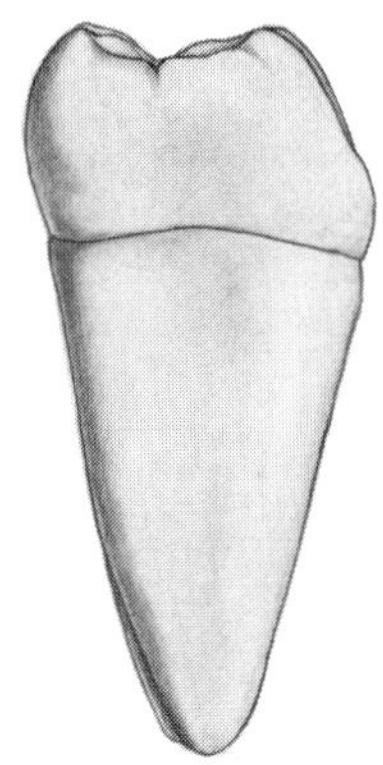

Distal

PROXIMAL (MESIAL AND DISTAL) VIEW

1. Crown wider faciolingually than long occlusocervically.
2. Cusp tips approximately equal in length.
3. Facial cusp tips about one third the faciolingual width of crown from facial height of contour.
4. Lingual cusp tips just facial to cervical line.
5. Central groove lingual to middle of crown.
6. Facial outline convex and leaning lingually with bulge in cervical third, denoting height of contour.
7. Lingual outline flattened convexity with height of contour in occlusal half.
8. Marginal ridges about level with middle of occlusal third.

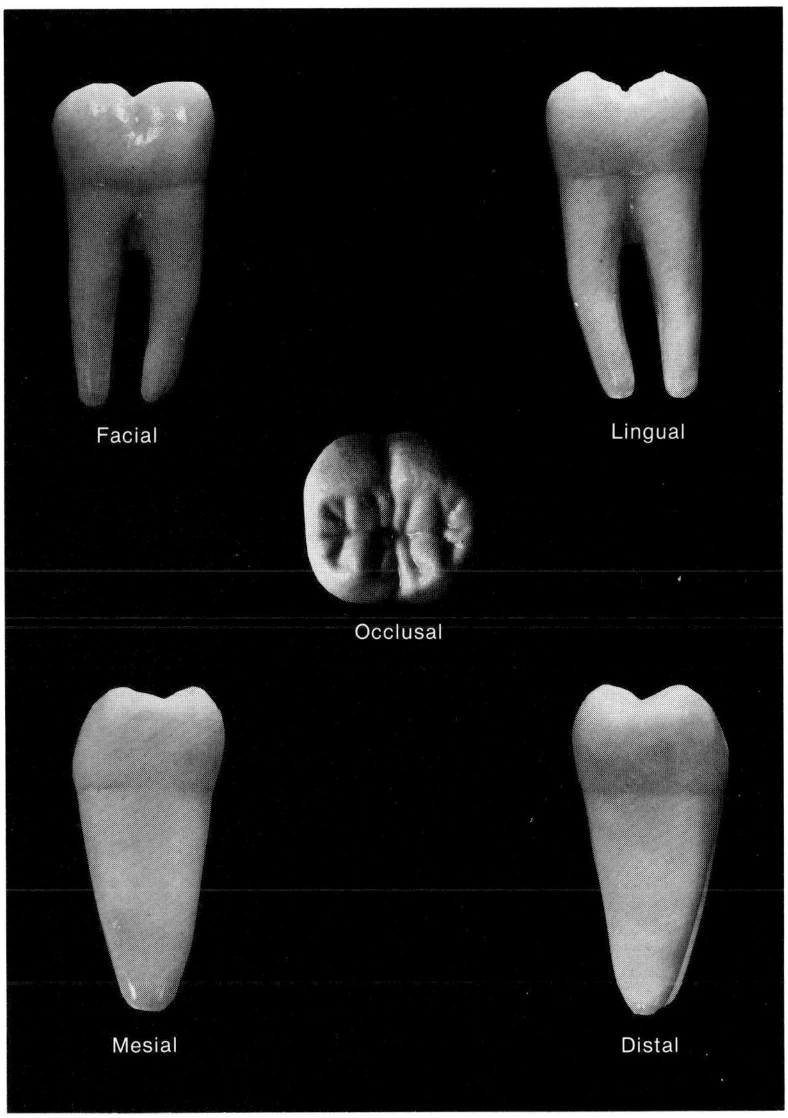

CHAPTER 4

VISUAL PERCEPTION AND TOOTH CONTOUR

HAROLD F. EISSMANN

Present technical procedures do not provide us with the possibility of "perfectly" duplicating the appearance of vital natural human teeth. This is due to the inability of industry to produce dental porcelain with the same light refraction and reflection present in translucent tooth enamel or the degree of opacity of the tooth dentin. Dentists also cannot exactly duplicate the very subtle color variations of hue, value, and chroma.

FACTORS INFLUENCING VISUAL PERCEPTION

The human visual system is not especially accurate or sensitive to finite minute color variations found in human teeth. We are, however, much more aware of their outline form and surface texture. This should not detract from any efforts to develop expertise regarding accurate shade selection and matching. This latter factor, regarding tooth form, emphasizes the importance of proper tooth contouring and positioning to enhance visual perception of the restorative effort.

Visual perception is the response of the eye to past experiences. Light, movement, outline form, surface form and texture, and color are all part of the recollection process of the brain to associate a past experience with a new stimulus.

Light

The high sensitivity of the eye to light is one of the causes for rapid fatigue to a continuous stimulus. For this reason the selection of tooth colors or evaluation of contour is best accomplished by five short repeated glances rather than a prolonged study.

The most important factor to consider is the reflection of light from a given surface. In ceramometal procedures, it is necessary to use procelain opaquing materials that allow minimal light transmission and provide blocking out of the metal casting surfaces with the least thickness of ceramic material. When this opaque masking is covered with a thin layer of translucent body/incisal porcelain, the restoration becomes highly reflective. This is the reason why many ceramometal restorations appear more prominent than their adjacent natural teeth. To compensate for high light reflection potential, some dentists select shades having a stronger chroma concentration, which often produces restorations that appear dull and unattractive once they are placed in the mouth. A more accurate and pleasing method would be to select shades that are slightly lower in value. Doing so will result in reduced brightness or brilliance of the restoration. The position of the restoration should be more lingual, and the incisal curvature should be increased to direct the light in various directions away from the observer's eye.

It is the opacity (degree of translucency) of the body porcelain that determines the reflection of light. The texture and gloss of the outer porcelain surface control the perception and character of light reflection. Contour and texture control of the outer porcelain surface will define the character form of the restoration and lend vitality to its appearance.

Movement

Visual sensitivity to the movement of an object will not be discussed, because it has little application to this discussion.

Outline form

The eye is extremely sensitive to the outline form of objects. This is readily demonstrated by the ease of identifying silhouettes of faces, ships, or airplanes. Outline form is especially noted when highly different and contrasting hue and chroma samples are involved. Each tooth is individualized and characterized by a distinct outline form. By comparison, human teeth are relatively weak in chroma and high in value and are surrounded, or framed, by the gingiva, interproximally by dark or stained embrasures, and incisally by the dark oral cavity. The incisal embrasures emphasize the particular character of the outline form and tooth position more than any other feature. This is because the incisal edge of the tooth is so prominantly silhouetted against the dark shadow of the oral cavity (Figs. 4-l to 4-3).

The outline form of restorations being contoured should be in harmony with the facial structure, sex, and temperament of the patient. The generally accepted prosthetic classifications are square, tapering, and ovoid with transitional modifications such as square tapering (Fig. 4-4). A true tapering outline form is not usually used in a fixed prosthesis because it causes uncosmetic, large, open gingival-interproximal embrasures. The strength or softness desired can be readily expressed by the square or ovoid forms on incisal edges of maxillary anteriors (Figs. 4-5 to 4-7).

The apparent size of the restored tooth is not necessarily determined on the basis of space available. A general guide for selecting removable prosthetic restorations is that the width of the maxillary central incisor be one sixteenth of the width of the patient's face. This guide should be modified. The maxillary central incisor can be larger than generally advocated, and this increase in size adds a very pleasant characteristic to the patient's smile (Figs. 4-8 and 4-9). The student must learn to visualize tooth form and tooth arrangement as they relate to the patient's facial architecture and personality. The study begins with the natural tooth, the arrangement of the natural anterior teeth in various patients, and the favorable or unfavorable effect of past restorative efforts (Fig. 4-10). These experiences are fundamental to treatment planning for cosmetic restorations. How the teeth appear, or how they should appear, is more art than science, and few rules can be applied. A removable prosthesis can be trial seated, and adjustment are readily made while the anterior teeth are set in wax. In fixed restorations, the plastic temporary coverage, a similar diagnostic step can be used to

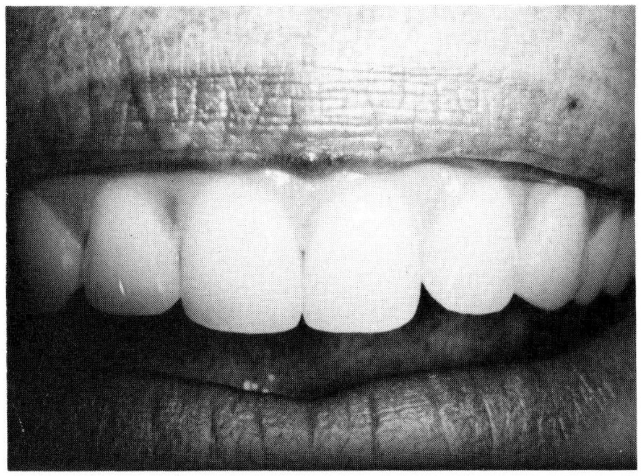

Fig. 4-1. Outline form of natural teeth framed by gingiva, interproximal embrasures, and dark oral cavity of 25-year-old woman.

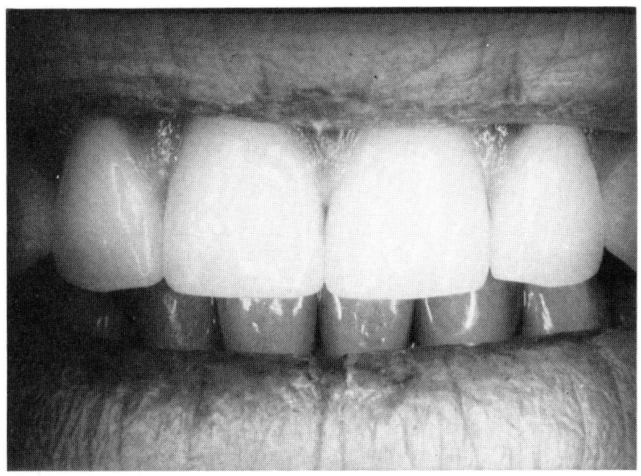

Fig. 4-2. Proper surface form and texture but improper incisal embrasure form on ceramometal restorations for 25-year-old woman.

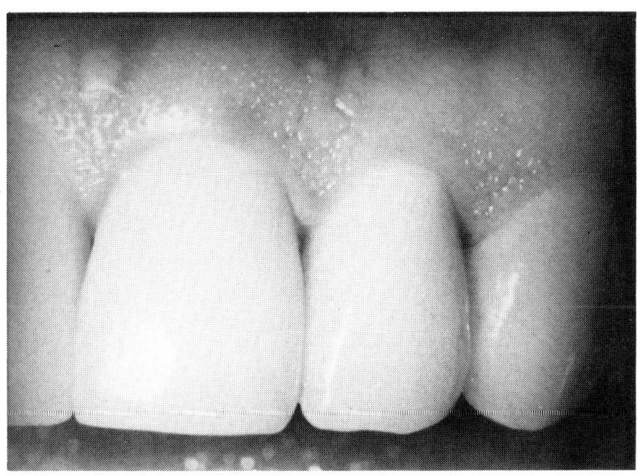

Fig. 4-3. Optimal outline form and surface form of central and lateral porcelain jacket crowns.

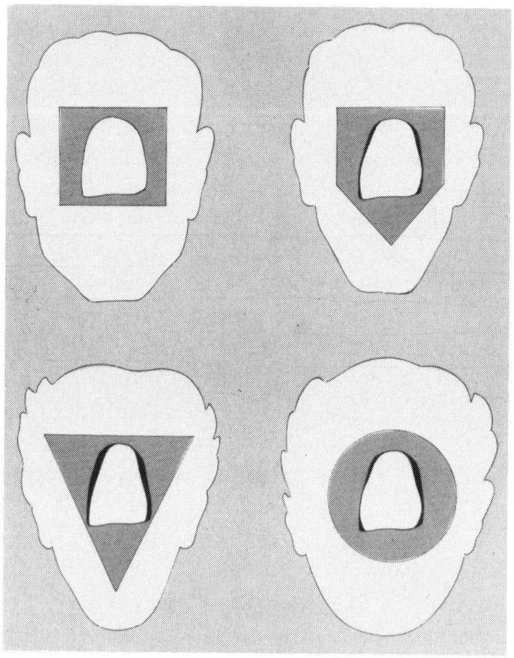

Fig. 4-4. Four classifications for facial outline form: square, square tapering, tapering, and ovoid.

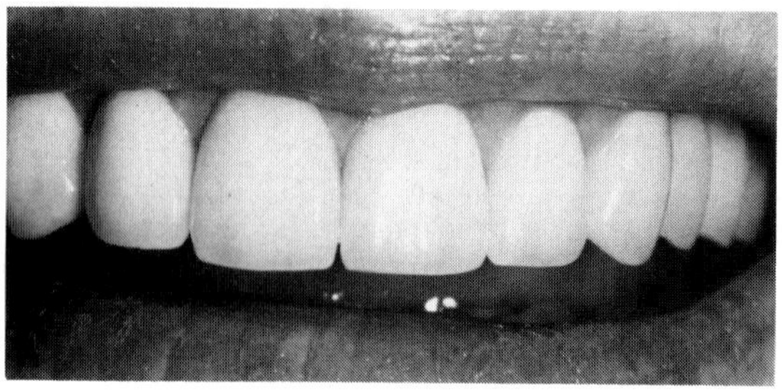

Fig. 4-5. Square-ovoid tooth form (female).

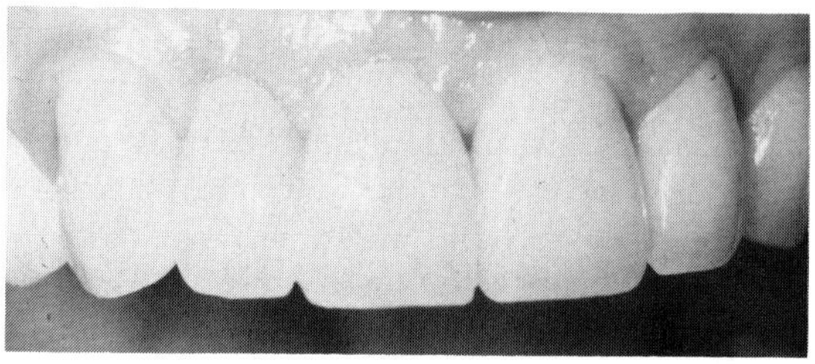

Fig. 4-6. Square-tapering tooth form (female).

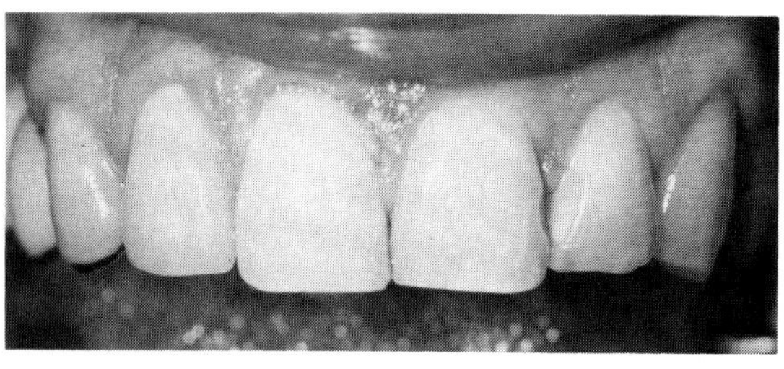

Fig. 4-7. Bold masculine tooth form. Note slight irregularity in positioning of central incisors and their size.

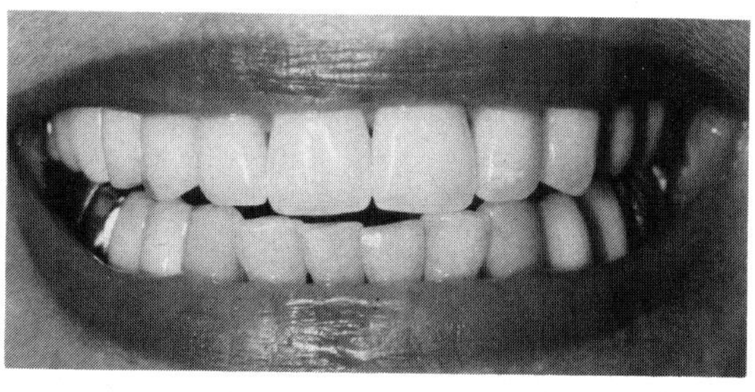

Fig. 4-8. Adverse effect of exceptionally large central incisors is softened by increasing size of lateral incisors.

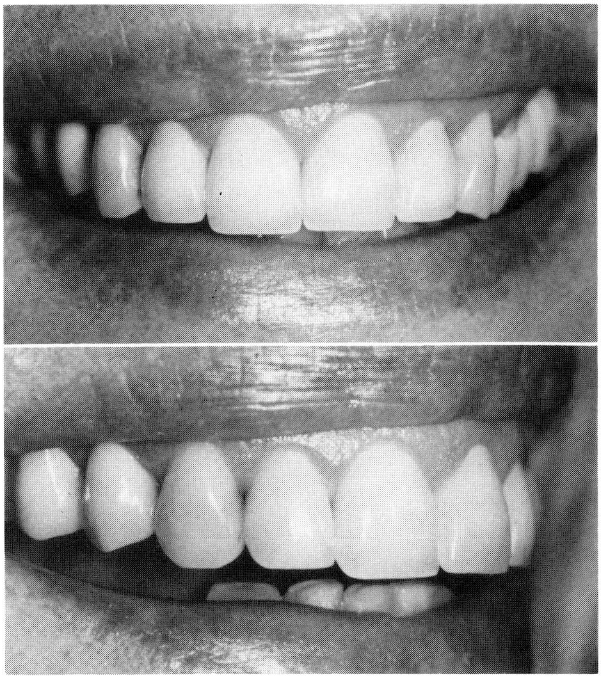

Fig. 4-9. Width of central incisors is accentuated by smaller lateral incisors.

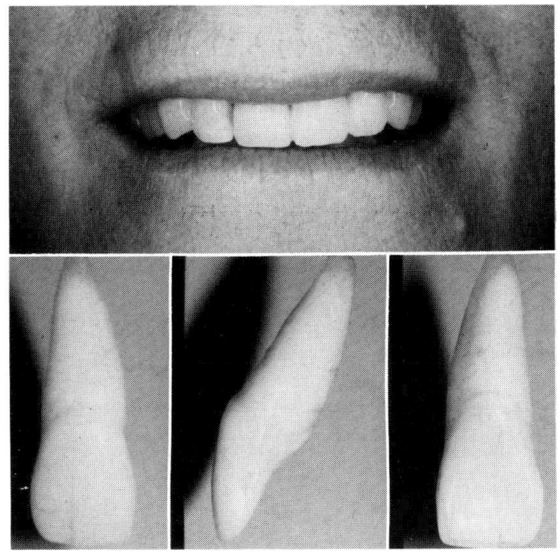

Fig. 4-10. Natural teeth should be studied individually to gain awareness and appreciation of tooth form and function, which is then expressed in restorative effort.

advantage (Fig. 4-11). The plastic is adjusted to satisfy the patient's cosmetic expectations. An impression is taken, and a model poured; this will serve as a three-dimensional laboratory instruction.

Surface form and texture

The surface form of a tooth can be classified, much the same way as an outline form, by examining the patient's facial features. The gingivoincisal profile of the tooth may be straight, convex, or slightly concave (Fig. 4-12). The mesiodistal profile can be straight, convex, or concave, depending on the prominence of the zygomatic arches (Fig. 4-13). Cosmetic anterior restorations will almost always have one characteristic in the gingivoincisal surface form, and that is a definite convexity in the incisal fourth. This reduces the forward reflection of light and prevents the possibility of the incisal edge appearing grossly protrusive (Fig. 4-14).

Surface texture is a most important feature of the restoration. A textured surface will diffuse and reflect (scattering) light in an irregular manner. The detection of slight color differences is greatly reduced under these conditions. Surface texturing of restorations that are similar to adjacent natural teeth produces an interplay of light and creates pleasant "color matching" experiences. Surface texturing the restoration should be slightly more emphasized than the texturing present on

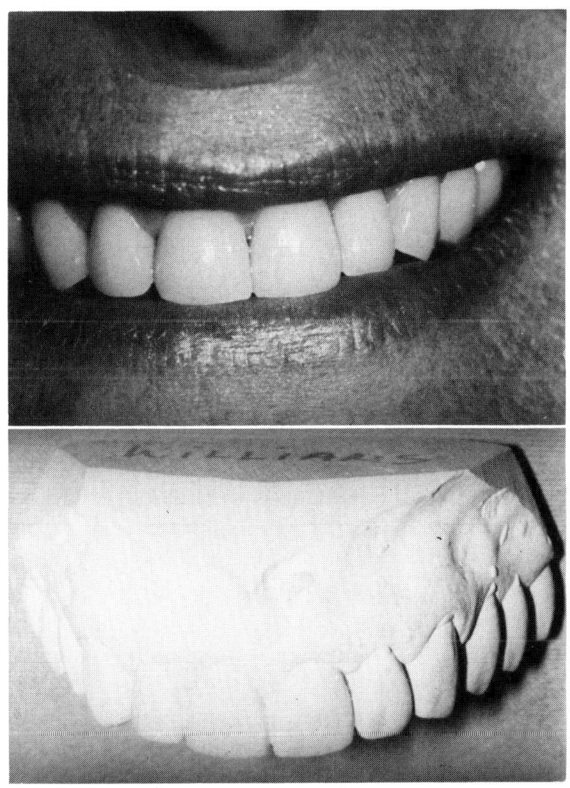

Fig. 4-11. Plastic temporary coverage is also diagnostic tool. Model of temporary will serve for dentist-technician communication.

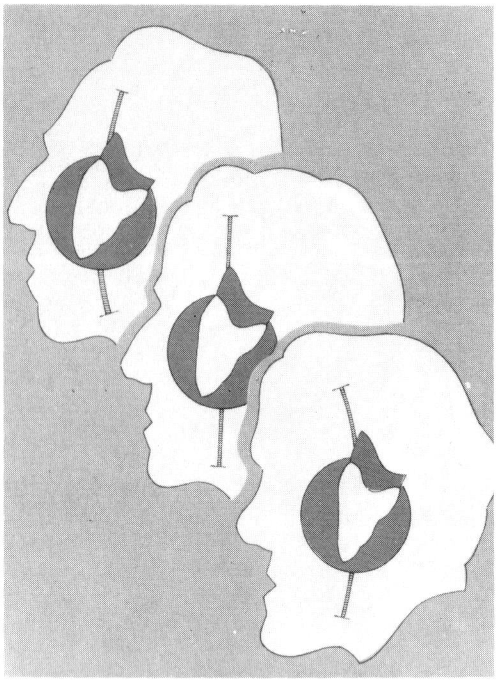

Fig. 4-12. Classifications of patient's profile may influence surface form of teeth.

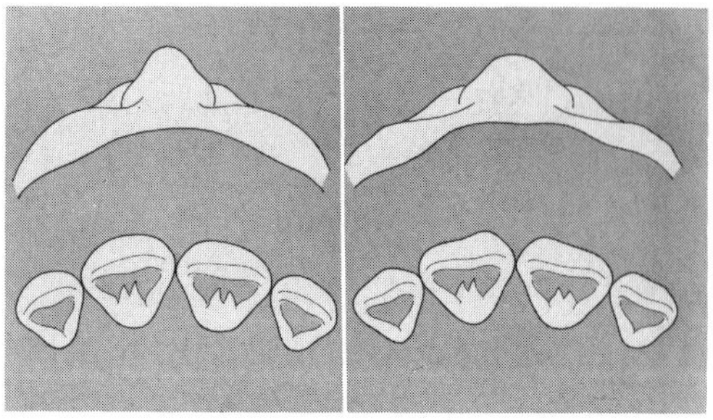

Fig. 4-13. Effect of prominence of zygomatic arches on surface form of teeth.

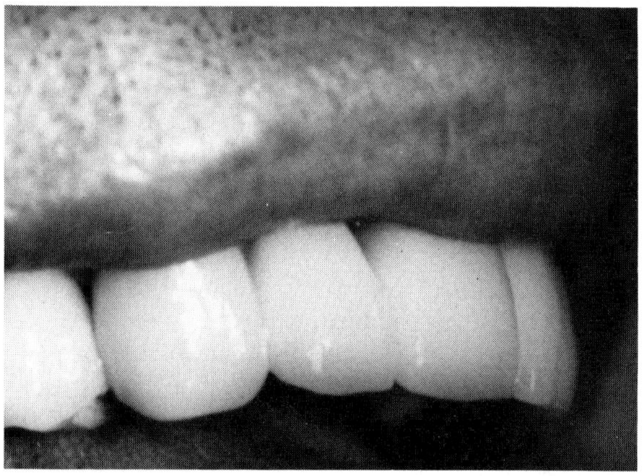

Fig. 4-14. To avoid "protruded" look, restorations are contoured lingually near incisal edge.

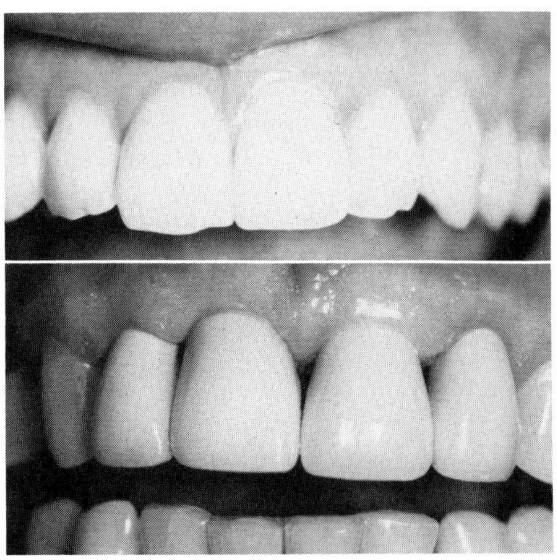

Fig. 4-15. Surface texture of natural dentition and "lackluster" texture of porcelain jacket crowns.

the adjacent tooth being matched. The choice of horizontal and vertical incremental lines will affect the apparent width or length of the tooth being fabricated (Figs. 4-15 to 4-18).

Color

In this discussion color will be considered only from the standpoint of how it can be used to enhance the effect of contouring.

In fixed prosthodontics the efforts to satisfy the patient's cosmetic requirements are frequently frustrated with problems caused by too little or too much available space in a horizontal and/or vertical dimension. Fortunately, the human visual system is susceptible to the trickery of lines, angles, and curvatures. Vertical lines accent height (length), horizontal lines accent width, shadows add depth, and angles add highlights and boldness. In contrast to angles, curved surfaces add softness and less definition to the outline of an object. The use of one or more of these subtle surface form variations is an invaluable tool that provides methods to effect necessary illusions. The illusions subsequently allow us to achieve apparent shade and outline matches.

Fig. 4-19 shows buildings of equal size. One appears larger because it is contrasted with a small object, whereas the large object diminishes the building beside it. This example demonstrates that small central incisors can appear larger if the size of the lateral incisors is proportionately reduced.

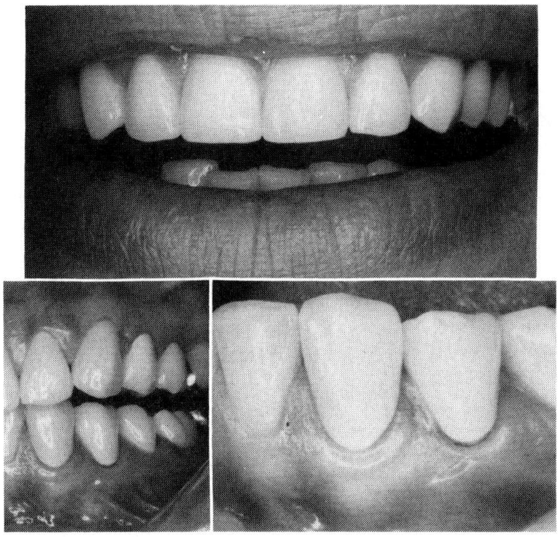

Fig. 4-16. Irregular or diffused light reflection from surface of properly textured teeth.

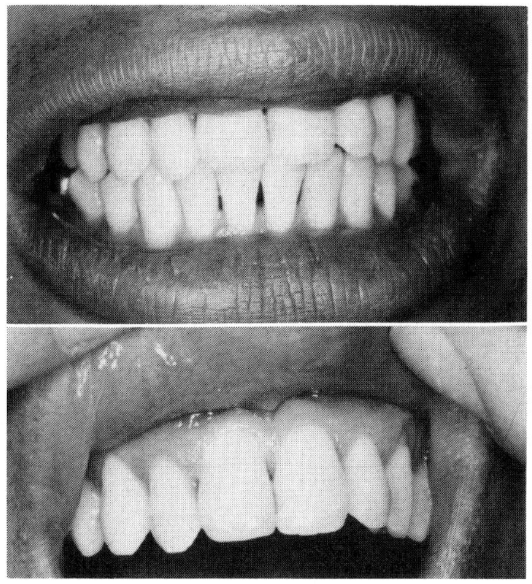

Fig. 4-17. Right central incisor crown matches its natural mate in outline, surface form, and texture.

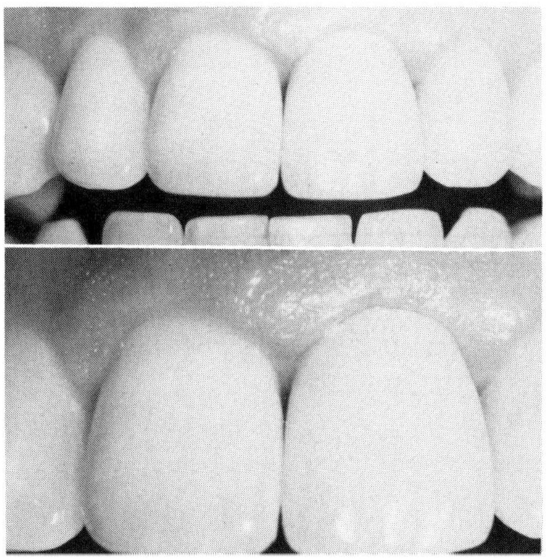

Fig. 4-18. Minute color differences defy detection when outline, surface form, and texture are matched to natural mate.

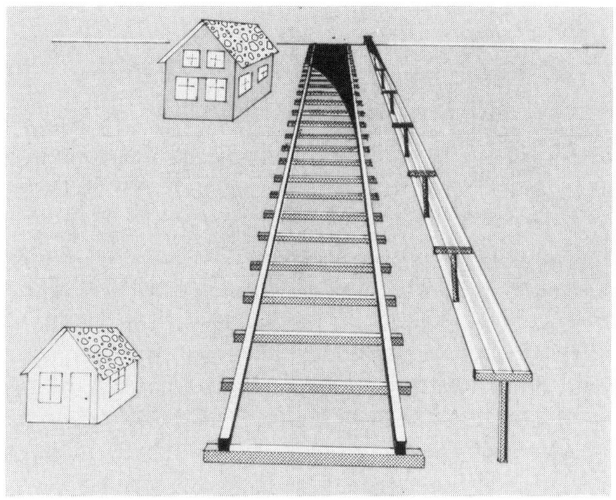

Fig. 4-19. Illusion of unequal-sized buildings when contrasted against unequal-sized objects.

The hat in Fig. 4-20 has a brim as wide as the hat is tall. The height is accentuated by additional vertical lines that tend to constrict the center, thereby emphasizing the illusion of height. The brim appears narrowed especially since the tips are darkened. Supplemental staining or mesiodistal hollow grinding for shadow effect can give the appearance of a narrow tooth or smile. Supplemental lines can accentuate height or width. The illusion used to narrow or broaden a smile is illustrated in Fig. 4-21. The two lines are identical in length, but one appears stretched. The broad smile results when the distal surfaces of lateral incisors and cuspids are flared out. Here, the cuspid should be kept light in color for an effect of maximum width. Conversely, a narrow smile is achieved by tucking-in the distal surfaces of lateral incisors and cuspids and by increasing chroma and lowering the value for cuspids and premolars. To apply these principles to solve common cosmetic problems, we will first consider procedures affecting tooth length and then those procedures which can be used to alter the width of the tooth.

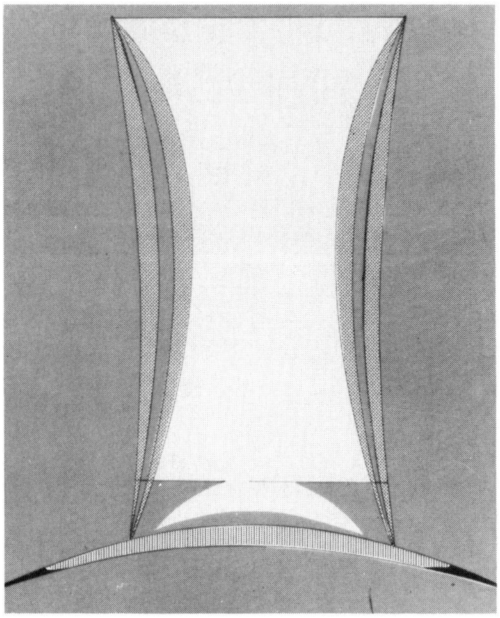

Fig. 4-20. Illusion of greater hat height than brim width effected by supplemental lines, which accentuate height.

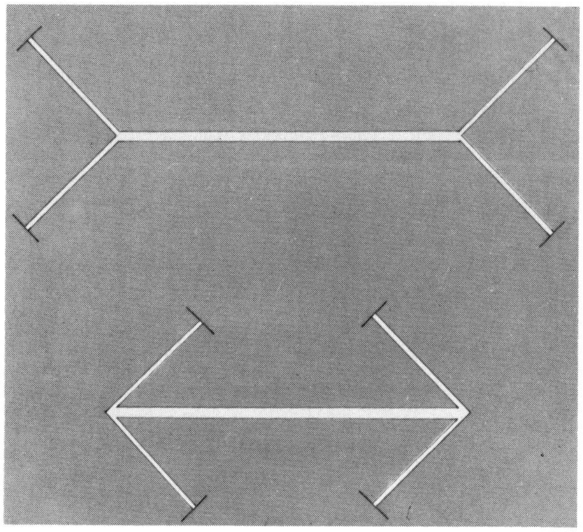

Fig. 4-21. Illusion of unequal length of lines caused by extending and contracting supplemental lines.

CHANGES IN TOOTH LENGTH

Recession of the gingiva or resorption of the edentulous ridge frequently poses a problem of excessive crown or pontic length. The contouring of a very definite cementoenamel junction will substantially shorten the apparent crown length. The root portion of the crown or pontic should be stained to further deemphasize the length of the anatomic crown, and the stain should be matched to exposed root surfaces of the patient's natural dentition (Fig. 4-22). In cases where the appearance of excessive gingival recession is undesirable, the addition of gingival color porcelain will replace the stained root portion (Figs. 4-23 to 4-25). The use of gingival pink stain is effective in masking subtle variations in crown length, or when a gradual transition of the crown and gingiva is desirable to minimize crown length (Fig. 4-26). This same effect is helpful to make pontics appear as though they blend into the edentulous ridge, when the pontics are merely resting against the epithelium.

Conversely, short teeth will appear longer when their weak chroma and high value contrasts strongly with the gingiva and when vertical incremental lines are added to the surface texture. A vertical concavity on the labial surface will tend to further enhance length (Fig. 4-27). These procedures will enhance the illusion of length, but only to a modest degree. Substantial increases in crown length must be done by surgical repositioning of the gingival margin (Figs. 4-28 to 4-30).

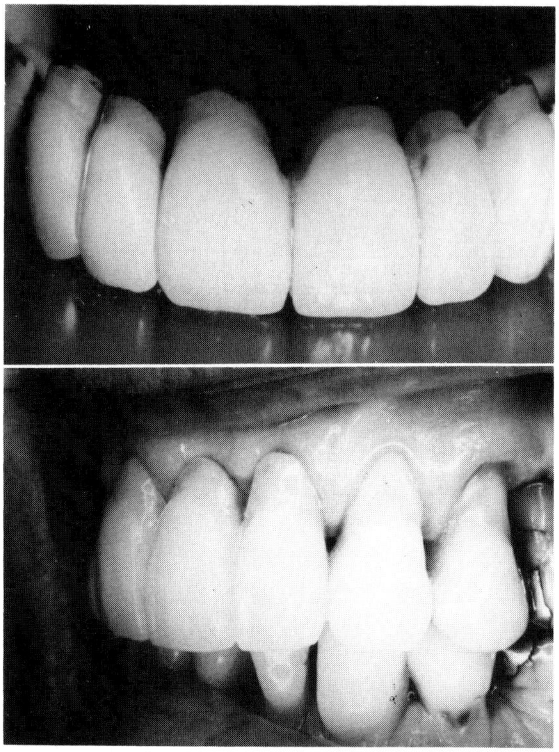

Fig. 4-22. Excessively long clinical crown can appear shorter by contouring very definite cementoenamel junction and by staining to color match exposed root surfaces.

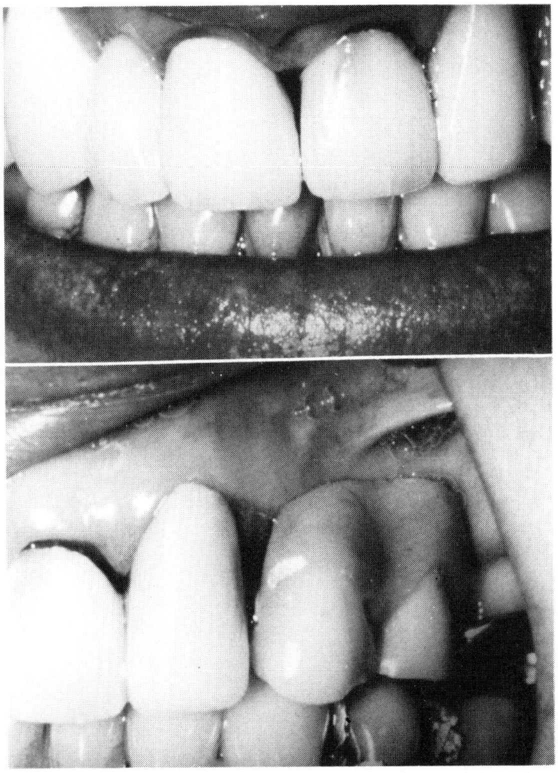

Fig. 4-23. Excessive crown length shown before restoration.

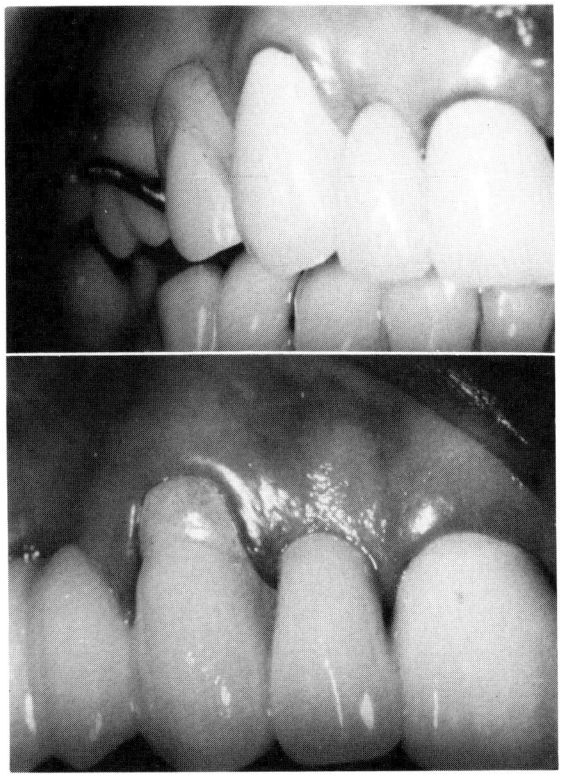

Fig. 4-24. Addition of gingival-colored porcelain.

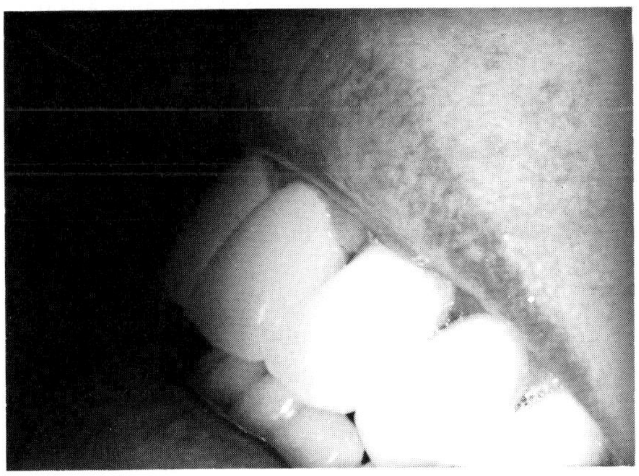

Fig. 4-25. Effected harmonious tooth outline form.

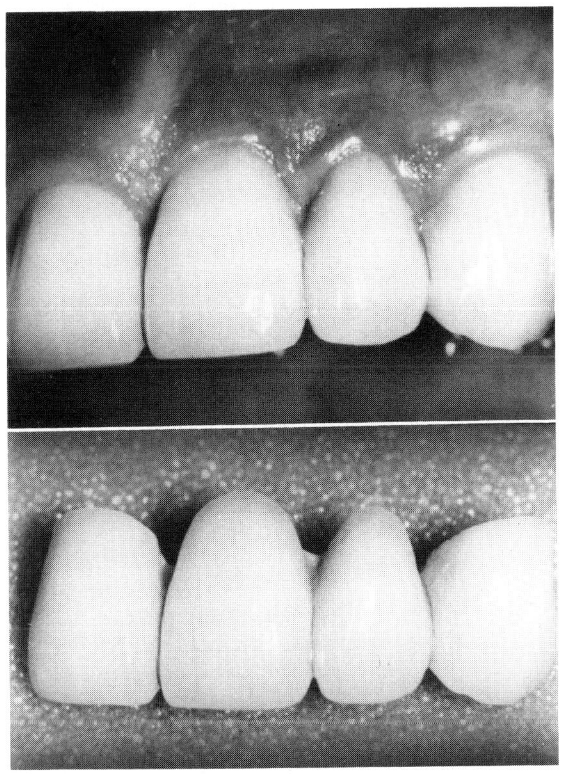

Fig. 4-26. Use of pink stain near gingival margin of crowns or tissue contact areas of pontics can visually soften transition from restoration to gingiva.

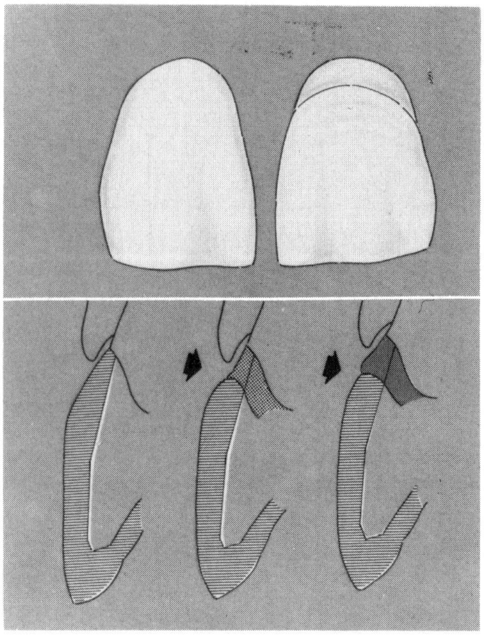

Fig. 4-27. Both incisors are equal in size, and supplemental anatomy will enhance height or width. Tooth will appear shortest when gingival pink is added to neck portion. Tooth will appear longest when high-value body porcelain is extended to gingiva.

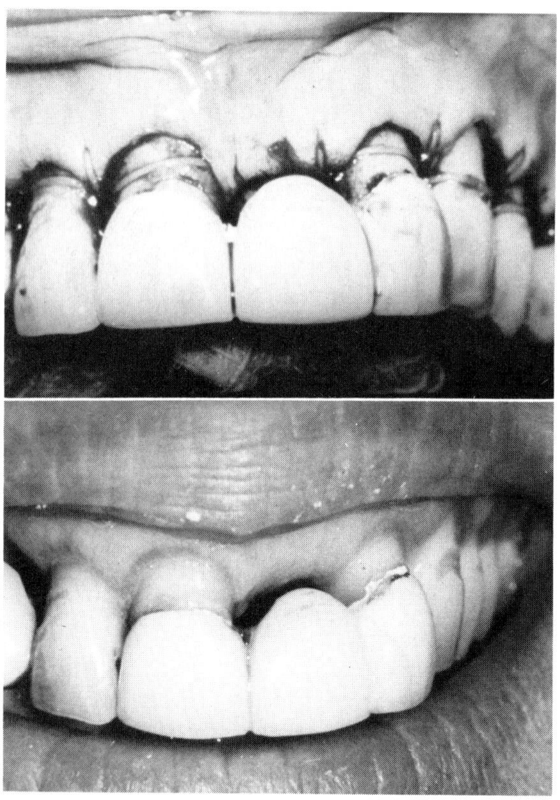

Fig. 4-29. Repositioned gingival margin at time of surgery and 3 weeks postoperatively.

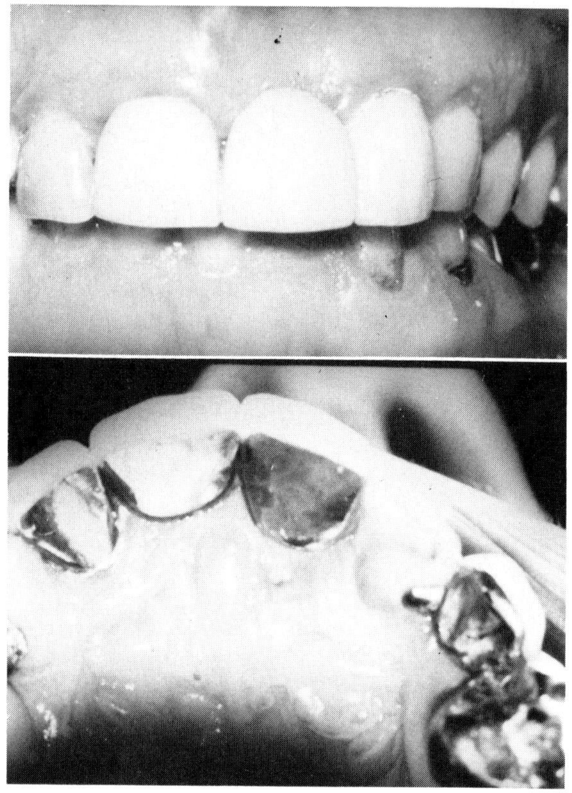

Fig. 4-28. When tooth has to be substantially lengthened, surgical procedure is indicated.

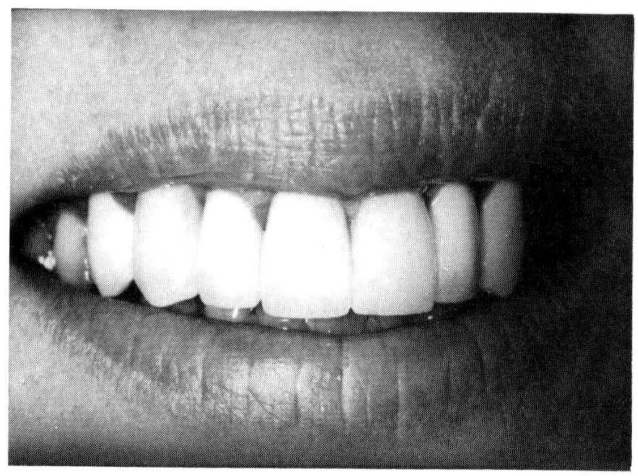

Fig. 4-30. Final restoration was placed 2 months postoperatively.

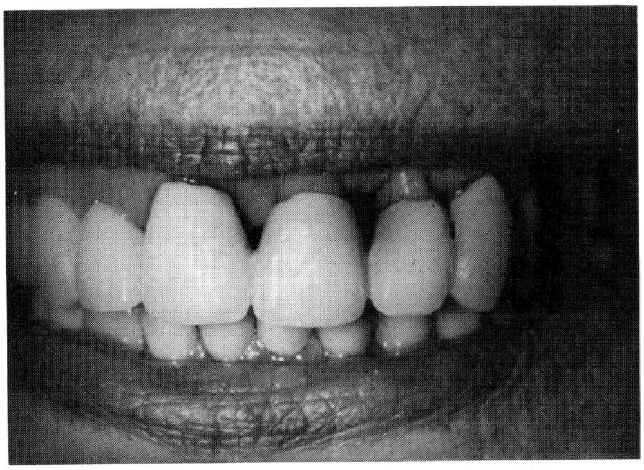

Fig. 4-31. Loss of gingival tissue was cosmetically repaired with removable plastic insert. Further restorative intervention was not indicated.

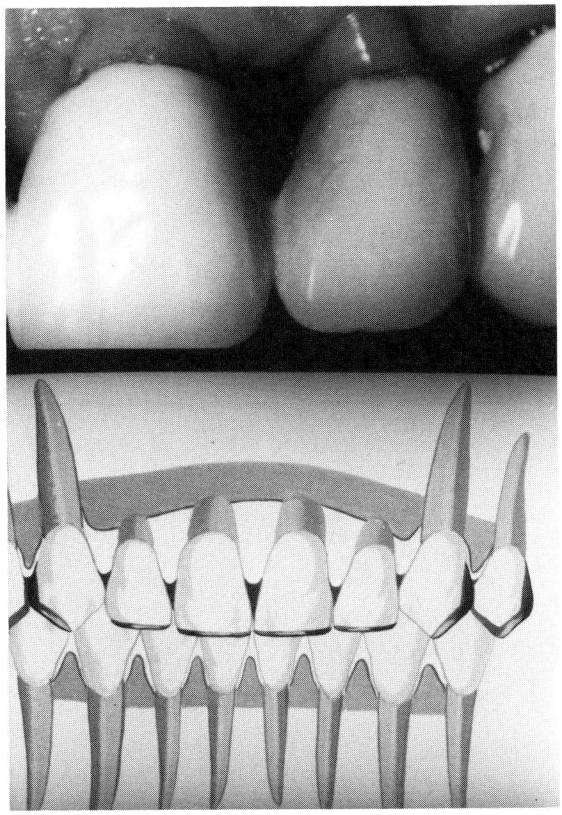

Fig. 4-32. Defect is treated with removable plastic insert that was occasionally advocated with use of long pin pontic facings.

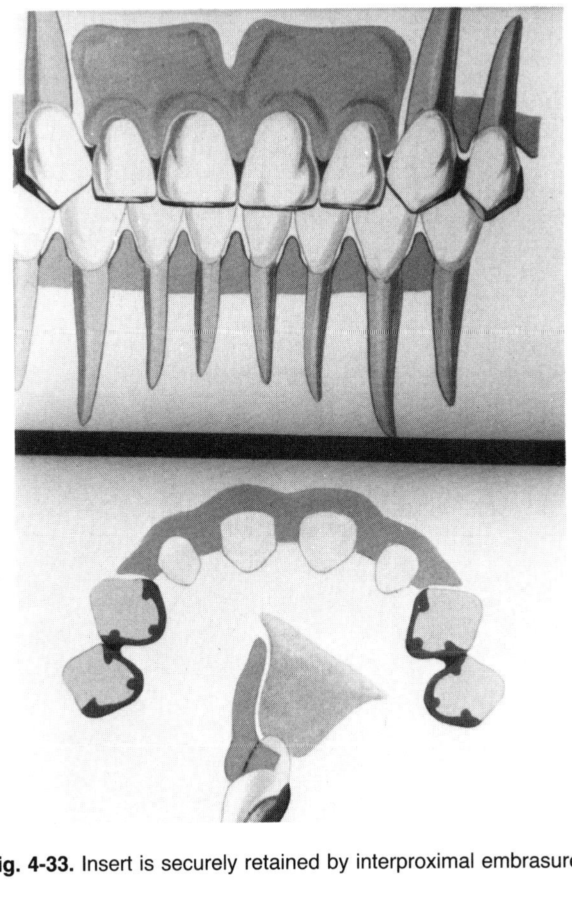

Fig. 4-33. Insert is securely retained by interproximal embrasures.

In the event of excessive tissue loss with an existing prosthesis in place, a removable plastic insert can be fabricated to restore a patient's lost cosmetic function (Figs. 4-31 to 4-33).

Single tooth restorations can appear deceptively natural when a normal healthy gingiva surrounds the crown margin (Fig. 4-34). The tissue architecture, however, may change abruptly when a tooth is lost. The subsequent tissue resorption and loss of the interdental papillae can cause an unacceptable display of the interproximal embrasure. Porcelain interdental papilla may have to be added. This is definitely a hygienic compromise, and the patient is instructed to use additional maintenance. Fig. 4-35 shows a lateral cantilever pontic with a porcelain interdental papilla added between the pontic and the cuspid abutment. A patient with a difficult space problem displayed a "toothy" smile with an existing prosthesis (Fig. 4-36). In constructing the replacement, one pontic was eliminated to balance the left side of the dentition. The patient has a high smile line, and unattractive interdental embrasures were displayed. Fig. 4-37 shows the addition of interdental papillae and the pleasing result.

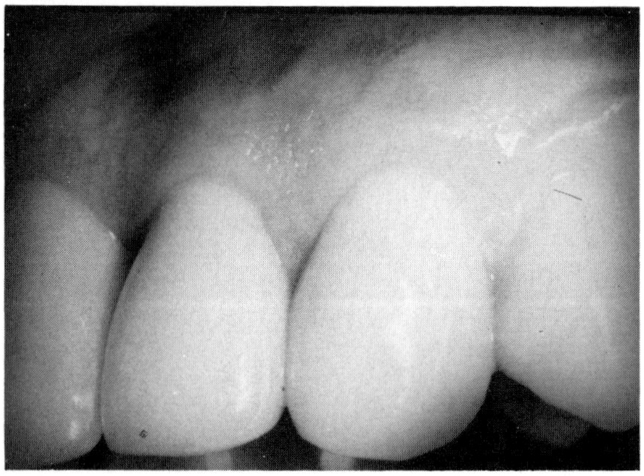

Fig. 4-34. Embrasures present no problems in single tooth restorations with optimal gingival architecture.

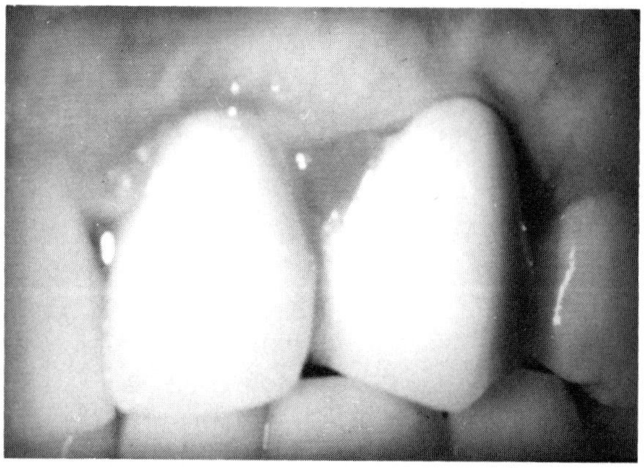

Fig. 4-35. When tooth is lost (here lateral incisor), tissue resorption may present unsightly embrasure problem that can be concealed with pink porcelain papilla.

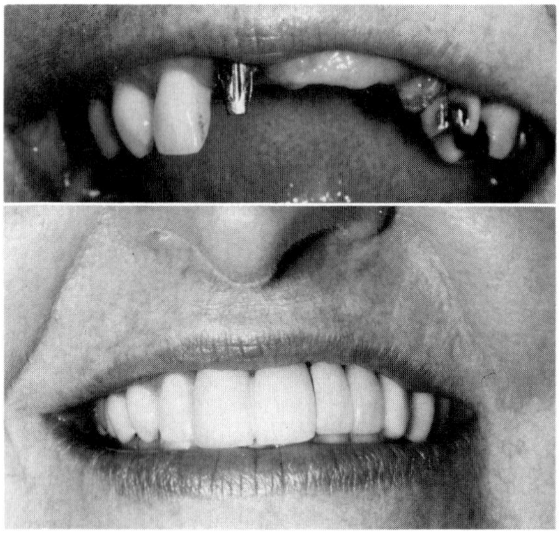

Fig. 4-36. Problem space was restored with prosthesis that gave patient unbalanced and "toothy" appearance.

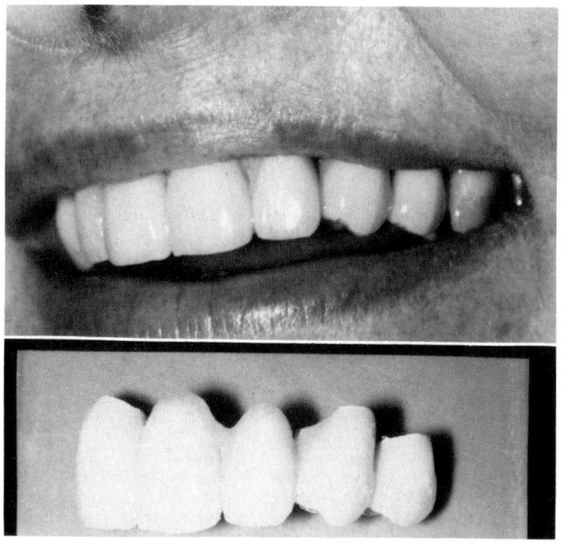

Fig. 4-37. Subsequent restoration restored optimal harmony. Embrasures had to be masked by slight additions of pink interdental papillae.

CHANGES IN TOOTH WIDTH

A diastema may be closed, without undue increase in visible tooth size, by altering the tooth position and by delicate interproximal contouring. The anterior teeth, from an incisal view, are positioned to describe a given curvature (Fig. 4-38). The greater the curvature, the larger the interproximal separation or diastema. In treating these cases, orthodontic measures should be explored to reposition the teeth lingually to effect minimal diastemas. To a minor degree, the curvature described by protruding anterior teeth can be reduced by maximal facial reduction during tooth preparation. The objective is to gain a tooth outline form as narrow as possible before supplemental contour adjustments. In preparation for these adjustments, the proximal contacts are placed lingually, which permits the contouring of large facial embrasures and aids in silhouetting the facial line angles of the tooth. In some instances, the tooth surface adjacent to the facial embrasure may be hollow ground incisogingivally to increase the shadow effect of the embrasure. The line angle formed will lend more definition to a highlighted tooth outline form. This procedure of hollow grinding the mesial and distal tooth surfaces can reduce the apparent tooth size by 1.5 mm or by 6 mm in the restoration of all maxillary incisors (Fig. 4-39).

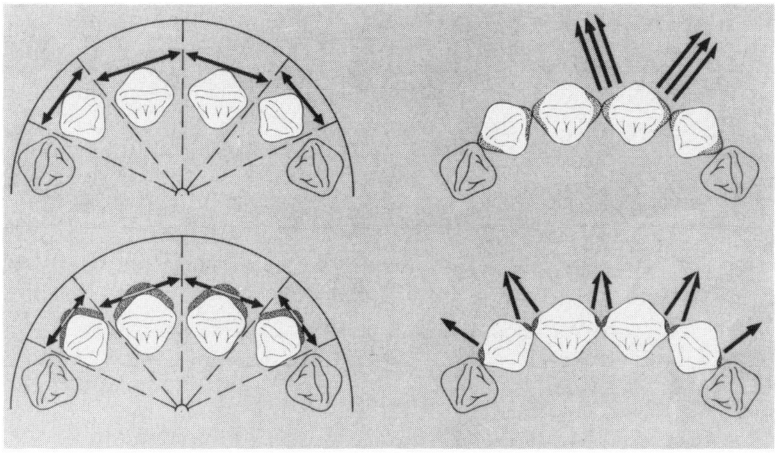

Fig. 4-38. To close diastemas teeth should be lingally repositioned and axial line angles hollow ground.

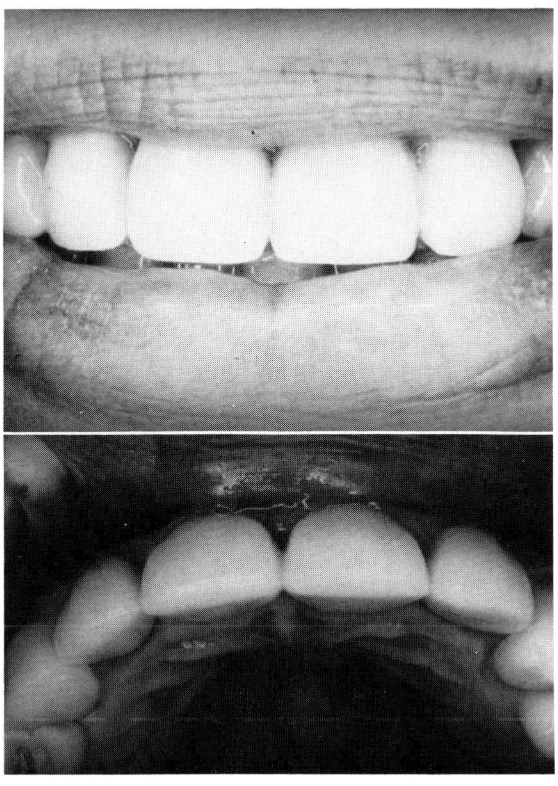

Fig. 4-39. Appearance of mesiodistal width of incisors was substantially reduced by proximal hollow-grinding technique.

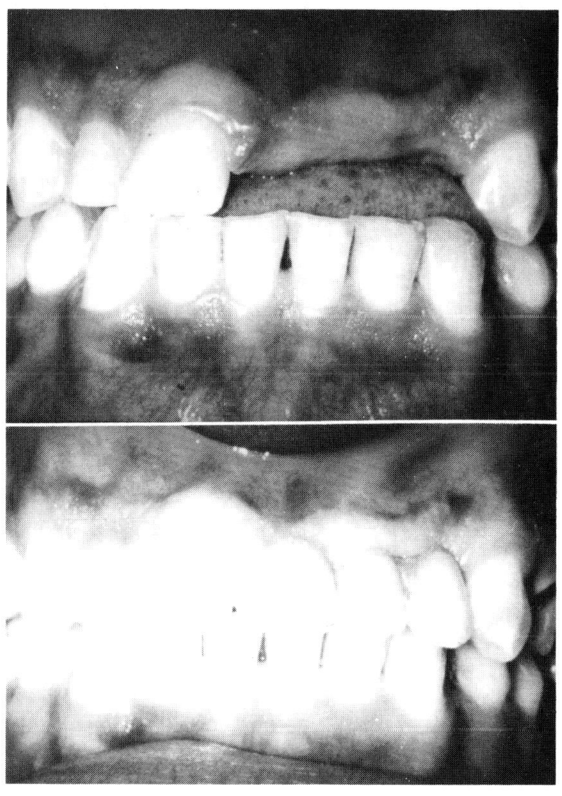

Fig. 4-40. Excessively wide spaces can be bridged by addition of supernumerary teeth. This was contraindicated for this patient.

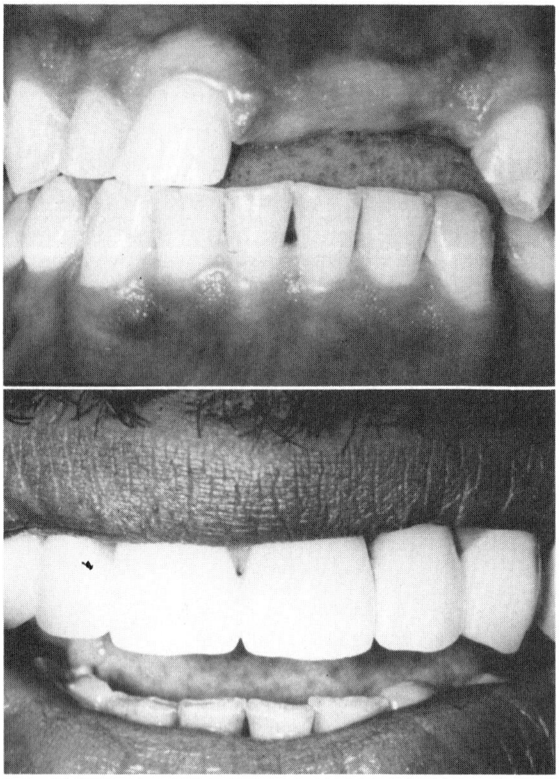

Fig. 4-41. Patient could tolerate larger tooth. Interproximal hollow-grinding gave optimal cosmetic effect.

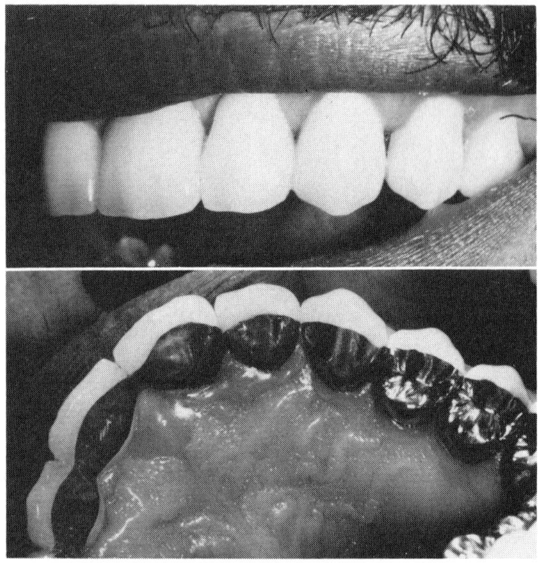

Fig. 4-42. Lateral and occlusal view of completed cast.

The use of a supernumerary tooth, frequently a maxillary lateral incisor, can be the most favorable solution of a "too much space" problem. For the patient in Fig. 4-40, the teeth, including his natural teeth appeared too small. Figs. 4-41 and 4-42 show the fixed partial denture, with supplemental interproximal contour modifications to effect a bold, masculine tooth form, but does not appear too large for the patient's strong facial architecture.

Fortunately, a supernumerary central incisor is rarely indicated; however, there was no better treatment alternative for this patient (Fig. 4-43). The pontic bridges the midline and consequently should be contoured to form a mesiofacial embrasure with the right and left central incisor abutment teeth (Fig. 4-44). As the patient smiles, the pontic can appear deceptively natural (Fig. 4-45).

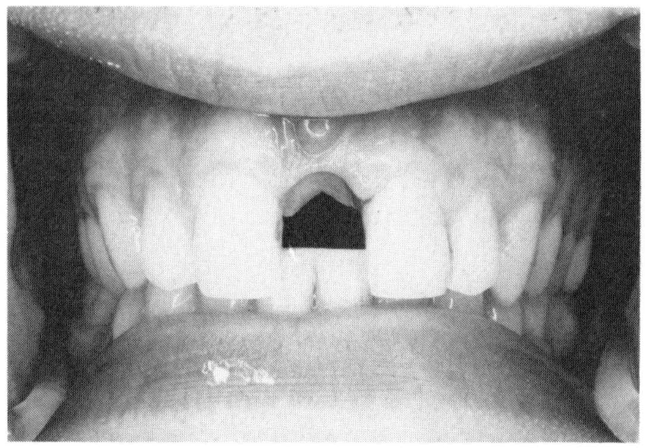

Fig. 4-43. Edentulous space centered over patient's midline.

Fig. 4-45 also illustrates the use of a solder connector or incisal papilla loop to effect a diastema. A few patients express a great desire to retain this characteristic when anterior teeth need replacement. A small separation between teeth (1 to 1.5 mm) can be effected with a V-shaped solder connector. The acute apex prevents unsightly display of the metal. The separation will appear like a space. For a larger diastema effect (1.5 mm

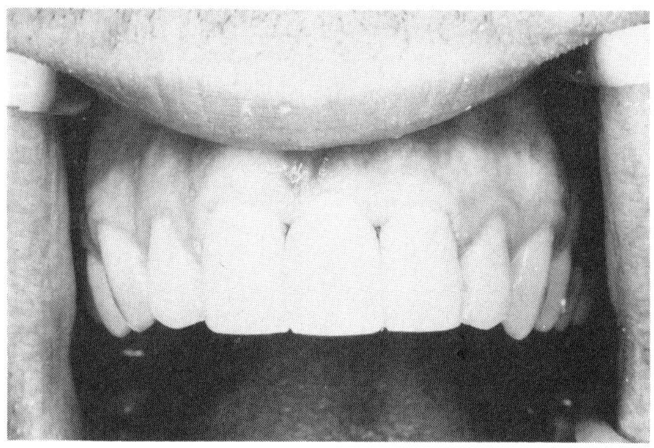

Fig. 4-44. Central incisor pontic forms mesiofacial embrasure with right and left central incisor abutment.

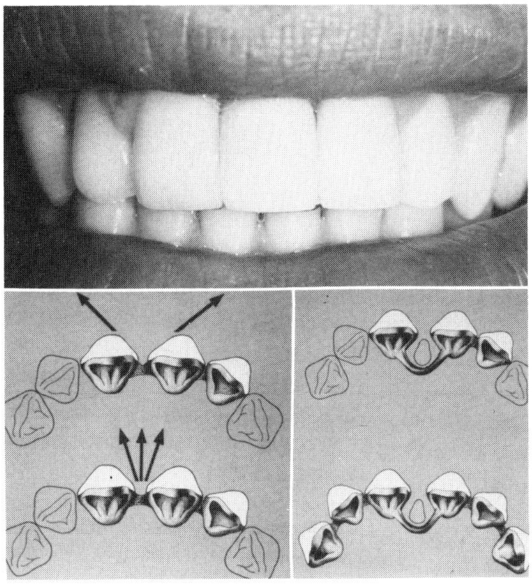

Fig. 4-45. To casual observer supernumerary central may appear deceptive. Small diastema may be effected by wide V-shaped solder joint or by incisal papilla loop for l.5- to 2.0-mm wide diastemas.

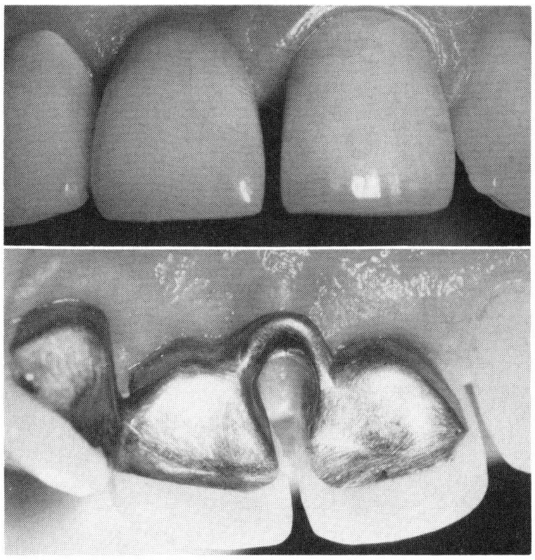

Fig. 4-46. Incisal loop connecter should rest against tissue, similar to pontic tissue contact area, to prevent lodgment of debris.

or more) an incisal loop should be used (Fig. 4-46). The working cast area contacted by the loop is relieved so that the loop will be ın tissue contact, but not sustain pressure.

To gain the effect of larger teeth, the tooth position must be more facial (Fig. 4-47). The proximal line angles are kept prominent and form minimal facial embrasures. The surface form of the tooth is relatively flat with a texture of predominantly horizontal lines (Fig. 4-48).

The patient in Fig. 4-49 has a prominent premaxilla and insufficient space for the large central incisors indicated by his strong facial features. The diagram superimposes the proper pontic size on the insufficient space, and two solutions are suggested. When the pontics are prominently displayed the teeth appear largest. In this case it was contraindicated because of the patient's prominent premaxilla. The optimal solution was to position the pontics lingually with the lateral incisors overlapping. This caused the laterals to appear relatively small and emphasized the size of the central incisors (Fig. 4-50).

An edentulous space too small to accommodate two maxillary premolar pontics can be occupied with a molar pontic (Fig. 4 51). The molar is recontoured by deepening the buccal groove and accentuating its depth with stain. The distobuccal slope is dramatically shortened on the first premolar and may be totally absent on the second premolar. The effect will be the appearance

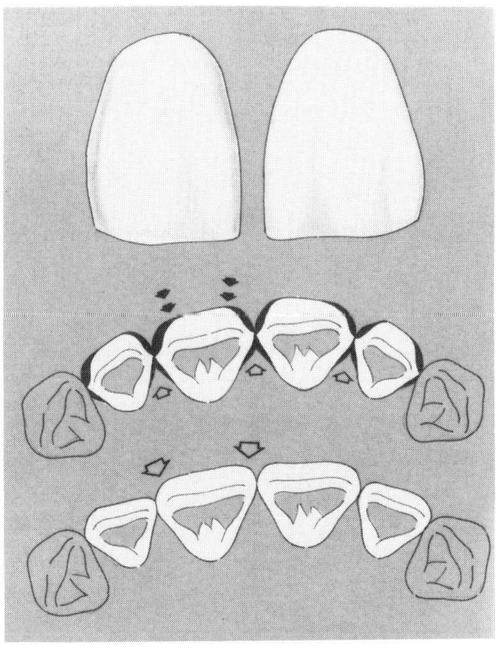

Fig. 4-47. Central incisors are equal in size but not appearance. So tooth can appear narrowed by proximal hollow-grinding, its width can be emphasized by prominent proximal line angles, flat surface form, and horizontal incremental lines.

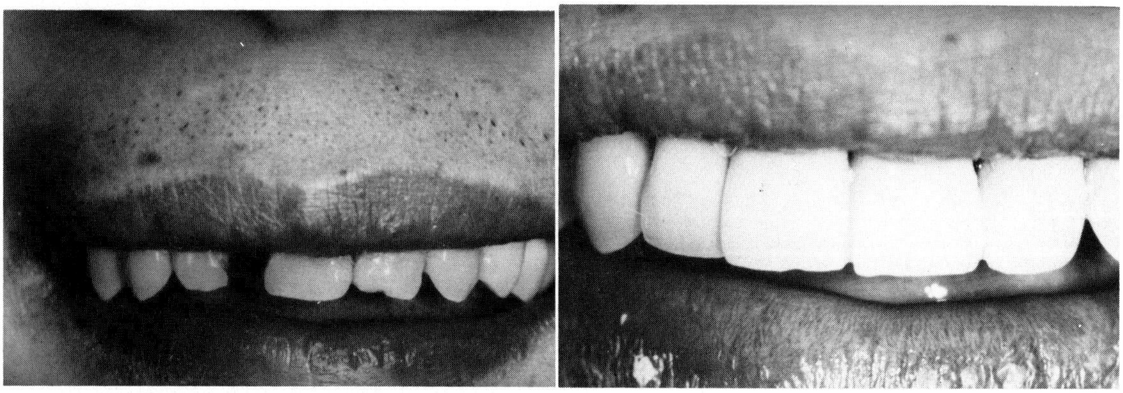

Fig. 4-48. Patient's mouth with insufficient space was restored without additional tooth extractions. Principles of emphasizing tooth width were applied.

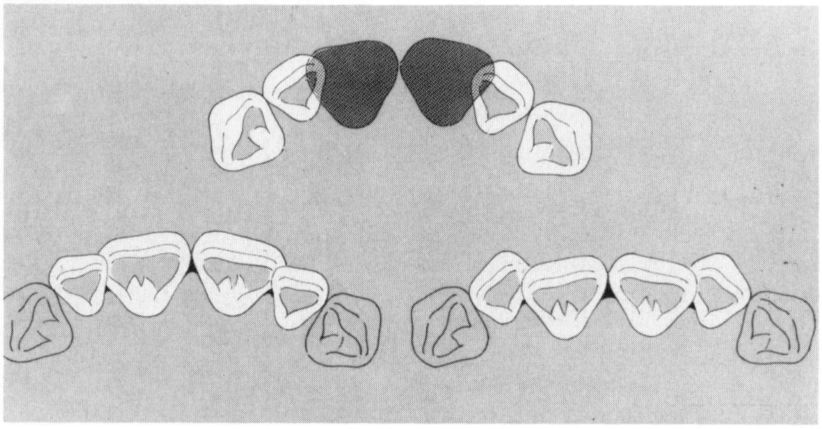

Fig. 4-49. Prominent premaxilla and insufficient space for two properly proportioned central incisor pontics require overlapping. Illustration offers two choices.

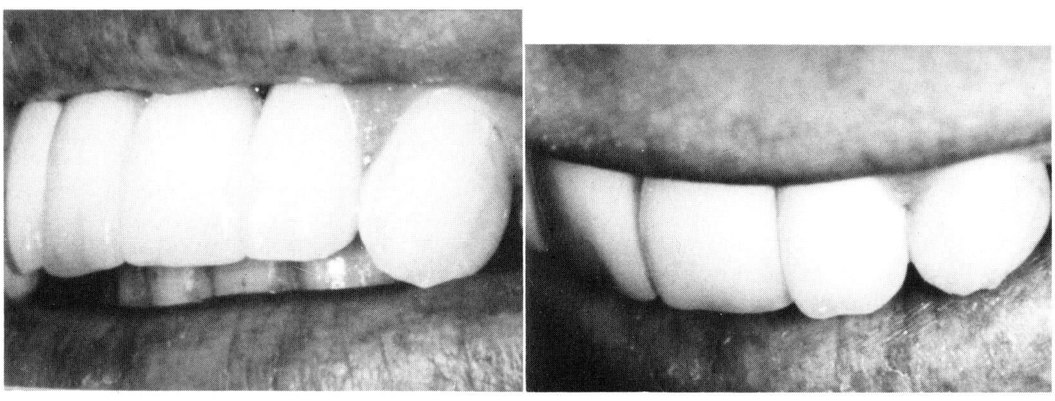

Fig. 4-50. Pontics should be recessed because of prominent premaxilla.

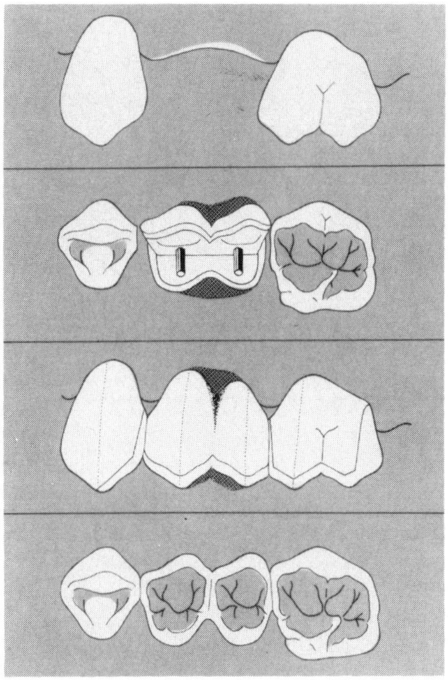

Fig. 4-51. Molar pontic may be fluted to give appearance of two premolars. Note longer mesioaxial slopes.

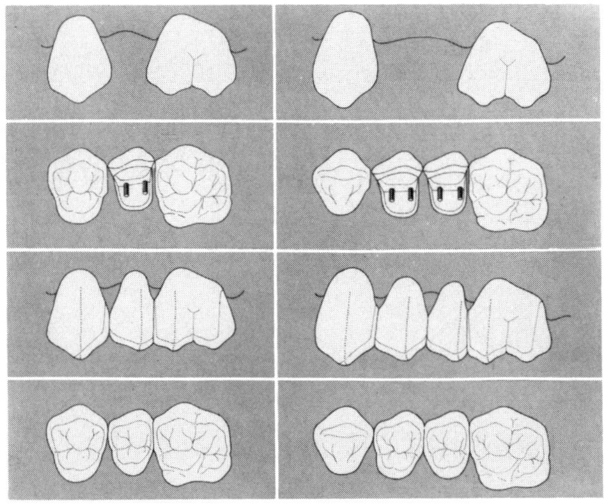

Fig. 4-52. When one or two premolar pontics are contoured for narrow edentulous space, mesial slopes are longest to give appearance of normal tooth.

of the mesiobuccal surfaces of two premolars that are "close to" normal size. In place of a molar pontic two premolars can be contoured with the same favorable illusion (Fig. 4-52).

CHANGES IN TOOTH POSITION

A constricted area can be visually expanded by variations in tooth positioning. This is done by turning the distal surfaces (line angles) of laterals and canines outward (labially). Color will further enhance the effect of a broader smile if the canines and premolars are shaded as light as the incisors. The patient in Fig. 4-53 has a prominent premaxilla with both central incisors remaining. The missing lateral incisors and canines are replaced with pontics. Tooth position and color effect give the patient a broadened smile. The "toothy" smile can be narrowed and minimized by a dominant display of the mesial angles of laterals and canines and by using a relatively dark shade for canines and premolars.

Fig. 4-54 shows a patient with disproportionately small central incisors and a "toothy" smile; also shown is the natural dentition of a male patient with very similar physical characteristics. The centrals predominante, and their dominance is enhanced by the relatively small size of the lateral incisors. The canines are positioned to decrease the width, and their color is one or two shades darker than the incisors. It would take little

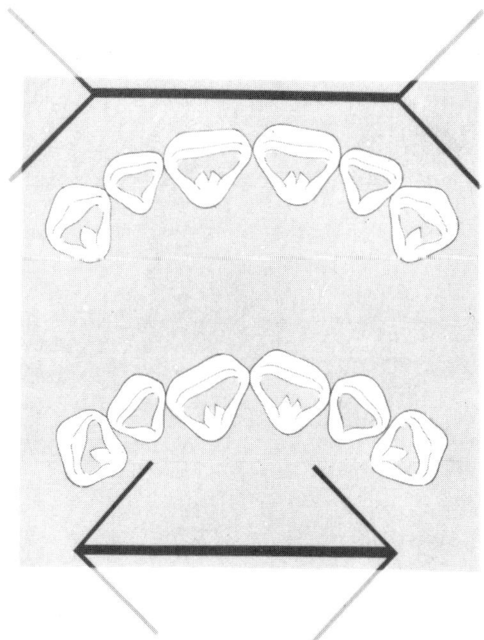

Fig. 4-53. Patient with missing laterals and canines. Central incisors were very prominent. By applying principles of tooth positioning and coloring for widened smile effect, patient was optimally restored.

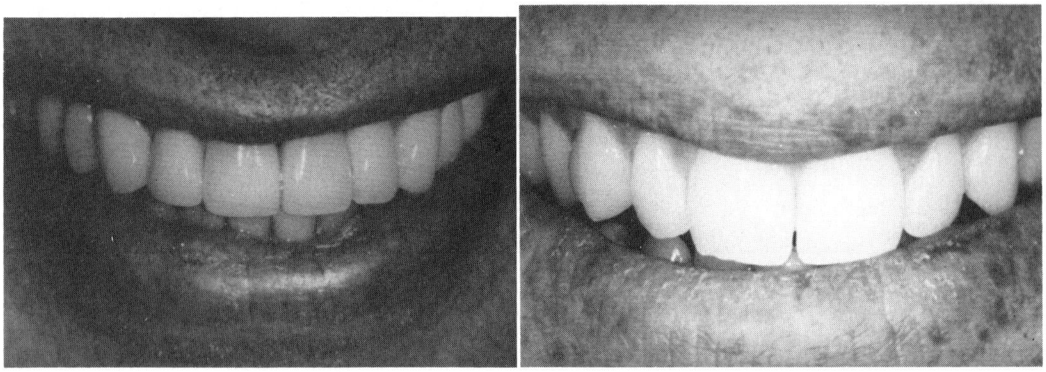

Fig. 4-54. Central incisors are disproportionately small, appearing too "toothy." With some imagination restoration can give patient pleasing smile illustrated here.

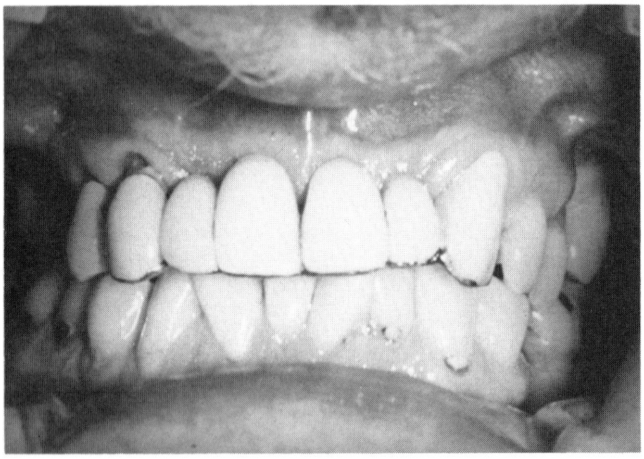

Fig. 4-55. Pontics should not be contoured to fit edentulous space.

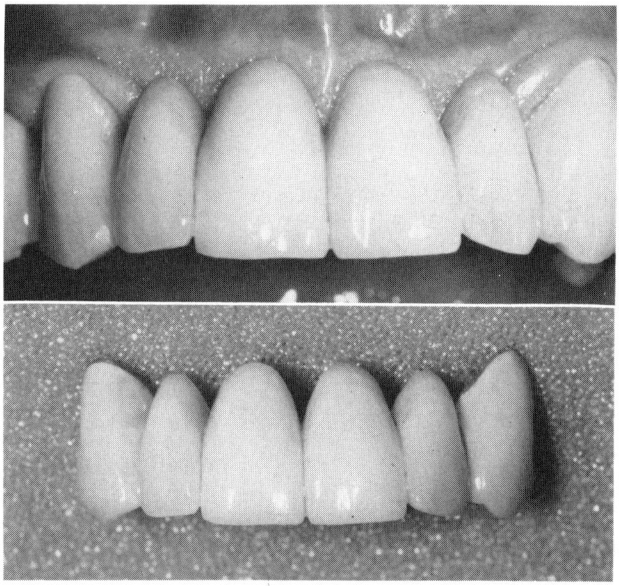

Fig. 4-56. Restorations should be contoured, from cosmetic standpoint, to harmonize with patient's physical characteristics.

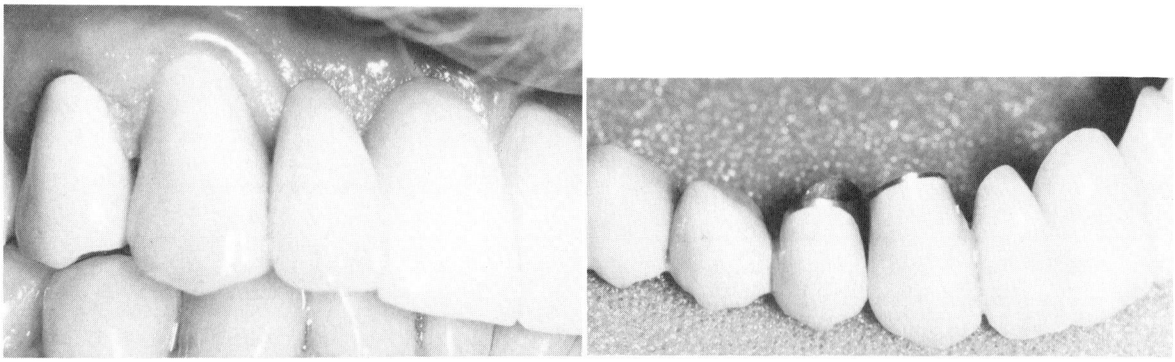

Fig. 4-57. There are various means by which tooth form and position can be modified to satisfy patient's cosmetic function.

imagination to offer a similar attractive tooth arrangement to our "toothy" patient.

In reviewing the suggestions presented in this chapter, the problem space should offer a challenge instead of frustration. In restoring the anterior region of the mouth, we are aided by materials that offer great flexibility for design and fabrication, and it is hoped that in our cosmetic endeavor we do not carve or shape teeth to fill a space (Fig. 4-55), but rather to artistically customize the teeth to fit the patient (Figs. 4-56 and 4-57).

SUMMARY

Patients with problem spaces will be the rule rather than the exception in constructing fixed partial dentures. Therefore an understanding of the phenomena of light and color, the use of illusion-creating custom color characterizations, and special contouring of tooth form are all important parts of developing the expertise and skill needed to create ceramometal restorations that optimally fulfill the patient's cosmetic requirements.

ACKNOWLEDGMENT

I wish to express my appreciation to Mr. Paul A. Lemire, author of *Color in Dentistry*.

BIBLIOGRAPHY

Blancheri, R. L.: Optical illusions, J. Calif. Dent. Assoc. **17**:24, 1950.

Boucher, C. D., editor: Swenson's complete dentures, ed. 6., St. Louis, 1970, The C. V. Mosby Co.

Brecker, S. C.: The porcelain jacket crown, St. Louis, 1951, The C. V. Mosby Co.

Frush, J. P., and Fisher, R. D.: Introduction to dentogenic restorations, J. Prosthet. Dent. **5**:586, 1955.

House, M. M.: Form and color harmony in denture art, Whittier, Calif. 1939, House & Loop.

Koper, A., and Gordon, D. C.: Esthetics in oral restorations (course), San Francisco, Dec. 3, 1971, University of California.

Krajicek, D. D.: Dental art in prosthodontics, J. Prosthet. Dent. **21**:122, 1969.

Lemire, P. A.: Color in dentistry, Bloomfield, Conn., 1975, The J. M. Ney Co.

Pincus, C. L.: Building mouth personality, J. Calif. Dent. Assoc. **14**:125, 1938.

Pincus, C. L.: Cosmetics—the psychologic fourth dimension in full mouth rehabilitation, Dent. Clin. North Am., March, 1967, p. 71.

Pound, E.: Esthetics and phonetics in full denture construction, J. Calif. Dent. Assoc. **26**:179, 1950.

Pound, E.: Applying harmony in selecting and arranging teeth, Dent. Clin. North Am., March, 1962, p. 241.

Shelby, D. S.: Esthetics and fixed restorations, Dent. Clin. North Am., March, 1967, p. 57.

Swenson, H. M., and Hanson, N. M.: The periodontist and cosmetic dentistry, J. Periodontol. **32**:82, 1961.

CHAPTER 5

ARTICULATION AND OCCLUSAL MORPHOLOGY

NILES F. GUICHET

A challenge or prosthodontic service is to restore occlusion with esthetically pleasing cuspal forms that facilitate efficient mastication and concurrently function in harmony with condylar paths of movement. There are many acceptable procedures by which this can be accomplished. However, in this chapter, rather than presenting a specific technique to accomplish the desired objective, a general specification for occlusal development concerning vertical and horizontal loading of teeth is first presented. Then specific relationships that exist between condylar paths of movement and occlusal anatomy are reviewed. An understanding of these relationships will aid the dentist or technician in effectively developing articulation with any of the popular techniques. The use of a pantograph and fully adjustable articulator in diagnosis and therapy to more efficiently develop the prescribed occlusion is also presented.

SPECIFICATIONS FOR OPTIMAL OCCLUSION

Consideration of vertical and horizontal stresses as applied to teeth and how the resultant proprioceptive stimuli affect muscle function dictates the criterion of an optimum occlusion.

Specification one

In considering the reduction of vertical stress, the first specification is to incorporate in the occlusion the following factors:

1. Provide for simultaneous even contact of the teeth in the most intercusped position.
2. Maintain cusp height as far as possible within the esthetic requirements of the patient for maximum masticatory efficiency.
3. Provide for a proportionate area of the food table relative to periodontal support. (This implies providing for proper axial contours and proximal contacts.)
4. Incorporate supplemental grooves.

Specifications for horizontal stresses must also be considered. Teeth can be subjected to horizontal stresses if the patient executes a bruxing movement by moving the mandible retrusively, protrusively, or laterally.

If the dentist provides for maximum intercuspation of the teeth with the condyles anterior to the terminal hinge position, and, if tooth inclines are disposed to prevent the horizontal retrusion of the mandible, the patient could contract the powerful retractor muscles of the mandible and subject the teeth to damaging horizontal loads that they are least capable of withstanding (Fig. 5-1).

Specification two

Specification two provides for maximum intercuspation of the teeth with the condyles in centric relation. It gives consideration to horizontal stresses induced by retrusive bruxing movements of the mandible.

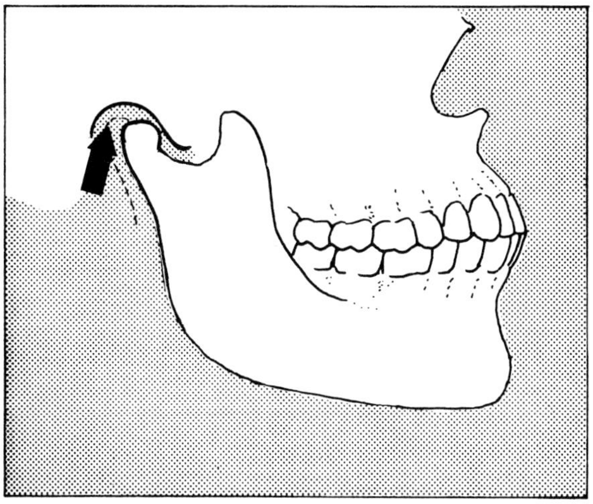

Fig. 5-1. Condylar displacement when maximum intercuspation of teeth is provided with condyles anterior *(arrow)* to terminal hinge position.

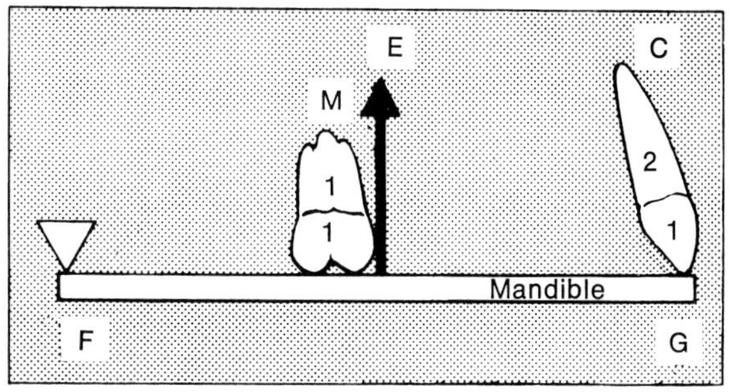

Fig. 5-2. Diagram of mandible as lever *(FG)* and effect of force *(E)* on maxillary canine *(C)* and second molar *(M)*.

Specification three

Specification three provides for horizontal movement of the mandible from the centric-related intercuspal position until those teeth most capable of bearing the horizontal load come into function. It gives consideration to protrusive and lateral bruxing movement.

Specification three merely states not to place the horizontal load on the teeth least capable of bearing the load. When, then, are the teeth most capable of bearing the horizontal load? Imagine a restorative challenge in which the patient is entirely edentulous in the maxillary right quadrant, except for the second molar and canine. Should the restoration be constructed so that the horizontal load in a right lateral bruxing movement would be borne by the canine, by the second molar, divided equally between the two, or distributed in some other manner?

To make this decision it would be valuable to know the relative ability of the canine versus the second molar to bear the load. An evaluation of the relative mechanical advantage or disadvantage each tooth has in relation to the vector of force applied to the mandible by the bruxing muscles, positions of the teeth, length and configuration of their roots, crown-root ratios, and character of their supporting bone dictates the best alternative.

Fig. 5-2 shows the mandible *(FG)* as a lever as it projects from the temporomandibular joint fulcrum *(F)*. Disposed along the mandible is a maxillary second molar *(M)*, a maxillary canine *(C)*, and an arrow *(E)*, representing the force vector of the bruxing muscles. In computing mechanical advantages, the arrow represents the effort, and the *M* and *C* represent resistance.

In considering the ability of the molar *(M)* to resist bruxing stress, note that its relative position on the lever with regard to the effort force vector *(E)* puts the molar at a mechanical disadvantage. The canine *(C)* has a mechanical advantage over the force vector *(E)*. Because of its relative position on the lever with regard to the force vector and fulcrum, the canine has approximately two times the capacity of the molar to resist lateral stress. The crown-root ratio of the canine is more favorable than that of the molar by approximately two times.

An entirely different consideration is the relative length of each root, not in regard to their crowns but in regard to each other. The canine root is approximately two times longer.

The foregoing is merely a biomechanical evaluation of what D'Amico (1958) has shown anthropologically and what we have all seen clinically. Clinical, anthropologic, and biomechanical evaluation indicates that in a normal healthy mouth, the canines are most capable of bearing horizontal stress. It appears that next in order are the first molars, first premolars, second premolars, and, last, the second molars. However, the occlusal scheme cannot be empirical. No one occlusal scheme is optimal for every patient. Consequently, the dentist must prescribe the optimum distribution of stress for each gnathostomatic system based on the result of the examination, evaluation of existing conditions, treatment potentials, and knowledge of the biomechanics of the gnathostomatic system.

MANDIBULAR MOVEMENT

To illustrate the various movements the mandible makes, an articulator is used as a teaching aid. A dental articulator is a mechanical equivalent of the lower half of the head; it is a mechanical jaw, so to speak. A completely adjustable articulator is capable of being adjusted to simulate the mandibular movements of any given patient.

Dental articulators are constructed to be reasonable facsimiles of their anatomic counterparts because this construction provides the most convenient means of producing the desired movements. However, the relative complexity of the posterior control areas of the articulator, the condylar controls, encourages overemphasis of their importance.

Better perspective and understanding can be achieved if the motion produced by the articulator is visualized as a motion that occurs between a beam running anteroposteriorly, which is movable (one member of the articulator), relative to a second beam running in the same direction, which is fixed (the other member of the articulator)(Fig. 5-3).

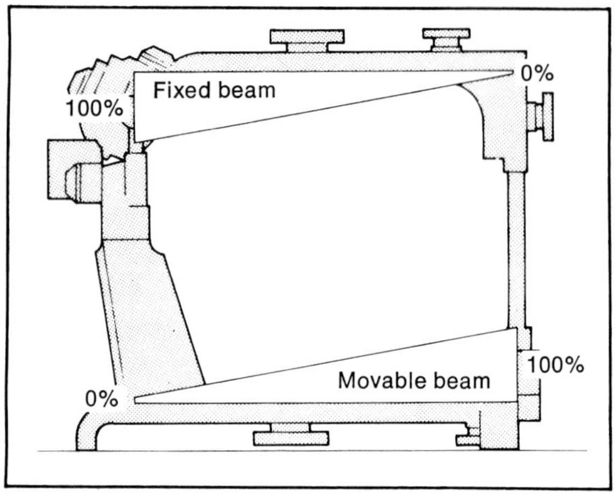

Fig. 5-3. Dental articulator is represented as fixed and movable beam with posterior and anterior controls and relative effect of these controls on articulator movement.

The motion produced by the movable beam is determined by the direction in which each of its two ends, the anterior and posterior, is guided. That is, the anterior and posterior guides have equal influence on the motion produced by the beam, regardless of the relative complexity of the guiding controls.

The posterior controls of the articulator are adjusted in consideration of the patient's condylar paths of movement. These paths may be recorded with a pantograph and diagnosed with an adjustable articulator. The anterior control area of the articulator is adjusted to the vertical and horizontal overlap of the anterior teeth (Pound, 1966). In edentulous mouths the vertical and horizontal overlap of anterior teeth is determined by esthetic and phonetic measurements.

The anterior and posterior control areas of an articulator have 100% influence on the articulator movement produced at each control area. However, the influence of one control area (the posterior, for example) on mandibular movement becomes progressively less when moving from that control area to the opposing area, at which point the influence of the prior control area on the movement produced is zero.

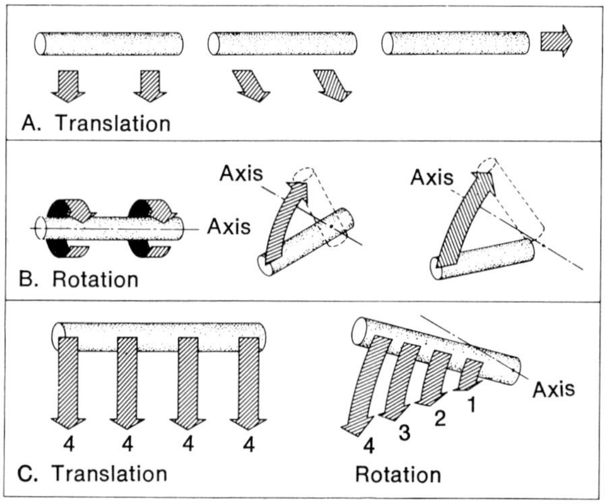

Fig. 5-4. Types of motion. *A,* Translation; *B,* rotation; and *C,* distance one point on beam moves in relation to another point on beam.

Types of motion

The study of mandibular movement can be a very complex study particularly when studying the composite of all movements made simultaneously by the mandible. However, if the complex movements of the mandible are separated into their basic components, the study of mandibular movement becomes a more simple study. The mandible makes two basic types of motion: rotation and translation.

movement Any change of place or position of a body.

mandibular movement Any change in position made by the mandible.

translation (translatory movement) The motion of a body that occurs when all points within the body are moving in the same direction at the same rate of speed (Fig. 5-4, *A).*

rotation (rotary movement) The motion of a body that occurs around an axis. A rotational movement may occur around an axis within the body or outside the body (Fig. 5-4, *B).*

In translatory movement, the distance one point in a body moves relative to another point in the body is a ratio of one to one (Fig. 5-4, *C*). In rotary movement, the distance one point in a body moves relative to another point in the body is directly proportional to their distances from the center of rotation (Fig. 5-4, *C*).

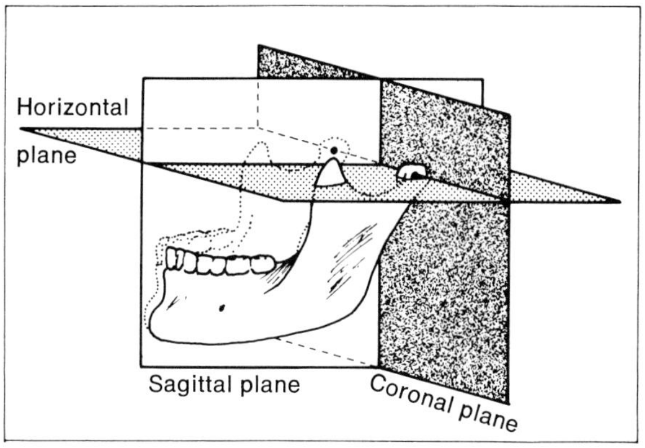

Fig. 5-5. Horizontal, sagittal, and coronal reference planes.

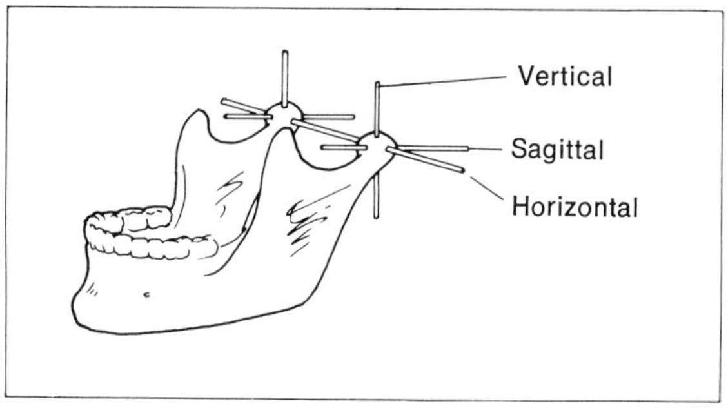

Fig. 5-6. Vertical, sagittal, and horizontal axes of rotation.

Planes of movement

The basic movements of the mandible can be described or studied in three planes, horizontal, sagittal, and coronal, which are mutually perpendicular to each other (Fig. 5-5).

plane An imaginary surface formed by extension of a flat surface through any three definite points of reference that are not in a straight line.
horizontal plane A plane that extends anteroposteriorly and mediolaterally, which is parallel to the horizon and perpendicular to the sagittal and coronal planes.
sagittal plane A vertical plane that extends anteroposteriorly and superoinferiorly, which is parallel to the sagittal suture of the skull and perpendicular to the horizontal and coronal planes.
coronal plane A vertical plane that extends mediolaterally and superoinferiorly, which is parallel to the coronal suture of the skull and perpendicular to the horizontal and sagittal planes.

Classification of mandibular movements according to type and plane

The two basic types of motion, rotation and translation, made by the mandible are studies in three planes: horizontal, sagittal, and coronal. The studies of these movements are therefore classified into the following categories:

1. Sagittal plane translation
2. Sagittal plane rotation
3. Horizontal plane translation
4. Horizontal plane rotation
5. Coronal plane translation
6. Coronal plane rotation

sagittal plane translation of the mandible A translatory movement of the mandible in which each point in the mandible moves within its own respective sagittal plane (e.g., a protrusive movement).
sagittal plane rotation of the mandible A rotary movement of the mandible in which each point in the mandible moves within its own respective sagittal plane (e.g., a centric relation opening or closing of the mandible).

Axes of rotation

In studying mandibular movement, it is important to distinguish between and "axis" and an "axle."

axis An imaginary line described by a rotary movement.
axle A physical part or pin designed to effect a predetermined rotary movement.

The clinical significance of these definitions is that the movement describes an axis. If the motion does not occur, the axis is nonexistent. An axle, on the other hand, is a physical part constructed in such a manner that a predetermination can be made as to what motion will be effected when movement does occur and where the axis (imaginary) will be located when the motion occurs.

Rotary movements of the mandible occur about axes that are perpendicular to the plane in which the motion is described (Fig. 5-6). Following are the rotational movements of the mandible:

1. Sagittal plane rotation occurs about a horizontal axis.
2. Horizontal plane rotation occurs about a vertical axis.
3. Coronal plane rotation occurs about a sagittal axis.

Since the mandible may pivot about either the right or left condyle in lateral excursive movements, vertical and sagittal axes are described in each condyle. However, the horizontal axis is common to both condyles. Following are five axes about which rotational movements of the mandible occur:

1. Horizontal axis (hinge axis)
2. Right vertical axis
3. Left vertical axis
4. Right sagittal axis
5. Left sagittal axis

When studying mandibular movements it must be remembered that the planes in which the motions are

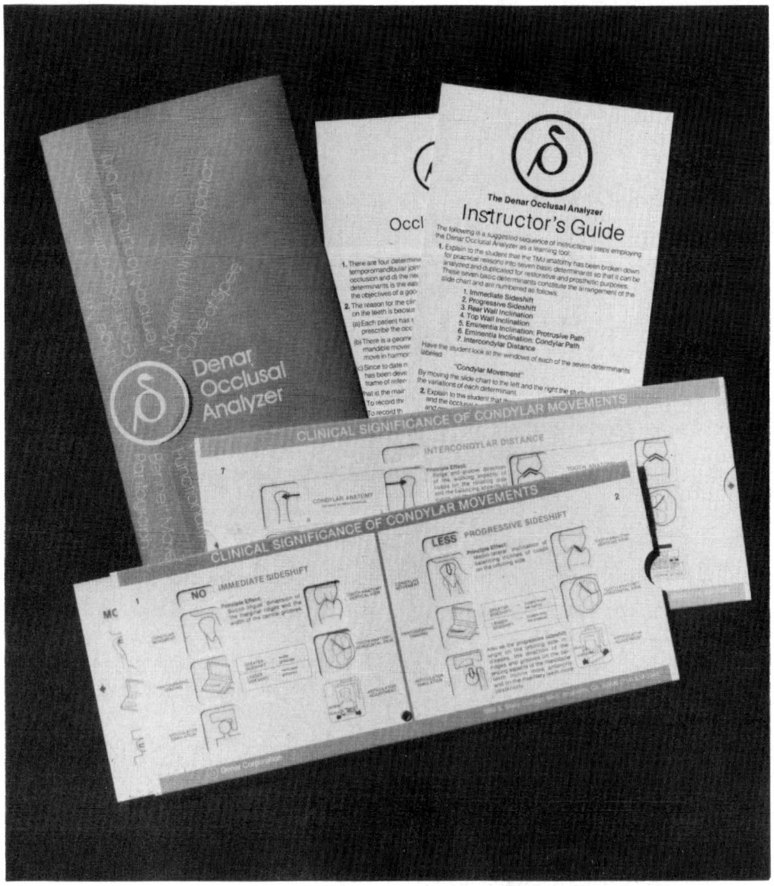

Fig. 5-7. Denar Occlusal Analyzer.

described are fixed reference positions like the points on a compass. The motions are described relative to these fixed planes. For example, a sagittal plane rotation does not imply that the sagittal plane rotates, but that the points rotating are described relative to the fixed sagittal plane.

Following are five general factors of the motion to consider:

1. Type (rotation or translation)
2. Direction (in which plane)
3. Degree of movement (how much)
4. Effect of the movement on occlusal form
5. Clinical importance

Study boards provide the most convenient means of studying the relationships of mandibular movement. They are available from various sources and range from simple plastic overlays that are included in teaching manuals on occlusion to more elaborate devices such as the Denar Occlusal Analyzer (Fig. 5-7).

Mandibular movement studies

Dr. B. B. McCollum is credited with developing the pantograph as a research tool in the 1930s when he and the members of the Gnathological Society were studying condylar paths of movement. The pantograph illustrates condylar paths of movements.

The principle employed with a pantograph is illustrated in Figs. 5-8 to 5-13. Fig. 5-8 is a horizontal plane view of the mandible with the condyles in centric relation. Lateral to each condyle is a rectangular record table that is by some means fixed to the cranium and immovable relative to the cranium. The points marked *C* on the record tables represent the records made by the tips of vertical styli, which are fixed to the mandible and move with the condyles. Anteriorly, the teeth are slightly disengaged by an intraoral center-bearing screw device to eliminate the influence contacting cusp inclines have on mandibular movements (Fig. 5-9). This is because the purpose of the pantograph is to record only the anatomic influence the temporomandibular articulations have on border paths of condylar movements when the movements are not inhibited or influenced by tooth contacts.

When the patient executes a protrusive excursion (Fig. 5-10), the condyles move along paths *CP*, and the styli simultaneously scribe path *C′P′* on the record ta-

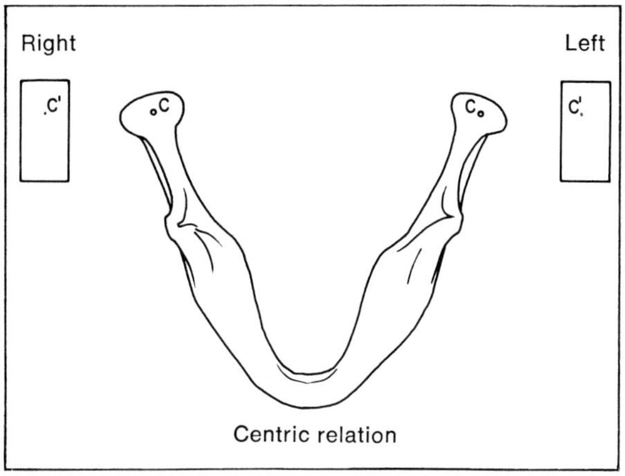

Fig. 5-8. Horizontal plane view of mandible with condyles in centric relation.

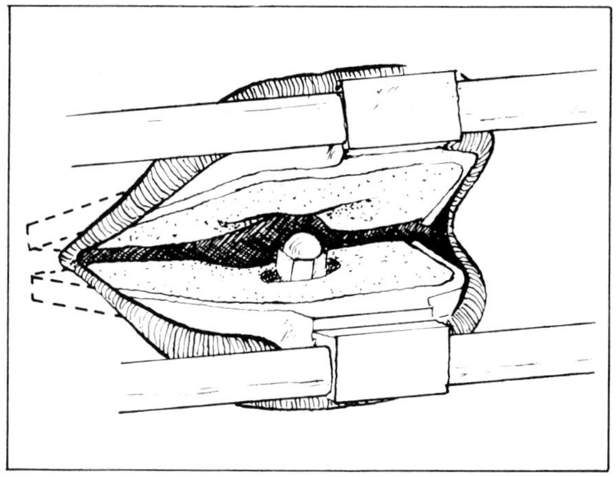

Fig. 5-9. Pantographic recording clutches with center-bearing screw device.

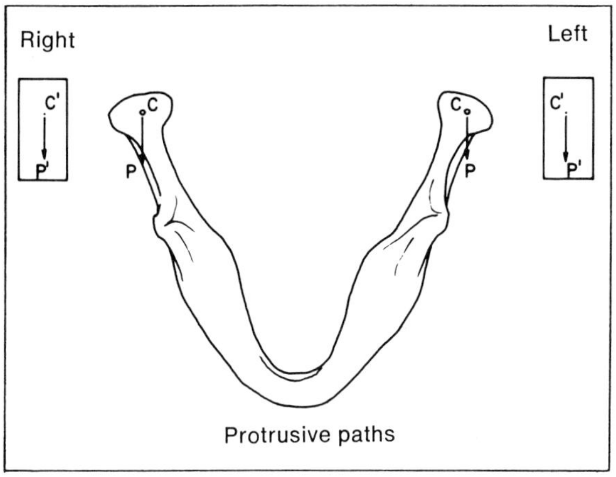

Fig. 5-10. Protrusive excursion. Protrusive condylar paths, *CP;* protrusive condylar path records, *C'P'*.

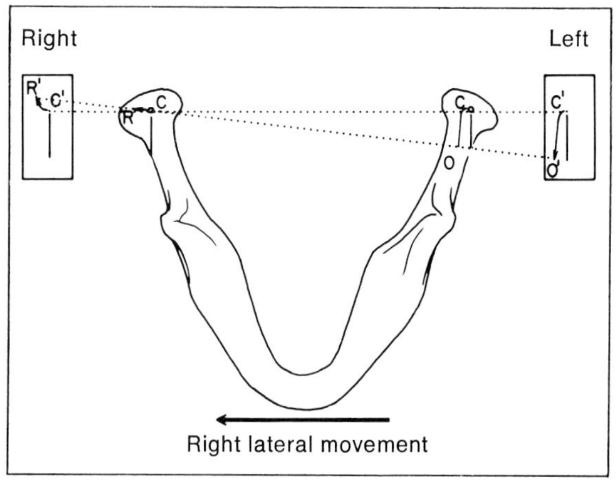

Fig. 5-11. Right lateral movement. Left orbiting condylar path, *CO;* left orbiting path record, *C'O';* right rotating condylar path, *CR;* right rotating condylar path record, *C'R'*.

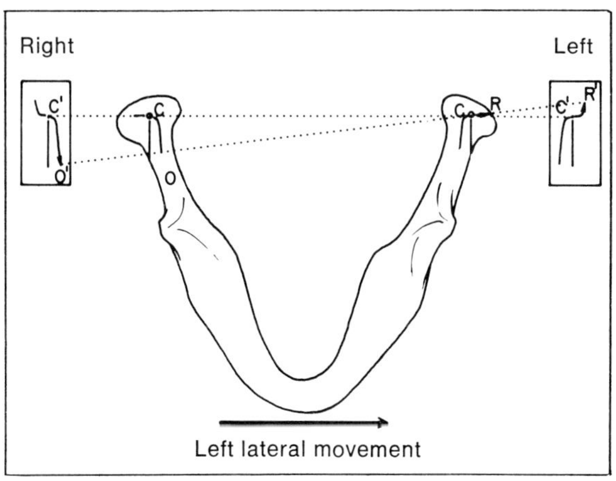

Fig. 5-12. Left lateral movement. Right condylar orbit, *CO;* left condylar rotation, *CR;* recording styli scribe *C'O'* and *C'R'* on recording table.

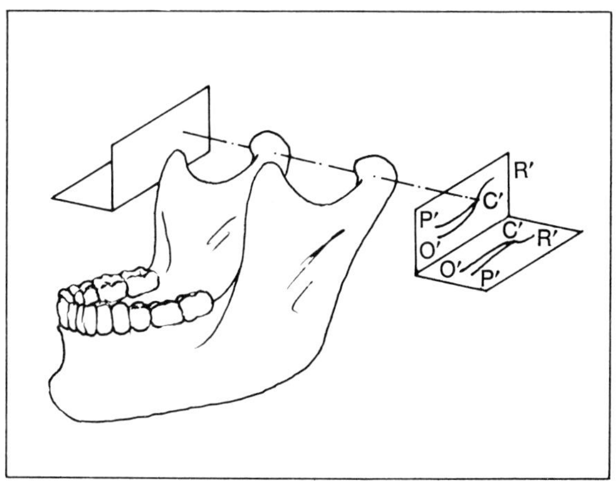

Fig. 5-13. Pantographic recording tables in horizontal and vertical planes.

bles. Paths *CP* are the protrusive condylar paths, and the recordings *C′P′* are the protrusive path records.

When the patient executes a right lateral bruxing movement (Fig. 5-11), the left condyle travels along path *CO* and begins to orbit around the right condyle, which simultaneously rotates and moves outward along path *CR*. Simultaneously the styli scribe lines *C′O′* and *C′R′* on the record tables. Path *CO* is the path of movement of the orbiting condyle and is called the *orbiting condylar path.* The recording *C′O′* is the orbiting path record. Path *CR* is the path of movement of the rotating condyle and is called the *rotating condylar path.* The recording *C′R′* is the rotating path record.

When the patient executes a left lateral bruxing movement (Fig. 5-12), the right condyle begins to orbit about the left condyle as the left condyle rotates and simultaneously moves outward. Concurrently, the styli scribe the record table to complete the recordings as illustrated.

The pantograph records in Fig. 5-12 illustrate condylar paths of movement as viewed in a horizontal plane and reveal important diagnostic information about the patient's condylar movement in the horizontal plane.

To study condylar paths of movement in the vertical plane, vertical record tables are placed in a fixed position lateral to the cranium, and horizontal styli that move with the condyles are used to register on the vertical record tables condylar paths of movement in the vertical plane. A pantograph constructed with recording styli and record tables in both the horizontal and vertical planes is shown in Fig. 5-13. This allows the vertical and horizontal movements of the condyles to be recorded simultaneously. As the left condyle advances along the protrusive path, the vertical and horizontal styli simultaneously track the protrusive path of movement of the left condyle in the vertical and horizontal planes and paths *C′P′* are recorded. The orbiting condyle paths *C′O′* and the rotating condylar paths *C′R′* are recorded in a similar manner.

orbiting condyle The condyle on the side opposite the side to which the mandible is located when the mandible is in a lateral position or movement.

rotating condyle The condyle on the side to which the mandible is located when the mandible is in a lateral position or movement.

protrusive condylar path The path the condyle travels when the mandible is moved forward of its centric relation position.

orbiting condylar path The path of movement of the orbiting condyle when the mandible is moved laterally from its centric relation position.

centric relation The relation of the mandible to the maxilla when the condyles are located in their midmost, uppermost position on the posterior aspect of the articulare tubercle.

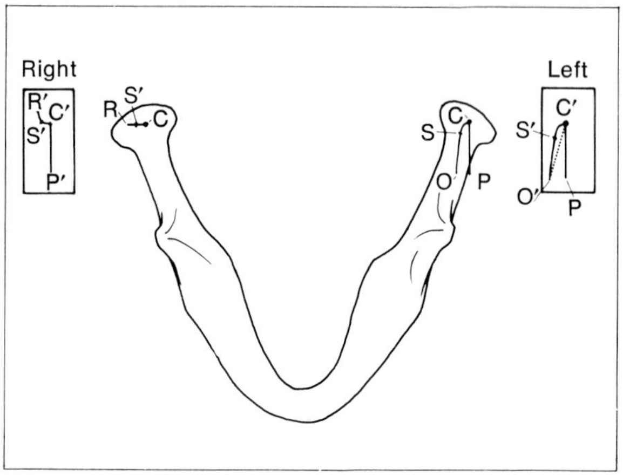

Fig. 5-14. Horizontal view of pantographic study of protrusive and right lateral movement.

Horizontal plane study

Fig. 5-14 illustrates a horizontal view of a pantograph recording of a protrusive and right lateral movement. The right tracing shows that as lateral excursion occurred, the rotating condyle did not stay at point *C*, but moved laterally to point *R*, indicating that the mandible bodily shifted to the side to which the lateral excursion occurred. This movement of the mandible is referred to as the *mandibular side-shift*, or *Bennett movement.*

Orbiting condylar path

The left horizontal tracing in Fig. 5-14 shows that the orbiting condyle did not move in a straight line as it moved from the centric relation position *C* to position *O*, but instead moved medially a relatively substantial amount as the left styli moved from position *C′* to position *S′* on the orbiting condylar path record *C′O′*. This indicates that the rotating condyle also moved laterally a considerable distance along path *CR*. When the left stylus is at point *S′* on the orbiting condylar path, the right stylus is at point *S′* on the rotating condylar path. Most of the mandibular side-shift has occurred by the time the left stylus reaches point *S′*. Subsequently, as the left stylus moves from point *S′* to point *O′* on the orbiting path, the right stylus moves laterally at a constant rate along path *S′R′*.

This study shows that the mandibular side-shift does not occur progressively at the same rate as the orbiting condyle advances in a lateral excursive movement, but it occurs at a greater rate or amount as the condyle leaves the centric relation position than it does later in the excursive movement. Orbiting path recordings are generally essentially straight after the stylus has advanced 4 or 5 mm from the centric relation position. The mandibular side-shift that occurs during the first 4

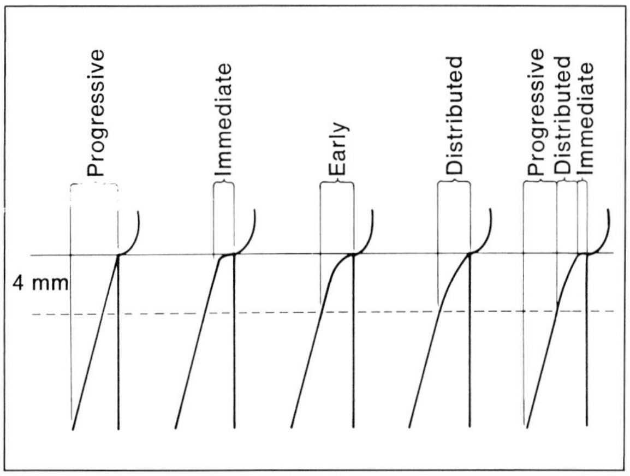

Fig. 5-15. Classifications of mandibular side-shift.

mm of forward movement of the orbiting condyle is classified as an immediate, early, or distributed side-shift, depending on the rate at which it occurs.

mandibular side-shift Bodily side-shift of the mandible that occurs during lateral jaw movement.

progressive side-shift Mandibular side-shift that occurs at a rate or amount which is directly proportional to the forward movement of the orbiting condyle (Fig. 5-15).

immediate side-shift Mandibular side-shift in which the orbiting condyle moves essentially straight medially as it leaves centric relation (Fig. 5-15).

early side-shift Mandibular side-shift in which the greatest rate of side-shift occurs early in the first 4 mm of forward movement of the orbiting condyle as it leaves centric relation (Fig. 5-15).

distributed side-shift Mandibular side-shift in which the greatest rate of side-shift is distributed throughout the first 4 mm of forward movement of the orbiting condyle as it leaves centric relation (Fig. 5-15).

A mandibular side-shift may be made up of more than one component. For example, Fig. 5-15 illustrates the character of an orbiting condylar path, which includes immediate, distributed, and progressive side-shift components.

There are various theories as to which anatomic structures determine the amount of mandibular side-shift. Today, many clinicians believe that the mandibular side-shift is an expression of slack or stretch in the ligaments of the articular capsule of the rotating condyle. The theory is that as the external pterygoid muscle on the orbiting side contracts to move the orbiting condyle medially, the rotating condyle moves out until some of the slack in its articular capsule is consumed (Fig. 5-16). Subsequently, the rotating condyle is braced in this position or moves outward slightly as the orbiting condyle advances.

A dental articulator is used to measure mandibular

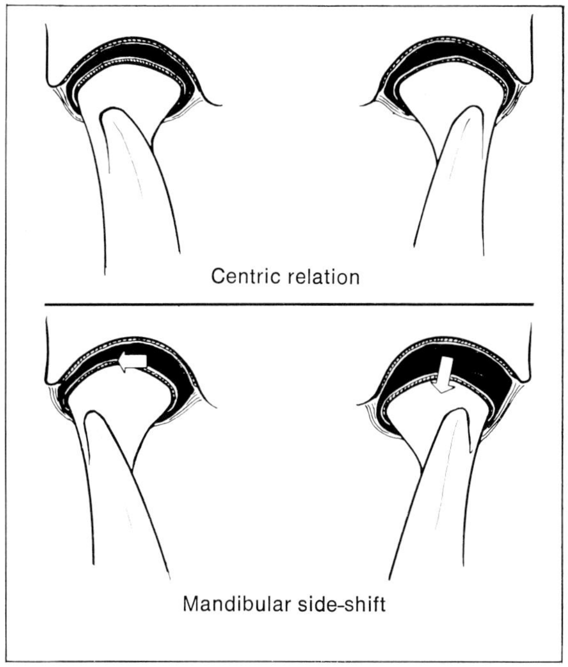

Fig. 5-16. Effect of articular capsule on side-shift.

side-shifts as well as other temporomandibular joint characteristics or condylar paths of movement. The immediate side-shift is measured on the horizontal plane orbiting path record and is expressed in units of tenths of a millimeter (Fig. 5-17, *A*). This value is almost always less than 2 mm.

The progressive side-shift component of the mandibular side-shift is measured relative to the sagittal plane and expressed in degrees (Fig. 5-17, *B*). This value is almost always less than 20 degrees.

The immediate side-shift has primary influence on the width of the central grooves of posterior teeth. The progressive side-shift of the mandible has primary influence on the mediolateral inclination of balancing inclines of posterior cusps on the orbiting side. It also influences the direction of the ridges and grooves of posterior teeth, primarily on tooth contacts on the orbiting side.

Rotating condylar path

As the rotating condyle moves outward along path *CR*, it does not necessarily move straight outward along a path coincidental to the horizontal axis passing through both condyles. The rotating condyle may move along a path that is inclined anteriorly or posteriorly to the horizontal axis.

The inclination of the rotating condylar path in the horizontal plane is measured on the rotating condylar

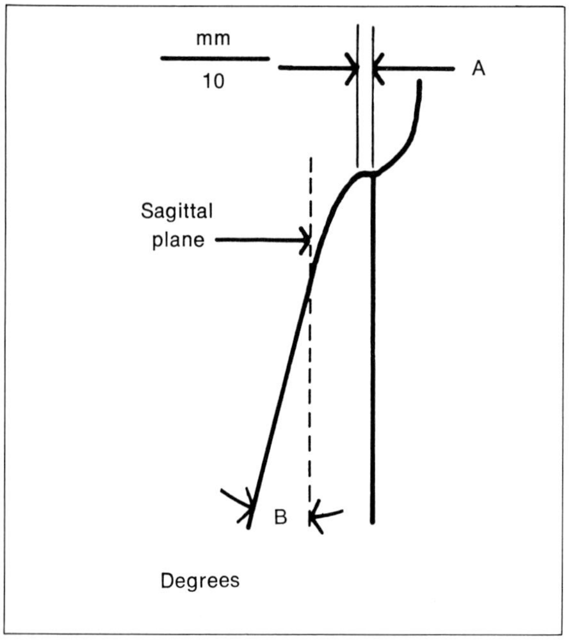

Fig. 5-17. On dental articulator *(A)* immediate side-shift is measured in units of tenths of millimeters. Progressive side-shift is measured relative to sagittal plane and expressed in degrees *(B).*

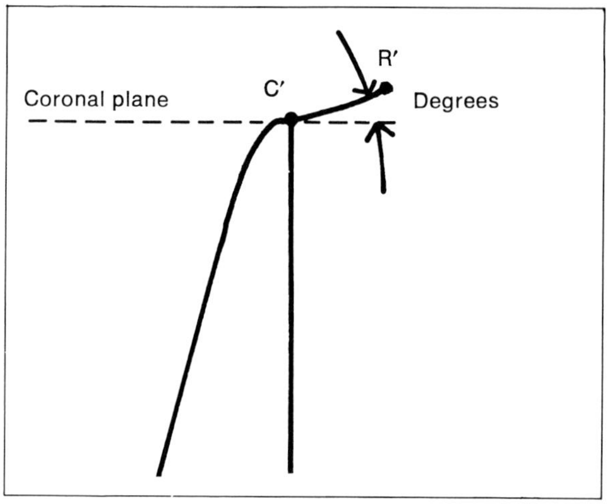

Fig. 5-18. On horizontal recording table, path of rotating condyle *(C′R′)* is measured relative to coronal plane and expressed in degrees.

path recording. This measurement is expressed as degrees of inclination of the rotating condylar path forward or backward relative to the coronal plane (Fig. 5-18). The rotating condylar path can incline as much as 15 degrees forward and 40 degrees backward of the coronal plane. In most patients the rotating condylar path is inclined backward. The rotating condylar path is generally less than 3 mm long.

Vertical axis

The location of each vertical axis is measured in millimeters from the midsagittal plane (Fig. 5-19). The average anatomic location of the vertical axis from the midsagittal plane is 55 mm. The average dimension at which the vertical axis is located medial to the surface of the skin on the side of the face is 12.5 mm.

If pure horizontal plane rotation were to occur in mandibular movement, the rotating condyle would stay in its centric relation position throughout a lateral movement. However, in lateral excursion movements of the mandible, horizontal plane rotation and translation occur. The location of a vertical axis and its translation are recorded on anterior bilateral record tables attached to the mandible, which move with the mandible beneath vertical styli fixed to the cranium (Fig. 5-20). The location of vertical axis *C* (left condyle, Fig. 5-20) and its outward translation influence the direction of the medial leg *CR* of the anterior Gothic arch record-

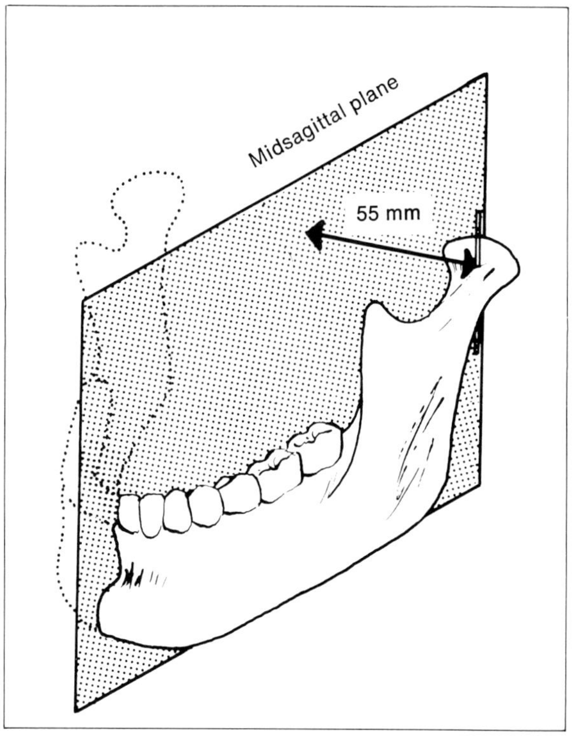

Fig. 5-19. Location of each vertical axis is measured in millimeters from midsagittal plane.

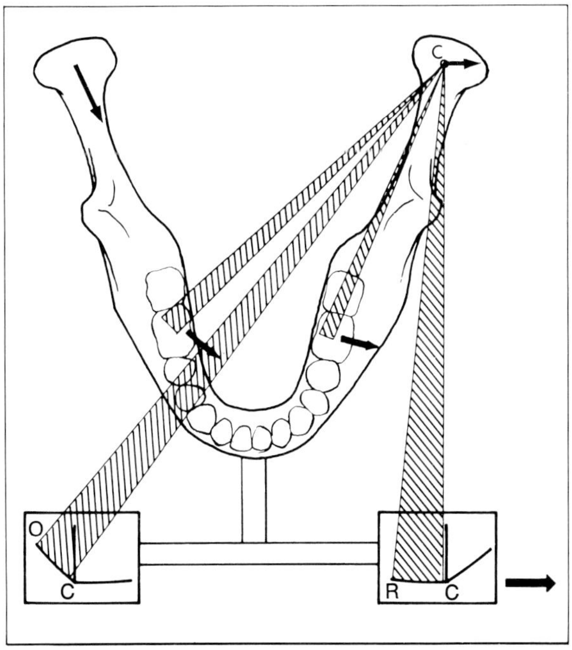

Fig. 5-20. Location of vertical axis *(C)* and its effect on anterior Gothic arch tracing *(CR)* and *(CO)*.

ing on the rotating side and the lateral leg *CO* of the anterior Gothic arch tracing on the orbiting side.

Fig. 5-21 illustrates various basic configurations of the medial leg of a right anterior Gothic arch recording. When there is no forward or backward displacement of the rotating condyle, the medial leg *CR* is straight (Fig. 5-21, *A*). If forward displacement of the rotating condyle occurs, the medial leg *CR* is bowed posteriorly (Fig. 5-21, *B*). If backward displacement of the rotating condyle occurs, the medial leg will be bowed anteriorly (Fig. 5-21, *C*).

The timing of the mandibular side-shift is reflected in an anterior bilateral Gothic arch recording. Fig. 5-22 shows posterior and anterior recordings of the jaw movement of a patient as recorded in the horizontal plane. It should be remembered, however, that in obtaining the posterior recordings, the styli were attached to the mandible, but in obtaining the anterior recordings, the writing tables were attached to the mandible.

As the patient moves from centric relation to the left lateral position, the right posterior vertical stylus records line *CIO*, while the right anterior stylus records line *C′I′O′*. The immediate side-shift occurs as the styli move from *C* to *I* and from *C′* to *I′*. The progressive side-shift occurs as the styli move from *I* to *O* and from *I′* to *O′*.

Sagittal plane study

Fig. 5-23, *A*, is a diagram of the superior limits of the condylar paths of movement as viewed from a position

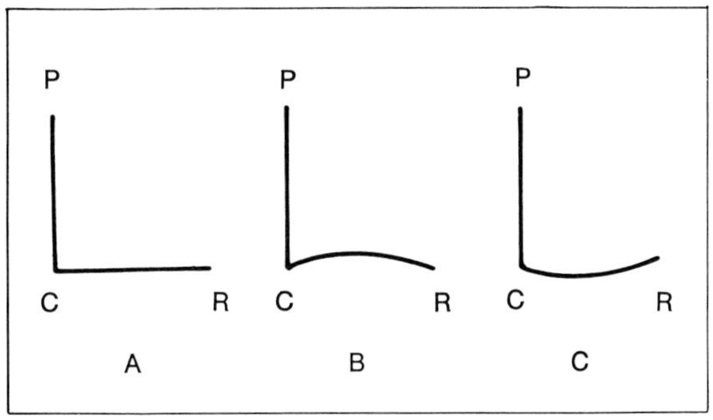

Fig. 5-21. Various basic configurations of medial leg of right anterior Gothic arch tracing recording displacement of rotating condyle.

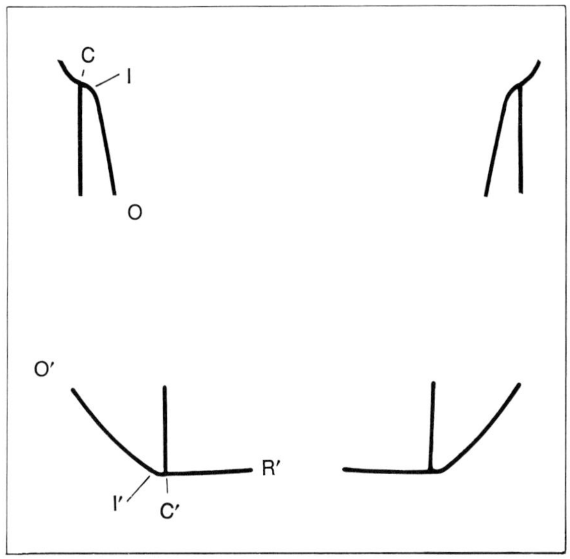

Fig. 5-22. Timing of side-shift *(CI)* as reflected in anterior Gothic arch recording *(C′I′)*.

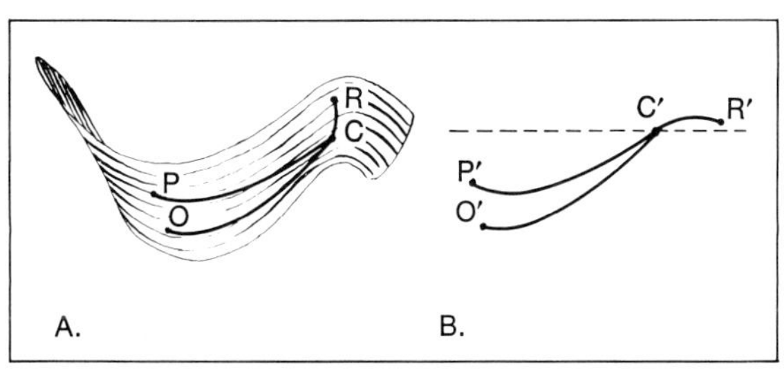

Fig. 5-23. *A,* Diagram of superior limits of condylar paths of movement. *B,* Sagittal plane condylar path recording of movements represented in *A.*

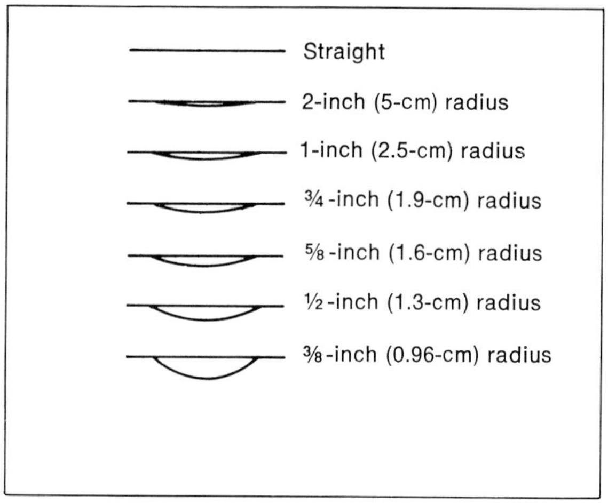

Fig. 5-24. Character of segments of protrusive condylar path may range from straight line to arc of circle of ⅜-inch (0.9-cm) radius.

lateral and inferior to the fossa. Fig. 5-23, *B*, is a sagittal plane pantograph of the condylar paths of movement illustrated in Fig. 5-23, *A*. Note in Fig. 5-23, *B*, that a surface contoured to simultaneously pass through the rotating, protrusive, and orbiting condylar paths has a curved and warped shape (similar to a potato chip).

It must be remembered that a condylar path of movement does not reflect any single temporomandibular joint characteristic. A condylar path of border movement is a composite of joint characteristics. The characteristics include the shape of the bearing surfaces of the disk, fossa, and condyle; degree of tautness and/or elasticity of the capsule and associated suspensory ligaments; and the way these component tissues function against each other when the muscles motivate the condyles to action.

Protrusive condylar path

The protrusive condylar path is generally convex in nature with the convexity facing downward. The character of the curvature of the path is generally flatter in that segment of the path nearest centric relation and becomes increasingly convex as the condyle advances. The character of segments of the protrusive condylar path as viewed in the sagittal plane may range from a straight line to the arc of a circle of ⅜-inch (0.9-cm) radius (Fig. 5-24). The protrusive condylar path is inclined downward from the horizontal plane. Protrusive condylar paths are classified according to their convexity and are measured relative to their degree of inclination from the horizontal plane (Fig. 5-25).

CLINICAL SIGNIFICANCE RULE

The protrusive condylar path inclination has its primary influence on the protrusive inclines of posterior teeth (mesial inclines of mandibular cusps and distal inclines of maxillary cusps).

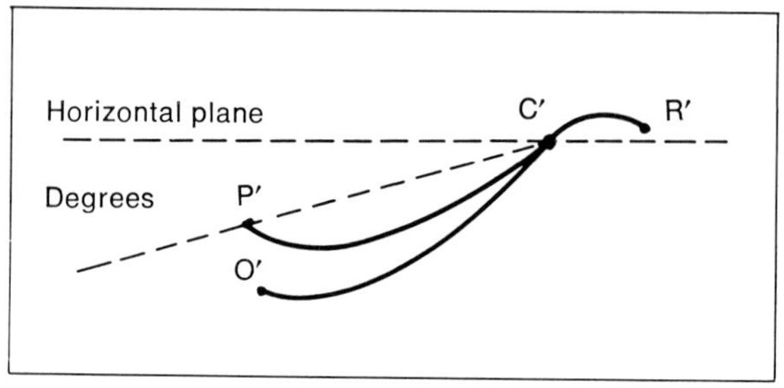

Fig. 5-25. Protrusive condylar path is classified according to convexity and measured relative to inclination from horizontal plane.

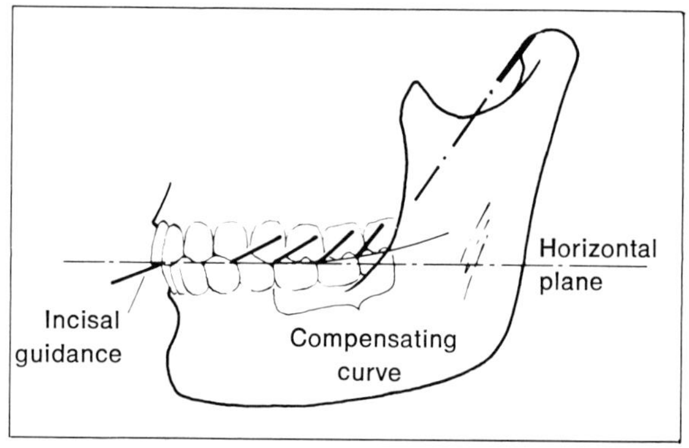

Fig. 5-26. Compensating curve formed by distal inclination of maxillary teeth and mesial inclination of mandibular teeth to harmonize protrusive cusp inclines with protrusive condylar path.

Compensating curve

In restorative procedures the maxillary molars are inclined distally, and the mandibular molars are inclined mesially in progressively greater amounts as the teeth are more closely located to the condyles. This progressively increases the degree of inclination of the protrusive cuspal inclines of posterior teeth relative to the horizontal plane (effective cusp angles), since the teeth are more proximate to the condyles to complement the protrusive condylar path of movement (Fig. 5-26).

compensating curve Anteroposterior curve of the plane of occlusion generated by orienting the plane of occlusion of each tooth in oral rehabilitation so as to provide for a pleasing esthetic effect and a coordinated occlusion.

Orbiting condylar path

In Fig. 5-27, as the condyle protrudes it moves anteriorly along path *C′P′*. However, as the condyle orbits it moves along a more medial path, *C′O′*. The or-

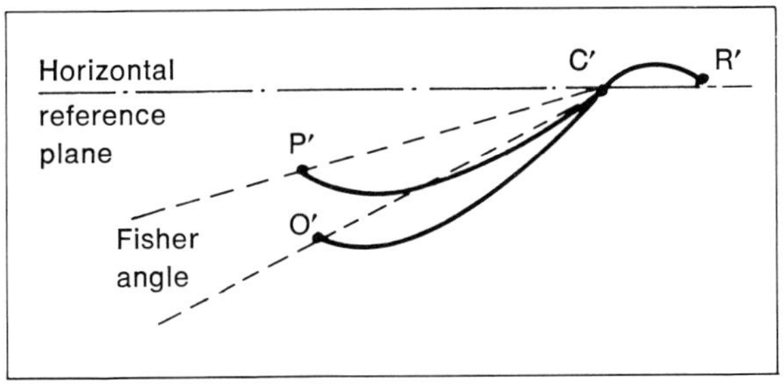

Fig. 5-27. Fisher's angle formed by inclination of protrusive and orbiting condylar paths *(<P′C′O′)*.

biting condylar path is always more medial to the protrusive condylar path and almost always has a steeper inclination. However, it can have the same degree of inclination as the protrusive condylar path. (It very rarely has an inclination that is less than the protrusive path just anterior to centric relation, which suggests derangement of the interarticular disk.) In all other respects the character and inclination of the orbiting condylar path is comparable to the protrusive condylar path. Orbiting condylar paths are classified according to their convexity and are measured relative to their degree of inclination from the horizontal plane.

CLINICAL SIGNIFICANCE RULE

The orbiting condylar path has its primary influence on the balancing inclines of the posterior teeth on the orbiting side—the mesiolingual aspects of the mandibular buccal cusps and the distobuccal aspects of maxillary lingual cusps.

Fisher's angle The angle formed by the inclinations of the protrusive and orbiting condylar paths (Fig. 5-27).

Rotating condylar path

If the paths of movements of the rotating condyle could be observed from a position on the horizontal axis a few inches lateral to the rotating condyle, the rotating condyle would advance toward the observer as it traversed the rotating condylar path. If the rotating condyle traversed a path coincidental to the horizontal axis, the condyle would appear to advance directly toward the observer, and no sagittal plane movement would be observed. However, as the rotating condyle travels laterally, it may track a path that is inclined upward, downward, forward, or backward from the transverse horizontal axis. The movements of the rotating condyle as studied in a sagittal plane view are termed *sagittal displacements of the rotating condyle.* These movements can be of great clinical significance. Sagittal plane rotation of the mandible occurs about the horizontal axis, which translates into normal jaw movements.

horizontal axis An axis that is perpendicular to the sagittal plane described by sagittal plane rotary movement of the mandible.

terminal hinge axis An axis that is perpendicular to the sagittal plane, which is described by sagittal plane rotary movements of the mandible when the condyles are in centric relation.

terminal hinge axis reference points Points on each side of the face through which the terminal hinge axis passes.

posterior reference points Two points located one on each side of the face in the area of the terminal hinge axis or on each side of the articulator on the terminal hinge axis, which together with a third anterior reference point establish a horizontal reference plane from which measurements of the anatomic determinants of occlusion are made.

The posterior reference points are starting positions that are located on the patient by means of hinge axis–locating instruments or by average anatomic measurements. When locating the hinge axis, the posterior reference points are the terminal hinge axis–reference points. The location of the horizontal axis is influenced by and has influence on motions that occur about that axis—sagittal plane rotations (opening and closing movements).

CLINICAL SIGNIFICANCE RULE

The relation of the horizontal axis to the mandibular dental structures of the patient or to casts of the mandibular dental structures on the articulator influences the path or arc of opening and closing that the mandibular structures follow relative to the maxilla in opening and closing movements.

Therefore if the vertical dimension is in any way changed on the articulator (as occurs when casts of the dental structures are mounted in an articulator at an increased vertical dimension and then restored to the vertical dimension at which the restoration is to be constructed), the relation of the mandibular dental structures to the horizontal axis of the patient must be coincidental to the relation of the mounted mandibular cast to the horizontal axis of the articulator. This is necessary so that the mandibular cast will have the same relation to the maxillary cast as the mandibular dental structures of the patient have to the maxilla at any vertical dimension.

Coronal plane study

Fig. 5-28, *A*, illustrates condylar paths of movement as they would appear from a frontal view. The condyle moves up and down and mediolaterally as its movements are studied in the coronal plane. Fig. 5-28, *B*, illustrates the coronal plane record of condylar paths of movement. The record table is positioned parallel to the coronal plane and the stylus parallel to the sagittal axis.

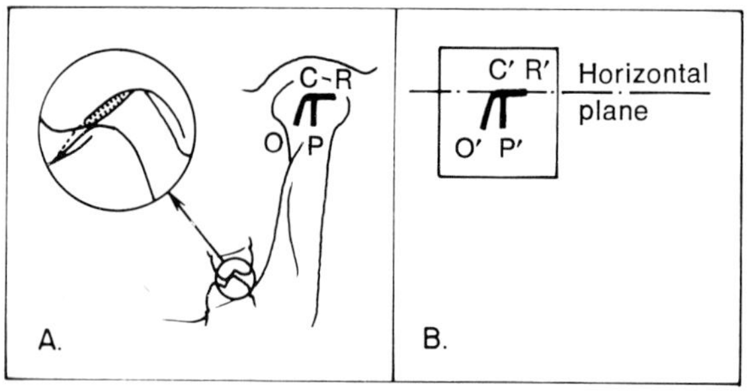

Fig. 5-28. *A,* Condylar path movements as they appear from frontal view. *B,* Coronal plane record of condylar paths of movement.

A single plane recording of mandibular movement (i.e., sagittal plane) will record movement of the condyle in two directions (i.e., up and down and backward and forward). By adding a second record table (i.e., horizontal) movement of the condyle in the third direction (mediolaterally) can be recorded. Note that only two record tables are necessary to record movements in all three directions. Since the sagittal and horizontal plane studies provide the largest recordings, coronal plane recordings of condylar paths of movement are not done in practical clinical procedures. However, a coronal plane record most effectively illustrates the upward or downward inclination of the rotating condylar path in occlusal studies.

Protrusive condylar path

Line *C'P'* in Fig. 5-28, *B,* reflects the amount of downward movement of the condyle as it advances from centric relation in the protrusive excursion. The character and amount of this movement is most effectively illustrated and studied in the sagittal plane.

Orbiting condylar path

Line *C'O'* reflects the character and amount of downward and medial movement of the orbiting condyle as it traverses the orbiting path. The amount of character of this movement is best studied in the sagittal and horizontal planes. However, the character and amount of the immediate side-shift is reflected in the orbiting path record *C'O'* (Fig. 5-28, *B*).

By studying Fig. 5-29 and simultaneously visualizing condylar paths of movement during a right lateral excursive movement, one can understand the relationship between the immediate side-shift and the width of the central groove of the teeth. Also as the orbiting condyle traverses the progressive side-shift portion of the orbiting path *CO,* one can appreciate why the progressive side-shift has a primary influence on the mediolateral inclination of the balancing inclines of cusps on the orbiting side.

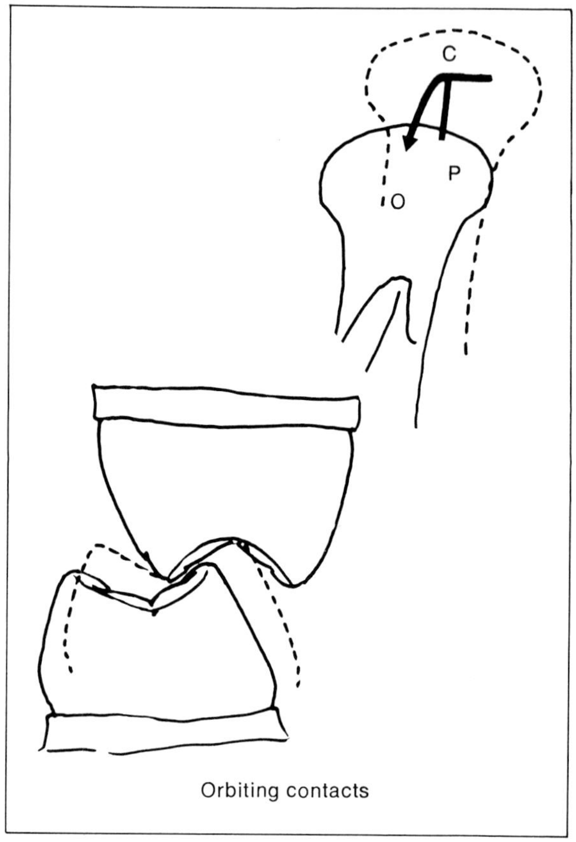

Fig. 5-29. Influence of immediate side-shift and orbiting condylar path on width of central grooves and balancing inclines of cusps on orbiting side during right lateral excursion.

Rotating condylar path

As the rotating condyle moves laterally along the rotating condylar path *CR* (Fig. 5-28, *B*), it may move straight laterally in the mandibular side-shift, or it may traverse a path that may be inclined upward or downward from the horizontal axis. The amount of mandibular side-shift may be as much as 3 mm. The rotating condylar path may be inclined up to 30 degrees upward or downward as measured relative to the horizontal plane.

By studying Fig. 5-30 and simultaneously visualizing condylar paths of movement during a left lateral excursion, one can understand the relationship between the inclination of the rotating condylar path in the coronal plane on the height of working cusps of posterior teeth on the working (rotating) side.

CLINICAL SIGNIFICANCE RULE

The degree of upward or downward inclination of the rotating condylar path has its primary influence on the mediolateral inclination of the working bite inclines of posterior cusps on the rotating side. This affects the

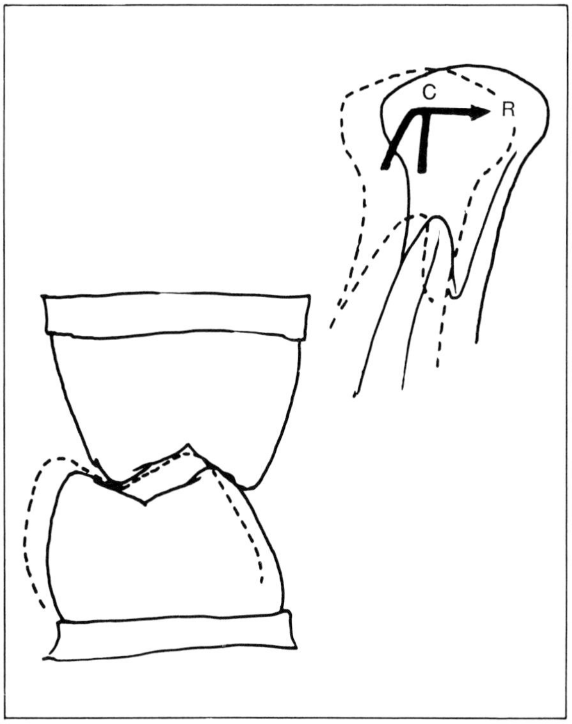

Fig. 5-30. Influences of rotating condylar path *(CR)* on height of cusps on working side.

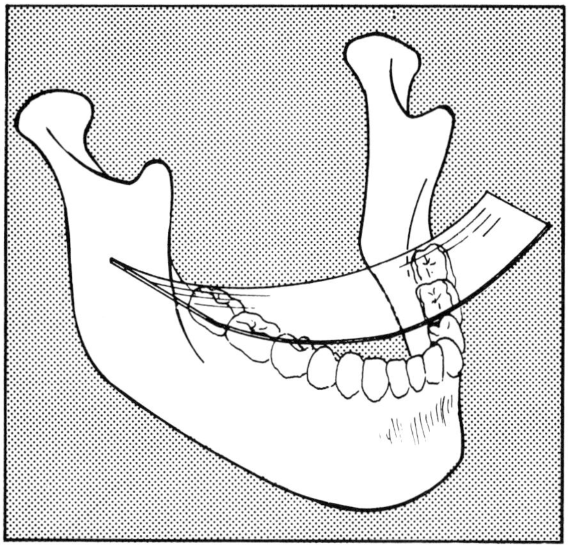

Fig. 5-31. Mediolateral curvature of plane of occlusion (curve of Wilson).

height of these cusps and/or the buccolingual inclination of posterior teeth.

Curve of Wilson

As one progresses more posteriorly in the dental arches, the mandibular teeth incline more lingually, and the maxillary incline more bucally (Fig. 5-31). This anatomic arrangement of posterior teeth provides an intimate shearing relation of the balancing inclines as the orbiting condyle traverses the orbiting condylar path. When the same condyle traverses the rotating condylar path, the shorter maxillary buccal and mandibular lingual cusps provide for an intimate shearing relation between the working inclines of posterior teeth.

curve of Wilson The mediolateral curvature of the plane of occlusion to complement condylar paths of movement (Fig. 5-31).

Sagittal axis

The sagittal axis is perpendicular to the coronal plane, described by coronal plane rotations of the mandible. Of the three types of rotary movements of the mandible, coronal plane rotations occur in the smallest degree, and the precise location of the sagittal axis is of the least clinical significance.

CLINICAL SIGNIFICANCE DISCUSSION

When simulating mandibular movement on an articulator, the horizontal and vertical axes of rotation are located in their approximate positions by anatomic measurements. The sagittal axis is automatically located at the intersection of the horizontal and vertical axes within the condylar element of the articulator.

In the skull it is doubtful that the three axes passing through a condyle ever intersect at a common point. In the condylar element of an articulator, the three axes always intersect. However, rotational movements that occur about the sagittal and vertical axes are so imperceptibly influenced by slight changes (3 mm or less) in the location of these axes relative to each other on the articulator that their influence on occlusal morphology is of no clinical significance. Precise location of the horizontal axes, however, is of greater clinical significance if there will be a change of vertical dimension of the casts on the articulator after mounting the casts.

CONDYLAR PATHS OF MOVEMENTS: PANTOGRAPHIC RECORDS AND OCCLUSAL ANATOMY

The pantographic records described previously in this chapter were made with a pantograph with tracking styli (posterior styli moved with the condyles). The records obtained with this type of instrument facilitate the study of mandibular movement. However, a pantograph constructed with tracking tables (posterior record tables move with the condyles) offers advantages that facilitate its routine clinical use. The following discussions present a study of recordings obtained with a pan-

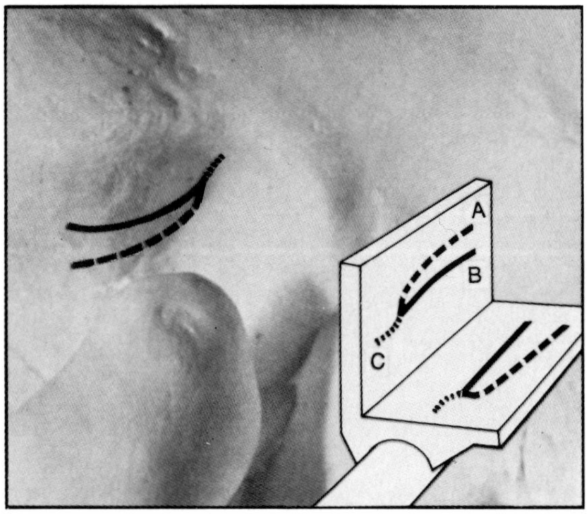

Fig. 5-32. Left condyle and posterior record table.

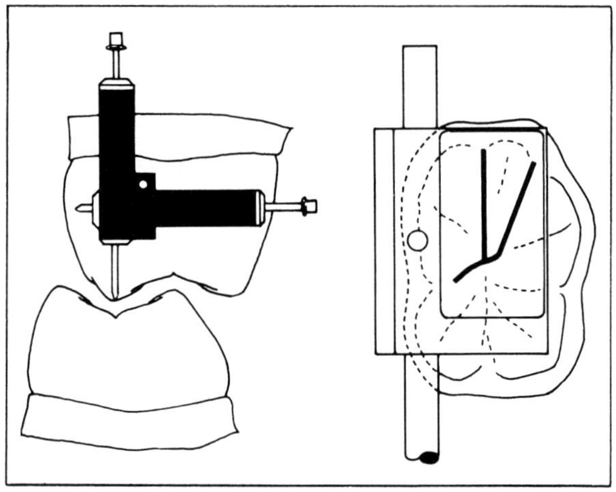

Fig. 5-33. Recording styli are visualized as maxillary cusps and recording tables as occlusal surfaces of mandibular teeth.

tograph that has tracking tables. The illustrations correlate condylar paths of movement, pantographic recordings, and occlusal anatomy.

Fig. 5-32 shows a left condyle and posterior record tables that move with the condyle. By studying this illustration and visualizing the record tables moving with the condyle, the protrusive, orbiting, and rotating condylar paths of movement of the condyle can be correlated with their respective recordings. The vertical record table can be interpreted as follows:

1. Line *A* is the orbiting path record that correlates with balancing inclines on the orbiting side.
2. Line *B* is the protrusive path record that correlates with protrusive contacts of the posterior teeth.
3. Line *C* is the rotating path record that correlates with working cusp inclines on the rotating side.
4. The lines on the horizontal record table correlate primarily with the direction of the ridges and grooves of the posterior teeth.

When using a pantograph with tracking tables, it is helpful to visualize the styli as maxillary cusps and the record tables as the occlusal surface of mandibular teeth (Fig. 5-33).

Sagittal plane records

Protrusive condylar path

Fig. 5-34 diagrams three potential protrusive path inclinations: shallow path *A*, medium path *B*, and steep path *C*. The paths of movement of the record tables, resultant protrusive path records, and influence on the effective cusp angles mesiodistally are also illustrated. NOTE: A shallow protrusive condylar path results in a shallow recording and a shallow cusp angle. Fig. 5-35 is helpful for recalling the relation of the protrusive condylar path to occlusal anatomy.

Orbiting condylar path

Fig. 5-36 shows a steep orbiting condylar path *A* and a shallow orbiting condylar path *B*. The resultant orbiting condylar path records and the influence these paths of movements have on the balancing contacts are also illustrated. A steep orbiting path of movement provides for steep balancing cusp inclines on the orbiting side, and, conversely, a shallow orbiting path allows for shallow balancing cusps inclines on the orbiting side. Orbiting path inclines are the mesial aspects of the lingual inclines of the mandibular buccal cusps and the distal aspects of the buccal inclines of the maxillary lingual cusps.

Rotating condylar path

Fig. 5-37 illustrates potential rotating condylar paths in the coronal plane, which are inclined as follows: *A*, outward and upward; *B*, straight laterally; and *C*, outward and downward. The resultant rotating condylar path records recorded on the sagittal record table and the influence these movements have on working bite inclines are also illustrated.

Fig. 5-37 shows that if the rotating condylar path is inclined upward, the sagittal record table concurrently moves upward with the condyle, resulting in a lower recording on the record table *(A)*. This is correlated with lower working bite inclines and shorter working bite cusps. If the rotating condylar path inclines downward, the rotating condylar path record is located higher on the record table *(C)*, which allows for higher working bite cusps and steeper inclines.

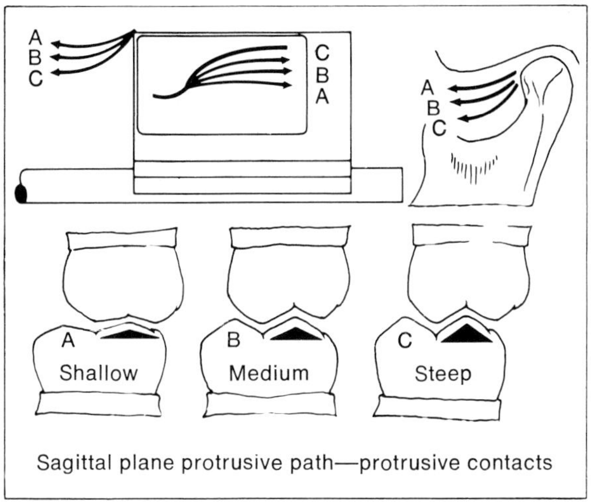

Fig. 5-34. Three potential protrusive path inclinations and their effect on cusp height.

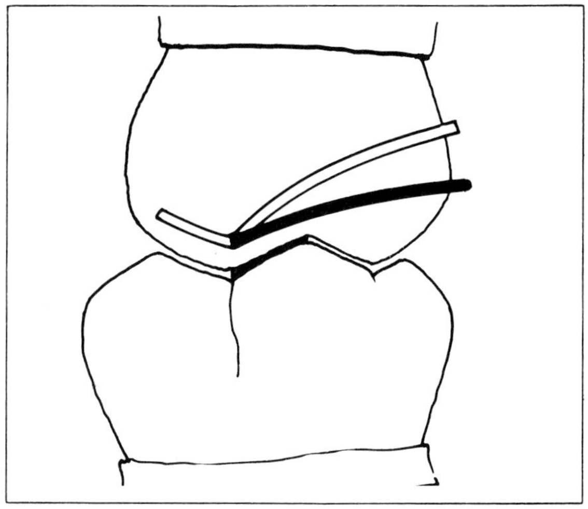

Fig. 5-35. Influence of protrusive path on occlusal anatomy.

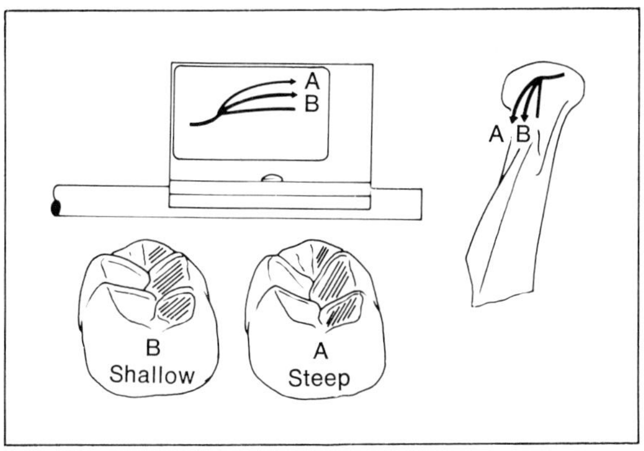

Fig. 5-36. Comparison of steep and shallow orbiting condylar path and its effect on balancing contacts.

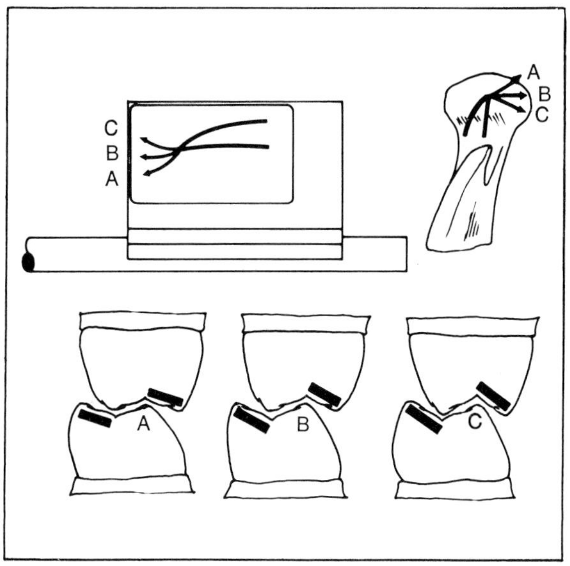

Fig. 5-37. Influence of displacement of rotating condylar path in coronal plane on height of cusps on working side.

Horizontal plane records

Rotating condylar path

Fig. 5-38 illustrates rotating condylar paths in the horizontal plane, which are inclined outward and backward *(A)*, straight laterally *(B)*, and outward and forward *(C)*.

The resultant rotating condylar path records recorded on the horizontal record table and the influence these condylar movements have on groove direction (and the ridges between the grooves) on the working side are also illustrated (Fig. 5-38). If the rotating condylar path is inclined outward and backward *(A)*, the horizontal record table concurrently moves outward and backward, and the resulting rotating condylar path record is inclined more forward *(A)*. This is correlated with a lingual groove on a lower molar *(A)*, which is positioned more forward. If the rotating condylar path is inclined forward *(C)*, the rotating condylar path record is positioned more distally.

Orbiting path record

In Fig. 5-39 the orbiting condylar paths in the horizontal plane exhibit *(A)* little mandibular side-shift and *(B)* increased mandibular side-shift. The resultant influences that these condylar paths of movement have on the orbiting path record on the horizontal record table

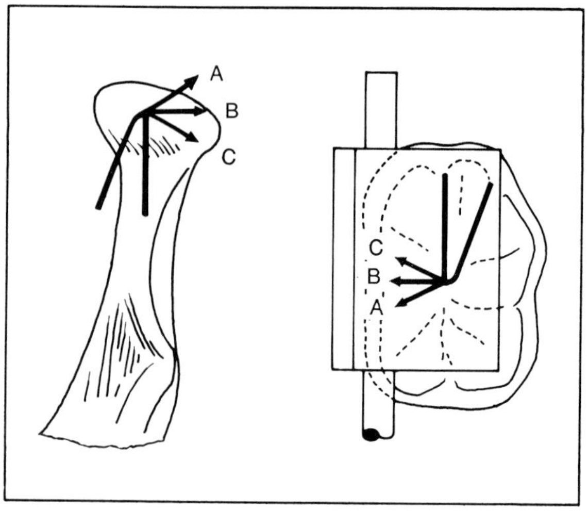

Fig. 5-38. Influence of displacement of rotating condylar path in horizontal plane on ridge and groove direction.

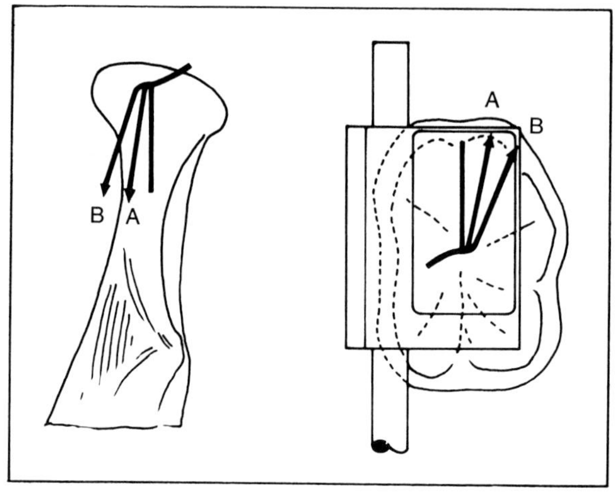

Fig. 5-39. Influence of orbiting condylar path on occlusal anatomy.

and on the direction of the grooves and ridges of the lower buccal cusps on the orbiting side are also illustrated.

When there is little mandibular side-shift *(A)*, the orbiting path record and grooves *(A)*, through which the maxillary lingual cusps escape, will be located more distally. Increasing the mandibular side-shift *(B)* locates the orbiting path record and grooves on the lower teeth through which the maxillary lingual cusps escape more mesially.

CLINICAL SIGNIFICANCE OF PANTOGRAPHIC RECORDS AND THE PRACTICAL APPLICATION OF INSTRUMENTATION

The pantograph

Fig. 5-40 is a horizontal view of a recorder transferred to the lower bow of an articulator. Note that on this patient, the scriber was attached to the maxilla, and the styli were stationary like the lingual cusps of maxillary teeth. The recorder was attached to the mandible and moved with the condyles. The record tables and occlusal surfaces of the mandibular teeth moved with the mandible beneath the cusps and styli attached to the maxilla. The record tables on the right side of the articulator demonstrate the lines scribed by the patient that are most conveniently used to analyze temporomandibular joint characteristics on that side of the patient (set the articulator).

The mesial leg of the anterior Gothic arch tracing is used to locate the position of the vertical axis of rotation on the same side. The lateral leg of the posterior horizontal scribing is used to interpret the amount of mandibular side-shift of the mandible that occurred during the lateral excursion. This line is almost always a curve, being most acute near the centric relation position. On a Denar articulator, this line is divided into two components: the immediate side-shift and progressive side-shift (articulator adjustments). On the left side of the articulator, tooth anatomy is superimposed over the scribings to assist in visualizing and understanding the clinical significance of these determinants of mandibular movements.

The anterior record table illustrates the influence the vertical axis of rotation has on determining the direction of grooves that will allow opposing cusps and ridges to travel without interference.

The immediate side-shift of the mandible has an influence on occlusal anatomy near the centric position, and the progressive side-shift of the mandible has an influence on the inclination of the balancing inclines of cusps on the orbiting side as well as on ridge and groove direction.

When a dental articulator is adjusted to follow the lines of the pantographic recordings of the patient, a diagnostic function of the articulator is performed. The recordings are interpreted in the calibrated control areas of the articulator, and the temporomandibular joint characteristics, which determined the motion that produced the recordings, are identified. These are diagnostic data.

To assist in understanding the function of a dental articulator in efficient occlusal treatments, assume a situation in which a dental articulator is set to the pantographic recordings of the patient. Anteriorly, and equally important, the incisal guide assembly is set to accommodate the horizontal and vertical overlap of the anterior teeth. This completes the diagnostic function of the articulator, and information on the patient's man-

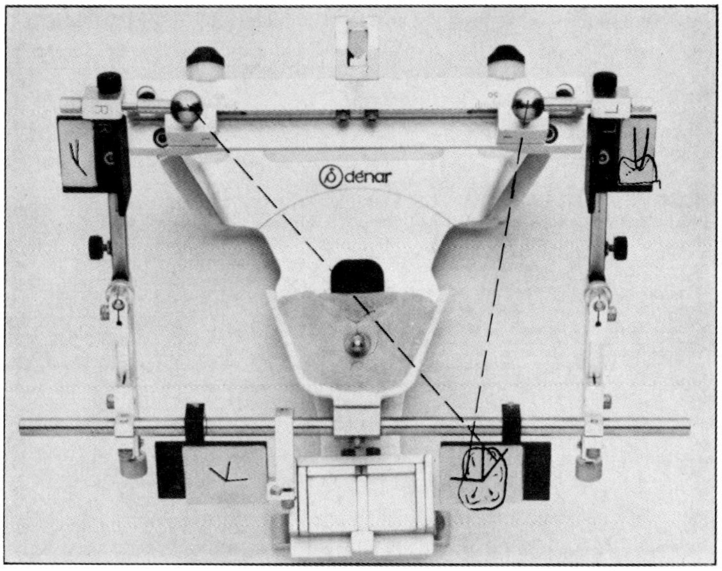

Fig. 5-40. Horizontal view of recorder transferred to lower member of articulator.

dibular movements is stored in the calibrated control areas of the articulator.

The articulator is now programmed for its treatment function: the efficient fabrication of the desired occlusion. The occlusal prescription is consulted, and the articulator is adjusted to produce a movement that is a specification of the occlusal scheme prescribed.

Laboratory procedure

In the laboratory, the anatomy of the maxillary teeth is developed and carried to completion with consideration for esthetics: the plane of occlusion, location of the vertical axes, and inclination of the articulator control areas. As wax is added to the mandibular preparations and the instrument is closed and moved in accord with its control areas, the information programmed in the articulator controls is automatically reflected in the occlusal anatomy and sheared in the mandibular occlusion. The direction of the grooves is established as determined by the location of the vertical axes of rotation and the side-shift adjustments. Planes are established as influenced by the condylar and incisal guide inclines. In between the grooves, ridges will appear as allowed by the spaces between the cusps of the maxillary teeth. These wax forms established by the motion programmed in the control areas of the articulator are then perfected to include those details of occlusal anatomy which have to do with the reduction of vertical stress, such as proper axial contours and inclusion of supplemental grooves.

In this manner, the laboratory time and effort required to fabricate occlusions with this directed approach will be no more than required to fabricate the same number of wax patterns on a simple straight-line articulator. However, the advantages of a directed approach will be apparent when the restorations are seated in the mouth.

In this example, a wax shearing technique was employed for efficiency and is practical in most treatments. However, in reconstructing badly mutilated occlusions or for the ultimate in esthetics and occlusal efficiency, the drop wax method of fabricating occlusions is preferred.

THE DENTAL ARTICULATOR

In restorative procedures, a jaw movement simulator, a dental articulator, is frequently used to facilitate the fabrication of the desired occlusion. The articulator is programmed to produce a motion that is a determinant of the occlusal anatomy being developed. The motion produced by the instrument is dictated by the settings of its three control areas, the two condylar controls and the incisal guide control.

Dental articulators are conventionally constructed to be reasonable facsimiles of their anatomic counterparts because this construction provides the most convenient means of producing the desired movements. However, the complexity of the posterior control areas in relation to the anterior control area tends to overshadow the relative importance of the incisal guide or anterior control area.

Better perspective and understanding can be achieved if the motion produced by the articulator is visualized as a motion that occurs between a movable

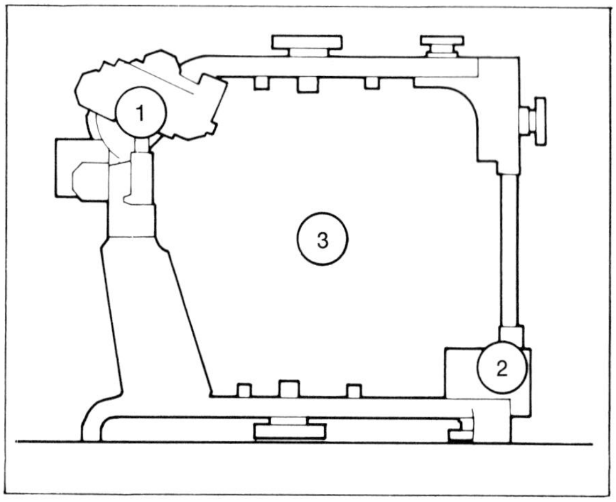

Fig. 5-41. Diagram of dental articulator with location of posterior control areas, *1;* anterior control area, *2;* and central occlusal position of mounted casts in proper orientation to control areas, *3.*

beam extending anteroposteriorly (one member of the articulator) relative to a second beam running in the same direction, which is fixed (the other member of the articulator) (Fig. 5-41). The motion produced by the movable beam is determined by the direction in which each of its two ends, anterior and posterior, is guided. The anterior guide and the posterior guide of the beam have equal influence on the motion produced, regardless of the relative complexity of the guiding controls.

The clinical significance of the guide control areas of an articulator is found in the motion produced, not in the manner in which the motion is produced. That is, the incisal guide control area is of equal importance to the condylar control areas.

In practical application, the tremendous clinical significance of these control areas is their capacity to be precisely readjusted after the diagnosis so that the instrument will produce a motion which facilitates the efficient accomplishment of the prime objective: fabricating the desired occlusion. The ability of the motion programmed in the articulator to be interpreted in calibrated control areas and expressed in numeric values permits the same instrument or another instrument in a remote location to be programmed subsequently without the expenditure of additional time and expense. This is clinically significant in that it encourages the treatment sequence to be accomplished according to the dentist's or patient's desires rather than to be dictated by instrument limitations. In using an articulator to facilitate the fabrication of the desired occlusion, the following three general areas should be considered:

1. *Posterior control areas (condylar controls).* These control areas are adjusted according to the patient's temporomandibular joint characteristics, which can be identified by a pantograph or other means.

2. *Anterior control area (incisal guide control).* This control area is of equal importance to the posterior control areas. In existing occlusions it is adjusted in consideration of the vertical and horizontal overlap of the anterior teeth. In edentulous mouths the vertical and horizontal overlap of anterior teeth is determined by esthetic and phonetic measurements.

3. *Centric occlusal position of the mounted casts in proper orientation to the control areas.* This is the most important of the three general areas of consideration. Accurate orientation of the mandibular cast to the maxillary cast at the centric occlusal position is of paramount importance and is often the most difficult and time-consuming accomplishment of these three areas of occlusal treatments. This may be especially true in full denture construction. A pantograph is not used in accomplishing this procedure. Here the dentist must rely on his knowledge of neuromuscle physiology, principles of occlusion, and on equilibration, checkbite, and laboratory technique.

REFERENCES

D'Amico, A.: Functional occlusion of the natural teeth of man, J. Prosthet. Dent. **11**:899-915, 1961.

Guichet, N. F.: Procedures for occlusal treatment, Anaheim, Calif., 1969, Denar Corp.

McCollum, B. B., and Stuart, C. E.: A research report, South Pasadena, Calif., 1955, Scientific Press.

Pound, E.: The mandibular movements of speech and their seven related values, J. So. Calif. Dent. Assoc. **34**:435-441, 1966.

Stuart, C. E.: Good occlusion for natural teeth, J. Prosthet. Dent. **14**:716-724, 1964.

Thomas, P. K.: Syllabus on full mouth waxing technique for rehabilitation, San Diego, 1967, Instant Printing Service.

CHAPTER 6

PREPARATION DESIGN FOR CROWNS AND RETAINERS

ROBERT S. STAFFANOU

preparation The selected form given to a natural tooth when it is reduced by instrumentation to receive a prosthesis (e.g., an artificial crown or a retainer for a fixed prosthesis). The selection of the form is guided by the clinical circumstances and physical properties of the materials.

retention The inherent property of a restoration to maintain its position without displacement under stress.

resistance form The shape given to a preparation to enable the restoration and remaining tooth structure to withstand masticatory stress.

The preparation design of any cast restoration must include the following principles (Shillingburg, Hobo, and Whitsett, 1976):

1. Preservation of tooth structure
2. Retention and resistance form
3. Structural durability
4. Marginal integrity

The purpose of any tooth restoration is to restore lost or destroyed tooth structure. Conversely, a restoration should also attempt to preserve the remaining tooth structure within the limits of resistance and retention form of the preparation. Teeth should not be subjected to needless removal. Likewise, the restoration should reinforce the tooth against further fracture or destruction.

GENERAL CONSIDERATIONS

For any restoration to be successful, it must restore the form and function of the tooth as well as remain intact without dislodgment. To prevent dislodgment, the preparation must possess a configuration that ensures retention and resistance for the casting. Retention is the quality that prevents removal in the long axis of the tooth preparation. Resistance is the quality that prevents dislodgment due to apically or obliquely directed forces. Retention is a function of height, diameter, and convergence of the preparation, as well as the texture of the prepared surface and the use of intracoronal retentive devices. The most critical retentive factor within the dentist's control is the convergence of the preparation. When convergence changes from 1 to 5 degrees, 40% of the retention of the opposing walls is lost (Kaufman, Coelho, and Colin, 1961). If a preparation is compromised by lack of sufficient tooth structure, resistance and retention can be increased by addition of intracoronal retentive devices such as grooves, pins, or box forms. Retention and resistance form are closely interrelated, but of the two, resistance form is the most critical in preventing dislodgment of the restoration.

To counteract the torquing or twisting forces applied in the horizontal plane, groove walls must be placed perpendicular to the direction of the dislodging forces. Structurally, the restoration should possess enough bulk and therefore rigidity to withstand functional and nonfunctional stressing. This requires careful preparation design. Correct preparation design is also essential to establish contour, resistance, and retention form (Fig. 6-1).

Marginal integrity of the casting is also essential to

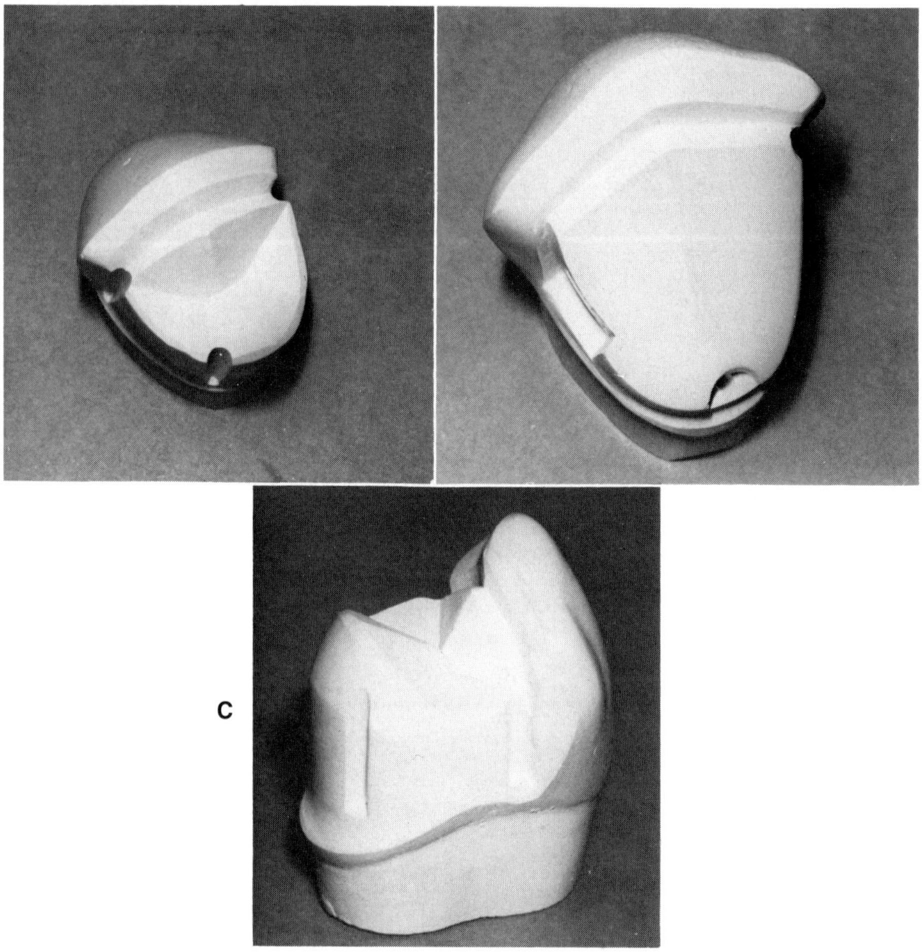

Fig. 6-1. A, Grooves provide additional retention and resistance form to preparations. **B,** Box forms and pins can be used for additional resistance and retention. **C,** Three-quarter crown with accessory groove for resistance and retention.

ensure a favorable prognosis for the restoration. Margins must be closely and completely adapted to seal the underlying tooth from the external environment. Whenever possible, cavosurface bevels should be established, since this allows even closer marginal adaptation. In addition to the marginal design, gold restorations can be burnished to further enhance marginal integrity. Generally, a chamfered gingival margin is indicated for metal restorations, a shouldered margin for ceramometal and porcelain margins, or a shoulder with a bevel can be used for ceramometal restoration.

The shoulder with a bevel is best for ceramometal restorations, since the bevel can produce the closest fitting margin. This design, however, compromises esthetics since the restoration must incorporate a metal band, or collar, on the faciogingival margin. If esthetic demands are high, the sloping shoulder is the desired marginal design. Margins on the occlusal outline should also be closely adapted to protect the enamel of the tooth in this area (Fig. 6-2). The placement of the gingival margin has a direct bearing on the success of the cast restoration. Certainly the best results are obtained with margins that are as smooth as possible and in an area where the patient can adequately maintain them. In placing a margin, the need for atraumatic duplication of this margin by impression techniques must also be considered. Mesially, on posterior teeth, partial veneer restorations should be placed well back into the interproximal space where esthetics will be optimal. Distally, on posterior teeth, metal margins can extend almost to midfacial without altering esthetics. All margins should end in enamel whenever possible. Anteriorly it is often necessary to extend margins subgingivally for esthetic considerations and to obtain enough preparation height for adequate resistance and retention form. The consequences of placing margins subgingivally is open to question. Margins that are kept well above (3 to 4 mm) the tissue in posterior areas are the least trau-

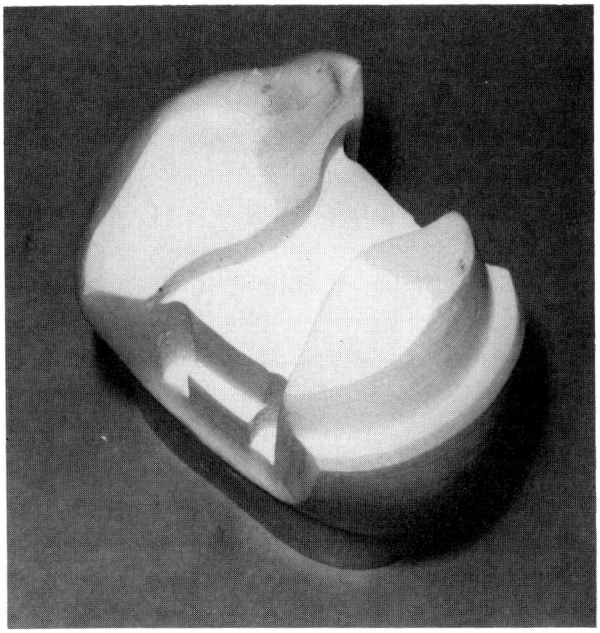

Fig. 6-2. Cavosurface bevels are essential for marginal integrity.

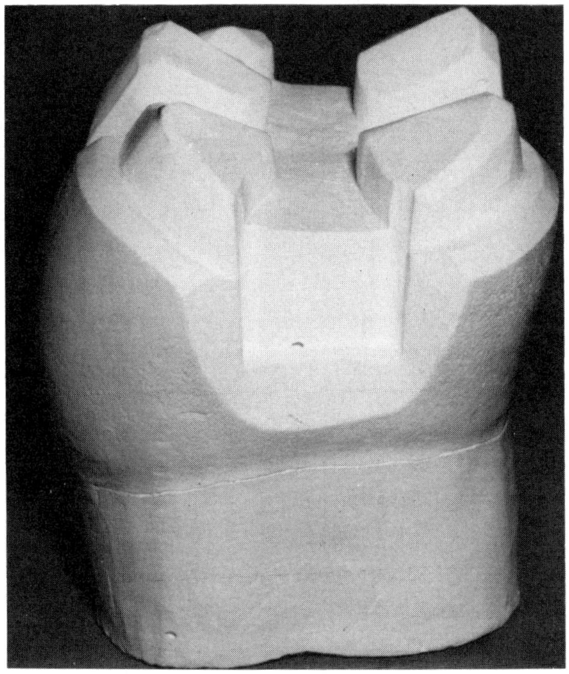

Fig. 6-3. Onlays afford protection to fracture-susceptible cusps.

matic to the surrounding tissues. Margins that end within 1 mm above the crest of the gingival tissue are in an area of high plaque concentration and are difficult for the patient to maintain. These margins may become secondarily involved by caries, or the tissue may remain clinically inflamed from the stasis of bacterial plaque concentration in the area. The rule of thumb, then, is to leave margins 3 to 4 mm above the tissue when compatible with resistance and retention forms of the preparation; otherwise, they should be extended subgingivally.

CLASSIFICATION OF RESTORATIONS BY PREPARATION DESIGN

Inlays and onlays

Inlays are cast restorations that gain their retention through parallel internal box forms prepared within the coronal portion of the tooth. Inlays are generally considered to be individual restorations for reestablishing coronal integrity that was lost because of carious destruction of the tooth. Due to the phenomenon known as *deflection*, inlays generally are not acceptable retainers for fixed partial dentures. The amount of deflection in a beam that spans a space varies directly with the cube of the thickness of the beam. Therefore a fixed partial denture that replaces two teeth will deflect eight times that of a one-tooth replacement, and a three-tooth replacement will deflect twenty-seven times that of a single-tooth replacement. Retainer selection therefore must be predicated on ability to resist displacement due to deflection. Two surface inlays are inadequate because when deflection occurs the occlusal portion will tend to lift up, and the proximal flanges will tend to flare. Mesial-occlusal-distal (MOD) inlays exhibit the same tendency and, in addition, the external proximal flanges will tend to move out of their seat. Joining the mesial and distal flanges by covering the lingual surface of the tooth with a veneer of metal and thereby creating the three-quarter crown can counteract deflection. Thus the strength and rigidity of the retainer is enhanced. If necessary, structural reinforcement can be carried a step farther by including the facial surface. This constitutes full coverage, which affords maximum strength and rigidity.

The use of inlays to restore MOD lesions is highly questionable, since there is no protection for the unsupported buccal and lingual cusps. An inlay, in reality, increases the cusp height of the tooth by the depth of the occlusal box, making these heightened cusps more vulnerable to fracture. The onlay is a modification of the MOD inlay, which covers the entire occlusal surface and provides protection and reinforcement of the cusps (Fig. 6-3). An onlay functions best (1) for broken-down teeth with buccal and lingual cusps still intact, (2) when half or more of the buccolingual dimension of a crown is involved in the isthmus of an MOD restoration, and (3) in endodontically treated posterior teeth with sound buccolingual tooth structure. Onlays usually

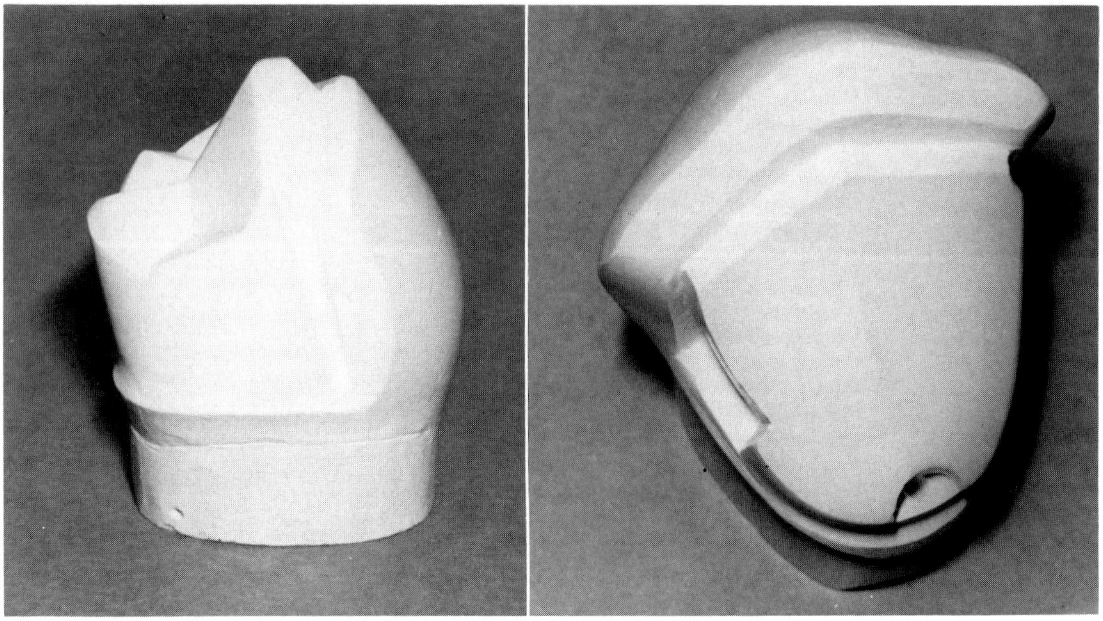

A B

Fig. 6-4. A, Posterior partial veneer crowns are conservative and provide adequate support for fixed partial dentures. **B,** Anterior teeth must have sufficient bulk and thickness to be amenable to partial veneer construction. Partial veneer preparations must be accurately and precisely machined to be successful.

lack adequate retention for bridge retainers, although occasionally they may be used on short-span fixed partial dentures. Onlays are usually less resistant to torquing stresses applied to fixed partial denture retainers. The onlay must be carefully and accurately prepared to establish maximum retention and resistance form. Onlays are prepared with proximal boxes as well as an occlusal box form. Buccal and lingual cusps are covered for protection and prevention of fracture. The circumference of the onlay margins should be adequately beveled for fit. All sharp edges or angles are rounded.

Partial veneer crowns

Partial veneer crowns, or three-quarter crowns, are used primarily as fixed partial denture retainers but are occasionally indicated as a single restoration. This preparation usually covers the proximal, lingual, and occlusal (or incisal) surfaces of the involved tooth. The facial surface is left untouched, except along the proximal and the faciocclusal or facioincisal margins. When conditions permit minimal facial extension, esthetics can be readily achieved. The partial veneer crown requires far less tooth reduction than the full veneer crown, while still providing maximum retention for the fixed prosthesis. If the abutment tooth is well supported periodontally and the crown has sufficient length for resistance and retention form, the partial veneer will provide adequate support for even the longest fixed partial denture (Fig. 6-4).

Partial veneer crowns are well suited for maxillary centrals, canines, premolars, and molars and for mandibular canines, second premolars, and molars. These teeth have ample thickness to allow sufficient reduction for casting rigidity. In addition, posterior teeth, by virtue of their occlusal surface configuration, provide a corrugated effect that increases rigidity. Partial veneer crowns are contraindicated for (1) short teeth, grossly carious teeth, and (excepting lower molars) teeth with a poor long-axis relationship with the path of insertion; (2) upper canines that have long cusps, contact areas at the gingival margin, and very short mesial and distal surfaces (the grooves will be too short to hold the prosthesis); (3) teeth that are too small or thin for proper groove placement; (4) teeth with extensive cervical caries (since grooves would extend into partially disintegrated tooth structure); and (5) mouths with a high caries index because of the long margin line.

Advantages of partial veneer crowns

Partial veneer crowns have the following advantages: (1) preservation of tooth structure; (2) much of the margin is accessible for finishing and oral hygiene; (3) they intrude less on the gingival crevice, reducing tissue irritation; (4) they are more easily cemented because of generous escape areas for cement; (5) seating is easily verified by direct vision; and (6) the tooth can be tested for vitality because of the intact facial surface; and (7) tooth contours are better maintained.

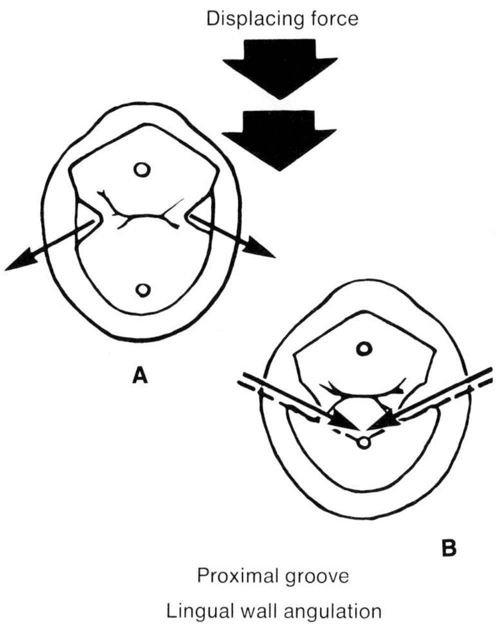

Fig. 6-5. A, With V-shaped groove, displacing force spreads casting laterally, away from preparation. **B,** With acute or flat lingual wall, displacing force creates medial force that causes closer adaptation of casting to preparation.

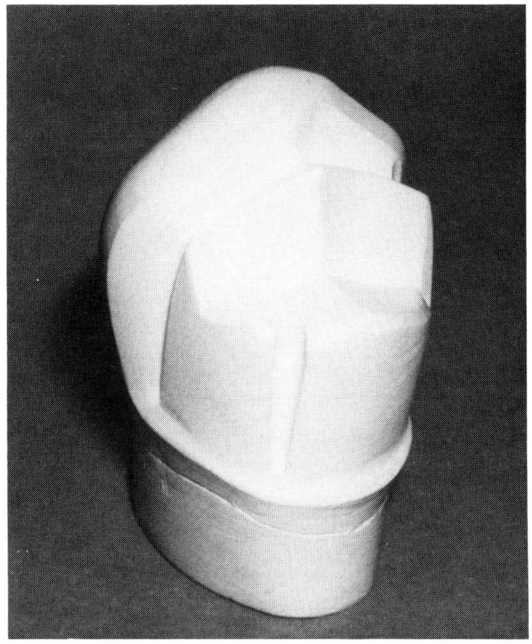

Fig. 6-6. Partial veneer margins are kept lingual to the buccal cusp height for esthetics.

Design

The design of the partial veneer crown must be carefully and exactly executed to obtain maximum retention and resistance form. Because one surface (facial) is left uncovered, a groove must be supplied to compensate for the retention and resistance lost by eliminating that wall. This groove must be accurately machined into the preparation. It must have a definite lingual wall that is parallel to the vertical height of the lingual wall of the preparation. To prevent proximal opening under function and to resist the effects of torquing, the lingual wall of the groove should be perpendicular, or slightly acute, to the sagittal plane when viewed incisally or occlusally (Fig. 6-5). These walls should be on a line with an imaginary center located in the cingulum of the anterior teeth or in the lingual cusp area of posterior teeth. By establishing this hooking or locking effect, the groove is more retentive and resistant to displacement. When a V-shaped groove is used, the inclined plane effect will cause opening of the proximofacial margins, which is critical on anterior teeth. Any force applied vertically along the long axis of the anterior preparation is translated to a lingual displacing force. This is due to the inclined plane configuration of the lingual surface. To compensate for this force and prevent gingivofacial opening, the lingual wall must resist this displacing force direction. If the groove is V shaped, the casting will want to slip laterally along the lingual wall inclined plane, resulting in an opening force being applied to it. If, however, it is acute to the sagittal plane, and force is applied incisally, the casting will still tend to slip along the inclined plane but in the opposite direction. Because of the direction of the lingual wall, then, the casting will slip axially or medially and actually grip or adapt to the tooth more tightly, rather than be spread laterally and away from the tooth. Grooves should be placed so that the buccal plate is not undermined, which can lead to enamel fracture during placement or, later, during function. If the grooves are too far lingually, there is less resistance form to the preparation, and the beveled margin will result in a long, thin casting margin that is susceptible to deformation.

For esthetics, the upper three-quarter crown should not be reverse beveled along the buccoocclusal margin, nor must the vertical height of the buccal plate of enamel be reduced. The bevel should be flat or knife-edged (Fig. 6-6).

Full veneer crowns

Full veneer crowns are indicated for maximum retention or for esthetic considerations. Full coverage can be an excellent restoration modality under the right conditions, but it should not be used indiscriminately. Reproduction of tooth form is decidedly more difficult

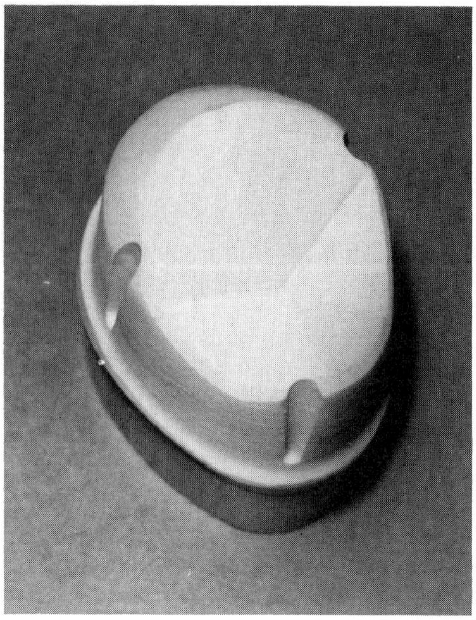

Fig. 6-7. Full veneer crown preparation.

with full coverage, and pulpal involvement occurs more frequently with the full veneer crowns. The most conservative full coverage restoration is the full gold crown. Usually minimal preparation is needed to cover the tooth with a thin veneer of metal. It should be remembered that although they can rebuild or restore function to a damaged or destroyed tooth structure, full crowns do not protect teeth from caries. Plaque control must be established for favorable prognosis of any restoration.

Design

The design of the preparation should incorporate the following design features:

1. Sufficient axial reduction to establish retention, resistance form, and proper axial contour.
2. Sufficient occlusal reduction to provide thickness and rigidity to the casting. The occlusal should be reduced uniformly along the triangular ridge planes and in the groove areas. By maintaining these planes intact, a corrugated effect is established, and rigidity is increased.
3. A light, smooth, and evenly symmetrical chamfered margin should be developed. If a tooth is exceptionally short, a knife-edged margin should be considered to allow maximum vertical height of the preparation.
4. A secondary bevel in the occlusal third of the buccal and lingual surfaces allows proper contour of the axial surfaces, occlusal diameter, and cusp size.
5. Buccal and lingual grooves can be added to improve retention and resistance form of the preparation if desired. This is particularly indicated on long bridge spans and on short teeth.
6. All sharp angles should be rounded (Fig. 6-7).

Esthetically veneered full crowns

Esthetically veneered full crowns are more radical in tooth reduction than complete metal crowns. The restoration consists of a metal substructure with a layer of bonded porcelain over it. It combines the strength and fit of the metal with the esthetics of porcelain.

DESIGN

The esthetically veneered full crown has the following mandatory design features:

1. Adequate reduction of the tooth to prevent overcontour of the final restoration.
2. Two planes of reduction on the facial surface (corresponding to the contour of the uncut tooth) are necessary for adequate retention, resistance, and contour of the facial surface.
3. Adequate lingual reduction for rigidity of the metal and/or placement of porcelain veneering of adequate thickness.
4. Proper marginal design based on esthetic and/or functional requirements.
5. The vertical portion of the cingulum on anterior teeth should be maintained as high as possible and parallel with the facial surface.
6. The proximal walls should be parallel with each other.
7. All sharp angles on the preparation should be rounded.

Facial margin designs include the following forms: shoulder, shoulder with a bevel, chamfer, 45-degree shoulder.

COSMETIC RESTORATIONS

Cosmetic restorations include the ceramometal restoration with a porcelain labial margin and the porcelain jacket crown. The porcelain-margined ceramometal crown is prepared exactly like the conventional ceramometal crown except that a labial shoulder is required. The metal is then finished short of the shoulder when the casting is made.

The porcelain jacket restoration requires even more aggressive tooth reduction than the ceramometal restoration (Fig. 6-8). The major difference is that it does not have a cast metal substructure. The porcelain jacket is probably capable of producing the best cosmetic results of all dental restorations. Since it is made entirely of porcelain, it is brittle and susceptible to fracture. The development of the aluminous core porcelains, which are stronger than conventional porcelains, has renewed the interest in these restorations. They are still used

A

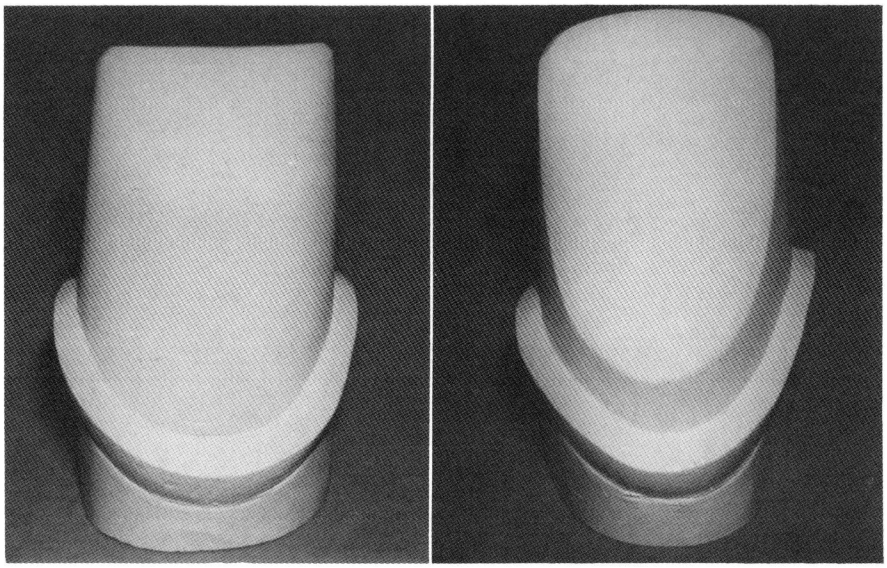

B

Fig. 6-8. A, Labial reduction for procelain jacket crown preparation. **B,** Lingual reduction for porcelain jacket crown.

primarily where maximum esthetics are required. McLean (1974) has reported a technique using a twin platinum foil procedure, which results in a restoration that is reportedly three times stronger than a conventional aluminous core porcelain jacket restoration. All porcelain jackets require that a platinum foil be burnished closely to the die in order to support the porcelain for firing. This foil is removed just prior to final cementation of the restoration. With the twin foil technique, a platinum foil is burnished over the die as described. Over this foil, another foil is burnished with the incisal end left open and the opposite edge trimmed short of the gingival margin. This second foil cylinder is then galvanized, which enhances the chemical bond of the porcelain to metal. The restoration is fired, using an aluminous core porcelain over the galvanized foil for strength. The difference is that the second (galvanized) foil cylinder becomes an integral part of the restoration, imparting strength to the jacket crowns. The first foil is removed prior to cementation. Although the galvanized foil adds considerable strength to the restoration, it may detract from the esthetics. Recent developements in the field of dental ceramics, such as the Cerestore* system, which employs a shrink-free ceramic core, impart new dimensions in fit and technique.

Preparation design

A porcelain jacket preparation is left as long as possible to provide maximum support for the porcelain. An overshortened preparation will result in stress concentration in the labiogingival area, which can cause the classic half-moon fracture in this area. A shoulder of uniform thickness, which encompasses 360 degrees of the preparation, is used to provide a flat gingival seat to support the restoration. The incisal edge is flat and placed at a slight lingual inclination to meet the incisal forces and prevent shearing. All sharp edges of the preparation must be rounded to prevent stress concentrations. When considering a porcelain jacket preparation, tooth position, occlusion, and tooth morphology must be considered. This restoration should be used only on incisors, and an edge-to-edge incisal relationship should be avoided. Likewise, it should not be used when opposing teeth occlude on the cervical fifth of the lingual surface. Short teeth are also contraindicated for porcelain jackets, since there is not enough preparation height to provide adequate resistance and retention form.

*Cerestore, Ceramco Inc. A Johnson and Johnson Company. 20 Lake Drive, CN 7065, East Windsor, N.J.

COPINGS

Copings are used effectively in the following situations:

1. Rebuilding grossly defective vital teeth
2. In combination with dowels to provide firm, stable restoration foundations
3. In extensive treatment cases with multiple abutments and in splinting
4. To support removable superstructures

When vital teeth are carious, fractured, or present isolated margins that are deeply subgingival, it is often simpler to restore the coronal and/or root integrity with

A 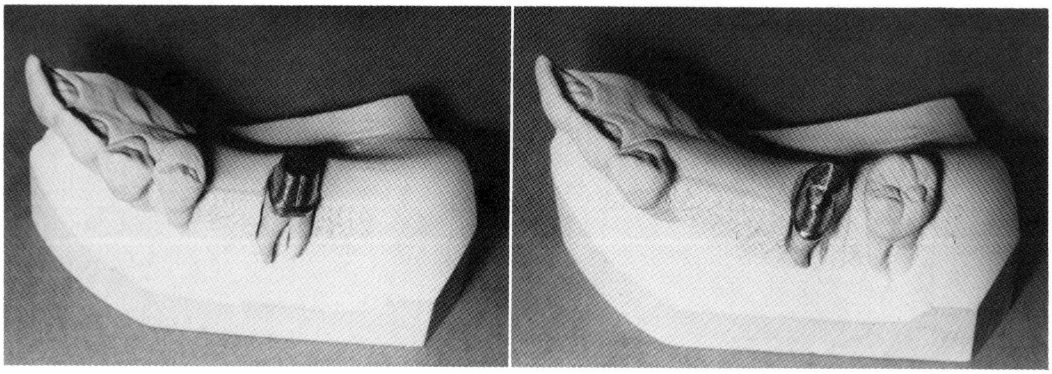 B

Fig. 6-9. A, Coping design for restoration foundation on intact tooth. **B,** Coping used to establish coronal integrity to tooth that has had root amputation.

A 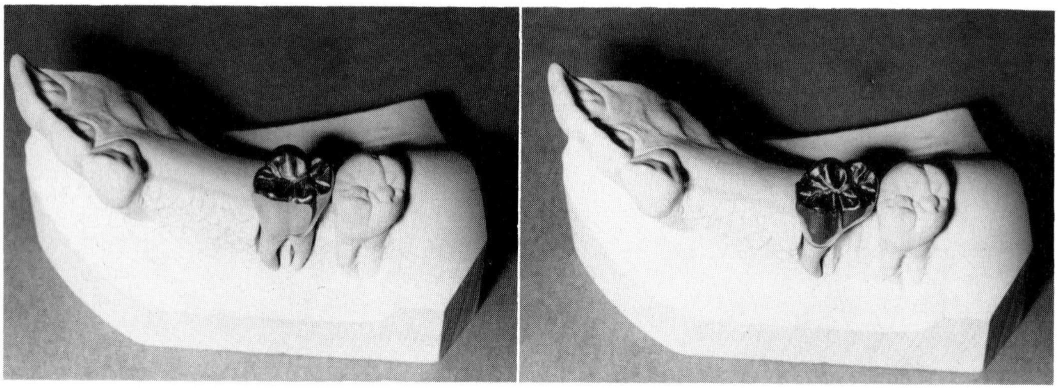 B

Fig. 6-10. A, Placement of final restoration on intact tooth. **B,** Final restoration of root amputation case.

a coping and then construct the final restoration with normal marginal extensions (Fig. 6-9). This metal coping provides minimum bulk for contour as well as presents the smoothest possible marginal transition from tooth structure to metal restoration. By establishing the margins of the final restoration at the normal gingival level, the restoration causes the least possible tissue abuse (Fig. 6-10).

Endodontically treated teeth can present little or no coronal tooth structure, weakened tooth structure, or distorted tooth contours because of root amputation or periodontal procedures. By first restoring tooth form and contour with a coping and then constructing the final restoration over this coping, tissue health is better preserved, and marginal extension and tooth form are easier to accomplish. If a tooth is weakened and needs reinforcement as well as coronal reestablishment, the coping can be used in conjunction with dowel construction. In addition, a coping used in conjunction with the dowel provides the ferrule effect so necessary for root reinforcement. When teeth are rebuilt with copings, a gold margin must be incorporated below the final restoration margin. This gold band may require an esthetic compromise for some patients.

Many times the abutment teeth for extensive rehabilitation cases are stabilized with copings prior to fabrication of the final restorations. This allows the final restorations to be temporarily cemented and removed without sensitivity and discomfort to the patient and without interrupting the integrity of the supporting abutments. This is particularly useful in splinting situations, where the restoration can be removed periodically for periodontal therapy, inspection, maintenance, or remount procedures without jeopardizing the supporting foundations. This technique greatly simplifies the necessary follow-up treatment on complicated and compromised restorative problems.

Copings can also be used as foundations for removable superstructures in the form of an overdenture support, which provides a vertical stop for a tissue-borne removable appliance, or as a preparation form to support a tooth-borne removable appliance. The overdenture is self-explanatory, but the tooth-borne case is more complicated. The abutment teeth are first recon-

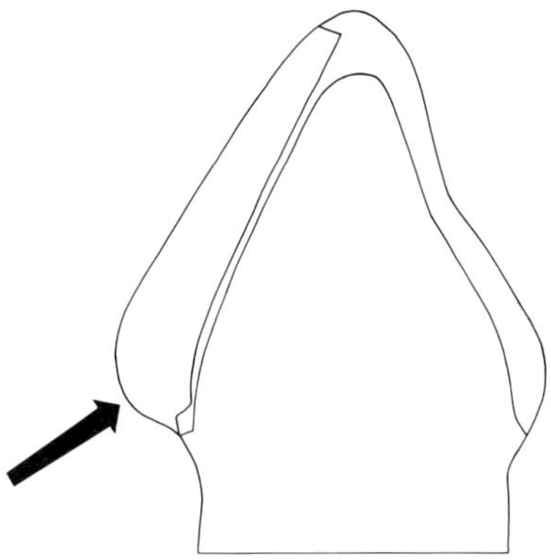

Fig. 6-11. Underpreparation gingivally results in a grossly overcontoured crown.

structed and restored to a retentive preparation form with metal copings. Over these metal coping abutments a fixed partial denture is constructed. This appliance can then be placed over the abutments, with external or frictional retention, as a removable partial denture that the patient can easily remove for oral physiotherapy procedures. These work quite well in maintaining abutment tissue integrity while supplying the comfort of a fixed appliance.

Occasionally coping restored abutments can be used in conjunction with a combination tissue-borne and tooth-borne removable partial denture for greater stability and patient comfort. In these cases the remaining teeth are restored with metal copings, crown restorations are made, and then a removable appliance is constructed for the edentulous areas. The individual crowns, along with the partial denture framework, are then joined into a single unit restoration that gains its retention and stability from the coping-abutment foundation. Copings are useful in dentistry, particularly with complications in compromised patients, requiring multiple treatment modalities.

Special considerations

Crown contours are essential to tissue health and the ultimate success of the restoration. This is as important, if not more important, than the esthetics of the restoration, because poor contours will lead to destruction of the supporting structures of the tooth. Contours also play an important part in esthetics.

Facial contours

Facial surfaces should have long, flatly convex contours with no bulges or marked convexities in the gingival third (Fig. 6-11). The gingival third of the tooth should be a straight line continuance of the facial root surface as it emerges occlusally from the tissue (Fig. 6-12, *A*). Stein has termed this contour the "emergence profile" (Fig. 6-12, *B*). At the junction of the middle and gingival thirds of the facial surface of the tooth, the surface changes direction to the occlusal or incisal surfaces. It is important to visualize this configuration in order to establish essential contour. If an esthetic veneer is to be placed on this surface, there must be sufficient reduction of the tooth structure in the proper places to accommodate the veneer without creating an overcontoured surface. REMEMBER: overcontouring of the finished restoration directly predisposes to periodontal disease of the adjacent supporting structures of the tooth. Contour, especially of the labial surface, is essential for esthetics.

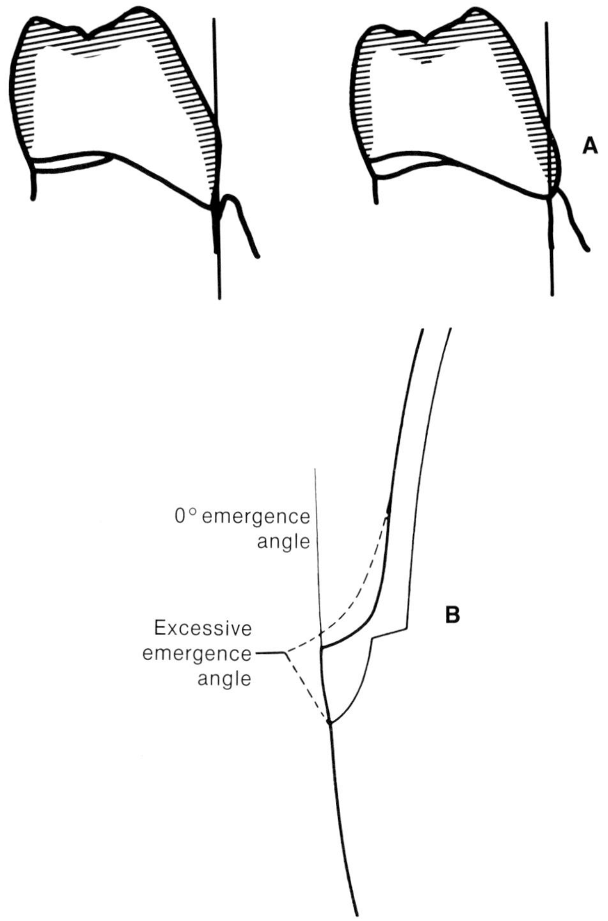

Fig. 6-12. A, Gingival third is direct continuation of root surface plane as it emerges from gingival sulcus. **B,** Emergence profile cannot be excessive if tissue health is to be properly maintained.

The first thing the eye perceives when viewing a restoration is the outline form (i.e., contour). This is the first condition that must be satisfied. The second perception is value (i.e., grayness or brightness) of the surface. The next area to be satisfied is the chroma (i.e., hue) of the restoration. This may not be as critical if the first two problems are properly addressed.

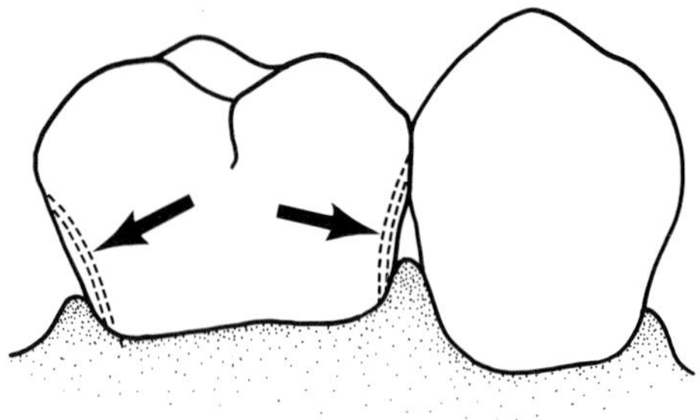

Fig. 6-13. Below contact area tooth must have subtle concavities to provide proper space for interdental papilla.

Lingual surfaces

Lingual contour of the restoration is as important as labial contour. These surfaces should imitate the contours of the axial surfaces of the original teeth. Posteriorly, they should be flatly convex and present no marked bulges. They should represent a linear extension of the lingual root surface of the tooth. Anteriorly, their inclined planes should be smooth and sloped to create open, obtuse embrasures lingual to the contact areas. Central incisors should be relieved to avoid impingement on the incisive papilla.

Interproximal surfaces

These are probably the most neglected areas in the fabrication of restorations. The natural tendency is to construct crowns with convex proximal surfaces. Proximal surfaces *are* convex through the contact area, but they become concave occlusogingivally from below the contact to the gingival margin (Fig. 6-13). This area is occupied by the interdental papilla. The space created by this architecture is nature's way of subtly providing space for this tissue without undue pressure and irritation. If space is not provided in our restorations, the tissue will be constricted. This, in turn, can lead to loss of soft tissue health and ultimate failure of the restoration. Contours, then, are extremely important from the standpoint of both esthetics and tissue health, two essential factors for the success of any restoration.

The above factors can be satisfied only by proper preparation of the tooth. If enough tooth structure is not removed in the right place, then neither contour nor esthetics can be properly accomplished.

Teeth must be prepared in two distinct planes. There must be a vertical retentive wall in the gingival two thirds of the tooth and the incisal or occlusal third must converge toward the incisal or occlusal surface for proper contours and esthetics (Fig. 6-14). The natural contour of the labial surface of anterior teeth should be imitated in tooth reduction. If the preparation does not allow the restoration to be properly contoured, it will

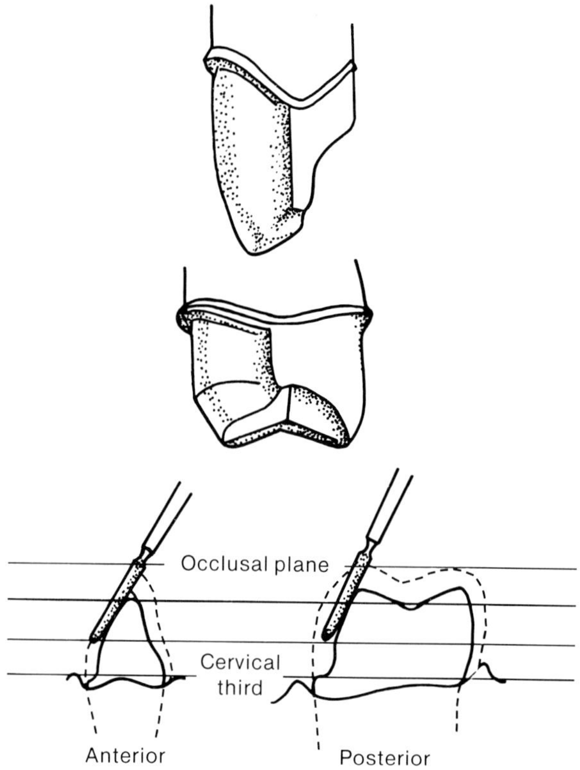

Fig. 6-14. Teeth must be prepared in proper dimension and proportion to allow contours, retention, resistance, and esthetics.

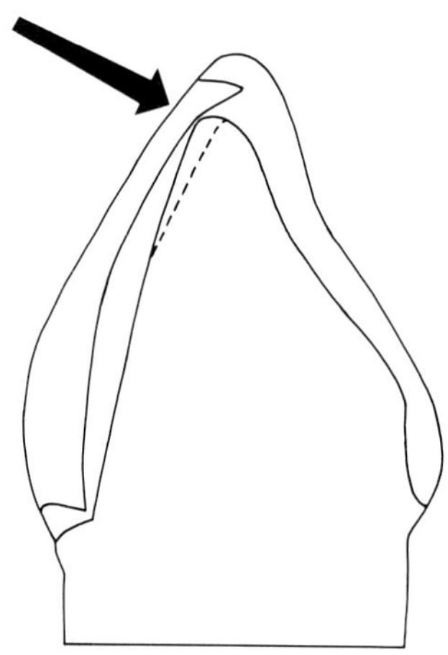

Fig. 6-15. Without proper incisal plane reduction, contour and esthetics are compromised by opaque show-through.

result in the restoration being too large, creating difficulty in the control of esthetics. The usual consequence of an improper preparation is the presence of a bright spot (high value) in the middle third of the tooth. The reason for this is opaque show-through from thinness of the veneer when trying to establish proper labial contour (Fig. 6-15).

Posteriorly the tooth must be prepared in a similar basic manner. The occlusal third should be contoured toward the occlusal in order to control the size of the occlusal surface. Large occlusal surfaces result in greater contact area and tend to overload periodontal support of the tooth, contributing to deterioration of supporting structures. Without this functional cusp bevel, the size of the occlusal surface cannot be controlled within proper limits.

Proper preparation is essential for tissue health, esthetics, surface area of the occlusal surface, and space for ease in laboratory fabrication of the restoration.

SUMMARY

The preparation is an essential link in the chain of success of our restorations. Without proper preparation we will not have proper retention form, resistance form, contour, tissue health, esthetics, or durability of our restorations. On the other hand, if the restoration does not meet proper criteria it will not succeed even on the otherwise most perfect preparation. Partial veneer restorations, while the most difficult to prepare, create the fewest problems and have the best longevity. They preserve natural tooth contours and create the fewest tissue problems. They do, however, compromise esthetic requirements in some cases.

Porcelain veneered restorations require more effort on the part of the practitioner and technician to provide a trouble-free restoration. Proper tooth preparation is essential to allow construction of a well-contoured esthetic restoration. The technician, then, must incorporate the design criteria necessary to produce a successful restoration. There are many variations in esthetic restorations. These include porcelain to metal, metal ceramic with a porcelain butt joint, metal collared ceramometal crowns, and porcelain jackets that include conventional jackets, aluminous core jackets, twin foil jackets, and cast ceramic restorations.

No matter what type restoration is used, it must contain certain basic preparation elements in order to be successful. It must incorporate resistance, retention, proper tooth reduction (in the right places), marginal integrity through proper impressions and die preparation, proper occlusion, and, in the final analysis, proper laboratory fabrication.

This chapter has described designs of various fixed prosthodontic preparations. These preparations, when properly executed, will produce optimal treatment results for partially edentulous patients as well as success with single-tooth restorations.

REFERENCES

Bassett, R.W., Ingraham, R., and Koser, J.R.: An atlas of cast gold procedures, Buena Park, Calif. 1964, Uni-Tro College Press.

Johnston, I.F., Dykema, R.W., and Phillips, R.W.: Modern practice in crown and bridge prosthodontics, ed. 3, Philadelphia, 1971, W.B. Saunders Co.

Kaufman, E.G., Coelho, D.H., and Colin, L.: Factors influencing the retention of cemented gold castings, J. Prosthet. Dent. **11**:487-502, 1961.

McLean, I.W.: The science and art of dental ceramics, Baton Rouge, La., 1974, Louisiana State University Press.

Schillingburg, H.T., Hobo, S., and Whitsett, L.D.: Preparations for cast gold restorations. In Die Quintessenz, Berlin, 1974, Buch- und Zietschriften—Verlag.

Shillingburg, H.T., Hobo, S., and Whitsett, L.D.: Fundamentals of fixed prosthodontics. In Die Quintessenz, Berlin, 1976. Buch- und Zietschriften—Verlag.

Stein, R.S., and Glickman, J.: Prosthetic considerations essential for gingival health, Dent. Clin. North Am., pp. 177-188, 1960.

Stern, R.S., and Kuwuta, M.: Current ceramometal procedures, Dent. Clin. North Am. **21**(4):729-749, 1977.

CHAPTER 7

DENTAL CASTINGS

PART ONE

Wax

The crown or fixed partial denture should resemble the natural dentition in form and function so the patient can enjoy the use of the prosthesis without being reminded of the loss that necessitated restorative intervention. To achieve this goal, one must be familiar with the composite form and nomenclature of the natural teeth, understand the determinants of occlusion and their effect on the occlusal surface of the teeth, and be able to interpret the harmonious relationship of axial and interproximal tooth surfaces with the adjacent teeth and architecture of the gingival tissues.

The objective of this chapter is to give theoretic and technical guidelines for the fabrication of cast restorations which, by their design, reflect the principles of optimal biomechanics and hygiene. The first of several materials used in this fabrication is wax.

Dental waxes are organic polymers consisting of hydrocarbons and their derivatives (e.g., ether and alcohols). Dental waxes are blends of natural and synthetic waxes, natural resins, oils, fats, and gums. Their molecular weights may range from 400 to 4000. The dental waxes melt over a range of 5° C to 30° C, rather than at a single temperature, because their components consist of a wide distribution of molecular weights.

Waxes used for the fabrication of patterns for dental castings (e.g., crowns and inlays) are divided into three types, as described in the third revision of the American Dental Association Specification No. 4. The intended uses for the three types are: Type A, hard or low-flow wax used in selected indirect techniques; Type B, used for direct techniques (fabricated in the oral cavity); and Type C, for direct techniques in the fabrication of crowns, inlays, and onlays.

Waxes have the highest coefficients of thermal expansion of any dental material; therefore, care must be exercised to minimize distortion of the pattern through extreme temperature changes. Waxes are partly elastic in behavior and tend to return to their original shape after deformation. Elastic recovery is slower at low temperatures, so if immediate investing is not practical, storage in a refrigerator is advised. If a wax pattern is refrigerated, it should be allowed to warm to room temperature before investing.

Softened or melted wax applied to the surfaces of a gypsum die tends to adhere. To allow for a clean separation of the wax pattern from a gypsum die or cast, a die lubricant must be applied to the gypsum surface prior to placement of the softened or molten wax. The common die lubricants are oil based and should be applied sparingly. Excess lubricant may obscure detail on the die and/or may be adsorbed to the wax, with similar consequences.

Wax placement must be controlled for obtaining both contours and accurate fit. The wax-added technique or functional waxing is a method of dripping hot wax on a die or cast to develop occlusion and contours in the wax pattern. When hot wax cools, it shrinks toward the center of the mass, generally pulling away from the lubricated surface to which it is applied. Care must be taken to establish proper adaptation and fit, which is usually accomplished by compression of the newly placed wax to the surface of the die or cast. Care to establish proper adaptation and fit is particularly important during margin adaptation. This is described in detail later in this chapter.

Functional occlusal wax-up

EVERITT V. PAYNE

To apply the principles of articulation when waxing the occlusal surface or opposing occlusal surfaces of posterior teeth, the wax-added technique for functional waxing was developed. Its advantage over the carving technique is that it provides an organized step-by-step procedure to develop the occlusal anatomic form. Furthermore, the wax-added technique offers a better understanding of the effects of articulation on the individual elements of the occlusal form: the height and distribution of cusps, ridge and groove direction, and fossa depth. The student can interpret mandibular movement as it relates to the occlusal surfaces of the teeth (Fig. 7-1).

THE WAX-ADDED TECHNIQUE

STEP 1: BUILDUP OF CONES. The cones are the buccal and lingual cusps of the maxillary first premolar (Fig. 7-2, *A*). The initial buccolingual position of the cusps is determined by dividing the distance from the lingual height of the contour to the tip of the buccal cusp in thirds (Fig. 7-2, *A*). On mandibular posterior teeth, the measurement starts at the buccal height of the contour. Also, note that the lingual cusp is located slightly anterior to the buccal cusp and on the maxillary molars. The mesiolingual cusp appears to be framed between the mesial and distal buccal cusps when viewed buccally. However, these are arbitrary considerations for the position of the cusps. The opposing occlusion and its dynamic function will influence modifications to the cusp height and placement. These are discussed later in the text (Figs. 7-7 to 7-9). The armamentarium used for the wax-added technique includes a wax spatula for bulky additions and for the buildup of cones, and a No. 23 explorer modified by flattening the tip and two sides so it will hold a drop of wax for minor additions and refinement of the wax-added occlusal surface.

STEP 2: ADDING THE TRIANGULAR RIDGES. A wax ridge is formed from the tip of the buccal cusp to the central developmental groove (approximately centered between the tips of the buccal and lingual cusp). This linguotriangular ridge of the buccal cusp should contact the distal cusp ridge of the opposing first premolar, but disclude any excursive movement (unless a working group function occlusion is indicated). At this point the

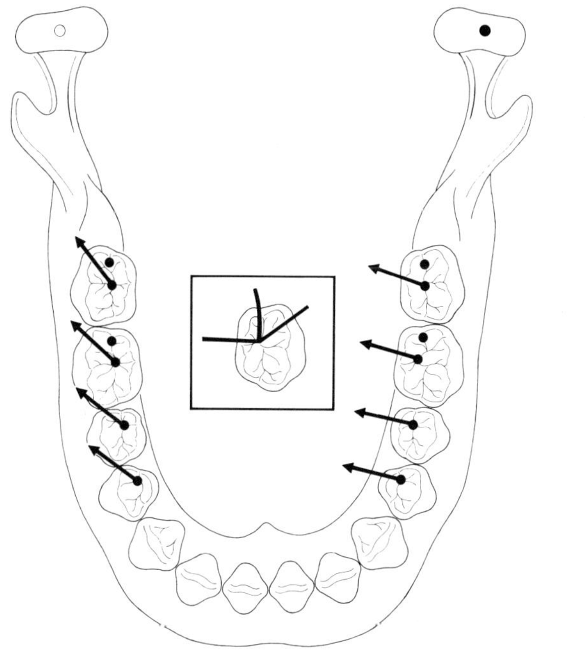

Fig. 7-1. Mandibular dental arch showing working and non-working paths of maxillary stamp cusps.

A

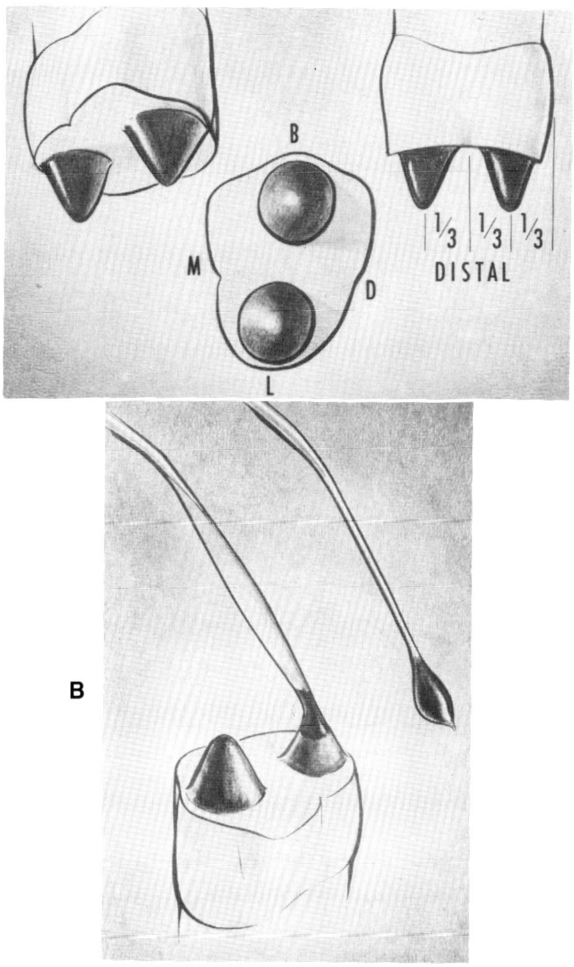

B

Fig. 7-2. Step 1: **A,** buildup of cones. Armanentarium used for wax-added technique. **B,** Wax spatula and modified No. 23 Sichel explorer.

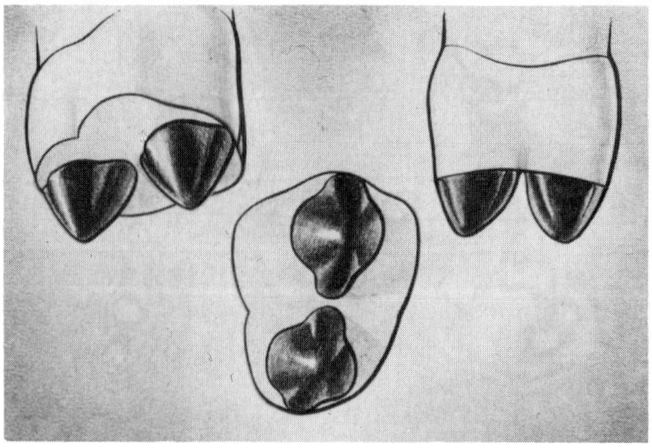

Fig. 7-3. Step 2: adding triangular ridges, and step 3: adding axial contour ridges.

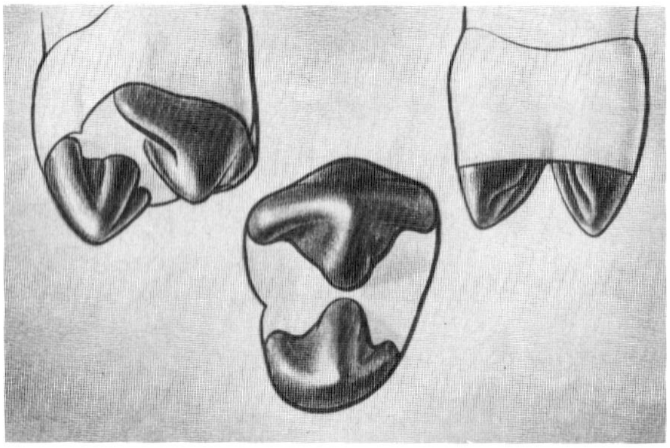

Fig. 7-4. Step 4: adding mesıodistal cusp ridges.

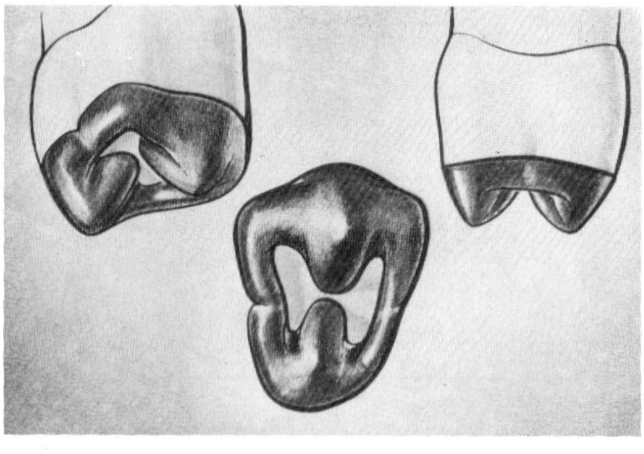

Fig. 7-5. Step 5: adding marginal ridges.

buccal triangular ridge of the lingual cusp is added. It is angled to meet the triangular ridge of the buccal cusp. There should be no interference when the articulator is moved into eccentric excursions (Fig. 7–3).

STEP 3: ADDING AXIAL CONTOUR RIDGES. Buccal and lingual contour ridges are added to complete the axial tooth form.

A

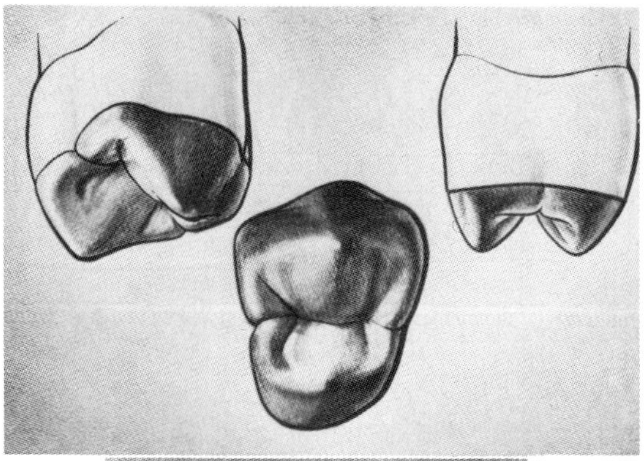

B

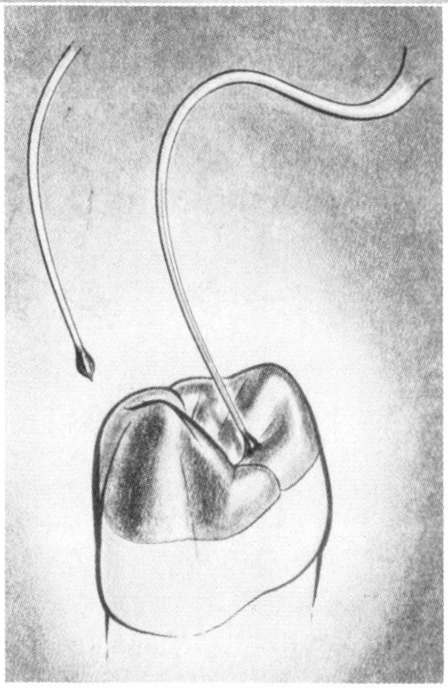

Fig. 7-6. Step 6: **A,** fill-in and refinement to complete occlusal form. **B,** Modified No. 23 Sichel explorer used to add supplemental ridges.

STEP 4: ADDING MESIAL AND DISTAL CUSP RIDGES. These ridges complete the buccal and lingual outline form of the tooth. There should be no contact in eccentric excursions except when a working group function is indicated (Fig. 7-4).

STEP 5: ADDING THE MARGINAL RIDGES. The mesial and distal marginal ridges complete the occlusal outline form of the tooth and form the occlusal interproximal embrasure. As the articulator is closed, the opposing cusp will determine the height of the marginal ridge. From this centric contact, escape channels for the noninterfering passage of the opposing cusp should be provided in an excursion (Fig. 7-5).

STEP 6: FILL-IN AND REFINEMENT. All working elements of the occlusal surface were established in steps 1 to 5. The supplemental anatomy and refinement of the final occlusal form (Fig. 7-6, *A*) is now completed. The modified No. 23 sickle explorer is shown as it is used to add minute supplemental ridges and grooves (Fig. 7-6, *B*).

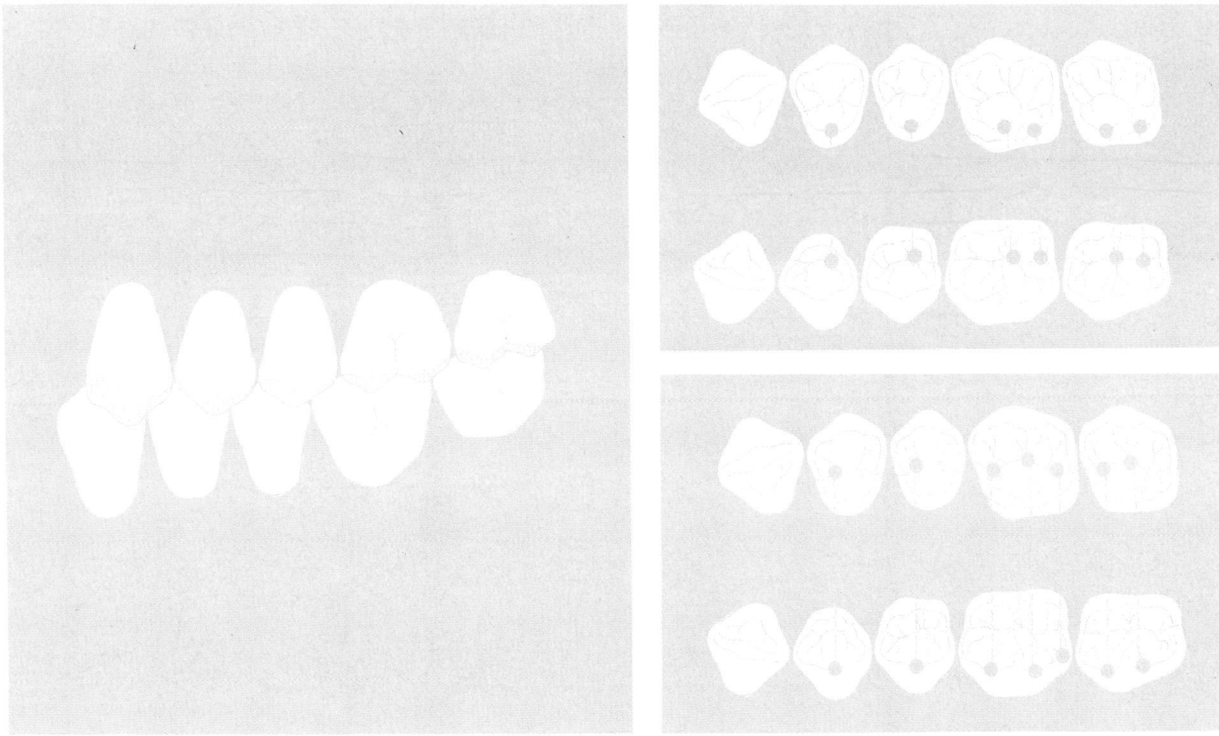

Fig. 7-7. Cusp-to-fossa relationship of opposing teeth. Cusp height decreases from first premolar to second molar.

The wax-added technique for the development of occlusal surfaces is readily adaptable to any occlusal scheme. Originally, the technique was developed to establish cusp-to-marginal ridge relationships and a balanced occlusion. The technique, with minor modifications only, was equally useful in establishing a cusp-to-fossa relationship and posterior disclusion.

CUSP-TO-FOSSA WAXING

A cusp-to-marginal ridge, or cusp-to-embrasure, relationship between opposing natural teeth is more prevalent than a cusp-to-fossa relationship (Lundeen, 1969). So why is the cusp-to-fossa relationship so widely accepted? It is because biomechanically the (1) most stable tooth contact in the position of maximum intercuspation can be established, (2) occlusal forces can be most axially directed, (3) "wedging effect" of a cusp articulated over the occlusal embrasure is avoided (Thomas, 1967).

The restored tooth cannot and need not be in appearance an exact reproduction of the natural tooth. The restoration should be an expression of the functional principles of tooth morphology applied to the altered conditions that inevitably exist when restorative intervention is indicated.

Fig. 7-7 shows a standard for the concept of cusp-to-fossa tooth position and, from a lateral view, the decreasing cusp height from first premolar to second molar. The second molar is the most vulnerable to excessive parafunctional forces, due to its position in the dental arch. The shorter cusp height and correspondingly shallow fossa minimize the potential stress resulting from nonaxial forces.

An illustration will convey only a stylized interpretation. Biomechanically, the fact that the lingual cusp of the maxillary second premolar articulates with the distal fossa of the mandibular second molar (Fig. 7-7) is meaningless, unless, in a given situation, this particular tooth-to-tooth contact distributes the occlusal force in the most axial direction. In other words, it is the skeletal position of the teeth that can cause a variety of combinations of cusp-to-fossa contacts. The biomechanical principle, however, requires that a stamp cusp articulate within a fossa of an opposing tooth and that with this contact the occlusal forces are transmitted to the supporting tissues in the most axial direction.

To complete the picture of the dynamic occlusal form, the excursions of the stamp cusps must be considered and escape ways emphasized in the occlusal form (Fig. 7-8). These escape ways are, in addition to grooves, definite concavities in the cusp ridges and marginal ridges. The mesiolingual cusp of the maxillary molar may, in a working excursion, escape through the lingual groove of the opposing mandibular molar. This

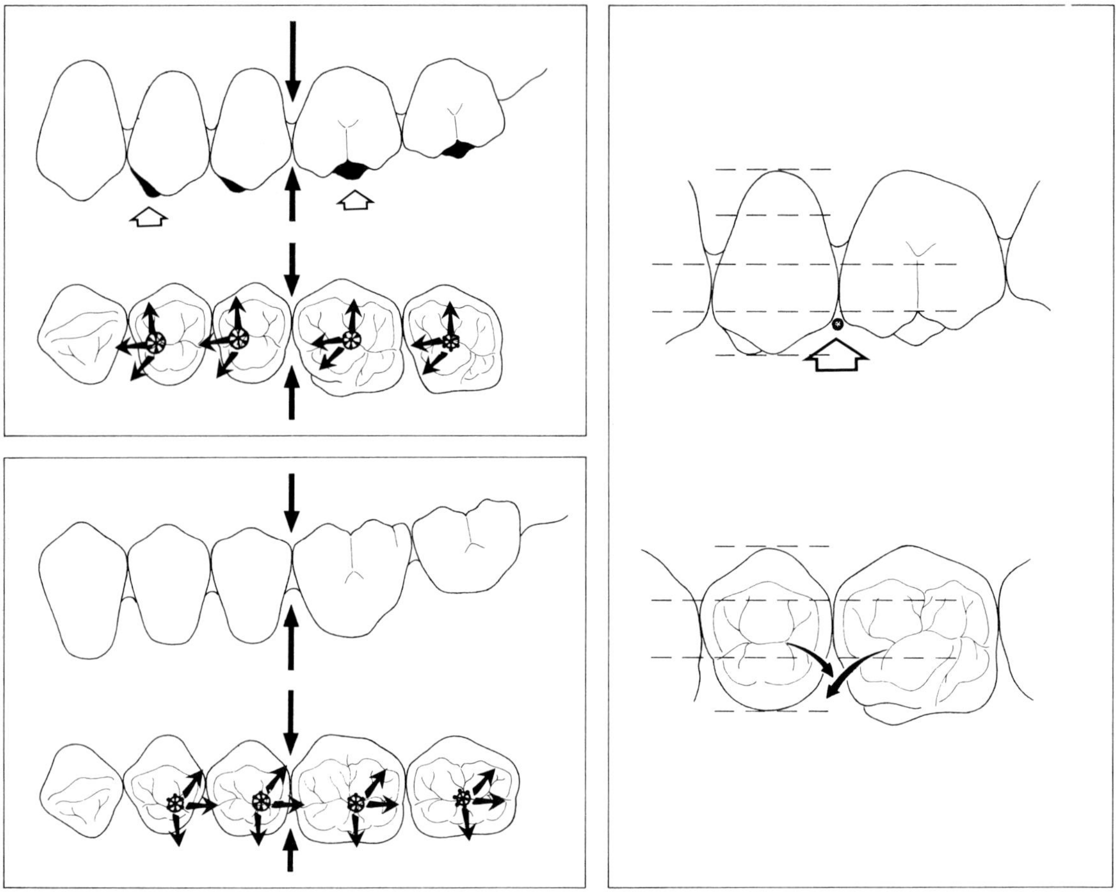

Fig. 7-8. Excursions of stamp cusps warrant placement of concavities, which act as escape ways for stamp cusps.

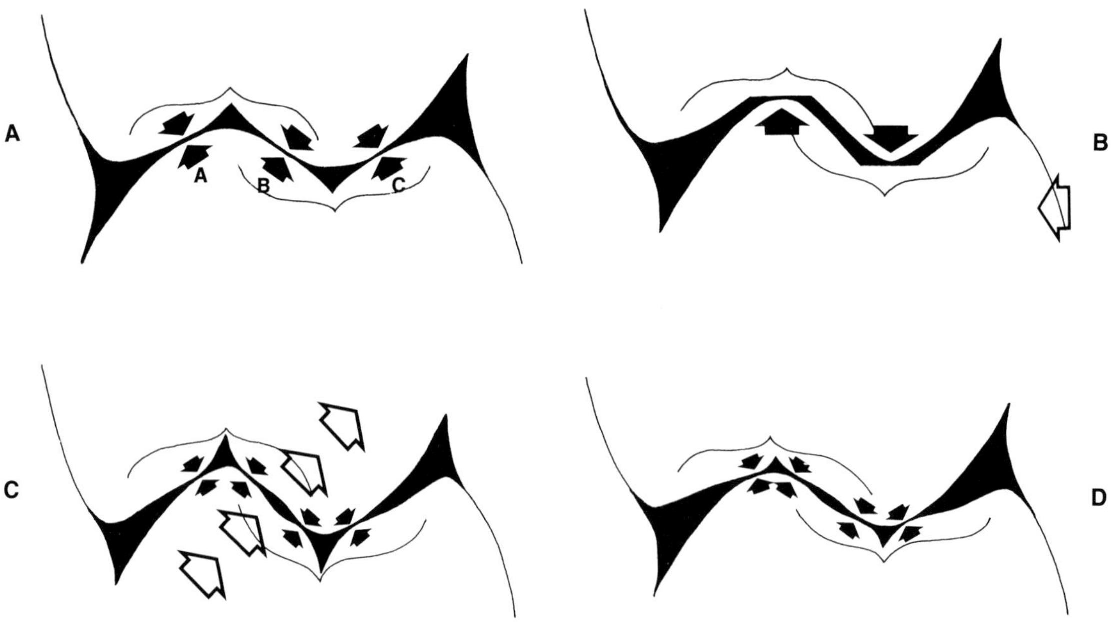

Fig. 7-9. Cusp-to-fossa relationship in anteroposterior cross section. **A,** Convex triangular ridges or "ball-mill" effect. **B,** Wide centric principle. **C,** Effect of increased cusp height. **D,** Relatively shallow but effective cusp height.

is a glide path, not a slide path (Stuart, 1969). No eccentric tooth contact is desired. As an additional guard against potential contact because unassisted mandibular excursions do not follow a precise path, the escape way is widened to form a funnellike path extending from the fossa to the marginal ridge. In the case described, the mesial and distal cusp ridges, which form the lingual groove, are concave rather than convex. The opposing cusp can travel without interference. The use of subtle concavities in the occlusal form and in the axial contour will continue to be emphasized throughout this text because of the biomechanical and hygienic importance of these features.

Fig. 7-9 is a cross section of the cusp-to-fossa relationship in anteroposterior opposing molars. When convex triangular ridges are used, an *A*, *B*, *C* contact is established (Fig. 7-9, *A*). In theory a uniform contact at points *A*, *B*, and *C* was advocated. Also in theory, it appeared to offer a stable occlusion with minimal tooth contacts (approximately 4 sq mm at maximum intercuspation) and be highly effective during mastication. This design, however, offers little compensation for irregularities of the patient's eccentric movements and frequently wear facets formed at points *A*, *B*, but especially at *C*.

A relatively small cusp, articulated within a larger fossa, seemed to offer a favorable solution (Fig. 7-9, *B*). The stamp cusp of opposing teeth can be centered over the respective fossa to transmit axial forces. The "freedom in centric" concept compensates for irregular mandibular movements. The disadvantage here is lack of stability. An excessive lingual or buccal musculature force could alter adversely the tooth position and with it the occlusal scheme.

Fig. 7-9, *C*, shows that modification to the triangular ridges (concavities) centers the stamp cusps over the opposing tooth and provides better escape ways. The steep inclines of the triangular ridges, caused by maximum cusp height, can contribute to excessive lateral forces during parafunctional muscular activity.

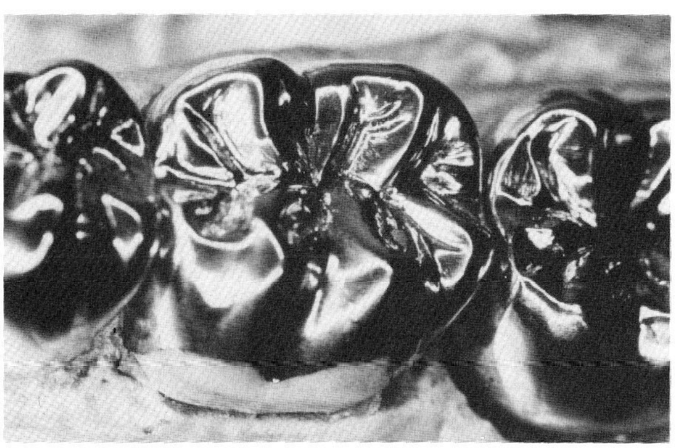

Fig. 7-10. Occlusal tooth morphology as described in Fig. 7-9, *D*.

A combination of the most advantageous occlusal features is illustrated in Fig. 7-9, *D*. A relatively short stamp cusp is nestled within a fossa for optimal stability. The concave arrangement in the triangular ridges assures minimal tooth contact in centric relation and ready disclusion in eccentric excursions. Even during parafunctional activity the potential for lateral forces is minimized.

Cusp height is often lauded for better masticatory efficiency; however, the destructive potential of resultant steep inclines must be considered. The science of physics has given us a law that applies here: a force exerted at a point is inversely proportional to the square area. Therefore with skillful arrangement of subtle concavities in the triangular and cusp ridges, a short stamp cusp (Fig. 7-10) can function as efficiently as a long cusp with a lesser stress potential.

Waxing to a functional core

G. ROGER TROENDLE

The functional generated path technique for use in fixed prosthodontics, first discussed by F.S. Meyer in 1938, has been popularized by the Pankey Mann Institute. The technique consists of generating a wax occlusal path in the mouth (Fig. 7-11) and replicating the wax path in stone (Fig. 7-12). The generated path captures selected mandibular movements in wax. These mandibular movements are then replicated in the stone core.

The functionally generated path technique will be discussed relative to five parameters:

1. Type of guidance
2. Placement of cusp tip contacts
3. Relationship of occlusal tooth contacts to the temporomandibular joint
4. Number of contact points
5. Waxing technique

Any one or combination of these parameters can be applied when waxing either to a functional core or to an anatomic cast.

TYPE OF GUIDANCE

Three types of guidance are used: (1) bilateral balanced posterior occlusion, (2) unilateral balanced posterior occlusion, and (3) anterior guided posterior occlusion.

Bilateral balanced posterior occlusion

A bilateral balanced posterior occlusion is not considered an acceptable type of occlusion for fixed prosth-

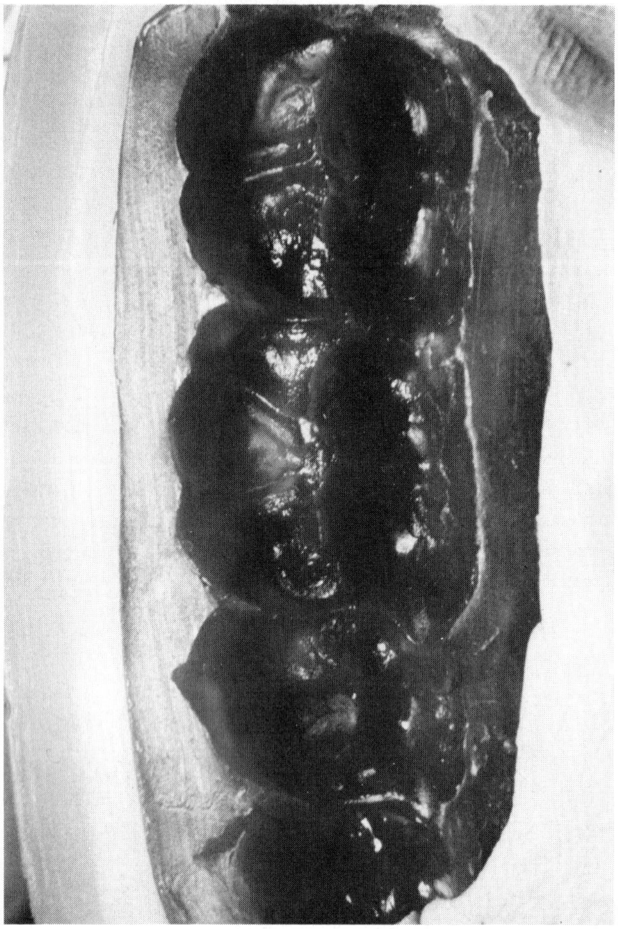

Fig. 7-11. Generated wax path.

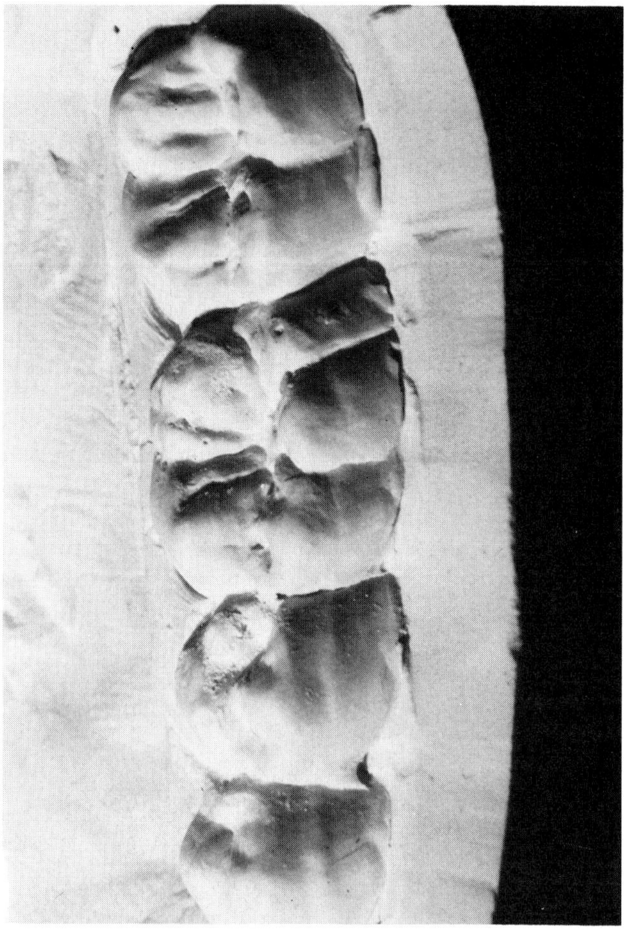

Fig. 7-12. Functional core poured from generated wax path in Fig. 7-11.

odontics and is reserved for removable prosthodontics. This concept of occlusion will not be discussed further here.

Unilateral balanced posterior occlusion

In a unilateral balanced posterior occlusion, the posterior teeth on the working side disclude the teeth on the nonworking side. It is with this type of occlusion that the functionally generated path technique is most applicable. Fig. 7-13 is a cross-sectional diagram of a maxillary right molar wax pattern adapted to a functional core. The functional core is a three-dimensional representation of selected mandibular movements recorded in wax and replicated in stone. Wherever the wax pattern contacts the functional core, the final restoration will contact the mandibular tooth in that movement. The working inclines (inner inclines of the maxillary buccal cusps) contact the functional core, whereas the nonworking inclines (inner inclines of the maxillary lingual cusps) are relieved to eliminate balancing contacts. Outlined on the functional core is the actual shape of the mandibular tooth.

The amount of contact desired on the working inclines for the first and second molar region is less than that desired for the cuspid-bicuspid region. This is dictated by two biomechanical principles. First, the mandible is a Class III lever system. Fig. 7-14 compares the mandible to the classic Class III lever, a nutcracker. Notice that in this system any force applied creates a greater stress on an object placed closest to the fulcrum. Therefore, the teeth farthest from the fulcrum can guide the mandible with the least amount of stress being applied to them. Second, during lateral movement the teeth closest to the center of rotation will travel less distance than those farthest from the center of rotation (Fig. 7-15). Therefore, if the working inclines of the molar teeth on an anatomic cast are waxed to contact the complete length of these inclines, then in extreme working movements only the molar teeth will guide the mandible. This is an extremely unfavor-

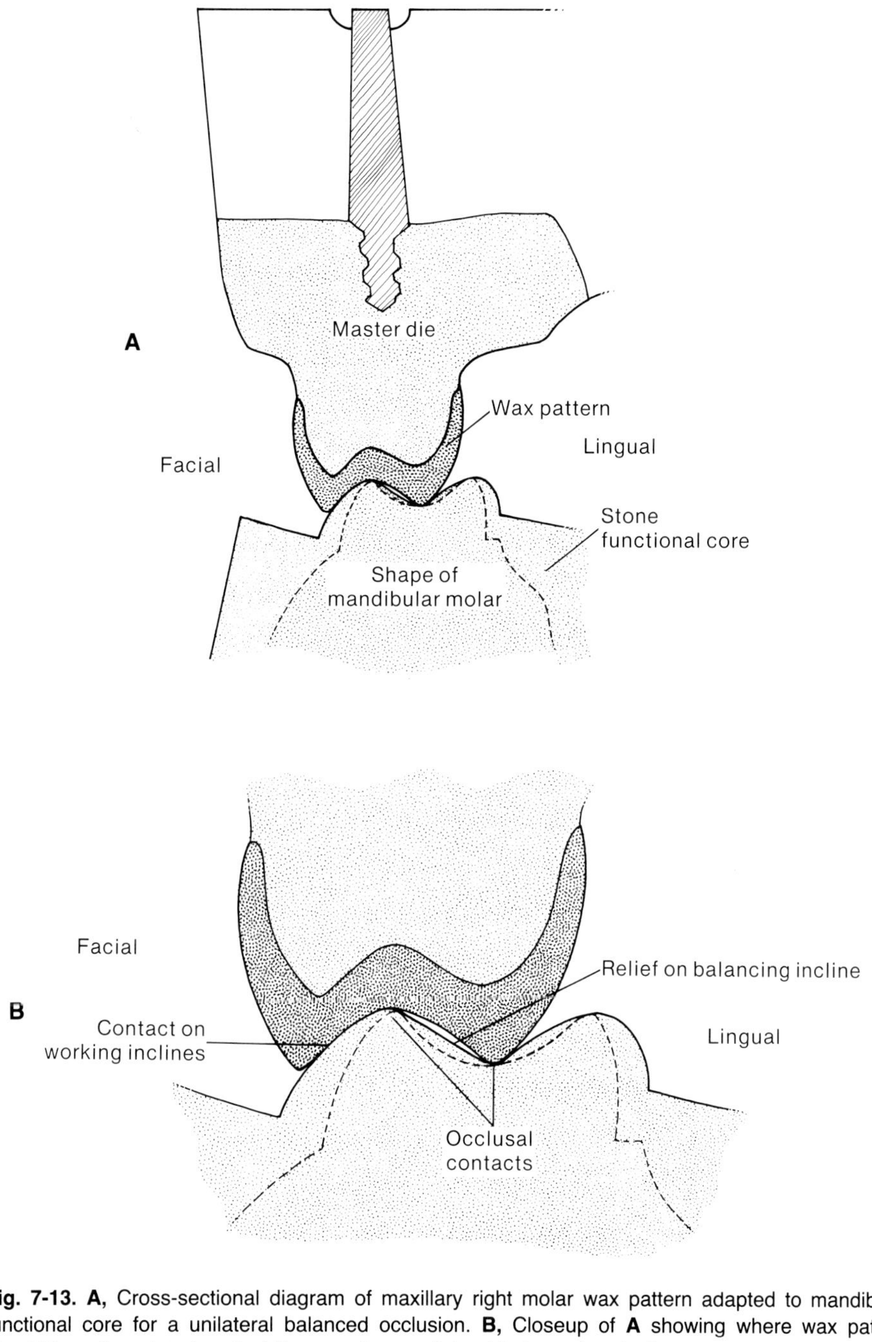

Fig. 7-13. A, Cross-sectional diagram of maxillary right molar wax pattern adapted to mandibular functional core for a unilateral balanced occlusion. **B,** Closeup of **A** showing where wax pattern should be relieved and contact the core for a unilateral balanced occlusion.

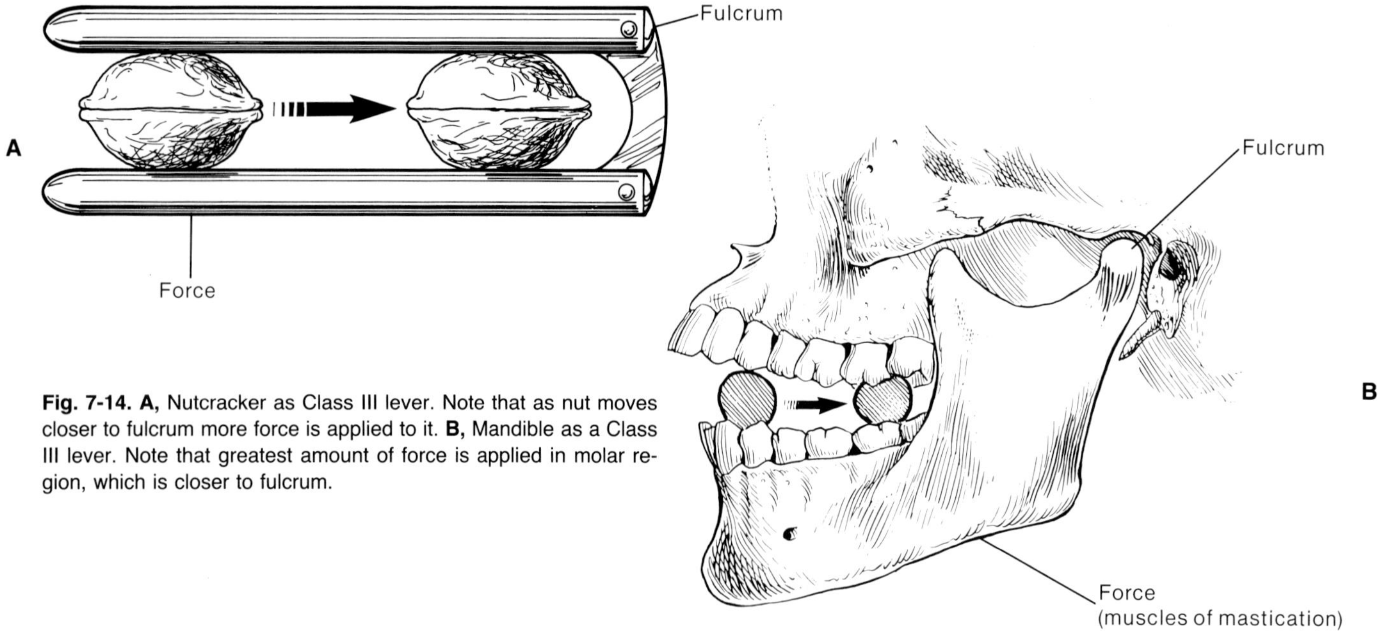

Fig. 7-14. A, Nutcracker as Class III lever. Note that as nut moves closer to fulcrum more force is applied to it. **B,** Mandible as a Class III lever. Note that greatest amount of force is applied in molar region, which is closer to fulcrum.

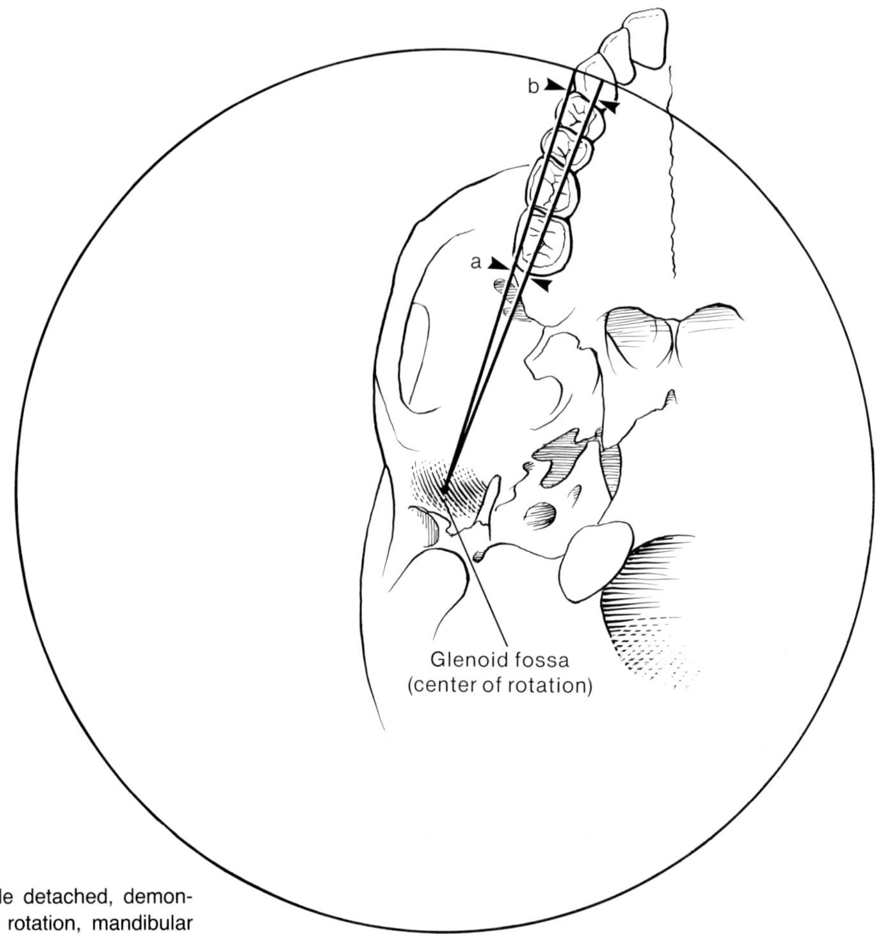

Fig. 7-15. Inferior view of skull with mandible detached, demonstrating that with glenoid fossa as center of rotation, mandibular molar teeth will track less distance across the working inclines of the maxillary molar teeth *(a)* than the cuspids *(b)*.

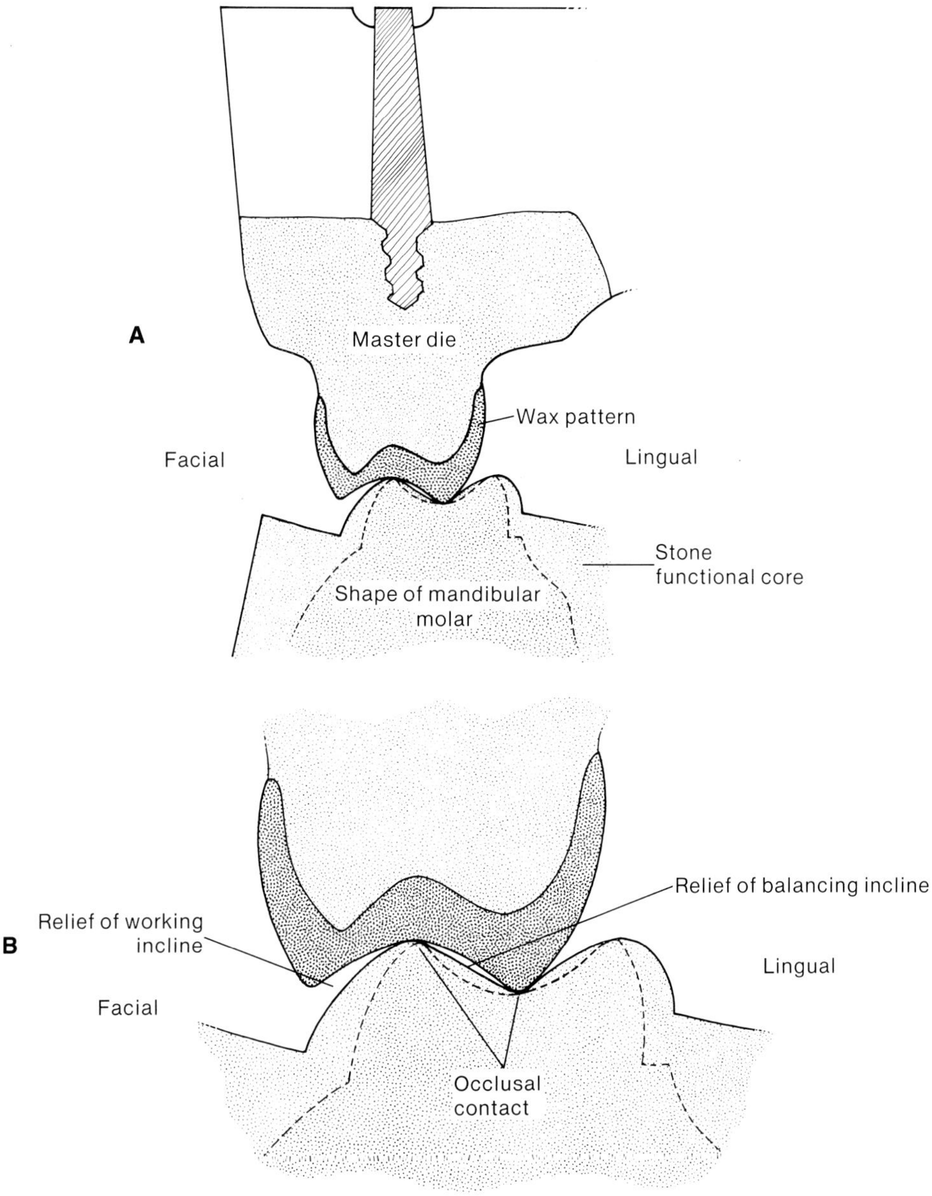

Fig. 7-16. A, Cross-sectional diagram of maxillary right molar wax pattern adapted to functional core for an anterior guided posterior occlusion. **B,** Closeup of **A** showing where the wax pattern should be relieved and contact functional core.

able situation, since the molar teeth are closest to the fulcrum point and maximum force is applied here. However, if the molar teeth are waxed to the complete length of the working incline of the functional core, the mandible will not be guided by the molar teeth since the functional core is a stone replica of mandibular movements captured in wax using the glenoid fossa as the center of rotation.

Anterior guided posterior occlusion

In an anterior guided posterior occlusion one or more of the anterior teeth discludes the posterior teeth in working and nonworking movements. Fig. 7-16 is a cross-sectional diagram of how the wax pattern should be adapted to the functional core to accomplish a posterior disclusion. Both the working and balancing inclines are relieved and only the cusp tips are in contact.

PLACEMENT OF CUSP TIP CONTACT

A cusp can have one of three possible relationships with an opposing tooth: (1) cusp-to-marginal ridge, (2) cusp-to-fossa, or (3) cusp-to-embrasure. Any of these three relationships can be accomplished when waxing to a functional core. However, it is advantageous to

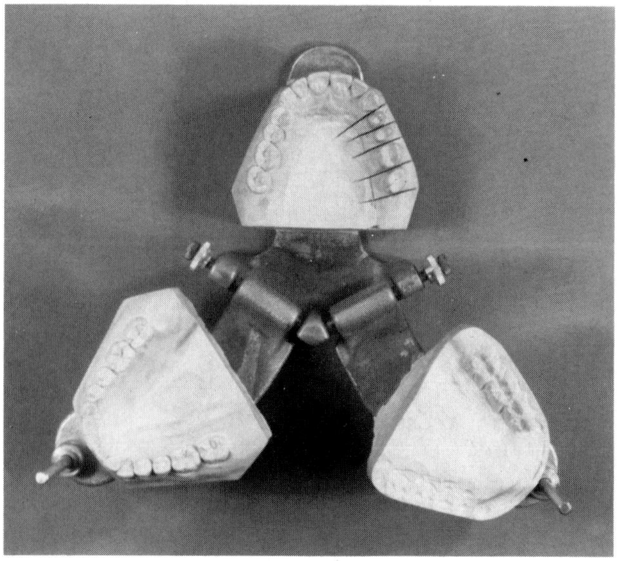

Fig. 7-17. Twin-stage occluder. Note master cast die is always mounted on lower member.

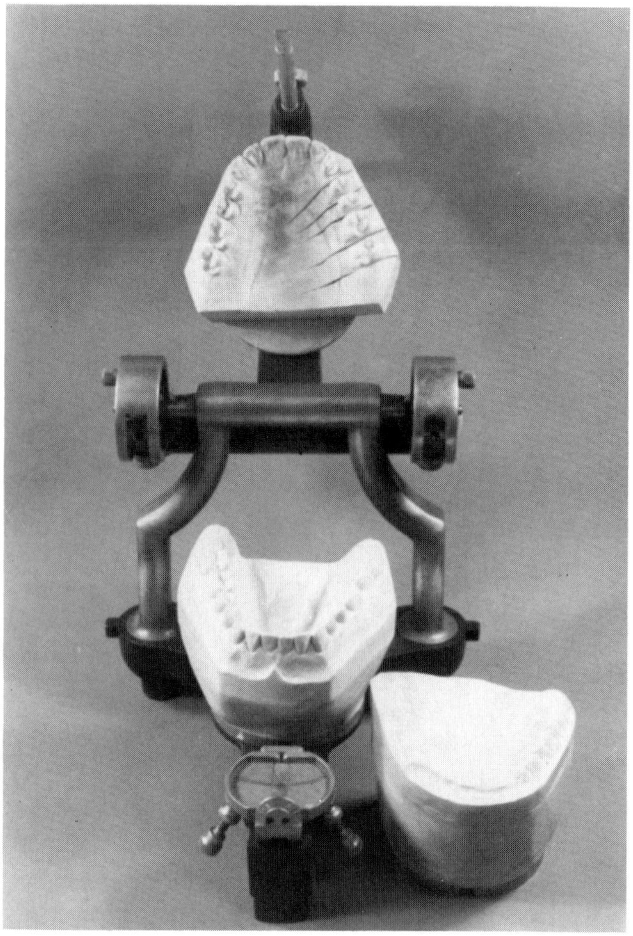

Fig. 7-18. Hanau 158 with anatomic cast mounted in articulator and a functional core that can be interchanged with mandibular anatomic cast.

have both the functional core and an anatomic cast mounted to the master die to facilitate cusp placement. The twin stage occluder permits the mounting of the functional core and the anatomic cast in the same instrument (Fig. 7-17). This may also be accomplished with a conventional semiadjustable articulator; however, the functional core and the anatomic cast must be inter-changed in the instrument (Fig. 7-18). The steeper the anterior and condylar guidance, the more the functional core resembles the anatomic cast, and the less an anatomic cast is needed for cusp placement. Fig. 7-19 shows three functional cores made from the same anatomic cast with different condylar and anterior guidances: *A* and *C* illustrate functional cores made with a condylar and anterior guidance of 10, 30, and 60 degrees, respectively; *D* is the cast used to generate these paths; *C* resembles the anatomic cast, *D*.

RELATIONSHIP OF THE OCCLUSAL CONTACTS TO THE TEMPOROMANDIBULAR JOINT

The teeth can be waxed in relation to the TMJ in one of three positions: (1) intercuspal position (ICP), (2) centric relation-occlusion (CR-O), or (3) long centric (LC).

With an anatomic cast, the functionally generated path technique can be used to wax the tooth-condylar position in any of these positions. However, the functional core itself is not mounted in ICP or CR-O but is rather a stone matrix made from a wax path that captures selected mandibular movements including ICP and CR-O. The functional core is a means for ensuring that there are no interferences between ICP and CR-O and, therefore, establishes a long centric position. The functionally generated path technique is most applicable where a long centric occlusion is established.

NUMBER OF CONTACT POINTS

Three types of occlusal contacts may be established in wax: (1) point-to-point, (2) three-point to three-point, or (3) point-to-surface.

Establishing an occlusal relationship with three-point contacts is most applicable when it is desirable to have the teeth establish the condylar position at one point. The position chosen can be CR-O or ICP. However, when a long centric concept of occlusion is established, it is not desirable to have the teeth position the condyles at one location. The mandible should be able to move from ICP to CR-O or vice versa without interference. A long centric relationship is best maintained by a point-to-point or point-to-surface contact.

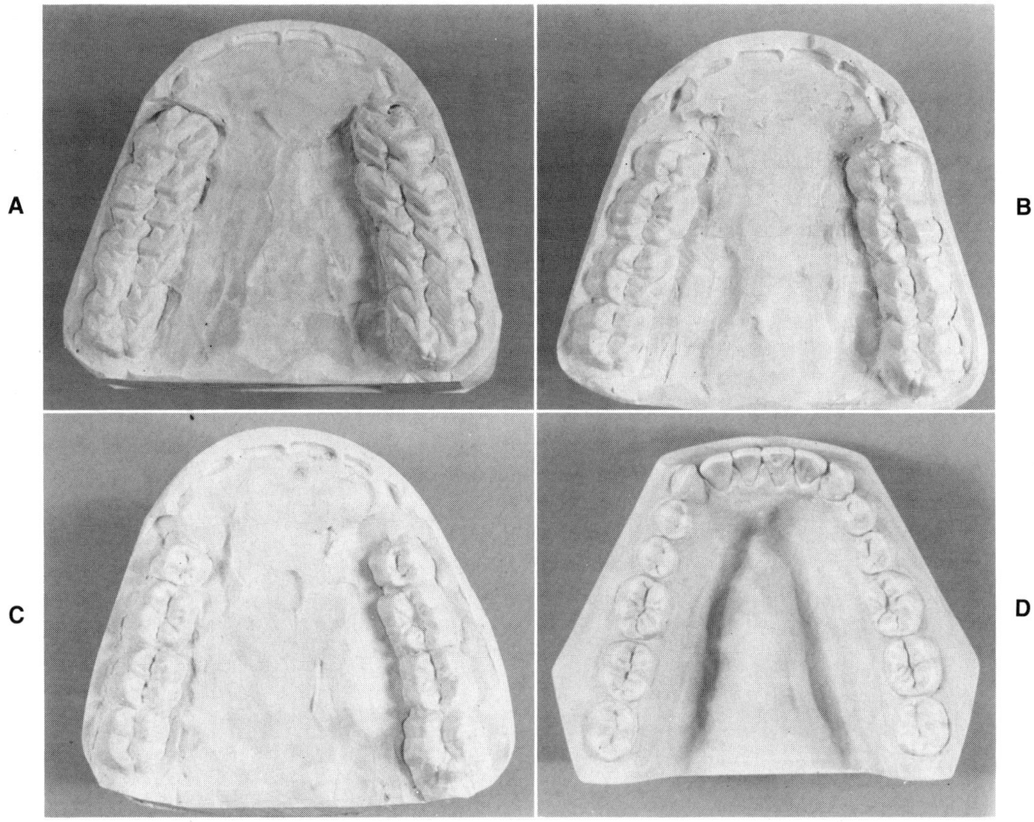

Fig. 7-19. Comparison of three functional cores, generated at different anterior and condylar guidances, to the anatomic cast that generated the paths. **A,** Anterior guidance, 10 degrees; condylar guidance, 10 degrees **B,** Anterior guidance, 30 degrees; condylar guidance, 30 degrees **C,** Anterior guidance, 60 degrees; condylar guidance, 60 degrees **D,** Anatomic cast that generated paths.

WAXING TECHNIQUE

The two methods of developing occlusal anatomy in wax are: (1) the additive technique and (2) the subtractive technique. Either technique is an acceptable method of waxing to a functional core. The wax additive technique was discussed earlier (pp. 171-175). The same principles apply when waxing to a functional core. Again, it is useful to have a mounted anatomic cast as well as the functional core for verifying cusp placement.

The remainder of this section will discuss the procedures for developing anatomy against a functional core by the wax subtractive technique. The maxillary left quadrant will be waxed to establish a long centric occlusion with a unilateral balanced occlusion.

PROCEDURE

1. Mount the maxillary master die in the twin-stage occluder along with the functional core and an anatomic cast. Be sure the pin is touching the incisal table (Fig. 7-20).

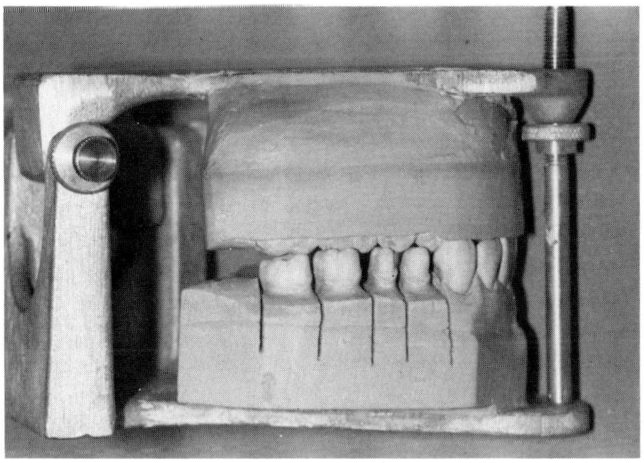

Fig. 7-20. Functional core mounted in twin-stage occluder with pin touching table.

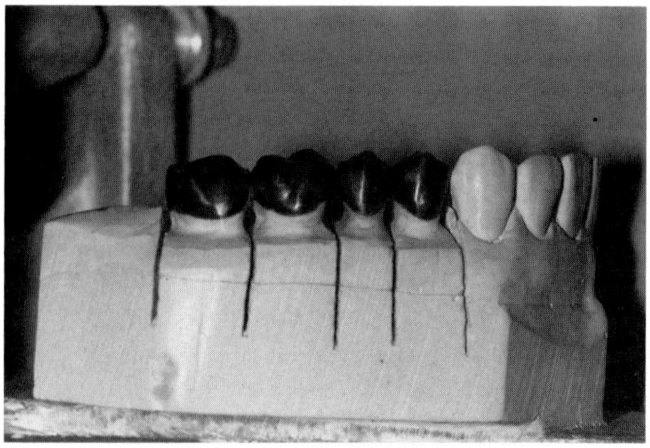

Fig. 7-21. Axial contours of wax patterns developed.

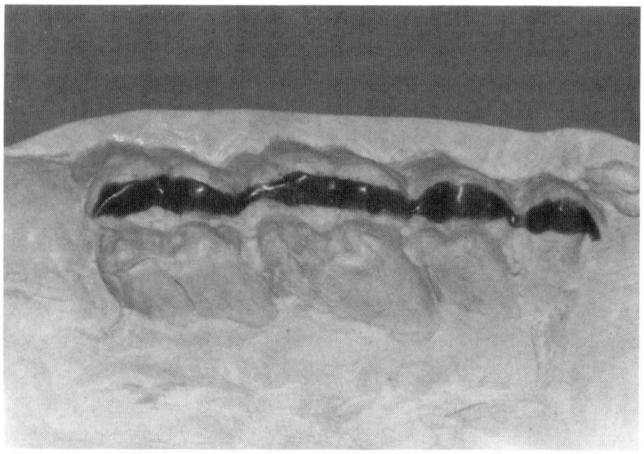

Fig. 7-22. Functional core with inner inclines of mandibular buccal cusps blocked out to prevent balancing contacts.

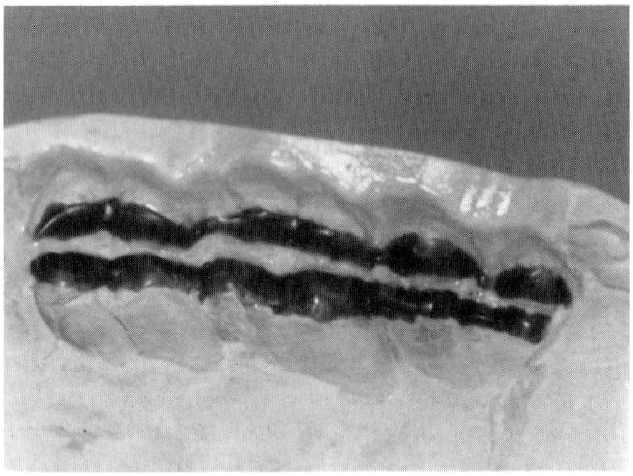

Fig. 7-23. Functional core with inner inclines of mandibular lingual cusps blocked out to prevent unwanted working contacts.

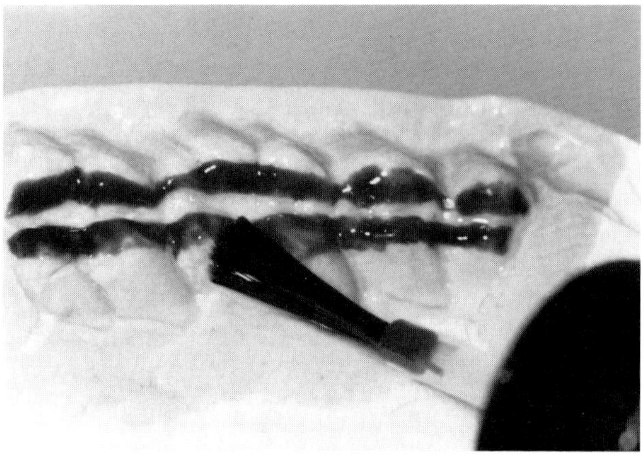

Fig. 7-24. Lubricating blocked-out functional core with die lubricant.

2. Develop the axial contours in wax on the dies (Fig. 7-21).

3. Block out areas of the functional core that should not be in contact with inlay wax. Here a unilateral balanced occlusion is being developed; therefore, block out the inner inclines of the mandibular buccal cusps on the functional core to prevent balancing contacts (Fig. 7-22), and block out the inner incline of the mandibular lingual cusp on the functional core to prevent unwanted working contacts (Fig. 7-23).

4. Lubricate the blocked out core with die lubricant (Fig. 7-24).

5. Warm the tip of a chip blower (Fig. 7-25).

6. Heat each occlusal surface separately with warm air stream from the chip blower (Fig. 7-26).

7. Close the lubricated functional core into the soft occlusal wax and observe the wax pattern (Fig. 7-27).

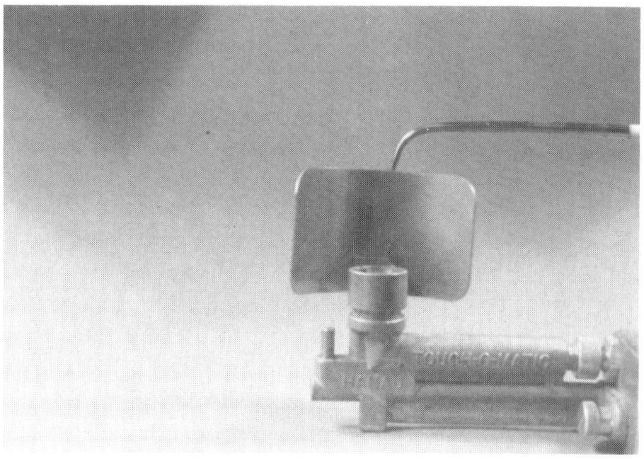

Fig. 7-25. Heating chip blower in flame.

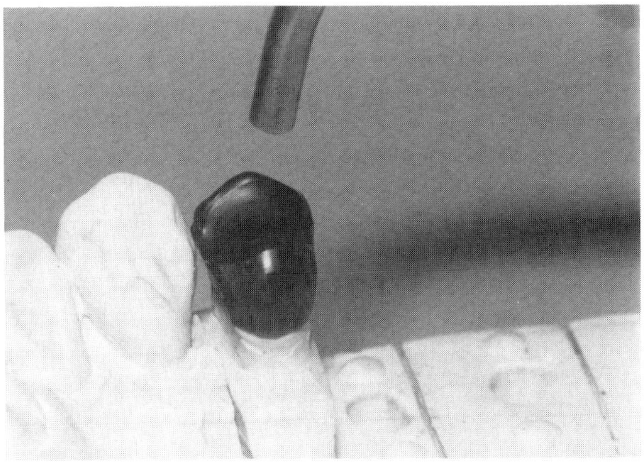

Fig. 7-26. Heating occlusal of wax pattern with heated chip blower.

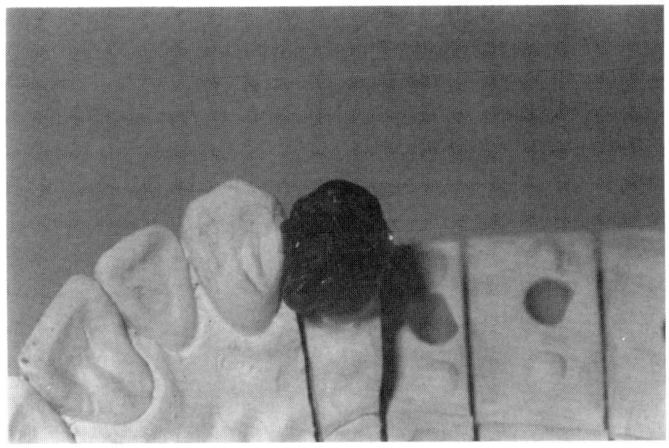

Fig. 7-27. Maxillary left first premolar after functional core has been closed into excess heated occlusal wax of pattern.

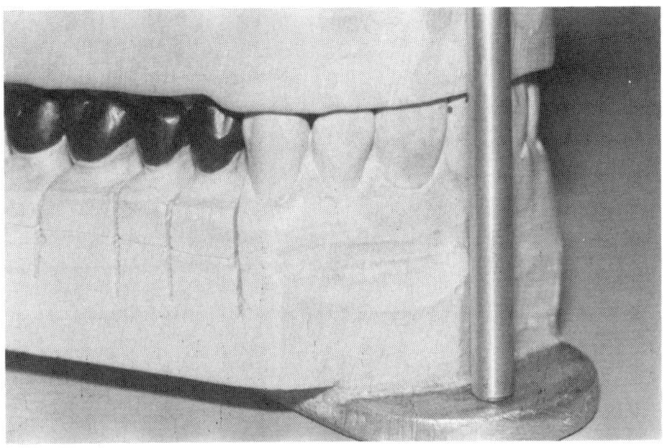

Fig. 7-28. Functional core closed into wax patterns after extruded wax was removed. Note that pin is touching table.

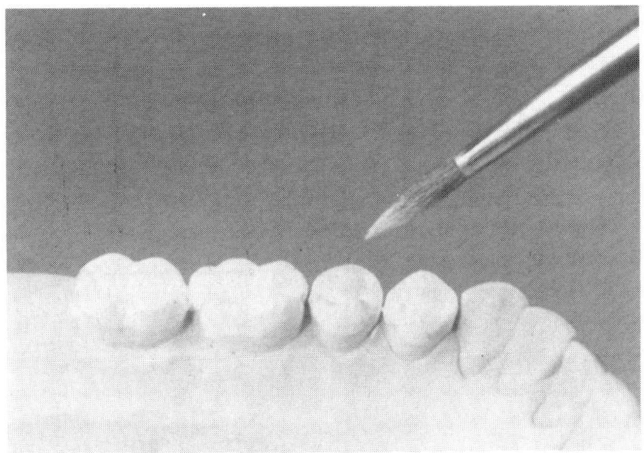

Fig. 7-29. Mandibular anatomic cast with occlusal surface being painted with white shoepolish.

Be sure the core is adequately impressed in the wax pattern and the pin is touching the table.

8. Repeat the above procedure for each wax pattern separately.
9. Remove the extruded wax until all the dies will seat in the master cast.
10. Close the functional core into all of the wax patterns at the same time, making sure the guide pin touched the table (Fig. 7-28).
11. Coat the occlusal of the anatomic cast with white shoe polish (Fig. 7-29).
12. Close the anatomic cast into the wax patterns, making the contacts in white on the wax patterns (Fig. 7-30).
13. Carve anatomic contours into the occlusal surface, taking care to avoid carving away the white occlusal contacts.

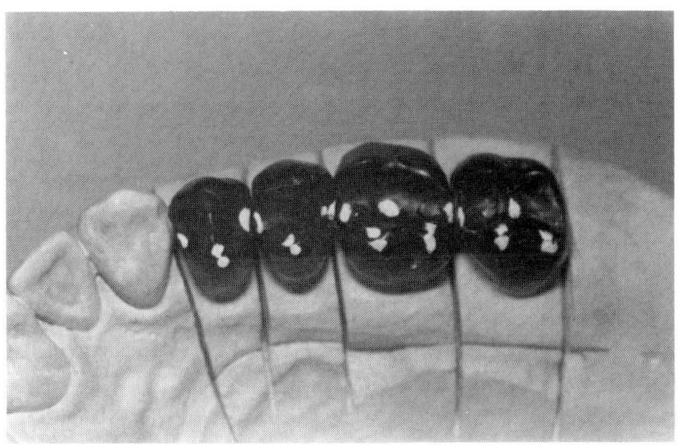

Fig. 7-30. Occlusal contacts after anatomic cast has been closed into wax patterns.

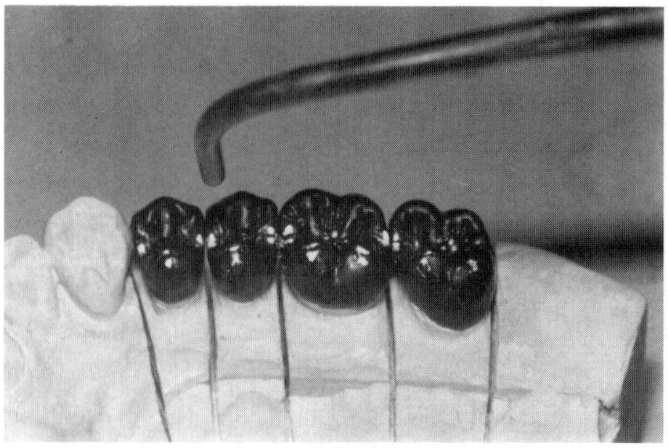

Fig. 7-31. Rounding carved occlusal wax with a gentle warm air stream from chip blower.

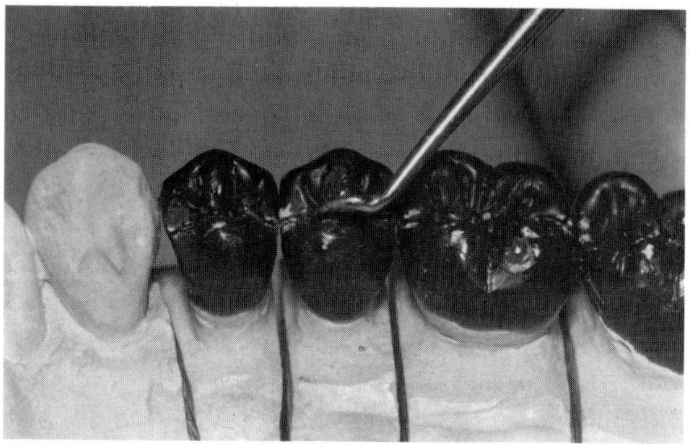

Fig. 7-32. Rounding flattened areas with a carving instrument after closing functional core into heated occlusal wax.

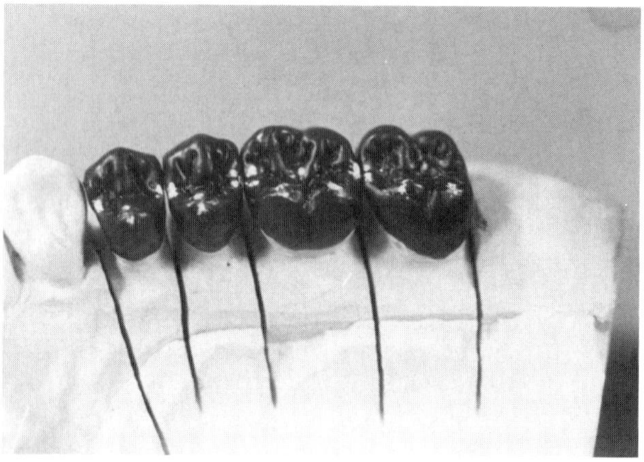

Fig. 7-33. Completed wax patterns after rounding with warm chip blower and checking with both anatomic cast and functional core.

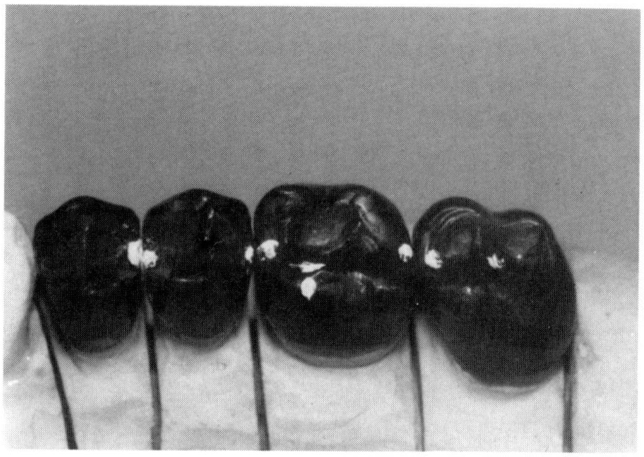

Fig. 7-34. Occlusal contacts after painted occlusal surface of anatomic cast has been closed into occlusal of wax pattern, which has already had functional core closed into it. Note that certain desired cusp tip contacts are not present on lingual cusp tips of wax patterns.

14. Round the carved occlusal of the wax pattern with a gentle, warm air stream from a heated chip blower (Fig. 7-31).

15. Close the functional core into the warmed occlusal of the wax pattern. Be certain the incisal pin touches the table. Repeat the procedure if the pin is not touching.

16. Remove any excess wax and round any flattened areas with a carving instrument (Fig. 7-32).

17. Smooth the occlusal of the wax pattern with a gentle, warm air stream from a heated chip blower and check the finished wax pattern with both the functional core and the anatomic cast (Fig. 7-33).

Axial contouring

HAROLD F. EISSMANN

The axial surfaces of fixed dental restorations must be contoured to afford protection as well as stimulation to gingival tissues, thereby providing an environment adverse to the formation of bacterial plaque. Protective contours are convexities, such as food deflection prominences, which prevent food impaction. Stimulating contours are concavities, such as embrasures and sluice gates, which provide ready access for cleaning tooth surfaces and massaging gingival tissues.

There cannot be a stereotype form for the facial sur-

Table 7-1. Waxing to a functional core

Problem	Probable cause	Solution
The wax pattern sticks to the inlay wax used for blockout when closing the functional core into the heated wax on the occlusal of the waxed restorations.	1. Core and wax used for blockout not lubricated. 2. Wrong kind of wax used to block out functional core.	1. Lubricate the core and wax used for blockout. 2. Use a hard inlay wax for blocking out the core.
Wax pattern fractures when closing the functional core into heated surface of the wax pattern.	Occlusal of the wax pattern not heated enough.	Reheat the occlusal of the wax pattern and gently close the core into it. Repeat the procedures as needed until the pin touched the table.
The anatomic cast with white shoe polish does not leave a white mark on the wax pattern impression of the functional core (Fig. 7-34).	1. The core or the anatomic cast is improperly mounted. 2. The cusp height of the mandibular teeth is steeper than the incisal guidance; therefore, centric holding cusps are obliterated in lateral movements when making the wax path and replicated in the stone core. 3. The patient did not have an occlusal contact when the wax path was generated.	1. Check the mounting of the anatomic cast and functional core and correct as necessary. 2. Reduce the cusp height of the mandibular teeth. 3. Make a decision either to adjust the remaining teeth in the mouth so that the teeth occlude or accept the occlusion as it is.
Wax patterns fracture when closing the anatomic cast into the wax patterns.	1. The functionally generated wax path was not seated completely on the teeth or dies when the functional core was poured. 2. The wax pattern was not seated on the die. 3. The die was not seated in the master cast.	1. Remake the functionally generated wax path, taking care that the wax path is seated on the teeth or dies before the core is poured. 2. Seat the wax pattern on the die. 3. Seat the die in the master cast.
Occlusal anatomy is obliterated when heating the occlusal wax with the chip blower.	Too large a volume of heated air from the chip blower is being used.	Recarve the anatomic contours and use a gentle stream of air from the chip blower.

face of a lower first molar or for any tooth surface. The contour must represent a functional interpretation of protective versus stimulating features, an interpretation that is relative to (1) clinical crown length, (2) tissue architecture, (3) contour of adjacent teeth, and (4) character of opposing occlusion.

Axial tooth contouring is directed toward minimizing plaque retention by exposing the largest possible area of the clinical crown and the surrounding gingival tissues to the cleansing and stimulating action of the food-flow pattern, musculature, and mechanical devices.

FACIOLINGUAL SURFACES

The principle of food flow over the faciolingual tooth surfaces is illustrated in Fig. 7-35. Axial prominences are sufficient to effect food deflection from the gingival sulcus, but subtle enough to afford a gentle stimulating action to the marginal gingiva. The bulk of food sub-

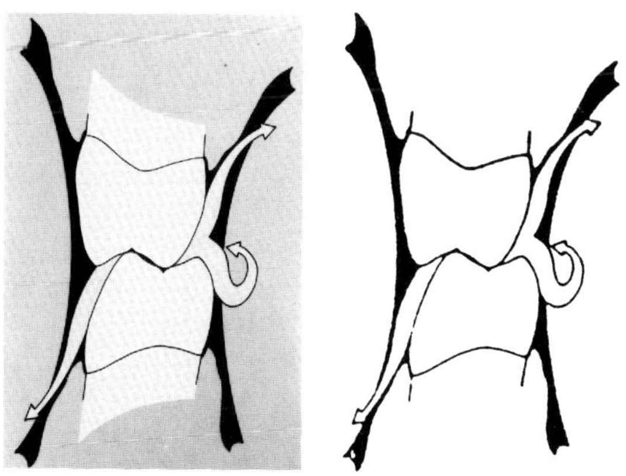

Fig. 7-35. Deflective prominences and their relationship to food-flow pattern.

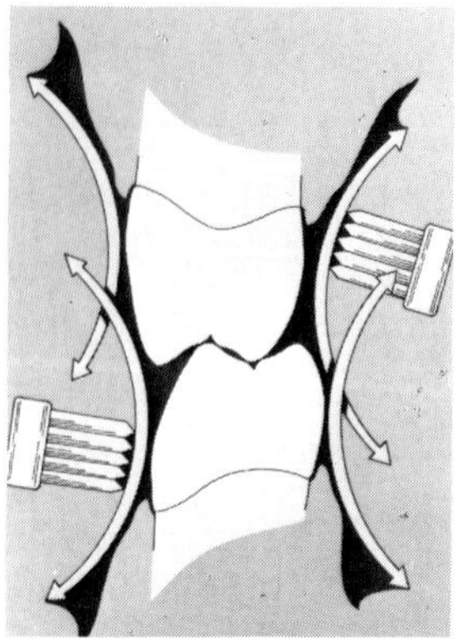

Fig. 7-36. Action of mechanical hygiene devices against axial surfaces.

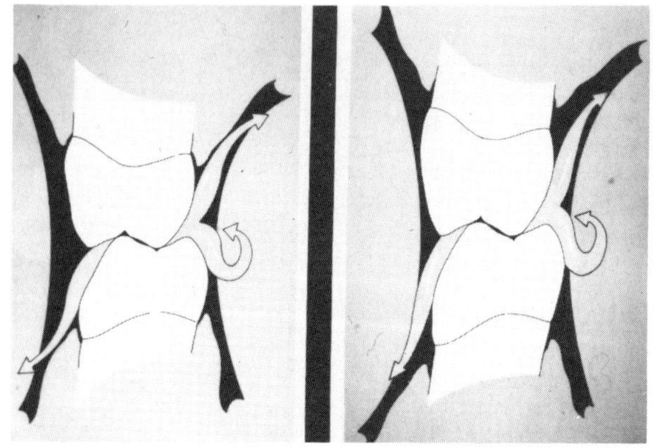

Fig. 7-37. Deflective prominences related to gingival architecture for short and excessively long clinical crowns.

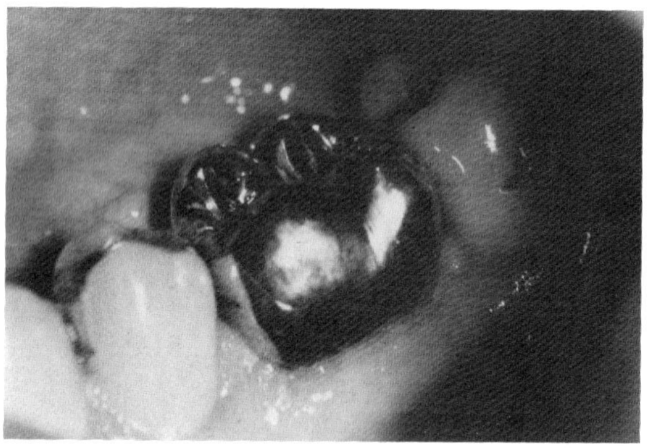

Fig. 7-38. Unsatisfactory restoration because of bulky, overprotective contours.

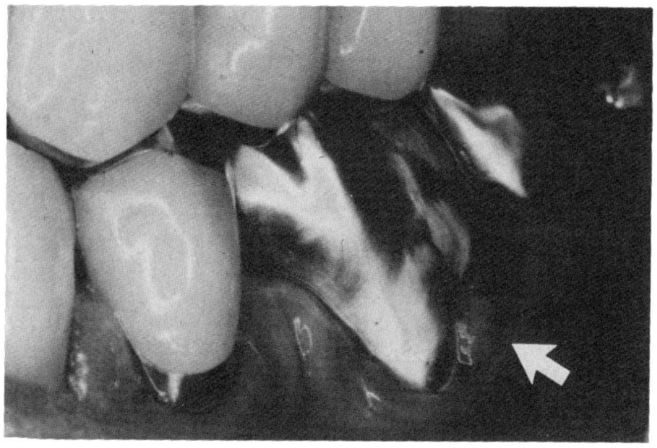

Fig. 7-39. Overprotected bifurcation area *(arrow)* contributes to adverse gingival changes.

stance shedding lingually is deflected near the occlusal third of the lingual surface of the lower posterior teeth onto the dorsum of the tongue and returned to the occlusal table for further mastication.

Mechanical hygiene devices provide the most effective cleansing for all crown surfaces (Fig. 7-36). Once the principles of hygienic crown contours are understood and a flow pattern about these contours is visualized, access channels to the gingiva can be arranged to allow for the most effective hygiene by mechanical devices.

To be truly effective, axial crown contours depend on a delicate relationship between clinical crown length and the gingival architecture. Fig. 7-37 shows two examples of this relationship: (1) the short, ovoid crown with prominent deflection contours harmonious with the bulky gingival architecture, and (2) the increased clinical crown length with diminishing contour prominences, to gain some stimulation to the gingival tissues.

Replacing occlusal and axial tooth enamel (Fig. 7-38) does not qualify as dental restoration. "Restoration" implies that optimum function has been restored; the occlusal surface generates the least amount of stress in the supporting tissues, and the design of the axial surfaces promotes continued health. The blunted form of the facial cusps increases their stress-gathering capacity; the convex contour of the facial surface tends to obliterate access to the interproximal area. The effectiveness of the facial cusps can be increased by the arrangement of concavities in the mesiodistal slopes. As these concavities are channeled gingivally, terminating interproximally below the contact area, a ready route is formed for access to the interproximal embrasures.

The concept of a "food deflection ridge" leads to placing prominent convexities at or near the faciogingival margin. These curvatures actually function like rounded ledges, which compounds the problem of plaque retention. Fig. 7-39 shows the proliferation of gingival tissue in response to bacterial toxins produced by organisms

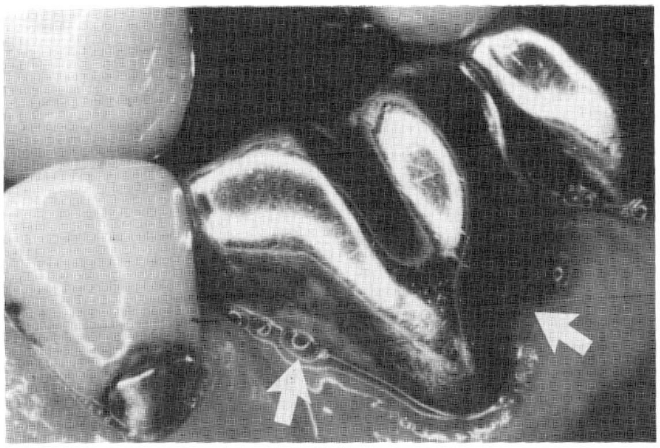

Fig. 7-40. Highlights emphasize overprotective contour prominences *(arrows).*

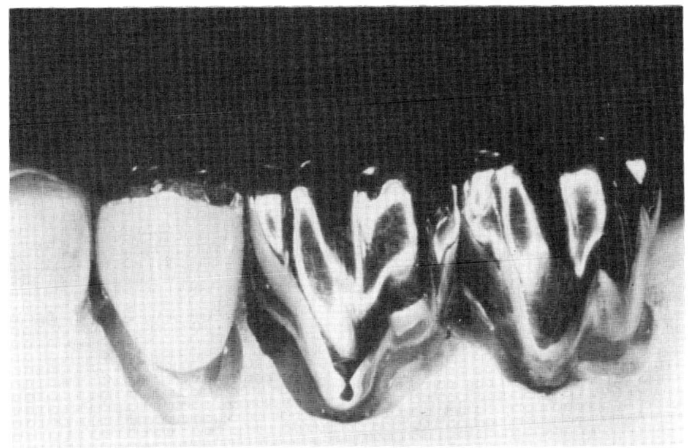

Fig. 7-41. Gentle concavities lead into interproximal embrasures to permit cleansing and stimulation.

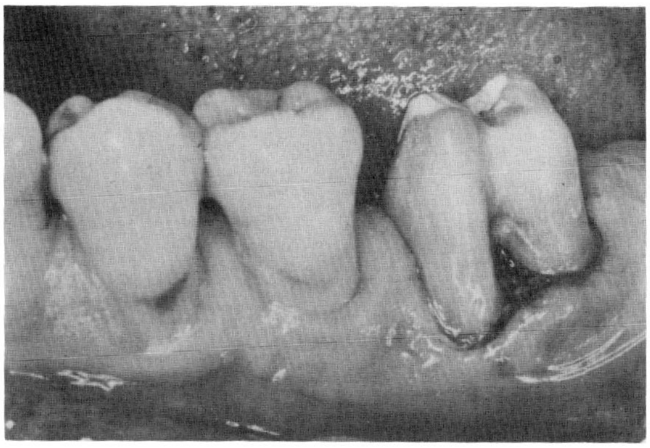

Fig. 7-42. "Fluted" preparation for ease of access to bifurcation.

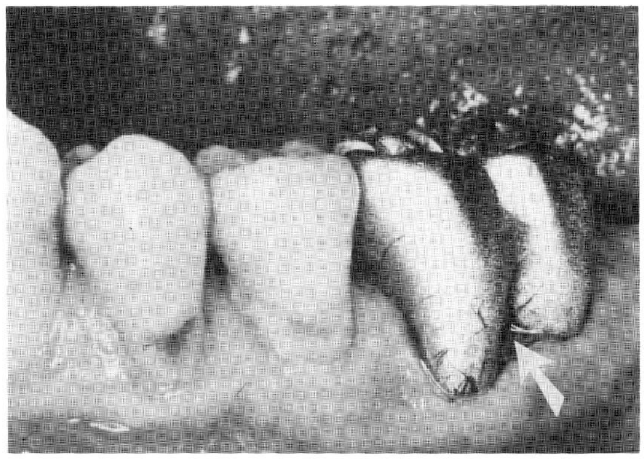

Fig. 7-43. Interrupted facial fluting in final crown contour *(arrow)* prevents convenient access to bifurcation.

sheltered in the overprotected bifurcation area of a crown.

Before the principle of protective contouring is applied, the area to protect should be carefully considered: the gingiva or bacterial plaque. Overly protective ridges are highlighted in Fig. 7-40 and show resultant plaque-retention areas. With decreased gingival convexity, the buccal groove extended to the bifurcation, and a gentle concavity contoured from the mesial slope of the facial cusp into the mesiogingival embrasure, the facial surface could function in a conveniently hygienic way. Fig 7-41 illustrates the arrangement for a favorable flow pattern except in the bifurcation area. Here the gingiva is overprotected. With the facial groove "fluted" from the occlusal table to the bifurcation, the marginal gingiva is accessible. When the bifurcation shows carious involvement, the tooth preparation is fluted to maintain a path of insertion (Fig. 7-42). This vertical concavity in the preparation wall permits subsequent fluting of the wax pattern. Any prominence placed into this facial groove constitutes an obstruction (Fig. 7-43) to the flow pattern and encourages plaque retention. Axial contours must be related to the gingival architecture, adjacent and opposing teeth, and adjacent musculature in a manner to promote continuing gingival health (Fig. 7-44).

The junction of the restoration and tooth should be the smoothest possible transition of restorative material to tooth structure (Fig. 7-45). This rule can be readily applied in cases where the preparation margin is placed in tooth enamel (Figs. 7-46 and 7-47). Here, to maintain a smooth transition, the curvature of the existing tooth surfaces is continued in the restoration. Fig. 7-48 *A*, shows how contouring in the margin area is facilitated when the margin is placed supragingivally and in tooth enamel. Difficulties are compounded when the margins are placed subgingivally, in cementum, and with a resultant excessively long clinical crown (Fig. 7-48, *B*). The tendency to overcontour is best resisted by applying some basic rules: (1) the occlusal table should

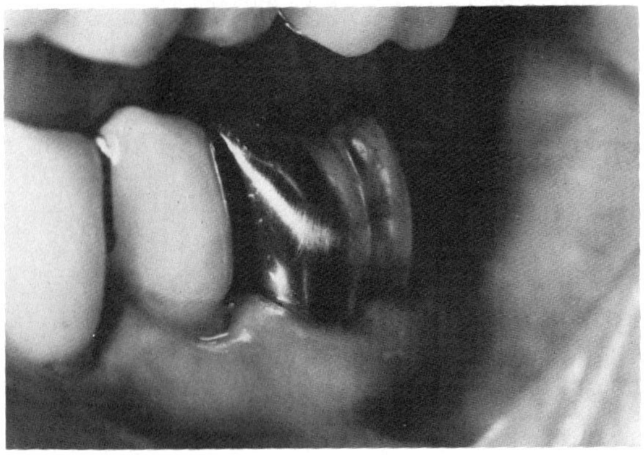

Fig. 7-44. Properly fluted molar crown; facial surface contoured harmoniously with adjacent teeth.

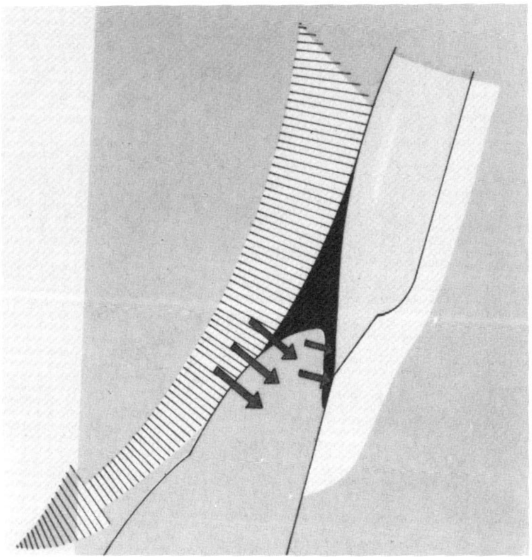

Fig. 7-45. Subgingival margin should be placed approximately 1 mm into gingival sulcus. Contour of restoration must allow stimulation to marginal gingiva.

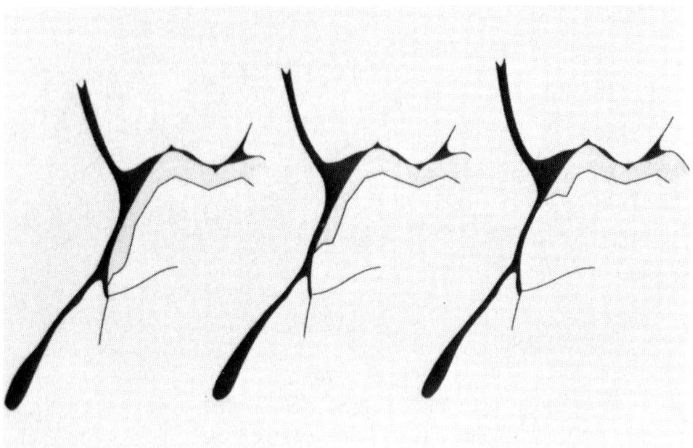

Fig. 7-46. Margins placed in tooth enamel facilitate axial contouring. No abrupt change from curvature of remaining tooth form should occur.

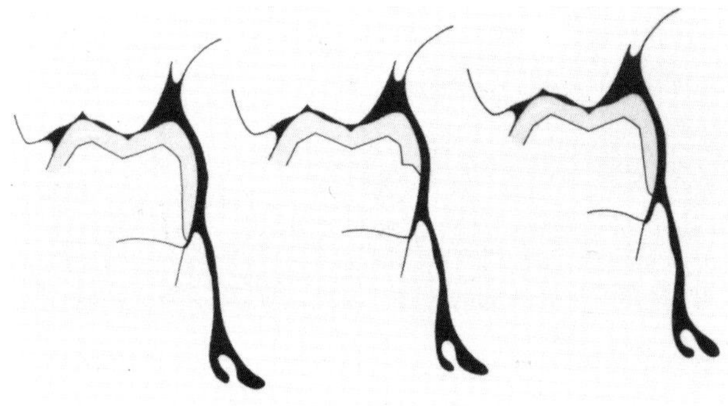

Fig. 7-47. Lingual margins placed at various levels show harmonious blending of restoration and tooth structure.

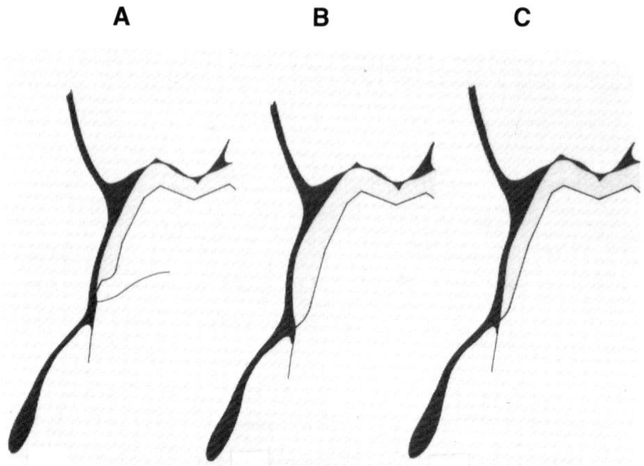

Fig. 7-48. A, Restoration contour in harmony with tooth form. **B,** Bulky, overprotective facial contour. **C,** At margin, restoration blends harmoniously with tooth structure.

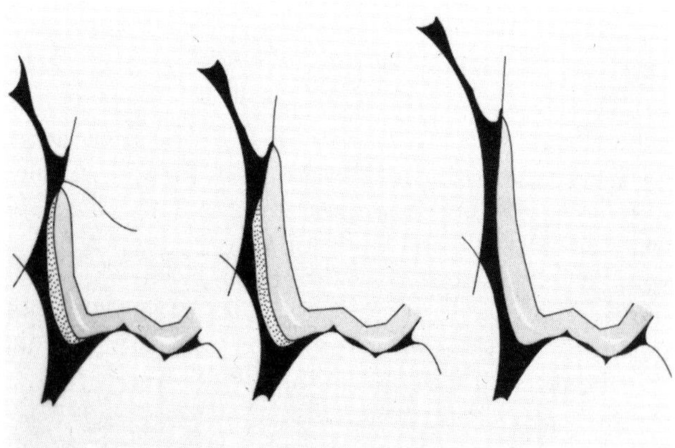

Fig. 7-49. As length of clinical crown increases, axial prominences decrease.

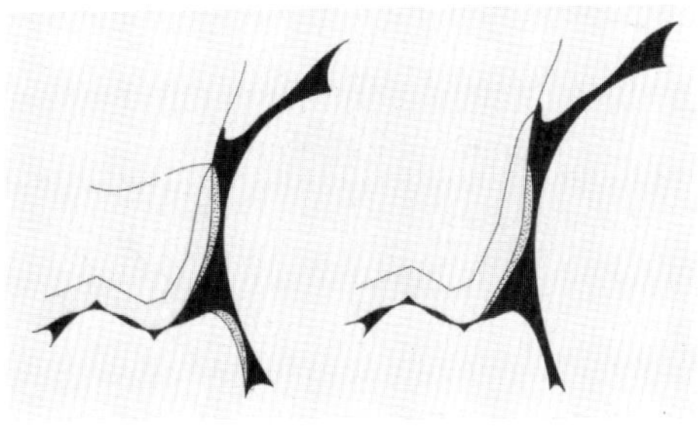

Fig. 7-50. When axial surfaces are reduced, sufficient horizontal overlap must be retained to avoid tongue and cheek biting.

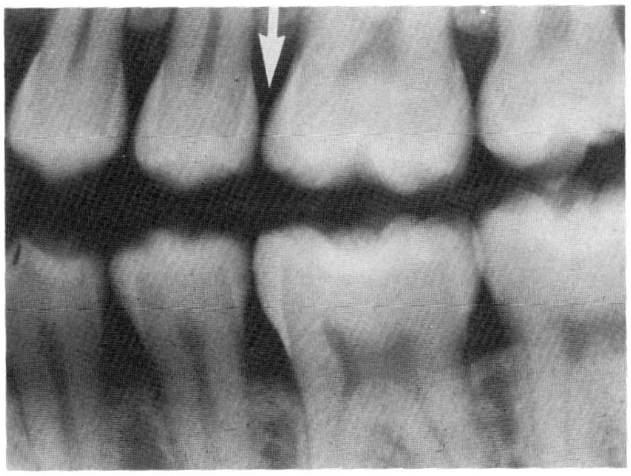

Fig. 7-51. Contact point *(arrow)* found in newly erupted dentition.

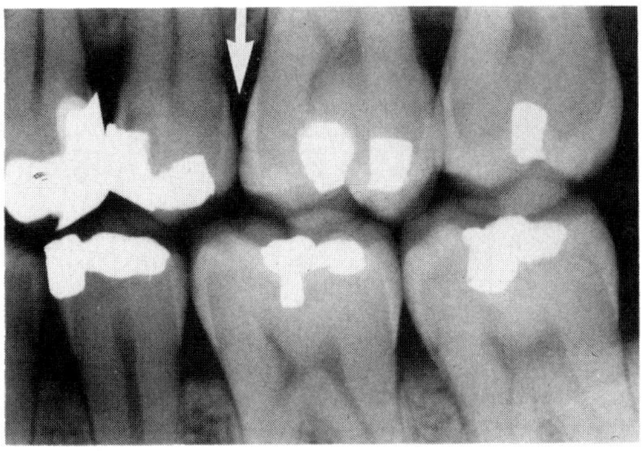

Fig. 7-52. Mature and stable dentition shows contact area *(arrow).*

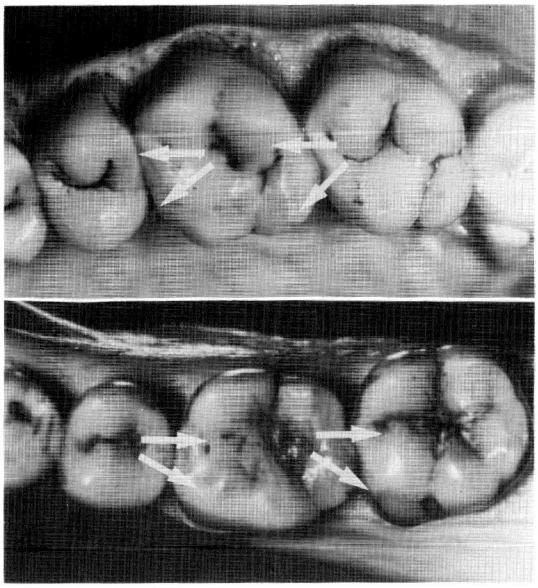

Fig. 7-53. Contact area is placed facially *(top arrows)* on mandibular posteriors and lingually *(bottom arrows)* on maxillary molars, coinciding with protrusive and idling excursion.

be narrower than the unrestored tooth, (2) deflection prominences diminish as the crown length increases, and (3) the margin constitutes a smooth transition (Fig. 7-48, *C*). The facial cusp of the maxillary posteriors (Fig. 7-49) and the lingual cusps of the mandibular posterior teeth (Fig. 7-50) may be reduced; however, a horizontal overlap must be maintained to avoid cheek or tongue biting. As the cusps are narrowed, the faciolingual axial surfaces are reduced to achieve conveniently hygienic contours.

INTERPROXIMAL SURFACES

Next to be explored are the contours of the interproximal tooth surfaces, contact between adjacent teeth, and embrasures formed occlusogingivally to this contact.

As teeth erupt, their proximal surfaces are convex. As these teeth adjust themselves against adjacent and opposing teeth, the contact point made by two contacting convex surfaces facilitates tooth alignment (Fig. 7-51). The young unblemished dentition is frequently accepted as the standard for proper tooth morphology, and with it the concept of the contact point. The contact point, however, is an important feature of an unstable dentition. As the dentition matures, it stabilizes itself, and interproximal contact points wear into contact areas (Fig. 7-52) that contribute to tooth stability. This may be described as physiologic splinting.

In restorations, the function of interproximal contact areas is twofold. First contact areas contribute to the stability of the dental arch. Second, by their width and location they prevent food impaction into the interproximal embrasure. For this reason the contact area is placed facially in the mandibular posterior region and lingually between maxillary molars (Fig. 7-53). The protective mechanism becomes evident when the travel of opposing cusps in a protrusive and idling excursion is reviewed. A more horizontal chewing path would indicate a broadened contact; correspondingly, a vertical chewing stroke indicates a relatively narrow contact area.

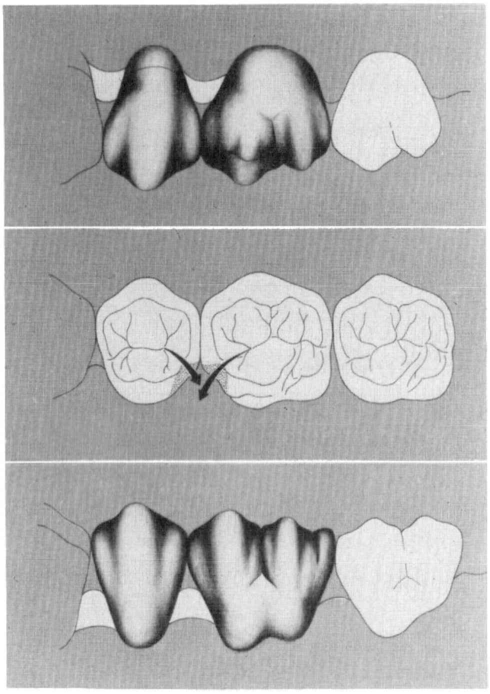

Fig. 7-54. Occlusal embrasures open lingually *(arrows)* into wide obtuse embrasure with ready access to interproximal tissues.

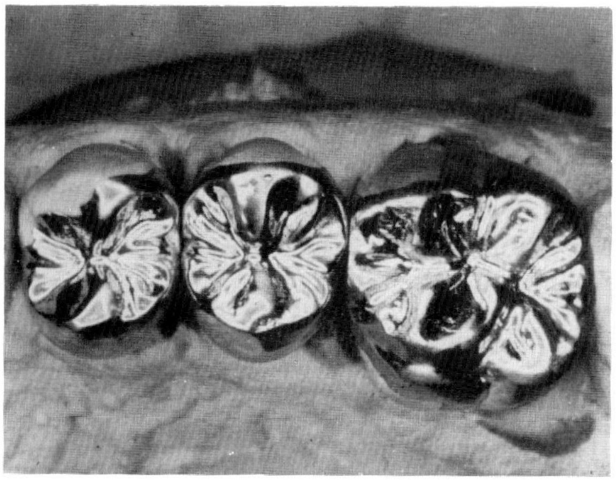

Fig. 7-55. Restorations that can function and are conveniently hygienic.

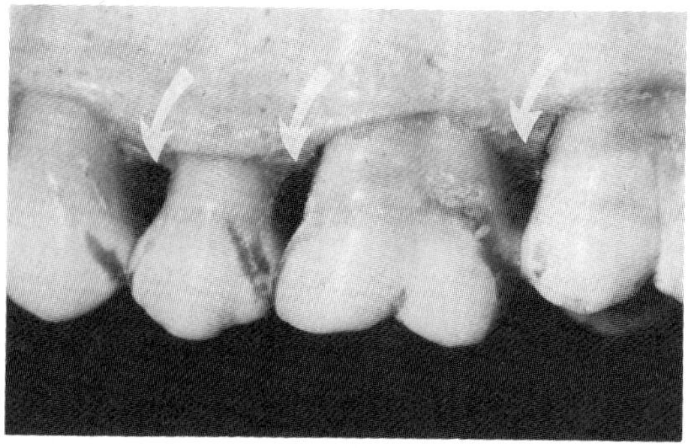

Fig. 7-56. Interproximal embrasure spaces *(arrows)* seen on human skull emphasize need for concave axial surfaces gingival to contact area.

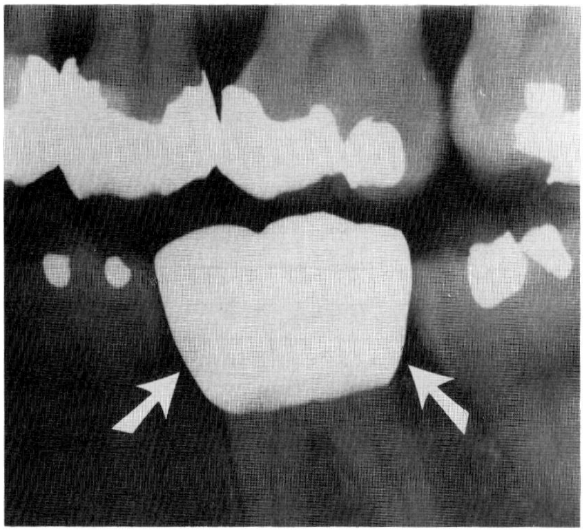

Fig. 7-57. Radiographs frequently show restorations with overcontoured interproximal axial surfaces *(arrows)*.

The occlusal embrasures, which channel food particles off the contact area, are formed by adjacent marginal ridges. Lingually, the occlusal embrasure is widened by sluice grooves that traverse the marginal ridges (Fig. 7-54). This forms an obtusely broadened embrasure in a gingival direction, becoming continuous with the gingival embrasure (Fig. 7-55). A pattern of flow is thereby established.

The occlusogingival length of the contact area may influence food retention. The embrasure space gingival to the contact area should allow ample room for the interdental papilla (Fig. 7-56). Bulky interproximal contours of restorations (Fig. 7-57) are not consistent with natural tooth form, and needlessly infringe on the tissues. Embrasures with acute apices must be considered trap embrasures (Figs. 7-58 and 7-59). Food debris and bacterial plaque find entrance into any crevice (Fig. 7-60), so ready access must be provided for cleansing and stimulation of the gingiva (Fig. 7-61).

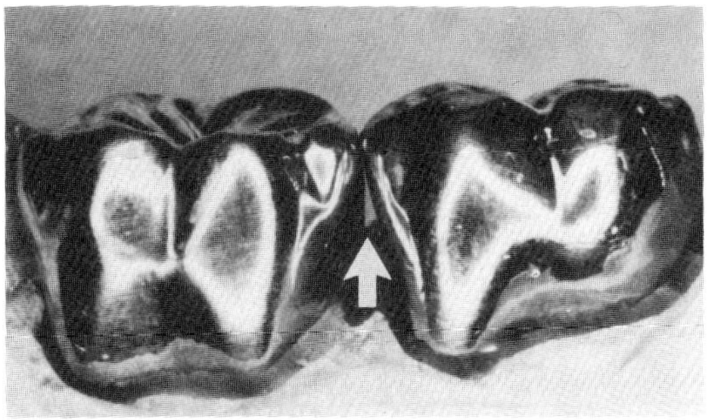

Fig. 7-58. Adjacent crown surfaces form narrow interproximal trap embrasure *(arrow)*.

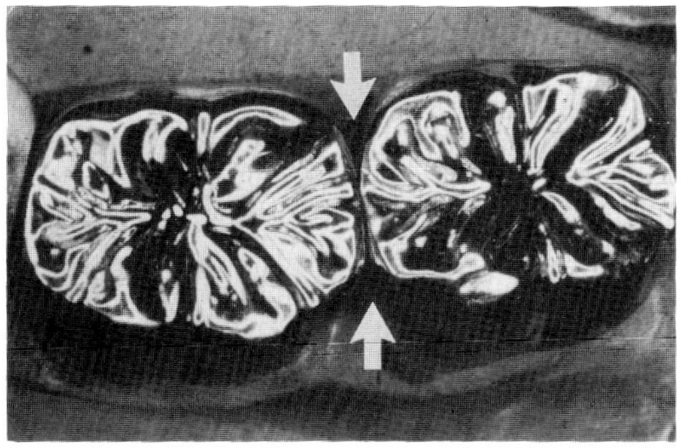

Fig. 7-59. Occlusal view of two molar crowns show facial and lingual trap embrasures *(arrows)* formed by gradually separating adjacent surfaces.

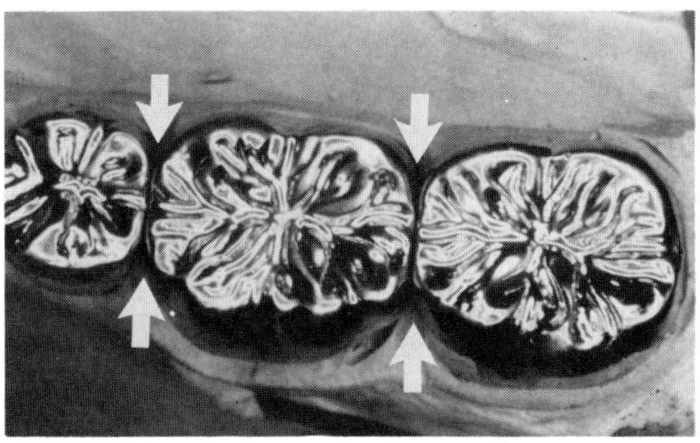

Fig. 7-60. Broad contact areas *(arrows)* function overprotectively to interproximal tissues.

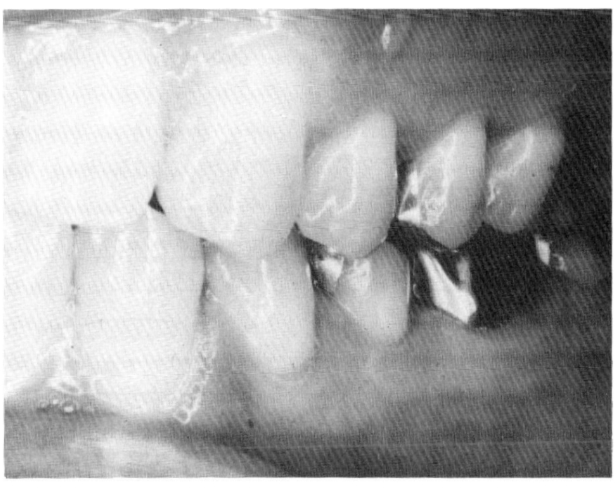

Fig. 7-61. Crown contours that function protectively and are conveniently hygienic.

Margin adaptation to die

HAROLD F. EISSMANN

When the wax pattern for a metal crown has been verified on articulated working casts for optimal occlusal function, and the axial contours have been tentatively carved, the wax pattern is transferred to the die for margin adaptation. The objective is to obtain a 2-mm border of smoothly adapted wax along the margin of the die to assure margin integrity of the casting and to minimize finishing procedures. The fabrication of a properly trimmed die is basic to margin adaptation and final axial contouring of the wax pattern.

TRIMMING AN INDIVIDUAL DIE

1. The stone cast (Fig. 7-62) is trimmed on a model trimmer to within 2 mm of the tooth preparation (indicated by line *a*). Multiple preparations are separated by initial vertical saw cuts through the interproximal papillae (line *b*) to prevent chipping of the stone cast near the margins. By making deep faciolingual cuts with a carborundum disk, the individual dies can now be freed (line *c*).

2. The base of the individual die (Fig. 7-63, *A*) is trimmed on the faciolingual surface to within 2 mm of the preparation and shortened to a length of approximately 20 mm (Fig. 7-63, *B*). The final trimming of the die is done with a large pear-shaped carbide trimming bur (Fig. 7-63, *C*). With this instrument, a gentle depression can be cut immediately apical to the margin of the preparation, which will facilitate the final contouring of the wax pattern.

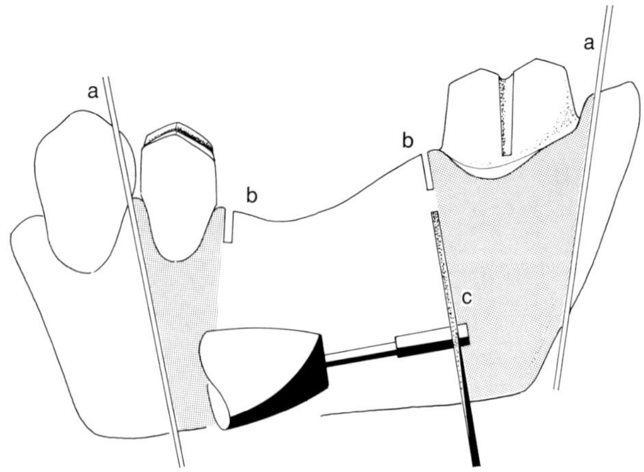

Fig. 7-62. Trimming stone cast. Remove portion with model trimmer *(a),* saw cut through interproximal papillae *(b),* and make buccolingual separation cuts with carborundum disk *(c).*

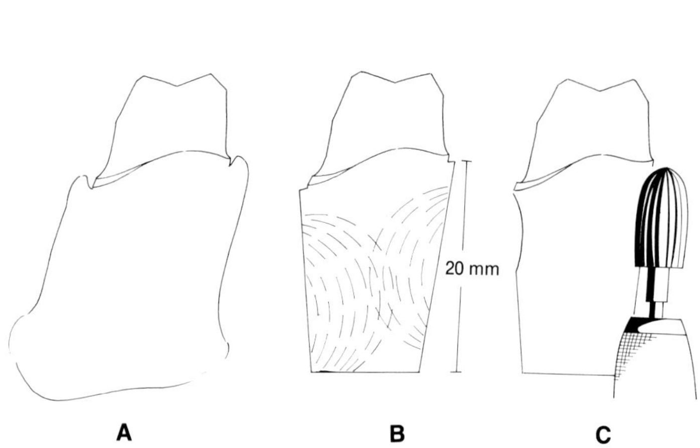

Fig. 7-63. Trimming die. **A,** Trim excess stone on faciolingual surface with model trimmer to within 2 mm of preparation. **B,** Shorten stone base to 20 mm, as comfortable die handle. **C,** Using large pear-shaped carbide trimming bur, cut gentle depression immediately apical to gingival margins.

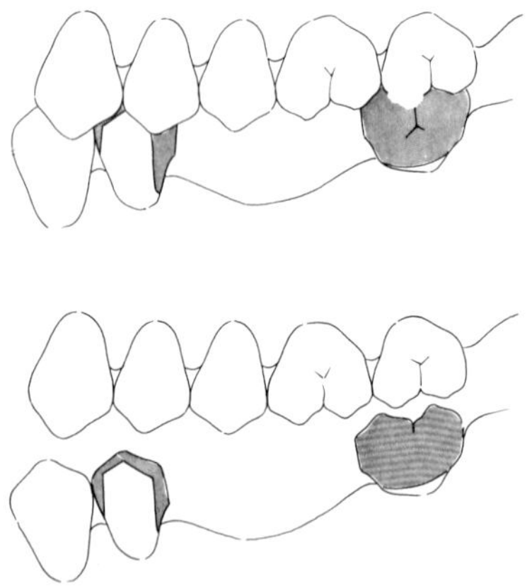

Fig. 7-64. Verify wax patterns on articulated working casts for optimal occlusal contacts and tentative axial contour.

MARGIN ADAPTATION OF WAX PATTERN

1. The wax pattern is verified on articulated working casts for optimal occlusal contact and initial axial contour (Fig. 7-64). The individual dies are properly trimmed and lubricated.

2. When transferred to the die, the wax pattern is cut to be 2 mm short of the preparation margins (Fig. 7-65, *A*). This space permits the addition of new wax, which is added quickly for a smooth internal adaptation (Fig. 7-65, *B*). A suitable (Hollenback) carver may be used to carve away the excess wax covering the margins and to finalize the axial contours. The carving instrument should be repeatedly warmed during the refining process. Keeping the point of the carver in contact with the die stone in the depression apical to the margin (Fig. 7-65, *C*) serves to control the instrument; it will

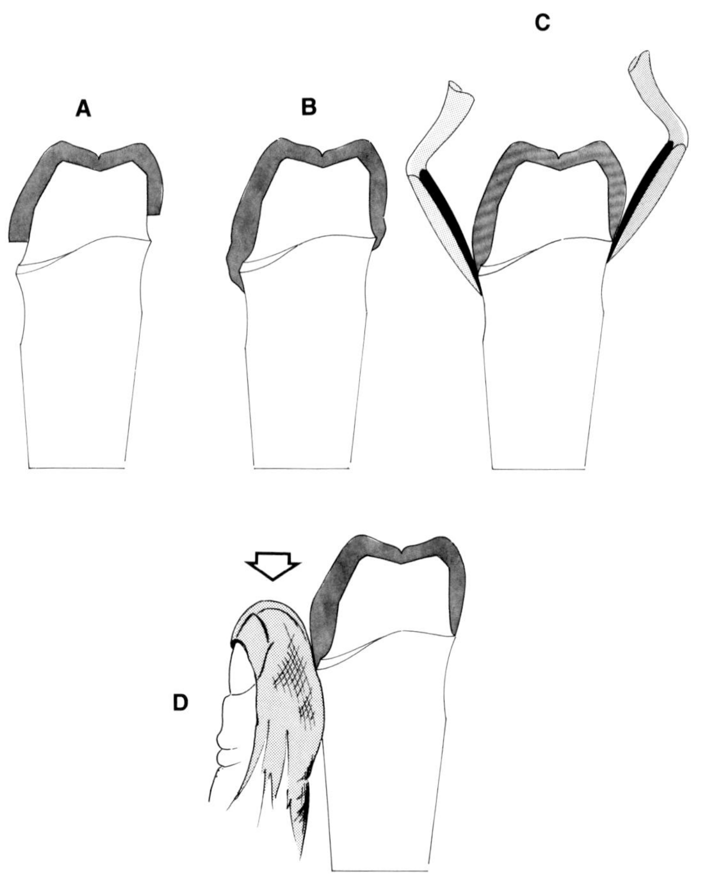

Fig. 7-65. Margin adaptation. **A,** Cut wax pattern 2 mm short of margins. **B,** Flow new wax quickly to cover margin with smooth internal adaptation. **C,** Remove excess wax with (Hollenback) carver in carving burnishing action with point of instrument resting against depression apical to margin. **D,** Smooth wax with silk or nylon cloth *(arrow)* by gentle apical strokes.

Table 7-2. Margin adaptation of wax pattern

Problem	Probable cause	Solution
Chipping of stone while trimming die	Use of dull, 6-fluted steel bur and/or excessive pressure	Use sharp, true-running, 12-fluted carbide bur with gentle pressure
Loss of detail after trimming of casts	Prolonged immersion in water	Soak cast in water saturated with calcine, or coat preparations with separating medium (Super-Sep)
Wax pattern has rough internal surface	Wax not hot enough or not flowed quickly	Add wax hot and quickly for even adaptation
Margins break when pattern is removed from die	Wax not carved out of undercuts in die, or die improperly lubricated	Start with properly lubricated die, and carve wax right to margin; use dead soft wax in problem areas
Crown is submarginal	Stone margin abraded during carving	Be sure die margin is always covered by wax

not rest against the wax being carved at the margin, and the chances of carving away delicate stone margins are minimized.

3. Once the margins are properly adapted, the axial contours can be carved with the same (Hollenback) carver. The carving edge of the instrument must be adjusted with a rubber wheel by the technician. A sharp carving edge cuts into the wax pattern and does not permit a smooth carving-burnishing action, and a too dull carving edge becomes ineffective.

4. Polishing is the final step in finishing the wax pattern. A silk or nylon cloth is stretched over the forefinger, and the wax is smoothed by gentle apical strokes (Fig. 7-65, *D*).

PROBLEM AREAS

A casting cannot be more accurate than the wax pattern from which it is made. Problems that could arise during the fabrication of a wax pattern, their probable causes, and solutions are given in Table 7-2.

1. The die should be the most accurate reproduction of the prepared natural tooth. It should be trimmed precisely to facilitate waxing and adaptation of wax to the margins. A stone die should never be immersed in water for longer than 2 to 3 minutes. Water acts as a solvent and sharp preparation detail is lost. Use air pressure to surface dry the die after the model trimmer has been used. The preparation portion of the die should not be touched or rubbed against. To avoid chipping while trimming near or at the margins, use a true-running, sharp No. 12 fluted carbide bur with gentle pressure.

2. Once the die has been properly trimmed (Fig. 7-63) and lubricated, apply hot wax quickly for even adaptation to the preparation. Modified cotton pliers are used as a carrying instrument to transfer molten wax efficiently from a heated metal reservoir to the preparation. When multiple restorations are to be waxed on the working cast, a large quantity of wax can be applied quickly with a glass eyedropper. The eyedropper can be prewarmed in the flame of a Bunsen burner, then filled with molten wax, and aspirated from a heated metal reservoir. The index finger and thumb are lubricated to contain the wax buccolingually as it is flowed onto the preparations.

3. When a wax pattern is transferred from a working cast to the die, the wax is cast 2 mm shy of the margins. Freshly molten wax is flowed around the margins for an even internal adaptation. A soft wax should be used for margin adaptation when the room temperature is relatively low and when there are problem areas in the preparation, such as a critical path of withdrawal.

SUMMARY

This chapter offered an interpretation of tooth form and function. The composite form and descriptive nomenclature served as an introduction to the morphology of the natural dentition. Beyond the static tooth form, the dynamic influences on the occlusal, axial, and interproximal surfaces were described as a guide for waxing. The wax pattern should be a precise model for the final restoration, and it is during the fabrication of the wax pattern that the design principles for optimal biomechanical and hygienic function are expressed in a crown or a fixed partial denture that resembles morphologically the natural dentition.

PART TWO

Pontic design

HAROLD F. EISSMANN

The full implication of hygienic pontic contour can best be experienced when the endentulous space is visualized in an anteroposterior cross section (Fig. 7-66). The boundaries of this space are the edentulous ridge, opposing occlusal surface, musculature of the tongue, and musculature of the cheek or lips. The task is to design within these boundaries a tooth substitute that favorably compares in form, function, and appearance with the tooth it replaces. The tooth substitute must provide comfort and support to the adjacent musculature, conformity to the food-flow pattern, conveniently hygienic contours, and a cosmetic value, if indicated.

A rationale for hygienic pontic design can best be explored by considering the mandibular molar region. Here the cosmetic requirement is minimal and does not compromise hygienic design.

MANDIBULAR POSTERIOR PONTIC

Fig. 7-67 illustrates an edentulous mandibular molar region for which numerous pontic forms have been proposed. Three popular concepts in pontic design are shown (Fig. 7-68): *(A)* saddle pontic, *(B)* sanitary pontic, and *(C)* modified sanitary pontic. These pontic

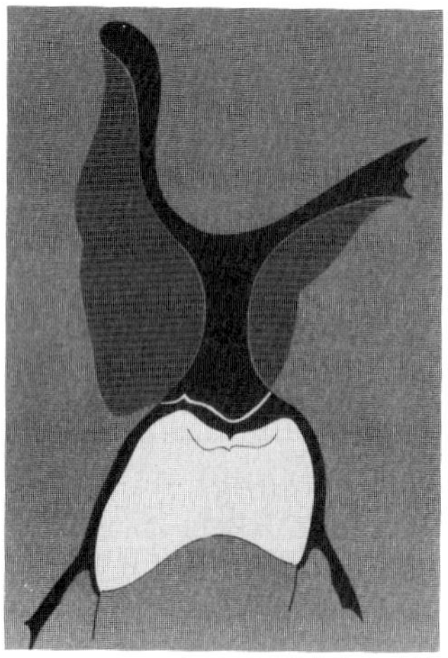

Fig. 7-66. Maxillary posterior edentulous space defined by its boundaries; edentulous ridge, opposing occlusion, tongue, and cheek.

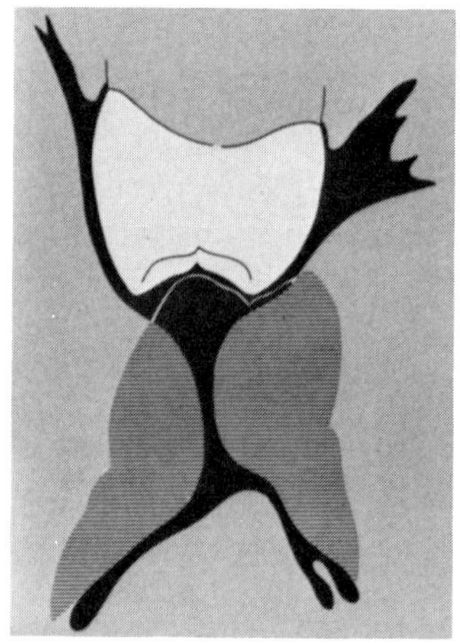

Fig. 7-67. Mandibular posterior edentulous space. Shaded area shows hard and soft tissues that are lost.

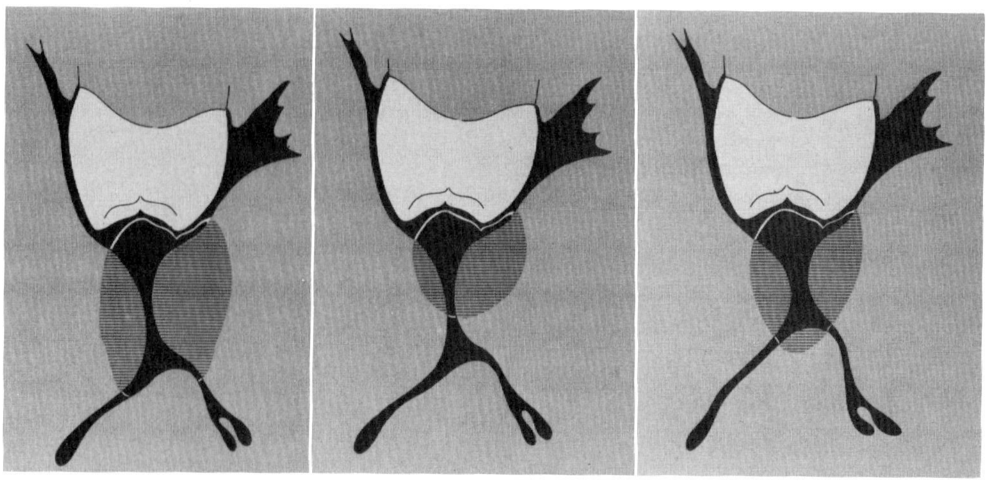

Fig. 7-68. Three most widely used pontic designs for mandibular posterior region: **A,** saddle pontic, **B,** sanitary pontic, **C,** modified sanitary pontic.

forms and others that have been proposed should be tested by the two major influences on pontic contour: the shape of the edentulous ridge and the length of the pontic span. For example, a short pontic span and a broad blunted ridge would preclude the use of a ridge-lap or sanitary tip pontic (Fig. 7-69). The lingual and buccal embrasures would trap food particles and interfere with the food-flow pattern.

The various shapes of edentulous ridges can be grouped into three categories (Fig. 7-70): normal, blunted, and excessive resorption. The merit of a proposed pontic design should be measured by its adaptability to each ridge category.

The saddle pontic (Fig. 7-71) is the original and widely used pontic form. It appears and feels much like the tooth it replaces; however, since the large concavity of the tissue contact area cannot be maintained by hygienic measures, the saddle design is unacceptable. Modifications to the contour of the saddle pontic led to the sanitary design, which appeared as a simple solution to the septic problems caused by the saddlelike tissue contact. The sanitary pontic avoided tissue contact, or contact was confined to a point contact only. When a rounded sanitary pontic is kept 2 to 4 mm above the edentulous ridge (Fig. 7-72, *A*), it can be conveniently maintained, does not interfere with the food-flow pattern, and affords comfort and support to the adjacent musculature. A pontic with less than 2 mm

A 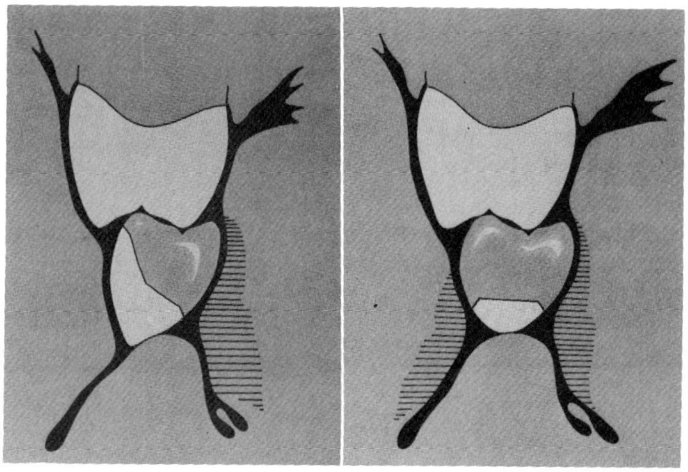 B

Fig. 7-69. A, Ridge-lap design with resultant unhygienic linguogingival embrasure. **B,** Sanitary tip design with faciolingual trap embrasures.

A B C

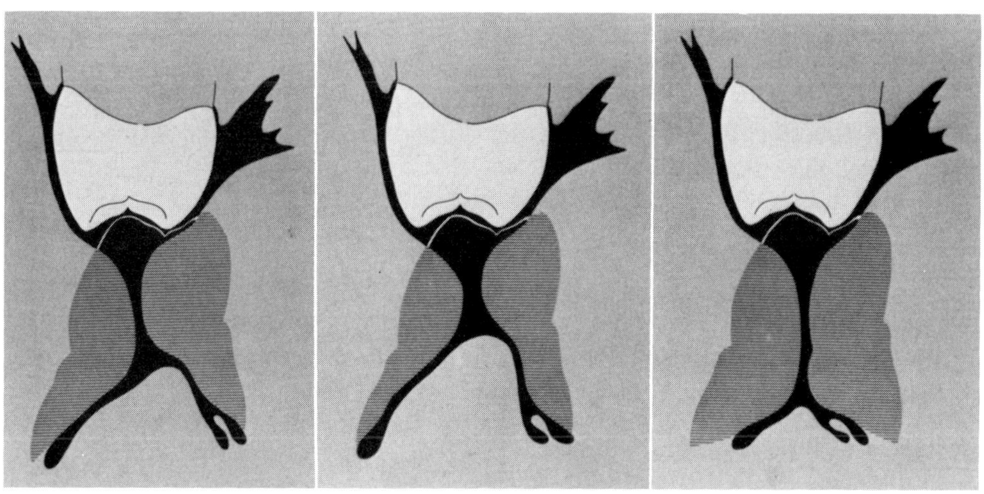

Fig. 7-70. Three types of mandibular edentulous ridges. **A,** Normal resorption. **B,** Minimal resorption. **C,** Excessive resorption.

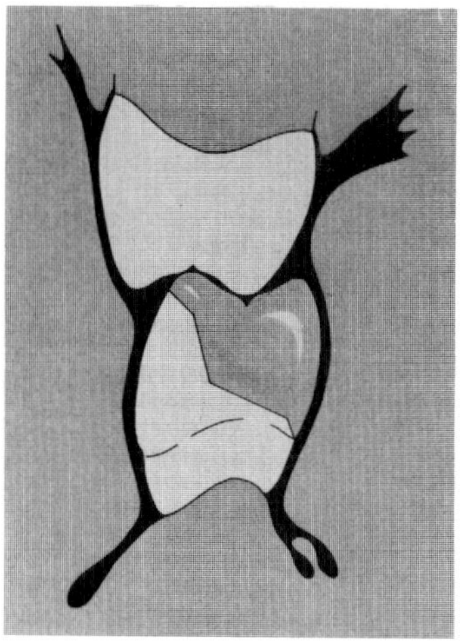

Fig. 7-71. Saddle pontic with unacceptable excessive tissue contact.

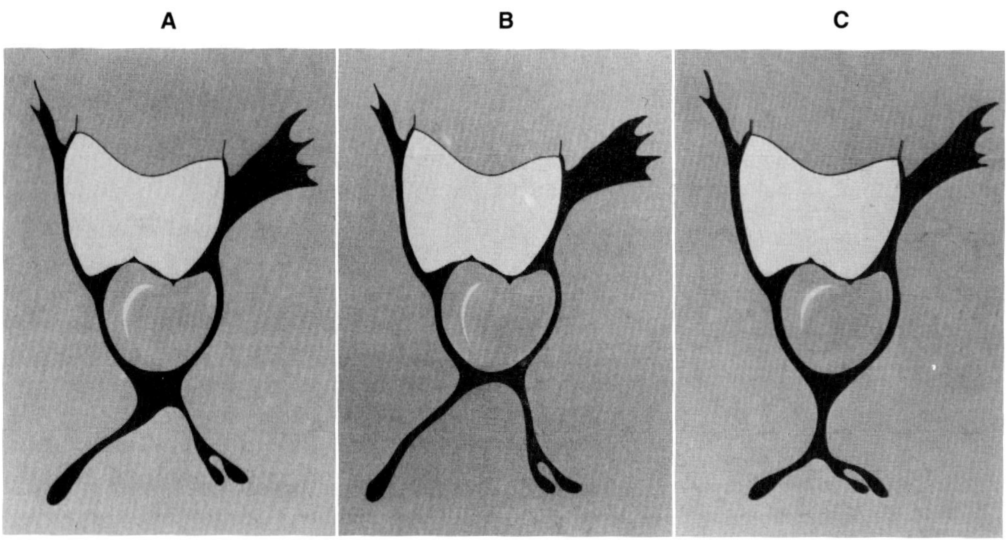

Fig. 7-72. Sanitary pontic related to three ridge types. **A,** Acceptable. Pontic is 3 to 4 mm from ridge and does not interfere with food flow. **B,** Unacceptable. Proximity of pontic to ridge causes food entrapment. **C,** Unacceptable. Pontic does not provide optimal support for adjacent musculature.

tissue clearance (Fig. 7-72, *B*) contributes to food lodgment; also, the rounded sanitary form does not adequately support the adjacent musculature in cases of excessive ridge resorption (Fig. 7-72, *C*).

The shortcomings of the sanitary pontic can be corrected by the modified sanitary design. Fig. 7-73 illustrates this design superimposed on the various ridge contours. The rounded sanitary form has been extended to an egg shape to improve the flow pattern which minimizes the entrapment of food debris, and to facilitate the adaptation of the adjacent musculature to a maximum surface area of the pontic (Fig. 7-74). A tissue contact area may result; however, there should be only the slightest concavity, and the angle formed by the buccal or lingual surface and the edentulous ridge should be obtuse to avoid trap embrasures. The technician's objective is to develop the area of least tissue contact without trap embrasures (Fig. 7-75). In a facial view (Fig. 7-76) the same principle is demonstrated. Where tissue contact is unavoidable, the master cast is reduced 0.5 mm in the contact area. If this area is marked with graphite, a porcelain pontic can be precisely adapted. As described for the buccal and lingual axial surfaces, the mesial and distal interproximal surfaces should leave the edentulous ridge at the most obtuse angle possible to gain a conveniently hygienic embrasure.

Pontics may be fabricated entirely from metal or a combination of metal and a cosmetic veneering material such as porcelain or plastic. The material must not in-

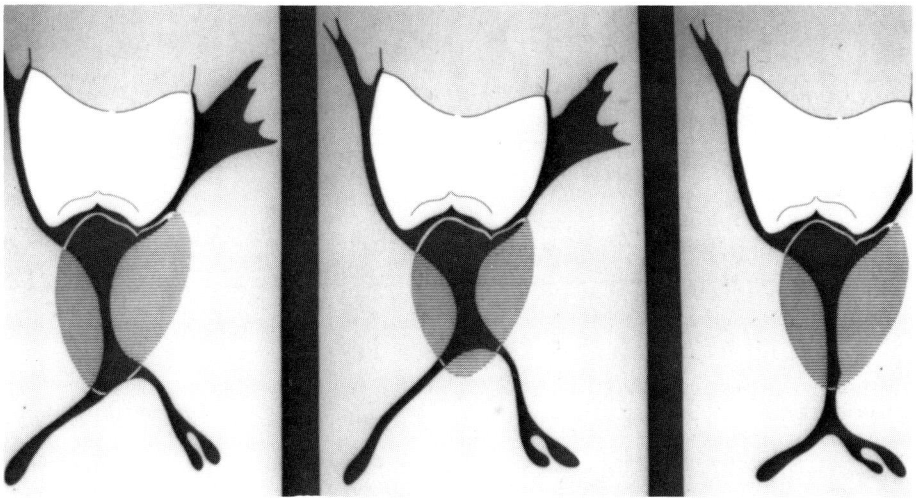

Fig. 7-73. Outline form of modified sanitary pontic is superimposed on three ridge types.

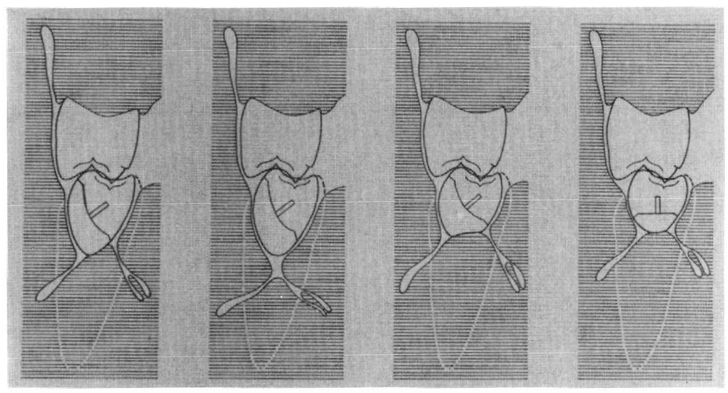

Fig. 7-75. Optimal pontic design illustrated in faciolingual cross section.

A

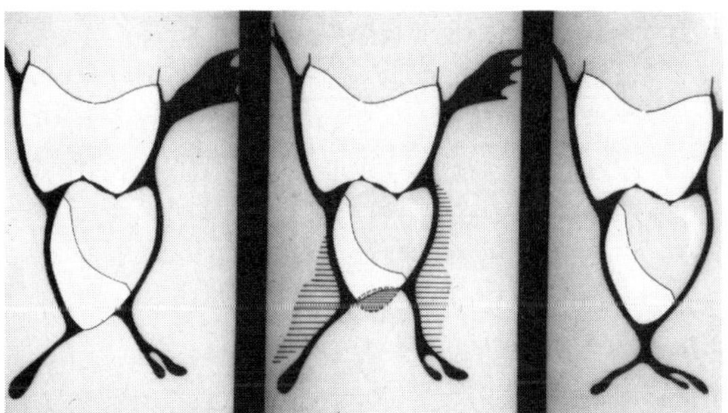

B

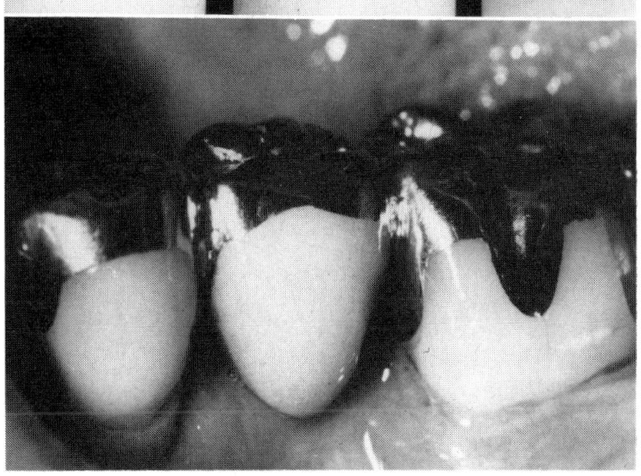

Fig. 7-74. A, Modified sanitary pontic design related to the various contours of mandibular ridges. **B,** Pontic adjusted to blunted ridge.

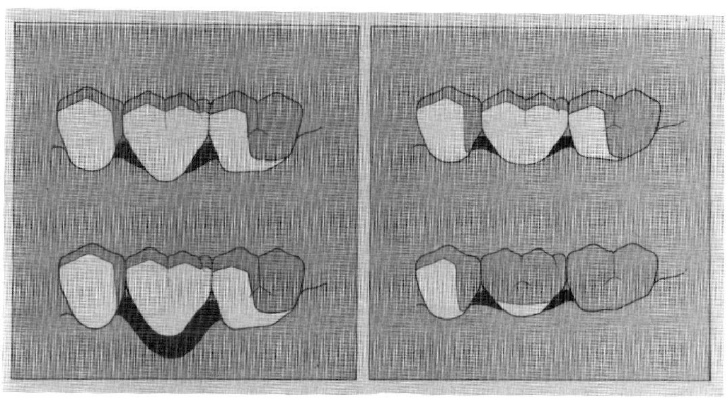

Fig. 7-76. Facial view of various acceptable pontics related to ridges with different degrees of resorption.

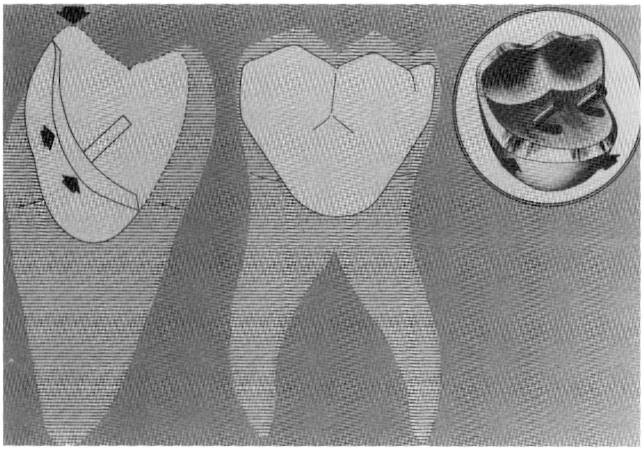

Fig. 7-77. Molar pontic superimposed on tooth it replaces illustrates needed changes in contour. Manufactured pin facing is shown properly beveled and hollow ground *(arrows, inset).*

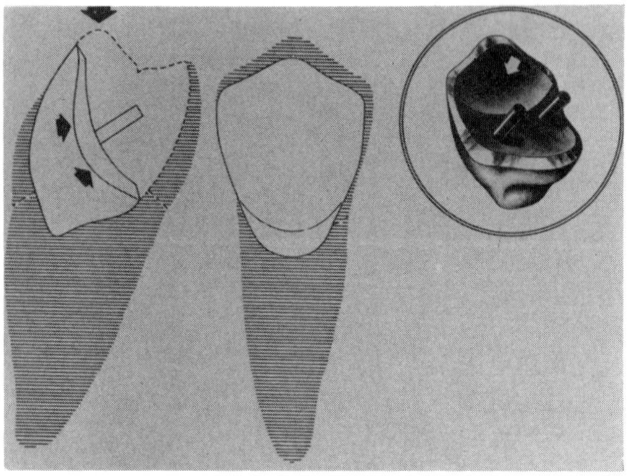

Fig. 7-78. Premolar pontic superimposed on tooth it replaces. Pin facing is beveled and hollow ground *(arrow).*

fluence the contour of the pontic. The all-metal pontic is used in noncosmetic areas and is best when tissue contact can be avoided. In short-bite case with tissue contact, the metal pontic may have to be used as a compromise if the addition of a porcelain facing to the pontic would weaken the rigidity of the bridge span.

Plastic facings can provide a cosmetic veneer with the least reduction of metal bulk. This is a definite advantage when the requirement for strength and cosmetics is high. Also, since plastic will wear rather than fracture, it is used as a veneer in cosmetic anterior restorations for patients with abusive bite patterns.

Vacuum-fired porcelain, with natural glaze or highly polished, is biologically most compatible with the attached gingiva that must cover a proposed contact area. For this reason a number of preformed porcelain facings have been developed, with different methods of attachment to the supporting gold backing: those with a tubular slot (Trupontic), those with pin retention (Harmony), and those with reverse pin retention (Shooshan). All manufactured facings need to be modified to the needs of the individual cast. The pin-retention pontics can be most conveniently adjusted so that the facing is mechanically joined to the metal backing by pin retention and long interproximal bevels (Figs. 7-77 and 7-78). To gain additional metal support against occlusal forces, the porcelain bulk near the occlusofacial margin is reduced by hollow grinding.

The reverse pin retention is used to alter any porcelain denture tooth into a pontic facing (Fig 7-79). A porcelain tip must be added before the tooth can be contoured to the requirements for pontic design. Then the pin retention should be distributed over the entire facing where the bulk of the porcelain allows for a pin length of 3 to 4 mm. As specified for the pin facing,

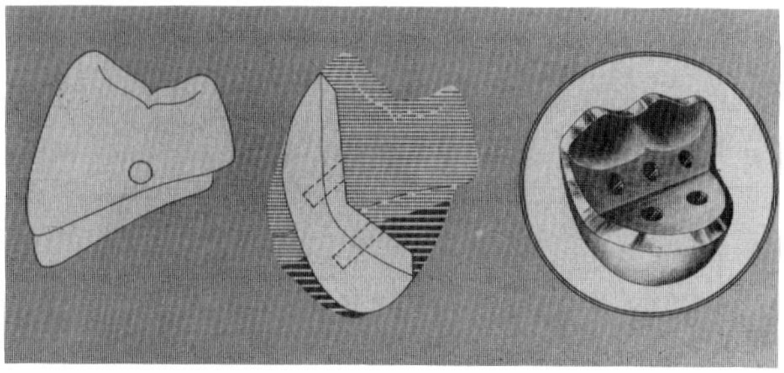

Fig. 7-79. Molar denture tooth altered to serve as reverse pin pontic facing, by addition of porcelain tip, removal of excess porcelain, beveling, and drilling of five pinholes *(inset).*

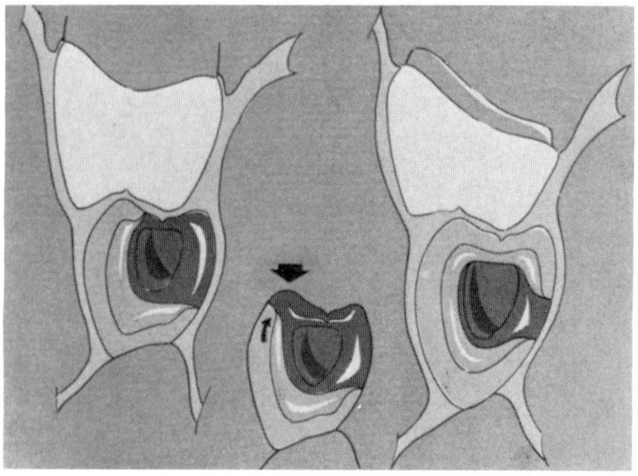

Fig. 7-80. Acceptable distribution of metal and porcelain *(arrows)* is illustrated for ceramometal pontics.

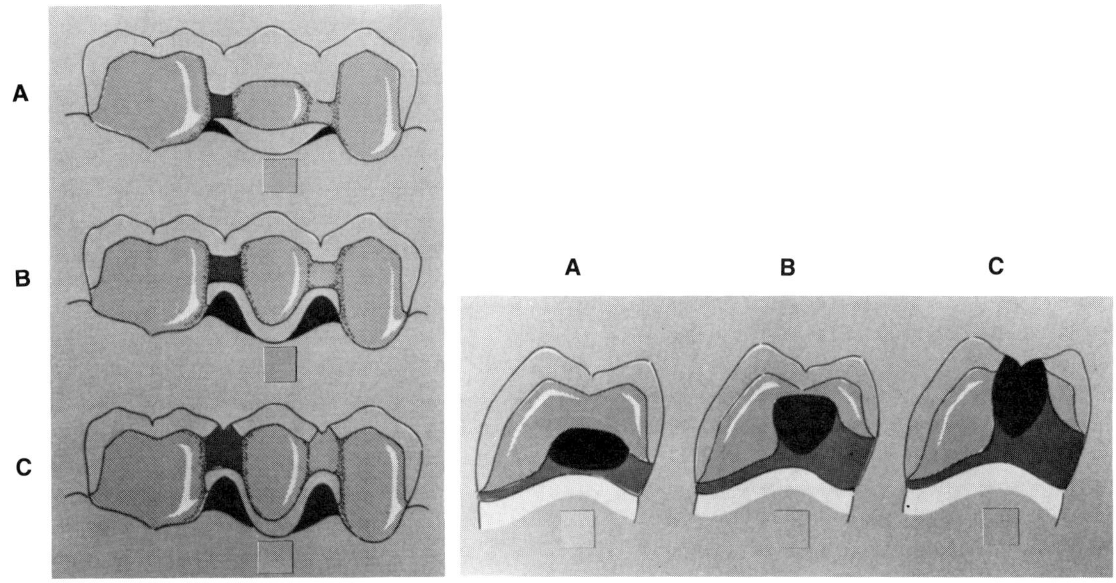

Fig. 7-81. Position and form of interproximal connectors for ceramometal restorations. **A,** Insufficient embrasure space and unsupported porcelain. **B,** Proper position and form. **C,** Optimal connector design for "short-bite" cases.

interproximal beveling and occlusofacial hollow grinding are very important for long-range resistance to fracture of the porcelain facing.

The popularity of the ceramometal technique has greatly reduced the demand for prefabricated pontic facings, but none of the principles of pontic contour should be changed (Fig. 7-80). Also, when a metal occlusal surface is used, the facial stamp cusp is reinforced with an additional bulk of metal, similar to the strengthening effect gained by hollow grinding the pin facing.

Placement and size of the solder connector has a special effect on the ceramometal pontic contour (Fig. 7-81). A connector placed gingivally for misinterpreted cosmetic reasons will prevent hygienic embrasure form (Fig. 7-81, *A*). Fig. 7-81, *B*, shows proper connector shape and position. As the occlusogingival dimension of the edentulous areas decreases, the connector can be extended to the marginal ridge (Fig. 7-81, *C*); the result is a rigid connector and adequate space for optimal interproximal contouring.

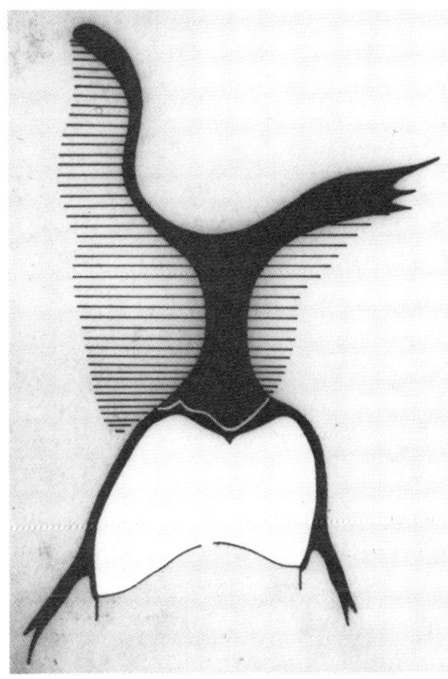

Fig. 7-82. Maxillary posterior edentulous space. Shaded area represents lost hard and soft tissues.

MAXILLARY POSTERIOR PONTIC

Design requirements for maxillary posterior pontics differ from mandibular posterior pontics in two areas: (1) the maxillary edentulous ridge is usually broad and blunted and (2) cosmetic considerations are important. For these reasons, tissue contact is necessary. The objective is to design a tooth substitute within the edentulous space that will function and appear similar to the lost soft and hard tissues indicated by the shaded outline in Fig. 7-82. The saddle pontic (Fig. 7-83) was most commonly used until 1936. At that time the sanitary conditions of fixed dental restorations were explored. Dr. D.E. Smith advanced a concept for hygienic pontic design: (1) the modified sanitary pontic for narrow and highly resorbed ridges and (2) the modified saddle pontic for broad, blunted ridge contour (Fig. 7-84). Many investigators believed that the modified saddle pontic contacted too large a tissue area, and the ridge-lap pon-

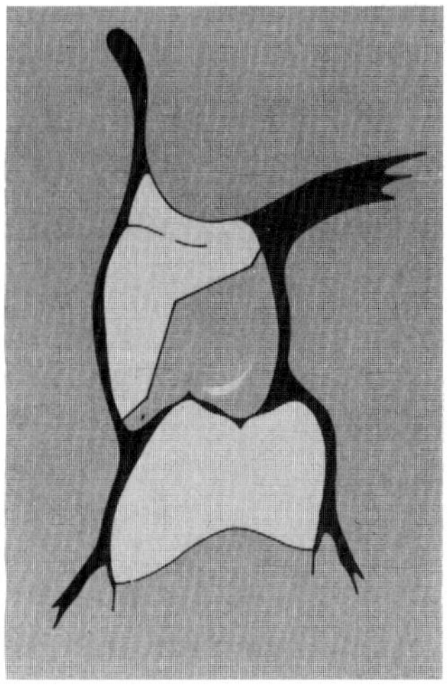

Fig. 7-83. Saddle pontic resembles missing tooth closely; however, excessive tissue contact is unhygienic.

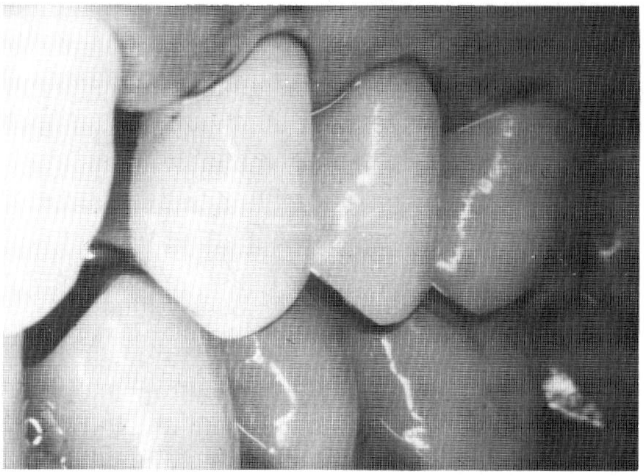

Fig. 7-84. Modified saddle pontic offers least possibility of food lodgment.

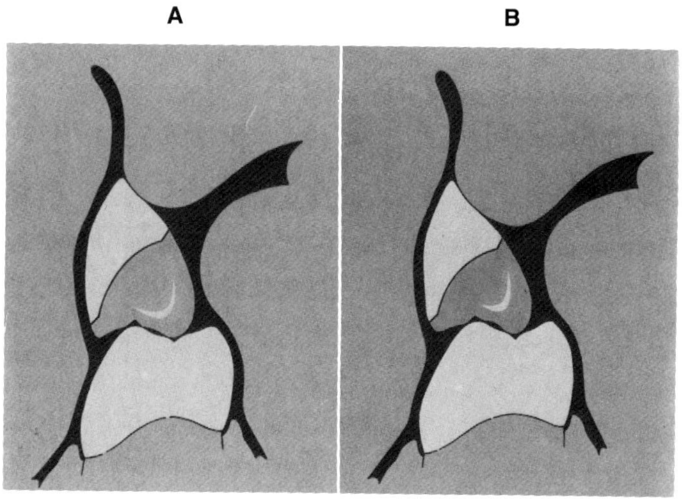

Fig. 7-85. Ridge-lap pontic has potential gingivopalatal trap embrasure. **A,** Adequate intermaxillary space with minimal gingivopalatal trap embrasure. **B,** Inadequate intermaxillary space with unhygienic gingivopalatal embrasure.

tic (Fig. 7-85, *A*) was developed. The tissue contact at the facial curvature of the edentulous ridge only satisfies cosmetic requirements with a minimal area of contact; however, in a "short-bite" case the angle formed by the palatal wall of the pontic and the ridge becomes increasingly acute (Fig. 7-85, *B*) and does not qualify as a conveniently hygienic embrasure. The design concept which mandates that the tissue-contacting surface of the pontic must always be convex is most widely accepted in present fixed prosthodontics. A convex pontic surface placed against the convex surface of a broad, blunted edentulous ridge can make a point contact only from which acute embrasures radiate (Fig. 7-86, *A*). To avoid these trap embrasures, it is advocated that the ridge should be surgically prepared to receive the convex pontic (Fig. 7-86, *B*). Only meticulous flossing can maintain this tissue contour, because a healthy edentulous ridge is convex, viewed in an anteroposterior cross section. The modified saddle concept takes into consideration the contour of the edentulous ridge; therefore the pontic is adjusted to form a definite contact area, with only the slightest concavity (Fig. 7-86, *C*). During function, the movement between tissue and pontic is adequate to maintain a healthy tissue tonus.

In Fig. 7-87 a modified sanitary pontic is superimposed onto the edentulous space. This illustrates that only minor adjustments are necessary to the pontic and ridge to develop a satisfactory pontic form (Fig. 7-88); that is, a modified saddle contact to a blunted ridge. An extensively resorbed ridge (Fig. 7-89) or an excessively resorbed ridge (Fig. 7-90) permits use of the unaltered egg shape of the modified sanitary pontic. In a facial view (Fig. 7-91), the relationship of tissue contact and interproximal embrasure space can be observed by con-

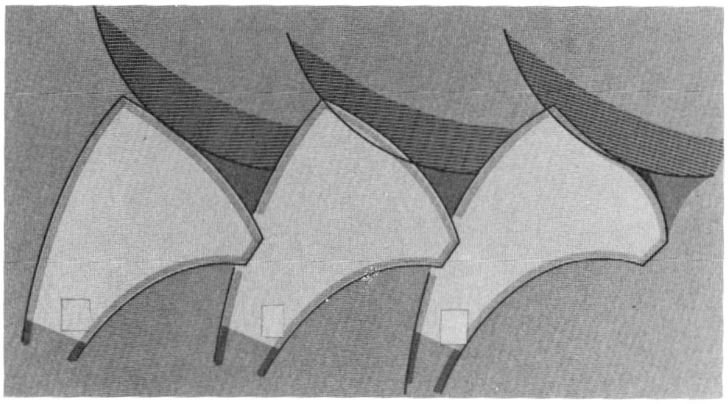

Fig. 7-86. Convex tissue-contacting surface of pontic should be recontoured for adaptation to broad blunted ridge. **A,** Facial and palatal trap embrasures are not acceptable. **B,** Surgical modification of ridge frequently causes tissue proliferation. **C,** Optimal modified saddle adaptation.

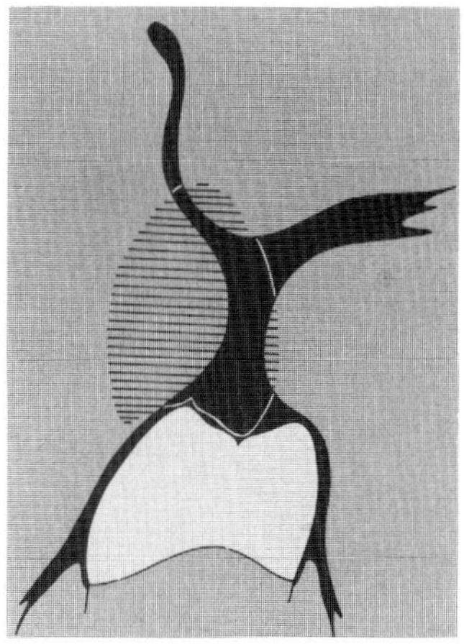

Fig. 7-87. Outline form of modified sanitary pontic superimposed on maxillary posterior edentulous space.

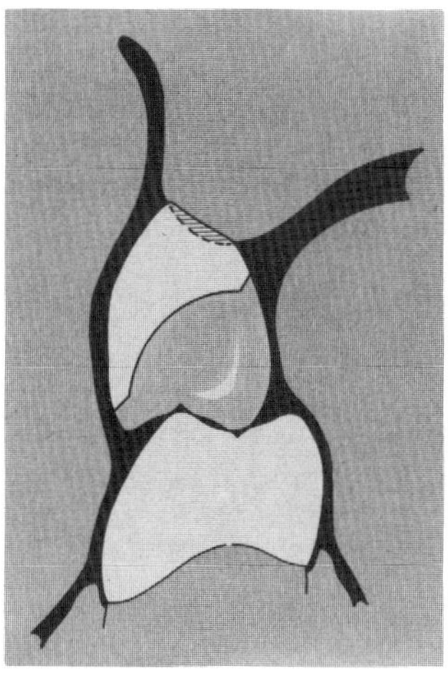

Fig. 7-88. Adjustment to modified sanitary pontic in case of broad blunted ridge.

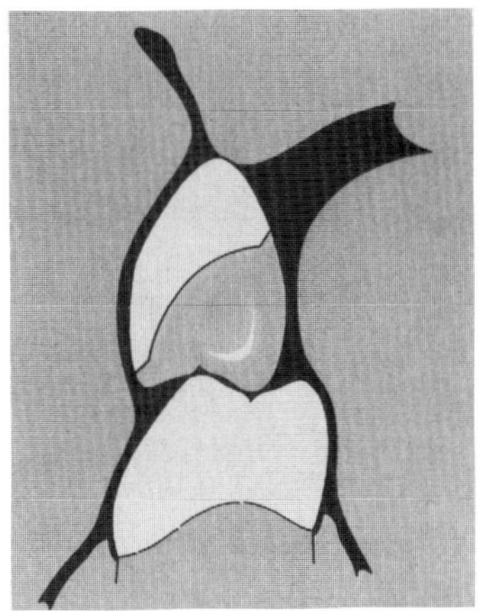

Fig. 7-89. Modified sanitary pontic related to highly resorbed ridge.

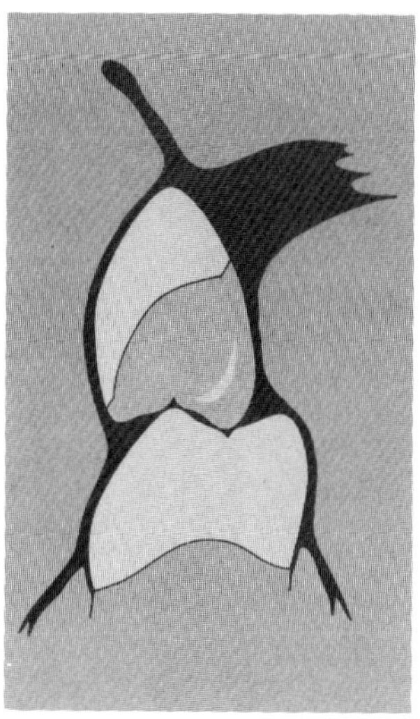

Fig. 7-90. Modified sanitary pontic related to excessively resorbed ridge.

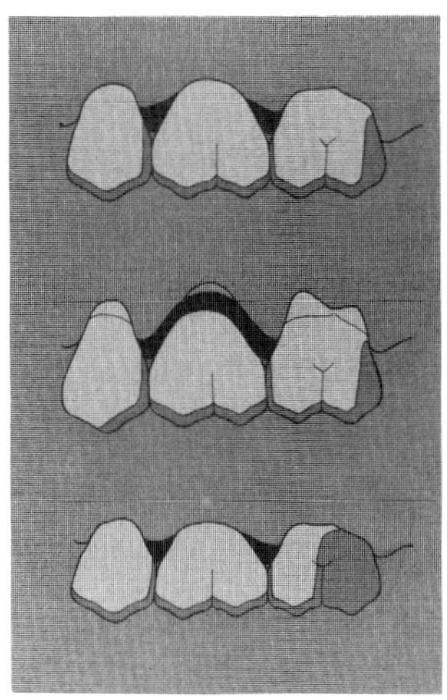

Fig. 7-91. Facial view of acceptable pontic contours related to ridges with various degrees of resorption.

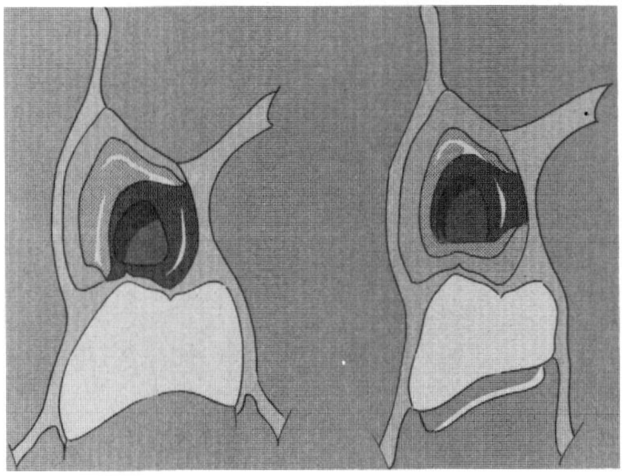

Fig. 7-92. Acceptable distribution of metal and porcelain for maxillary ceramometal pontics.

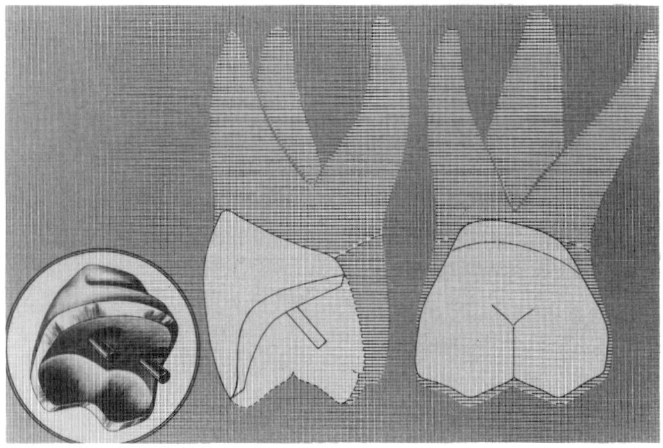

Fig. 7-93. Maxillary molar pontic is superimposed on natural tooth to illustrate change in contour. Manufactured pin facing is beveled and hollow ground *(inset).*

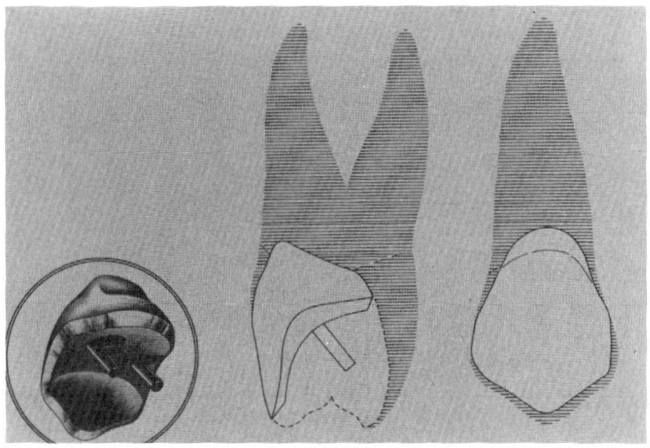

Fig. 7-94. Premolar pontic shows distinctly changed form from natural tooth it replaces.

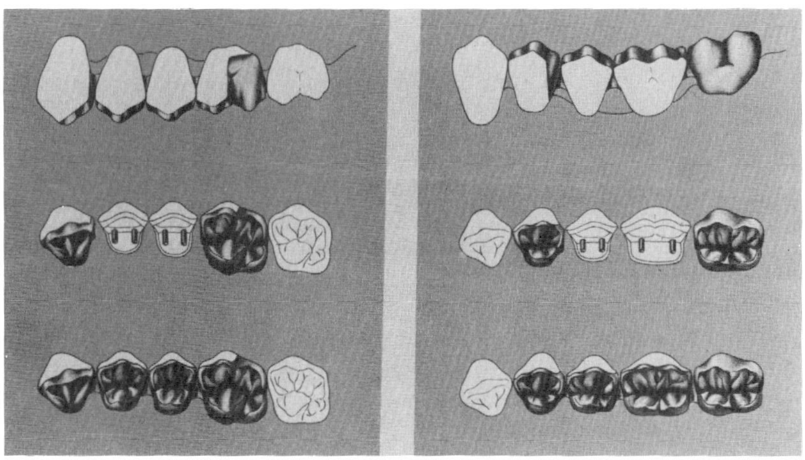

Fig. 7-95. Straight and narrow span of posterior fixed bridge best resists forces of deformation.

touring gentle concavities into the proximal surfaces. Hygienic embrasures may be developed even in cases with minimal occlusogingival dimension.

Fig. 7-92 illustrates the two most frequently used designs for ceramometal pontics. (See Chapter 13.) Pin pontics from manufacturers of porcelain pontic facings are shown in Figs. 7-93 and 7-94. The pontic is superimposed on the outline form of the natural tooth it replaces to illustrate the modifications in pontic contour necessary to satisfy optimal design requirements for a maxillary molar and premolar pontic adapted to a broad blunted ridge.

The continued optimal function of a fixed bridge is substantially enhanced by the cosmetic, hygienic, and mechanical design of the pontic span. These design requirements are shown in Fig. 7-95. Cosmetically, the pontic should have the appearance of the tooth it replaces. Hygienically, the pontic contour should ensure convenient maintenance; mechanically, the pontic span should have adequate strength, gained from metal support, to resist deformation. The metal support provides the mechanical integrity of the pontic span; plastic pontic facings are used only to satisfy cosmetic needs, and porcelain is used as a cosmetic and hygienic veneering material.

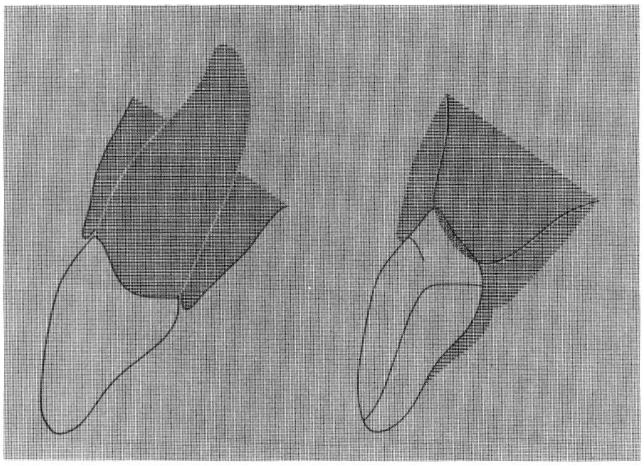

Fig. 7-96. Maxillary central incisor and pontic for this tooth with modified saddle-type ridge contact. Working cast should be relieved 0.5 mm.

ANTERIOR PONTIC

In restoring the anterior region of the mouth, the overriding requirement is that of cosmetics. There is no question that restorations fabricated by the metal-ceramic technique can satisfy the cosmetic requirement best.

In selecting and contouring the anterior pontic, every effort is made to artistically reproduce the facial characteristics of the natural tooth. The maxillary pontic, in high lip lines, is adapted to the edentulous ridge to achieve an outline form identical to the natural teeth. In cases with moderate ridge resorption, a modified saddle tissue contact will result (Fig. 7-96). The cingulum prominence of the pontic can be reduced to minimize tissue contact, but this prominence should not be entirely lost, since the cingula of the maxillary anterior teeth serve an important phonetic function. In cases of high ridge resorption, the tissue contact can be progressively minimized, and the desired tooth outline form may be emphasized by cervical contouring and supplemental staining.

The mandibular incisor pontic is shown in a relationship to one edentulous ridge with minimal resorption and one that is excessively resorbed (Fig. 7-97). The first condition requires a modified saddle tissue contact; the second condition permits a sanitary design. Both pontics fulfill equally all functional requirements. There simply is no stereotype in pontic design, and similar examples could be given for the maxillary anterior region as well as for the posterior quadrants of the mouth.

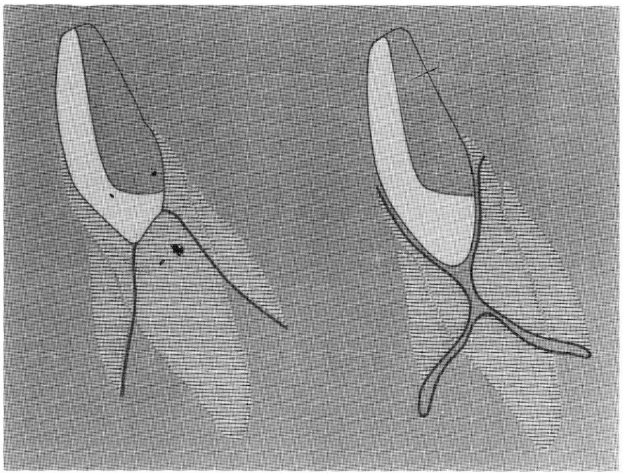

Fig. 7-97. Mandibular anterior pontic shown adapted to one moderately resorbed ridge and one excessively resorbed ridge.

The ceramometal technique greatly expanded the potential for cosmetic pontic design. The pontic contour principles are time proven and remain unaltered (Fig. 7-98). With the understanding of these principles, which find their expression in the final form of the prosthesis, the technician will be able to design the mechanical elements (Fig. 7-99) to be structurally sound and to permit optimal cosmetic and hygienic contouring of porcelain.

PROBLEM AREAS

The problems most frequently encountered in the fabrication of pontics, their probable causes, and solutions are identified in Table 7-3.

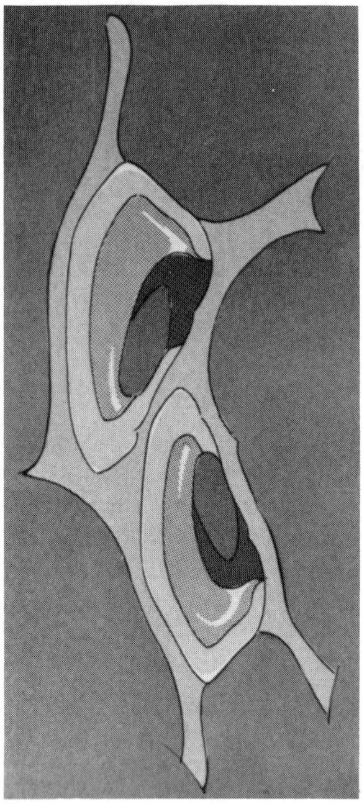

Fig. 7-98. Proper distribution of metal and porcelain for maxillary and mandibular ceramometal pontics.

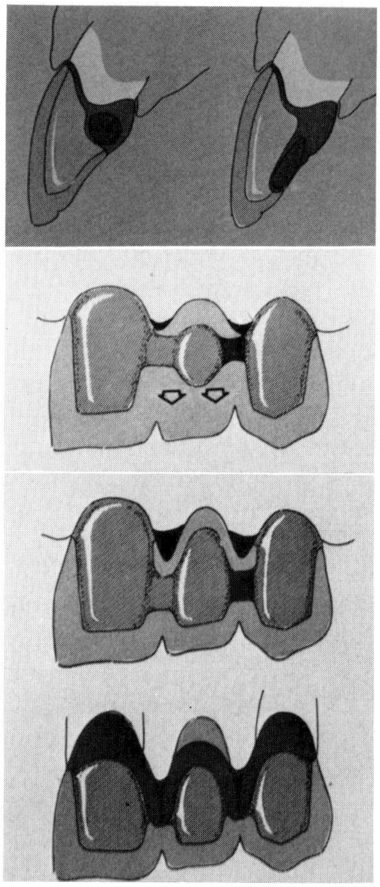

Fig. 7-99. Position and form of interproximal connectors for ceramometal restorations. **A,** Insufficient embrasure space and unsupported porcelain. **B,** Proper position and form.

1. The incomplete seating of a porcelain pin facing into the cast metal backing is a common source for frustration. Care must be exercised to reproduce pin channels in the casting of equal dimension as formed in the wax pattern. This is best accomplished by selecting graphite pins or pencil lead with the same diameter as the metal pins of the facing. Once the facing is withdrawn from the waxed backing, the pin channels are slightly lengthened (1 mm) by hand reaming with a No. 1 round bur. Graphite pins, approximately 10 mm long, are now pushed into the pin channels, and the wax pattern may be processed for casting. The graphite is best removed from the pin channels in the cast metal backing with a No. 588 fissure bur; also, the entrance to the pin channels is lightly recessed with a No. 2 round bur.

2. The porcelain pin facing may become wedged to the backing during trial seating. This is the case when the facing was forced to seat without proper enlargement of the pin channels. To separate the facing and backing, attach the facing to a large wax spatula with sticky wax; with the backing upward, tap the spatula rapidly with a metal instrument. The repeated forceful tapping near the pontic will cause the heavy backing to rise off the pontic. Now, hand ream the pin channels with a No. 588 fissure bur before the facing is reseated.

3. Improper ridge adaptation is the result of too little or too much relief of the working cast. The working cast is an expanded reproduction of the edentulous ridge. A pontic precisely adapted to the unaltered ridge of a working cast will be slightly shy of ridge contact in the mouth. The resultant crevice between the pontic and gingiva can needlessly harbor bacterial plaque or can be cosmetically unacceptable. To compensate for the expansion of gypsum used in cast fabrication, the ridge area should be relieved approximately 0.5 mm. The area to which the pontic is to be adapted is marked with a soft lead pencil, then scraped clean with a Bard-Parker knife blade. This procedure is repeated six times for optimal relief.

The porcelain pontic should then be adapted precisely to the altered ridge area. The cast is marked again with a soft lead pencil to indicate any premature contact on the porcelain for adjustment. Excessive tissue contact when the pontic is seated against the gingiva will cause blanching of the tissue. Here the edentulous ridge can be marked with lipstick to indicate those tissue contact areas of the pontic which are to be adjusted.

Table 7-3. Pontic design

Problem	Probable cause	Solution
Incomplete casting of pinholes	Nodules or broken investment	Use graphite pins or pencil lead of comparable size
Pinholes too tight for easy seating of facing	Undersized graphite pin used	Hand ream pinhole with No. 588 fissure bur
Facing does not seat completely into backing	Nodules or incomplete seating of graphite pins into wax pattern	Remove nodules if present; deepen pinholes with No. 1 round bur
Facing stuck to backing	Overretentive pinholes	Attach spatula to facing with sticky wax; with backing upward, tap spatula rapidly with metal instrument
Improper ridge adaptation	Ridge inadequately relieved	Relieve stone of working cast approximately 0.5 mm; pencil tissue contact area with soft lead; porcelain will be marked for premature contact
Gingival porcelain fractured when facing is trial seated to backing	Retention pins and gingival wall of porcelain almost parallel	Avoid parallelism or relieve gingival floor on metal backing
Facing fractures during occusal function	Insufficient metal support	Hollow grind facing for stronger metal protection
Entire facing dislodged during occlusal function	Inadequate retention	Increase boxed-in effect by longer mesial and distal bevels; burnish metal to facing during cementation
Porcelain fractures when drilling pinholes	Excessive pressure and heat generated by drill	Use sharp bibevel drill, ample lubricant (50% kerosene and 50% olive oil), and light pressure
Porcelain fracture of ceramometal pontic	Improper bonding, excess bulk of porcelain, improper occlusal adjustment, too rapid temperature change, incompatible combinations of porcelain and metal	Review metal conditioning and manufacturer's porcelain-firing procedures; porcelain thickness should not exceed 2 mm

4. The fracture or dislodgment of porcelain facings during functions is due to inadequate metal support and retention form. The porcelain is used only for cosmetic and hygienic reasons. The strength of the pontic span, its resistance to deformation, is entirely the function of the metal backing. For this reason, the occlusal or incisal portion of the porcelain facing must be hollow ground to ensure sufficient bulk of metal to resist deformation.

Retention pins that are parallel to the gingival floor on the metal backing can concentrate stresses in the porcelain where the pins are embedded and cause horizontal fracture of the porcelain facings. The gingival wall of the facing should form an obtuse angle with the retention pins.

When the reverse pin retention technique is used, an irregular pattern of pin placement is advised to avoid forming lines of stress along which the facing could fracture.

The incidence of facing dislodgment is minimized by proper pin retention. Retention pins must not be shortened to obtain complete seating of the facing, and the pin channels must not be enlarged to cause loosely fitting pins. In addition to pin retention, the facing is prepared with long interproximal bevels. These mesial and distal bevels are almost parallel to each other. The boxed-in effect gained within the subsequently fabricated metal backing and the burnishing of metal to the facing during cementation will add considerably to the retention of the facing.

5. Porcelain fracture of ceramometal pontics is caused by improper bonding and/or by insufficient metal support. If properly bonded, porcelain gains its greatest strength near the interface of metal and porcelain. The greater the bulk of porcelain, the less the resistance to the shear stresses. For optimal pontic design, the thickness of porcelain should not exceed 2 mm. This rule is frequently violated by excessive bulk of porcelain for gingival extension of the pontic. Stresses induced into the porcelain may cause fracture of the porcelain tip during function and deformation of the pontic span. It is advisable to wax the entire contour of the pontic, following by a cutback of the wax, to allow for the desired porcelain veneer. The cutback must not exceed the 2 mm rule.

In addition to chemical bonding, there must be physical retention. During firing, porcelain will shrink, a characteristic that offers a mechanical advantage if the metal substructure contoured to the porcelain veneer can, at least in part, surround it.

With the large number of porcelains and metal alloys currently available, the technician should verify the compatibility of these products with the manufacturers before selecting a particular combination. High-expansion porcelains bonded to low-expansion metals often result in fracturing during cooling or during post-soldering procedures. Special rapid cooling or investing techniques may be required to prevent fracture with these combinations.

SUMMARY

No phase of restorative dentistry requires as much imaginative interpretation to supplement basic knowledge as does the design of pontics for the large variety of edentulous ridge shapes. To suggest a rationale for the contouring of axial surfaces of pontics, the various forms of the edentulous ridges were divided into three groups according to the amount of tissue resorption.

The relationship of pontic form to ridge contour was demonstrated for each group with emphasis on the hygienic requirements that determine the form of the pontic and its harmonious function with associated oral tissues. These restorations will then contribute to a state that can be maintained with relative immunity to disease.

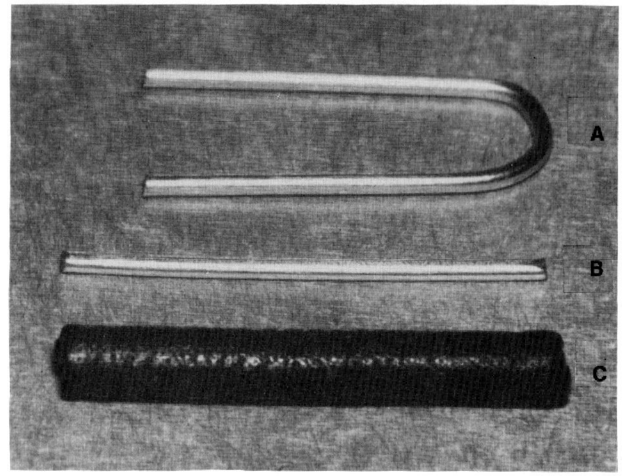

Fig. 7-100. *A,* Bent paper clip for use with MOD inlays. *B,* Straight paper clip for use with small inlays. *C,* Eight- to twelve-gauge wax sprue for use with onlays and crowns. Paper clips should be coated with film of wax to increase diameter of sprue former and facilitate removal from set investment. Reservoir should be added to decrease shrinkage porosity.

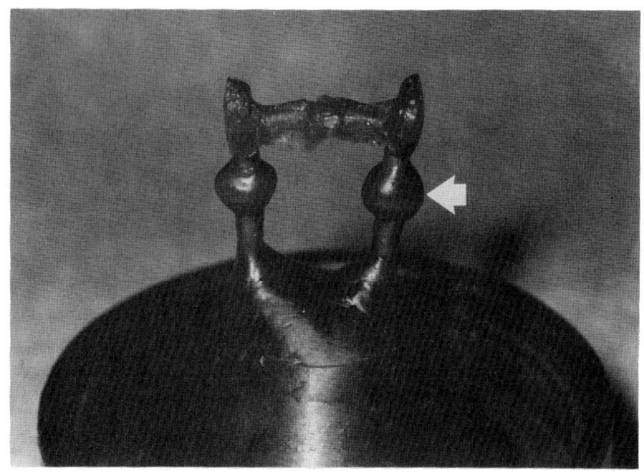

Fig. 7-101. When small patterns need long sprues, wax reservoir *(arrow)* placed approximately 1/16 inch (1.5 mm) from pattern provides bulk of molten alloy from which cooling, shrinking pattern can draw. These reservoirs should have diameter greater than thickest portion of pattern.

PART THREE

Spruing principles and techniques

MALCOLM D. JENDRESEN and CLIFFORD L. STOCKS

Accurate dental castings are produced by the lost wax process whereby the wax pattern is used to produce a precise refractory mold into which molten alloy is cast. After cooling, the casting will reproduce exactly the size and shape of the original wax pattern. The first step in the production of the refractory mold is termed spruing the pattern, whereby the wax pattern is attached to a conical base by a short extension of wax, plastic, or metal (which is later removed). This connector is termed the sprue former. Proper selection of size and configuration of the sprue former is critical to the production of a dense, complete, and accurate casting.

SPRUING THE PATTERN

The method and care used in spruing the pattern prior to investing can substantially affect the quality of the cast restoration. Selection of the sprue former depends on the type and size of the pattern and the size of the ring to be used. The sprue former should be at least 1.7 mm in diameter (14 gauge) unless the pattern is extremely small, and sprue formers up to 2.5 mm in diameter (10 gauge) may be used for very large patterns such as bulky full crowns (Fig. 7-100). Long and thin sprue formers are likely to cause internal porosity, commonly called *shrinkage porosity.* If a long, thin sprue is used, the metal will freeze in the sprue before it freezes in the inlay or crown, thus preventing more metal from entering the mold. This may be overcome by using a reservoir or larger sprue. If a reservoir is used, it must have greater bulk than the adjacent portion of the pat-

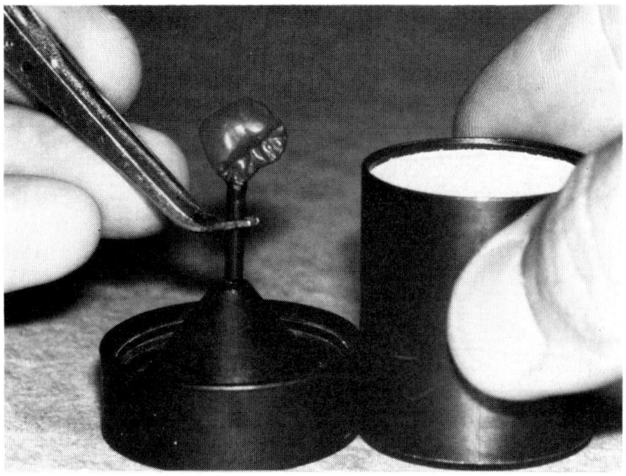

Fig. 7-102. Wax sprue-former length is checked before attachment to ensure that pattern is at least ⅛ to ¼ inch (3 to 6 mm) from end of ring.

tern into which the sprue former is inserted (Fig. 7-101). The length of the sprue former should be adjusted so that the pattern is approximately 3 to 6 mm from the open end of the ring (Figs. 7-102 and 7-103).

If a greater thickness of investment is present, "back pressure" porosity may result. When the investment is too bulky, air in the mold cannot escape through the investment, and the gold is prevented from completely filling the mold.

Either wax, plastic, or metal sprue formers may be used. Metal should be rust resistant to prevent contamination of the mold. The sprue former is generally attached to the most bulky part of the pattern (Fig. 7-104). Any overheating of the wax, which could distort the pattern, must be avoided. For this reason hollow metal (e.g., orthodontic tubing) or hollow plastic sprue formers are preferred, since they hold less heat than a solid sprue former. The sprue former should be smooth and produce no sharp angles at the juncture of the wax pattern or the crucible former (Fig. 7-105).

MOD patterns are best sprued centrally on the occlusal surface. However, the sprue former should also be attached in a position to minimize the effect on the occlusal contours of a restoration (Fig. 7-106). The orientation of the pattern in the ring also plays a role. For example, if an MOD pattern is sprued on the occlusal surface, the mesiodistal expansion is reduced by the confining action of the ring. The expansion may be increased a bit in such a case by attaching the sprue on the proximal surface so that the mesiodistal expansion is in the direction of the open ring. The distance between the end of the pattern and the unlined portion of the ring will significantly affect the size of the resultant castings. To eliminate this variable, position both

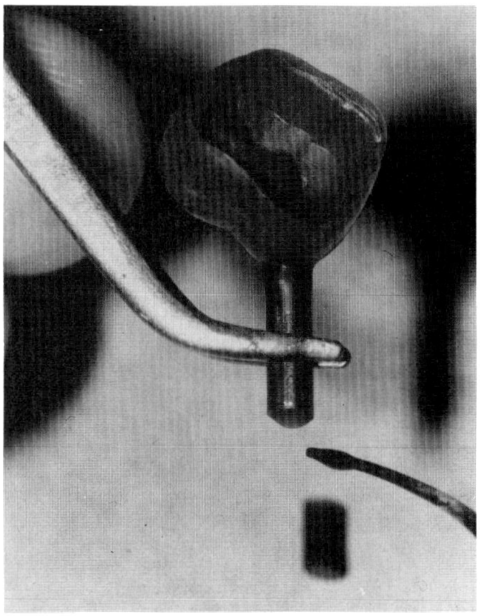

Fig. 7-103. Wax sprue-former length is adjusted by small hot instrument. Wax spatulas or other large instruments radiate excessive heat and may distort pattern.

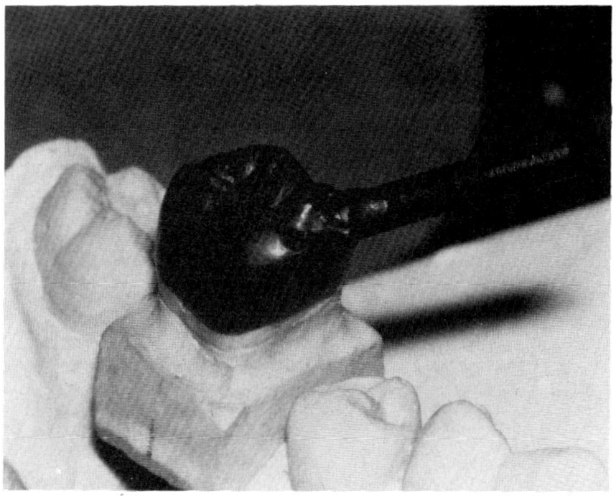

Fig. 7-104. Sprue former is attached to thickest portion of pattern before pattern is removed from die to prevent distortion caused by heat from fingers holding pattern.

the pattern and lining accurately in the ring. The pattern is best placed at a constant distance of 3 to 6 mm from the open end of the ring (Fig. 7-107).

Prefabricated sprue formers are available in a variety of sizes and configurations (Fig. 7-108). These plastic sprue formers are more rigid than those of wax and decrease the chances of distorting the pattern. Fig. 7-109 illustrates a three-unit bridge and sprues with the "gate" technique, using prefabricated plastic formers. This is particularly useful for long-span multiple castings.

Poor sprue designs can result in poor castings (Fig. 7-110). The sprue former must provide a proper ingate,

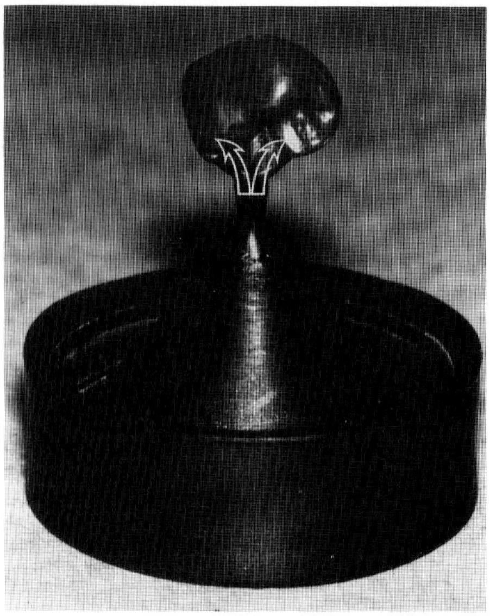

Fig. 7-105. Sprue former placement should provide smooth-flowing entry of gold into mold *(arrows),* with no sharp angles in path of incoming gold.

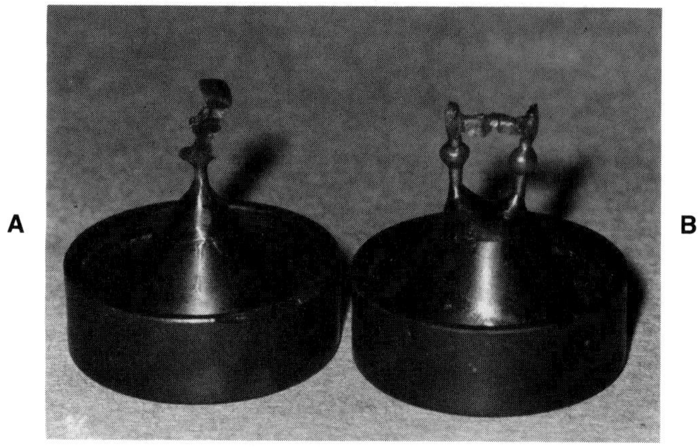

Fig. 7-106. MOD patterns may be sprued in either of two ways. Sprue former placed in contact *(A)* preserves occlusal anatomy and will result in increased expansion in mesiodistal direction due to mold expansion out end of casting ring. Sprue former placed on marginal ridges *(B)* preserves contacts at expense of some occlusal anatomy and provides for equal expansion in all directions.

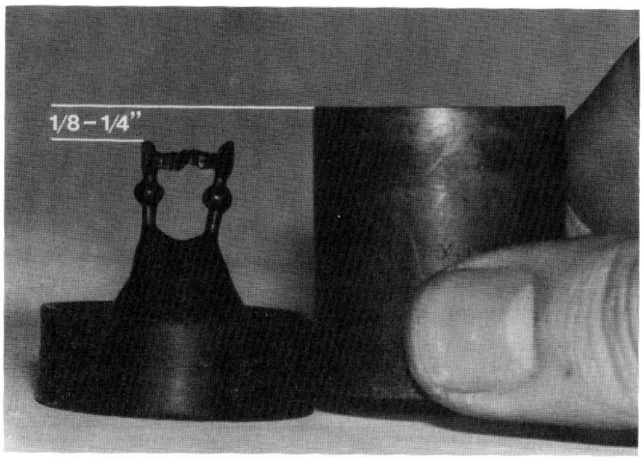

Fig. 7-107. Space of 1/8 to 1/4 inch (3 to 6 mm) between pattern and end of ring provides adequate bulk of investment to withstand force of inrushing gold, yet still allows gases to escape from end of mold. Distances greater than 1/4 inch (6 mm) tend to increase incidence of back pressure porosity in casting.

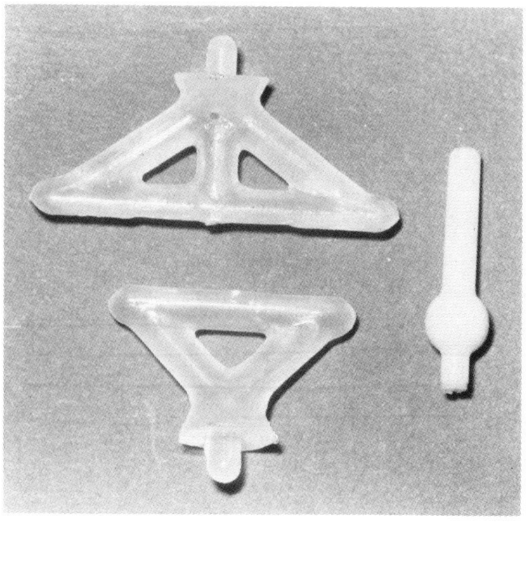

Fig. 7-108. Prefabricated plastic sprue formers are more rigid than wax sprue formers and decrease chance of distorting pattern.

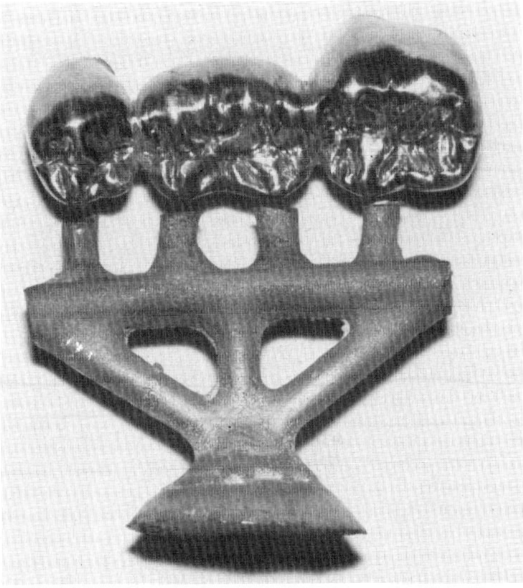

Fig. 7-109. Three-unit bridge and sprues with "gate" technique, using prefabricated plastic sprue former. This minimizes distortion in long-span restorations.

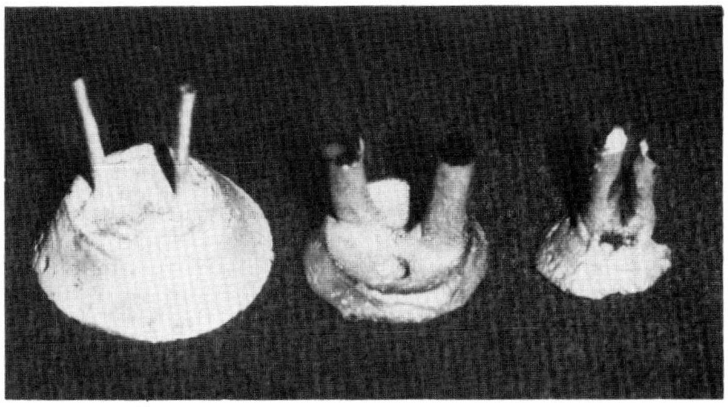

Fig. 7-110. Poor sprue designs such as these can lead to casting failure.

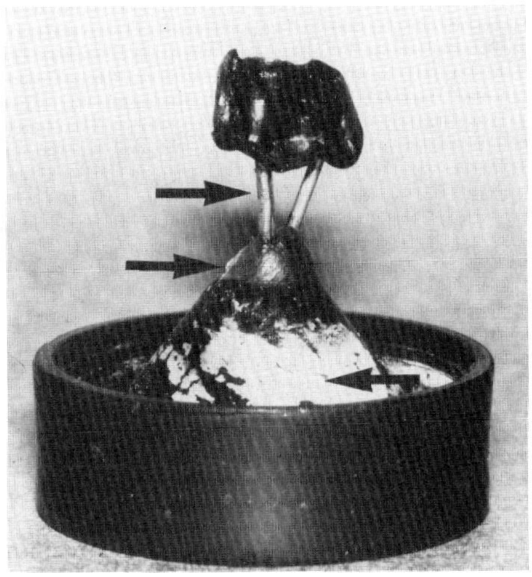

Fig. 7-111. Poorly sprued pattern. No wax relief around wire sprues that are also dirty *(top arrow).* Poorly contoured wax surface around sprues *(bottom arrow).* Each could result in poor casting.

A

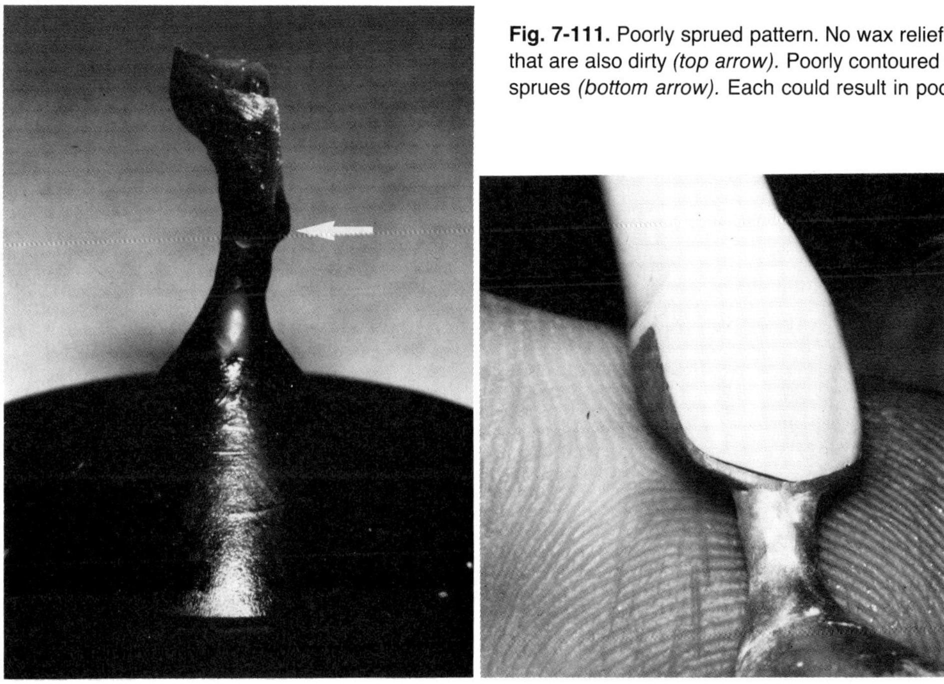

B

Fig. 7-112. A, Sprue former placed too close to margins *(arrow).* Bulk of wax in sprue former shrinks as it cools and distorts margin. **B,** Resulting casting exhibits open margin in area close to sprue.

allowing for smooth unobstructed flow of the molten gold into the mold. Figs. 7-111 and 7-112 illustrate additional considerations, each of which can cause poor castings.

SPRUING METAL-CERAMIC UNITS

Spruing the metal-ceramic coping or framework is similar to spruing conventional inlays and crowns. For small crowns a short, 8-gauge wax sprue former should be placed on the incisal edge so that the gold may flow directly into the thinnest section of the casting (Fig. 7-113). The investment mold is generally about 1000° F (540° C) cooler than the molten alloy, and solidification occurs very quickly. Movement of the liquid metal to the most distal margins of the casting (Fig. 7-114) must not be obstructed. There should always be sufficient bulk of the sprue and associated button to allow for contraction of the metal during solidification without introduction of shrinkage porosity. For larger castings (e.g., posterior crowns or small bridge units) an additional auxiliary sprue may be placed to facilitate filling the mold. However, very small-diameter primary or auxiliary sprue formers (e.g., 14 to 16 gauge) attached to thicker sections of the casting (Fig. 7-115) will often cause shrinkage porosity, since they provide no reservoir from which to draw the solidifying alloy.

Large units (e.g., bridges cast as a single unit) are best sprued by the "gate" method, whereby a series of short 8-gauge wax sprue formers are attached to a con-

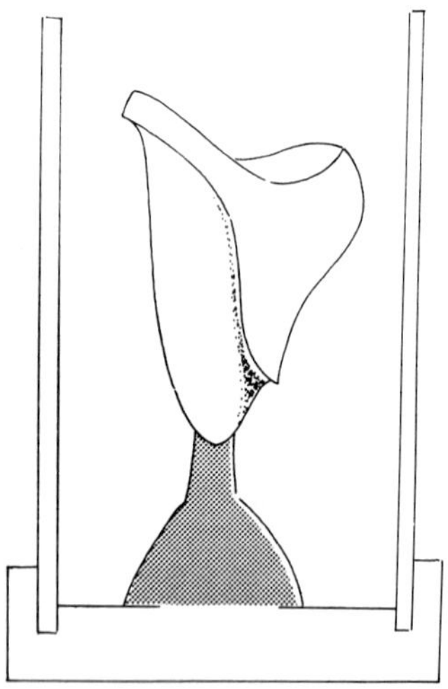

Fig. 7-113. Small units are easily cast by attaching short 6- or 8-gauge wax sprue former at incisal tip of wax pattern.

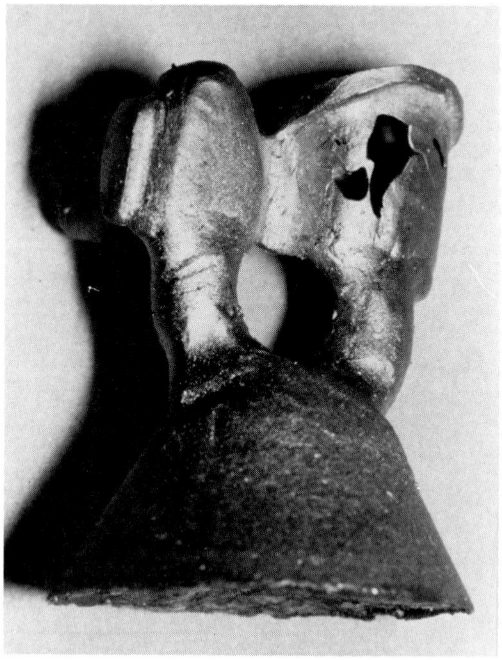

Fig. 7-114. Incomplete casting caused by excessively thin wax patterns and obstruction of gold flow in facial area of coping.

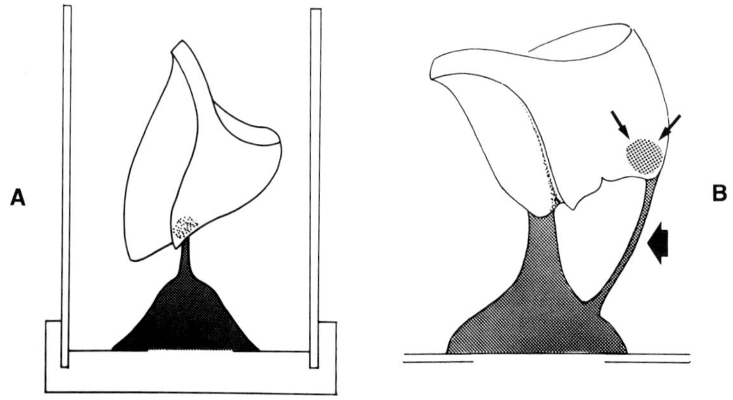

Fig. 7-115. A, Small primary sprue formers can create shrinkage porosity in casting. **B,** Very thin auxiliary sprues *(bottom arrow)* can create regions of porosity *(top arrows)* in thicker sections of larger castings.

tinuous 6- or 8-gauge "runner bar" of wax or (preferably) plastic (Fig. 7-116). This runner bar in turn is attached to the crucible former by two or more large sprue formers, providing (1) a minimum of distortion of the wax pattern, (2) a fairly uniform reservoir of metal near the entire casting, and (3) even distribution of the alloy to all parts of the casting to minimize porosity.

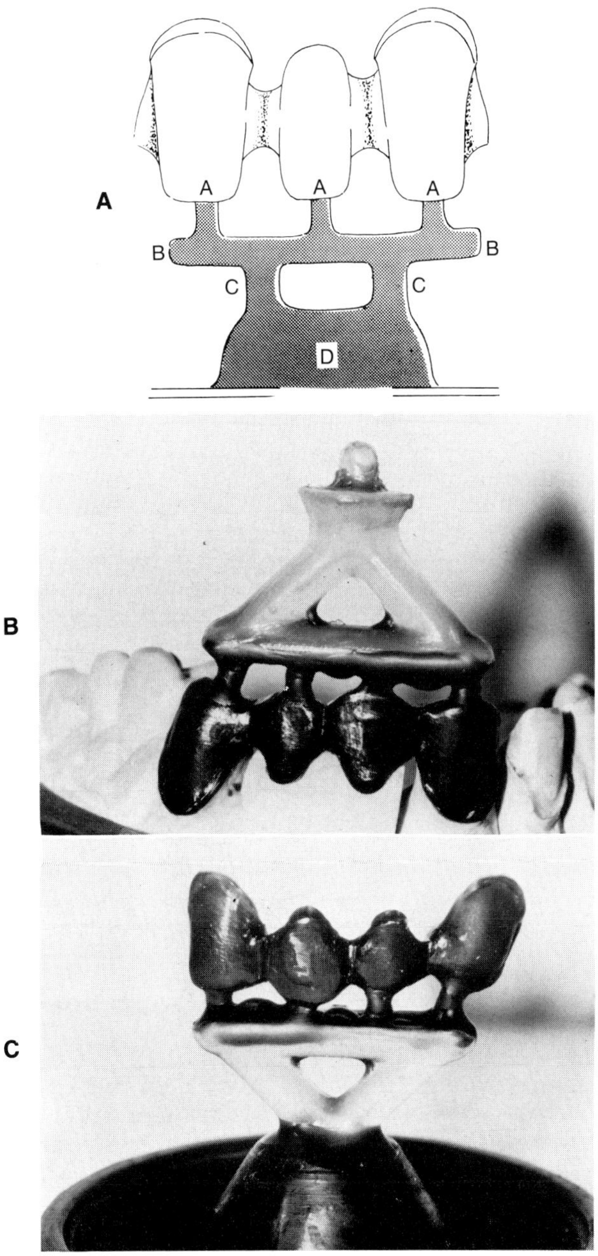

Fig. 7-116. A, "Gate" spruing. Six- or eight-gauge sprue formers *(A);* runner bar, 6-gauge or larger *(B);* feeder sprues, 6-gauge or larger *(C);* crucible former *(D).* **B** and **C,** Four-unit bridge to be cast using prefabricated plastic "gate" sprue former. These rigid patterns help minimize wax distortion during investing procedures.

When constructing such an arrangement, care must be taken not to distort the large pattern during handling or by heating and softening the large bulk of spruing wax so that shrinkage on cooling stresses the pattern. The use of rigid plastic sprue formers and runner bars will reduce this problem.

Porosity will always occur in that portion of the casting that cools last. For large castings such as multiple unit bridges, it is critical that the spruing arrangement provide a bulk (or reservoir) of metal that is external to the dental unit but positioned at the heat center of the investment mold. Generally the alloy immediately adjacent to the walls of the mold will solidify first, the exposed surface of the button will solidify second, and the alloy internal to the mold will cool last. In the gate sprue technique illustrated in Figs. 7-117 and 7-118, the runner bar will usually be the last part to solidify and will contain porosity. If bulky pontics are placed at the heat center of the mold or are cast without a res-

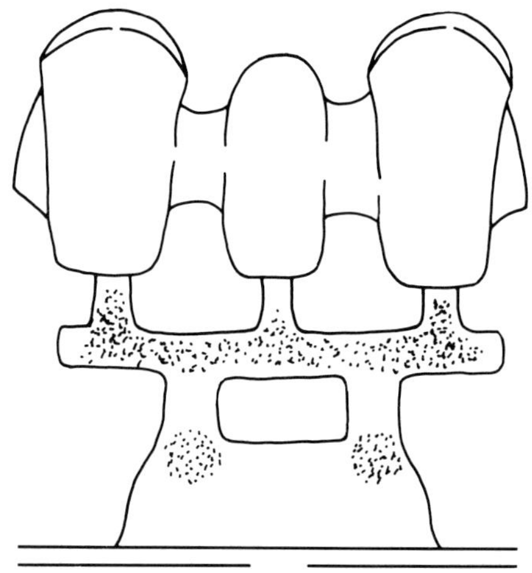

Fig. 7-117. Proper gate spruing. Reservoir is in heat center of mold.

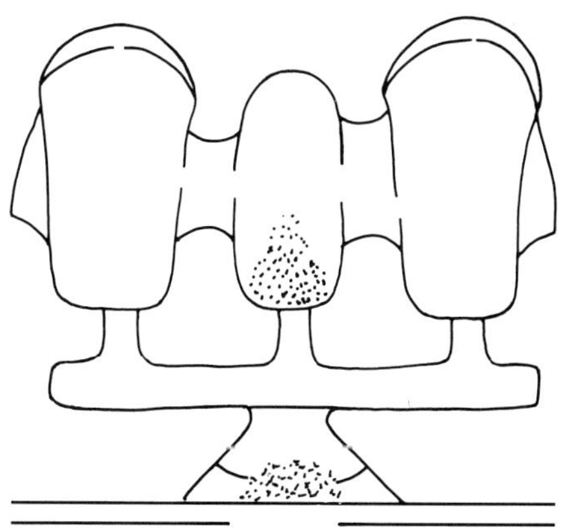

Fig. 7-118. Improper spruing. Dental unit is placed at heat center, resulting in porosity in casting.

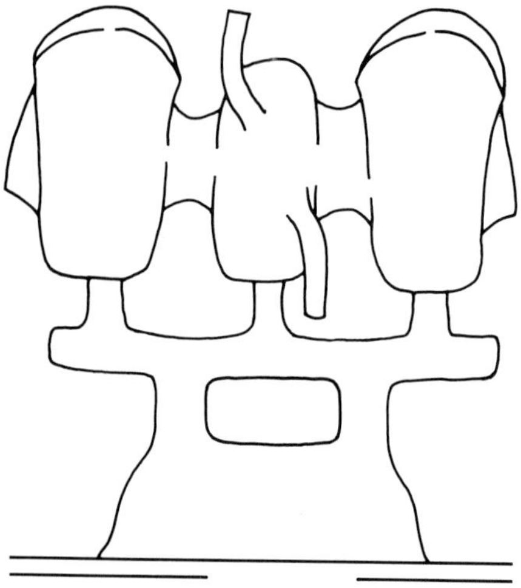

Fig. 7-119. Addition of chill vents to bulky dental units may speed solidification and minimize porosity in the thick pontic or connector areas.

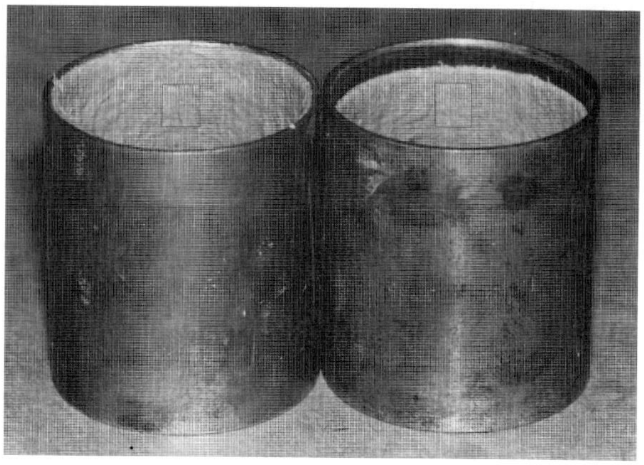

Fig. 7-120. Placement of liner. *A,* Liner set flush with top of ring to allow increased expansion out open end of ring. *B,* Liner set in ⅛ inch (3 mm) to provide "lock" at end of ring; this equalizes expansion in all directions. Both techniques can be used, depending on individual needs of casting.

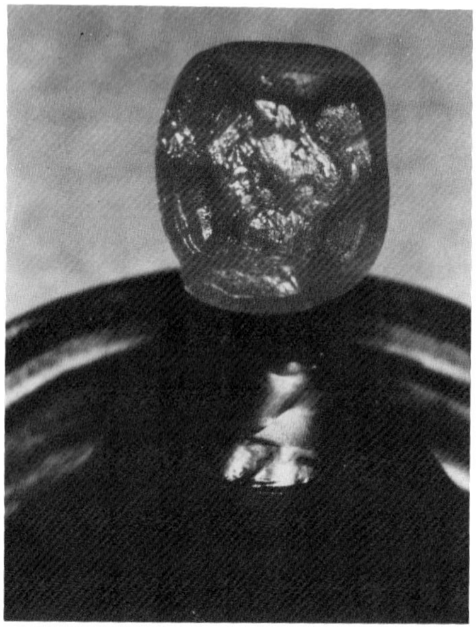

Fig. 7-121. Shiny oily layer of die lubricant often adheres to wax pattern and should be removed before investing.

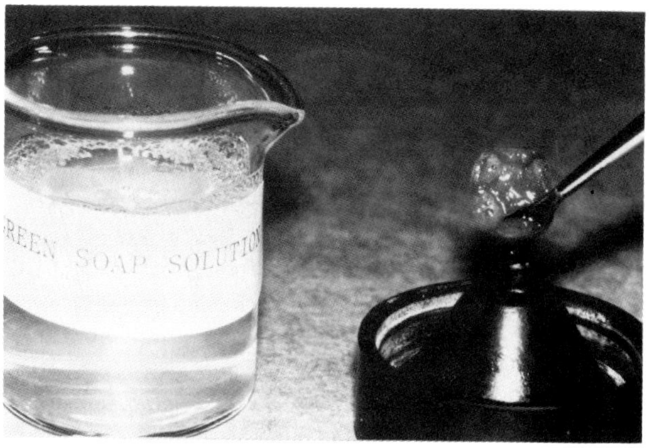

Fig. 7-122. Green soap solution or commercial wax pattern cleaner is used to remove any residual oily die lubricant.

ervoir within the investment, porosity is very likely to occur in the pontic itself or at the connector between the pontic(s) and the abutments, resulting in a weak bridge. Where a dental casting contains both thick and thin elements, porosity can be minimized by the addition of chill vents (Fig. 7-119) that accelerate the cooling of the pontic relative to the parts of the casting external to the dental unit itself. These cast extensions are cut off after retrieval of the casting from the investment.

The casting ring must be lined with sheet asbestos or ceramic paper to permit a greater freedom of expansion of the investment, which would otherwise be restricted by the ring. The compressible property of the liner helps offset the contraction of the more rapidly cooling ring while the gold alloy is being melted. When a wet liner is used, the water in the liner affords a certain amount of hygroscopic expansion.

Placement of the liner within the ring influences expansion of the mold. When maximum expansion is required, a liner flush with the open end of the ring should be used. A liner that is 3 or 6 mm short of the

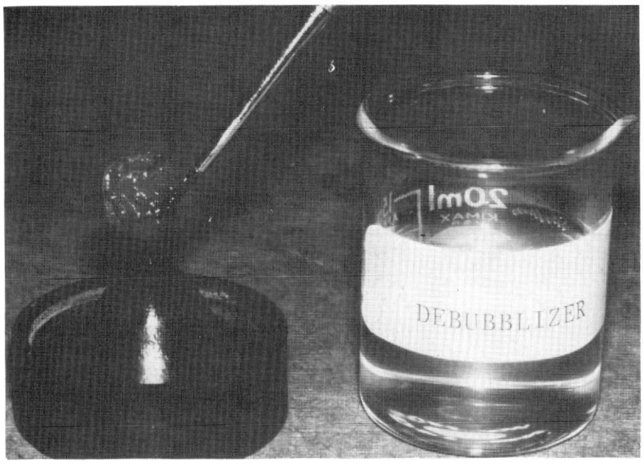

Fig. 7-123. Debubblizers reduce surface tension of wax and promote wetting of surface by investment. Pattern is blown dry with gentle stream of air to remove excess liquid that would weaken investment.

open end of the ring will produce a smaller casting. The greater the unlined portion of the ring, the greater the restrictive effect; thus the distance by which the liner is short should be carefully controlled (Fig. 7-120). The liner should be attached firmly to the ring by wax to prevent it from "riding up" during the investing procedure and inadvertently affecting the size of the casting.

Using a liner flush with the end of the ring eliminates the need to measure the distance of the liner from the open end of the ring and may simplify standardization of the procedure. A liner that is 3 mm short of the open end of the ring promotes a more equal expansion of the casting in the axial and horizontal directions. Because of potential health hazards from asbestos in the dental laboratory, many manufacturers now offer ceramic lining materials for lining the casting ring. These materials absorb water much less readily than asbestos, and their use in combination with certain gypsum-bonded investments may result in a significant incidence of fins on the castings. They will generally give a slightly higher expansion of the mold than asbestos, and they should be thoroughly wetted before investing the wax pattern. They are most compatible with phosphate-bonded investments (discussed in the next section). Cleanliness is essential throughout the entire investing procedure. The wax pattern must be free of any oil film or debris before investing (Figs. 7-121 and 7-122).

The surface tension of the wax pattern can be improved by using a commercial debubblizer. This procedure promotes better wetting of the pattern surface by the investment material, thereby providing a smooth and accurate reproduction of the surface (Fig. 7-123).

The sprued pattern should be positioned so that there will be ⅛ to ¼ inch (3 to 6 mm) of investment covering it when the ring is filled (Fig. 7-124). After spruing, the pattern should be thoroughly cleansed to remove residual die lubricants. Gentle washing with a soft No. 2 point brush and liquid soap is effective. The soap should be thoroughly rinsed off with room-temperature water, and the pattern dried with a stream of clean air.

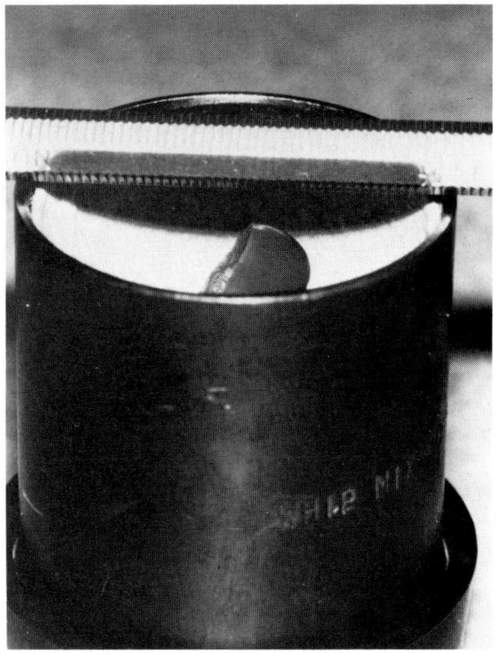

Fig. 7-124. There should be at least ⅛ inch (3 mm) of investment covering pattern when coping is cast.

After cleansing, the pattern may be treated (according to manufacturer's directions) with any one of a number of commercial debubblizing solutions. They are painted on the pattern and dried with a gentle airstream. It is important that they not be allowed to pool in internal line angles of the pattern. Debubblizing solutions increase the wettability of the wax surface so as to reduce the entrapment of air bubbles on the surface during investing. They are useful but not essential to obtaining an acceptable casting.

PART FOUR

Investing

MALCOLM D. JENDRESEN and CLIFFORD L. STOCKS

Once the wax pattern is positioned within the ring, the refractory mold is formed by filling the ring with an investment material, two types of which are used for dental casting—gypsum-bonded and phosphate-bonded. All investments, irrespective of type, are composed of a refractory material and a binder. The refractory material imparts thermal expansion and durability at high temperatures, while the binder contributes setting expansion and structural integrity for the refractory mold.

PROPERTIES OF GYPSUM-BONDED INVESTMENTS

Low-heat investments are composed of gypsum binders and are known as *gypsum-bonded investments.* These investments may have as their refractory materials different allotropic forms of silica, such as cristobalite or quartz. In one form or another, silica is a source of mold expansion when heated. The gypsum binder is a source of mold expansion during its setting reaction. The combined expansions of investment materials give rise to the total expansion of the mold. Mold expansion is necessary to compensate for shrinkage of the cast metal as it cools to room temperature. Total shrinkage of the cast inlay gold alloy, on cooling from its casting temperature to room temperature, has been calculated to be approximately $1.4\% \pm 0.2\%$. In low-heat investments mold expansion can be controlled or managed by various procedures and conditions. Following are three types of expansion associated with the use of gypsum-bonded investment materials.

1. *Setting expansion* is caused by the normal crystal growth of gypsum on dissolution and recrystallization during the setting reaction.
2. *Hygroscopic expansion* is caused by water being added to the setting investment, which provides a greater volume into which the gypsum crystals can realize their full growth potential. Hygroscopic expansion can only be realized after growing crystals have made contact. If additional water is added to the initial mix, a thinner mix is produced, and the expansion is not increased. Hygroscopic expansion is a continuation or form of setting expansion. The final (total) setting expansion depends on the number of crystals per unit volume of setting investment.
3. *Thermal expansion* occurs when the silica is subjected to high temperatures. A phase transformation occurs in the silica, producing a slightly different atomic configuration, which is accompanied by an expansion. The amount of thermal expansion depends on the allotropic form of silica used; for example, the thermal expansion of cristobalite is greater than that of quartz at most temperatures. Thermal expansion is also related to the quantity of silica in the investment material and the water-powder ratio; for example, thick mixes have greater thermal expansion than thin mixes.

On heating, the set gypsum exhibits a slight shrinkage because of dehydration; however, overall expansion negates this event. Additives such as sodium chloride or boric acid will reduce or eliminate this shrinkage.

The particle size of the silica and gypsum binder influences the surface texture of the mold, which in turn contributes to the smoothness of the cast restoration. The finer the particle size, the smoother the surfaces. The particle size distribution also influences the porosity of the set investment. The set investment must be porous enough to allow mold gases to escape when the gold is forced into the mold; therefore maintaining a fairly uniform particle size will reduce packing of the particles and prevent reduction in porosity. When dental personnel mix different investments together to create their own blend, they encounter the hazard of increasing the density of the investment. The setting time for low-heat investments is similar to that of dental stone and plaster.

Strength characteristics of gypsum-bonded investments are reflected by the type of gypsum used and the initial water-powder ratio. When the correct water-powder ratio is used, these materials are sufficiently strong to withstand the forces associated with the molten alloy entering the mold.

All porcelain-bonding alloys melt at temperatures several hundred degrees higher than inlay gold. It is important when making castings that: (1) the investment does not react with the alloy and thereby contaminate it and (2) the expansion of the investment compensates for the shrinkage of the molten alloy from freezing temperature to room temperature. Gypsum-bonded investments should not be used for casting high-fusing alloys, since the gypsum binder breaks down at temperatures near 1350° F (730° C) and liberates sulfur dioxide (SO_2). Not only is the strength and accuracy of the investment mold reduced by this disintegration, but sulfur dioxide can contaminate the alloys. The need for stable high-temperature investments has been met by development of phosphate-bonded, high-heat investments. Phosphate-bonded investments have the following approximate composition according to Allan and Asgar (1966) and Mabie (1973):

Quartz, cristobalite	75% to 90%
Monoammonium phosphate ($NH_4H_2PO_4$)	7% to 10%
Magnesium oxide (MgO_2)	3% to 5%

Unspecified amounts of carbon are often added to these powders, giving them a black color, to minimize oxidation of the alloys cast into them. Base metals may react with carbon, however, forming carbides that can embrittle these alloys; carbonfree (white) phosphate investments are available for fabrication of copings and frameworks from these metals.

Most commercial phosphate investment powders are mixed with a liquid (supplied by the manufacturer) that is predominately water with a proportion of colloidal silica, sufficient to add about 2% silica (SiO_2) to the investment mix. Other ionic salts may be present in the liquid in small amounts. Since silica will precipitate out of the colloidal solution on freezing, manufacturers issue cautions against subjecting the liquids to extremely cold temperatures. These liquids are sometimes artificially colored by the suppliers to facilitate measurement and dilution.

The purpose of silica is to give high strength to the mass at elevated temperatures by the formation of a silicophosphate glass binder. Mixing phosphate investments with pure water or precipitated liquid will produce a weaker mass at high temperatures, which may not be capable of sustaining the forces of casting without cracking. The liquid supplied by the manufacturer is usually diluted with pure water to regulate expansion of the mold. High liquid-water ratios increase the proportion of silica in the set investment (i.e., decrease the water-powder ratio) and thereby increase the thermal expansion of the mold.

Some phosphate-bonded investments use only water as a reactant, the silica presumably being incorporated in the powder mix. The setting reaction of phosphate-bonded investments involves reactions between magnesium, water, and monoammonium phosphate to form a hydrated gellike ammonium magnesium phosphate ($NH_4MgPO_4 \cdot H_2O$) and magnesium phosphate ($Mg_3(PO_4)_2 \cdot 4H_2O$), which bind together unreacted components to form a rigid mass. On heating, water is lost at 212° F (100° C), and ammonia (NH_3) is released at 480° F (250° C), forming magnesium phosphate ($Mg_2P_2O_7$). Also, at about 390° to 500° F (200° to 260° C), excess monoammonium phosphate ($NH_4H_2PO_4$) decomposes and forms phosphorous pentoxide (P_2O_5), ammonia, and water. At 903° F (500° C) there is a further loss of water from crystallization of $Mg_3(PO_4)_2 \cdot 4H_2O$, forming magnesium phosphate $Mg_3(PO_4)_2$. All these decomposition reactions result in shrinkage (which is offset by expansion of the quartz and cristobalite) of these components and a decrease in crushing strength of the investment mass.

At temperatures from 930° to 1800° F (500° to 1000° C), phosphates ($Mg_3P_2O_7$ and P_2O_5), silica (SiO_2), ionic salts, and minor impurities react to form liquid silicophosphate glass (which serves to glue all constituents together). The resulting investment achieves great strength and becomes relatively difficult to remove from castings (as compared with gypsum-bonded investments). Since the escape of gas through open pores in the investment is necessary for a dense casting, these investments should not be heated much beyond 1800° F (1000° C) for extended periods. To do so will produce excessive fusion of the investment components, thereby sealing the possible escape routes of gas as molten alloy enters the mold. The likelihood of back-pressure porosity or incomplete castings increases as the investments are heated to these temperatures. Liquefaction within the investment also increases the reactivity between the molten alloy and the investment itself (particularly with nonprecious nickel-chromium and cobalt-chromium alloys). Overheated base metal alloys cast into overheated molds can initiate chemical reactions (particularly between chromium and the magnesium components) that produce a tenacious green scale and rough casting surfaces. The presence of free carbon in these investments can reduce these scale-forming reactions; however, it can also induce carbide formation in the alloy, which may adversely affect its mechanical properties by embrittling it. In general practice, phosphate-bonded investment molds are heated to approximately 1400° F (760° C) for ½ to 1 hour and receive molten alloy cast at approximately 2400° to 2600° F (1315° to 1425° C).

INVESTING

The technique of investing a wax pattern does not require undue haste, but all materials and equipment needed should be at hand, so there will be no delay after the wax pattern is removed from the die. Gypsum-bonded investments require very specific water-powder ratios. The manufacturer's direction for any given investment product should be followed carefully.

A variation of only 1 ml of water can significantly alter the setting expansion and also affect the manipulation of the investment and the character of the casting surface. Although increasing the water-powder ratio makes the investing process somewhat easier, the investment will lose strength. The reduced strength may cause cracks to occur during heating, and the surface of the casting will be inferior. For these reasons the water should be accurately measured in a graduated measuring cylinder, and the powder weighed.

The powder and water must be mixed thoroughly to properly wet all particles (Fig. 7-125). Further mixing under a vacuum is recommended even when a paint-on technique is used for applying the investment material to the wax pattern (Fig. 7-126).

When a brush or small instrument is used to apply the investment material to the pattern, the wet material should be gently applied, pushed ahead of the applicator (Fig. 7-127, *A*). When the pattern is completely covered in this manner, the remaining investment is poured into the ring carefully to avoid entrapping air, and the investing procedure is completed (Fig. 7-127, *B*).

Mechanical investing under a vacuum is easier for the inexperienced operator (Fig. 7-128). Excessive vibrating during this procedure may cause bubbles in the investment and on the surface of the pattern, resulting in nodules on the casting.

After the casting ring has been filled with the investment material, any excess should be removed before

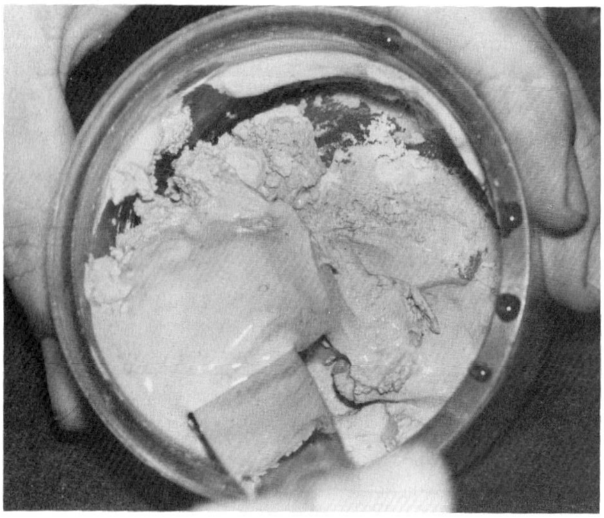

Fig. 7-125. Hand mixing prior to vacuum investment ensures complete wetting of all investment particles.

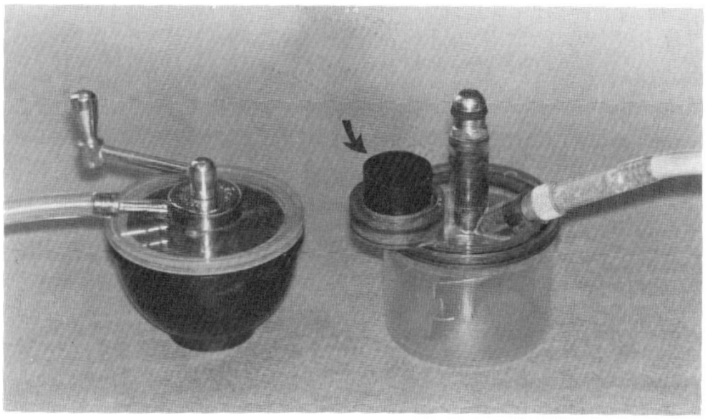

Fig. 7-126. Paint-on investment technique uses vacuum mixer, hand or mechanical, with ring hole plugged. Plastic 35-mm film container seals open ring hole *(arrow)*.

A

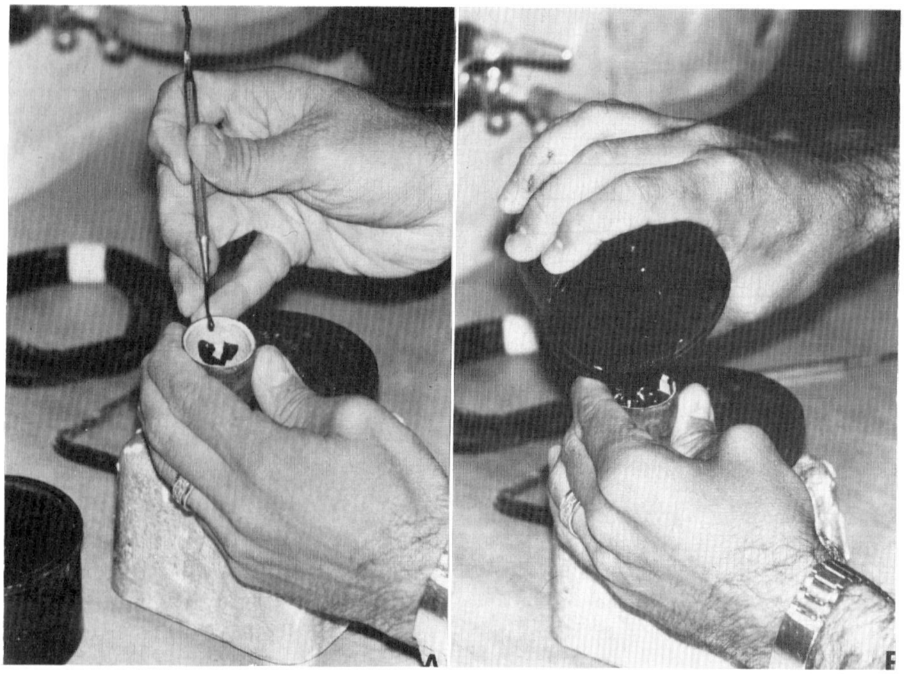

B

Fig. 7-127. A, Paintbrush or small instrument is used to apply initial layer of investment over pattern; this procedure decreases chances of bubble entrapment inside pattern. **B,** Remaining investment is then poured into ring, carefully, so as not to create voids in ring.

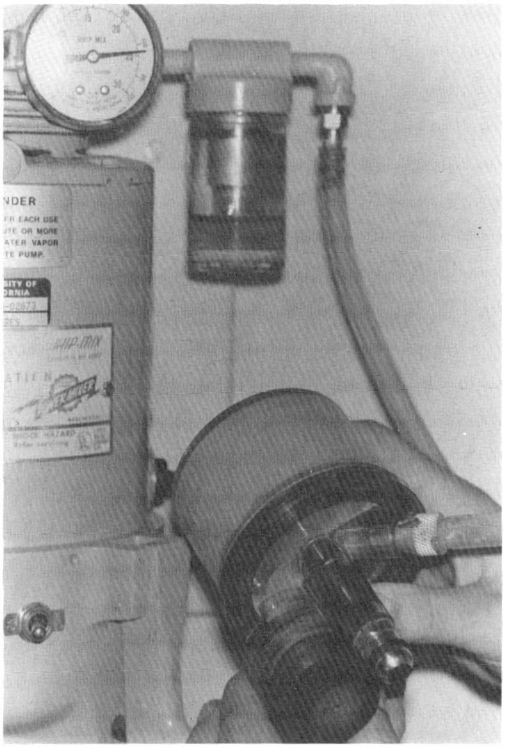

Fig. 7-128. With mechanical vacuum investing technique, ring is filled while still under vacuum, greatly decreasing amount of "micro-bubbles."

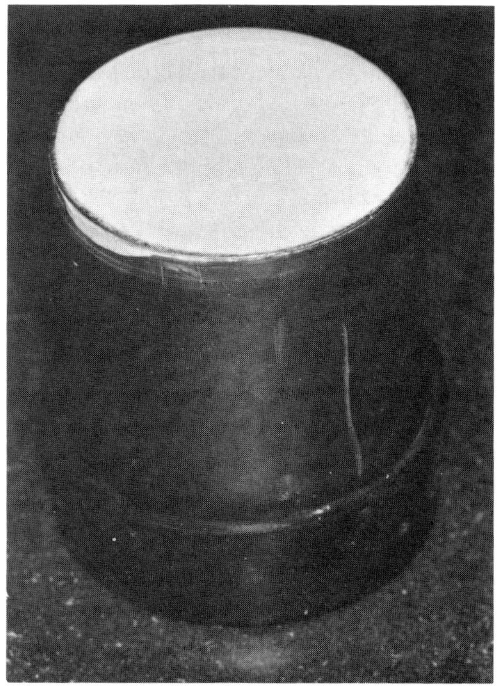

Fig. 7-129. Before it starts to set, investment is wiped flush with top of ring. Any scraping attempted after set may fill in pores and inhibit gas escape from mold during casting.

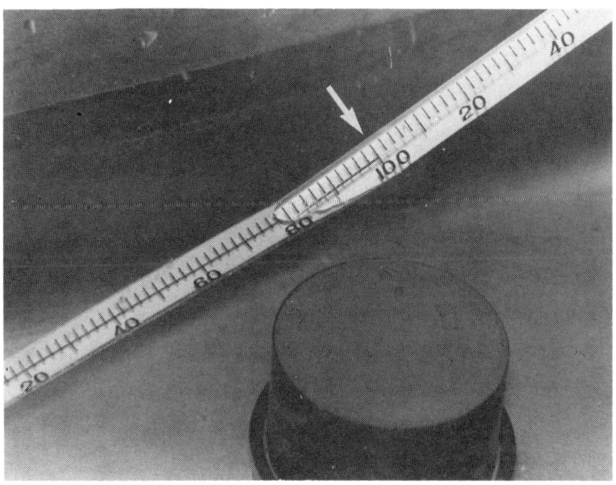

Fig. 7-130. Hygroscopic technique relies mainly on setting expansion to gain proper expansion of mold. After being filled, ring is immediately placed in constant temperature water bath at 100° F (38° C) for at least 30 minutes.

the material sets (Fig. 7-129). The filled ring is now set aside to allow the investment material to complete its setting reaction and the accompanying setting expansion. In most instances the setting is complete in 30 to 40 minutes, at which time it may be placed in a burnout oven to eliminate the wax and obtain the remaining required thermal expansion.

When a hygroscopic technique is used, the freshly filled investment ring is immediately placed into a water bath for 30 minutes and kept at 100° F (38° C) (Fig. 7-130). As previously discussed, this allows for additional expansion of the mold during the setting reaction.

INVESTING WITH PHOSPHATE-BONDED INVESTMENTS

The techniques described for investing with gypsum-bonded investments apply as well to porcelain-metal castings. Expansion of the mold cavity can be increased as follows:

1. *Increasing* the number of layers of asbestos or fibrous ceramic lining the casting ring.
2. *Increasing* the special liquid-water ratio.
3. *Decreasing* the total liquid-powder ratio.
4. Placing the investment in contact with water during setting.

5. Burning out the mold at a higher temperature.

The mold cavity may accordingly be decreased in size by the reversal of any or all of these methods. It is not possible to prescribe a single "correct" technique in a text such as this, since many variables are involved in casting. The following method has been shown to produce very suitable castings and is given as a guide.

The metal casting ring is lined with one layer of damp asbestos or fibrous ceramic liner, which covers all of the inner surface of the ring except for ⅛ inch (3 mm) at each end. This serves to lock the investment within the ring and equalize radial and axial expansion.

A phosphate-bonded investment is selected and its liquid diluted according to manufacturer's instructions. The diluted liquid and the powder should be accurately dispensed in a calibrated measure, and the powder should be similarly weighed out according to the manufacturer's liquid-powder ratio (Fig. 7-131). All investments are available in preweighed packages (generally 60 gm). These packages are occasionally improperly filled and/or weighed by the supplier, so the powder should be weighed before mixing it with the liquid.

The mixing apparatus must be clean. Residual, hardened investment in an unclean mixing bowl will greatly accelerate the set of newly mixed investment. Phosphate investment should not be mixed in an apparatus that has been used for gypsum investments (unless the apparatus has been *very* thoroughly cleaned). Residual gypsum will also accelerate the set and will break down at temperatures above 2400° F (1300° C), liberating sulfurous gases that can be detrimental to the casting.

First, the liquid is added to the mixing bowl, then the powder. The investment should be vacuum mixed according to manufacturer's recommendations at slow to moderate (not high) speed, usually for 15 to 45 seconds. Ammonia gas is given off during mixing, and it is important to hold the mixed investment under the vacuum after mixing ceases to dissipate some of this gas and thereby reduce the incidence of bubbles adhering to the wax pattern. (This additional holding time will vary from 15 to 45 seconds, depending on the brand of investment used.) Bubbles in the investment will cast as many little spheres on the coping surface and will have to be ground off later (Fig. 7-132).

The casting ring can be filled while attached to certain types of vacuum apparatus or filled by hand over a vibrator after the investment has been vacuum-mixed. Some technicians prefer to hand-paint investment into complex patterns to assure complete coating of the pattern without entrapment of large air bubbles.

The initial set of phosphate-bonded investments is generally rapid, with the liberation of noticeable heat. If for some reason the pattern is only half covered when set occurs or if there was insufficient investment, the operator has no choice but to quickly prepare more investment and fill the ring. Enough heat is liberated by setting the investment to distort the patterns, and delay in filling the ring will result in a casting that does not fit. This procedure is very risky, and the technician should know the quantity of investment needed and its setting time in advance of the actual investing.

The invested pattern should rest at least 45 minutes before burnout procedures commence. If the invested pattern cannot be burned out within 1 hour or 2, the ring should be stored in a humidor at 100% humidity; it should not be soaked in water, since excessive hydro-

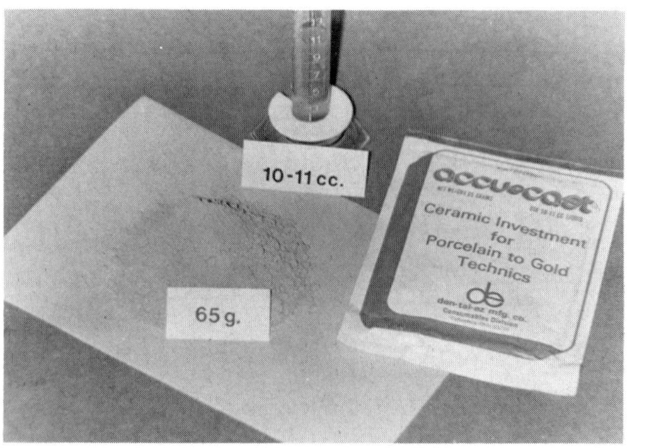

Fig. 7-131. Although investments come in preweighed packages, it is good policy to weigh and measure required amounts of powder and liquid before investing.

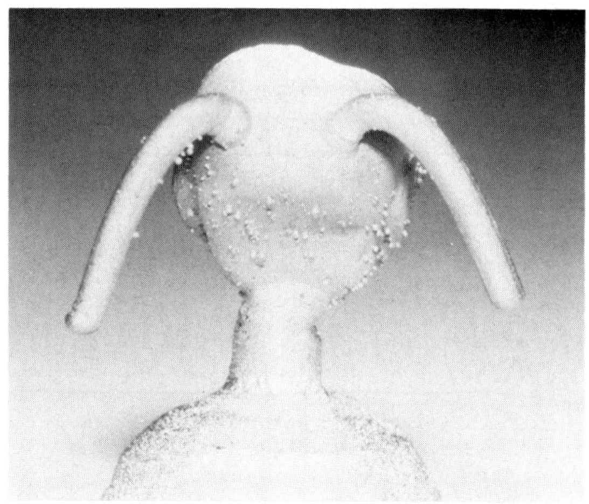

Fig. 7-132. Bubbles cast to copings formed in phosphate-bonded investment molds are result of gas generation during initial mixing. Problem can be minimized by prolonging mixing and holding times of investments, by using mixes with higher liquid/powder ratios, and by proper use of debubblizer liquids on wax patterns.

scopic expansion may result. A slight amount of residual water within the investment will facilitate wax removal by forming steam that flushes molten wax from the internal pores of investment. Loss of water because of crystallization from the investment binder will have the same effect, and soaking a properly stored ring prior to burnout is not necessary. Rapid steam release from a water-saturated ring can fracture the investment (Fig. 7-133), although phosphate-bonded investments have high set strength and are less susceptible to fracture from thermal or mechanical shock than are gypsum-bonded investments.

Carefully grinding (on a model trimmer) or scraping the shiny "skin" off the end of the investment just prior to burnout (Fig. 7-133) is advisable. This removes a relatively impervious layer, opening the pores of the investment and facilitating gas release as the alloy is cast into the mold.

PROBLEM AREAS

Problems associated with spruing and investing the pattern do not usually become apparent until the casting is recovered from the mold and tried on the die.

Problems with the fit of the casting, either too large or small, can usually be traced to failure to follow the investment manufacturer's instructions. Alteration of the water-powder ratio, number and placement of the asbestos liners, and mixing rate can all alter the size of the casting.

Lack of attention to neatness when spruing and investing the pattern can cause such problems as porosity, bubbles, incomplete margins, or rough surfaces.

To prevent problems, it is important to develop and maintain a consistent investment technique.

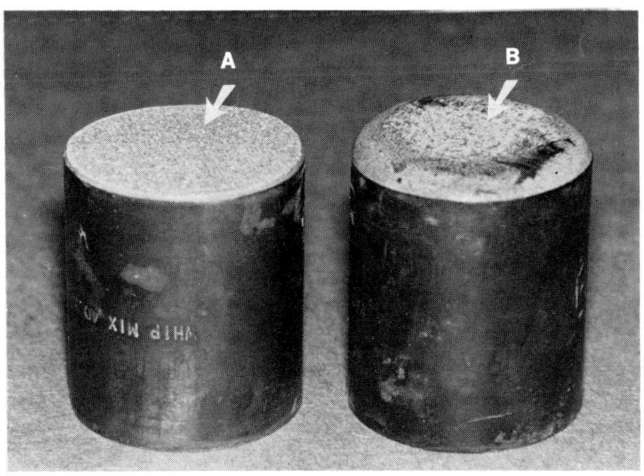

Fig. 7-133. Grinding *(A)* shiny, set "skin" of investment *(B)* at end of ring opens porosity to facilitate gas escape as alloy is cast into mold.

SUMMARY

Successful casting procedures require meticulous attention to detail during the spruing and investing procedures to ensure production of an accurate mold. Proper choice of the type of investment and knowledge of the properties of the investment can aid in controlling the size of the final restoration. Proper sprue size, placement of the liner, position of the pattern in the ring, and cleanliness and neatness of equipment all aid in production of a clean, well-fitting final restoration.

PART FIVE

Casting procedures

MALCOLM D. JENDRESEN and CLIFFORD L. STOCKS

BURNOUT PROCEDURES

Elimination of the wax pattern from the mold of set investment material is referred to as the burnout. The burnout procedure should not be started until the investment has set for at least 30 minutes, preferably 45 to 60 minutes. Ideally the casting ring containing the investment should be placed into the oven approximately 1 hour after investing the wax pattern. If the burnout procedure must be delayed for several hours or overnight, it is advisable to place the invested pattern into a humidor to prevent excessive drying (Fig. 7-

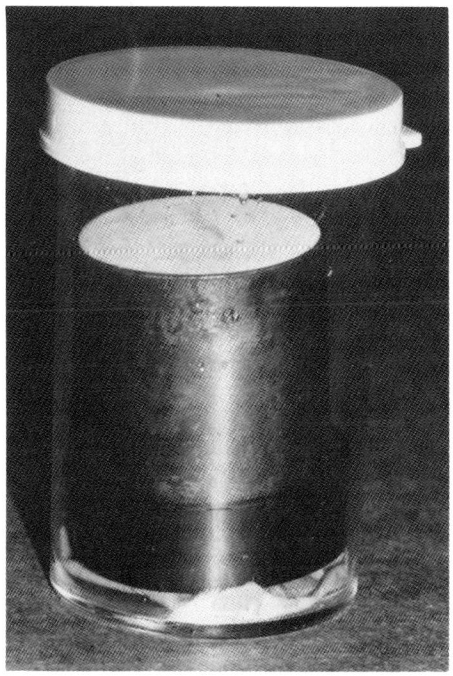

Fig. 7-134. Investment rings should be placed in humidor to prevent drying if it is anticipated that pattern will not be burned out for several hours or overnight. Plastic vials, as seen here, serve well as humidors when damp piece of paper towel is placed on bottom.

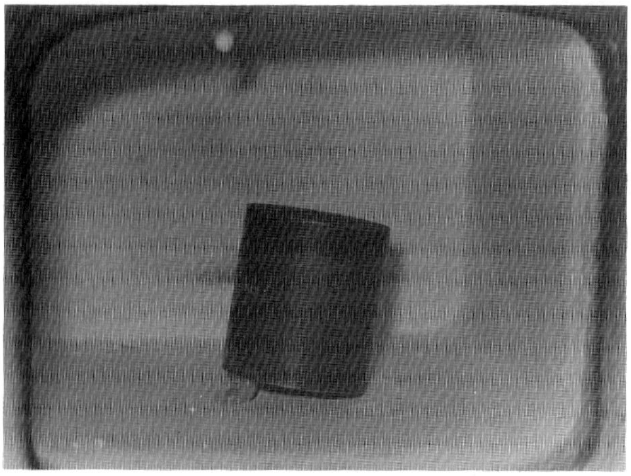

Fig. 7-135. Porcelain tooth placed in bottom of oven provides good support for one edge of ring, allowing molten wax and gases to escape freely.

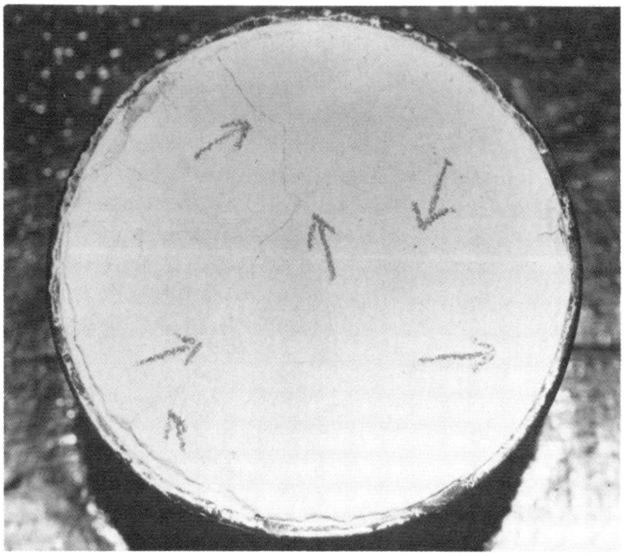

Fig. 7-136. Cracks, caused by expanding steam, occur when damp investment is heated too rapidly. This is major cause of fins on castings

134). If the investment dries out, molten wax produced during burnout will be absorbed into the dry investment, making complete wax elimination from the surface of this mold more difficult.

To facilitate a rapid and clean burnout, the ring may be placed on a raised object within the oven (Fig. 7-135). A burnout started prematurely may cause fine cracks in the gypsum-bonded investment (Fig. 7-136). Cracking of the investment may also occur from too rapid heating. Once the heating is initiated, the casting should be completed without permitting the mold to cool. Although the investment will expand if reheated, a significant loss in strength will occur.

The mold should be placed in an oven preheated to approximately 900° F (480° C), held at that temperature for 20 minutes, and the temperature then raised slowly to 1290° F (700° C) and held for 30 minutes. A cold furnace may be used to start the burnout if the mold temperature is raised slowly and uniformly and the ring held at 1290° F an adequate time to assure a complete wax elimination. Care should be taken to avoid prolonged heating above 1290° F. Dental gypsum-bonded investments will break down at this temperature, and the sulfur and chlorine in some investments may be liberated and contaminate the gold alloy as it enters the mold.

With a quartz investment, the rate of heating should be carefully controlled, since rapid heating will produce a larger casting than will slow heating. For such investments care must also be taken not to initiate heating in a preheated oven on one occasion and then use a cold oven for another casting. The differences in the initial burnout temperatures can produce variation in the size of the castings. Apparently this variable is not important in a cristobalite investment.

The burnout oven should be equipped with an accurate pyrometer to assure that a well-controlled burnout is occurring. Chemical templates that melt at designated temperatures may be obtained from dental alloy manufacturers and should be used to check the accuracy of the oven pyrometer periodically.

Alloys for dental use

PHYSICAL AND CHEMICAL PROPERTIES OF CAST GOLD ALLOYS

The dentist and dental laboratory personnel should be aware of selected physical and chemical properties inherent to the different gold alloys they use. These properties depend on the composition of the gold alloys cast for dental use.

Alloying metals used with gold have specific effects on the cast restoration; also, the amount of each constituent in the final alloy is a major factor in the physical and chemical behavior of that alloy. The American Dental Association Council, through Specification 5, classifies alloys be composition ranges (Table 7-4). Modern dental casting golds, excluding the special gold alloys used with porcelain, contain up to seven different metals. Each metal contributes certain qualities to the final alloy (Table 7-5).

Ideally, the composition is dominated by the gold or noble metal content, such as platinum and palladium. Resistance to tarnish and corrosion in the oral cavity is an important consideration that is determined by the noble metal content.

Other important aspects of alloy composition are its

Table 7-4. Composition of dental casting gold alloy: component percentage range*

Type of alloy	Gold	Silver	Copper	Palladium	Platinum	Zinc
I	80.2 to 95.8	2.4 to 12.0	1.6 to 6.2	0 to 3.6	0 to 1.0	0 to 1.2
II	73.0 to 83.0	6.9 to 14.5	5.8 to 10.5	0 to 5.6	0 to 4.2	0 to 1.4
III	71.0 to 79.8	5.2 to 13.4	7.1 to 12.6	0 to 6.5	0 to 7.5	0 to 2.0
IV	62.4 to 71.9	8.0 to 17.4	8.6 to 15.4	0 to 10.1	0.2 to 8.2	0 to 2.7

*From the American Dental Association Council on Dental Materials, Instruments and Equipment, Chicago, Ill.

effects on melting and handling characteristics in the dental laboratory. Each metal included in an alloy contributes certain qualities to the final alloy.

GOLD. The major contribution of gold in the alloy is to increase the tarnish and corrosion resistance. The gold content should be approximately 75% by weight to be effective against tarnish in the oral cavity. Gold influences the color of the alloy and also its ductility.

PLATINUM. Platinum, like gold, increases the resistance to tarnish and corrosion. Platinum is the best hardener in the alloy, superior to copper. However, even in small amounts platinum raises the melting temperature severely and is therefore rarely used in amounts greater than 3% to 4% of the total composition.

PALLADIUM. Palladium has a profound effect on the color of the alloy. It is used in place of platinum because of cost and its ability to contribute similar physical properties to the alloy.

COPPER. Copper, one of the most important metals in the dental gold alloys, increases the strength and hardness of the alloy. In an alloy of 6% copper and 94% gold, the hardness is more than double that of pure gold. Copper also allows the gold alloy to be successfully heat treated. A hardening heat treatment can be obtained from dental gold alloys when as little as 8% copper is combined with the gold. Copper does reduce the resistance to tarnish and corrosion of the alloys and is therefore used in amounts up to 20%. Excessive amounts of copper will redden the alloy. Copper reduces the melting range of the alloy and when combined with gold increases the ductility of the alloy in the presence of other metals.

SILVER. Silver modifies the color of the alloy. It neutralizes the redness from copper and tends to enrich the gold appearance of the alloy. Silver has little effect on the strength of dental alloys, although it increases somewhat the ductility when used with palladium.

ZINC. Zinc is added to the molten alloys as a scavenger for oxides. Its only beneficial property to the alloy is its ability to reduce oxidation during the casting procedures.

INDIUM. Indium is added in small amounts to reduce grain size and increase the fluidity during the casting procedure. Iridium is also used in the alloys for a similar effect. Both metals have a tendency through smaller grain size to increase ductility. This generally aids in finishing the castings made from such alloys.

Physical and chemical properties of alloys for ceramometal restorations

The metals to which porcelain is fused fall generally into three classes, popularly termed *precious*, *nonprecious*, and *semiprecious* (more recently: high noble, low noble, and base metal). Low-fusing porcelain may be bonded to any of these alloys, but chemically and physically they bear little resemblance to each other.

PRECIOUS (HIGH NOBLE) ALLOYS

Precious alloys are composed of approximately 85% gold, 5% to 8% platinum, 5% to 8% palladium, and 2% to 4% indium and tin, with less than 1% iron. Gold and platinum are chemically noble; that is, they do not oxidize under conditions of porcelain application. Palladium oxidizes minimally, and tin and indium oxidize readily. The tin and indium oxide forms the chemical linkage between porcelain and the underlying metal. Platinum and palladium are used in gold alloys to elevate their melting temperatures and to lower their coefficients of thermal expansion to values compatible with the overlying porcelain. Platinum and palladium also whiten the alloy. Precious alloys have the highest density of all dental casting alloys and consequently a low specific volume. The comparative cost per unit is therefore highest for these alloys.

These alloys have hardness and stiffness values similar to conventional type III inlay gold and can be manipulated by the technician using instrumentation similar to that for the type III. They have, however, less ductility (percent of elongation) than inlay gold alloys, and although margins can be burnished and thinned,

Table 7-5. Role of alloying elements in dental gold alloys*

	Gold (Au)	Platinum (Pt)	Palladium (Pd)	Copper (Cu)	Silver (Ag)	Zinc (Zn)	Indium (In)
Specific gravity	19.32	21.45	12.0	8.96	10.49	7.31	7.31
Melting point (°F)	1945	3224	2829	1981	1761	787 (1663 boiling point)	313 (2642 boiling point)
Atomic diameter	2.88	2.77	2.74	2.55	2.88	2.66	3.24
Space lattice	Face-centered cubic	Face-centered cubic	Face-centered cubic	Face-centered cubic	Face-centered cubic	Close-packed hexagonal	Face-centered tetragonal
Chemical action	Inert	Inert	Mild	Very active	Active	Very active	Active
Color	Yellow	White	White	Red	White	White	White
Approximate content	50% to 95%	0% to 20%	0% to 12%	0% to 17%	0% to 20%	0% to 2%	0% to 0.5%
Density (specific gravity)	Increases markedly	Increases markedly	Lowers slightly	Lowers	Lowers	Lowers	Lowers
Color	Lends yellow color	Whitens slowly; 12% required; not pure white	Whitens rapidly; as little as 5%	Lends red color; dark plate high in copper	Whitens very slowly, counteracts redness of copper; creates green and gold color	Percentages too low to have effect	Very low percentages
Melting	Raises melting range mildly	Raises melting range fairly rapidly	Raises melting range rapidly	Lowers melting range even below its own	Slight effect; may raise or sometimes lower mildly	Lowers melting range rapidly in most solders	Lowers melting range rapidly; can be used in solders
Tarnish resistance	Essential to good tarnish resistance	Contributes importantly to tarnish resistance	Increases tarnish resistance, but less than gold and platinum	Contributes to tarnish in flame, or with sulfurous food	Tarnishes in presence of sulfur	Will tarnish, but in low percentages has little effect	Tarnishes, but less than zinc
Heat hardening	Contributes importantly with copper	Increases with copper	Some increase with copper	Essential if alloy heat hardens	Increases with copper	Slight with copper	Little effect
Gas absorption			Rather high for hydrogen		Rather high for oxygen	Good deoxidizer	Good deoxidizer
Castability	(Effects are not critical)					Decreases surface tension and increases fluidity	Same effect as zinc, slightly milder

*From Brumfield, R.C.: New Rochelle, N.Y., 1955, J.F. Jelenko Co.

precious porcelain-bonding alloys work harden and flake easily.

All precious bonding alloys should be melted with a gas-oxygen torch, because they have melting ranges from 1950° F (1066° C) to over 2500° F (1370° C). At elevated temperatures they have the poorest sag resistance of all the porcelain-bonding alloys, and the framework design of long-span bridges must account for this by appropriate placement of metal bulk in high stress areas.

NONPRECIOUS ALLOYS (BASE METALS)

On the other end of the chemical, physical, and economic spectrum is a class of alloys, composed of base metals, which have become popular within the profession, since the dramatic increase in the price of gold. These alloys are chemically composed primarily of nickel and chromium, with other alloying elements added to refine the physical and chemical properties. Dozens of brands are available to the profession, and the manufacturers or distributors usually provide a listing of physical properties for each particular alloy.

These alloys usually contain no noble metals and are readily oxidized at elevated temperatures. They are also capable of alloying with carbon, which is found in certain investments. Such alloying may alter the physical properties of the alloy or liberate gases during porcelain addition. For these reasons, base metal alloys are often recommended to be cast into carbon-free, phosphate-bonded investments.

The ease of oxide formation has led to much controversy within the profession over the ability of these alloys to actually bond to porcelain. Evidence is cited in some literature showing cleavage of porcelain from the base metal, leaving no attached porcelain. Such poor bonding raises questions of clinical acceptability of base metal restorations. In fact, the porcelain readily bonds to the oxide of base metals, but excessive oxide formation promotes fracture, either through the interfacial oxide layer or at the oxide-metal interface (Fig. 7-137). Because of this high oxidizing ability, the techniques for metal preparation and porcelain addition are considerably different from those used with precious alloys. These will be discussed in some detail later in the chapter.

Physically, nonprecious alloys differ significantly from the precious alloys. No two alloys will exhibit the same properties, but as a class, nonprecious alloys are much stiffer, harder, and more sag resistant at elevated temperatures than are the precious gold-bonding alloys. Their higher yield strengths and hardness require using high-speed handpieces to generate the forces necessary to burnish and finish the metal. Once sufficient stresses are applied, nonprecious alloys exhibit a ductility (or

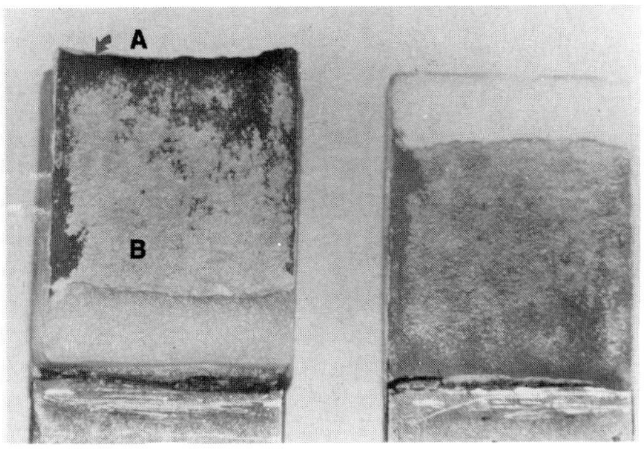

Fig. 7-137. Fracture of porcelain bonded to nickel-chromium test specimen revealing cleavage of porcelain from excessively oxidized metal surface along edge *(A).* Good porcelain bonding is in central area *(B)* where superficial oxide was removed before opaque porcelain was added.

elongation) greater than the precious alloys and therefore can be burnished without tearing under appropriate laboratory conditions. They are very difficult to adjust intraorally. Nonprecious alloys may be useful in situations where long-span, thin frameworks are necessary and/or in situations where economy is a prime consideration. The low density of these alloys (roughly half that of precious alloys), coupled with the low cost of the metal, provides a large volume of metal framework at a comparatively low cost. Typically the dental laboratory can produce at least five times more castings per dollar from nonprecious than from precious alloys.

SEMIPRECIOUS (LOW NOBLE) ALLOYS

Semiprecious alloys encompass a large variety of primarily silver-palladium alloys; some also contain gold. Gold and palladium are relatively noble, but silver is easily oxidized. The melting ranges of these alloys are comparable to precious alloys, and the physical properties are generally intermediate to precious and nonprecious (base metal) alloys. Semiprecious alloys are somewhat more workable than nickel-chrome alloys, but are generally more difficult to finish than gold-platinum-palladium alloys. The generally high chemical reactivity of semiprecious alloys dictates special techniques specific to each alloy so that excessive oxidation does not form on the porcelain bonding surface. The alloys that contain silver, although very suitable when properly manipulated, are occasionally associated with discoloration of porcelain at the porcelain-metal junction when porcelain is baked to copings that have been overheated during casting (Lacy, Hirose, and Jendresen, 1977). Semiprecious alloys are generally selected on the basis of their relative economy and stronger mechanical properties (compared to precious alloys) that make them suitable for long-span bridgework and more delicate metal substructures.

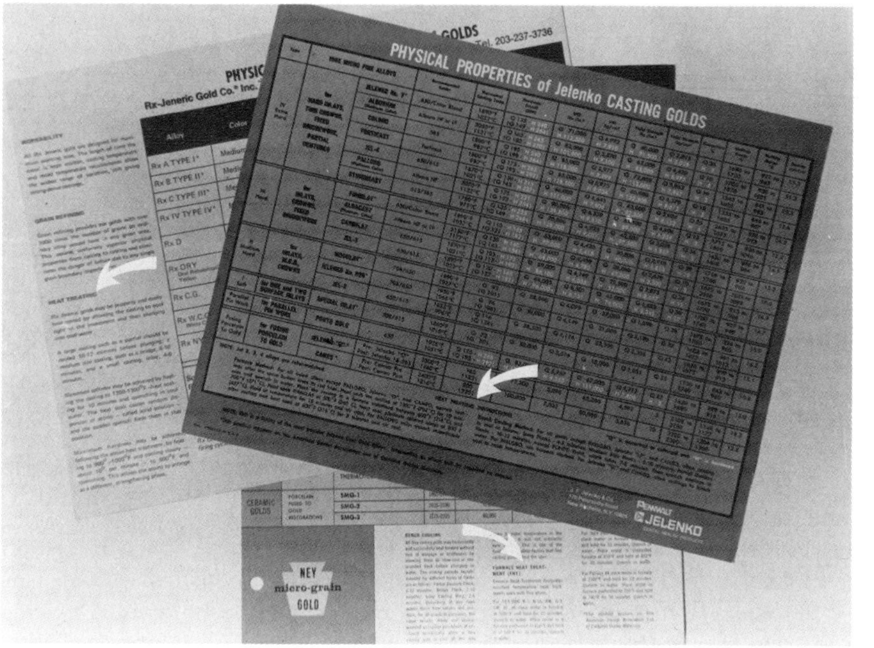

Fig. 7-138. Instructions for proper heat treatment of various alloys can be found on physical property charts supplied by manufacturers. Charts contain valuable information about handling characteristics and treatment of many alloys produced.

All physical properties of the casting alloys are affected by their composition. Certain of these properties are more important to the dentist and laboratory technician than others. The selected physical properties influencing fabrication, handling, and clinical performance of the cast restoration are of primary concern when deciding which alloy to use. These properties are as follows:

1. *Modulus of elasticity* indicates the relative stiffness of the alloy. The higher the modulus, the stiffer the alloy.
2. *Yield strength* is similar to the proportional limit or useful strength of the alloy. The higher the yield strength, the more difficult it will be to permanently deform the casting. Also, when margins of a casting are to be finished or altered with a hand or rotary instrument, an alloy with a low yield strength will be easier to finish or burnish than an alloy of high yield strength.
3. *Percent of elongation* is a measure of ductility. The higher the percent of elongation, the more the metal will yield when pulled or burnished. The combination of yield strength and percent of elongation provides a degree of workability to an alloy. Relative low yield strength and a high percent of elongation allow an alloy to be cold worked quite easily, whereas a high yield strength and low percent of elongation in a cast alloy make it more difficult to finish margins and adjust clasps or attachments.
4. *Hardness* in an alloy indicates its resistance to indentation. As the value for hardness increases, resistance to wear increases.

The values for these properties are readily available in the manufacturers' alloy charts. The major suppliers of dental casting alloys provide physical property charts for their alloys (Fig. 7-138). These charts also include valuable information as to the recommended heat treatment for their alloys.

The classification of dental casting gold alloys is based on their composition and physical properties. The American Dental Association, in Specification 5, divides these alloys into four types:

1. Type I alloys are soft and very ductile; they are normally used in nonstress-bearing restorations.
2. Types II and III alloys are the most widely used. Type II alloys are popular for inlay restorations in which burnishability is preferred to high hardness. Type III alloys are used for inlays, onlays, and crowns in which occlusal stresses are a major clinical consideration.
3. Type IV alloys are extra hard and generally used for removable partial denture frameworks, not for individual tooth restoration.

HEAT TREATMENT

Working with a complex casting in a softened condition may be helpful to the dentist or laboratory techni-

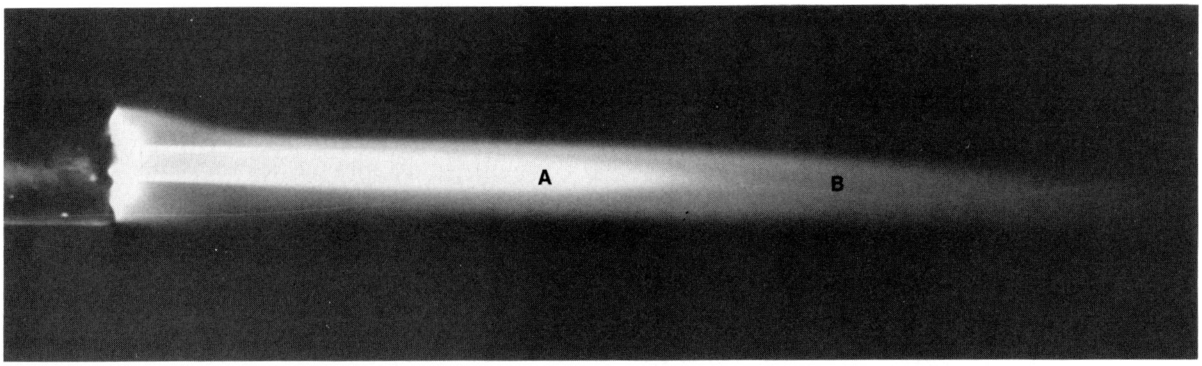

Fig. 7-139. Properly adjusted torch. Reducing zone *(A)* is used to melt gold. Oxidizing zone *(B)* is cooler than reducing zone and will not heat gold to proper casting temperature.

cian while finishing margins. To adequately resist excessive wear, however, the restoration must be returned to a hardened state prior to its clinical use.

The physical properties, specifically the mechanical properties of some gold alloys, may be modified by heat treatment. Gold alloys containing 7% or more copper will respond to heat treatment by changes in microstructure, and consequently in their handling properties. Specific information from manufacturers for the heat treatment of gold alloys and their physical properties is given in Fig. 7-138.

Softening heat treatment consists of heating the alloy to 1290° F (700° C) and maintaining that temperature for approximately 15 minutes, followed by quenching in room-temperature water.

Hardening heat treatment may be conducted in either of two ways: (1) heat soaking at a constant temperature of approximately 840° F (450° C) for 15 minutes or (2) slow cooling from 840° to 480° F (450° to 250° C) over a period of 15 minutes, followed by quenching in water. To provide a homogenization of the metallurgical structure prior to the hardening treatment, all gold alloys should be heat softened before being heat hardened.

CASTING PROCEDURES: LOW-FUSING GOLD ALLOYS

To melt low-fusing gold alloy for the casting procedure, three methods are available: compressed air and gas, oxygen and gas, or an electric casting machine. When a torch is used with compressed air and gas, the valves should be adjusted until the reducing cone is approximately 40 mm. The tip of the reducing cone is used to make a rapid and clean melt. Fig. 7-139 illustrates a properly adjusted torch.

When an oxygen and gas combination is used, a hotter flame is produced. A small multiorifice oxygen-gas tip is ideal for rapid melting of the gold ingots. With this tip caution must be exercised not to overheat the alloy. Single orifice tips may also be used if they are large enough. The small soldering tips should not be used to melt the casting alloy.

Before any torch is lit, each hose must be bled separately by opening and closing each torch valve before opening the cylinder valves. The oxygen cylinder valve must always be opened slowly to prevent sudden high pressure from hitting the regulator and producing high recompression heat. The gas is ignited first and extinguished last.

The use of an electric furnace casting machine eliminates the need for a torch and the judgment required in heating the gold alloy. This method is well controlled, accurate, and precise (Fig. 7-140).

When a torch is used the alloy should be preheated before the mold is removed from the burnout oven. This will reduce the time the investment has to cool before the molten alloy is forced into the mold. If the investment cools prior to the casting, the mold will become smaller through cooling contraction of the investment. This is particularly true of quartz investment materials.

The amount of gold alloy used to produce the cast restoration is an important consideration. Castings produced with large amounts of alloy in the remaining sprue and button will usually produce better detail and definition than will castings made with minimum amounts of metal. The larger amounts of molten alloy, times the force generated by the casting machine, create more pressure on the metal in the mold. When casting a restoration that requires 2 pennyweight (dwt) of alloy, casting with 8 to 10 dwt is advisable. The remaining alloy in the sprue and button can of course be combined with a new alloy for future castings.

When a previously cast alloy is reused, different types should never be mixed. If types II and III alloys are mixed, an entirely different alloy with unknown

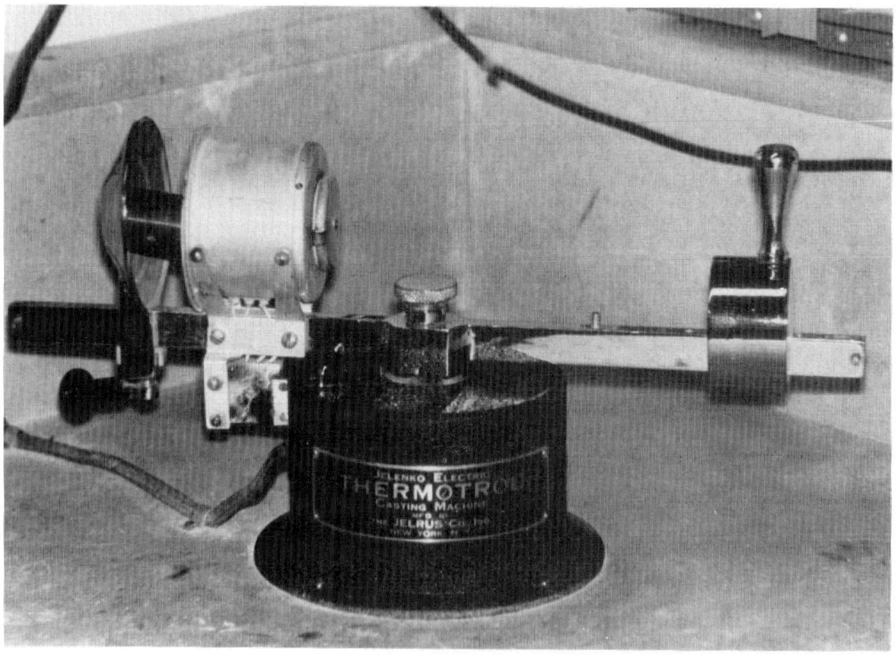

Fig. 7-140. Electric casting machines permit accurate determination for casting temperature of gold alloy and provide clean, reducing atmosphere for melting alloy.

properties will be created. If melted in a reducing flame, molten gold alloy that has reached the proper temperature for casting will appear shiny with a mirror-like surface (Fig. 7-141). When the alloy is melted by the oxidizing portion of the flame, a dull film will appear. The color of the properly melted alloy should be quite light, and the alloy will appear to be spinning.

A reducing flux should be used in melting the alloy. The flux (50% boric acid powder and 50% fused borax) increases the fluidity and reduces the potential for oxidation. If a pressure machine is used, the casting pressure should be between 7 to 9 kg (15 to 20 pounds). With a centrifugal machine, a minimum of four turns is necessary (Fig. 7-142). There is no evidence that too much casting pressure, within reasonable limits, can be used, but insufficient pressure is a common cause of casting failure.

When the alloy has solidified and cooled for approximately 1 minute, the investment may be placed into room-temperature water, and the alloy quenched. This will aid in removing the adhering investment, which can be cleaned from the casting with a laboratory brush, toothbrush (Fig. 7-143), or an air abrasive (Fig. 7-144).

Nonfuming pickling solutions are available to assist in the final removal of investment particles. Dilute acids such as 50% hydrochloric acid or 50% sulfuric acid also may be used to dissolve the gypsum (Fig. 7-145). The casting is submerged into the solution and heated until near boiling, then the porcelain or glass crucible is set aside for 30 seconds. The casting should be its characteristic gold color and is now ready to be rinsed with copious amounts of water prior to further finishing.

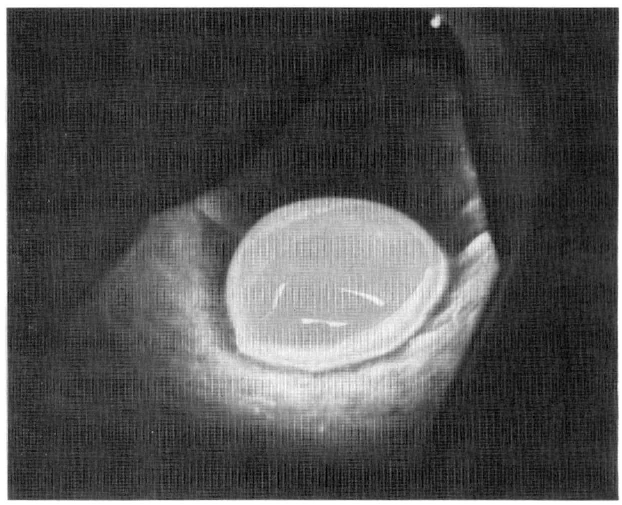

Fig. 7-141. When gold has reached proper temperature for casting, it will be elliptic with well-rounded edges, yellow-orange in color, and will appear to be "spinning."

Pickling solutions that have changed color from pre-

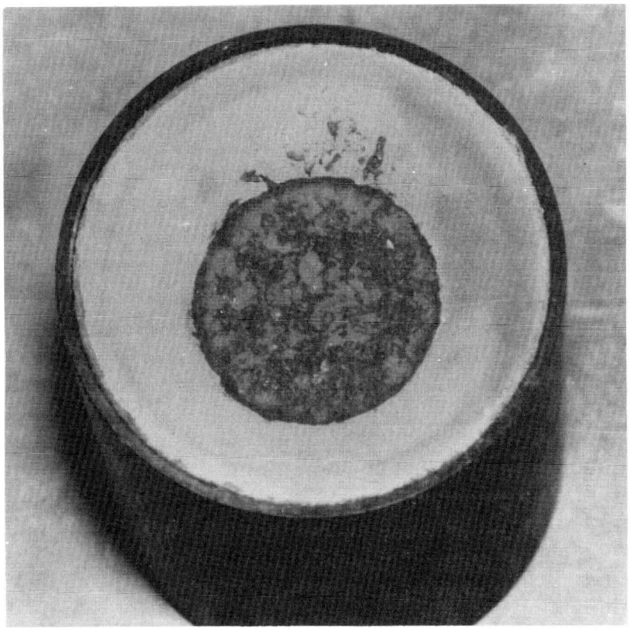

Fig. 7-142. If gold is cast in centrifugal casting machine at proper temperature and force, button will exhibit flat or concave surface with sharp edges. If gold alloy is cast at temperature that is too cold, button will appear rounded with dull edges.

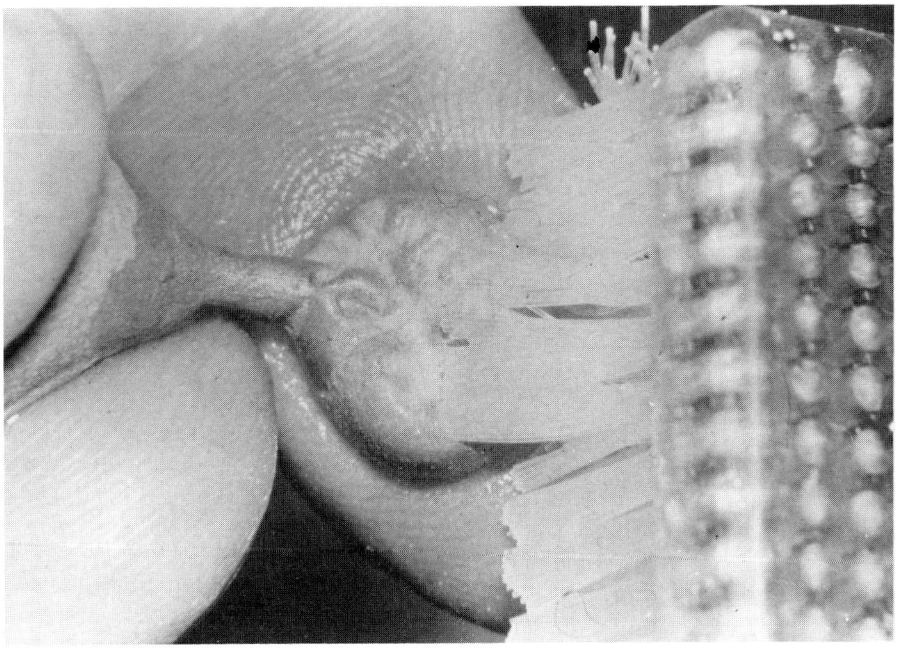

Fig. 7-143. Most of investment can be removed from casting with toothbrush.

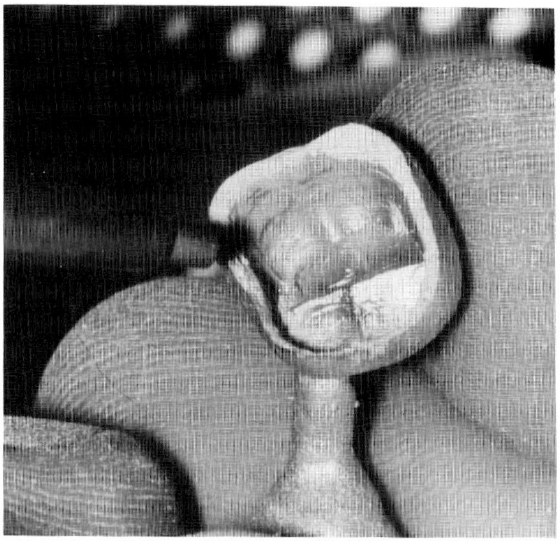

Fig. 7-144. Pencil-type abrasive blasters can be used to remove investment and oxides from casting without appreciable danger of damaging margins.

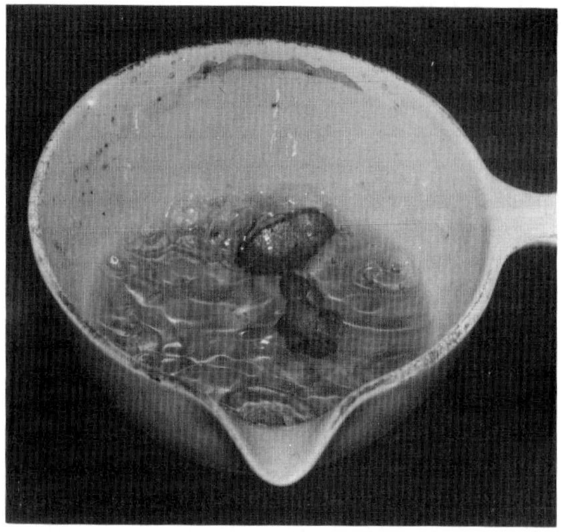

Fig. 7-145. Surface of casting may be coated with layer of oxides and tarnish. This layer normally can be removed by pickling (heating casting in dilute acid solution). Recently introduced commercial pickling solutions can be boiled without danger of noxious fumes being released.

vious use should not be reused. Nor should metal tongs be used with casting and pickling solutions, because it is possible to inadvertently plate the casting with unwanted copper. The casting should never be heated in a flame and then dropped into pickling solution. This may distort the casting, the margins may become rounded, and grain growth may occur, weakening the casting and making the surface difficult to polish.

Proper attention to details and a well-controlled reproducible technique should produce accurate, smooth, troublefree castings (Fig. 7-146).

PROBLEM AREAS

Problems arising during the casting procedure can usually be traced to errors in technique (Table 7-6).

Failure to maintain proper temperature control either during burnout or in the casting torch can cause incomplete castings, holes in castings, rough surfaces, or rounded margins. It is essential to maintain scrupulous neatness and cleanliness of the mold, crucible, and gold. Problems such as pitted castings, incomplete margins, and rough surfaces are caused by debris and dirt in the mold.

As with the investing technique, the best way to prevent problems during casting is to maintain a consistent sequence of procedures.

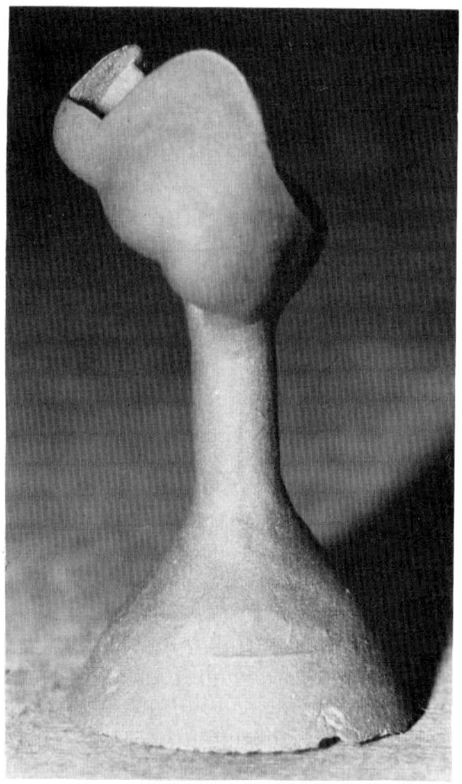

Fig. 7-146. Clean, smooth, dense casting is easily obtained by proper attention to cleanliness and observing basic rules of technique.

Table 7-6. Investing and casting procedures

Problem	Probable cause	Solution
Incomplete castings (Fig. 7-147)	Inadequate spruing	Sprue former too small to allow mold to fill completely before alloy freezes in ingate; use 10-gauge sprue former for average castings
	Alloy not hot enough	Have casting temperature at least 150° F (57° C) above indicated fusion temperature of alloy
	Mold too cold	Oven too cold—check pyrometer; mold should heat soak 1 hour at burnout temperature
	Ingate obstructed	Ensure that debris (loose investment) is not in ingate
	Insufficient casting force	Force alloy into mold rapidly; use centrifugal machine with good springs and several winds; use air pressure and vacuum machines with proper force
	Insufficient gold	Cast enough gold to allow for good button
Rounded margins (Fig. 7-148)	Incomplete burnout of wax pattern	Carbon residues in mold create atmosphere producing shiny rounded margins; smooth surface occurs when mold surface is filled with this carbon residue; heat soak mold for 1 hour at minimum of 950° F (510° C) to ensure elimination of carbon residue
	Insufficient heating of alloy before casting (Fig. 7-149)	Heat alloy to 150° F (57° C) above fusion temperature at moment of casting alloy
	Margins melted while attaching pattern to sprue or former	Keep pattern and sprue former in horizontal position when attaching, so that heat rising from instrument does not soften pattern
	Improper diameter/length of sprue restricts flow of alloy into mold; metal freezes before margins are complete	Average casting should have 10-gauge sprue approximately 6 mm long
Porosity (Fig. 7-150)	Improper sprue former, size, length, or placement	Shrinkage porosity caused by insufficient bulk in sprue former; sprue cooled before casting; diameter of sprue former must be greater than thickest part of pattern and should be attached to thickest part of pattern; use 10-gauge sprue former no longer than 6 mm
Rough surface on casting (Fig. 7-151)	Excess moisture on pattern	Remove all moisture from pattern, sprue former, and ring
	Water-powder ratio too high in mixing investment	Use correct water-powder ratio
	Too much casting pressure, causing investment breakdown from force of alloy	Do not wind machine too tightly
	Prolonged overheating of gypsum-bound investment (Fig. 7-152)	Use correct heating cycle for burnout procedure; do not heat above 1290° F (700° C)
Pits in casting (Fig. 7-153)	Debris in mold	Join ingate, sprue former, and pattern with continuous smooth surface with no jagged areas of investment to be broken off and pushed into mold ahead of alloy
	Dirty wax	Use only clean, new wax for patterns and sprue formers
	Loose debris in crucible	Use clean crucible for each casting
	Mold temperature too hot	Lower burnout temperature since too high temperature causes investment breakdown, producing weak surface easily abraded by alloy
Fins on castings (Fig. 1-154)	Overvibration during investment or disturbing ring during set	Avoid overvibration and place investment ring in area free from disturbances until investment is completely set
	Heating ring too rapidly causes moisture in mold to form steam and rupture out mold	Heat mold slowly (1 hour for 1290° F [700° C] temperature rise)
Bubbles or nodules on casting (Figs. 7-155 and 7-157)	Investment not mixed under enough vacuum to remove entrapped air bubbles	Thoroughly mix investment under vacuum to eliminate air bubbles; apply investment carefully to pattern to allow proper wetting
	Air leak between crucible, sprue former, and casting allowed bubble to form and become trapped under pattern	Obtain good seal between ring and sprue former prior to introducing investment

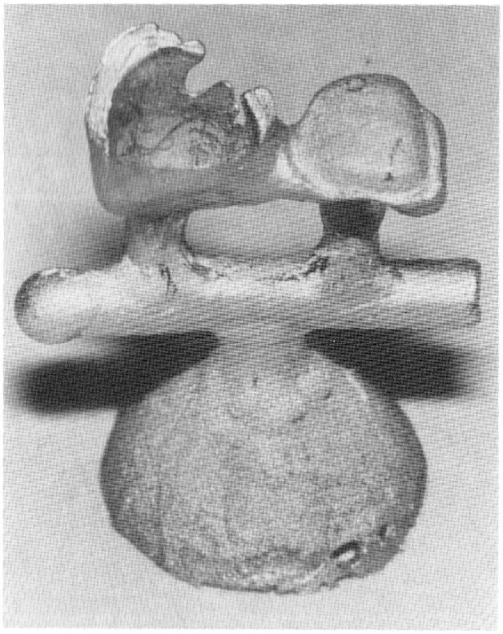

Fig. 7-147. Probable causes of this incorrect casting: gold too cold, mold too cold, insufficient casting force, incomplete wax elimination.

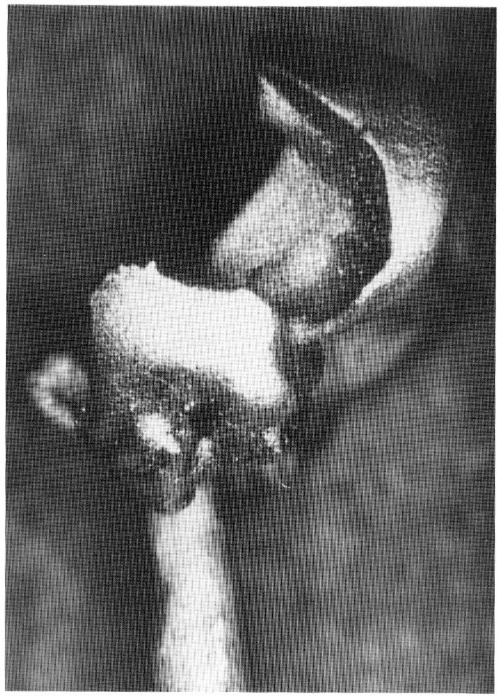

Fig. 7-148. Shiny rounded margins are indications of incomplete wax elimination from casting mold during burnout.

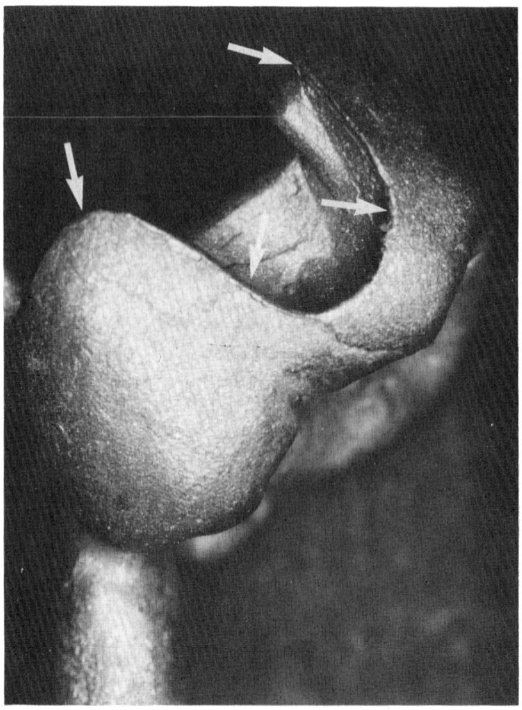

Fig. 7-149. Rounded margins *(arrows)* are due to insufficient heating of alloy at moment of casting or mold temperature too low, causing premature solidification of alloy before reaching extremes of mold.

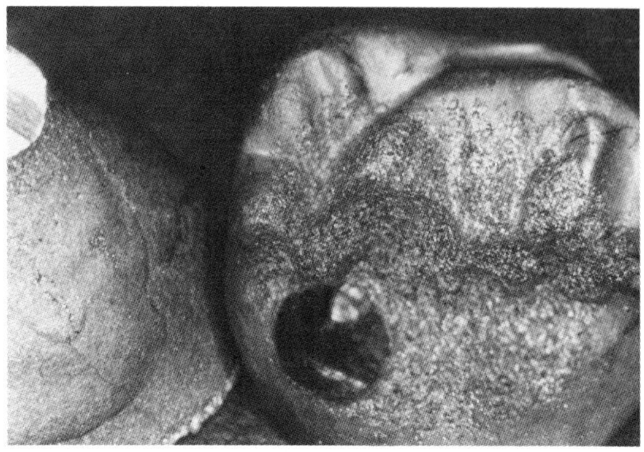

Fig. 7-150. Shrinkage porosity. Improper sprue former size and placement.

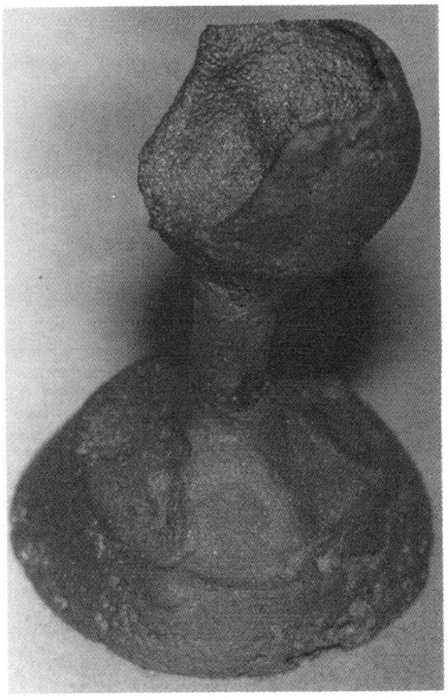

Fig. 7-151. Rough casting can occur from too high water-powder ratio or casting with underheated gold.

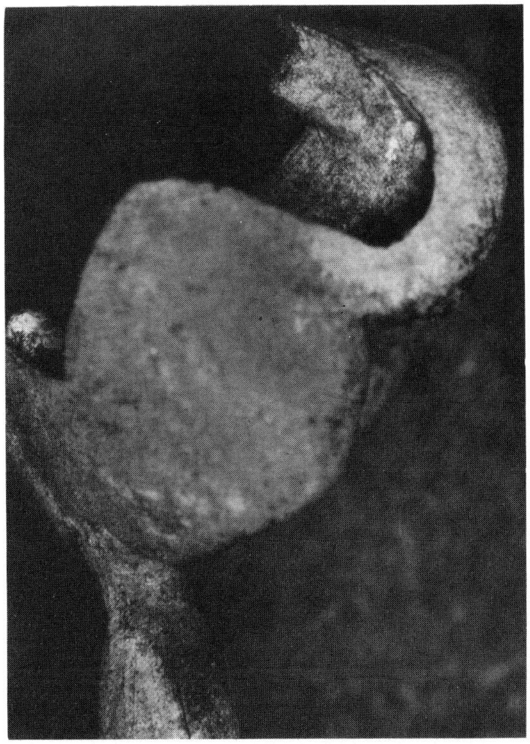

Fig. 7-152. Discolored and rough castings result from prolonged overheating of gypsum-bound instruments. Overheating causes gypsum to break down and release sulfides, which cause surface contamination.

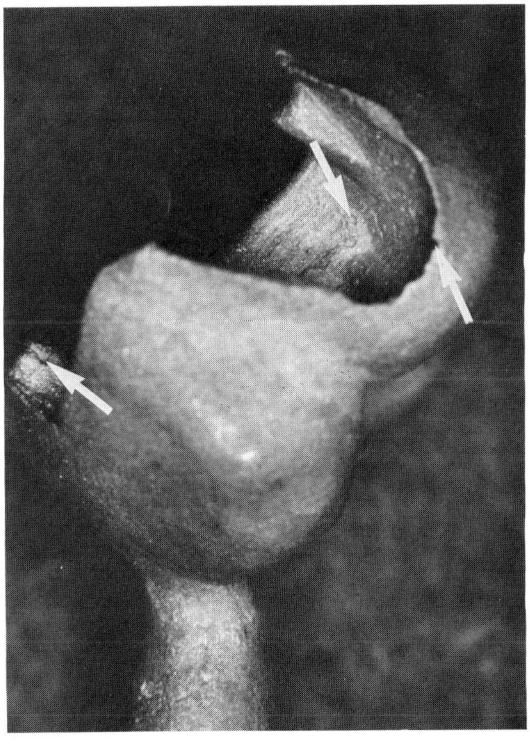

Fig. 7-153. Keep mold free of debris, which, when present in mold, may cause pitted surface and pitted margins *(arrows).* Debris may come from dirty wax, loose gypsum particles in mold or ingot, and dirty crucible.

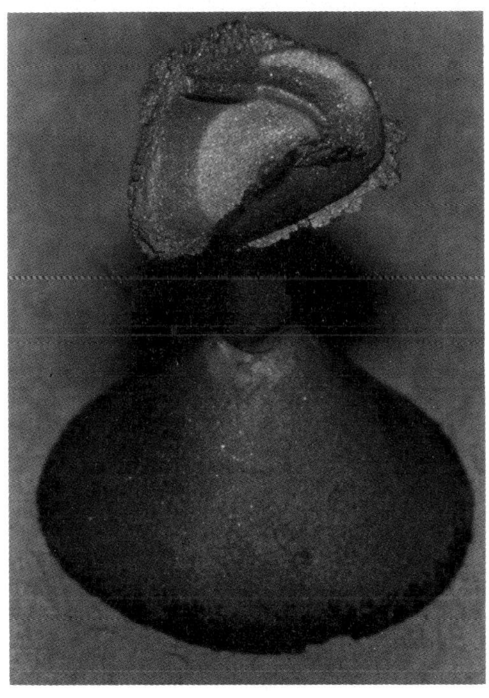

Fig. 7-154. Fins are sometimes caused by excess vibration, water-powder ratio, high pressure during casting, and/or too rapid burnout. Too rapid burnout allows steam to form, causing investment to crack in area of mold.

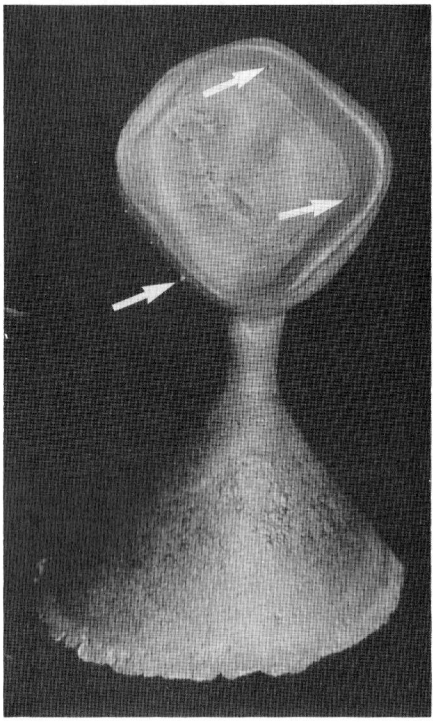

Fig. 7-155. Small bubbles *(arrows)* can occur on surface due to air entrapment. Thoroughly mix investment under vacuum to remove bubbles.

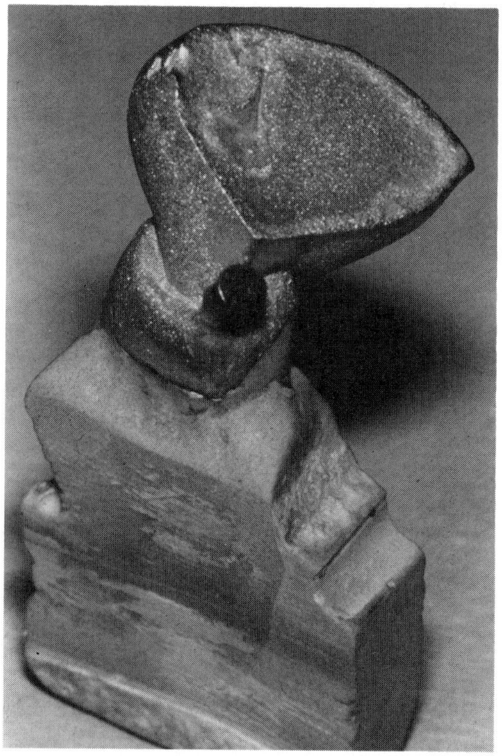

Fig. 7-156. Improper seal between casting ring and crucible former lets air enter investment, travel to undersurface of pattern, and form large bubble.

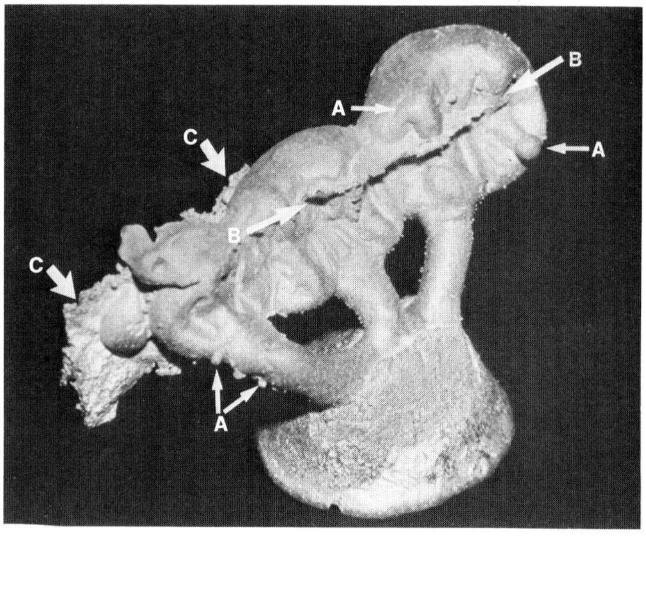

Fig. 7-157. Compound mistakes can lead to compound failures. Investment was not vacuum mixed, resulting in many bubbles *(A)*. Insufficient investment was mixed initially, so second mix was needed to completely fill ring, resulting in line between layers *(B)*. Investment was air dried overnight, then soaked for ½ hour and heated rapidly to 1100° F (594° C), resulting in fins on casting *(C)*.

CASTING HIGH-FUSING METAL-CERAMIC ALLOYS

Casting of porcelain-bonding alloys requires that the metal be heated approximately 200° F (100° C) higher than its upper melting point. This is generally in the range of 2200° to 2500° F (1200° to 1370° C). These temperatures can be achieved with either a gas-oxygen torch or by induction heating.

Induction casting

Induction casting can be used for alloys of any composition and provides for excellent control of the casting temperature. The alloy is rapidly melted in a carbon crucible, heated by electrical induction. The atmosphere is reducing, and at casting the molten alloy temperature is centrifugally cast into the mold. The apparatus for induction casting is expensive and is best adaptable to laboratories that make many castings.

Torch casting

All alloys can be cast with a gas-oxygen or oxyacetylene torch. The operator variables for this technique are more numerous than for induction casting, but generally this is the only practical method available to the small laboratory or individual practitioner. The casting of porcelain-bonding alloys differs from casting low-fusing gold alloys in the following respects:

1. No asbestos is used in the high-heat crucibles, since it may react with the alloy constitutents at high temperatures.
2. The technician should have one high-heat crucible for each brand of alloy being cast in order to avoid cross-contamination.
3. No casting flux is used on porcelain-bonding alloys, since flux may alter its composition and diminish the bond strength. This is particularly true of gold alloys.
4. The visual cues for assessing casting temperatures are different from low-fusing gold alloys, since high-fusing alloys are heated white-hot before they are released into the mold. Base metal alloys, for instance, should not "pool" like gold alloys; rather, at casting temperature the ingots only slump and round over at the corners.
5. Greater casting pressures (i.e., the number of turns of a centrifugal machine) are generally required to force the porcelain-bonding alloy into the mold. This is dictated by (1) the greater degree of chilling found with high-fusing alloys (as compared to inlay gold), (2) the very thin sections often have to be cast in copings, and (3) the lower density of the semiprecious and, particularly, the base metal alloys.

The gas-oxygen flame, generated with a single orifice tip, should form an inner reducing cone about ¾ to 1

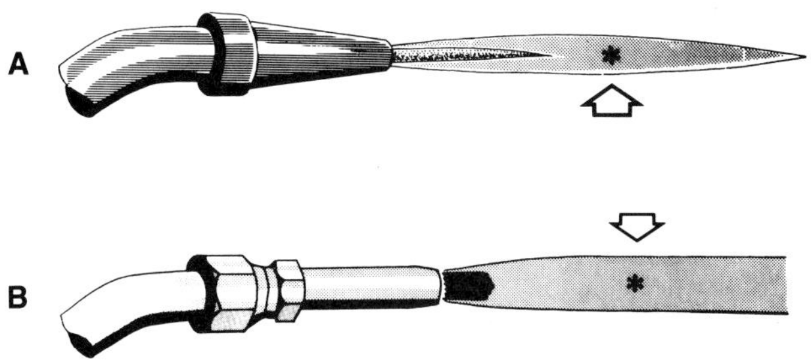

Fig. 7-158. A, Proper single orifice. **B,** Multiorifice flames for casting high-fusing alloys. Alloy should be at positions indicated.

inch (2 to 2.5 cm) long. The multiorifice tip will have inner cones about ½ inch (1.3 cm) long (Fig. 7-158). Oxygen pressure will vary according to manufacturers' specifications, but it is generally 2 pounds per square inch (psi) for single orifice tips and 4 to 10 psi for multiorificed tips. The latter produce a larger flame, which is well suited for melting base metal alloys and larger quantities of gold alloys.

When a multiple-sprue technique is used, the inlets should be aligned for the fastest and most uniform distribution of alloy within the mold. This means placing the inlets vertically in a horizontal casting machine. The mold or the ring should be marked so that aligning the units in the machine is easy. A mark ground into the outside of the ring or small bits of wax placed at the distal end of the ring (which leave indentations in the investment when burned out) are quite useful. As a rule, 8 to 10 dwt (12 to 16 gm) of gold alloy are used for casting a single coping. The average premolar coping alone will consume approximately 1 dwt (1.6 gm) of high-fusing gold alloy. The sprue and button should be sufficient to provide for cooling dynamics that do not lead to shrinkage porosity. For casting bridges, 3 to 4 dwt (5 to 6 gm) of high-fusing gold alloy should be added for each additional unit. A three-unit bridge, sprued with a "gate" technique (Fig. 7-159) should therefore be cast with 14 to 18 dwt (20 to 28 gm) of gold alloy to assure a dense casting. Base metal alloys, having twice the specific volume of gold alloys, will require about half this amount of alloy. For large masses of alloys, the casting force (i.e., number of turns of a centrifugal machine) may be reduced by 1 or 2, since the force pushing the metal into the mold is proportional to both the mass of alloy and the number of turns (acceleration) of the machine. Excessive casting pressure can blow the alloy through the distal end of the ring, thereby ruining the casting.

High-fusing gold alloys (both precious and semiprecious) are generally supplied as flat tabs and will melt into a pool that is cast when it has reached a white-hot, almost vaporous state (Fig. 7-160). Nonprecious nickel-

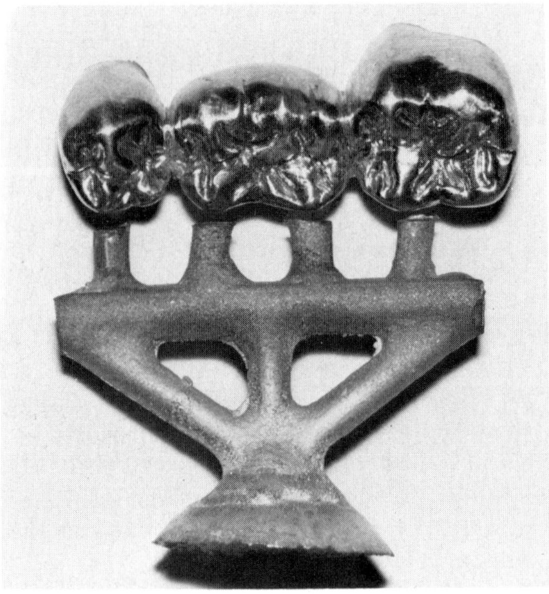

Fig. 7-159. This casting arrangement will require approximately 16 to 20 dwt (25 to 30 g) of gold alloy or 8 to 10 dwt (12 to 15 g) of nickel chromium alloy.

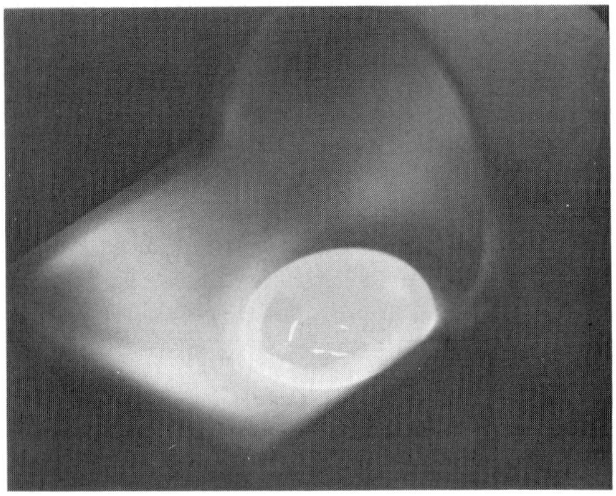

Fig. 7-160. When gold alloy is ready to cast it will be white hot, forming smooth oxide-free elliptical pool.

A B C D

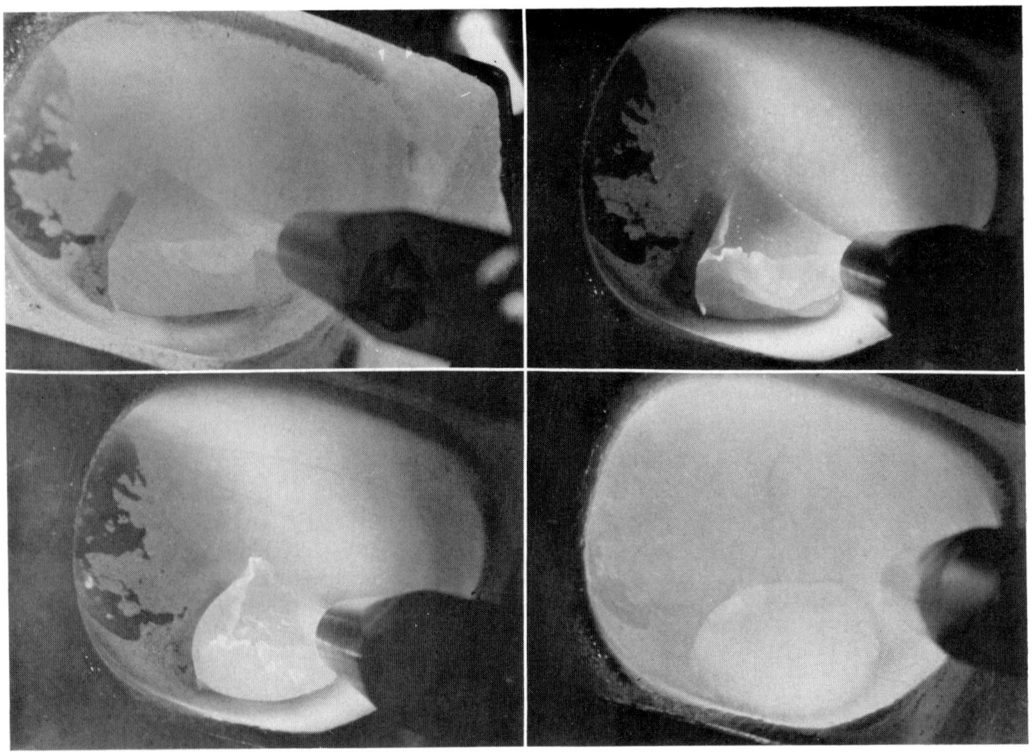

Fig. 7-161. A, Base metal ingot—beginning of melt with gas-oxygen flame. **B,** Ingot continues to melt. **C,** Base metal ingot ready to cast. Corners and sharp edges have rounded. **D,** Base metal ingot overheated. Heating to this point produces changes in composition and excessive oxidation.

chromium alloys are generally supplied as sharp-cornered ingots of various shapes and are heated until the corners round over (Fig. 7-161). They are cast at this point and should not be allowed to "pool," which would overheat this alloy. Nickel-chromium alloys are highly oxidizable and form an oxide skin, which tends to encapsulate the molten metal. There is little change in external shape. When cast, the molten metal breaks through the skin and quickly fills the mold, with oxide trailing it.

All alloys should be melted as quickly as possible to avoid excessive oxidation, which can interfere with both the porcelain-metal bond and the color of the overlying porcelain. This is particularly meaningful for semiprecious alloys, since overheating the alloy often leads to peripheral yellowing of the porcelain-metal junction, particularly when using custom trays made from refractory investment materials. High-fusing gold alloys are least sensitive to overheating or prolonged heating.

After casting, the machine should be allowed to spin freely until it has nearly stopped. It may then be braked still, and the ring removed and promptly quenched in water. Phosphate-bonded investments do not burst apart when quenched, as gypsum investments do, and they will remain warmer longer. The investment is initially removed by carving and breaking it off the casting, taking care not to damage the casting (Fig. 7-162).

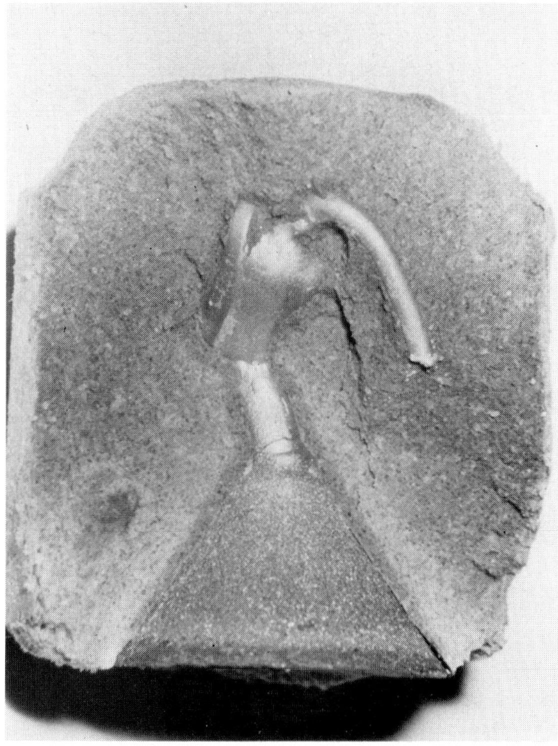

Fig. 7-162. Phosphate-bonded investments must be carefully broken away from casting. Attention to proper investing and casting procedures will allow for clean separation of casting from investment.

CLEANING THE CASTING

The first step is to thoroughly clean the surfaces of all residual investment. Abrasive blasting is effective for this, although the thin marginal regions must not be heavily blasted (Fig. 7-163). The blasting medium can become embedded in the surface and be a source of contamination if the abrasive is not thoroughly removed. Alloy manufacturers recommend a variety of techniques to prepare the metal for the addition of porcelain, and some of these techniques are very specific for the alloy of interest. All investment should be removed before further surface refinement. Traces of investment can easily be ground into the metal surface and act as sources of gas at the porcelain-metal interface when porcelain is added.

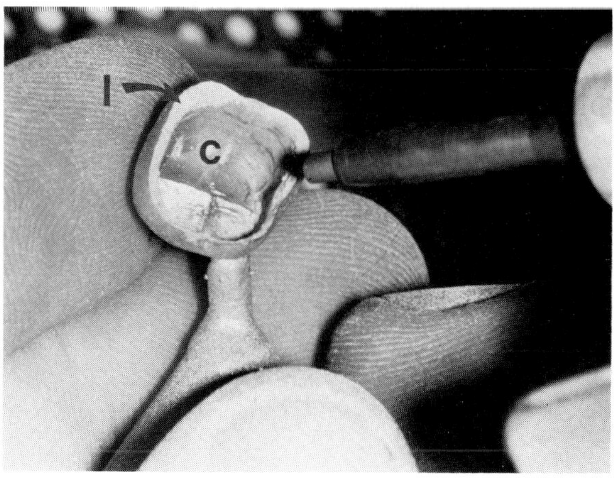

Fig. 7-163. Residual investment *(I)* is easily removed from casting *(C)* by use of Al_20_3 or glass bead powders in pencil-tip air-abrasive units. Margins are easily protected by using this type apparatus.

Precious (gold-platinum-palladium) gold alloys can be soaked in hydrofluoric acid or substitutes to help remove investment. Semiprecious alloys (gold-silver-palladium or silver-palladium) should only be acid treated according to the manufacturer's suggestions; nonprecious nickel-chromium alloys must never be placed in acid because of their high reactivity.

The part of the casting *not* to be veneered with porcelain should be finished first (Fig. 7-164), and can be polished to a smooth finish by conventional techniques;

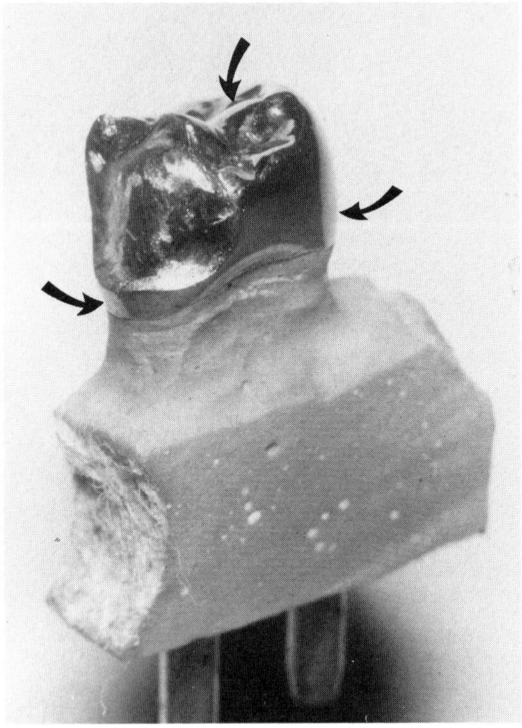

Fig. 7-164. Areas of coping that are not to be veneered with porcelain should be finished to smooth surface *(arrows)* before any other metal finishing is done.

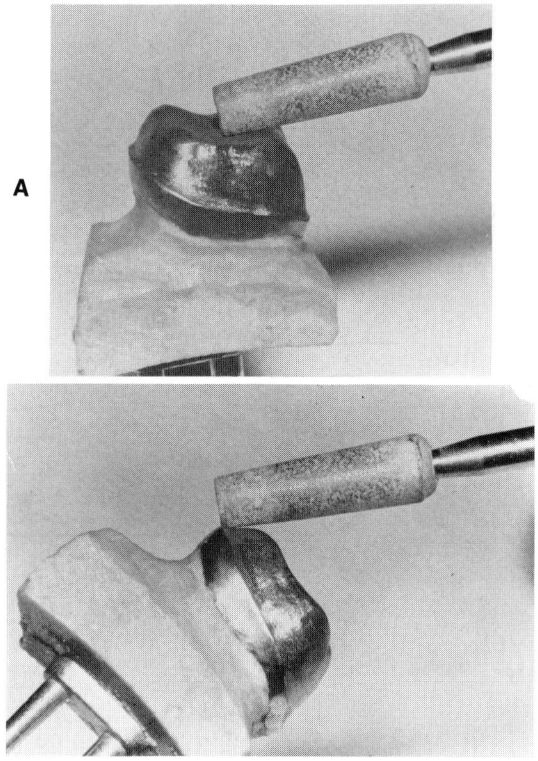

Fig. 7-165. Ceramic-bound white stones are useful for removing superficial bubbles **(A)** and for defining butt-joint porcelain-metal finish lines **(B)**.

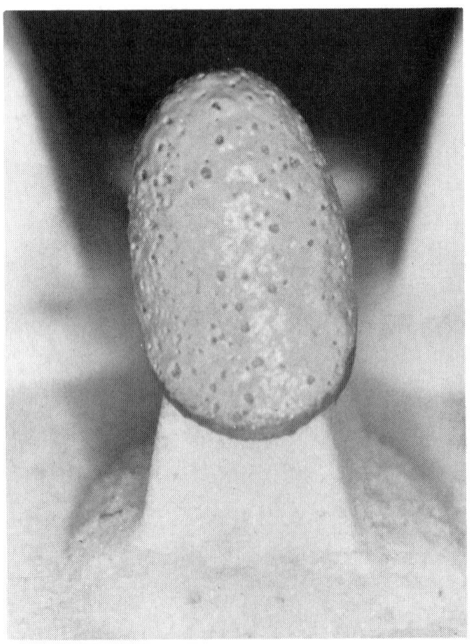

Fig. 7-166. Contamination of metal surface by finishing with resin-bound abrasives can lead to severe bubbling in porcelain. This layer must be removed with hydrofluoric acid and metal refinished with noncontaminating, ceramic-bound abrasives.

but grease-based agents (rouge sticks, tripoli, etc.) must not contact the surface to which porcelain is added because the organic residue could easily lead to gas bubbles, porcelain detachment, and discoloration as it is baked. Greasy films are generally removed by cleansing the casting with household ammonia, followed by *thorough* rinsing with distilled water.

Small nodules and residual oxidation on the porcelain-bearing surface can be removed by rotary carbide burs and ceramic-bound stones. These instruments can also be used to thin the coping, if necessary, and to define porcelain-metal finish lines. For best cosmetic results, the porcelain should meet the metal surface at butt joints wherever possible (Fig. 7-165). Resin-bound abrasives (e.g., some carborundum or paper disks) can contaminate the metal surface with resin, leading to severe bubbling when porcelain is added (Fig. 7-166).

Once the porcelain-bearing surface is clean, it may optionally be sandblasted with a clean 25 to 50 μm aluminum oxide abrasive to texturize it. This will increase the area of bonding and improve the wettability of the metal (Fig. 7-167). Surface roughness is not necessary to achieve a satisfactory porcelain-to-metal bond, since the main mode of attachment is chemical, not mechan-

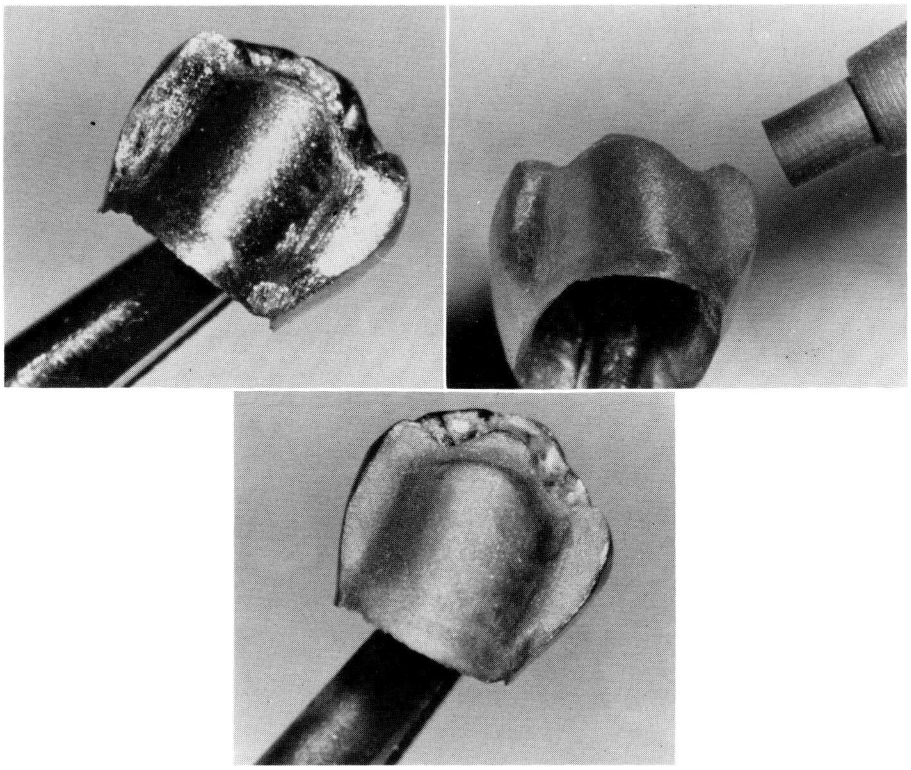

Fig. 7-167. Aluminum oxide air-abrasion of metal surface after finishing with ceramic-bound stones will produce uniform texture and improve wettability by opaque porcelain.

ical. Some operators prepare the metal surface with rubber wheels, although this increases the risk of embedding abrasive and gas-forming organic particles in the coping surface. The casting can now be cleaned in distilled water in an ultrasonic cleaner.

When the metal surface is absolutely clean—free of oxides, investment, and organic films—it is ready for the next stage of metal conditioning.

DEGASSING CERAMOMETAL CASTINGS

After the coping or framework is cleaned, it should be subjected to a degassing or surface-conditioning treatment. During degassing the unit is heat treated to remove contaminants from the surface or possibly to remove entrapped gas from the alloy. In addition, a thin oxide film is formed on the surface. This film is essential to porcelain bonding.

Precious gold alloys should be supported on a refractory sagger tray and rapidly heated in air to 1950° F (1065° C), held there 5 to 10 minutes, and rapidly cooled to room temperature. The unit will have darkened due to surface oxidation. Some recently introduced gold alloys melt near 1950° F. For each of these, the manufacturer will recommend a lower degassing temperature.

Semiprecious and base metal alloys are generally heated to 1950° F, and held at this temperature in a 25- to 28- inch (64- to 70- cm) mercury vacuum for 5 to 10 minutes. At this temperature the vacuum can be broken and the unit then cooled quickly. This procedure will produce a thin but sufficient oxide coating on the metal surface. A second aluminum oxide (Al_2O_3) abrasive blasting of the surface is recommended for base metal alloys to remove excessive oxidation.

SUMMARY

Production of an accurate casting requires development of a precise casting procedure that produces consistent results. Many variables are encountered in the burnout and casting steps: the amount and type of metal chosen, oven temperature, time in the oven, temperature of alloy at the time of casting, and casting pressure. Failure to control one or more of these variables can result in defects in the casting, ranging from porosity to pitting, incomplete margins, or no casting at all. Adherence to the casting procedures described will aid in the production of clean, well-fitting castings.

PART SIX

Dental soldering procedures

ROBERT A. MELI

soldering The joining of metals by fusion of a filler metal. The bond is created by wetting the parent metals with the solder, not by melting or diffusing the parent metals.

solder A metal filler alloy that, when melted, flows into intimate contact with (wets) the metal surfaces to be joined.

soldering flux A material (typically borax and silica compounds) that increases the flow and wetting properties of solder by controlling the oxidation of parent and filler metals during soldering procedures.

soldering investment A compound of gypsum, cristobalite, and other materials that can be formed into a matrix for positioning parts of a prosthesis accurately during soldering.

It is common practice to assemble prostheses by soldering them. After cleaning the portions to be joined, the dentist aligns them properly and joins them by melting solder between them in the presence of the fluxing agent. Solder forms the connection by adhesion (primary metallic bonding). Although some atomic diffusion of the parent metal into the solder also can occur, it is neither necessary nor desirable. The quality of the resultant connector reflects not only the compatibility of the parent metals, solder, and flux, but also the specific technical procedures used.

PHYSICAL REQUIREMENTS FOR SOLDER MATERIALS

Phillips (1973) gives the following desirable characteristics for a dental solder: (1) resistance to tarnish and corrosion in dental fluids, (2) a fusion temperature 90° to 180° F (320° to 640° C) below that of the parts to be joined, (3) "free flowing" when melted, (4) resistance to pitting, (5) at least as strong as parts being joined, and (6) color compatible with the parts to be joined. To satisfy these requirements, the manufacturers compound solders for each alloy that they produce; for example, SMG-2 solder is recommended by the J. M. Ney Company for presoldering prostheses fabricated from their SMG-2 alloy. Use of the recommended alloys and solders in conjunction with precise laboratory techniques will produce solder connections of consistently high quality.

Soldering fluxes

Oxidation of metal surfaces during the soldering procedure can prevent both the flow and wetting of solder. Soldering flux controls this oxidation by flowing over surfaces to be joined, displacing atmospheric oxygen from contact with the metal, and forming soluble compounds with the oxides already formed. Fluid solder can displace the molten flux and wet the uncontaminated metal surface beneath.

Manufacturers also formulate fluxes that are compatible with their alloys and solders. As in the previous example, soldering SMG-2 alloy requires a flux such as Flux H* for the desired results.

Soldering investments

Positioning the parts accurately during the soldering procedure is of paramount importance. Sizable dimensional changes occur when heating the parts to be joined, connecting them with fluid metal, and cooling them to room temperature. The investment must allow completion of the solder connection as planned with respect to size and contour and with the least possible dimensional change. To satisfy these requirements a soldering investment should have the following characteristics: (1) dimensional changes with temperatures compatible with those of the parts to be joined, (2) sufficient strength to maintain its integrity throughout the heating and cooling cycles without fracture, (3) noncontamination of surfaces being joined, that is, constituents compounded to facilitate solder flow by producing a reducing environment, and (4) ready removal from the prosthesis once assembled.

Fundamental considerations

Soldering procedures in their various applications to dentistry are remarkably similar to those used elsewhere. The procedures are as follows: (1) position accurately the uncontaminated parts to be joined; (2) determine the solder joint gap and configuration; (3) place the flux and solder *within* the joint space, if possible; (4) heat the parent metal and solder until the solder flows, filling the joint space; (5) remove the heat as soon as possible; and (6) inspect the connection and correct it as necessary. The source of heat is a torch or an oven, but the selection of fluxes and solders depends on the alloys being joined and their intended application.

Solder joint configuration

The size and shape of the completed solder connector must satisfy the requirements of the prosthesis for strength, cosmetics, and hygiene. In general, the larger the buccolingual and occlusogingival dimensions are, the stronger the joint will be. The occlusogingival dimension is particularly significant (Fig. 7-168).

The realities of the oral environment limit freedom in design of the solder joints because it is essential to: (1) size the tooth/connector compatibly with adjacent and opposing teeth, (2) control the metal display in anterior regions, and (3) provide access for hygienic procedures. In response to these demands, modification of rectangular configurations, which afford maximum strength, is necessary (Fig. 7-169).

*Vita Zahnfabrik Sackingen, Germany.

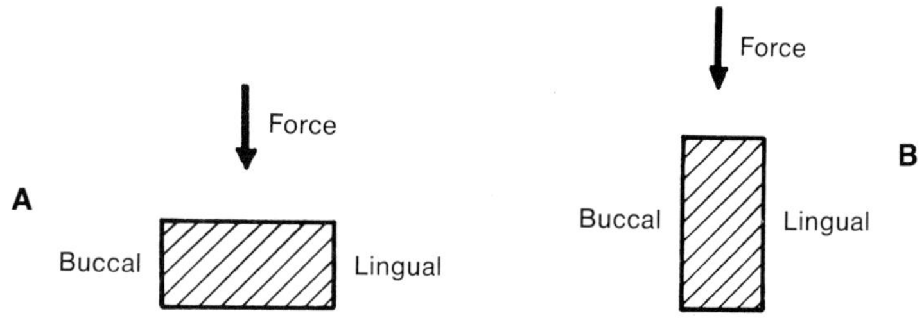

Fig. 7-168. For joint configuration shown, **B** is stronger than **A,** all other factors being equal.

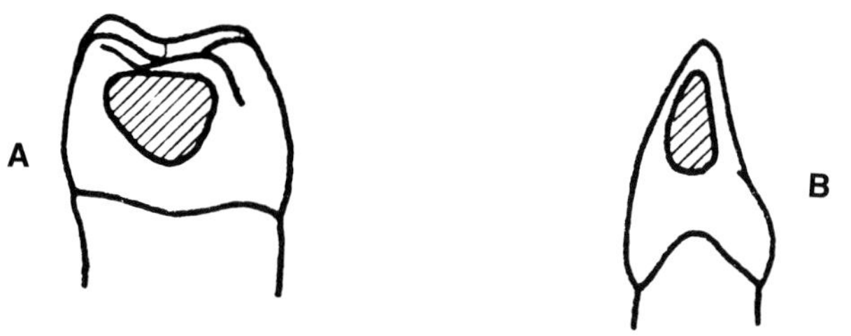

Fig. 7-169. Representative solder joint configurations *(shaded areas).* **A,** In posterior regions, rounded triangular shape provides adequate strength with gingival access for hygienic purposes. **B,** In anterior region, limited labiolingual dimensions of these teeth and their cosmetic prominence make oval shape necessary, but strength is minimal.

Solder joint gap

If solder is to flow between adjacent metal surfaces, a specific amount of space, or gap, is necessary; however, opinions as to its dimensions vary. Phillips (1973), for example, recommends a 0.1 mm separation between units to be joined. Stade, Reisbick, and Preston (1975), on the other hand, recommend a gap of at least 0.31 mm, though less than 0.76 mm. I recommend that the joint gap be sufficient for placing the solder *within* the joint prior to melting. Since the strip solder commonly available is approximately 0.3 mm thick, the joint gap should approximate that dimension as well. However, if the amount of space is not available, it is possible to narrow the solder by grinding or to add the solder to the joint after heating the parent metal parts.

The actual dimension of the joint gap is relatively unimportant; it need only allow for complete wetting of the planned joint area. If the dimension is inadequate, the joint will be pitted, whereas if it is excessive, it will exhibit voids and incomplete adhesion.

TORCH (FLAME) SOLDERING

An oxygen-gas or an air-gas torch is the preferred means of applying heat for dental soldering procedures because (1) access and visibility are maximal throughout the procedure; (2) the laboratory technician can apply heat differentially to the work, that is, to some areas more than others; (3) oxidation and reduction reactions can be controlled directly; (4) heat can be removed immediately after solder flow; and (5) the addition of solder to the partially completed joint can be made readily.

Torch soldering has the following disadvantages that also merit consideration: (1) the uneven distribution of heat created during soldering can warp or damage portions of the prosthesis; (2) the overall control of temperature is imprecise; that is, the laboratory technician must assess the procedure without the benefit of a thermocouple or temperature gauge; and (3) a pressurized supply of the necessary gases must be available. As explained later in the chapter, it is possible to overcome readily these potential shortcomings in soldering regular (type III) gold alloys. However, when postsoldering a porcelain-bonded-to-gold prosthesis, the rigid temperature control requirements of the porcelain make it essential to heat it only in the closely controlled environment of an oven.

Soldering type III gold alloys

PROCEDURE

1. Determine the necessary joint size and configuration while waxing the prosthesis on the working model (Fig. 7-170).
2. Separate the units of the prosthesis, invest the wax patterns, and cast. Check the fit of castings on dies.
3. Transfer the castings to the working model (Fig. 7-171). Adjust the joint interfaces as needed to create a joint space of approximately 0.3 mm into which the solder will fit (Fig. 7-172). Finish surfaces that will receive solder with a rubber wheel or suitable fine abrasive disk.
4. Confirm the marginal fit and proximal relationships of castings intraorally. Form a wax tray to cover the occlusal and lingual surfaces of the prosthesis (Fig. 7-173).
5. Fill the tray with impression plaster,* and place it over the occlusal and lingual surfaces of the prosthesis (Fig. 7-174). Once the plaster has reached the initial set (3 to 5 minutes), remove the template, and check it for accuracy. The castings should seat positively within the template in the same orientation as in the mouth.

*Snow White Impression Plaster No. 2, Kerr Manufacturing Co., Romulus, Mich., or equivalent.

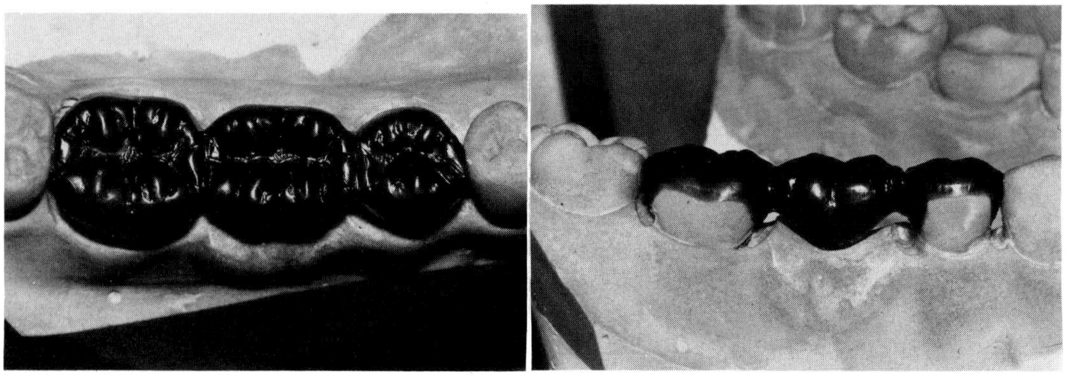

Fig. 7-170. Prosthesis is waxed to desired configuration. Joint areas are oversized to allow for finishing and polishing.

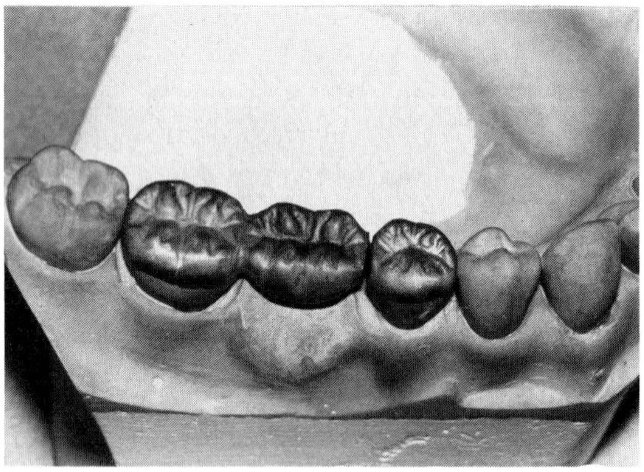

Fig. 7-171. Castings should seat on working model in same relationship as wax patterns.

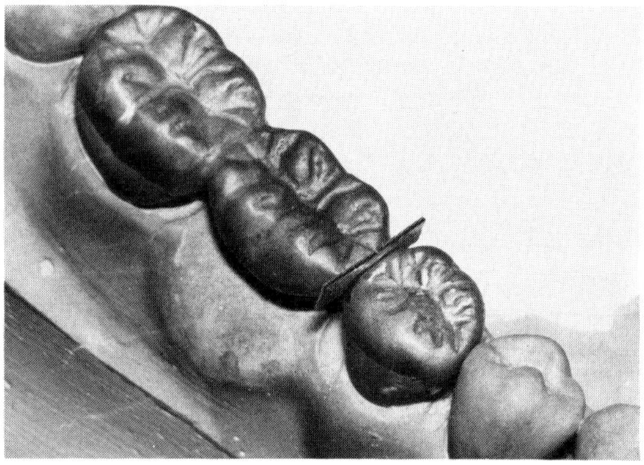

Fig. 7-172. Solder strip can be tapered to fit within joint gap. Excess solder is permissible at facial and lingual surfaces, but not occusal surface.

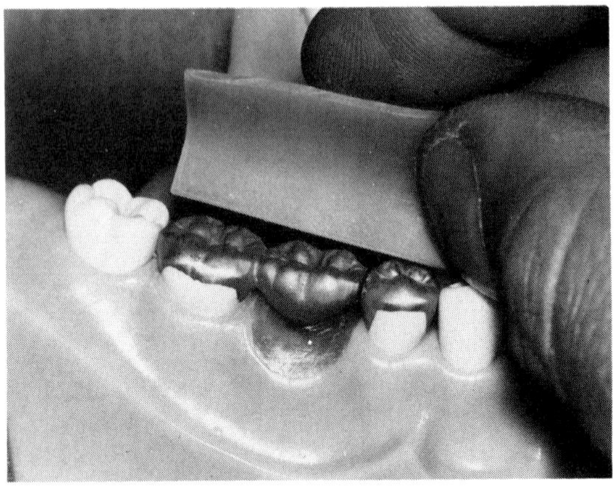

Fig. 7-173. Wax tray is cut slightly longer mesiodistally than prosthesis. Soft baseplate wax can be used.

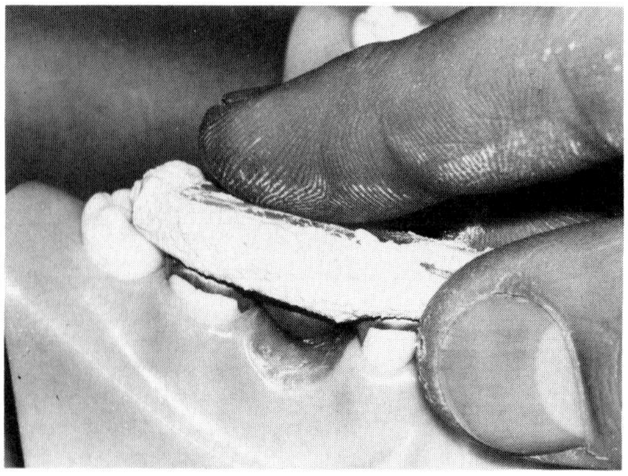

Fig. 7-174. Plaster-filled tray is protected from displacement by tongue during setting.

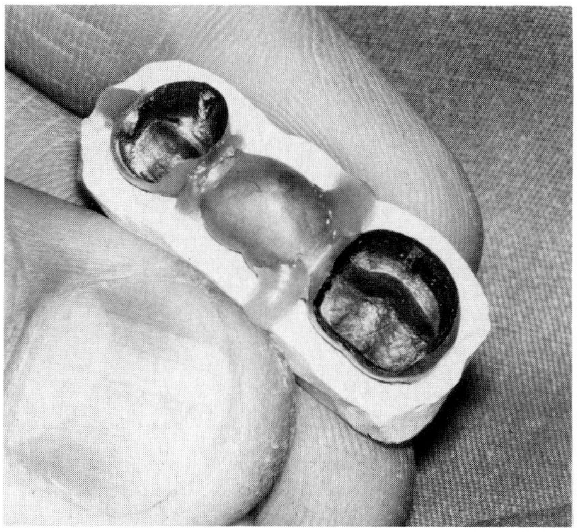

Fig. 7-175. Joint area is filled with white inlay wax to preserve adequate space for solder flow once prosthesis is invested.

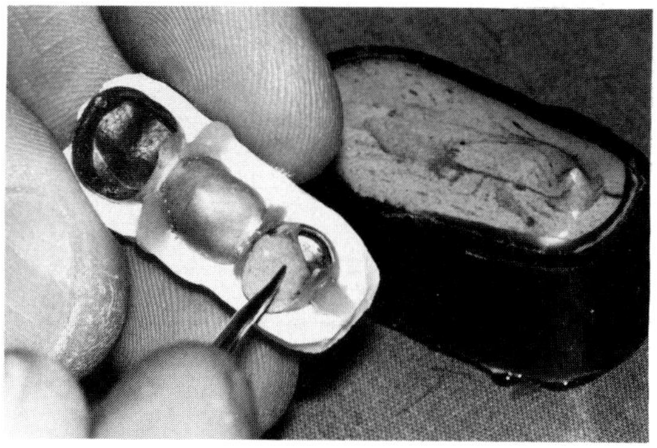

Fig. 7-176. Investment is flowed into castings, using wax spatula. Suitable mound of investment is created by placing it within form made of boxing wax.

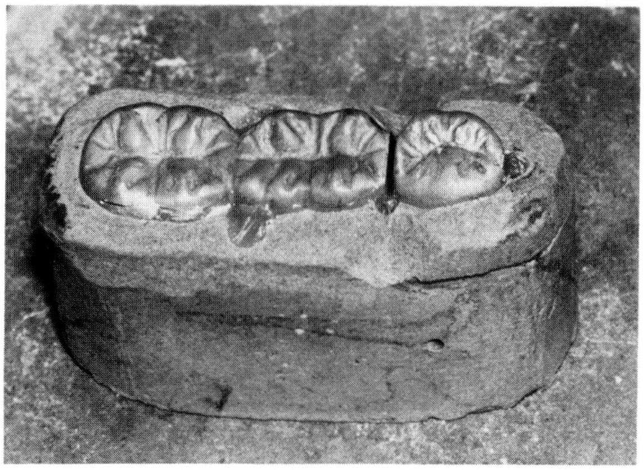

Fig. 7-177. Soldering model has been placed on soldering stand (block). Note V-shaped notches in investment at facial and lingual surfaces to facilitate flame access.

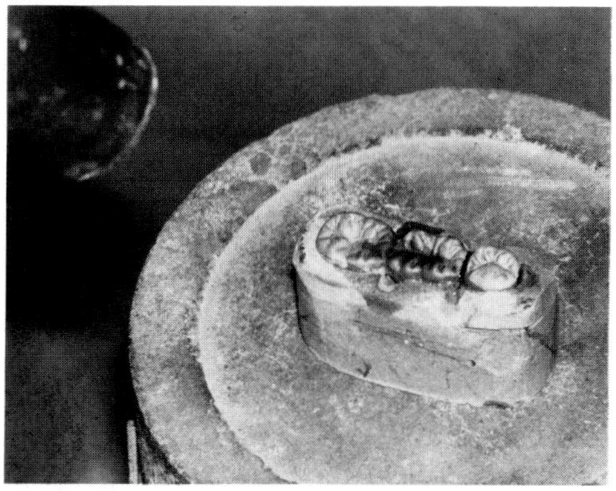

Fig. 7-178. Minimal heating with reducing brush flame before fluxing of joint minimizes oxidation.

6. Trim the excess plaster so that after seating the castings in the template, it is possible to cover their margins with soldering investment. Lute the castings into the template with sticky wax (Fig. 7-175). Make a final evaluation of the joint space before filling it with wax.

7. Mix the soldering investment* according to the manufacturer's directions. Completely fill the interiors of the retainer castings, and place them on a suitable mound of investment (Fig. 7-176). Exercise care to avoid "burying" the prosthesis in the investment, and allow the investment to bench set.

8. Remove the plaster template, and trim the investment so that the soldering model allows the ready access of heat to the joint areas (Fig. 7-177).

9. Heat the soldering model sufficiently to vaporize any wax remaining in the joint (Fig. 7-178). While the joint is still warm, coat the solder* with flux,† and place the solder in the joint (Fig. 7-179).

10. Reheat the soldering model until the solder flows; then remove the flame immediately (Fig. 7-180). Apply a brush flame in a circular manner around the soldering model to heat it as evenly as possible. As the solder is about to flow, it slumps and loses rectangular definition. Aim the flame into the joint to direct the solder

*R & R Soldering Investment, The Ranson & Randolph Co., Toledo, Ohio, or equivalent.

*.650 Fine solder, the J. M. Ney Co., Hartford, Conn., or equivalent.

†The J. M. Ney Co., Hartford, Conn., or equivalent.

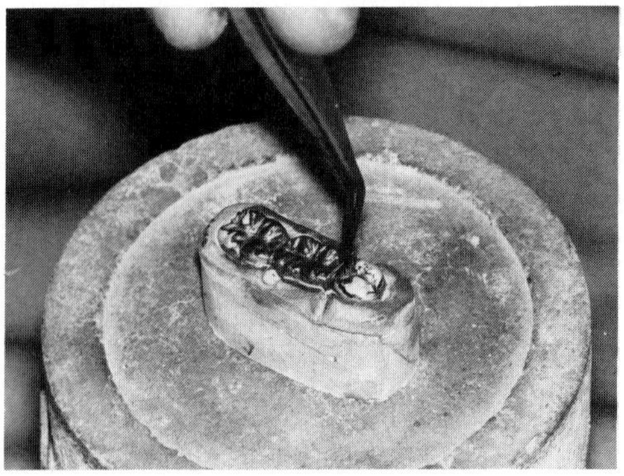

Fig. 7-179. When placing solder, avoid spattering flux on adjacent occlusal surfaces; solder can flow to fill occlusal features. Antifluxes, such as pencil lead, can be used to restrict solder flow to joint area.

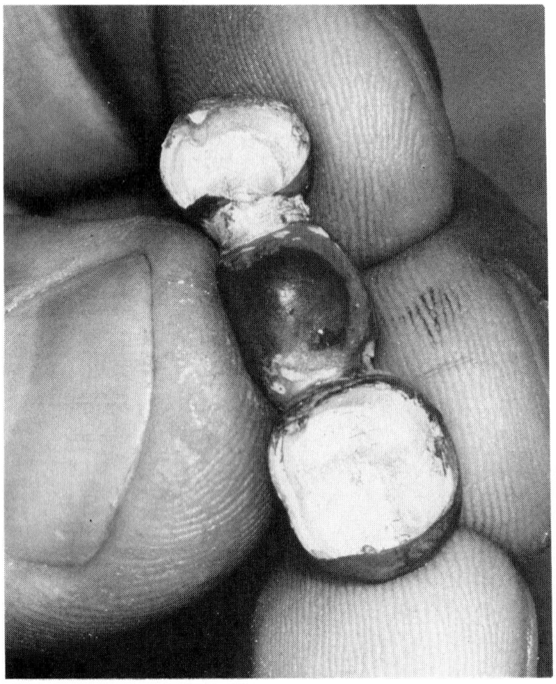

Fig. 7-181. Solder fills joint in configuration determined by white inlay wax (Fig. 7-175). Note unoxidized interiors of retainer castings produced by soldering investment.

flow. Use only reducing portions of the flame, characterized by bright, shiny areas on the metal directly under the flame.

11. Allow the prosthesis to bench cool to heat treat the metals properly. Remove the investment, and inspect the joint (Fig. 7-181). Make necessary corrections: for example, add solder to the joint after pickling the prosthesis and reinvesting it in a soldering model.

12. Try the assembled prosthesis in the mouth (Fig. 7-182). Finish and polish the prosthesis.

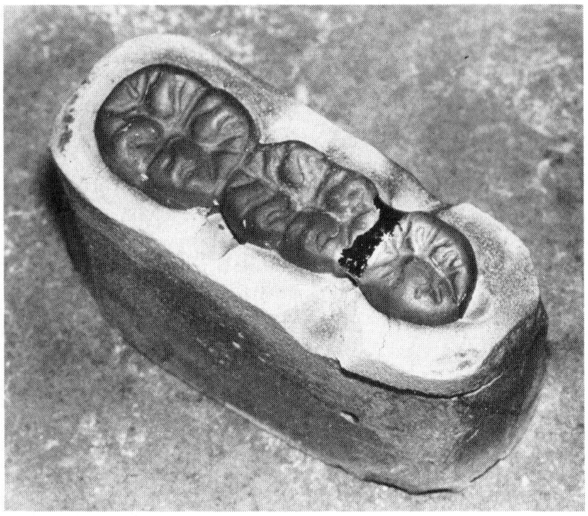

Fig. 7-180. When melted, solder becomes shiny fluid that rapidly fills joint space after use of properly directed reducing flame.

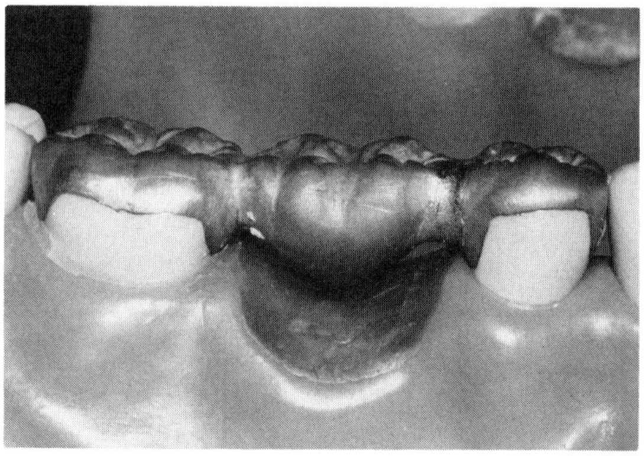

Fig. 7-182. Excess contour is noted, especially at gingival margin. Joint is finished and polished to provide access for necessary hygienic procedures, without undue weakening.

Soldering porcelain-to-metal frameworks

It is possible to solder metal frameworks prior to applying porcelain, that is, to presolder, with a torch almost in the same manner as type III gold alloys. As mentioned earlier, the solder and flux selected must be suitable for the alloys to be joined. Since the melting temperature of these alloys is so high (1925° F [1051.5° C] for SMG-2 solder), an oxygen-gas flame, and a high temperature investment* are essential.

Although it is feasible to solder noble porcelain bonding alloys (high gold, platinum, and palladium content by weight) without flux (Stade et al., 1975), the resultant porosity can reduce the strength of the joint ma-

*Hi-Heat Soldering Investment, Whip-Mix Corp., Louisville, Ky., or equivalent.

Table 7-7. Torch soldering

Problem	Probable cause	Solution
Soldered prosthesis unable to be reseated on teeth	Prosthesis warped during soldering	Break joint, check fit of castings, and resolder
	Inaccurate plaster template technique	Break joint, retake template, and resolder
Inadequate joint size	Insufficient amount of solder	Add solder to joint, or break joint and resolder
	Improper design for prosthesis	Remake prosthesis, and resolder
Pitted joint	Insufficient joint gap	Break joint, widen gap, and resolder
	Excess flux	Break joint, clean surfaces, and resolder
	Contamination or oxidation of solder	Break joint, clean surfaces, and resolder
	Overheating of prosthesis	Break joint, clean surfaces, and resolder
Voids and incomplete solder flow	Excessive joint gap	Break joint, remake prosthesis to narrow gap, and resolder
No solder flow	Contamination or oxidation of solder and/or parent alloys	Clean joint interfaces, add new solder, and resolder
	Inadequate heat in joint	Redesign soldering model for improved access of heat
Prosthesis melting	Solder incompatible with parent alloys	Check manufacturer's specifications, remake prosthesis, and resolder
	Inadequate thickness of metal	Remake prosthesis, resolder, and thin metal *after soldering*
	Margins inadequately protected by investment	Remake prosthesis, and resolder
Solder flow outside of joint	Excess flux	Add solder to joint if needed, and remove excess
	No antiflux adjacent to joint gap	Add solder to joint if needed, and remove excess
	Heat improperly applied	Add solder to joint if needed, and remove excess

terially. Since a suitable flux* appears to increase the wetting of these alloys and thereby eliminate most of the pitting, the routine use of a flux for presoldering is recommended.

Base metal alloys for porcelain-to-metal framework fabrication have attracted attention recently. The working properties of these alloys vary according to their melting temperatures and oxidation potentials, which are much higher than for noble alloys. Following closely the manufacturer's instructions as to materials and techniques makes it possible to obtain satisfactory results (Staffanou, 1977). However, the results are so "technique sensitive" that the prosthesis is often cast in one piece to circumvent the need for a soldered connection (Carrigan, 1977).

PROBLEM AREAS

As explained previously, there are exacting requirements for the design of soldering models. Trimming is essential to allow the prosthesis to be positioned and protected, yet exposed properly to the soldering flame. Excess investment drains heat from the joint, whereas an undersized model fractures under the stresses of heating and cooling. Strength considerations, such as those previously discussed (Fig. 7-168), apply equally well to the design of the soldering model.

Problems with torch soldering (Table 7-7) often center on the joint space. The interfaces must be smooth to let the solder flow readily and wet completely (Tylman and Malone, 1979). The gap must not be less than 0.1 mm for the solder to be directed through the joint without causing porosity. Polishing joint interfaces with rubber wheels and concomitantly enlarging the joint space to allow placement of the solder within it are the principal means of assuring the desired solder flow.

Inadequacies in the design of the model and/or excessive oxidation can lead to overheating of the prosthesis during soldering. The consequences may be readily apparent, as in the warping or melting of the prosthesis, or undetectable, as in the diffusion of the

*Flux H, Vita Zahnfabrick Sackingen, Germany, or equivalent.

parent metal into the solder joint. The latter defects may not become evident until the prothesis fails in service and shows a fractured "crystallized" joint. The soldering model requires only enough heat to cause the complete flow of the properly fluxed and positioned solder. Additional heat promotes the diffusion of the parent metal ions into the solder mass, thereby creating a different, weaker alloy. Detectable pitting of the joint also may result from overheating.

The means of relating the parts of a prosthesis for assembly deserves further consideration. Of the techniques available, plaster templates appear to be the most accurate and versatile when properly applied. Various waxes and plastics have been used in assembling the parts of a prosthesis prior to investment for soldering. However, these materials obscure the joint space until they burn off; even then they leave contaminating residues in the joint space. The plaster template permits the inspection and correction of the joint space *before* investment and the ready removal without residual contamination after investment of the prosthesis. Since this procedure reduces the quantity of residual material to be eliminated by subsequent heating, it has a similar effect on the potential for unwanted oxidation produced by such heating.

OVEN SOLDERING

Soldering in an oven offers the following advantages: (1) temperatures are more nearly uniform throughout the work, (2) temperatures are known at any point during the procedure, (3) application of vacuum can control oxidation, and (4) close monitoring of the procedure is feasible if the work is visible in the furnace. Although it is possible to use a vacuum oven for any soldering procedure within its temperature limits (Stade et al., 1975), it is particularly suitable for joining porcelain-to-metal prostheses after applying porcelain (postsoldering). The temperature sensitivity of the porcelain in relation to the bonding metal makes it essential to have precise control of temperature and heat distribution during soldering to avoid fracture and/or discoloration of the porcelain.

As in all soldering procedures, the solders and fluxes chosen must be compatible with the alloys to be connected. In addition, it is necessary to protect the bonded porcelain. Contact with fluxes and investments discolors porcelain; rapidly changing or uneven temperatures cause cracking and pitting. The presence of porcelain limits the soldering procedures and renders them more technique sensitive than those for joining metals alone.

Postsoldering in vacuum oven

PROCEDURE

1. Follow steps 1 to 6 used in torch soldering type III gold restorations. Add porcelain to the metal framework, and check for color and contour in the mouth. Make corrections, and stain and glaze the porcelain.

2. To prevent contact between the porcelain and the soldering investment, cover the porcelain surfaces with a layer of wax* before investing the prosthesis (Fig. 7-183). Invest the prosthesis, as described previously, and allow it to bench set.

*White Inlay Wax, Kerr Manufacturing Co., Romulus, Mich., or equivalent.

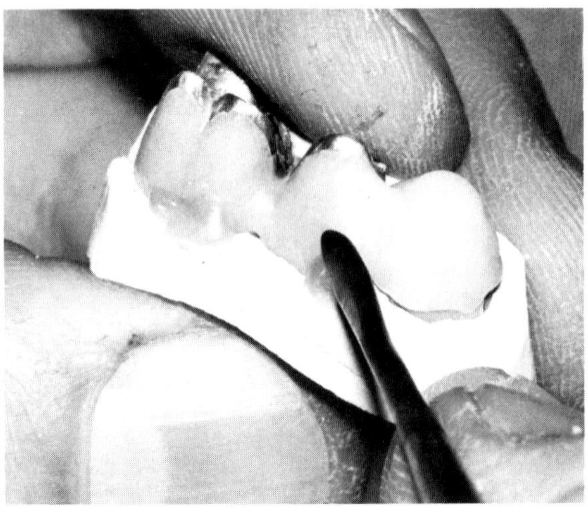

Fig. 7-183. Wax is added so that porcelain will be 1 to 2 mm from soldering investment. White inlay wax appears to leave least residue on porcelain when vaporized.

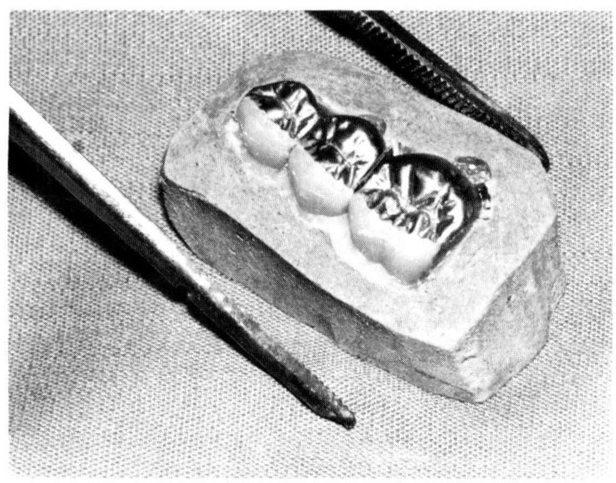

Fig. 7-184. Soldering model base is tapered to facilitate grasping with tongs. Note trial placement of solder *within* joint space, but without contact with porcelain.

3. Remove the plaster template, and trim the investment for ease in handling the soldering model with tongs (Fig. 7-184). Confirm that the joint gap is free of debris and accessible for solder placement.

4. Remove the residual wax, thereby allowing the least possible oxidation of surfaces that will receive solder. Boil out the soldering model in water, or heat it in an oven at 1200° F (640° C) for 5 to 10 minutes (Fig. 7-185). While the prosthesis is still warm, place a piece of fluxed solder within the joint. To join noble porcelain-to-metal alloys to similar alloys or to type III gold alloys, use the previously described .650 solder and flux for dependable results.

5. Move the soldering model to a position immediately adjacent to the muffle of a vacuum oven preheated to 1400° F (760° C) (Fig. 7-186). Allow time for heat accommodation by the soldering model before placing it in the muffle. This period of time should be the shortest required to raise the temperature of the prosthesis without heat shocking the porcelain, since oxidation of the parent metal and solder interfaces increases *with time.*

6. Place the model within the muffle and raise the temperature *under vacuum* until the solder flows (e.g., 1420° to 1490° F [770° to 810° C] for .650 fine solder). For ovens in which the contents of the muffle are not visible, raise the temperature from 1400° to 1500° F over a span of 3½ to 4 minutes. If the solder still does not flow, return the prosthesis to the muffle for 1 to 2 minutes more.

7. Remove the soldering model from the oven, inspect the joint, and allow the prosthesis to bench cool in air (Fig. 7-187). For some porcelains, the manufacturer recommends cooling under glass.

8. Remove the investment and inspect the joint (Fig. 7-188). If it is inadequate, usually it is necessary to separate the joint and repeat the entire soldering procedure. A fine saw (blade 0.01 inch thick) facilitates this procedure.

9. Try the assembled prosthesis in the mouth to confirm the clinical adequacy of the solder connection (Fig. 7-189). Finish and polish the prosthesis.

PROBLEM AREAS

As shown in Table 7-8, oven soldering can be both a demanding and a "technique-sensitive" procedure. Some aspects of the technique require careful consideration in order to satisfy the dual requirement of solder flow and porcelain protection with any reliability.

The potential for oxidation during oven soldering is high. It is impossible to control the distribution of heat and/or oxidation-reduction potentials *differentially* as in torch soldering. Therefore it is essential to exercise care during every heating step to expose the work to the

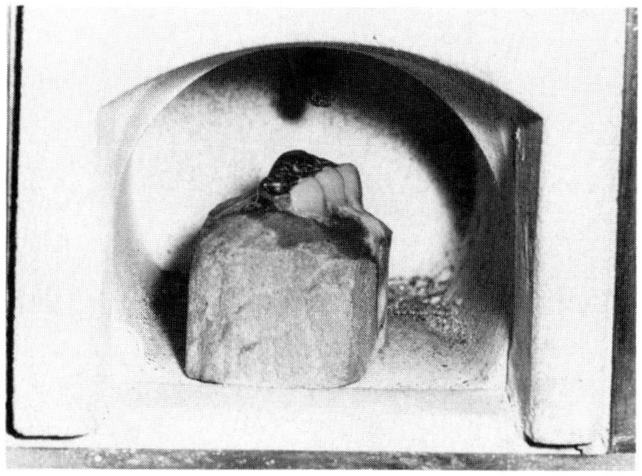

Fig. 7-185. Small glazing oven is used to vaporize wax, thereby preventing contamination of vacuum porcelain furnace. Prosthesis should remain in oven only long enough to vaporize residual wax.

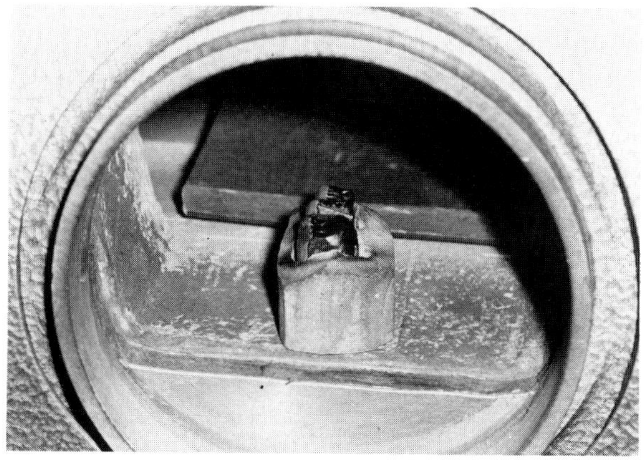

Fig. 7-186. Heating in air must be minimal to control oxidation. If technique is organized properly, heat loss during placement of solder is minimized, and prosthesis can be placed within muffle after 2 or 3 minutes.

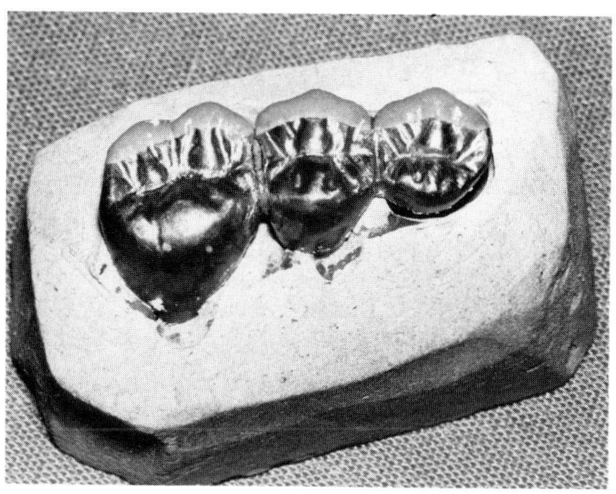

Fig. 7-187. Solder has flowed within joint space without apparent contamination of porcelain.

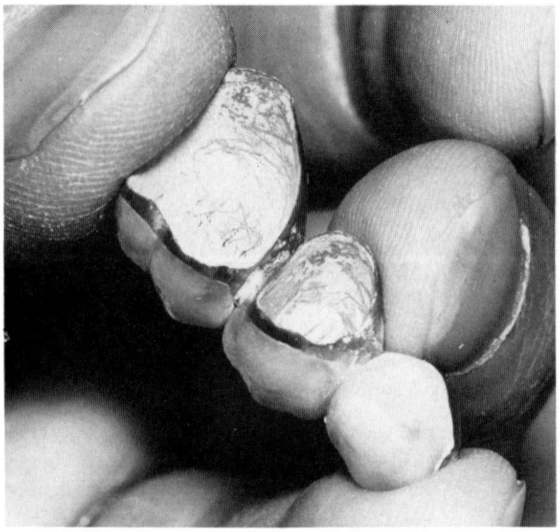

Fig. 7-188. Solder displays adequate gingival extension. Excess solder at buccal surface is removed to avoid possible compromise of esthetics.

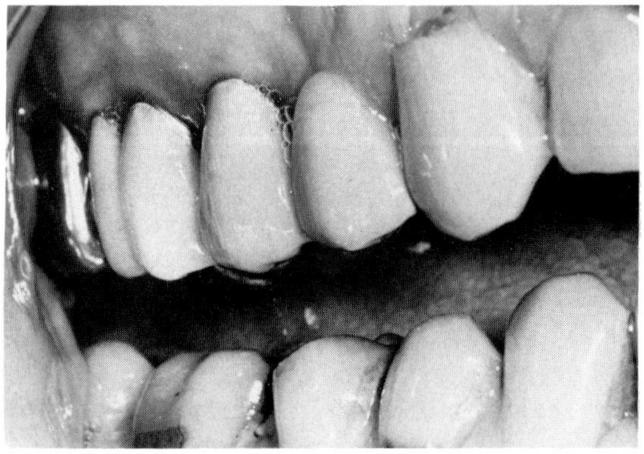

Fig. 7-189. Finished solder joint represents good balance between strength, cosmetics, and hygiene.

Table 7-8. Oven soldering

Problem	Probable cause	Solution
No solder flow	Oxidation or contamination of solder and/or parent metal	Clean joint interfaces, add new solder, and resolder
	Oven pyrometer reading higher than true temperature	Calibrate oven, clean joint interfaces, add new solder, and resolder
Incomplete solder flow	Joint space inadequate	Break joint, enlarge joint gap, and resolder
	Inadequate quantity of solder	Clean joint space, add solder, or break joint, and resolder
Discoloration of porcelain	Contact between porcelain and flux or investment	Break joint, correct porcelain, and resolder
Cracking and pitting of porcelain	Temperature variations excessive for brand of porcelain used	Check manufacturer's specifications for porcelain; rebake porcelain and resolder
Melting of porcelain and/or parent metal	Oven pyrometer reading lower than actual temperature	Calibrate oven, remake prosthesis, and resolder
	Incorrect solder for parent metal used	Recheck manufacturer's requirements for solder and parent metal; remake prosthesis and resolder
Size of joint inadequate	See Table 7-7	See Table 7-7
Pitted joint	See Table 7-7	See Table 7-7
Voids and incomplete solder flow	See Table 7-7	See Table 7-7
Solder flow outside of joint	See Table 7-7	See Table 7-7

least possible heat for the shortest possible time. Oxidation progresses rapidly in a few minutes at 1200° F (649° C) in air, even when using noble alloys. Therefore wax is preferable to plastics (DuraLay) for positioning parts and protecting porcelain; plastic elimination requires more heat than wax and is more likely to produce residual contamination. Even excessive quantities of flux will not control oxidation.

It can be difficult to direct solder flow in oven soldering, since there is no temperature differential to "draw" solder, as in torch soldering. It is essential to position the solder in the final location before heating. Widening the joint gap sufficiently to place the solder within the joint accomplishes this. Then it is necessary only for the solder to melt in place and not flow to distant areas through a narrow space.

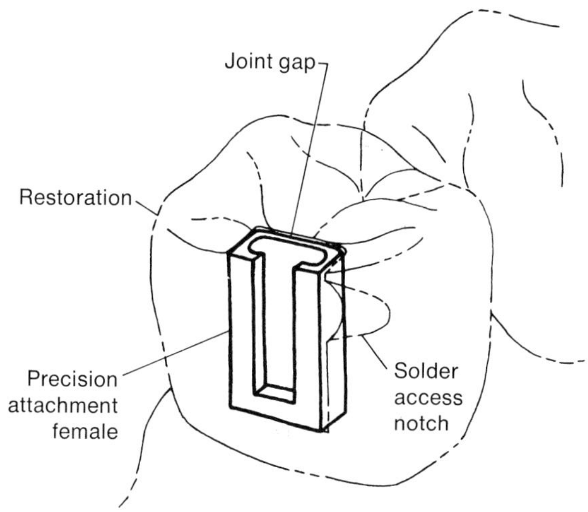

Fig. 7-190. When flowing solder into preheated joint through access opening, care must be exercised to avoid flowing solder into precision recess. Antifluxing agents, such as carbon or gold rouge in alcohol, are effective in limiting solder flow.

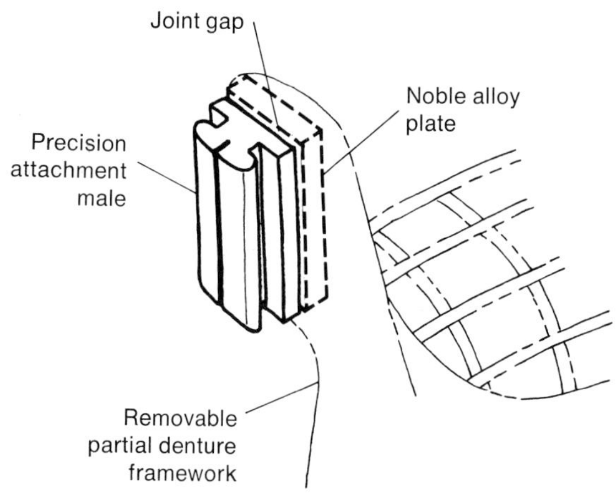

Fig. 7-191. Noble metal insert (plate) is roughened suitably to provide mechanical lock with base metal in which it is embedded.

Porcelain discoloration resulting from contamination by flux is difficult to control. When added to a warm soldering model, flux often spatters and comes into contact with the porcelain at a considerable distance from the site of application. Too little flux, on the other hand, virtually assures an inadequate flow of solder. This can be corrected by first applying a uniform, thin coating of flux to the solder and then adding the solder at the desired position within the joint space. However, if the flux contaminates the porcelain, refinishing and reglazing are essential to establish the necessary shading.

SOLDERING PRECISION ATTACHMENTS

It is possible to incorporate precision attachments in restorations or removable partial denture frameworks by including them within the parent casting or by making a soldered connection between them and the parent casting. The procedures are the same as those given previously, except for modifications required by the parent metals, solders, and joint configurations chosen.

When soldering the female portion of a precision attachment to a restoration, it is necessary to make a recess in the casting slightly larger than the attachment it is to contain (Fig. 7-190). The extra space is available for the solder joint gap. Since this space and access to it often are limited, preloading the joint with solder may not be feasible. Under these circumstances, the procedure is to flux the joint, heat the prosthesis to the melting point of the solder, and add the solder to the preheated joint. It should flow immediately, guided by the differential heating and the oxidation/reduction potential of the torch.

Joining the male portions of precision attachments to base metal chrome-cobalt removable partial denture frameworks requires special considerations. Since the melting temperatures and oxidation potentials of base metal alloys are so much higher than the corresponding values for the noble alloys used in making the precision attachments, soldering is difficult and unreliable at best (Carrigan, 1977). It is possible to simplify the procedure by casting the framework to a plate of suitable noble alloy, such as an alloy with high platinum content, placed to form a joint interface with the male portion of the attachment (Fig. 7-191). The problem becomes merely one of joining adjacent noble metal interfaces, as described previously.

Repairs

It is possible to repair minor surface defects in cast restorations by soldering. Generally, this repair includes filling small holes or pits and adding proximal contours to improve relationships with adjacent teeth. Since these corrective procedures have limitations, clinical judgment must determine when it is better for the patient to have the entire restoration remade than to have some defects, such as incomplete casting margins, repaired.

Type III gold castings

PROCEDURE

1. Clean the surface to be repaired (with a rubber wheel), and cover it with a fluxed piece of solder* of appropriate size (Fig. 7-192).

2. Grasping the restoration with soldering tweezers,

*.615 Fine solder, The J.M. Ney Co., Hartford, Conn., or equivalent.

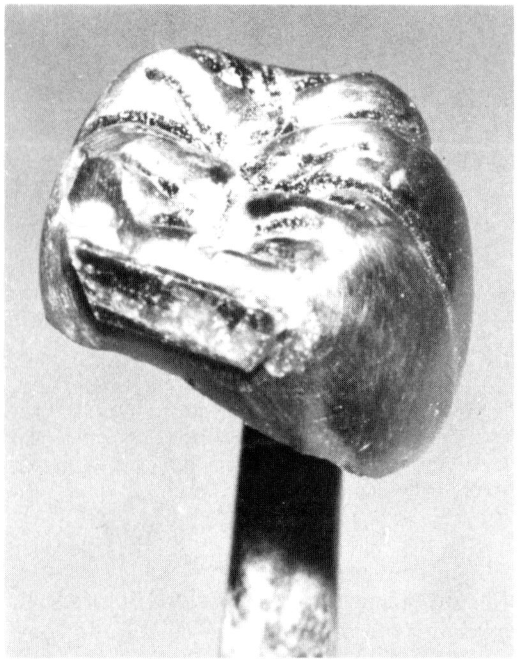

Fig. 7-192. Solder is cut to extend beyond area to be repaired to allow for subsequent finishing procedures.

A

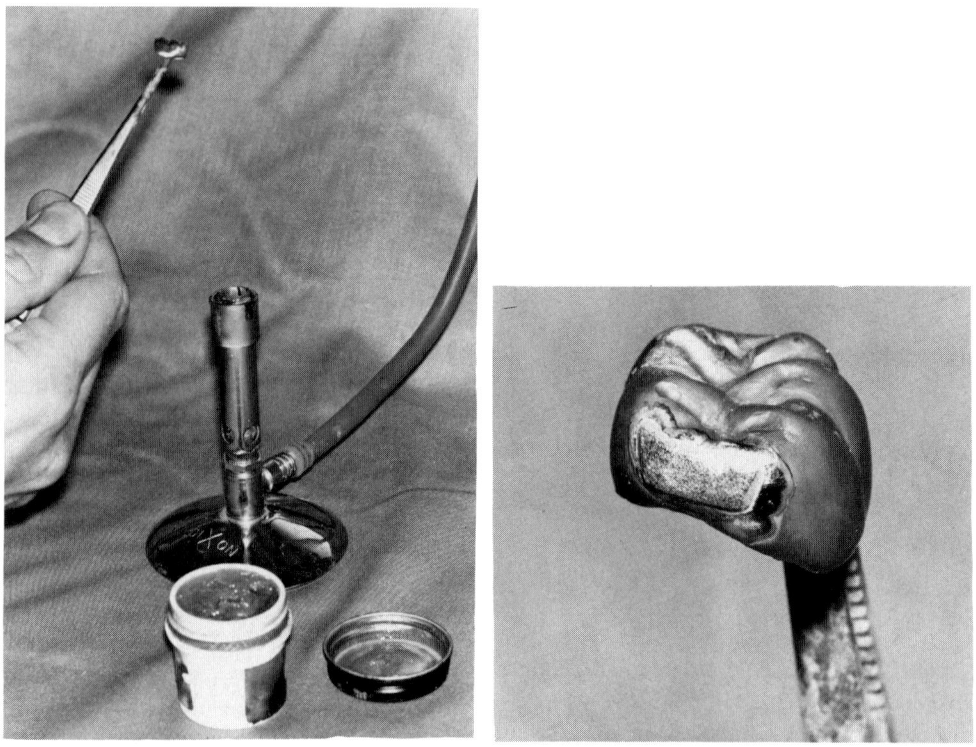

B

Fig. 7-193. A, Small repairs may be soldered freehand in Bunsen burner flame. **B,** Repair has been heated only until solder has slumped into intimate contact with restoration, and edges have begun to melt. Additional heating will "ball" solder and produce voids in repair.

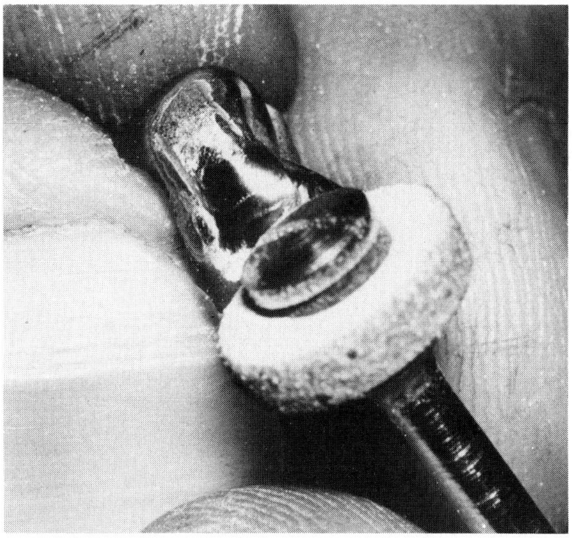

Fig. 7-194. Solder is feathered into restoration with separating disks and rubber wheels. Proper color compatibility between solder and restoration assures invisible repair.

heat it in the reducing portion of a gas-air flame until the solder begins to flow (Fig. 7-193). Then remove it from the heat immediately.

3. When cool, shape and polish the repair (Fig. 7-194).

These procedures are subject to defects, such as pitting of the solder and flow away from the desired location. Experimentation with a variety of materials and techniques may reveal refinements in these procedures that can minimize failure. Frequently, however, the technique of choice is to remake a defective restoration, rather than to solder on a repair.

SUMMARY

To provide the student with a reference for dental soldering procedures, this chapter defines the terminology and requirements for dental solders, fluxes, and solder investments. The step-by-step procedure for torch (flame) soldering of type III gold alloys is described. For precreamic and postceramic soldering procedures, the technique of oven soldering is outlined. The chapter further discusses the soldering of precision attachments and solder repair procedures.

PART SEVEN

Finishing techniques

HENRY N. YAMADA and CALVIN S. LAU

Ease in finishing a casting depends directly on the quality of the wax pattern, the investing technique, and the casting technique. The smoother the wax pattern, the smoother the casting; the denser the casting, the easier the finishing. Porosity in cast restorations makes it difficult to develop a proper finish. It can develop for several reasons discussed in previous chapters, but the primary cause of porosity is overheating the gold during the casting procedure.

The technique of finishing and polishing gold castings is a systematic reduction of surface irregularities. The purpose is to produce such a smooth surface that it is free of any roughness, scratches, or irregularities visible to the naked eye. The finished casting must maintain the fundamental requirements of fit, form, function, and marginal integrity.

FITTING CASTING TO DIE

The best time to check for nodules is immediately after removing the investment from the casting and before attempting any stripping. It is difficult to see small details and nodules in a stripped casting because of its shiny surface. However, after stripping a casting, use a 50 μm aluminum oxide pressure blast to dull the surface or, if unavailable, use a regular sandblast.

PROCEDURE

1. Carefully inspect the interior surface of the casting for nodules (Fig. 7-195). Use a 20-power binocular microscope with a reflective front surface light source because it is necessary to scrutinize the depths of the casting carefully. However, if the microscope is unavailable, use any magnifying glass.

2. Remove the nodules with a No. 1 round steel bur in a straight handpiece. The new steel burs are ideal for this type of work, since they cut off any projection or nodule and do not tend to push or burnish metal. A high-speed handpiece may tend to push metal rather than cut it unless operated with a light touch, but it is useful in large areas. Most often the nodules appear at the corners on the interior surface of the casting and along the grooves. If necessary, change to a smaller bur to work in small areas. A spear-shaped bur, cut from an old round bur, is the most efficient along the grooves.

3. Cut the sprue as close as possible to the casting with a separating wheel (Fig. 7-196). Use the palm-thumb grasp for maximum control of the wheel (Fig. 7-197). Bend the remaining uncut section until the metal becomes fatigued, and then smooth it to contour with the same wheel (Fig. 7-198 and 7-199). When grinding gold, remember to collect the shavings because of their scrap value.

4. While holding the casting over the collecting box, redefine the grooves with a half round, old steel bur or a small Busch bud finishing bur (Fig. 7-200). Note the use of the palm-thumb grip. It is advantageous to use a

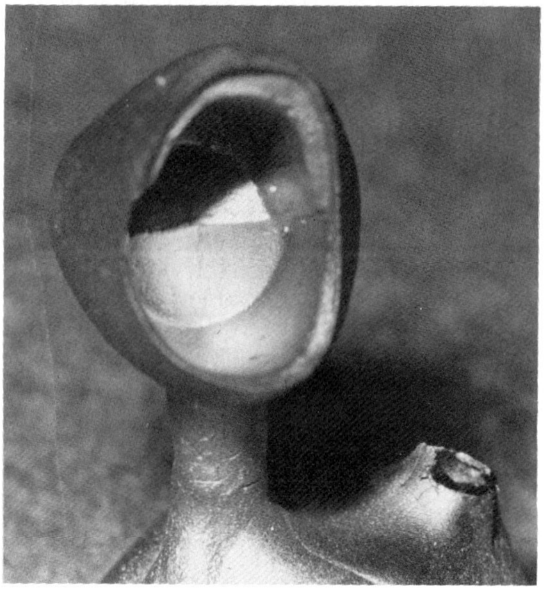

Fig. 7-195. Inspecting for nodules.

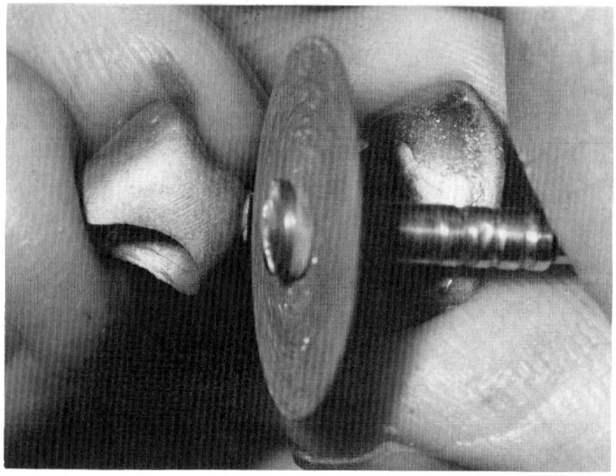

Fig. 7-196. Separating wheel.

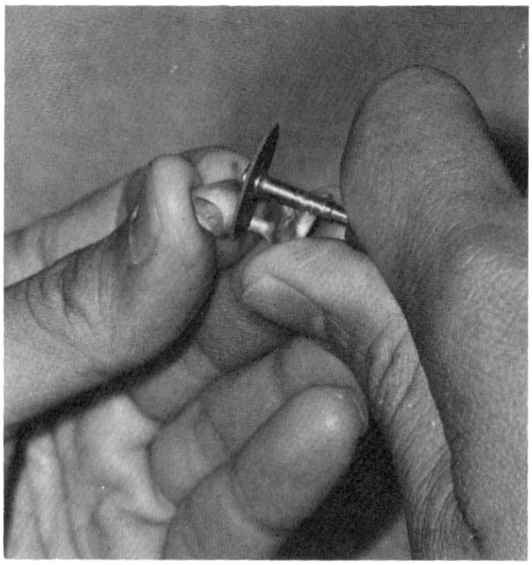

Fig. 7-197. Palm-thumb grasp.

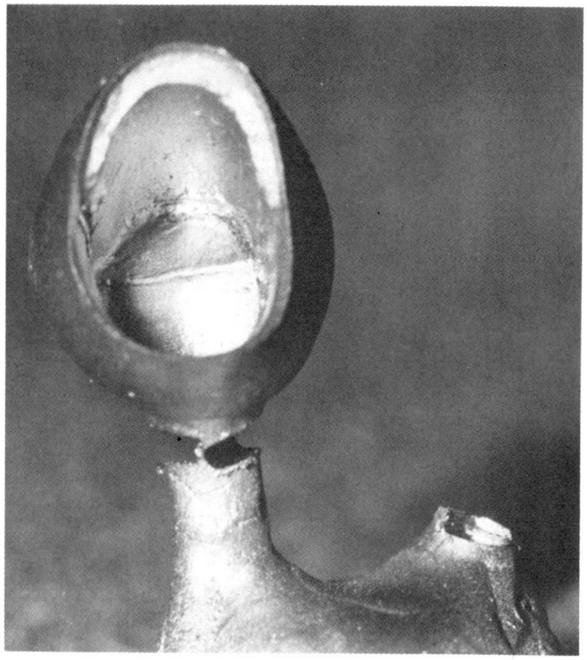

Fig. 7-198. Separating cut.

finishing bur because it is possible to vary the width of the cutting edge by changing the angulation of the bur. Use the tip of the bur where the grooves are small and the wider part of the bur near the axial surfaces where the grooves are wider (Fig. 7-201 and 7-202).

5. Check the fit of the casting by placing it carefully on the die, but do not apply force to the casting. It should be possible to smoothly seat the casting in place.

6. If there is any obstruction to complete seating and a careful visual inspection reveals no other nodules or imperfections, remove the casting, apply some type of marking liquid to the die, dry the die, and reseat the casting (Fig. 7-203). The liquid will mark any high spots on the interior surface of the casting. Marking liquids tend to show lateral discrepancies better than small residual nodules (Fig. 7-204). Therefore look carefully at the die for small white abrasion spots that indicate nodules or imperfections in the casting. When using a bin-

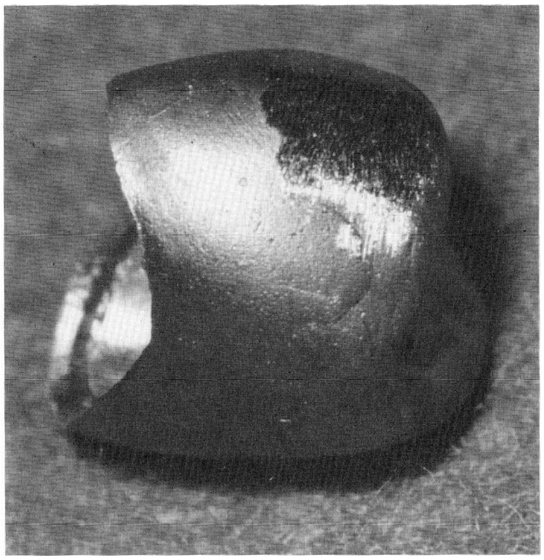

Fig. 7-199. Smooth to contour.

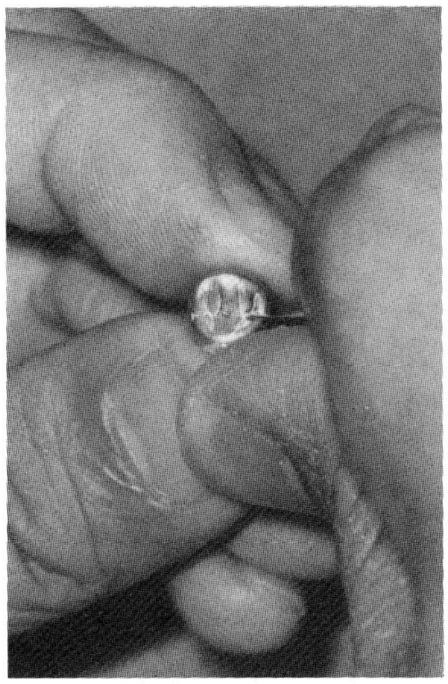

Fig. 7-200. Redefining grooves.

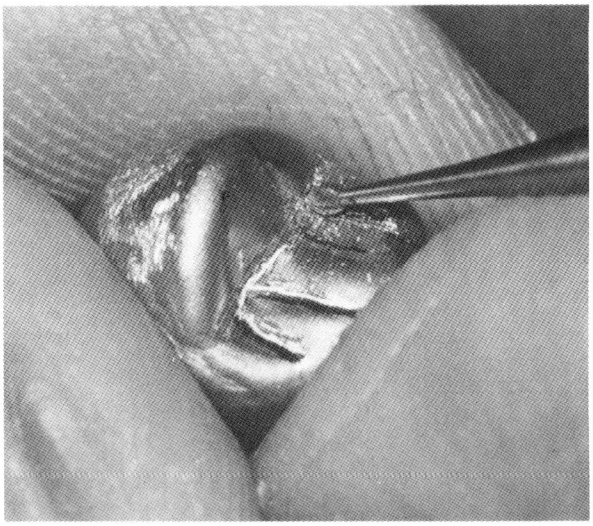

Fig. 7-201. Using tip of bud bur.

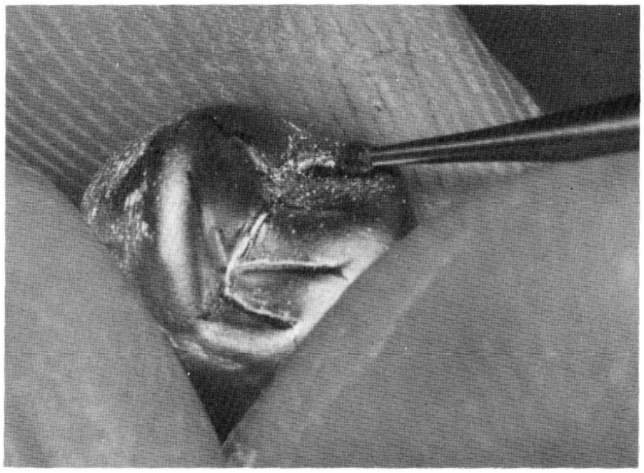

Fig. 7-202. Using body of bud bur.

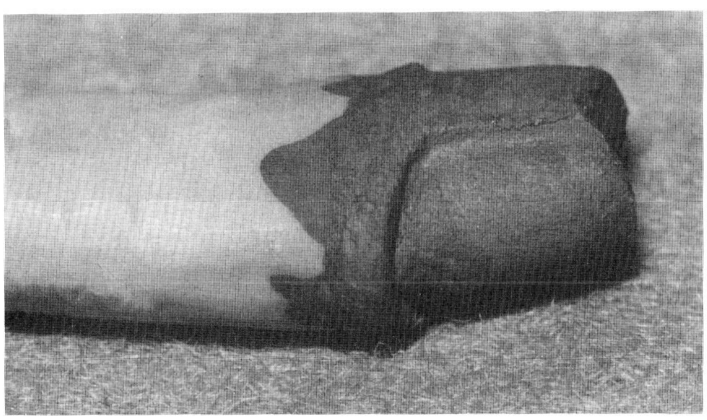

Fig. 7-203. Liquid marking on die.

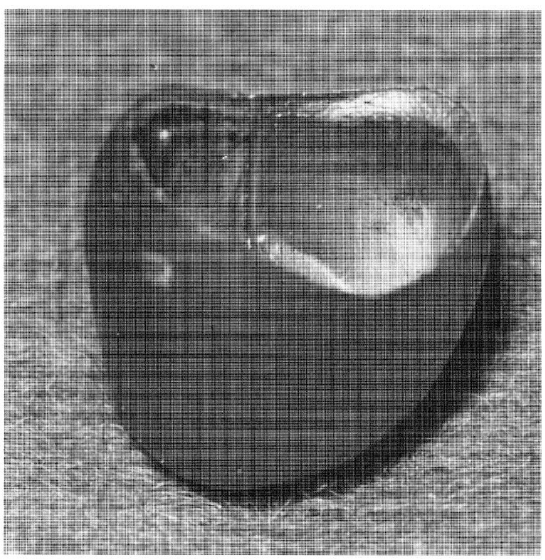

Fig. 7-204. Lateral spot on casting.

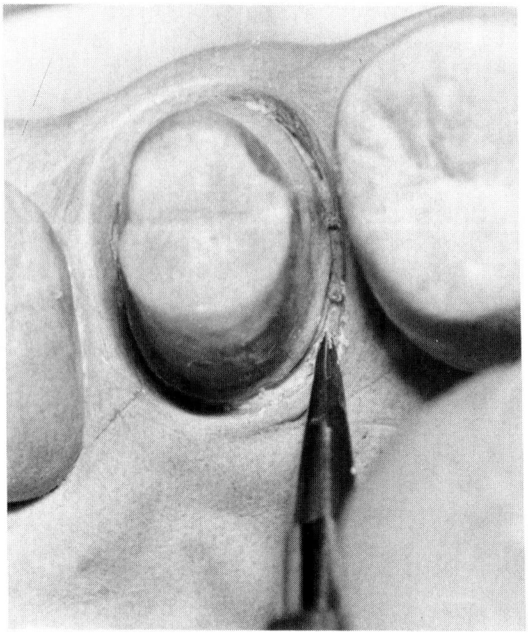

Fig. 7-205. Relieving margin areas.

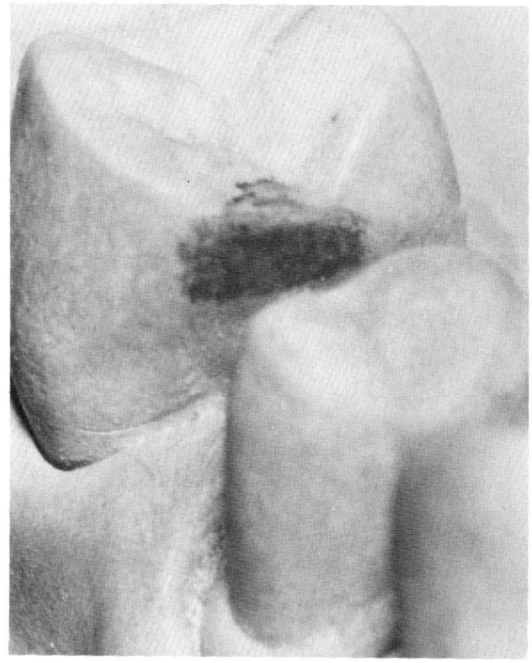

Fig. 7-206. Penciling adjacent contact areas.

ocular microscope to locate nodules, most likely this problem will not arise.

7. At this time determine whether the casting fits properly, or whether it is possible to seat it by judicious fitting. If not, rewax at this time to avoid having an inadequate casting. It may be possible to reuse the die and still obtain an adequate casting. Make the decision now to avoid considerable delay for the patient and dentist.

FITTING CASTING TO WORKING CAST

Before using removable dies, the margin areas are trimmed. However, when using separate working casts and dies, it is essential to relieve only the margin area with a No. 1 round bur, so that the casting can go into place (Fig. 7-205). One advantage of the separate die technique is being able to maintain the form of the gingival tissue and contour the casting to the tissues of the mouth. It is especially important when working with ceramometal restorations.

PROCEDURE

1. Use a pencil to mark the adjacent contact areas, and seat the casting carefully (Fig. 7-206). With proper use of the waxing technique there should be a slightly tight fit at this time (Fig. 7-207). Rely on visual keys to aid in adjusting the contacts correctly (Fig. 7-208). Do not reduce the marked areas of the casting arbitrarily. If there are two contact areas, find out which one is

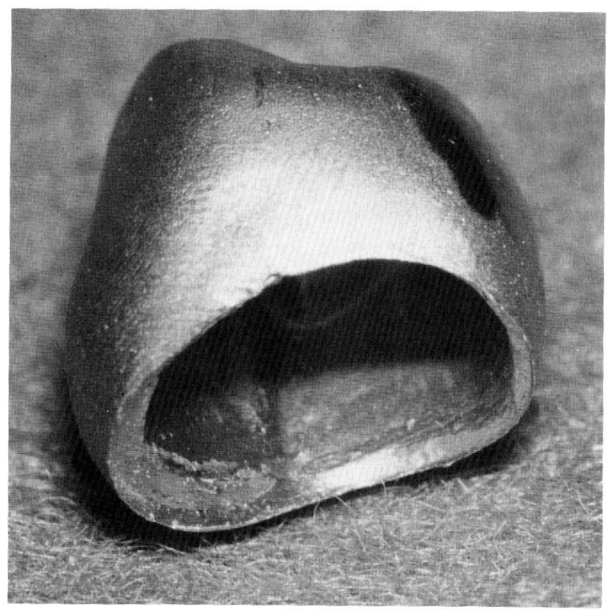

Fig. 7-207. Contact mark on gold crown.

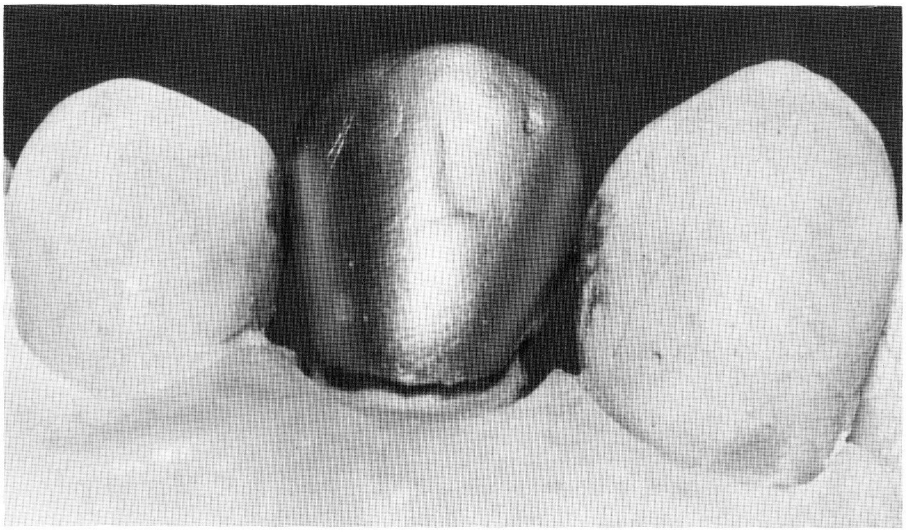

Fig. 7-208. Checking lateral displacement by contact area.

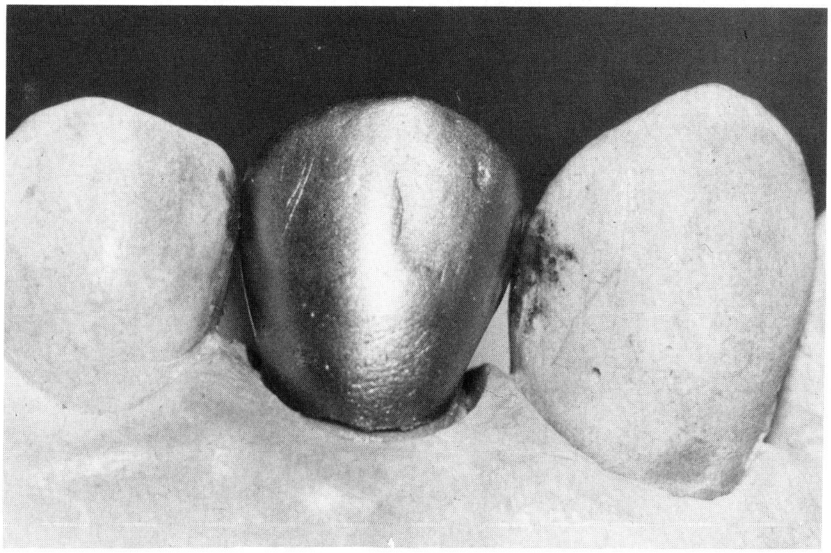

Fig. 7-209. Final seating of casting.

tighter, and relieve it with a rubber wheel.* Look at the casting from the buccal aspect, and observe as it goes into place. If the casting shows slight canting with relatively even seating, the opposite contact has caused the displacement and requires adjustment.

2. Adjust the contact areas until all of the margins are *almost* down, but the contacts still mark (Fig. 7-209). If a mesial or distal margin is completely down and the other is open, adjust the contact on the side of the open margin.

3. Relieve the adjacent contact areas gently by scraping them with a No. 15 Bard-Parker blade (Fig. 7-210). Scraping also will remove the pencil marks.

At this time a slight opening should be visible between the casting and adjacent teeth, but the casting should be completely seated (Fig. 7-211). Check to see that no marginal areas of the casting touch the stone cast; relieve them if necessary. If one contact area has a slight opening, as it should, and the area on the other side does not, relieve that contact area again with a rubber wheel until a slight opening is visible. A slight excess at the contact area is better than insufficient contact when the dentist tries the casting in the mouth (Table 7-9).

*White Flexie, Dedeco, Brooklyn, N.Y.

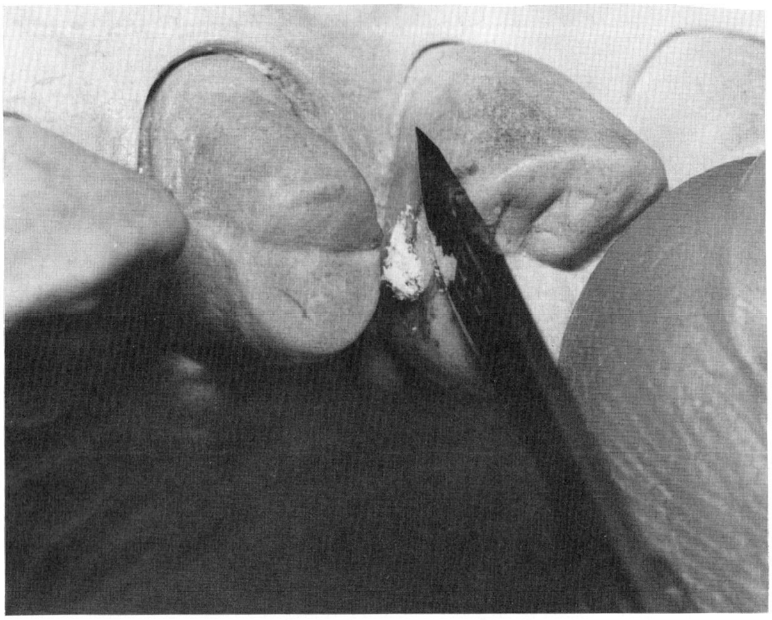

Fig. 7-210. Scraping of contact area.

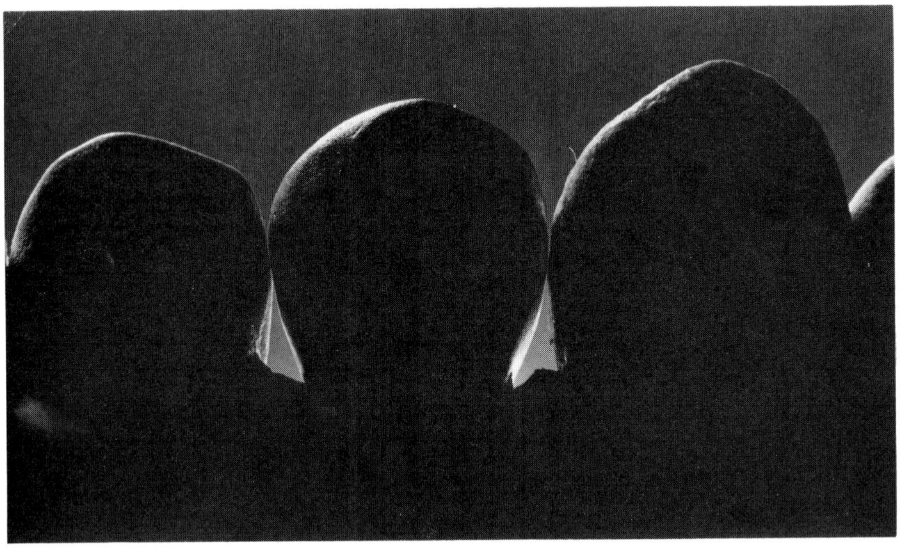

Fig. 7-211. Slight opening between casting and cast.

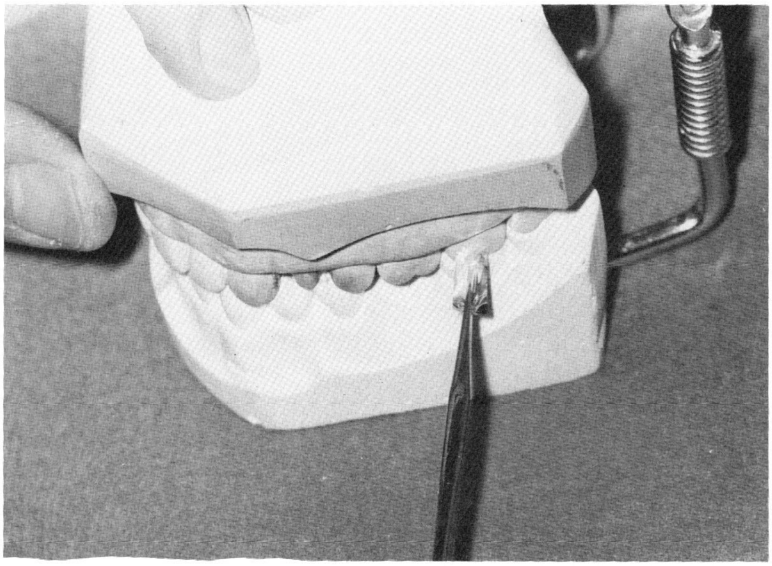

Fig. 7-212. Checking occlusion with plastic strips distal to casting.

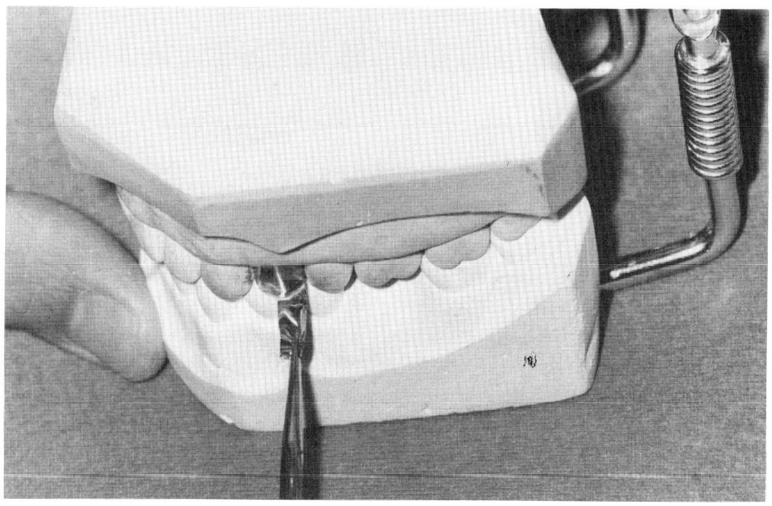

Fig. 7-213. Checking occlusion with plastic strips on casting.

4. With the same rubber wheel, smooth all axial surfaces of the casting to within 1 mm of the margins, replace the casting on the working cast, and check for occlusal accuracies. Avoid touching the occlusal surfaces with the rubber wheel because it is exceedingly difficult to see the markings on a shiny surface.

5. Before seating the casting on the working cast, check the adjacent tooth with a plastic strip (Mylar strip) only 0.0005 inch thick (Fig. 7-212). If it is a multiple unit case on an articulator with an incisal guide pin, use that area as a guide to check the accuracy of the occlusion.

6. Place the casting on the working cast, and check the adjacent teeth for occlusal contact with plastic strips. If they do not contact, determine that the casting is in supraocclusion and, if so, use a thin marking paper or ribbon to mark the contacting areas. After carefully carrying out all previous steps, especially the waxing, probably it will be possible to adjust the excessive occlusal contacts with a rubber wheel. Remember that any polishing sequence removes some of the gold. Therefore unless there are gross inaccuracies, do not use anything especially rough to remove the areas adjusted. If excessively roughened during adjustment,

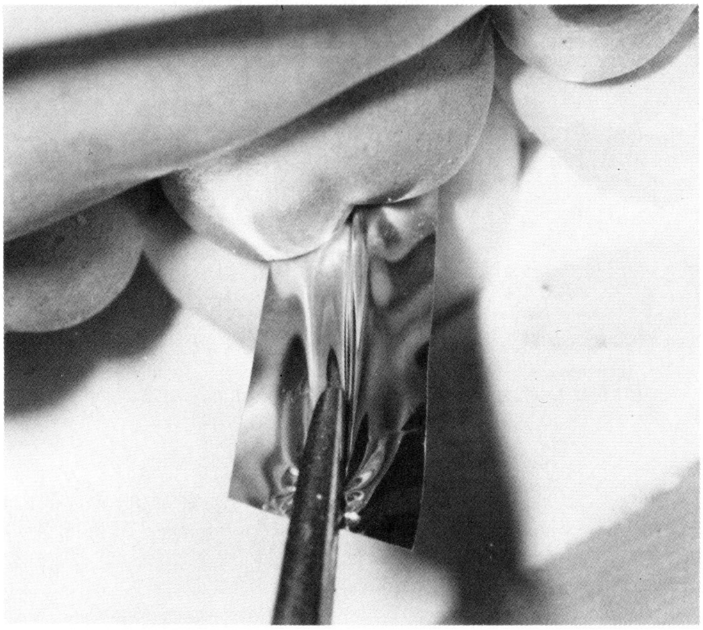

Fig. 7-214. Checking pull of plastic strips.

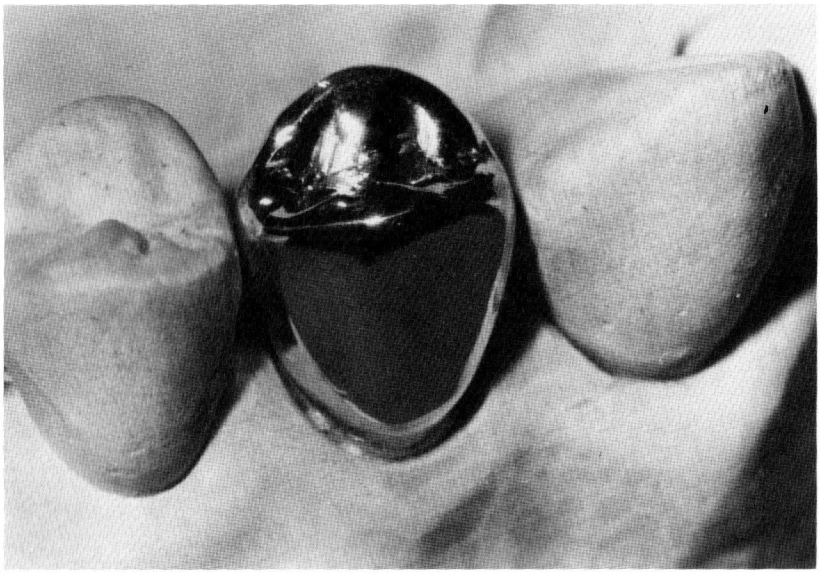

Fig. 7-215. Finished casting.

subsequent polishing may destroy the fine occlusal contacts that have been developed. Adjust the casting until it and the adjacent teeth make contact and both hold the plastic strip (Fig. 7-213). If the adjustment is correct, it will be possible to see and feel a definite pull of the plastic strip (Fig. 7-214).

FINAL POLISHING

The final polishing sequence is as important in achieving excellent results as any other previous procedure. Underpolishing can cause areas of plaque retention or make the casting prone to tarnish, whereas overpolishing can cause loss of centric contacts, inadequate contact areas, or obliteration of functional anatomy.

PROCEDURE

1. Use a soft bristle brush* with polishing compound† initially, and then with red rouge for polishing. Keep the brush moving back and forth over the casting, and use a bouncing motion on the occlusal surfaces in the direction of the grooves. Hold the casting in the fingers, and polish lightly toward the margin with the soft brush. Use the finger to help protect the margin from the brush. Do not use the die during the final polishing. It is too easy to overpolish these areas and cause submarginal areas, with the result that the casting may fit the die, but not the tooth. The final polishing is one of the most critical aspects of finishing the casting.

2. Change to a chamois wheel with red (jeweler's) rouge to finish the polishing, and use only a straight handpiece. Do the final cleaning of the casting with an ultrasonic cleaner and a liquid detergent or with an old toothbrush and hot soapy water. Any other aids, such as steam cleaning, are especially beneficial (Fig. 7-215).

MULTIPLE ADJACENT CASTINGS

In multiple casting, a few modifications of the technique described earlier will give superior results. After doing the entire wax-up, cast every other wax pattern, and follow the same steps up to the instructions for adjusting the contact area. Smooth the casting, and adjust the occlusion before developing the adjacent wax pattern contact area to the full contour; then invest and cast it. It is extremely difficult to adjust all contact areas of the castings at the same time. The procedure described will facilitate obtaining accurate contact areas for all castings. However, the advantage of scraping the adjacent tooth when adjusting the contact areas of multiple casting is lacking. Therefore extreme care is required to see that the finished casting has adequate contact.

*No. 11 Robinson brush.

†Buffing Bar Compound (B.B.C.), J. F. Jelenko & Co., New Rochelle, N.Y.

PROCEDURE

1. In complete mouth rehabilitation, the accuracy necessary for occlusal contacts generally makes it imperative to omit polishing. After a remount and the final occlusal adjustment, use a wire brush for a final finish. With a complete mouth rehabilitation, the high polish should be done before the final occlusal adjustment.

2. Many times the dentist prefers an abrasive blasted finish on the occlusal surfaces so that it is possible to read the markings in the mouth. In this instance, it is necessary to postpone the blasting process until *after* the final polishing. It is not a shortcut to the final step.

POLISHING CERAMOMETAL RESTORATIONS

The polishing technique for the ceramometal casting differs little from the one described for type III gold, except that ceramometal is more difficult to polish. Only by following the previously described step-by-step sequence is it possible to obtain an excellent finish. Each step requires more time than when working with type III gold, especially smoothing with polishing rubber wheels. A critical area when polishing ceramometal castings is the porcelain-metal junction. If any porcelain or glaze remains on the metal, the result will be a definite black shadow area (Table 7-9).

PROCEDURE

1. During the final stages of the porcelain finishing prior to glazing, grind both the porcelain and gold at the same time to make certain that no porcelain remains over the junction.

2. If an overglaze appears on the metal, use a rubber wheel* to remove it during the finishing; otherwise, the black shadow effect will remain.

PROBLEM AREAS

During the finishing procedures for castings, frequently encountered problems, their probable causes, and solutions are identified in Table 7-9.

1. Casting with a defective surface because of nodules or porosity requires unnecessary finishing time or possible remaking. A review of the investing technique (Part Four) and casting procedures (Part Five) is indicated.

2. Before castings are seated on the die, the internal

*No. 2 green, knife-edge rubber wheel, Craytex, Burlingame, Calif., or equivalent.

Table 7-9. Finishing techniques

Problem	Probable cause	Solution
Nodules	Poor investing techniques	Grind out nodules or redo casting if gross number of nodules exists
Porosity	Casting procedure not controlled and gold too hot	Redo wax pattern
	Poor spruing technique and sprue too small	Make sprue larger
	Pattern too far from top of ring, allowing no gas to escape	Redo casting (review Parts four and five)
Interior surface too shiny	Stripped before interior surface checked	Pressure blast with aluminum oxide or sand
Bur running off uncontrolled	Wrong rotation of bur and incorrect cutting direction	Run engine clockwise to pull bur toward operator if operator is right-handed
	Poor grasp of handpiece	Use palm-thumb grasp
Tight contacts in mouth	Too much relieved from adjacent contact	Remove contact areas carefully
Open or loose contacts	Contact areas overpolished or overreduced	Solder contacts with low-fusing solder
Occlusion too high	Wax-up too high Adjustments on casts incorrect	Make adjustment on cast or in mouth carefully
Occlusion too low	Wax-up too low Overpolished Casting not down on working cast when adjusting occlusion	Redo casting
Not polishing well	Porosity (see above)	Redo casting
Black shadow at porcelain-gold junction	Porcelain over margins	Grind off excess porcelain until porcelain and gold are reduced together; then refire
	Overglaze over margins	Use rubber wheel over metal until overglaze is removed; then polish
Margins short	Waxed short of margin	Redo (see discussion on waxing)
	Overpolished at margins	Redo (see discussion on final polishing)
	Incomplete casting	Redo (see investing and casting technique)

surface should be examined under magnification for surface irregularities. Abrasive blasting the metal surface with aluminum oxide or sand will reveal tiny nodules and interferences when the casting is seated on the die. When removing surface irregularities, be sure that the bur will run true and in a clockwise direction to maintain control.

3. Excessively tight or open contact areas can be avoided in single tooth restorations by slightly relieving the proximal contacts on the working cast prior to seating the casting. The adjacent contact area may be marked with a soft lead pencil and scraped lightly to provide a slight excess of metal in the contact area of the casting. The casting should be carefully relieved where marked by a thin articulating paper. The final contact adjustment is done with a rubber wheel.

When multiple castings are seated on the working cast, the adjacent metal contacts can be identified with thin articulating paper or by pressure blasting the proximal surfaces. Multiple castings should not be adjusted to seat completely on the working cast unless a removable die working cast is used. Stone casts are a slightly expanded reproduction of the mouth, and castings seated on a fixed cast usually will have looser proximal contacts when transferred to the abutment teeth.

4. Occlusal adjustments are the most time-consuming error when seating castings in the mouth. A minor amount of intraoral occlusal adjustment should be anticipated, but extensive grinding-in of a casting can be avoided by (1) mounting the working cast to accurate interocclusal records (Chapter 1), (2) finalizing the wax pattern by adjusting the occlusal contacts with zinc-free talcum powder, and (3) making sure that a wax pattern will seat properly when transferred to an individual die before adapting it to the margins. Waxing aids, such as tin foil adapted to the opposing occlusal surfaces, are entirely unnecessary and defeat precise laboratory techniques.

5. When castings are consistently submarginal, the technician should review the die trimming, waxing, and polishing technique. A die should be trimmed under magnification to avoid overreduction of the margins. In

carving wax that is in excess of the margins, a blunt instrument, slightly warmed should be used to avoid abraded die margins. A slight excess bulk of wax at the margin will assure a complete casting and lessen the chance for overpolishing as the casting is finished on the die.

SUMMARY

This chapter on finishing techniques described the laboratory procedures of preparing the cast restoration for insertion in the patient's mouth. Inspecting the casting, seating it on the die and working cast with proper adjustments to the proximal and occlusal surfaces and margins, redefining the occlusal anatomy, as well as polishing the casting were discussed.

Since the casting is a metal reproduction of the wax pattern, repeated references have been made to Part Four and Part Five, in which the investing and casting procedures are described.

The technician can be instrumental in minimizing the chairtime required for the insertion of restorations by meticulously adjusting these restorations on dies and working casts.

REFERENCES

Allan, F.C. and Asgar, K.: Reaction of Co-Cr casting alloy with investment, J. Dent. Res. **45**(5):1516-1528, 1966.

Carrigan, J.: Personal communication, 1977.

Lacy, A.M., Hirose, R., and Jendresen, M.: Observations on the discoloration of low-fusing porcelain, J. Calif. Dent. Assoc. **31**:44-49, 1977.

Lundeen, H.C.: Introduction to occlusal anatomy, Lexington, Ky., 1969.

Mabie, C.P., Jr.: Petrographic study of the refractory performance of high-fusing dental alloy investments. I. High-firec, phosphate-bonded investments, J. Dent. Res. **52**(1):96-110, 1973.

Meyer, F.S.: Can the plane line articulator meet all the demands of balanced and functional occlusion in all restorative work? Colo. State Dent. Assoc. J. **17**:6-16, 1938.

Phillips, R.W.: Skinner's science of dental materials, ed. 7, Philadelphia, 1973, W.B. Saunders Co.

Smith, D.E., and Potter, H.R.: The pontic in fixed bridgework, Dent. Digest **43**:16-20, Jan., 1937.

Stade, E.H., Reisbick, M.H., and Preston, J.D.: Preceramic and postceramic solder joints, J. Prosthet. Dent. **34**:527-532, Nov., 1975.

Staffanou, R.: Personal communication, 1977.

Stuart, C.E.: Good occlusion for natural teeth, J. Prosthet. Dent. **14**:716-724, 1964.

Thomas, P.K.: Syllabus on full mouth waxing technique for rehabilitation, San Diego, 1967, Instant Printing Service.

Tylman, S.D., and Malone, W.F.P.: Tylman's theory and practice of fixed prosthodontics, ed. 7, St. Louis, 1978, The C.V. Mosby Co.

CHAPTER 8

COLOR IN CERAMICS

ROBERT C. SPROULL

Ontogeny recapitulates phylogeny; the evolutionary stages of the development of the individual repeats racial history. In a way, this principle can be applied to our grasp of color. Just as our understanding of color slowly evolves as we learn to think and to talk, the human race has ever so slowly added to its comprehension of this complex phenomenon. Misconceptions abound. Color is both subjective and objective, and erroneous conclusions have confused the human race for thousands of years and can confuse an individual for a lifetime, (Sproull, 1973 and 1974).

DEVELOPMENT OF COLOR CONCEPTS

Primitive humans started without so much as the names for the various hues; they had no one to teach them and no references to study. How long was it before they became conscious of color differences? How long before these were named? An interesting study of primitive societies by Berlin and Kay (1969) showed marked similarity in how color terms evolved in such groups. In all the societies they studied, colors were first divided into two groups—black and white (Stage I). With a little more sophistication a third color was distinguished—always red (Stage II). The fourth color named was either green (Stage IIIa) or yellow (Stage IIIb) and, by the time five colors were named, they were always black, white, red, green, and yellow (Stage IV). From there, words for purple, pink, orange, and gray were developed (Stage VII). Berlin and Kay linked the "technological/cultural complexity" of cultures to the stages in the evolution of these basic color terms.

In 1858, William Gladstone (later prime minister of England) studied the color terminology of the ancient Greek literature of Homer's *Iliad* and the *Epic of Gilgamesh* (Kuehni, 1981). He concluded that the "organs of color impressions were but partially developed among the Greeks of the heroic age" because of the scarcity and limited number of color terms. Based on Berlin and Kay's study, a more likely explanation is that these ancient Greeks were in a stage where words for full color expression had not developed.

Aristotle (327-287 BC) gave considerable thought to color; based on the variety of color terms used in his writings, the Greeks of his time had entered Berlin and Kay's Stage VII of cultural development. In *De Sensu et Sensibili* he set down his general color theory and in *Meteorologica* he wrote of his rainbow color or spectral theory of color (Parkhurst and Feller, 1982). In *De Sensu* he arranged color in a linear scale with white at one end and black at the other; yellow, red, violet, green, blue, and gray lay between. These seven steps gave a fixed value of lightness/darkness to each of the colors and were used for centuries by artists to signify lightness (red), darkness (blue), and gradations between. The color circle and three-dimensional color solids can trace their ancestry to this linear scale, though admittedly it is a tortuous and ill-defined family tree.

In his *Meteorologica*, Aristotle spawned a mistaken concept that took over 2100 years to correct. In discussing the theory of the colors in the rainbow he states that there are three—red, green, and blue (the additive light primaries). From these three all others are formed by mixing. This is a remarkable insight written over 2300 years ago! His error was in then stating that these

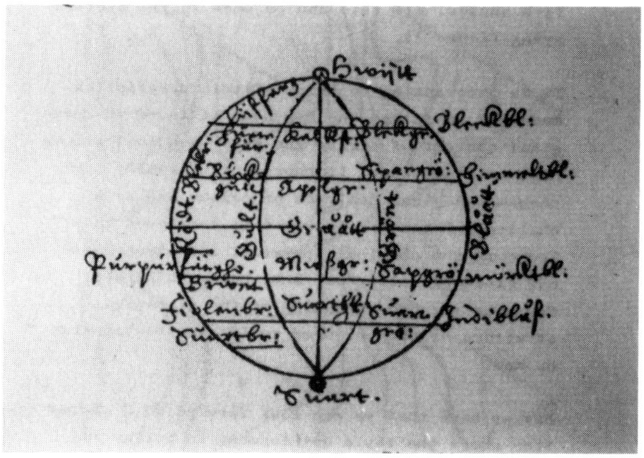

Fig. 8-1. Color sphere of Sigfrid Forsius, 1611.

were also the primary colors for artists and their pigments (subtractive primaries). Since anything Aristotle wrote was not questioned (and if he didn't write it and it couldn't be felt, heard, or seen with the unaided senses, it didn't exist) the confusion was perpetuated through the Renaissance and into the nineteenth century (MacAdam, 1983; Parkhurst and Feller, 1982).

The struggle to understand color through the ages is important for today's dentists and dental technicians, not from the standpoint of how our concepts developed, but from the knowledge available to us today of how to work with color. Color was recognized as a three-dimensional entity as early as the thirteenth century; a graphic depiction of a three-dimensional color sphere (published by Swedish Engineer Sigfrid Forsius in 1611) (Fig. 8-1) has survived to this date (Feller and Stenius, 1970). It is that three-dimensional quality of color that is an important key to successful manipulation of color in the twentieth century.

ESTHETIC RESTORATION

Color in everyday life

Color is playing an ever more important role in our lives. Today's patients are becoming more sophisticated in their ability to evaluate colors and whether they match. Books such as Carole Jackson's best selling *Color Me Beautiful* have sent hundreds of thousands of women into the marketplace with their personalized color swatches attuned to their skin, hair, and eye colors as they shop for clothes and accessories. The ability to perceive color differences is a skill that becomes better with practice and training, and the women with their swatches do have that! Recently the same author published *Color for Men.*

We must accept the fact that we are living in a society that is daily bombarded with idealized perfection of the body. Whether on television, in movies, in magazines, in newspapers, or on billboards, the constant message is there. It is small wonder that the demands for restorations to complement a photogenic smile are increasing, that the standards are getting ever higher.

Color in dentistry

Choosing or adjusting a color for a ceramic restoration requires a judgment call. The ability to make that judgment call depends upon the ability of the dentist or dental ceramist to analyze the differences seen and to know in which direction an adjustment needs to be made. This is possible because color *is* a three-dimensional phenomenon. A ceramic restoration or a tab from a shade guide, when compared to a tooth to be matched, can be more red or more yellow than the tooth, can be more saturated in color or less saturated, and can be darker or lighter. These are the ways colors can differ.

E. Bruce Clark first alerted dentistry to the importance of the dimensions of color in 1931 when he wrote: "In the study of color not only is an intimate acquaintance with its three dimensions the first requisite, but it is, without exception, the most important (Clark, 1931). This strong, positive statement was so completely ignored by the profession that in 1973 Dr. Clark felt that this concept was "an old horse that has been dead for 40 years." It is not dead and it is as valid today as it was in 1931.

A correct color match is admittedly just one of the essentials in creating an esthetic restoration (Eissmann et al., 1980; Goldstein, 1976; Sproull, 1973; Yamada, 1977). Outline form, surface anatomy, real and/or apparent translucency, texture, function, alignment, and other factors share in the total effect. And just as the total esthetic effect is composed of many elements, a correct color match is also a compound phenomenon. Visual response functions of the individual, the quality and quantity of the viewing lights, metamerism, the color of the surround, and past experiences are among those elements that enter into that correct color match (Beck, 1972; Billmeyer and Saltzman, 1981; Boynton, 1979; Burnham, 1963; Committee on Colorimetry, 1966; Evans, 1948; Frisby, 1980; Gregory, 1970; Hurvich, 1981; Keuhni, 1983; Verity, 1980; Yamada, 1977). This chapter will not discuss such elements of color matching but will be restricted to the perception of color as a three-dimensional phenomenon and how this information relates to practical color matching of dental restorations.

MUNSELL COLOR ORDER SYSTEM

The Munsell Color Order System is one of the many that can be used to organize our thoughts on color (Luke, 1980). It is not a perfect system, but then nei-

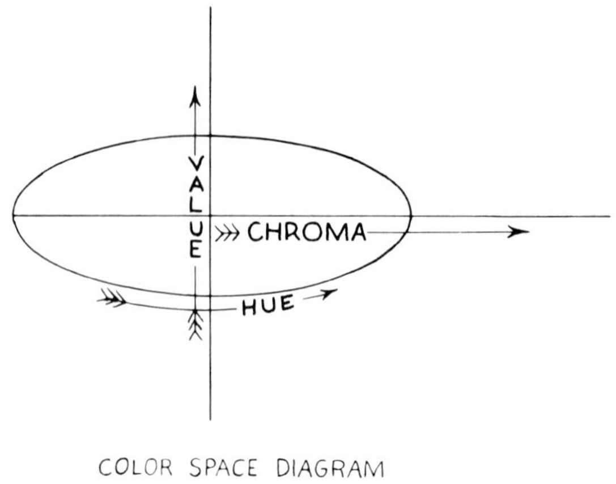

Fig. 8-2. Munsell color space diagram.

thei is any of the others. It was organized with the goal of creating equal perceptual steps from one color to another in whichever dimension of color one travels (Birren, 1969; MacAdams, 1983). It demonstrates good distribution when dealing with small color differences; it is noticeably uneven for large color steps. In dentistry we are working within its area of strength. For this reason and the fact that it is universally recognized, consistent, flexible, and easily learned, it is recommended as a starting point in gaining familiarity with color (Sproull, 1973).

Once the basic three-dimensional nature of color is understood, the dentist and the dental technician have the foundation to logically approach a color matching problem, *but not until then.*

The names of the dimensions of color in the Munsell Color Order System are hue, value, and chroma. The names of the dimensions vary from one color system to another, but not the dimensions themselves. Color can vary in color family, lightness/darkness, and purity or strength. This is the basis of the organization of three-dimensional color order systems (Billmeyer, 1981).

"Hue" presents not much of a problem, as we live with and understand color families. It refers to the distinct colors of the rainbow, the different colors of the color wheel, the difference between a red and a green and a blue (Billmeyer, 1981; Goldstein, 1976; Munsell, 1946; Sproull, 1973).

Fig. 8-2 is a diagrammatic representation of the relationship of hue, value, and chroma in the Munsell system. Plate 1 is a picture of the three-dimensional Munsell color tree. Each clear plastic leaf contains a single hue. The differences seen on any one leaf are value and chroma differences, not hue differences.

Value and chroma are the dimensions that cause problems: too often they are confused, making a correct evaluation of observed color differences an impossibility (Billmeyer, 1981; Goldstein, 1976; Munsell, 1946; Sproull, 1973).

"Value" refers to the lightness/darkness of a color and to no other quality. (It does *not* refer to the amount of gray in a color.) In the Munsell three-dimensional solid (the color tree) there is an achromatic (colorless) axis or trunk, extending vertically through the color solid. (See Plate 1.) Black, at the bottom, is assigned a value of 0; white, at the top, is assigned a value of 10; nine value levels ascend through the color solid. Value is the only dimension that can exist alone—it has no nue or chroma. Values are what we see on a black and white television set. The original scene on such a set has colors in three dimensions of hue, value, and chroma; only the values of the colors come through. The value of any color can be determined by how light or dark it would transmit on such a black and white television.

Values can be determined clinically by squinting the eyes and cutting down the amount of light reaching the retina. The scotopic vision of the rods (for dim lighting) then takes over. The rods transmit only a gray or white signal (Hurvich, 1981), as does the black and white television. This rod mechanism is fortunate, because it gives a means of determining with some degree of certainty the dimension of value—it is a starting point (Plates 2 and 3).

Chroma is the dimension that describes the strength or purity of a color. It describes the increased strength of the colors, at any given value level, as they depart from the central achromatic (value) axis that runs through the center of the color tree. On a Munsell chart (Plate 4), any of the colors in a given vertical row have the same chroma; the differences seen are those of value. Any of the colors in a given horizontal row have the same value; the differences seen here are those of chroma. In chroma, the amount of gray (an achromatic diluent) *is* important: the more gray, the weaker the chroma!

The identification of any color in the Munsell system is positive and can be understood worldwide. The Munsell notation places hue (H) to the left, value (V) next, and chroma (C) last—value and chroma are separated by a slash mark: H V/C. Each of the ten hues in the system is divided into ten subdivisions and a letter is used to designate the hue being identified. A middle red (R) (halfway between yellow red and red purple) would be 5R. The most saturated red in Plate 4 (at value 4 and chroma 14) would be identified as 5R 4/14. Every color in the system can thus be identified.

Many are already familiar with these concepts. For those wishing a more complete explanation, the references listed at the end of this chapter are excellent sources. At the risk of being overly repetitious: If the

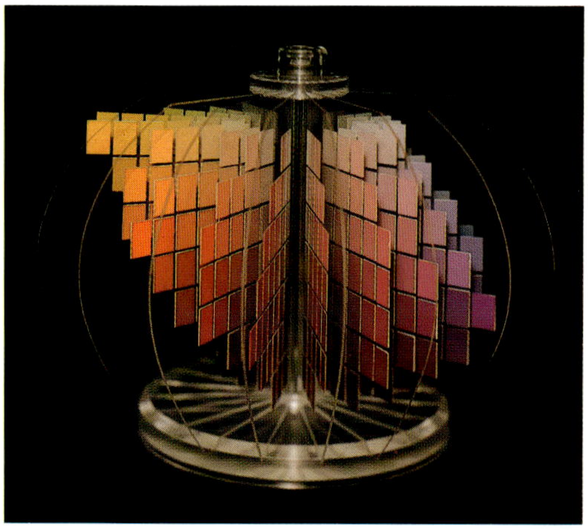

Plate 1. Munsell color tree.

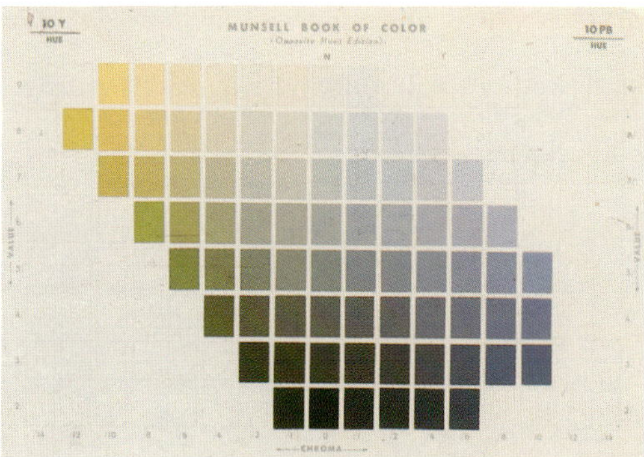

Plate 2. Yellow and purple blue pages of the Munsell Book of Color.

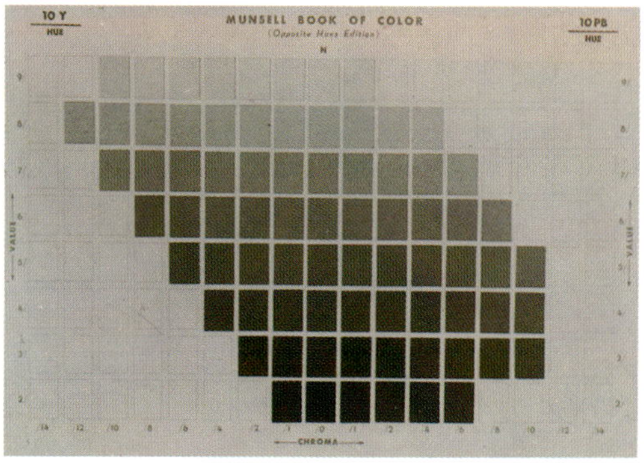

Plate 3. Yellow and purple blue pages of the Munsell Book of Color in a black and white photograph. This is similar to the effect obtained by squinting the eyes and going to rod vision.

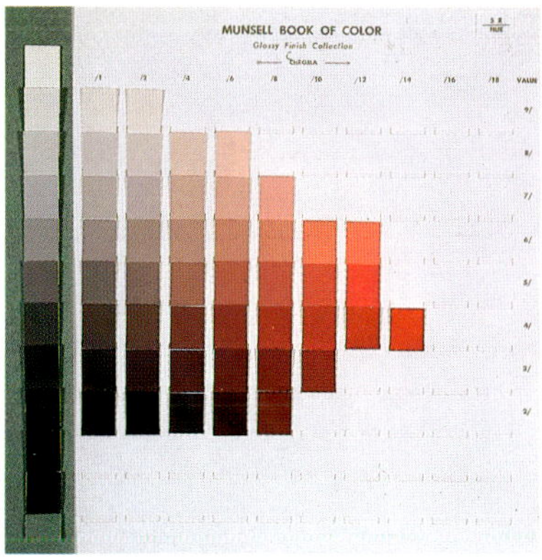

Plate 4. 5R page of the Munsell Book of Color. The achromatic value axis is shown to the left.

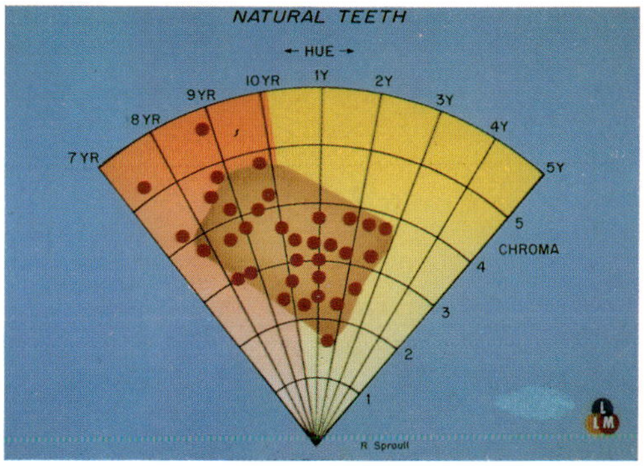

Plate 5. Hue-chroma plots of a spectrophotometric study of a series of natural teeth. The brown area indicates the range of most natural teeth. (Courtesy Dr. Lloyd L. Miller.)

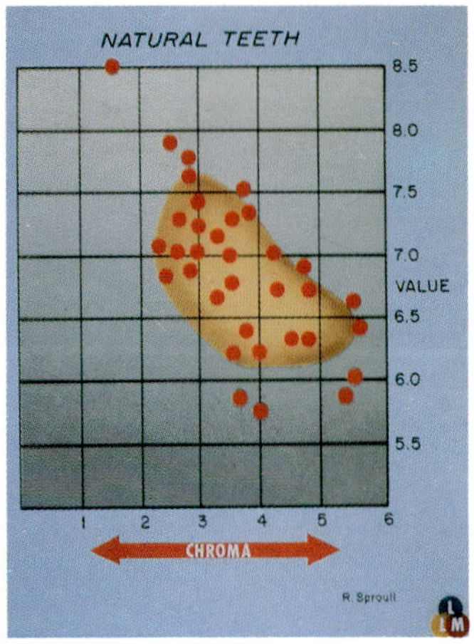

Plate 6. Value-chroma plots of a spectrophotometric study of a series of natural teeth. The brown area indicates the range of most natural teeth. (Courtesy Dr. Lloyd L. Miller.)

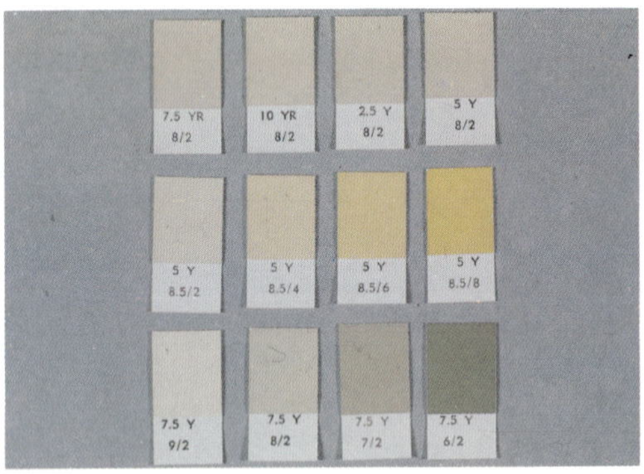

Plate 7. Hue, chroma, and value differences as shown by Munsell tabs from the Munsell Book of Color.

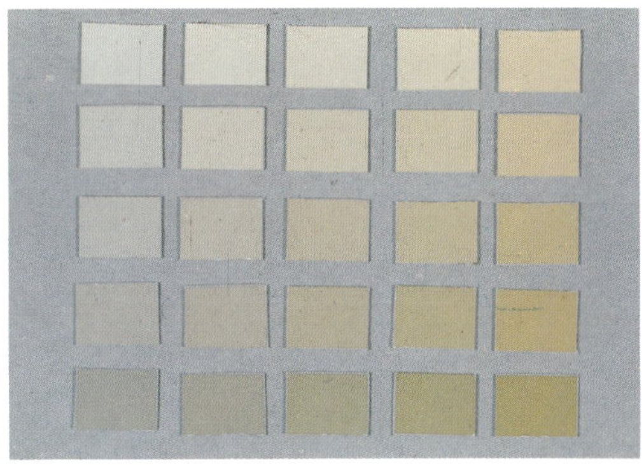

Plate 8. Depiction of a page from the "ideal" guide by Hayashi.

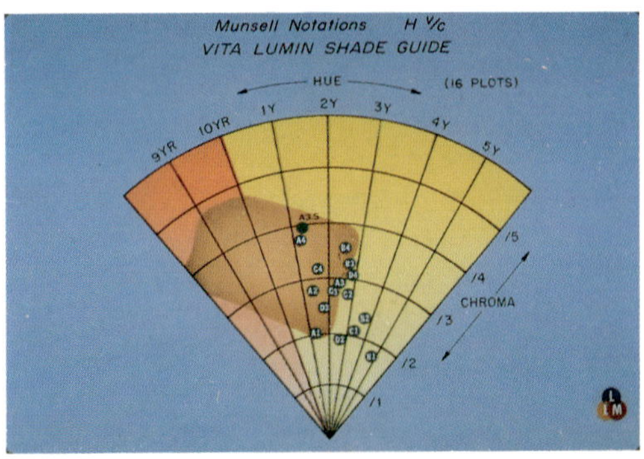

Plate 9. Hue-chroma range of the Vita Lumin shade guide. The brown area indicates the range of most natural teeth. (Courtesy Dr. Lloyd L. Miller.)

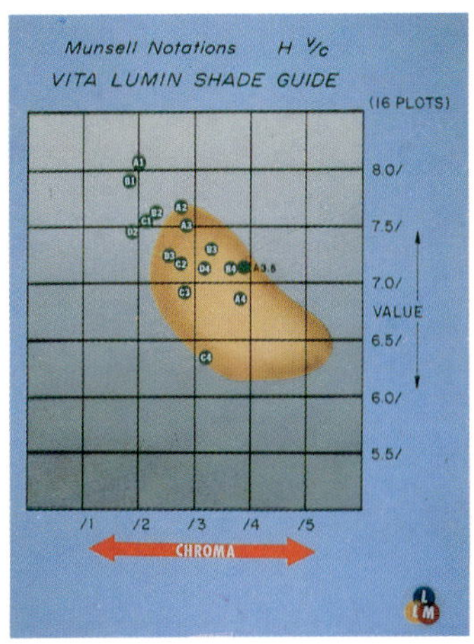

Plate 10. Value-chroma range of the Vita Lumin shade guide. The brown area indicates the range of most natural teeth. (Courtesy Dr. Lloyd L. Miller.)

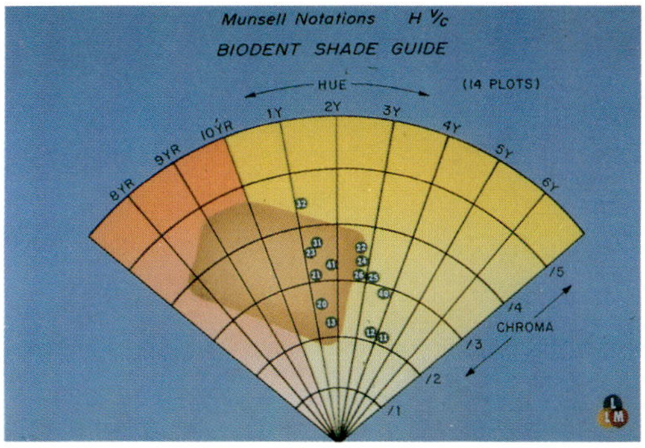

Plate 11. Hue-chroma range of the Biodent shade guide. The brown area indicates the range of most natural teeth. (Courtesy Dr. Lloyd L. Miller.)

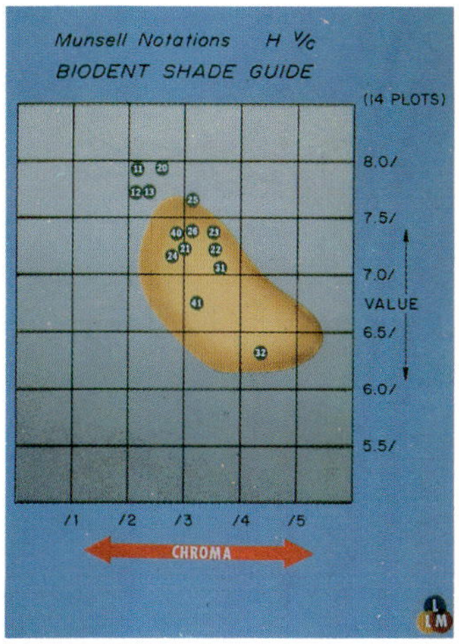

Plate 12. Value-chroma range of the Biodent shade guide. The brown area indicates the range of most natural teeth. (Courtesy Dr. Lloyd L. Miller.)

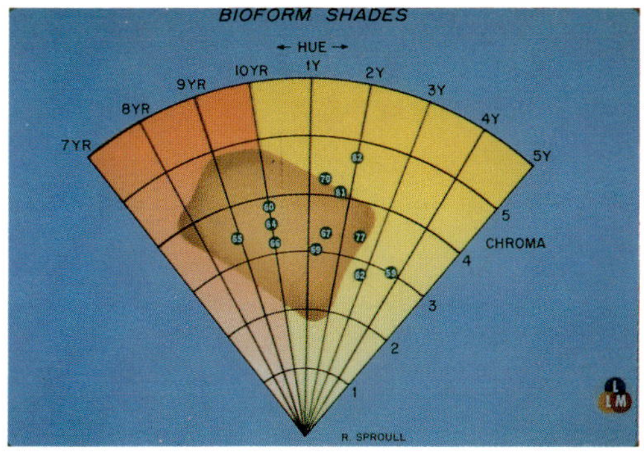

Plate 13. Hue-chroma range of the Bioform shade guide. The brown area indicates the range of most natural teeth. (Courtesy Dr. Lloyd L. Miller.)

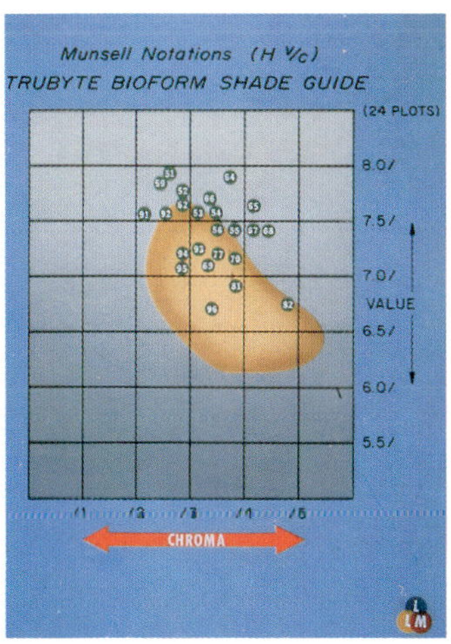

Plate 14. Value-chroma range of the bioform shade guide. The brown area indicates the range of most natural teeth. (Courtesy Dr. Lloyd L. Miller.)

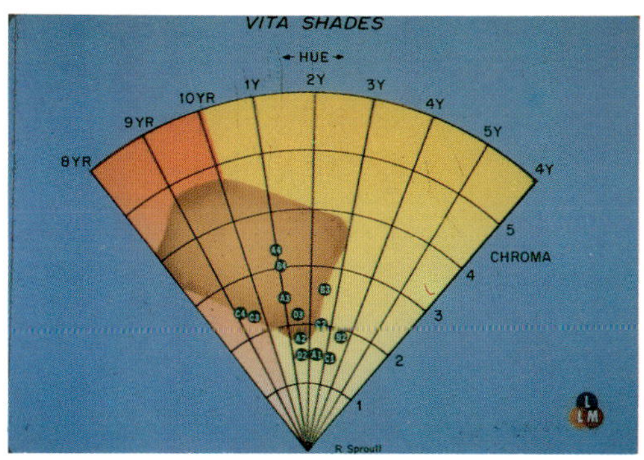

Plate 15. Hue-chroma range of the Vita shade guide. The brown area indicates the range of most natural teeth. (Courtesy Dr. Lloyd L. Miller.)

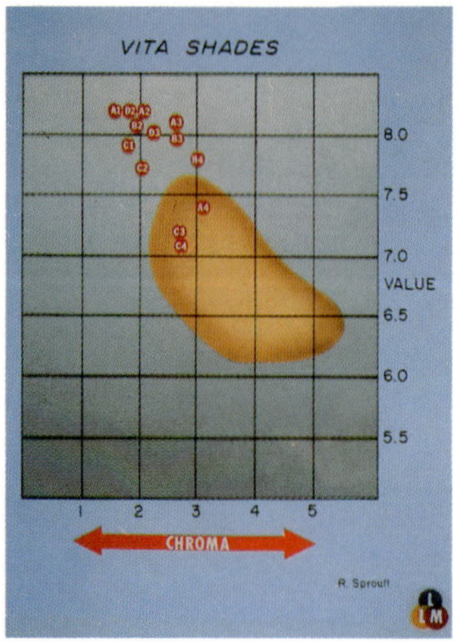

Plate 16. Value-chroma range of the Vita shade guide. The brown area indicates the range of most natural teeth. (Courtesy Dr. Lloyd L. Miller.)

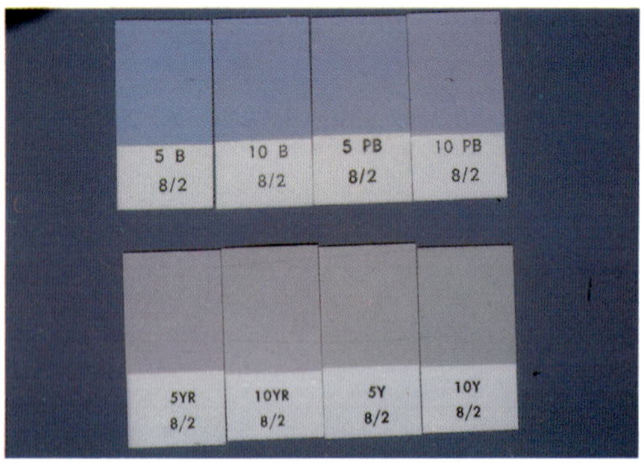

Plate 17. High value–weak chroma range of natural teeth and the high value–weak chroma complementary hues.

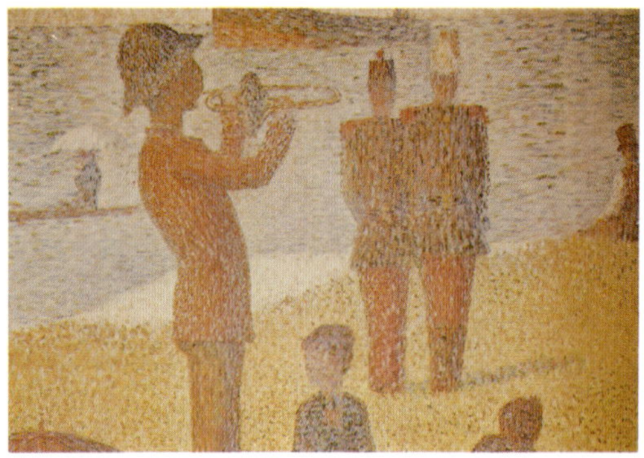

Plate 18. Pointillist art.

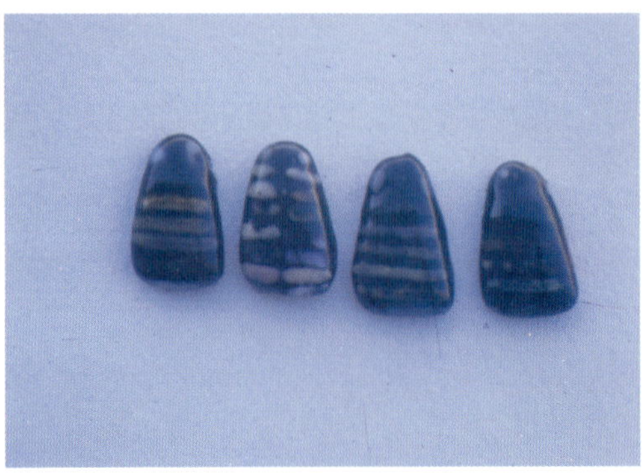

Plate 19. Porcelain stains fired on black porcelain chips. (From Sproull, 1979)

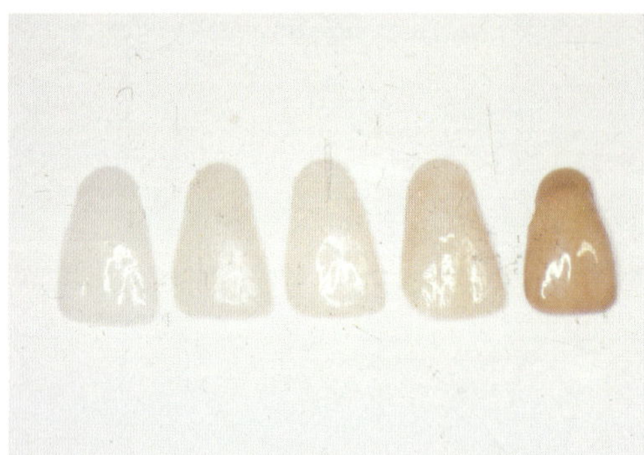

Plate 20. Effects of a single dark gingival stain varying from light application on the left to increasingly heavy applications to the right. The extreme right chip was fired several times.

concepts are not understood by an individual, logical color matching is not yet possible for that individual.

Shade guides

In choosing the color for a restoration, a shade guide is used. A more correct term would be a color standard; in color literature, "shade" can have at least seven different meanings (Little, 1969). In deference to common usage, shade guide will be used.

The inaccuracy in the name of the shade guides is less a problem than the guides themselves; they have historically been a weak link in an orderly approach to color matching in dentistry. The colors of shade guides, from a given manufacturer, vary from guide to guide. The porcelain for the guide is not necessarily the same as the porcelain used for the restoration. The guides do not duplicate the manner in which porcelain restorations must be constructed (thickness of opaque, thickness of body and incisal porcelain, metal bonding, etc.). The colors of the guides are illogically arranged and do not cover the volume of color space of the natural teeth.

In an earlier publication (Sproull, 1973) the prime requirements of a shade guide were listed as (1) a logical arrangement in color space and (2) an adequate distribution in color space. These requirements are still valid and, for the most part, unmet. A description of an ideal shade guide and how it could be used will illustrate the advantages of such a system.

An ideal shade guide

A shade guide based on the three-dimensional Munsell Color Order System would be a boon to dentistry and to the color matching of ceramometal restorations. In the Munsell system the relationship of any of the color chips to the chips surrounding it is instantly known by geographic location. If the achromatic axis is to the left, any color chip to the right will be more saturated in color, i.e., have a higher chroma. Any chip to the left will have a weaker chroma. Any chip above will be higher in value, and any chip below will be lower in value. Chips on the same level will be equal in value. Hue changes are predictable from the location ahead of or behind the chip on the hue circle.

As stated earlier, choosing the color for a ceramometal restoration requires a judgment call. In comparing a shade guide tab with a tooth, differences in hue, value, and chroma must be determined. If the value of the tab is too low, and the shade guide is arranged according to the Munsell Color Order System, all the tabs at or below the value level of the tab being used can be eliminated from consideration. Likewise, if the chroma is too strong, all tabs of that strength and stronger can be eliminated. If the hue is more yellow than that of the tooth, only tabs in the red direction of the hue circle will need to be considered. It is obvious that such a rational approach is impossible with shade guides in general use.

A look at the color space of natural teeth, as determined by spectrophotometric analysis,* will help in designing that ideal guide. Plates 5 and 6 show the hue, value, and chroma range of one such study (Sproull, 1973). They can be oriented by referring to the diagram of Munsell color space in Fig. 8-2.

One solution to a Munsell-based shade guide is diagrammed in Figs. 8-3 and 8-4. Fig. 8-3 (looking down at a segment of the color solid in the 7YR to 4Y hue range) shows a horizontal cut through the solid. Equally spaced dots indicate shade guide tabs at hues of 8.75YR, 10YR, 1.25Y, 215Y, and 3.75Y (1.25 step intervals), and chromas of 1, 2, 3, 4, and 5 (1 step intervals). Fig. 8-4 shows a vertical cut through the color solid at the position of the 8.75YR shade guide tabs. Values range from 6 to 8 in half-step intervals; the chromas repeat the steps seen in the horizontal cut. There would be similar vertical cuts through each of the five hues listed above. If porcelain tabs were available for each of the designated positions, a shade guide of 125 tabs would be available. Such a guide would cover the volume of color space of natural teeth in an orderly manner. Fig. 8-5 shows how such a guide could resemble the pages of a book.

A guide with 125 tabs instantly strikes one as an unwieldy, cumbersome, and unmanageable monster. If arranged (or disarranged) in the manner of guides in general use this would indeed be true. The key is the orderly arrangement according to hue, value, and chroma. The approach used with such a guide would enable the user to swiftly arrive at the closest color match available with the assurance that the correct tab had been chosen.

The user would first determine the value of the tooth to be matched. By squinting, stimulating the rods and not the cones, the value level of the tooth can be ascertained with some degree of accuracy. Once a tentative value level is chosen, the shade guide tabs remaining as candidates have been reduced from 125 to 25; five chroma steps on the five hue pages at the chosen value level.

Next a tentative hue is chosen. If the cuspids are present, their stronger chroma usually offers a good clue to the hue of the remaining teeth (Plate 7). The shade guide tabs to be considered have now been reduced from 25 to 5 the five chroma steps at the tentative value level of the tentative hue.

The chroma that looks most compatible with the

*Dr. Henry Hemmendinger, Belvedere, N.J.

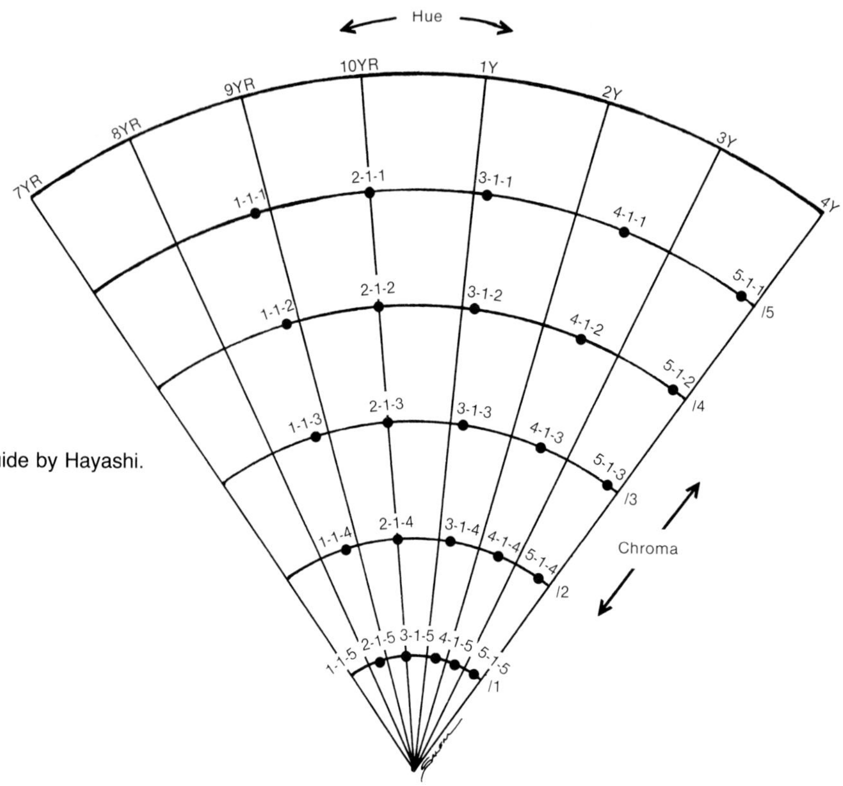

Fig. 8-3. Hue-chroma plots of an "ideal" shade guide by Hayashi.

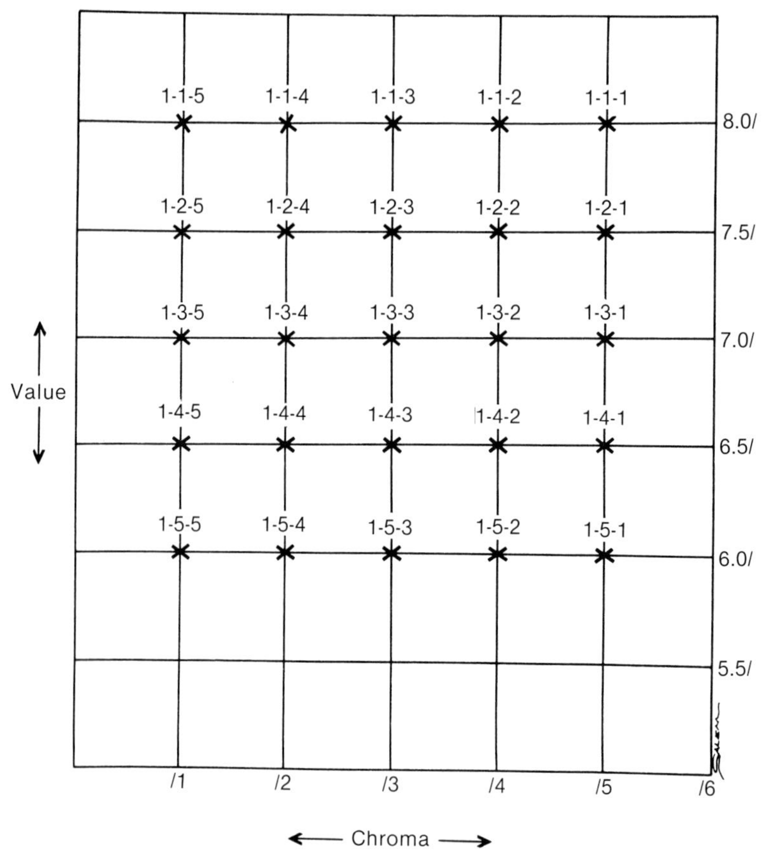

Fig. 8-4. Value-chroma plots of an "ideal" shade guide by Hayashi.

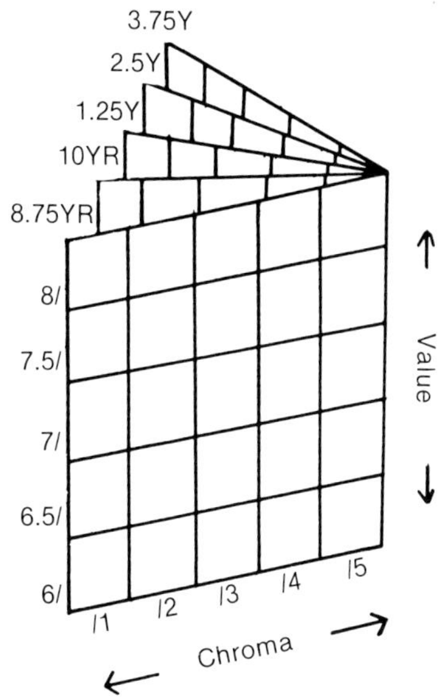

Fig. 8-5. Depiction of Hayashi's "ideal" shade guide as a book.

tooth to be matched is then identified. If differences are still evident, the user would probe in three-dimensional space to determine if a better match is available. The tab above will be lighter (higher in value); the tab below will be darker (lower in value); the tab to the right will be more saturated (higher in chroma); the tab to the left will be less saturated (lower in chroma) (Plate 8); the tab on the page ahead will be redder; the tab on the page behind will be yellower. Once such procedures were mastered, the choice of the closest match would be rapid and it would be accurate (Goldstein, 1976; Sproull, 1973).

In such a system the numbers of tabs could be doubled and the only result would be a more accurate choice, not an increase in time involved. Practicality dictates that the manufacturers of porcelain are not going to give the profession 125 tabs, let alone 250. The inadequacy of the guides in general use have been documented since 1973, with little noticeable reaction from the manufacturers (Sproull, 1973).

The theoretic shade guide is one with existing blueprints. Dr. Toshio Hayashi published such a guide in Japan in 1967. The guide is printed on paper. Metameric and specular differences between paper, porcelain, and teeth do not permit its use as an actual guide. The guide would need to be converted to porcelain, and the porcelain would need to be commercially available for ceramic restorations.

Additional spectrophotometric measurements of natural teeth by Dr. LLoyd Miller (1984) have refined this volume of color space of natural teeth, and the limits of Hayahsi's blueprint would need to be adjusted to reflect these measurements. A spectrophotometer (DCM-1000) being developed is programmed to be able to get spectrophotometric readings of teeth in vivo by means of a fiberoptic system (O'Brien, 1983). Data from such readings need to be compared to those obtained on extracted teeth. If it were found that vital pulpal tissues establish a different volume of color space, further adustments would be necessary.

Some of the tabs are in areas not needed to cover the volume of color space of the natural teeth. These could be eliminated.

Since there is an orderly gradation of colors from one tab to another, the number of porcelain colors needed could be reduced. Porcelain colors could be interpolated from formulas to match the tabs for which a specific porcelain did not exist. This was the system used by Dr. Clark for a similar guide system developed in the 1930s in porcelain.

Use of existing shade guides

The foregoing paragraphs describe the approach with an idealized shade guide. Although the guide does not exist, the general approach is still applicable. In any color-matching procedure, the dimensions of color must be analyzed before appropriate action can be taken. With the idealized guide described, the evaluation is made much simpler since the tentative choice can be rapidly checked for accuracy. With illogically arranged guides, this does present a problem (Plates 9 to 16).

IDENTIFYING THE HUE

With available guides, not too many choices of colors are offered. If the guide is arranged by color families, one can try to identify the hue. In the high-value, weak-chroma range of most natural teeth, this can be difficult (Plate 17), but it can also be an advantage. Hue differences in this volume of color space are least likely to be noticed. Also, if it is difficult for the dentist to see the differences in hue, it will be difficult for the patient as well. As discussed in the exercise with the ideal shade guide, the cuspids are many times the best clue to the correct hue. The higher the chroma, the easier it is to identify the hue.

IDENTIFYING THE VALUE

The most noticable and objectionable difference to the patient will be a difference in value. Fortunately, this is the dimension of color that is easiest to determine. By squinting, switching to scotopic rod vision, the optic system is converted to the equivalent of a black and white TV receiver that will show differences in value without the overlaying confusion of hue and chroma. Plate 7 shows a series of tabs from the Munsell Book of Color. The top row shows only hue differences in 2½-step increments. The middle row shows only chroma differences in two-step increments. The bottom row shows only value differences in one-step increments. This a good place to practice the squinting procedure, since the value of all tabs is known.

With available shade guides, the relative values of the tabs would need to be determined, and those tabs with acceptable values in the correct range of hue would be considered.

IDENTIFYING THE CHROMA

Once the approximate hue and value have been determined, the remaining difference seen will be that of chroma. If the individual attempting to analyze these color differences is confused as to what constitutes value and what constitutes chroma, the process breaks down. If a stronger chroma than needed is mistaken for a value difference, the chances for an eventual color match is destroyed. Value differences are most objectionable and must be identified, but chroma differences can also be deadly. The rule of survival in this choice is to choose a shade higher in value and weaker in chroma than the tooth to be matched. The reasons for this will be discussed in the section dealing with the rules of color mixing.

Part of the difficulty that arises from attempting to pick a workable color with current guides lies in the inability to logically zero in on the best available choice. If the color chosen leaves doubts, where is the next closest shade guide tab? Geographic location on the guide is not necessarily a clue. Until adequate shade guide–porcelain systems become available, the dentist and dental laboratory technician must learn to survive with what is available. The beautiful simplicity of zeroing in on the correct choice that would be possible with a well-ordered guide does not exist. This does not negate the importance of the ability to analyze differences in the dimensions of color—it makes such ability imperative!

ADJUSTING THE APPEARANCE OF THE RESTORATION

Practical considerations

Seldom will a shade guide tab be found to match the natural teeth without a modification of the ceramic restoration with mineral porcelain color modifiers or stains. With these modifiers the dentist and dental ceramist have the tools to manipulate the dimension(s) of color needing correction. Numerous kits are available (Preston and Bergen, 1980).

Internal staining or modification is possible, but the economics involved with remakes if the staining is incorrect is a factor that must be considered. This has to be tied into the fees received for the restorations by the dentist and the dental laboratory. (If the restoration must be stripped and rebaked, the laboratory should be paid for the additional work involved.) If the fees are sufficient to cover the cost of potential remakes, it is practical; if the fees are not sufficient, it is not. It is a decision the individual dentist must make. Quality results are possible using only external modifications but, once again, this is directly related to familiarity with the dimensions of color.

Refining the final outline form, surface anatomy, occlusion, etc. of a restoration is a "laboratory procedure" that must be carried out in the mouth of the patient. Attempts to carry this out in the dental laboratory with the patient not present will disappoint the discriminating dentist and patient (and dental ceramist, who may see his work in the mouth of the patient at a later date).

Final color modification of the restoration is likewise a "laboratory procedure" that requires the patient to be seated in the dental chair for ready reference. To expect the dental ceramist, located in a separate facility, to be able to match the patient's natural teeth is unrealistic. Treatments such as those involving a complete quadrant of posterior teeth or all of the maxillary or mandibular incisors (and/or cuspids) may have some chance for success, assuming that the restorations have been finessed in the mouth by the dentist. To place restorations on additional teeth to cover up inadequate color matching techniques is a gross dereliction of responsibility on the part of the dentist.

Treatments involving an individual anterior restoration, or an easily seen posterior restoration, present situations that frankly are not amenable to final color modification in a distant dental laboratory. How can the correct information be transmitted to the dental ceramist? Color photographs are notoriously inaccurate in conveying the true colors of the natural teeth. Even the dentist and the dental ceramist completely conversant in color language would find it most difficult to communicate all the nuances the human eye can perceive.

The dentist can meet the responsibilities in color matching in several ways. One is to have an in-house dental ceramist skilled in the art. Economics and space limitations make this a choice not open to all. The most practical situation, in the majority of cases, is for the dentist to have a fast-heating glazing oven in the dental operatory. Color modifications can then be rapidly carried out with the patient available for instant color reference. Preston and Bergen list the various "stain" kits available and give excellent step-by-step instructions on how to apply the stains and how to properly use a glazing oven (1980).

Modifying the color of a restoration is not a haphazard application of stains in the hope that one of them will be right. It is a matter of planned color manipulation.

It was mentioned earlier that the rule of survival in choosing a shade was to be certain that it was higher in value and weaker in chroma than the natural teeth to be matched. Once the principles involved are understood, the reasons for such a choice becomes clear.

Laws of color mixing*

Additive and subtractive mixing

Color mixing follows certain laws. It is not the purpose of this section to pursue this matter in depth; however, our actions should be based on an understanding of what is happening. Additive color mixing has as its primary colors red, green, and blue. The principles involve the mixing of lights and the resultant color is always lighter—higher in value—than either of the mixed colors. Mixing any two of the primary colors results in a hue that is the complementary color of the color not used. Thus red and green result in yellow (the complementary of blue), red and blue yield magenta (the complementary of green), and green and blue result in cyan (the complementary of red). These colors—magenta, cyan, and yellow—are the primary colors of subtractive color mixing and are typified in the pigments used by artists. The resultant color of mixing two of the pigment primaries is always darker—lower in value—than either of the mixed pigments. The resultant color is the complementary of the third primary not used. The complementary colors resulting from separately mixing magenta, cyan, and yellow are red, green, and blue (the additive primaries).

The subtractive color system is usually used to explain the results of applying porcelain mineral stains to the surface of a ceramic restoration. The laws of subtractive mixture, however, apply only if the colorants used are transparent. Transparent colorants must be applied to a white or a light background in order to work; if applied to a black background they are invisible (Kuppers, 1973). Testing the available porcelain stains by firing them on black porcelain chips does not reveal any transparent stains; all are easily visible on the black background (Plate 18). It must be concluded that instructions are in error if based on the supposition that the laws of subtractive mixture apply.

Complementary colors

Much emphasis has also been placed on the use of complementary colors in adjusting the hue, value, and chroma of a ceramic restoration. The frustration in attempting to do this can be understood after looking at the facts. It is extremely difficult to identify hue in the high-value, weak-chroma volume of color space in which the teeth lie (Plate 17). If the hue could be identified, a complementary stain would need to be identified. (Remember that this is a difficult exercise for artists working with identified hues of stronger chroma.) What are the chances of correctly identifying the hue of the tooth and its true complementary? If the complementary could be identified, what are the chances that such a mineral stain—of the correct spectrophotometric character—exists? What are the chances of applying the proper amount? Not good at all! The general conclusion must be that, if the color of the restoration requires manipulation of its dimensions by use of complementary stains, the wrong color was initially chosen.

If the laws of subtractive mixture do not apply, the question of what does happen in our correction of the ceramic restorations with mineral stains needs to be resolved. Unfortunately at this time a definitive answer is probably not possible. Research is needed to identify and understand the complex subtractive mixing that occurs. Some clues, based on clinical experience, offer guidelines.

Under the laws of subtractive mixture the value of the restorations will always be lowered as the stains are applied (Kuppers, 1973; Gerritsen, 1974). Since most mineral stains available are lower in value than the porcelain to which they are applied, this is generally true—but not for the reasons given in commercial brochures. Clinically the result most nearly resembles an averaging of the value of the restoration and the stain. If the stain is higher in value than the restoration, the resultant value will be a little higher; if the stain is lower in value than the restoration, the resultant value will be a little lower. How much higher or lower will depend upon the initial difference in values *plus* how heavy an application of stain is used.

Partitive mixing

Partitive color mixing predicts such an averaging of values (Gerritsen, 1974; Kuppers, 1973; Preston and Bergen, 1980). This is the system used by the pointillists in which, on their canvas, they juxtapose tiny dots of color that are too small to be individually resolved by the eye at the correct viewing distance (Plate 19). A combination of additive and subtractive mixing occurs. The small dots act as filters to subtractively remove certain wavelengths of light. The remaining wavelengths are reflected toward the observer where they are additively mixed by the eye. Thus tiny dots of magenta interposed with tiny dots of yellow, if proportioned correctly, are perceived as red. The resultant value will be the average of the value of the magenta and the value of the yellow. (It has not been determined if the parti-

*See Billmeyer, 1981; Burnham, 1963; Gerritsen, 1974; Kuehni, 1983; Kuppers, 1973; Lempire, 1975; Preston, 1980; Verity, 1980; Zakia, 1974.

tive system does or does not apply to our staining of ceramic restorations.)

Rational approach to color modifications

The recommendations to pick a shade higher in value and weaker in chroma than that of the teeth to be matched can now be more readily understood.

Most mineral stains are lower in value than the porcelain to which they are applied. It is logical to pick the desired color at a value level at which most stains will work. It is difficult to raise a value if the stains of the correct hue and chroma are all lower in value.

A chroma that is stronger than the chroma of the natural teeth must be weakened. In the discussion of complementary colors used to accomplish this lessening of chroma, it was pointed out that the chances of success are slim, sometimes nonexistent. If the value is correct and must be maintained, an additional requirement for the elusive complementary stain would be that it be of the same value as the color to be modified. Experience teaches that a chroma that is too strong usually requires the restoration to be remade.

A cookbook step-by-step procedure has not been offered on how to correct the dimensions of color. If the principles discussed in this chapter are understood, the dentist and ceramist have the necessary information to approach this complex problem. An attempt to cover all the variables that can be encountered would be impossible.

After the restoration has been adjusted in the mouth to the correct outline form, surface anatomy, occlusion, and compatibility with the soft tissues, etc., the color correction process begins.

First application of color modifiers

The restoration should be moistened and the general hue, value, and chroma observed. The value should be a little high, the chroma a little weak, and the hue fairly close to that of the natural teeth.

The hue, if different from that of the natural teeth, will either be a little more yellow or a little more red. The mineral stain to modify the restoration will be chosen based on this observation. Firing the different stains on tooth-shaped porcelain chips ahead of time serves as a reference guide and makes the operator more aware of the characteristics of the different stains available.

Once the color family is chosen, an estimate is made of the value change needed. The shade guide should permit a choice of a porcelain only a little higher in value. The chroma change needed must be considered in conjunction with the value change. The needed decrease in value and increase in chroma is a combined operation. Experience is the most important factor in the procedure. The same stain can assume a variety of roles, depending upon how heavily it is applied. A dark gingival stain sparingly applied can produce a very subtle change. The same stain thickly applied over several firings can be overpowering (Plate 20).

After the initial firing of the porcelain stains, the evaluation process is repeated. If a hue modification was necessary, was the change in the right direction? If a value change were required, are the values of the restoration and the natural teeth closer than before as they are viewed through squinted eyes? If the chroma needed strengthening, was the change sufficient? Too much? Too little? This initial firing is invaluable in enabling the dentist or ceramist to judge what additional modifications are needed.

Additional applications of color modifiers

Any second application of porcelain color modifiers is based on the evaluation of the results of the first firing. Modifying the color of the restoration is a repeat of the judgment calls regarding the dimensions of color exercised in picking the initial color with the shade guide and in applying the initial porcelain stains.

As experience is gained, confidence builds. Many times the needed color modification can be obtained in one firing; seldom are more than two or three modifications necessary. The fast-heating porcelain oven makes this a practical procedure in the dental office. Patients appreciate the personal attention their restorations receive, and the restorations are more likely to be an acceptable color match.

Commercial brochures offer helpful hints in characterizing restorations. Their discussions of color theory and means for modifying hues are best ignored.

SUMMARY

One of the best sources of practical information relating to color in ceramics is contained in Preston and Bergen's *Color science and dental art: a self-teaching program* (1980). It is aptly named. By following the text, answering the questions, and carrying out the practical exercises, the fundamentals of color manipulation *will* be understood.

Color is a complex phenomenon, but it need not be feared. Studying the three-dimensional nature of color places the dentist and the ceramist in a position to understand differences in observed colors and how to correct those differences. Hue, value, and chroma are the keys to the world of color as we see it.

REFERENCES

Beck, J.: Surface color perception, Ithaca, N.Y., 1972, Cornell University Press.

Berlin, B., and Kay, P.: Basic color terms, Los Angeles, 1969, University of California Press.

Billmeyer, F.W., Jr., and Saltzman, M.: Principles of color technology, ed 2., New York, 1981, John Wiley & Sons, Inc.

Birren, F., Editor: A grammar of color; a basic treatise on the color system of Albert Munsell, New York, 1969, Van Nostrand Reinhold Co.

Boynton, R.M.: Human color vision, New York, 1979, Holt, Rinehart & Winston.

Burnham, R.W., Hanes, R.M., and Bartleson, C.J.: Color: a guide to basic facts and concepts, New York, 1963, John Wiley & Sons, Inc.

Clark, E.B.: The color problem in dentistry, Dent. Dig. **37:** 6, 1931.

Clark, E.B.: Personal communication, January 29, 1973.

Committee on Colorimetry, Optical Society of America: The science of color, Ann Arbor, Mich., 1966, Edward Brothers, Inc.

Eiseman, L.: Alive with color, Washington, D.C., 1983, Acropolis Books, Ltd.

Eissmann, H.F., Rudd, K.D., and Morrow, R.M.: Dental laboratory procedures, Vol. II. Fixed partial dentures, St. Louis, 1980, The C.V. Mosby Co.

Evans, R.M.: An introduction to color, New York, 1948, John Wiley & Sons, Inc.

Feller, R.L., and Stenius, A.K.: On the color space of Sigfrid Forsius, Color Eng. **8**:48-51, 1970.

Frisby, J.P.: Seeing: illusion, brain and mind, New York, 1980, Oxford University Press.

Gerritsen, F.: Theory and practice of color, New York, 1974, Van Nostrand Reinhold Co.

Gladstone, W.E.: Studies on Homer and the Homeric Age, London, 1858, Oxford University Press.

Goldstein, R.E.: Esthetics in dentistry, Philadelphia, 1976, J. B. Lippincott Co.

Gregory, R.L.: The intelligent eye, New York, 1970, McGraw-Hill Book Co.

Hayashi, T.: Medical color standard, V. Tooth crown, Tokyo, 1967, Japan Color Research Institute.

Hurvich, L.M.: Color vision, Sunderland, Mass., 1981, Sinauer Assoc. Inc.

Jackson, C.: Color for men, New York, 1984, Ballantine Books.

Jackson, C.: Color me beautiful, Washington, D.C., 1980, Acropolis Books, Ltd.

Kuehni, R.G.: Color: essence and logic, New York, 1983, Van Nostrand Reinhold Co.

Kuehni, R.G.: Notes on the color terminology in the Iliad and the Epic of Gilgamesh, Color Res. Appl. **6**:233-236, 1981.

Kuppers, H.: Color: origin systems, uses, London, 1973, Van Nostrand Reinhold Co.

Lemire, P.A., and Burk, B.: Color in dentistry, Hartford, Conn., 1975, The J.M. Ney Co.

Little, A.: Shades of meaning, Color Eng. **7**:10, 1969.

Luke, J.T.: Compromises in color solids, Color Res. Appl. **3**:178-179, 1980.

MacAdam, D.L.: Discovery of the composite nature of white light, Color Res. Appl. **8**:123-124, 1983.

McJimsey, H.T.: Art and fashion in clothing selection, ed 2, Ames, 1973, Iowa State University Press.

Miller, L.L.: Personal communication, December 19, 1984.

Munsell, A.H.: A color notation, Baltimore, 1946, Munsell Color Co.

O'Brien, J.: Personal communication, October 12, 1983.

Parkhurst, C., and Feller, R.L.: Who invented the color wheel? Color Res. Appl. **7**:217-230, 1982.

Preston, J.D., and Bergen, S.F.: Color science and dental art: a self-teaching program, St. Louis, 1980, The C.V. Mosby Co.

Sproull, R.C.: Color matching in dentistry, Part I. The three dimensional nature of color, J. Prosthet. Dent. **29**:416-424, 1973.

Sproull, R.C.: Color matching in dentistry, Part II. Practical applications of the organization of color, J. Prosthet. Dent. **29**:556-566, 1973.

Sproull, R.C.: Color matching in dentistry, Part III. Color control, J. Prosthet Dent. **31**:146-154, 1974.

Verity, E.: Color observed, New York, 1980, Van Nostrand Reinhold Co.

Wyszecki, G., and Stiles, R.S.: Color science, ed 2, New York, 1982, John Wiley & Sons, Inc.

Yamada, H.N.: Dental porcelain: the state of the art—1977, Los Angeles, 1977, University of Southern California School of Dentistry.

Zakia, R.D., and Todd, H.N.: Color primer I and II, Dobbs Ferry, N.Y., 1974, Morgan & Morgan, Inc.

CHAPTER 9

METAL-CERAMIC CROWNS AND FIXED PARTIAL DENTURES

CALVIN S. LAU and HENRY N. YAMADA

A metal-ceramic or porcelain-fused-to-metal restoration consists of an esthetic porcelain veneer and an underlying metal framework. The design of the framework plays a vital role in the ultimate success of this restoration. Strength in restorations of this type, especially those with multiple units, depends greatly on the design of the framework, which should not be compromised. Not only does this foundation provide strength for the restoration and support for the porcelain, but it also contributes to the development of esthetics, contour, and occlusion.

It is important to understand the interrelationship of *strength, esthetics, contour,* and *occlusion.* For example, a framework with a minimal amount of metal and thick layers of porcelain may be too weak to withstand functional forces during a prolonged period. Conversely, a framework that is bulky at the gingival area can result in a completed restoration with an overcontoured axial surface.

Although esthetics may be the primary reason for using a metal-ceramic restoration instead of a complete gold crown, designing and constructing the framework with regard only for esthetic consideration may irreversibly compromise the clinical result. A restoration with an exact shade match is not a laboratory success if a factor under the control of the technician had led to breakage (strength), discolored gingival tissue (contour), or abnormal wear (occlusion).

Therefore it is important to be aware of the various design features necessary to achieve optimum results and consistent quality. It is possible to predict not only whether a metal-ceramic restoration will be esthetic, but also whether it will be physiologically contoured, harmonious in function, and able to withstand normal stresses.

FABRICATION OF FRAMEWORK

Optimum esthetics and strength in a metal-ceramic restoration are present when porcelain forms a relatively uniform layer on the metal framework. It is essential to design the framework to accommodate a nearly uniform layer of porcelain ranging from 1 to 1.5 mm in the completed restoration. Trying to accomplish this in the casting rather than in the wax-up will be either unnecessarily tedious (if the metal requires extensive adjustment) or impossible (if the metal is not thick enough to allow a uniform layer of porcelain).

The most reliable and predictable manner of obtaining a uniform porcelain layer in the wax-up is to start with the finished contours reproduced in wax, that is, the full-contour, wax-up. By starting here, it is simple to gauge accurately the removal of a uniform layer of wax, resulting in a framework that is properly designed to support an esthetic layer of porcelain. This procedure also enables the technician to predict whether or not it is possible to achieve a particular contour in the completed restoration.

This waxing procedure is the cutback technique for wax patterns of metal-ceramic restorations. This technique is especially useful in making multiple unit restorations, which can have critical esthetic considerations. The ceramist, especially, will find this technique of tremendous assistance in fabricating an esthetic restoration.

CUTBACK TECHNIQUE

The step-by-step procedure for fabricating a wax-up of a metal-ceramic restoration is relatively simple. It is important to understand how esthetics and strength play fundamental roles in the framework design.

PROCEDURE

1. Wax the framework to the form of the completed restoration (Fig. 9-1). This full-contour wax-up should duplicate the desired tooth form, axial contours, embrasures, and occlusion. A helpful option is an underlying thermoplastic coping that assures a wax pattern of sufficient thickness for casting. Swage a heated plastic coping disk onto the die, trim it short of the margins, and add wax in the usual manner. Maintaining a minimum thickness is equally important for the strength of the metal framework (Fig. 9-2).

2. Make a facial core of the completed full-contour wax-up with a silicone putty impression material* (Fig. 9-3). This core should include one or two teeth on either side of the wax-up and the opposing teeth (Fig. 9-4).

3. Pour the facial core with plaster or stone to make a permanent three-dimensional record of the wax-up for future reference by the ceramist. The cast shows not only the tooth form and spacing, but also the amount of horizontal and vertical overlap.

4. Section the facial core horizontally at a level immediately apical to the incisal edge with a sharp knife

*Optosil, Unitek Corp., Monrovia, Calif., or equivalent.

A 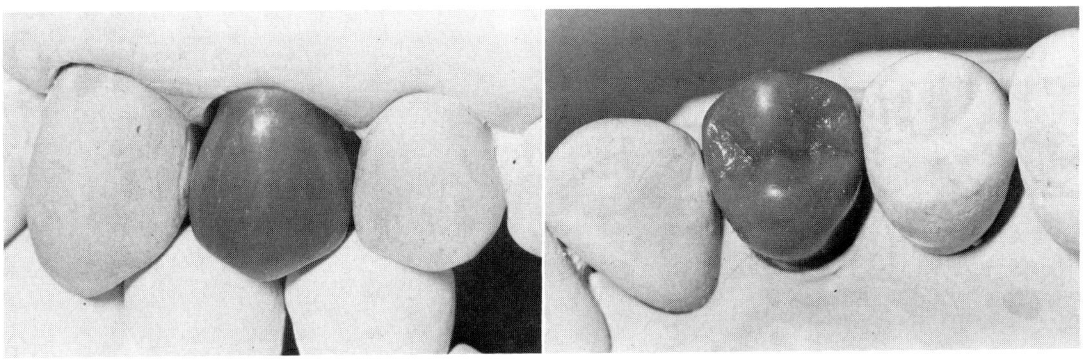 B

Fig. 9-1. Full-contour wax-up of maxillary first premolar. **A,** Facial view. **B,** Occlusal view.

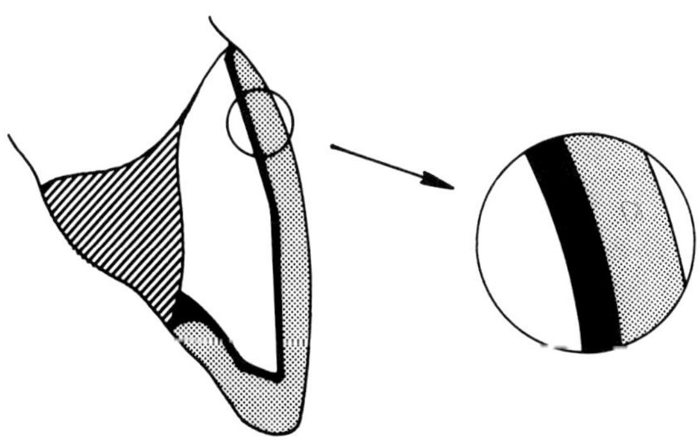

Fig. 9-2. Metal should be at least 0.3 mm thick *(inset).*

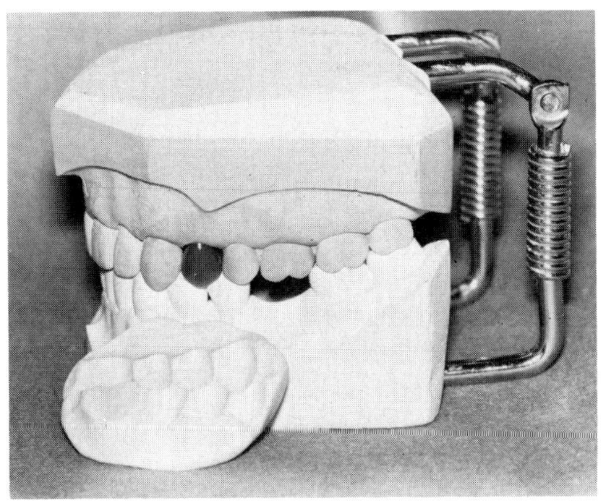

Fig. 9-3. Facial core of single-unit wax-up taken with teeth in occlusion.

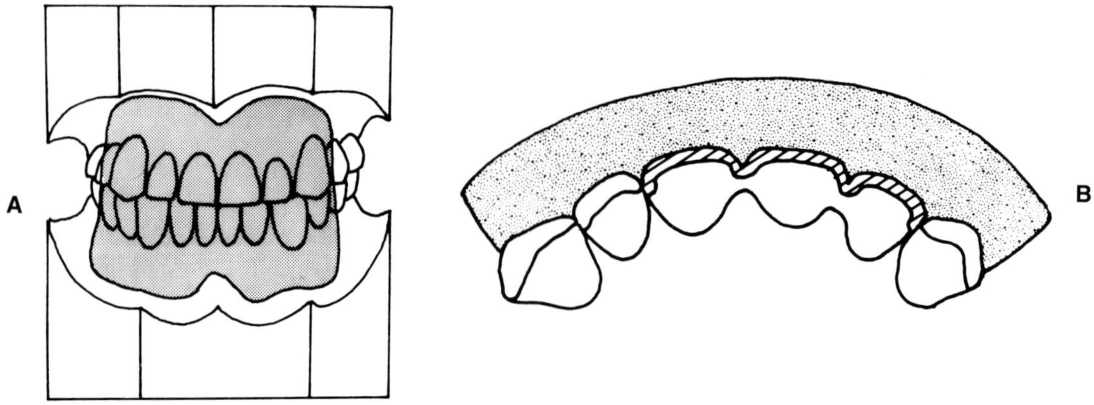

Fig. 9-4. Facial core for anterior wax-up of maxillary right lateral incisor to maxillary left central incisor. **A,** Facial view. **B,** Incisal view, indicating proposed design of framework.

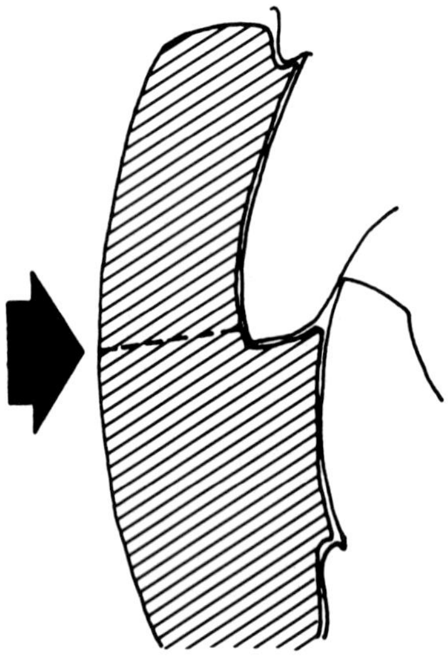

Fig. 9-5. Section core immediately below incisal edge *(arrow).*

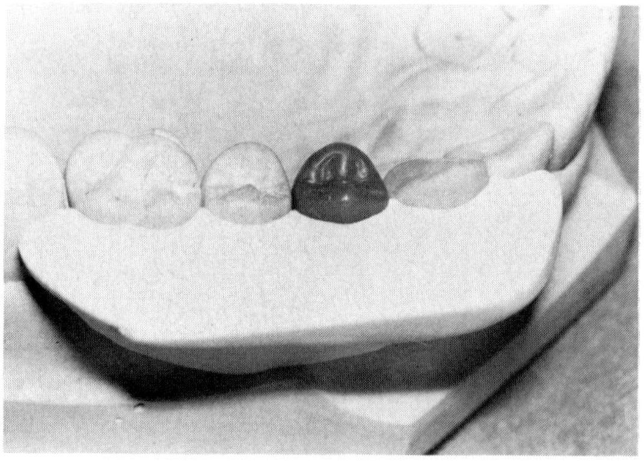

Fig. 9-6. Sectioned core back in place on working cast.

(Fig. 9-5). For a posterior tooth, section the core at the level of the occlusal embrasures (Fig. 9-6).

5. To visually determine whether the wax-up has enough space for both the metal and the porcelain, place the sectioned core on the working cast without the wax-up in place (Fig. 9-7). Generally, a total space of 1 to 1.5 mm is sufficient for a porcelain-fused-to-metal restoration. An absolute minimum for esthetic areas is 0.75 mm. More than 2 mm can compromise strength unless the framework is built up to allow for a nearly uniform layer of porcelain up to 1.5 mm thick.

If the space is less than 1 mm, it will require the utmost skill to fabricate a restoration with a natural translucent appearance. More than likely the restoration will lack translucency and appear dull, lifeless, or opaque. It may be advisable to consider alternative

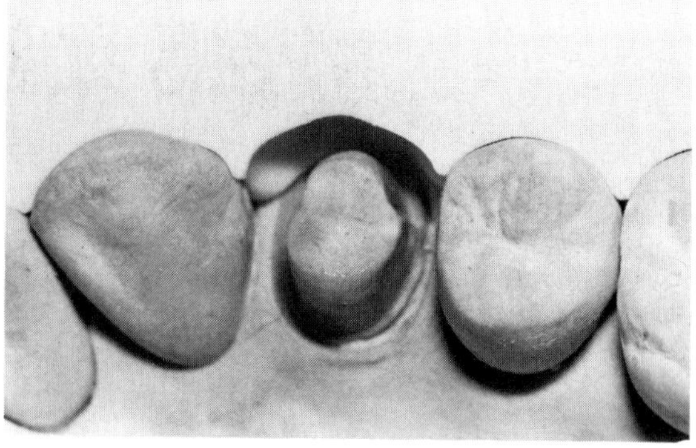

Fig. 9-7. Facial core gauges space available between prepared tooth and outer surface of wax-up.

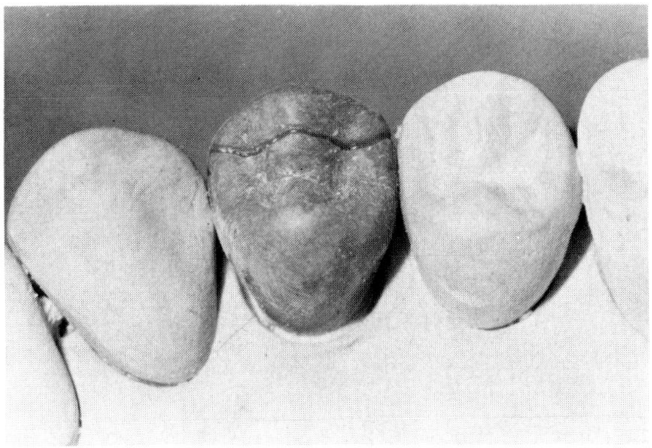

Fig. 9-8. Porcelain-metal junction is located away from any centric contact.

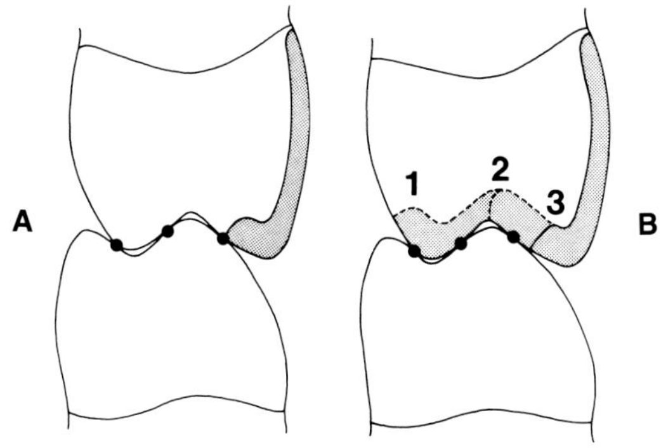

Fig. 9-9. A, Incorrect design places centric contact on porcelain-metal junction. **B,** With correct design, no contact occurs on porcelain-metal junction in following acceptable designs; *1,* porcelain occlusal; *2,* half porcelain and half metal; and *3,* metal occlusal. Note that porcelain wraps around from facial to occlusal surface.

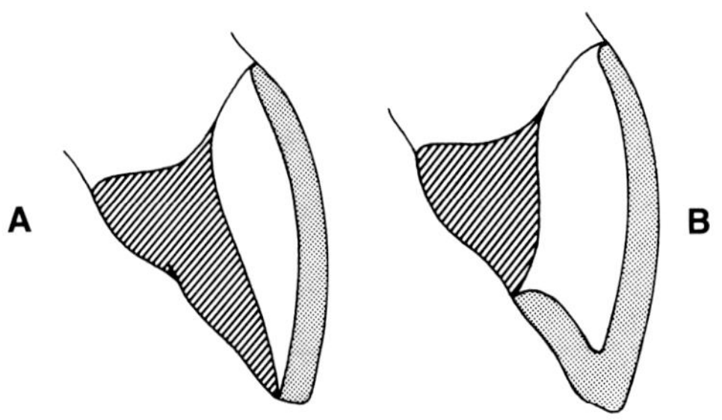

Fig. 9-10. A, Incorrect design covers only one surface. **B,** With correct design, porcelain wraps around to lingual surface.

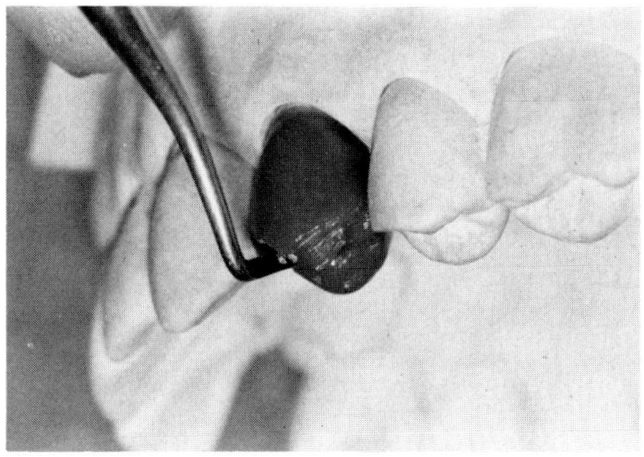

Fig. 9-11. Occlusal surface is cut back to junction.

contours and to consult the dentist about esthetic limitations.

6. Scribe a free-flowing porcelain-metal junction on the surface of the wax pattern with a pointed instrument such as an explorer (Fig. 9-8). The porcelain-metal junction is free of any centric contact and has a wraparound effect (Figs. 9-9 and 9-10).

Compressive stresses are important for the strength of porcelain. Although porcelain exhibits greater compression when it covers more of the occlusal surface, it manifests adequate strength in partial coverage of the occlusal surface when the porcelain wraps from the facial surface to the occlusal surface. The chief advantage of partial coverage is that a precious metal occlusal surface displays better long-term compatibility with the opposing dentition clinically than porcelain. Additionally, it is easier for the dentist to adjust and polish a metal surface than one entirely of porcelain.

7. Use an instrument with a blade 1 mm wide to cut back the wax-up. The sequence of cutback is as follows:

a. Reduce the incisal or occlusal surface 1.5 mm following the established contour (Fig. 9-11).

b. Reduce the proximal surfaces 1 mm (Fig. 9-12). Esthetically, it is advantageous to cut back through the proximal contact areas of single-unit anterior teeth to achieve lifelike translucence. On the other hand, it is more convenient to work on posterior teeth with metal proximal contact areas when esthetics is not critical.

c. Reduce the facial surface 1 mm (Fig. 9-13). Framework designs used for plastic veneer restorations are based on mechanical undercuts for retention and should not be used for metal-ceramic restorations. Although it is desirable esthetically to have maximum room for plastic, the result in a porcelain-fused-to-metal restoration would be unsupported porcelain subject to breakage and failure. The cutback technique gives assurance of a

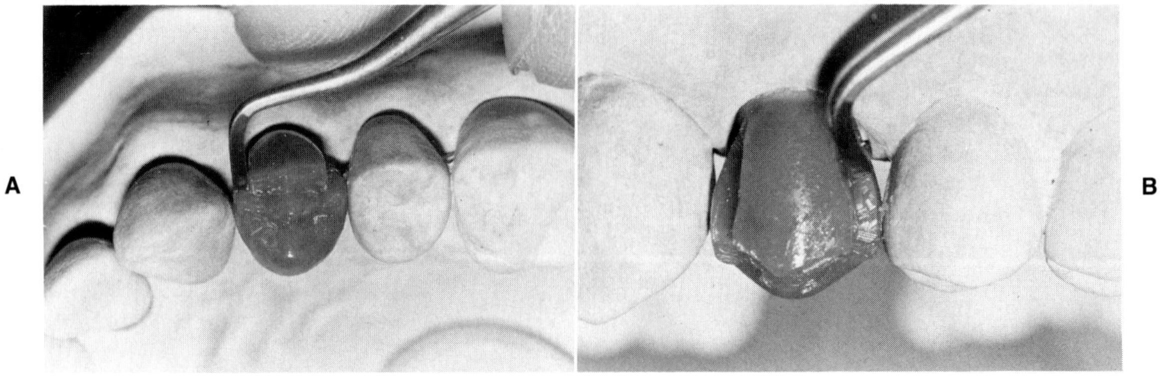

Fig. 9-12. Proximal surfaces also are cut back, **A,** Occlusal view. **B,** Facial view.

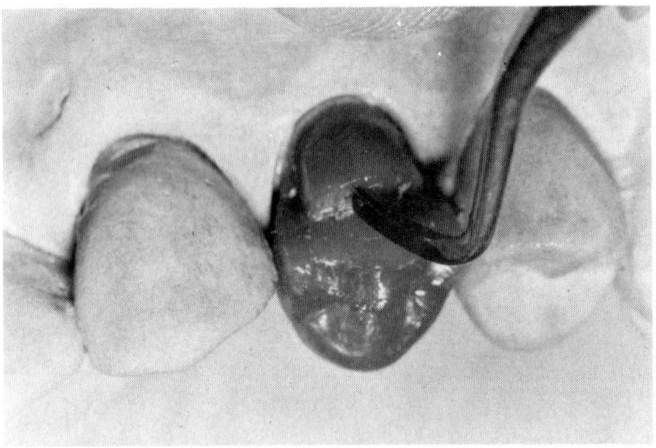

Fig. 9-13. Facial surface is cut back following established contour.

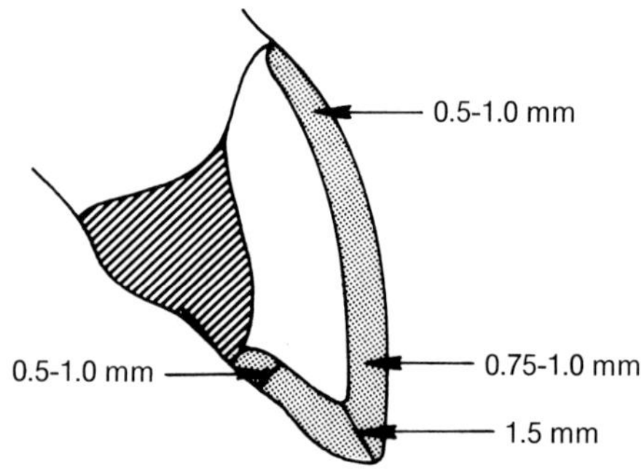

Fig. 9-14. Porcelain thickness varies from 0.5 to 1.5 mm. Minimum of 0.5 mm is necessary for esthetics, whereas maximum of 1.5 mm is allowable for strength.

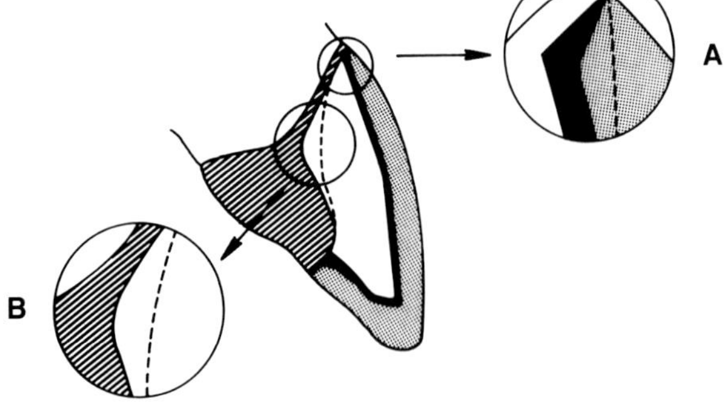

Fig. 9-15. Critical esthetic areas in which sufficient space is necessary for porcelain. Dotted line indicates which too much metal bulk often remains but is corrected. **A,** Gingival design. **B,** Proximal design.

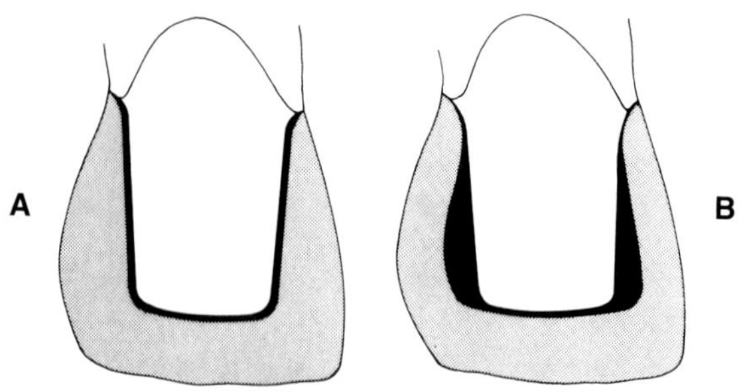

Fig. 9-16. A, Incorrect design has metal of minimal thickness, but porcelain that is unnecessarily bulky. This is of particular importance in teeth were buccal or lingual cusp or incisal edge is fractured. **B,** With correct design, porcelain is nearly uniform in thickness, but metal varies in thickness.

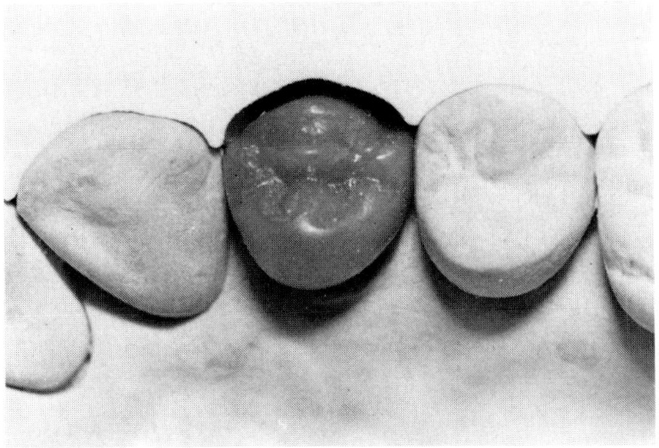

Fig. 9-17. Confirm evenness of cutback with facial core in place.

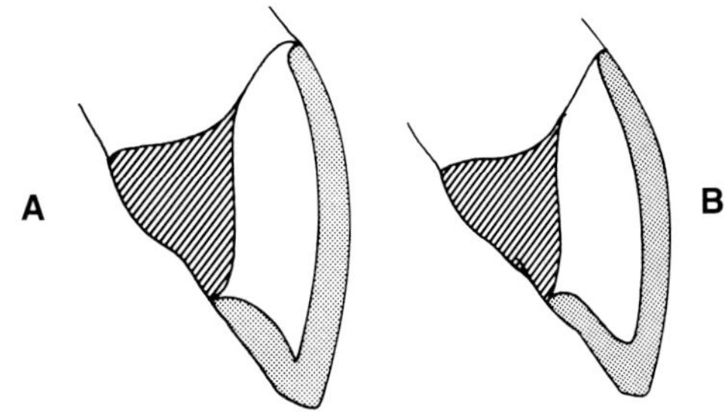

Fig. 9-18. A, Incorrect design leaves sharp, acute angle and area of undesirable stress concentration. **B,** With correct design porcelain-bearing areas should have no sharp edges or points.

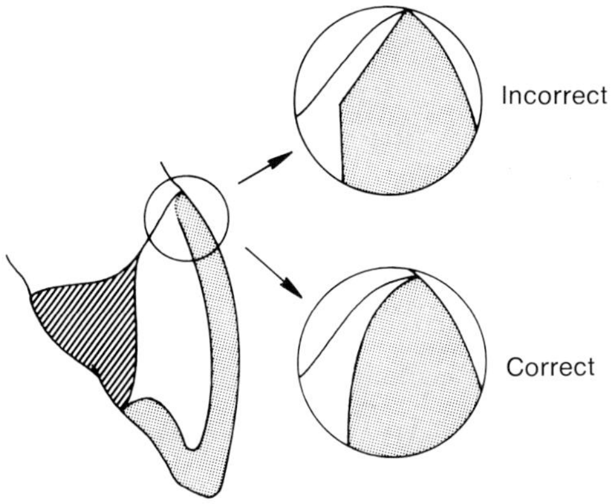

Fig. 9-19. Porcelain-bearing areas should have no sharp corners.

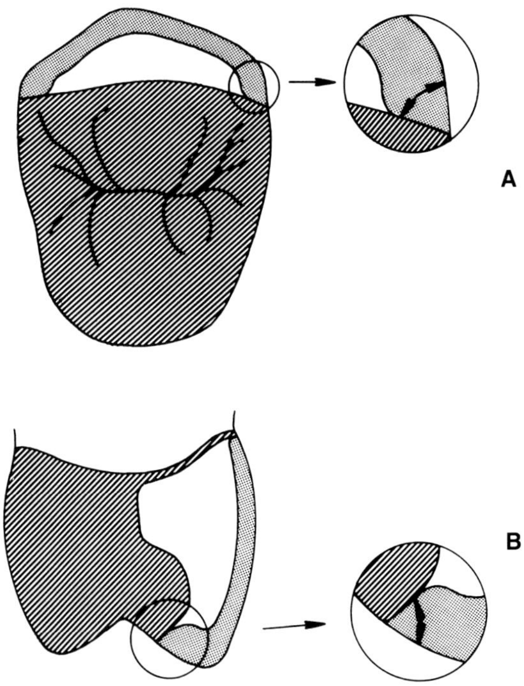

Fig. 9-20. Porcelain in cross section is 90 degrees or less. **A,** Proximal view. **B,** Occlusal view.

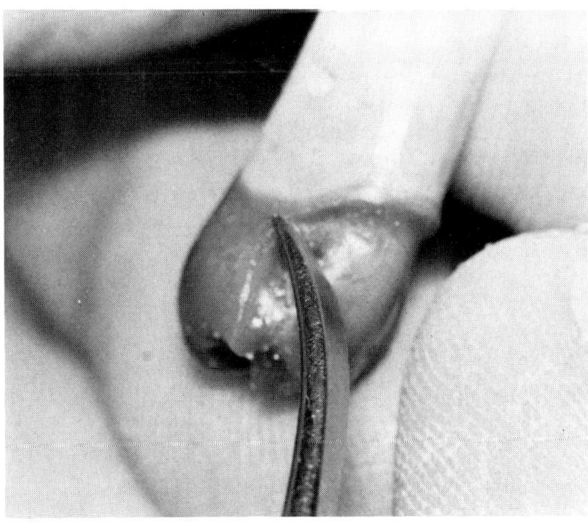

Fig. 9-21. Define porcelain-metal junction with beavertail burnisher.

well-supported, nearly uniform layer of porcelain for esthetic effect and allows sufficient space for porcelain near the gingival areas (Figs. 9-14 and 9-15). The thickness of the metal in porcelain-bearing areas usually varies (Fig. 9-16).

d. Check the amount of cutback with the facial core (Fig. 9-17).

8. Round any sharp angles or corners created during the cutback process (Figs. 9-18 and 9-19). Place the wax pattern on the die, use a slightly warmed beavertail burnisher No. 2 to define the porcelain-metal junction, and smooth any irregularities on the cutback areas (Figs. 9-20 and 9-21).

Leave a slightly bulky collar at the gingival margins for ease of casting. If there is to be a metal gingival collar in the completed restoration, do the final contouring just prior to glazing the porcelain (Fig. 9-22).

9. With the wax pattern back on the working cast, view the cutback from an oblique angle. Compare the profile of the adjacent teeth to that of the wax pattern. Roll back the incisal or occlusal edge of the wax pattern just lingual from the adjacent intact teeth (Fig. 9-23). Then finish the margins, and invest in the usual manner.

Framework design

Illustrated examples of typical anterior and posterior situations show the design features that contribute to the overall success for metal-ceramic restorations. The examples are as follows:

1. Maxillary anterior teeth (Figs. 9-24 to 9-29).
2. Mandibular anterior teeth (Figs. 9-30 and 9-31).
3. Maxillary posterior teeth (Figs. 9-32 to 9-35).
4. Mandibular posterior tooth (Fig. 9-36).
5. Multiple units (Figs. 9-37 to 9-39).
6. Pontics (Figs. 9-40 to 9-42).

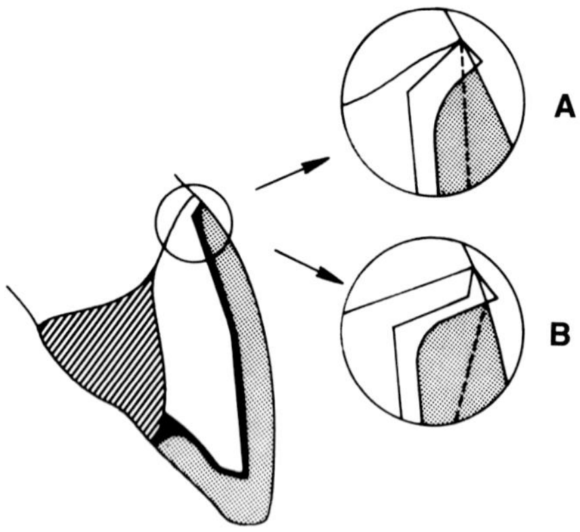

Fig. 9-22. Gingival collar is easier to cast and finish to nonconcave contour than knife-edged margin *(dotted line).* Leave slight additional contour on collar. **A,** Slanted shoulder preparation **B,** Shoulder-bevel preparation.

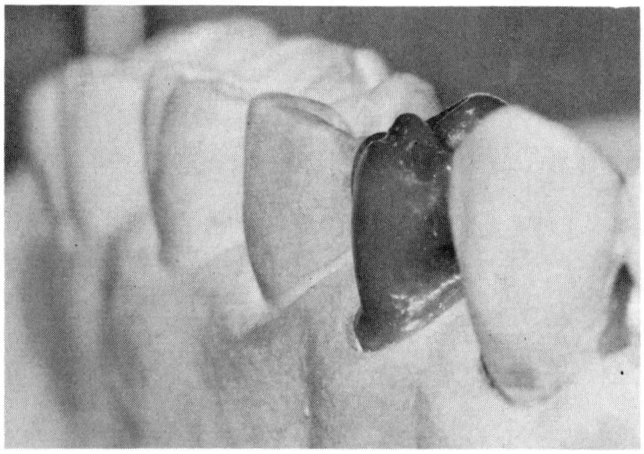

Fig. 9-23. Visually superimpose adjacent tooth contours over wax-up to assure adequate space for porcelain.

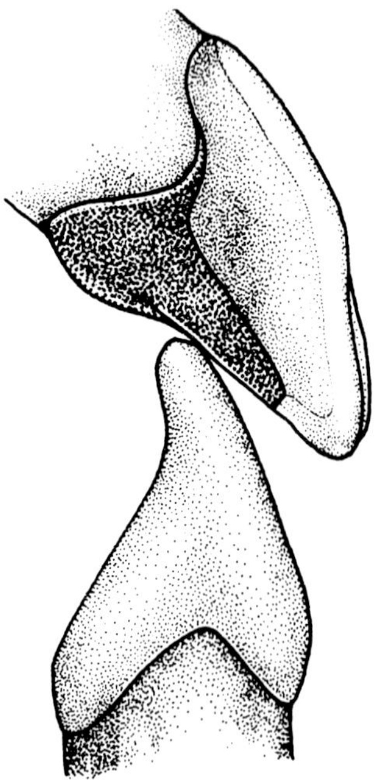

Fig. 9-24. This maxillary incisor occludes in metal (preferred) at middle third. Proximal contacts for anterior teeth are usually in porcelain to allow increased translucency and esthetics.

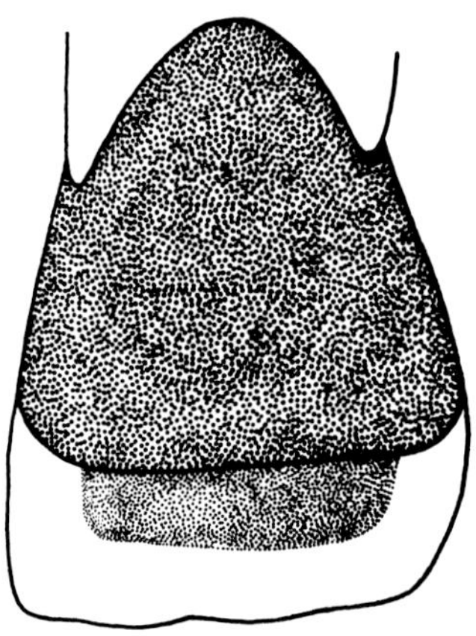

Fig. 9-25. Lingual view of incisor framework design for occlusion in metal at middle or gingival third.

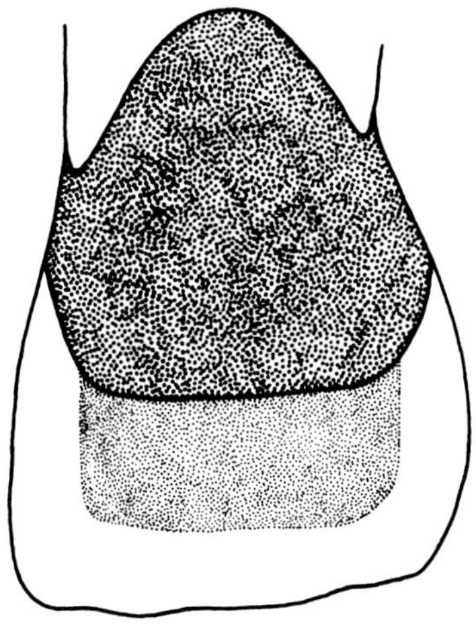

Fig. 9-26. Suitable design for occlusion in metal (preferred) at gingival third or in porcelain at incisal third.

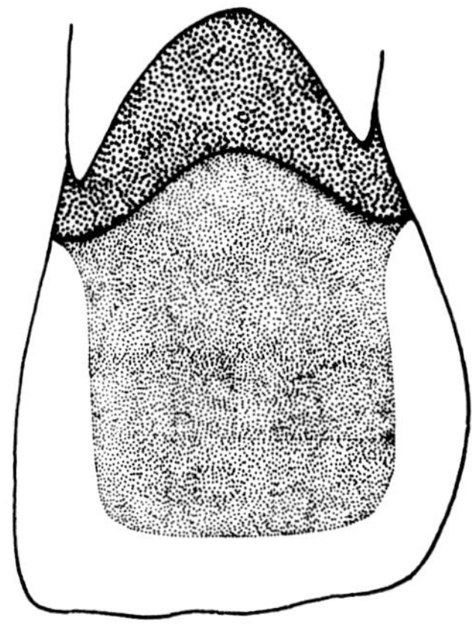

Fig. 9-27. Suitable design for occlusion in porcelain at middle or incisal third.

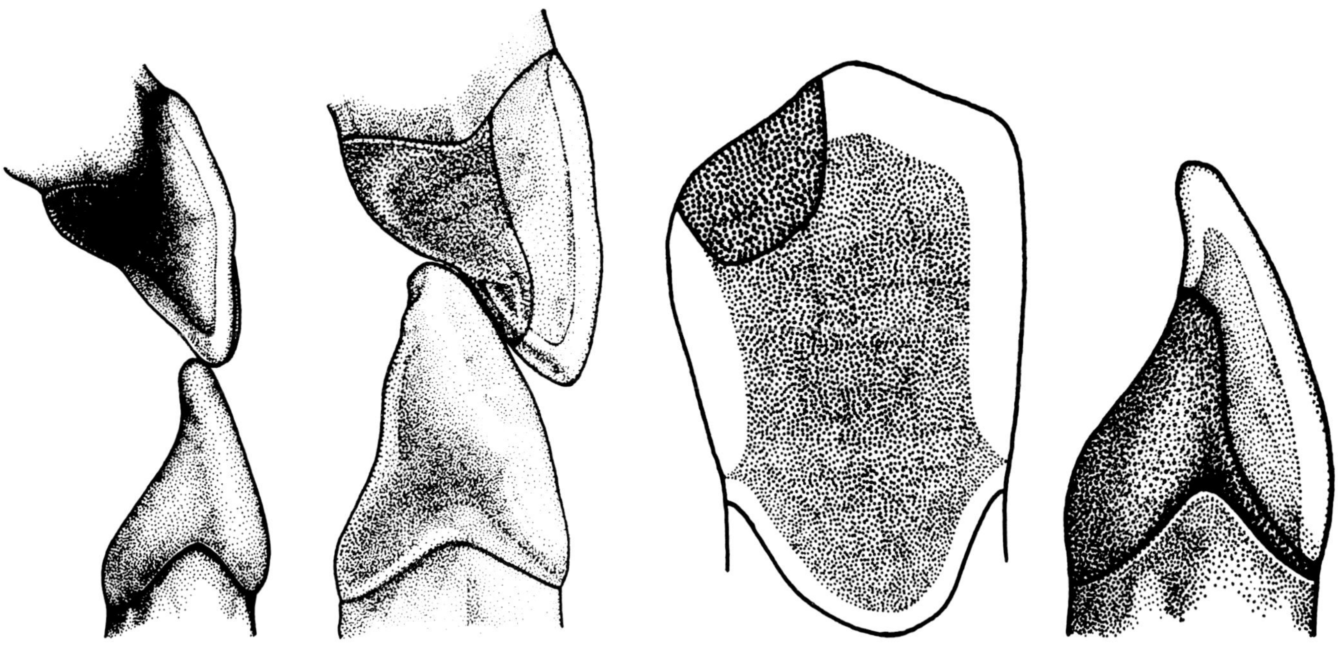

Fig. 9-28. Maxillary incisor with full veneer occludes in porcelain. Occlusion in metal would lead to stress and potential chipping of porcelain near incisal edge.
Fig. 9-29. Preferred design for maxillary canine. Centric contact and initial part of excursive movements are in metal.
Fig. 9-30. Preferred design for occlusion in metal on distal slope of cusp of mandibular canine if esthetics and function permit.
Fig. 9-31. Mandibular incisor often may have metal collar without esthetic impairment. Note wraparound to lingual surface.

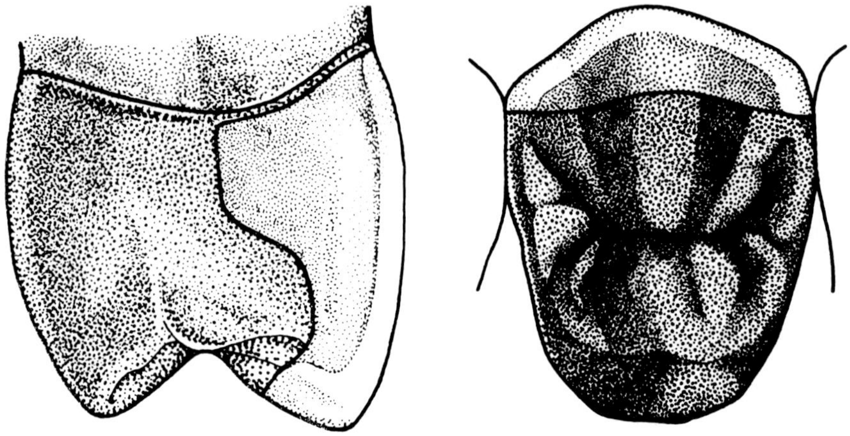

Fig. 9-32. Often maxillary posterior teeth are designed with occlusion, proximal contacts, and gingival collar entirely of metal. Porcelain-metal junction is halfway between tip of cusp and central groove. Note wraparound to occlusal surface, which is the preferred design.
Fig. 9-33. Occlusal view of preferred design for maxillary premolar.

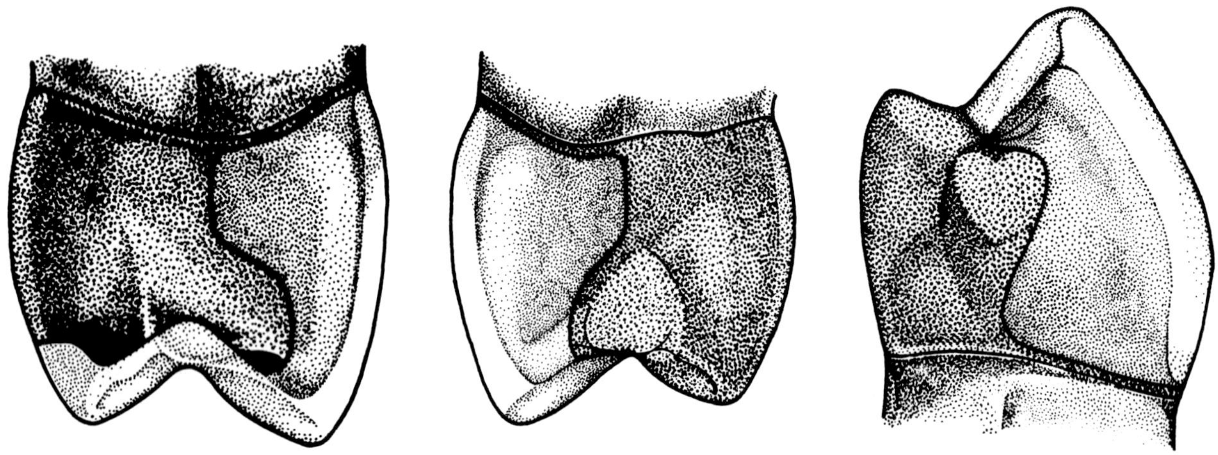

Fig. 9-34. Esthetics may dictate use of full porcelain occlusal surface for maxillary posterior tooth. Generally, it is easier to adjust metal proximal contact than one of porcelain.
Fig. 9-35. If occlusion on metal is preferable, but centric contact is on porcelain-metal junction in the design see in Fig. 9-32, place junction in central groove.
Fig. 9-36. Mandibular posterior tooth has different esthetic and functional demands than maxillary. Design leaving entire buccal cusp in porcelain reflects these demands. Gingival collar and proximal contact are in metal if esthetics permit. NOTE: Alternate design, other than one with full porcelain occlusal surface, is occlusal island of metal opposing contacting maxillary cusp. This design can be modified further to include distal slope of cusp similar to mandibular canine seen in Fig. 9-30. However, design using all-metal occlusal surface does not seem to be justified esthetically.

Fig. 9-37. Incisal view of this anterior framework shows several important points. Note even layer of porcelain across facial surface. In particular, design at connector areas is critical to assure sufficient metal bulk for strength and enough space for esthetic layer of porcelain at facial embrasures. This bulk is obtained at expense of the lingual embrasure. For lifelike translucency, proximal contracts are in porcelain.

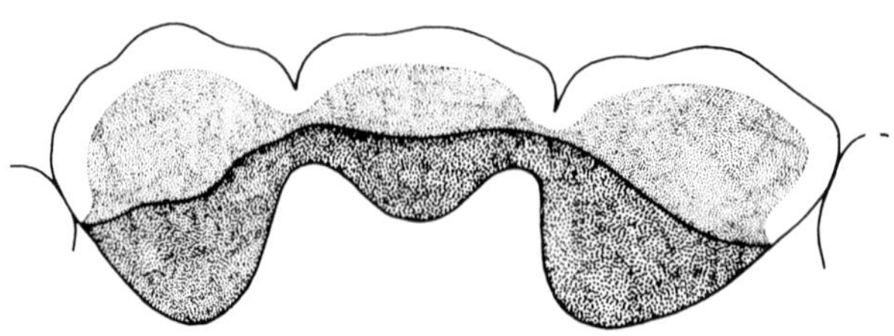

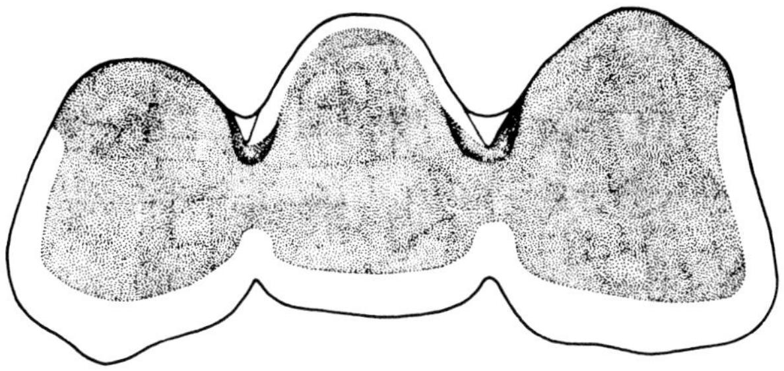

Fig. 9-38. From facial view, anterior framework shows similar important points. There is relatively even layer of porcelain from one proximal surface, across incisal edge, to other proximal surface. Note especially design at incisal embrasures for porcelain. Here, too, there is adequate metal bulk in connector areas. Bulk is at lingual embrasure. This is also known as strut type of design when lingual aspect of connector areas is maintained in metal.

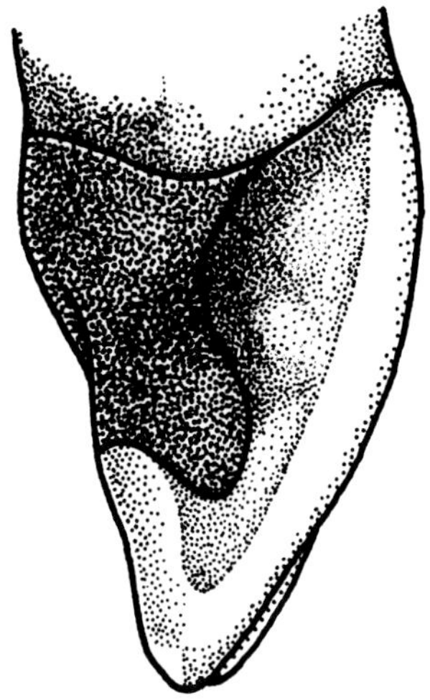

Fig. 9-39. Maxillary anterior tooth, when splinted or used as abutment, must have definite connector area. Note difference at proximal connector area between this design and design in Fig. 9-24.

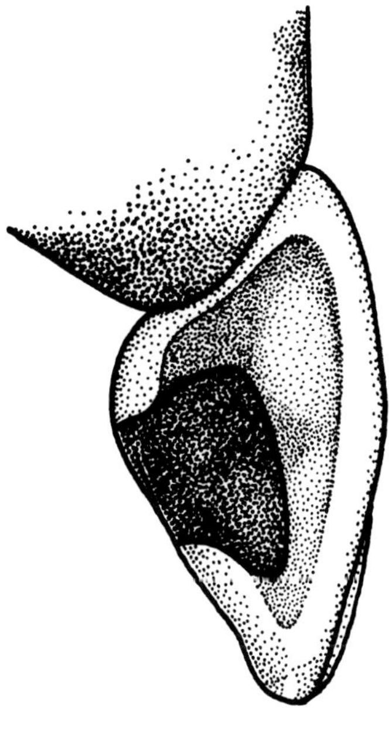

Fig. 9-40. Maxillary anterior pontic also has definite connector area, which is quite necessary for strength. Additionally, note nearly circumferential wraparound of porcelain. This design allows porcelain on ridge and occlusion in metal on middle third of lingual surface.

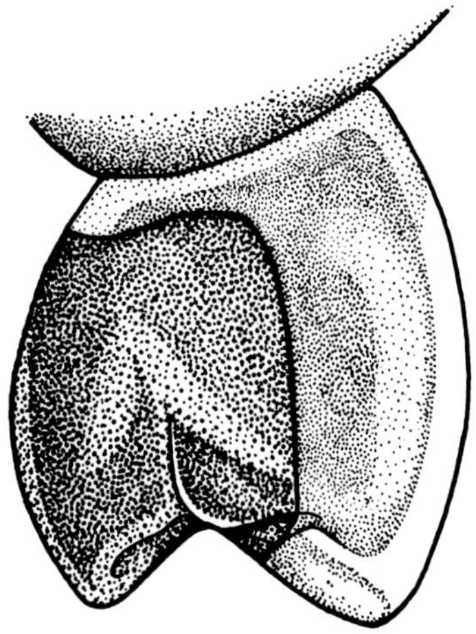

Fig. 9-41. Maxillary posterior pontic has characteristics similar to those of anterior. Note occlusion in metal, wraparound of porcelain, porcelain on ridge, and connector area.

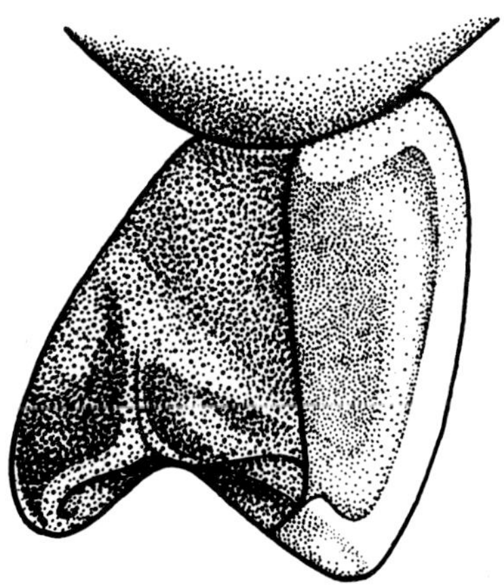

Fig. 9-42. This modification of maxillary posterior pontic is useful when occlusogingival height of pontic space is minimal, that is, "short-bite situation. Note that metal on ridge allows more occlusogingival bulk to framework and thereby increases rigidity.

CHOICE OF METAL

Nonprecious or base metal alloys have been gaining in popularity over precious or high noble alloys for fabrication of metal-ceramic restorations. The greater rigidity of the base metal-ceramic alloys make them better suited for long-span, multiple-unit restorations, especially those where limited occlusogingival space is available. Although it is true that the rigidity of metal is inversely proportional to the cube of the difference in thickness, the increased modulus of elasticity of the base metal-ceramic alloys allows them to be employed in thinner cross-section and still retain the necessary rigidity to serve in long-span restorations. It is essential to weigh carefully the advantages of additional space for porcelain against the disadvantages of increase in stress, especially for those alloys with high gold and platinum content.

PROBLEM AREAS

The function of ceramometal restorations is greatly influenced by the design of the metal framework. Design problems, probable causes, and their solutions are described in Table 9-1.

1. The color of the porcelain veneer may be compromised by opaque areas, inconsistent shade values between abutments and pontics, or lack of translucency, especially in interproximal areas.

These problems can be traced to improper frame design. The porcelain veneer must have a thickness of 0.75 to 1.5 mm for proper shade control. If the thickness of porcelain varies greatly from tooth to tooth, from the facial surface of the tooth to the interproximal contact area, or on the facial surface of a tooth, then the shade will be inconsistent. The design of the framework should provide for a relatively uniform veneer of porcelain of adequate thickness.

Table 9-1. Framework design

Problem	Probable cause	Solution
Opaque shows through body porcelain at desired contour	Insufficient thickness of body porcelain	If there is sufficient room (at least 0.75 mm) between preparation and surface of desired contour, reduce metal to 0.3 mm and rebake porcelain (Figs. 9-2 and 9-14) If there is insufficient room, consider alternate contour or consultation with dentist about tooth preparation and esthetic limitations
Color of porcelain varies from one tooth to the next, even though same shade is used	Nonuniform thickness of porcelain from tooth to tooth (especially abutment and pontic)	Use core to determine space available for porcelain and adjust framework so there is relatively uniform layer (Fig. 9-14)
Interproximal area appears dark	Metal is displayed at interproximal area because porcelain-metal junction is too facial	Design framework to include porcelain about halfway between facial and lingual surfaces at interproximal area (Figs. 9-15, B, and 9-21)
Anterior teeth lack translucency at interproximal area	Proximal contact area has too much metal	Design framework so contact area is all porcelain; this only applies to teeth without connector areas (Fig. 9-37)
Metal collar on facial aspect is undercontoured	Inadequate bulk in framework Too much reduction during contouring	Design collar with more bulk so that there is slight excess contour during initial porcelain firing (Fig. 9-22)
Porcelain has craze line or fracture	Porcelain is too thick	Design framework with more bulk for relatively uniform layer of porcelain (Fig. 9-16)
	Framework has sharp angle	Round sharp angles on any porcelain-bearing surface (Fig. 9-18)
Porcelain cracks on seating casting on die	Framework too thin, resulting in distortion and flexing	Maintain at least 0.3 mm thickness to metal in porcelain-bearing areas (Fig. 9-2)
Connector area fractures	Insufficient bulk to connector area	Use strut-type design for framework
Porcelain chips near porcelain-metal junction after restoration has been in place for awhile	Functional occlusion too close to porcelain-metal junction	Keep porcelain-metal junction away from centric contact and initial excursive movements (Fig. 9-24)

2. When the porcelain veneer is too thick (in excess of 2 mm), much of the bond strength, which is greatest at the ceramometal interface, is lost, and fracture of the porcelain can occur more easily.

The metal framework should permit the addition of a porcelain veneer with a thickness of 0.75 to 1.5 mm for proper shade and strength. Additional strength is imparted to the porcelain veneer if it is allowed to surround portions of the metal framework supporting the porcelain. Any porcelain-bearing metal surface must be rounded to avoid stress or fracture lines in the porcelain caused by sharp edges, corners, or recesses in the metal framework.

3. The metal framework is designed to resist deformation. Fractures of connector areas are not uncommon. A connector is the area that joins two adjacent teeth in a fixed partial denture. It is usually constricted compared to the bulk of a pontic. As the prosthesis flexes during function, stresses are concentrated at the connector area. These stress concentration areas have the potential of fatigue and subsequent fracture. To avoid fracture, adequate bulk must be provided without interfering with proper embrasure contour. The use of a strut-type connector design is advised.

If the metal frame is of insufficient strength to support the facial veneer of porcelain, chipping or cracking of the porcelain may result. A metal thickness of not less than 0.3 mm should be maintained in porcelain-bearing areas. Centric occlusal contacts and initial excursive movement should not be at the porcelain-metal junction.

ACKNOWLEDGMENTS

I wish to express my appreciation to Harvey L. Colman, D.D.S., formerly of the University of Southern California School of Dentistry, for his development of the *Manual for Pre-clinical Fixed Prosthodontics*, and to the Audio Visual Services, University of Southern California School of Dentistry, for the artwork.

CHAPTER 10

DENTAL PORCELAINS

ALTON M. LACY

PART ONE

Dental porcelain

Dental porcelains that are fused to a metal substrate are primarily powdered glasses with small amounts of residual, unreacted feldspar particles. They are generally classified as "low fusing" because they sinter into a relatively dense, rigid mass at temperatures several hundred degrees below those required to fuse the denture tooth and pontic porcelain. These latter porcelains are often referred to as high- or medium-fusing porcelains, and although they can be made visually similar to low-fusing "bake-on" porcelains, high-fusing porcelains are not designed to be powdered and re-fused. The proportion of glass in higher fusing porcelains is sufficient to allow for glazing of the surface when heated to temperatures in excess of 2200° F (1200° C), but such temperatures are unsuitable for metal veneering.

For a compatible metal-ceramic restoration, criteria other than fusing temperatures must be fulfilled by the porcelain: (1) it must be chemically and optically stable over a series of firing cycles and (2) it must have a coefficient of thermal expansion nearly equal to that of the substrate metal. These criteria can be met by production of nearly homogeneous glass powders that will fuse at temperatures around 1800° F (980° C) to form a solid mass that can subsequently be shaped and finished into a cosmetic restoration.

TYPES OF LOW-FUSING PORCELAIN

Basically, three types of low-fusing porcelain are used: (1) porcelains for metal veneering, (2) stains and glazes, and (3) aluminous porcelains for jacket crowns.

Porcelains for metal veneering

A kit of veneering porcelain contains a variety of low-fusing glasses whose thermal expansion closely matches that of veneering metal alloys. These include opaque porcelains and body porcelains.

Opaque porcelains are powdered glasses to which particles of relatively insoluble oxides such as titanium dioxide, zirconium oxide, and tin oxide are added. These oxides reflect the incident light; when fused to a metal substrate, opaque porcelain will block out the dark color of the metal (Fig. 10-1). The shade of the opaque porcelain is determined by the color of the opacifying oxide powder and the glass matrix. The color of the opaque is very important to the development of the final shade of the tooth, since a realistic effect is best created by overlaying this thin, highly pigmented layer with more translucent porcelains. Such a technique softens and diffuses the color of the opaque, creating a sense of depth to the restoration. The degree of gloss developed in the opaque is directly related to the brightness of the final restoration. Opaque porcelains are formulated to produce a pebbly texture when properly baked, and it is this texture that diffuses the reflected light as it passes through the overlying porcelain (Fig. 10-2). Colored opaque porcelains can be skillfully used to develop realistic internal coloration. These opaques are nearly chemically identical to the standard "tooth-colored" opaques and can be freely intermixed with them.

Body porcelains represent a variety of porcelains that generally can be subdivided into three groups: (1) gingival or dentin porcelains, (2) incisal or enamel porce-

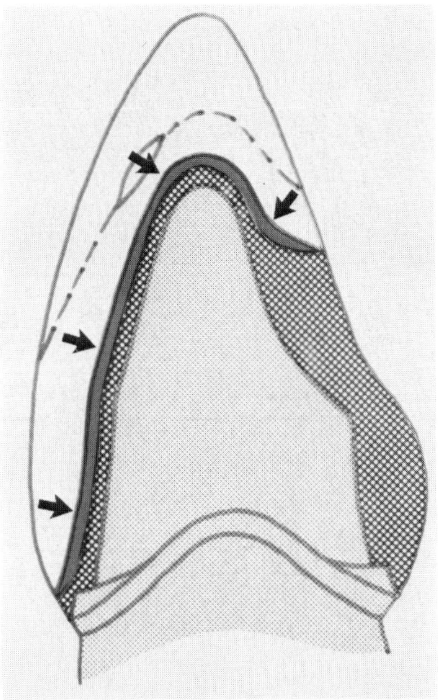

Fig. 10-1. Arrows show position of opaque veneer, which is generally 0.2 to 0.3 mm thick.

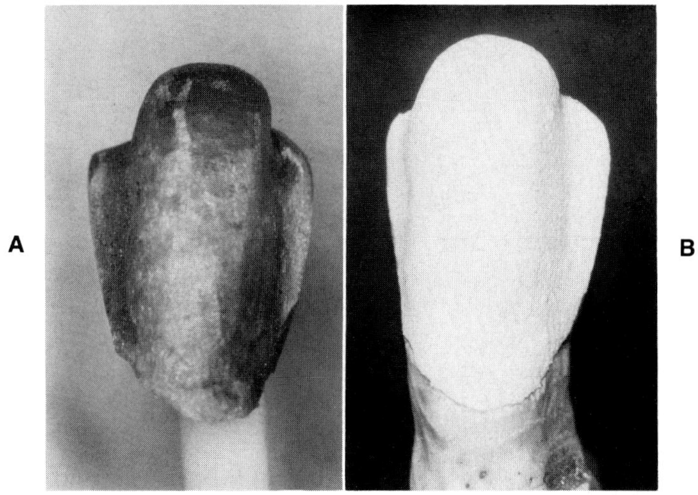

Fig. 10-2. A, Masking of dark metal surface by 0.3-mm coat of fired opaque porcelain. **B,** Pebbly texture will scatter reflected light through overlying porcelain.

lains, and (3) modifiers. These porcelains are almost exclusively powdered glass with a very small content of insoluble mineral additives. As such, they are relatively translucent and are always fused over opaque porcelain (Fig. 10-3). The body porcelains have a very limited ability to mask underlying metal. They are all chemically similar, the only difference being small additions of color oxides that have little effect in their fusion range or thermal expansion. These three body porcelains can be freely mixed and fused together to create a desired cosmetic effect. They are sometimes compounded for use at slightly lower temperatures than opaques, although they are often baked at the same temperature. The comparative fusion temperatures will vary among manufacturers. When properly fused in a vacuum, they form a dense, smooth body that can be ground into proper form with ceramic-bound rotary abrasives, diamond cutting instruments, or carbide burs.

Incisal porcelains are relatively colorless (clear gray) and are used to imitate the enamel of the incisal edge of natural teeth (Fig. 10-4). Gingival porcelains are generally dentin (yellowish) colored, and when baked over appropriate opaques, they can closely mimic that portion of tooth where enamel is supported by dentin.

Modifiers are fairly intensely colored and are fused within the body porcelains (Fig. 10-5) to create special cosmetic effects or to add color dimension to restorations that attempt to replace teeth not well matched by the available shade guides.

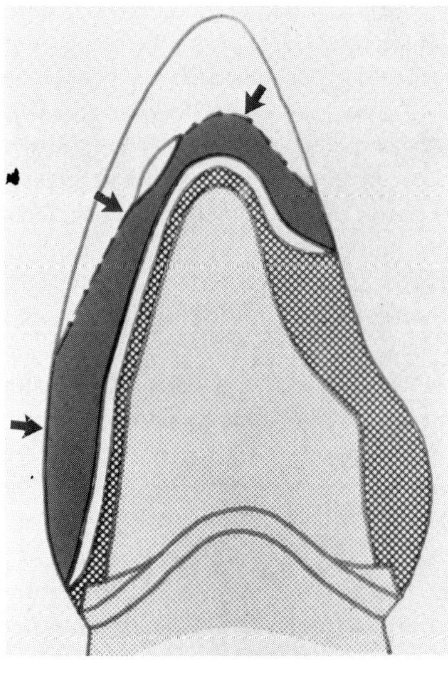

Fig. 10-3. Arrows show position of "gingival" or "dentin" porcelain veneer.

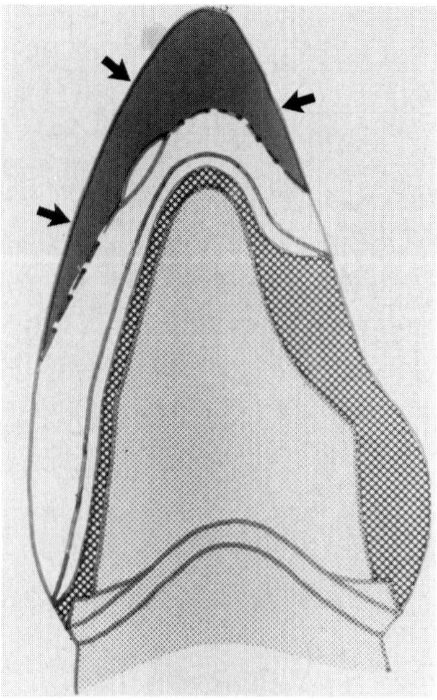

Fig. 10-4. Arrows show placement of "incisal" or "enamel" veneer over other body porcelain.

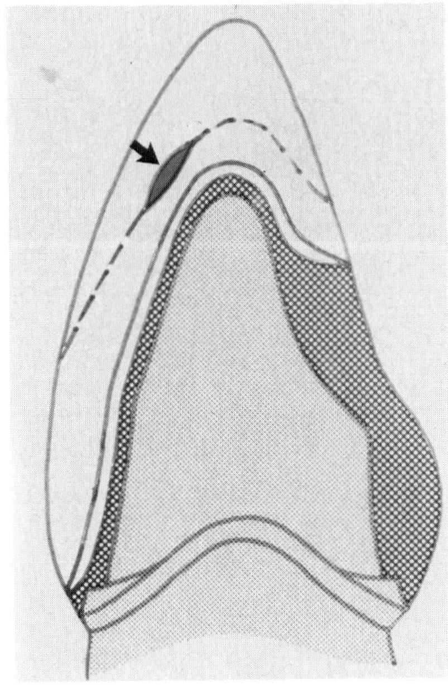

Fig. 10-5. Colored modifying porcelains are built up with other body porcelains *(arrow)* to enhance color effects in final restoration.

Stains and glazes

These glass powders are provided to the technician in kits separate from other porcelains. Stains and glazes fuse at temperatures approximately 150° F (83.3° C) lower than body or opaque porcelains. Their thermal expansion coefficients are probably nearly equal to or slightly lower than low-fusing body porcelains. Stains are highly colored glasses that are added superficially (Fig. 10-6) to porcelain restorations to adjust the shade or create special effect such as craze lines, shadows, simulated restorations, hypoplasia, etc. Glazes, although chemically similar to stains, are uncolored (clear) and are used to provide a glassy surface after occlusal, cosmetic, or morphologic corrections have been made by grinding a previously glazed surface. The lower fusion temperature of stains and glazes minimizes the risk of further morphologic change in the restoration as they are baked.

Aluminous porcelain

Aluminous dental porcelain, developed by McLean and Hughes (1965), is composed of a mixture of low-fusing powdered glass and powdered aluminum oxide (alumina). Its principal use is in the construction of porcelain-jacket crowns or special jacketlike crowns of porcelain fused to an oxidized tin-plated platinum foil, which remains in place as an integral part of the restoration (Fig. 10-7). This technique can produce a highly cosmetic crown that resembles the classic porcelain jacket, but has greater strength.

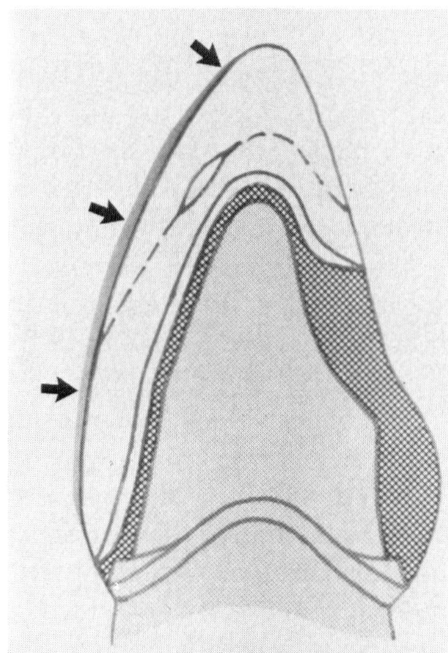

Fig. 10-6. Stains and glazes are used to create superficial color on restorations *(arrows)*. They are sometimes added internally for small effects, but because of differences in thermal expansion coefficients, they should be used sparingly as body "modifier."

Alumina is partly soluble in low-fusing glass, and its presence strengthens the glass, making it less sensitive to crystallization and elevating its fusion temperature. Aluminous porcelains are fired at temperatures up to 200° F (110° C) higher than bake-on porcelains and are usually held at maximum temperature for several minutes to allow for densification. They are less susceptible

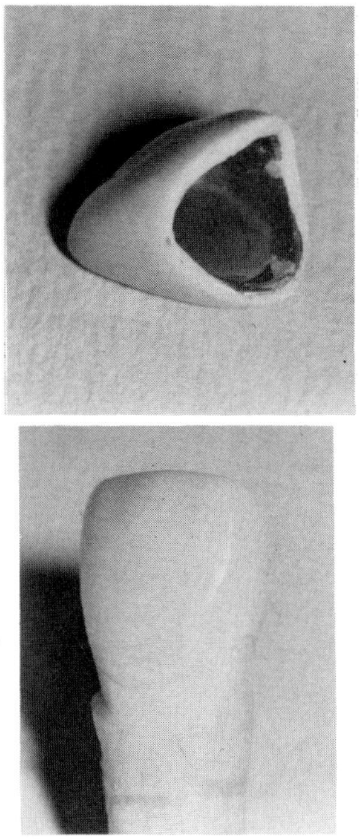

A

B

Fig. 10-7. A, Aluminous porcelain jacket made by "twin-foil" technique. Internal platinum foil is tin-coated, oxidized, and bonded to aluminous porcelain, making it stronger crown than nonaluminous jacket porcelain. **B,** Aluminous porcelain jacket crown seated on master die.

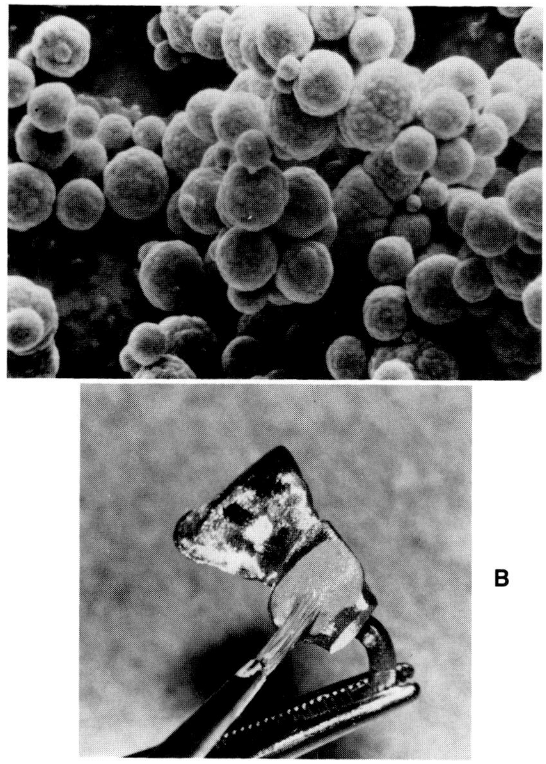

A

B

Fig. 10-8. Spherical gold powders **(A)** are mixed with their special liquids (which contain lithium borates and other oxide-forming ingredients) and then thinly painted onto prepared metal surfaces **(B).** Unit is then dried and fired to 1950°F (1065°C) in air for 5 to 10 minutes.

to overfiring and loss of contour than are bake-on porcelains. Aluminous porcelain kits contain opaque body and modifying porcelain powders, which are analogous in purpose to other low-firing porcelains.

PART TWO

Surface conditioning of metal

As an alternative or as a procedure intermediate to degassing and the addition of opaque porcelain, one or more of a variety of so-called *surface conditioners* may be applied. These commercially available products are generally of two types: gold powders (sometimes with additives) and porcelain powders. The use of both is an optional procedure, since porcelain can bond adequately to a properly cleaned and degassed alloy without such intermediate treatment.

GOLD POWDERS

Gold powders are made to seal the surface to supress or mask the liberation of gases that could create bubbles within the porcelain. Gold powders should be used only with precious and semiprecious alloys of high gold content (not previously degassed) metal surface, using the liquid supplied, and dried in front of the furnace (Fig. 10-8). The unit is then rapidly heated in air to 1950° F (1065° C). Since pure gold does not bond to porcelain, it is essential that the coating not be thick. The unit should be held at 1950° F for 5 to 10 minutes so that the gold may diffuse into the underlying alloy and allow for outward diffusion of oxidizable elements (e.g., indium and tin) so that a bond to porcelain can be established. The liquids contain soluble tin and lithium-borate compounds, which form tin oxides and lithium borates on the surface at high temperatures. These compounds presumably contribute to glass-metal bonding (Fig. 10-9). At this point the initial mirrored golden finish will have dulled to a matte yellowish surface. The coping can be rapidly cooled in air.

Insufficient firing of the gold coat will significantly reduce the porcelain-metal bond strength (Fig. 10-10). Also, excessive amounts of superficial gold can set up interfacial stresses, leading to fracture of the veneer. This results from the differences in thermal expansion among the porcelain, gold coating, and substructural alloy. "Pooling" of gold surface conditioners should be removed with a noncontaminating abrasive (Fig. 10-11).

Overfiring of the gold coat will cause loss of golden

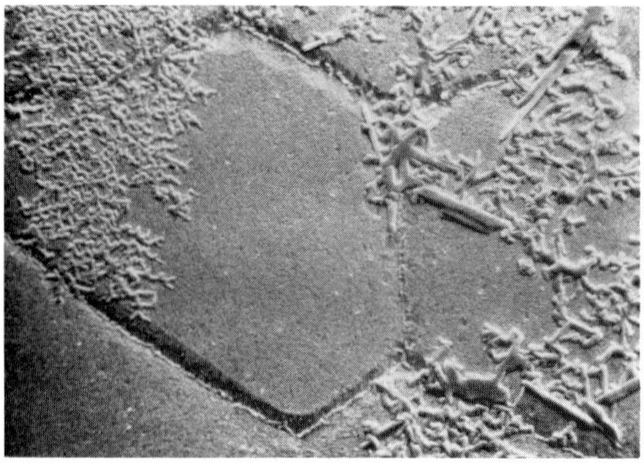

Fig. 10-9. Scanning electron micrograph of heated metal surface heavily coated with gold-powder surface conditioner. Hexagonal crystals are nonbonding gold. "Residue" on surface is presumably lithium borate and tin oxide—factors necessary to establish bond with porcelain.

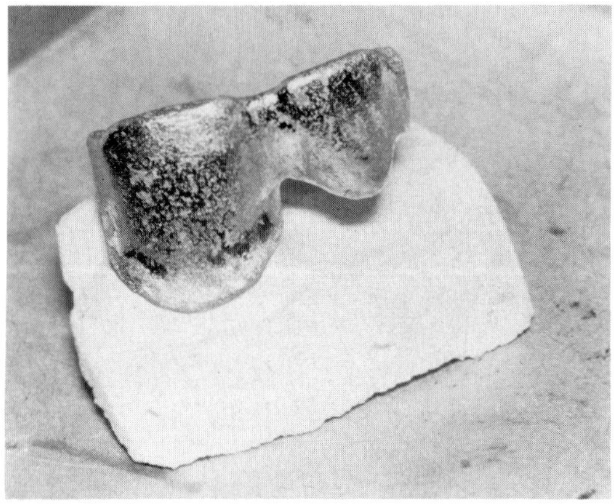

Fig. 10-10. This unit has been fired to 1950°F (1065°C) but held at that temperature for insufficient time. Shiny gold areas will form very weak bonds with overlying porcelain.

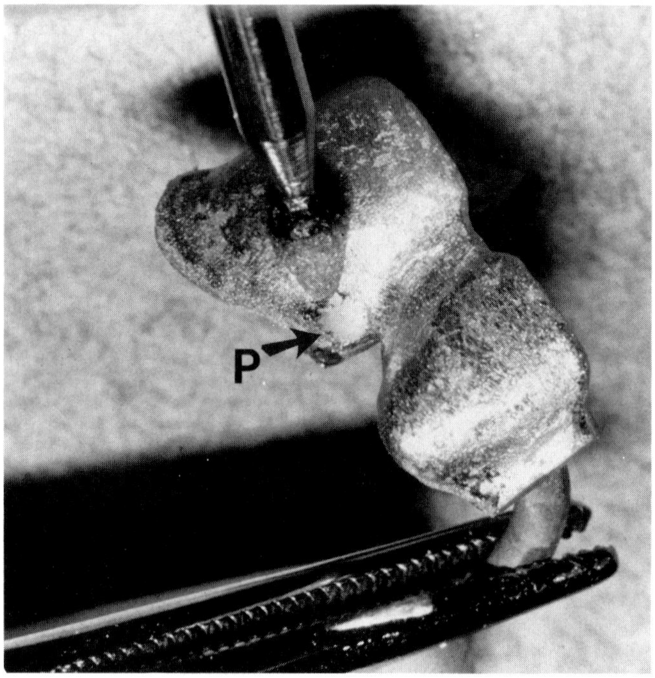

Fig. 10-11. When properly fired, gold surface conditioner will have dull-yellow color with matte texture. Areas of pooling *(P)* should be removed with noncontaminating abrasives, since they can act as sites of stress generation and poor porcelain bonding.

yellow color, but will not impair the porcelain bonding. Undercoating and overfiring the gold coatings is preferred to overcoating and underfiring.

PORCELAIN POWDERS

Porcelain powders, referred to as ceramic metal-bonding conditioners, are available for application to porcelain-bearing metal surfaces. Their stated purpose is to improve the strength of the porcelain-metal bond by sandwiching a layer of glass between the metal and opaque porcelain. This layer is composed of a glass somewhat more fluid than the opaque, and it supposedly results in better adaptation of the porcelain to the metal. Microscopic viewing of opaque porcelain fired without the use of these conditioners often shows poor coalescence of the particles and spotty metal contact

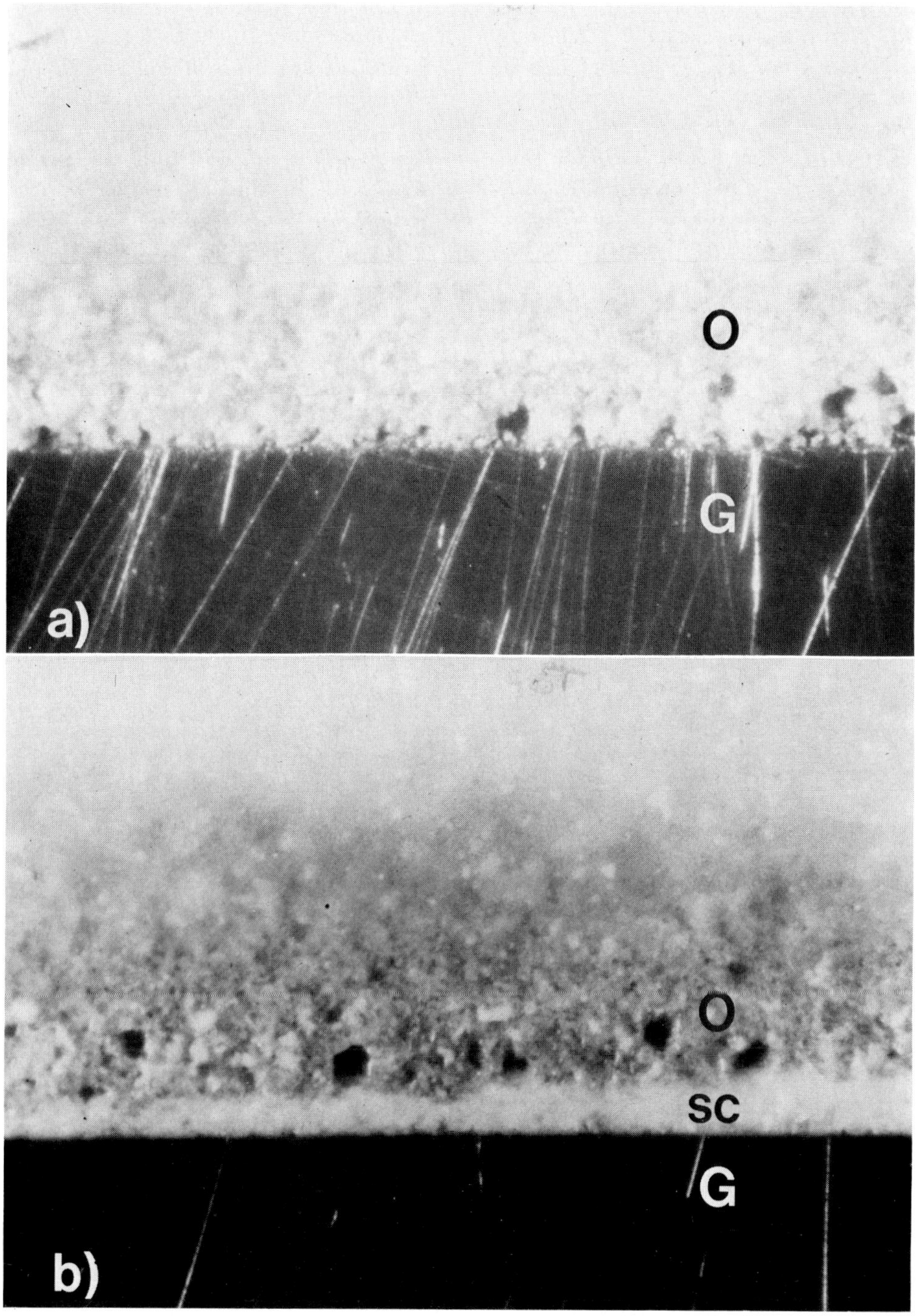

Fig. 10-12. A, Opaque porcelain *(O)* baked to gold alloy *(G)* without any surface conditioning treatment. *B,* Opaque porcelain *(O)* baked to gold alloy *(G)* with interfacial "sandwich" of porcelain surface conditioner *(SC)*. There is better apposition of glass to metal, although this may not be clinically significant.

(Fig. 10-12, *A*), although the degree of bonding is usually clinically satisfactory. Interposing a thin layer of the porcelain surface conditioner appears to improve glass-metal contact, although the degree of improvement of bond strength has not been conclusively established (Fig. 10-12, *B*). These bonding conditioners can be used on all alloys and can be applied over surfaces that have first been treated with gold-powder conditioners. Some manufacturers of base metal alloys insist on their use prior to the addition of opaque porcelain. The surface-conditioner color may easily interfere with the determination of proper color of the overlying opaque and will add to the total thickness of the opaque layers.

The conditioning porcelain is mixed with its appropriate liquid to a thin, paintlike consistency and painted onto the metal. Puddling or thick application must be avoided. The unit is dried at the entrance of the furnace at about 1470° F (800° C) until it looks powdery white. At this time it is inserted into the furnace, a mercury vacuum 25 to 28 inches (64 to 70 cm) is drawn, and the furnace temperature is raised at 50° to 100° F (28° to 56° C) per minute to about 1832° F (1000° C). Here it is held 1 minute, then air is introduced into the furnace, and the unit is withdrawn. The glassy surface will have a slight sheen. Opaque porcelain can now be added over the "conditioned" surface.

The use of these surface conditioners is generally optional and is not essential to success with the porcelain-fused-to-metal restoration if all other procedures are done properly.

CHAPTER 11

COSMETIC FULL VENEER CROWNS

RUSSELL T. DeVREUGD and HAROLD F. EISSMANN

PART ONE

Metal-ceramic crown with porcelain margin

Since the complete veneer porcelain crown was first described by Charles H. Land in 1902, there has been a steady progression in technique for the cosmetic restoration and replacement of missing or mutilated anterior teeth. Various types, styles, and methods have been devised to produce cosmetic facings of resin or porcelain. A marked development was the porcelain-faced crown as advocated by Dr. D.E. Shooshan in 1954. The technique was a decided improvement over existing types of treatment and became a viable alternative to the resin-faced cast gold crown. Since that time the development of metal-ceramic systems for crown and fixed partial dentures, along with marked improvement in porcelains for complete porcelain crowns, has given new impetus to and has created intense interest in cosmetic restorations.

Public demand for improved esthetics in metal-ceramic crowns has resulted in the development of techniques to eliminate the unsightly metal collar at the facial margin. In instances where thin translucent gingival tissue is present, the use of a porcelain margin is advisable to satisfy esthetic demands. It must be remembered that such a restoration is a compromise to achieve a demanding cosmetic result. Mechanics of the technique require that the prepared tooth have a shoulder from proximal to proximal contact which is at least 1.0 mm in width (Fig. 11-1).

PROCEDURE

The technique involves combining the conventional metal-ceramic crown technique with the use of a platinum foil matrix to reproduce the facial margin in porcelain.

1. To prepare the die for waxing, apply a thin application of cyanoacrylate cement in the area around the shoulder of the margin where platinum foil will be burnished. This will protect the margin from erosion during handling of the die. For best results silver-plated or copper-plated dies are preferred.

2. Apply a liberal amount of die lubricant, and allow it to soak in for 15 to 30 seconds. Blot the excess lubricant with soft tissue. Do not rub the die.

3. Use a soft brush dipped in zinc stearate, or an equivalent substitute, and apply it liberally to pick up excess lubricant from the die. Blow off the excess powder. This is especially useful on plated dies.

4. Soft wax should be used for initial application to the die. Specially compounded waxes are available for "wax-pot" dipping to produce a thin layer of uniform thickness upon which the remainder of the frame wax-up can be developed. Such wax should be of contrasting color to other waxes used so that proper wax thickness can be determined during subsequent cutback procedures. Thermoplastic resin sheet of appropriate thickness can also be adapted to produce a 0.3 mm base matrix to which additional wax can be applied in fabrication of the frame.

5. Proceed with the wax-up, using a harder inlay wax. It is useful to wax to complete contour to determine if the preparation design is sufficient to fulfill the

A 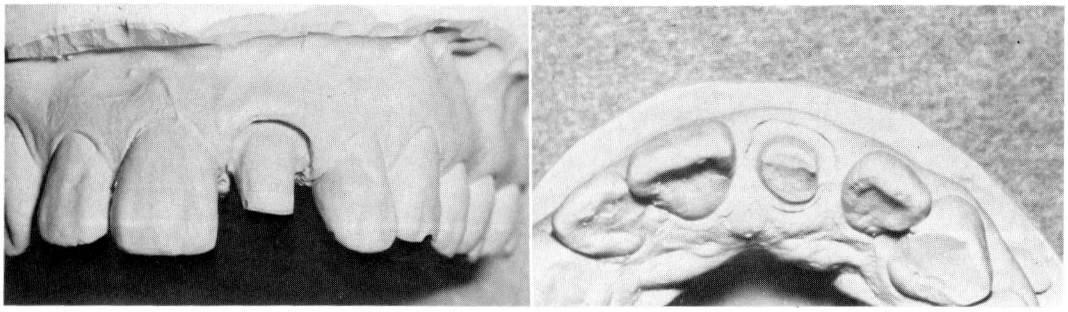 B

Fig. 11-1. A, Fontal view of preparation showing shoulder. **B,** Incisal view showing proper labial reduction.

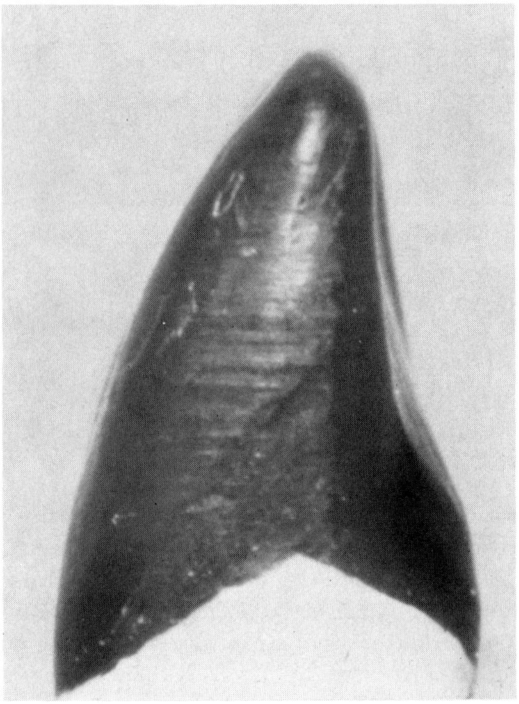

Fig. 11-2. Proximal view of full wax-up.

requirements (form, function, and esthetics) (Fig. 11-2).

6. Cut back the wax-up to complement good metal design (Fig. 11-3, *A*).

7. The facial wax thickness is reduced to approximately 0.3 mm. The shoulder of the preparation that is to receive the porcelain margin is exposed (Fig. 11-3, *B*). The pattern is placed on the master cast and checked for clearance (Fig. 11-3, *C*).

An alternate technique is that of casting the frame with the metal margin complete to be used in the subsequent adaptation of the platinum foil matrix to the shoulder of the die. After adaptation of the platinum, the cast metal margin is cut away.

8. Invest and cast the pattern using the manufacturer's instructions. Proper seating of the casting on the die is a critical step. The procedure follows:

a. Apply a thin coat of marking liquid on the die. Allow it to dry or blow dry.
b. Seat the casting gently, and stop when the casting does not seat freely.
c. Remove the casting, and using appropriate burs, relieve any areas that show red on the internal portions of the casting. Continue this procedure until all internal interferences are removed and the casting seats without force (Fig. 11-4, *A*).

PREPARING CERAMIC ALLOYS FOR PORCELAIN

All the separating disks and grinding stones used on ceramic alloys must be kept separately and should be used only for this purpose. Do not grind the casting with any stone that has previously been used on other alloys; indiscriminate use can cause contamination by

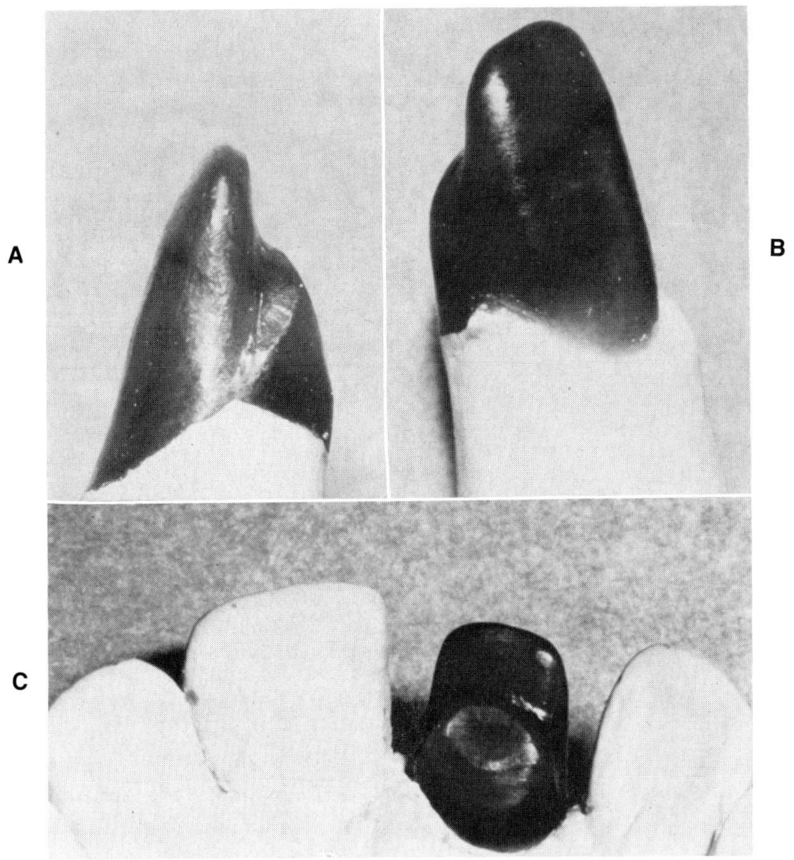

Fig. 11-3. A, Cutback of wax-up. **B,** Removal of wax at facial margin. **C,** Check for incisal and lingual clearance.

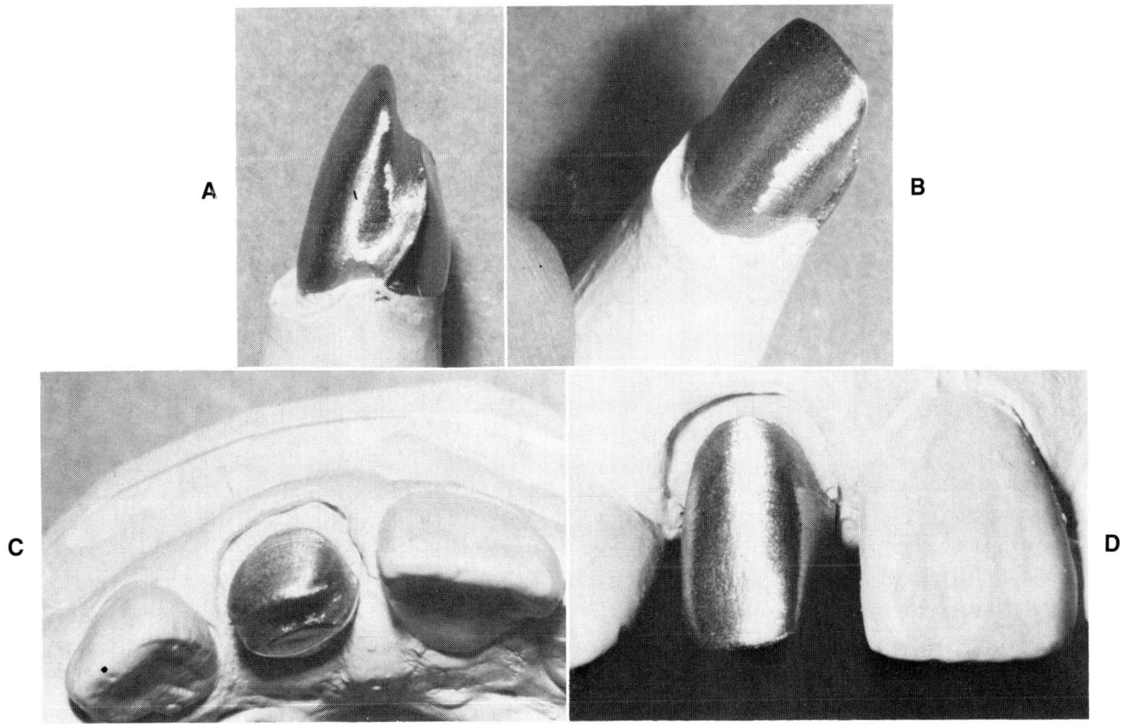

Fig. 11-4. A, Casting seated after internal interferences removed. **B,** Facial view of final metal design. **C,** Incisal view of casting seated. **D,** Check for incisal reduction.

A 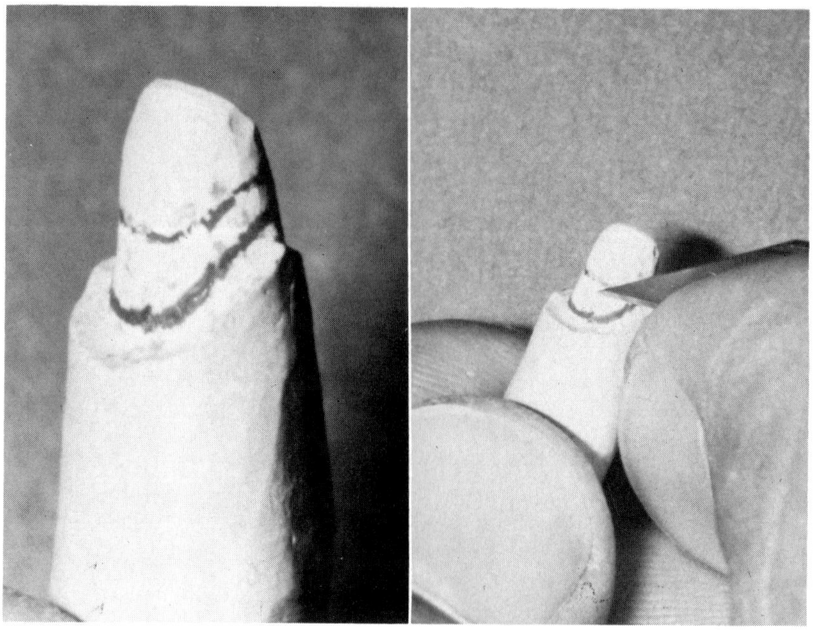 B

Fig. 11-5. A, Mark outline for internal portion of platinum. **B,** Scrape die to relieve platinum.

copper, silver, or zinc. Those disks and stones used on cobalt-chromium alloys can also cause contamination. Do not pickle ceramic alloys in acids that have been used for crown and bridge alloys.

The use of vitrified stones or carbide burs in conjunction with the metal-ceramic technique is advised. The metal-ceramic restoration has an important place in dentistry. It is a process that must be handled properly and used with discretion. Because of the nature of the materials involved, there are exacting technical considerations that must be understood. The importance of adhering to recommended procedures when fabricating a metal-ceramic restoration cannot be overemphasized. To gain a better insight into this form of restoration the following information and literature is helpful: *Metal Design for Porcelain to Gold Restorations* and *Quality Control for Porcelain to Metal Restorations** and *Crown and Bridge Construction.*† It is important to follow the manufacturer's suggestions.

METAL DESIGN

PROCEDURE

1. Remove excess metal with noncontaminating disks or burs.

2. Finish all surfaces of the casting to receive porcelain with a fine mounted stone to achieve uniform smoothness. Finish the metal in one direction to avoid trapping particles in folds of metal that would surface during baking procedures (Fig. 11-4, *B*). It has also been recommended that the surfaces that are to receive porcelain be treated by abrasive blasting with 50 μm aluminum oxide to remove any minute wire-like folds or drawn areas of metal in which particles of abrasive or binder from grinding stones could be trapped.

3. There should be no sharp points, corners, or angles on the porcelain-bearing surface. All areas should be gently rounded and convex. Mechanical retention should not be used on the coping substructure. After preparing the porcelain-bearing surfaces, place the casting on the working model to verify proper seating and adequate clearance for application of porcelain (Fig. 11-4, *C* and *D*).

Cut out an arcuate piece of platinum foil, as shown in Fig. 11-6, approximately 5.0 mm in width and long enough to reach well into the interproximal areas mesially and distally. A tool made from an orangewood stick, tapered to a rounded point on one end and with a chisel-shaped edge on the other, will serve to adapt the platinum foil to the appropriate die surfaces. Adapt the platinum matrix, first with finger pressure and then with the orangewood burnishing tool before seating the casting (Fig. 11-7, *A*). Seat the casting over the foil matrix and finish burnishing for final adaptation (Fig. 11-7, *B*).

Prepare the die by placing an outline of the area where the platinum will be formed on the axial and interproximal portion of the preparation (Fig. 11-5, *A*). Using a sharp instrument, relieve the stone in this area

*The J. M. Ney Co., Bloomfield, Conn.

†J. F. Jelenko & Co., New Rochelle, N.Y.

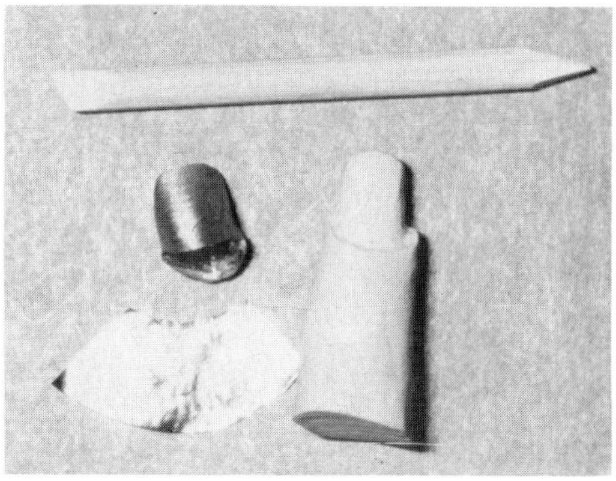

Fig. 11-6. Cutout of platinum to form margin.

A

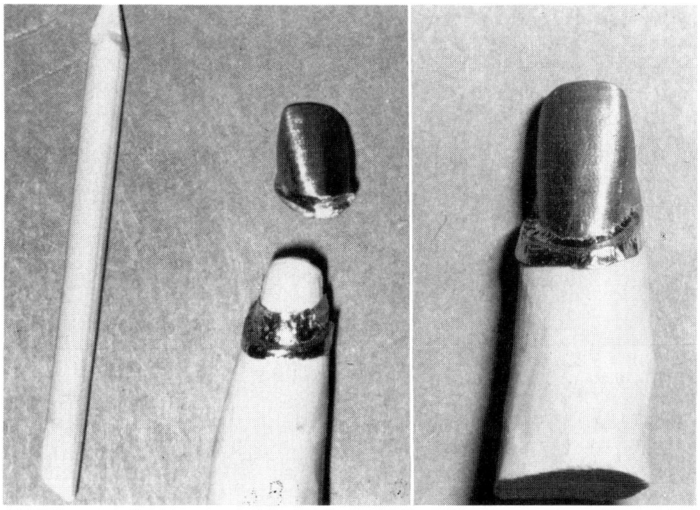

B

Fig. 11-7. A, Adapt platinum to die. **B,** Seat casting over platinum and burnish.

carefully to allow the casting to seat completely on the die when the platinum is placed inside (Fig. 11-5, *B*).

4. Remove the casting, and clean the metal coping prior to the application of opaque. Leach the metal by applying a coat of opaque and firing as recommended by the manufacturer. After cooling place the coping in a stripping solution. When all the material is removed, clean the coping in distilled water. Be sure to not touch the surface that will receive the porcelain. The casting is now ready for porcelain applications.

PORCELAIN APPLICATION

PROCEDURE

1. Apply the first application of opaque with a brush, spatula, or airbrush (Fig. 11-8, *A*). The airbrush is preferred because of the controlled uniform thickness of opaque. When using an airbrush, heat the coping by placing it in front of the muffle or by using a hot dryer. This will keep the opaque under control. Be sure to place the coping on the die while spraying to keep the opaque from entering the internal portion of the coping (Fig. 11-8, *B*).

2. Remove the casting, and, using a soft bristle brush, remove the opaque as shown in Fig. 11-9, *A*. Be sure to clear the porcelain from proximal-to-proximal contact (Fig. 11-9, *B*). This will give a clean surface for spot welding the platinum margin to the coping.

3. Select the appropriate temperature as directed by the manufacturer for the first opaque application and fire at a rate of 58° F/min (32° C/min).

4. After the casting has cooled, place it on the die with the platinum collar in place (Fig. 11-10). Readapt the platinum, and use sticky wax to hold the platinum to the casting in an area that is not to receive opaque.

5. Using an orthodontic spot welder, weld the platinum to the coping (Fig. 11-11, *A* and *B*) about 3 mm from proximal-to-proximal contact. Return the coping to the die, and burnish it around the margins (Fig. 11-11, *C*).

6. Apply the opaque with an airbrush (Fig. 11-12, *A*),

A B

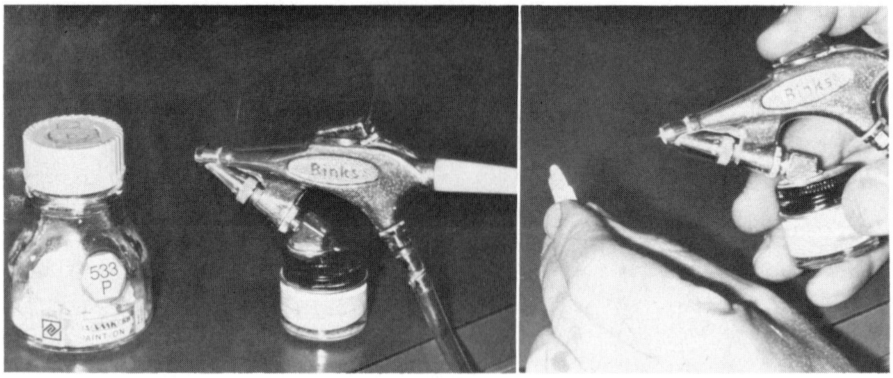

Fig. 11-8. A, Artist's airbrush for opaquing, **B,** Application of first opaque with airbrush.

A B

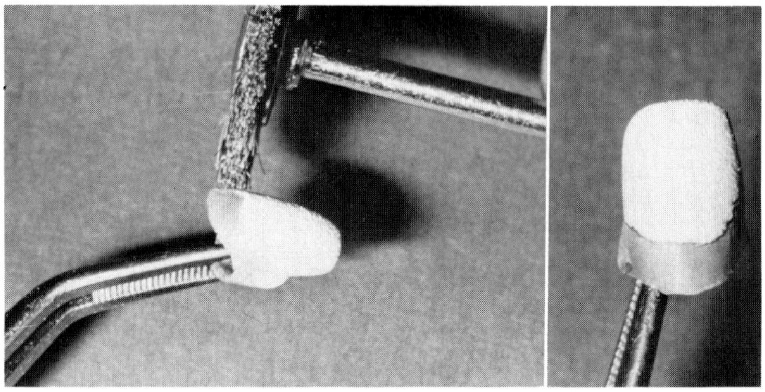

Fig. 11-9. A, Removal of opaque at margin before baking. **B,** Opaque cleared from mesial to distal interproximal areas.

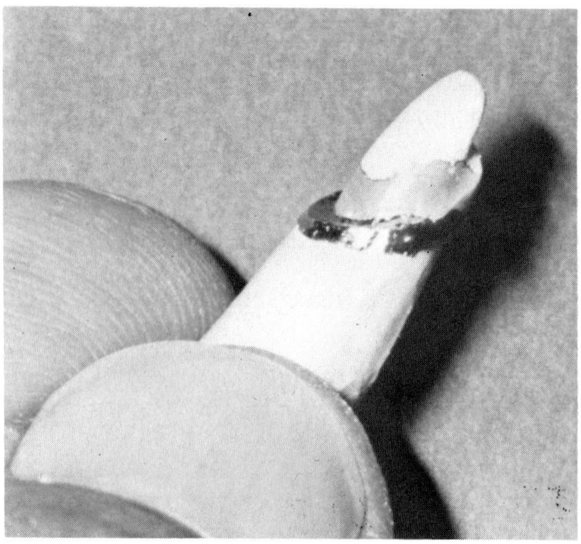

Fig. 11-10. Casting and platinum sticky waxed together.

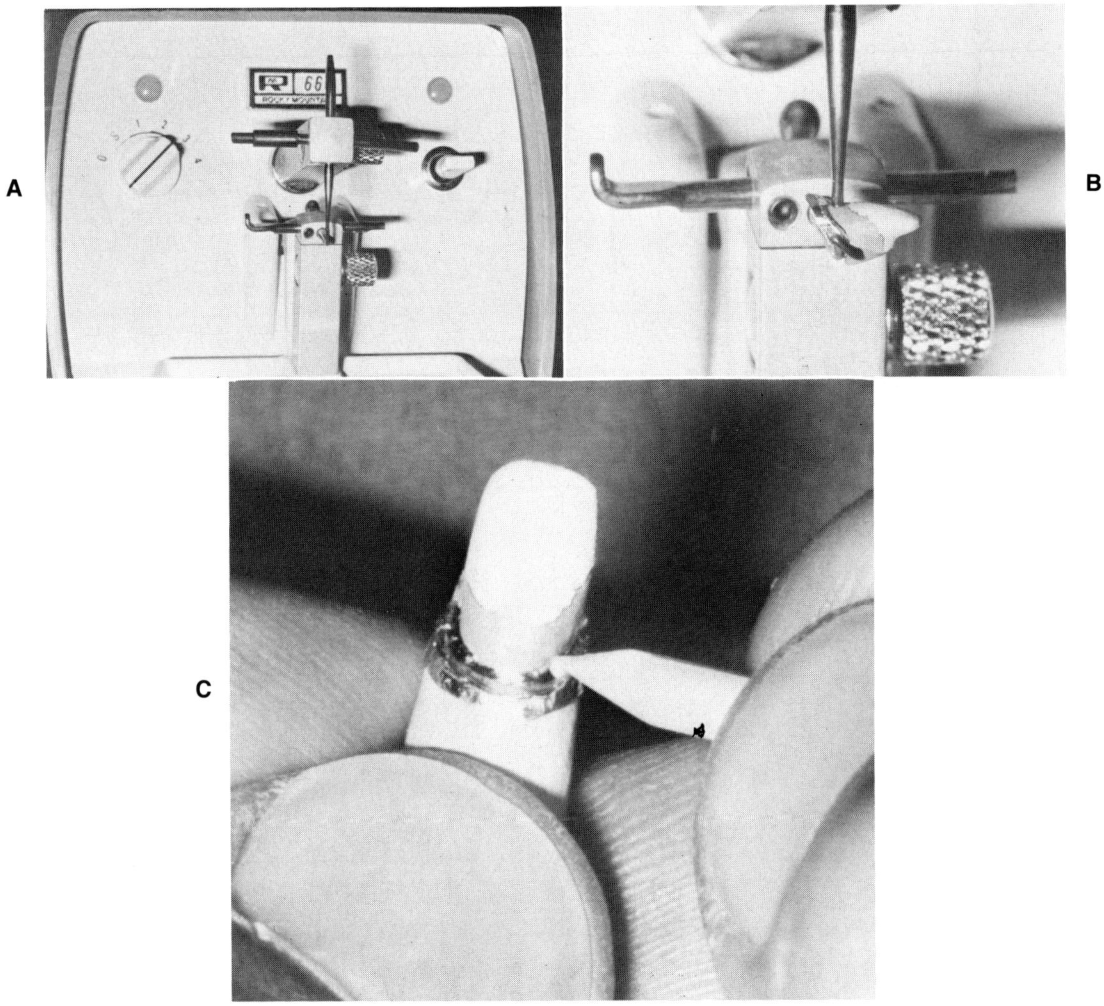

Fig. 11-11. A, Orthodontic welder. **B,** Spot weld platinum to casting. **C,** Adapt platinum to margin.

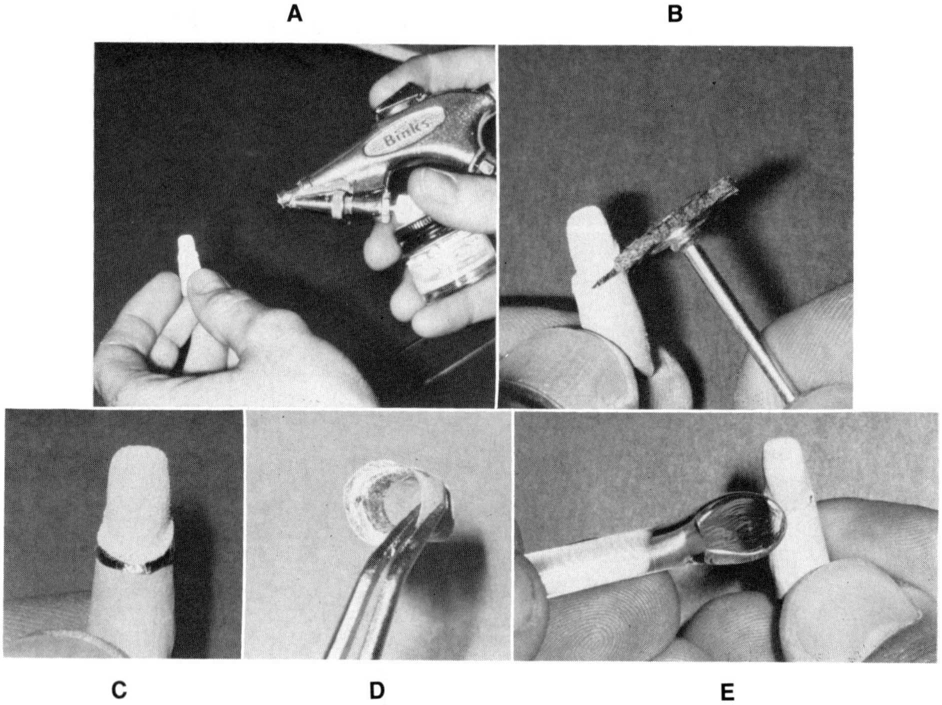

Fig. 11-12. A, Airbrush opaque at margin. **B,** Remove opaque around platinum apron. **C,** Ready for furnace. **D,** Check inside for opaque before baking. **E,** After cooling, check coping for marginal defects, and readapt foil if necessary.

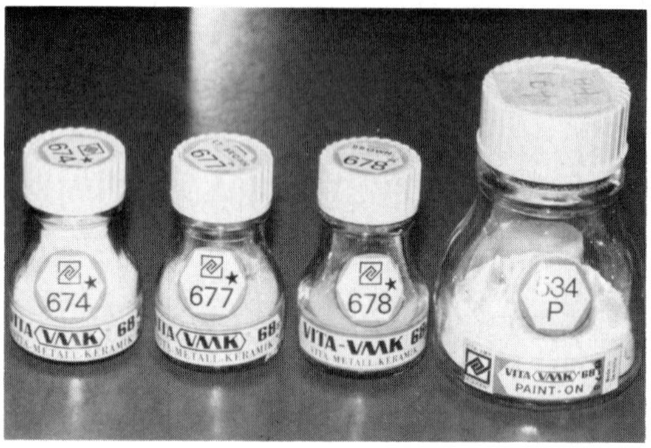

Fig. 11-13. Base opaque with colored modifiers.

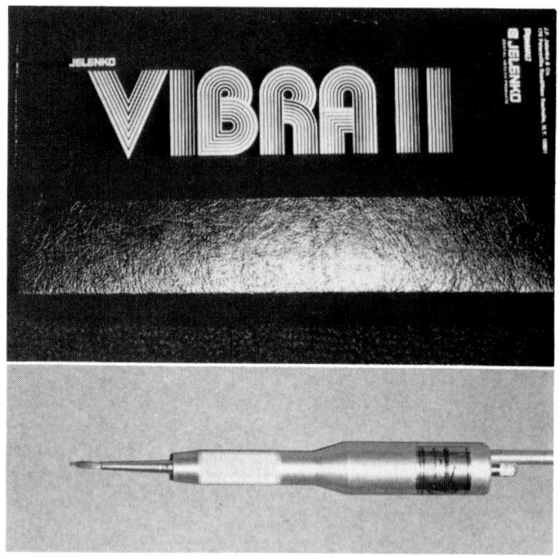

Fig. 11-14. Jelenko Vibra-Brush.

and remove the porcelain excess around the platinum apron (Fig. 11-12, *B* and *C*). Inspect the inside of the coping, and remove any opaque residue (Fig. 11-12, *D*). The coping is now ready for the first opaque bake. After cooling check the coping on the die for any marginal warpage. Readapt if necessary (Fig. 11-12, *E*).

To achieve a good shade match without the use of surface staining, routinely use opaque modifiers (Fig. 11-13). The modifiers also help to create the three-dimensional effect of natural dentition.

7. Apply a thin mix of dark brown opaque mixed with the body shade opaque to a color that gives the desired contrast (Figs. 11-14 and 11-15, *A*). Experience in mixing modifiers will aid in achieving the best results for all shades (i.e., darker shades require more modifications than lighter shades). Add a lighter amount of this mix around the margin and up the center of the tooth to enhance the shade from within (Fig. 11-15, *B* and *C*). Because metal design may allow only 0.5 mm of

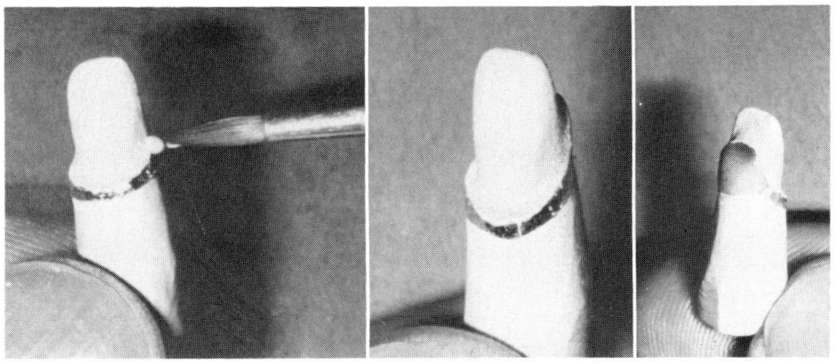

A B C

Fig. 11-15. A, Applying mixture of base opaque and dark brown modifier to proximal contact with Vibra-Brush. **B,** Modifier added around margin and cervical third of facial surface. **C,** Modifier added to lingual surface.

A B C

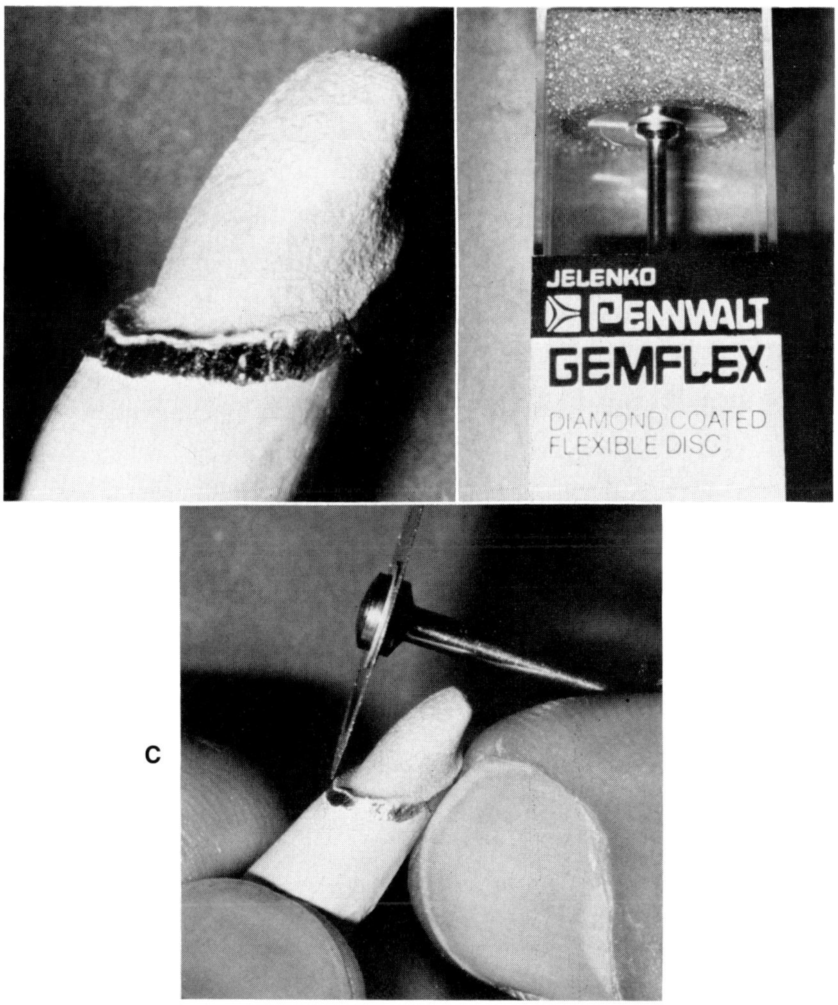

Fig. 11-16. A, Texture of opaque after firing. **B,** Thin diamond disk. **C,** Removal of platinum apron.

porcelain on the lingual side, this area should be similarly modified to lower the value. Use a violet modifier to reduce value at the incisal edge. At this time note the texture of the final opaque bake (Fig. 11-16, *A*). An application of the opaque with the airbrush gives a final surface texture that minimizes specular reflection. The texture on the surface is also an important part of this restoration and will be covered at the glazing stage.

8. Use a thin flexible diamond disk (Fig. 11-16, *B*), and carefully go around the collar to remove the platinum apron (Fig. 11-16, *C*). This will allow the crown to seat on the solid working cast without destroying the stone tissue landmarks. Reexamine for marginal adaptation of platinum.

DENTIN AND INCISAL BUILDUP

PROCEDURE

1. Mix the dentin, enamel or incisal, color modifiers, and translucent powders with the modeling fluid. Be sure to mix a sufficient quantity of porcelain for the entire buildup (Fig. 11-17).

2. Begin by applying a thin wet wash to the entire coping (Fig. 11-18, *A*). At this time use color modifier, based on the shade selected, mixed with the dentin, and apply this mix to the center gingival area (Fig. 11-18, *B*).

3. Next build out the body contour at the facial margin (Fig. 11-18, *C*).

4. Apply brown modifier mixed with the dentin shade to the interproximal surfaces (Fig. 11-18, *D*).

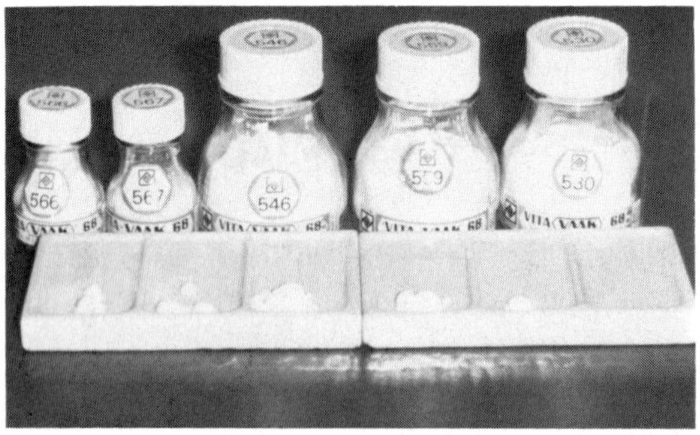

Fig. 11-17. Dentin, enamel, and colored body modifiers.

A B C D

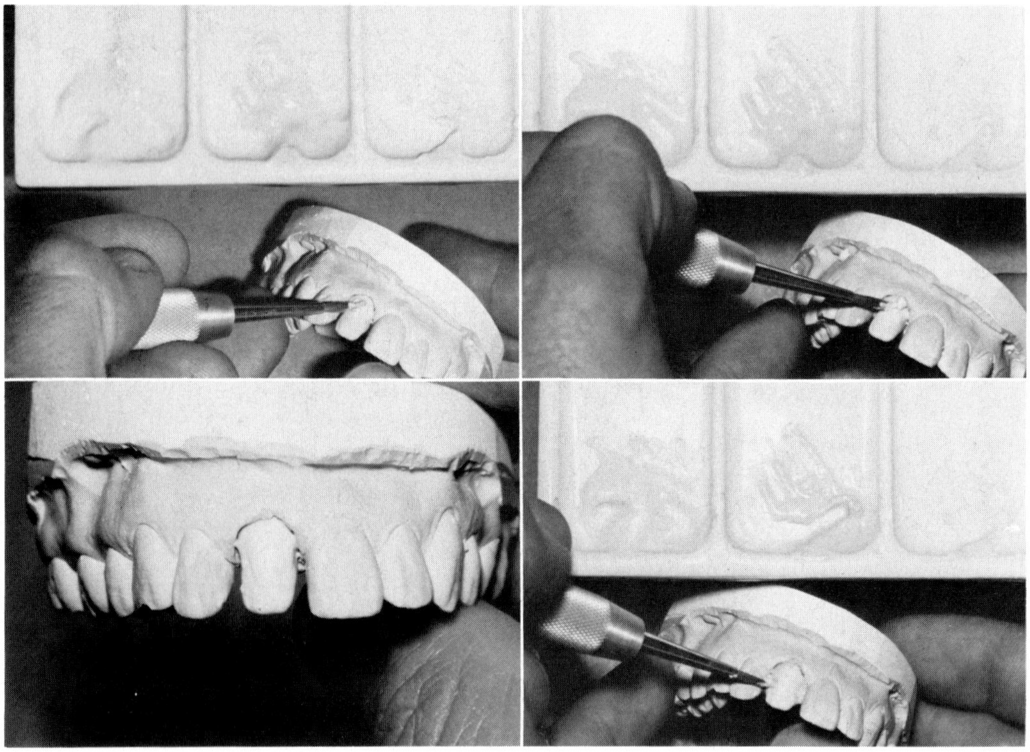

Fig. 11-18. A, Apply thin slurry body mix over entire coping. **B,** Apply dentin and light modifier mix on facial surface. **C,** Build out facial margin. **D,** Apply dentin and dark modifier mix into interproximal surface.

5. Remove moisture from the linguoincisal area with an absorbant tissue. Do not allow the porcelain to dry out totally. Apply the tissue to the facial margin, and build up the lingual surface to contour (Fig. 11-19, *A*). Be sure to extend the incisal length at least 1 to 1.5 mm to allow for shrinkage on baking (Fig. 11-19, *B*).

6. Apply a tissue to the lingual area, and proceed to build up the facial contour, starting with the mesial lobe (Fig. 11-20, *A*).

7. Build the distal lobe next (Fig. 11-20, *B*), and fill in the center using a modeling tool or brush to obtain the desired contour (Fig. 11-20, *C* and *D*).

INCISAL CUTBACK

PROCEDURE

1. Starting at either the mesial or distal bevel, slice into the interproximal area (Fig. 11-21, *A*). Create a gradual bevel incisofacially down to about the middle third of the tooth (Fig. 11-21, *B*).

2. Thin transparent ceramic rods can be embedded within the porcelain buildup in the area of the developmental grooves to give the finished porcelain greater translucence and depth of color. The rods should be applied as illustrated in Fig. 11-21, *C*. If two rods are employed, one (the distal) should be made slightly

A
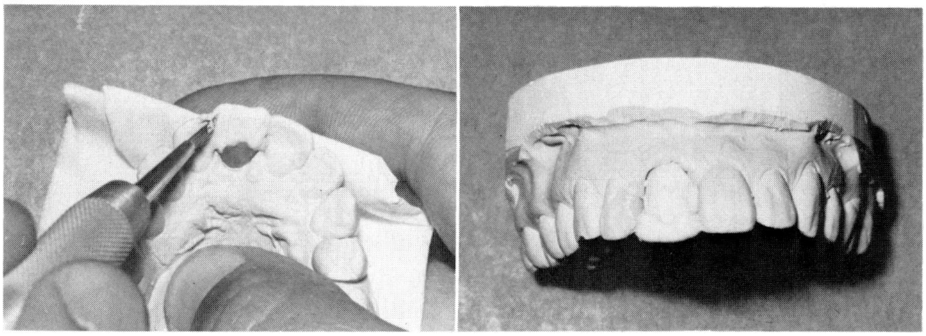
B

Fig. 11-19. A, Build up lingual contour. **B,** Extend incisal length at least 1 to 1.5 mm.

A
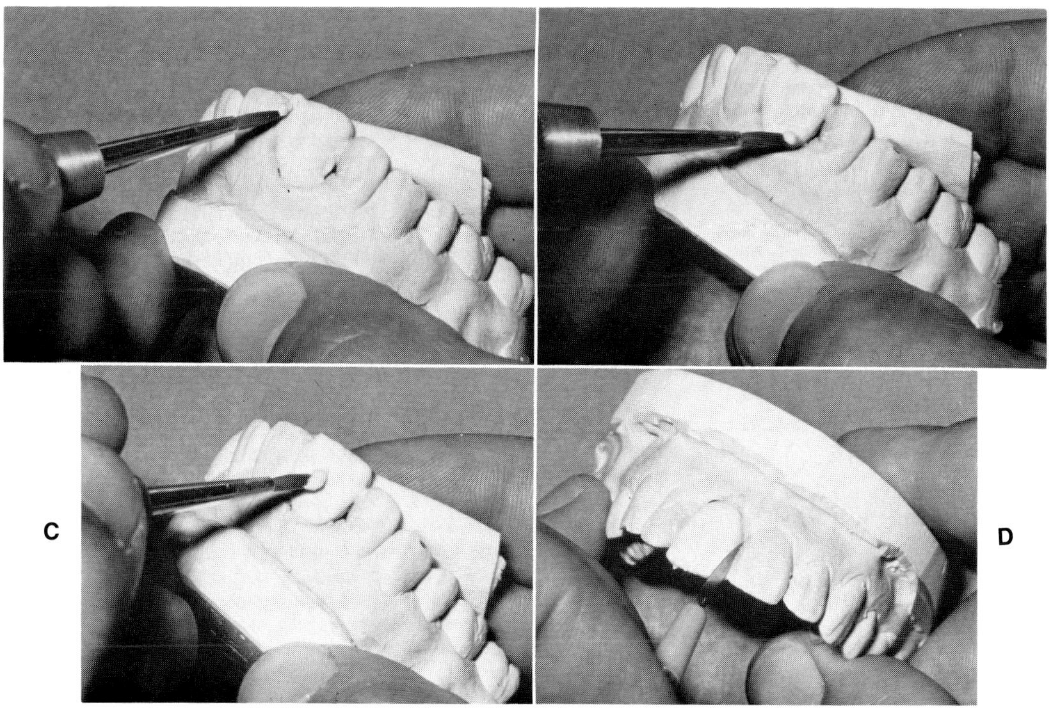
B

C
D

Fig. 11-20. A, Build up mesial lobe. **B,** Build up distal lobe. **C,** Fill in center of tooth. **D,** Shape tooth form with tool.

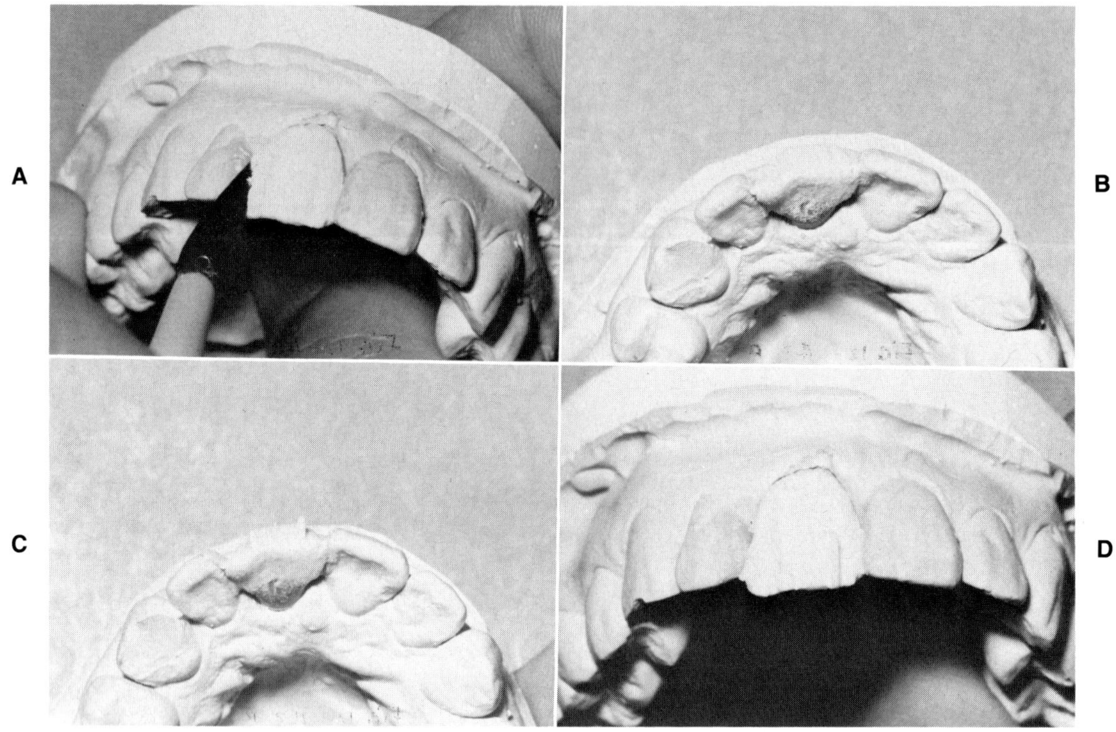

Fig. 11-21. A, Bevel mesial, distal, and proximal surfaces. **B,** Make gradual bevel incisofacially down to middle third of tooth. **C,** Apply transparent rods. **D,** Mesial rod longer than distal rod.

shorter than the other (Fig. 11-21, *D*). At this stage of the porcelain build-up, any desired "wet-staining" of the incisal region should be applied to achieve a more natural effect.

3. Moisten the dentin porcelain slightly to receive the enamel overlay, and apply enamel first between the two rods to hold them in place (Fig. 11-22, *A*).

4. Complete the enamel buildup on the mesial and distal lobes, and shape with a model tool (Fig. 11-22, *B*).

5. Using a soft artist's brush, drag all surfaces to give a good incisal-body blend (Fig. 11-22, *C*).

6. Remove the crown, and add contacts (Fig. 11-23, *A*).

7. Using a fine-bladed instrument, ditch the margin to prevent shrinkage from lifting the margin (Fig. 11-23, *B*).

8. Bake according to the manufacturer's directions.

9. After the crown has cooled, use thin (0.00075) articulating paper, and adjust contacts to seat the crown on the solid model (Fig. 11-24, *A* and *B*).

10. Use a porcelain grinding wheel, and adjust the width as necessary (Fig. 11-24, *C* and *D*).

11. Seat the crown, and examine it for any voids on the facial surface or contacts (Fig. 11-24, *E*).

12. Reseat the crown on the single die, and burnish the platinum margin if necessary (Fig. 11-25, *A*).

13. Add a mixture of dentin plus modifier around the collar, and bake (Fig. 11-25, *B*).

14. Using a fine diamond disk, finish the marginal contour on the single die (Fig. 11-26, *A*).

15. Seat the crown on the working model, and rough in the facial contours and incisal length (Fig. 11-26, *B* and *C*) with a bulk grinding wheel. For the final contour and texture use fine diamond points (Fig. 11-27, *A*), such as a barrel-shaped diamond for facial reduction, the short tapered diamond for rolling out the embrasure over facial surfaces, and the long thin tapered diamond for final surface texture (Fig. 11-27, *B*, *C*, and *D*).

Texture is very important when using material such as porcelain to create the optical illusion of the surface reflection and absorption of light in natural teeth. A mirror-smooth surface will reflect much of the light source back to the observer. The results may be too high a value or too bright a tooth, which in turn decreases chroma. The opposite can happen by putting in too much texture. The most natural looking restorations in the mouth are those which are textured by the dentist in the environment in which they will be seen . . .

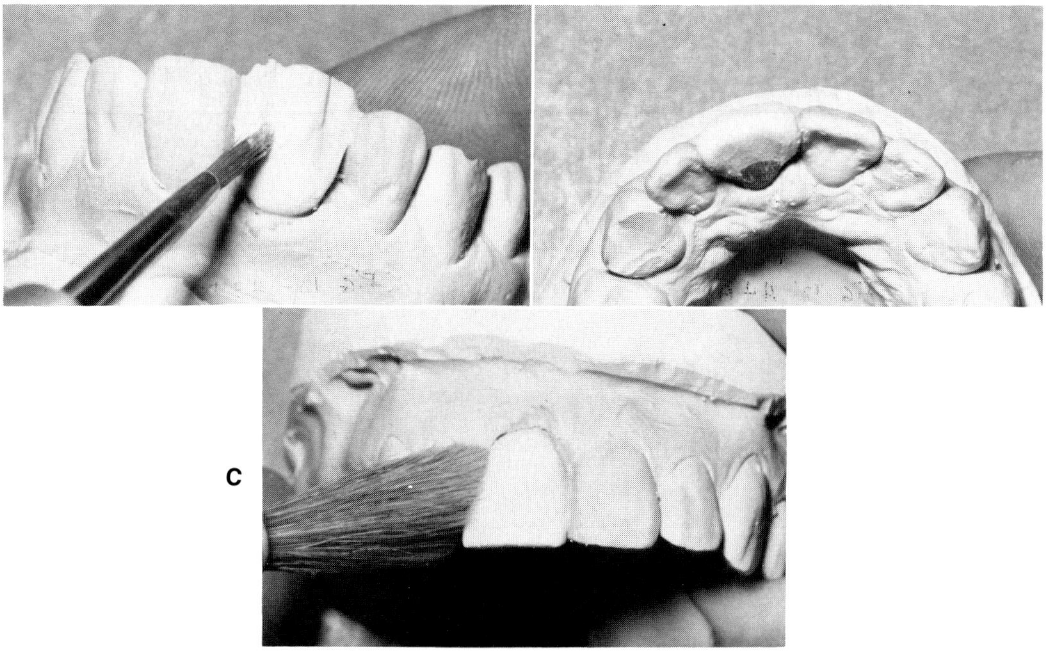

Fig. 11-22. **A,** Lay enamel between two rods. **B,** Complete enamel buildup. **C,** Blend incisal porcelain to body with soft artist's brush.

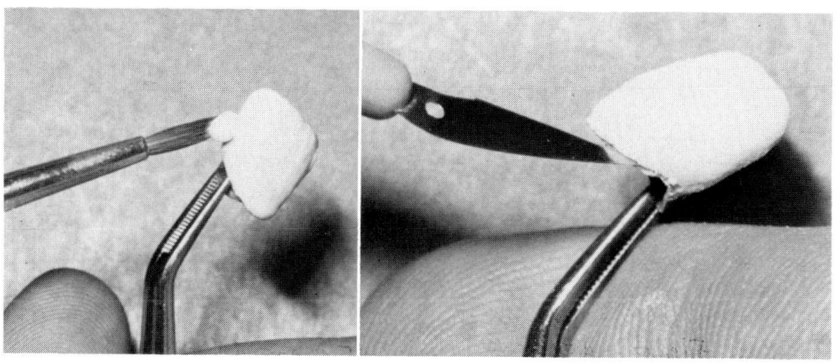

Fig. 11-23. **A,** Remove crown, and add contacts. **B,** Ditch margin before first bake.

A B C D E

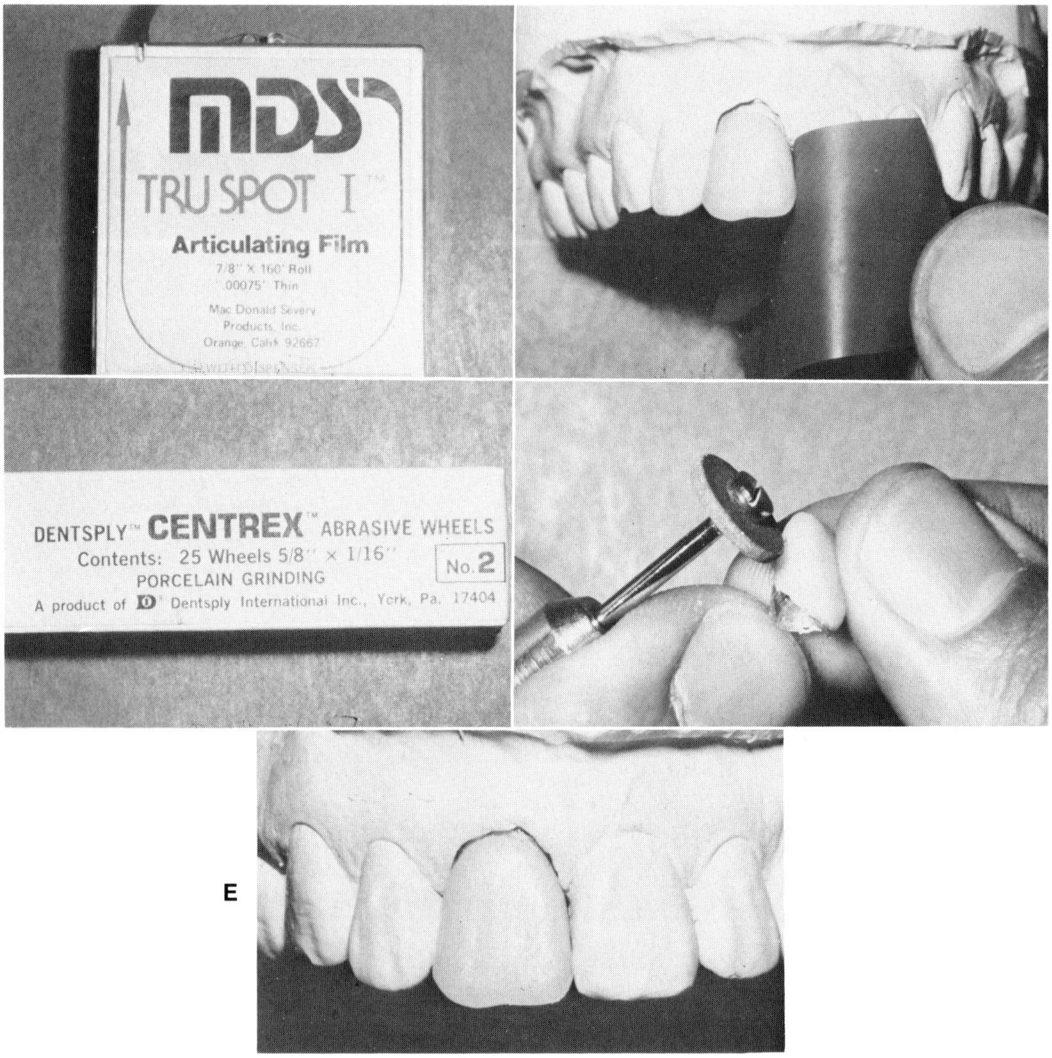

Fig. 11-24. A, Thin articulating film. **B,** Check for tight contacts. **C,** Procelain grinding wheels. **D,** Adjust contacts. **E,** Check for additional buildup.

A B

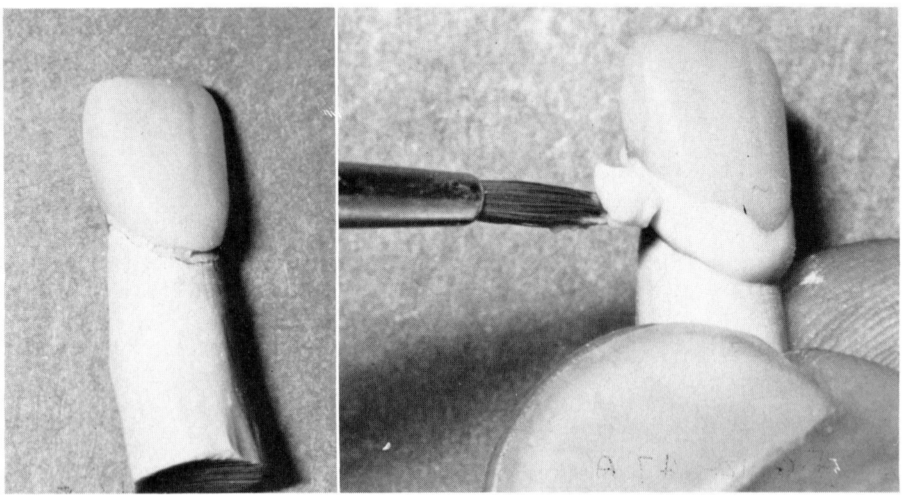

Fig. 11-25. A, Recheck margins and burnish. **B,** Cervical blend added at margin.

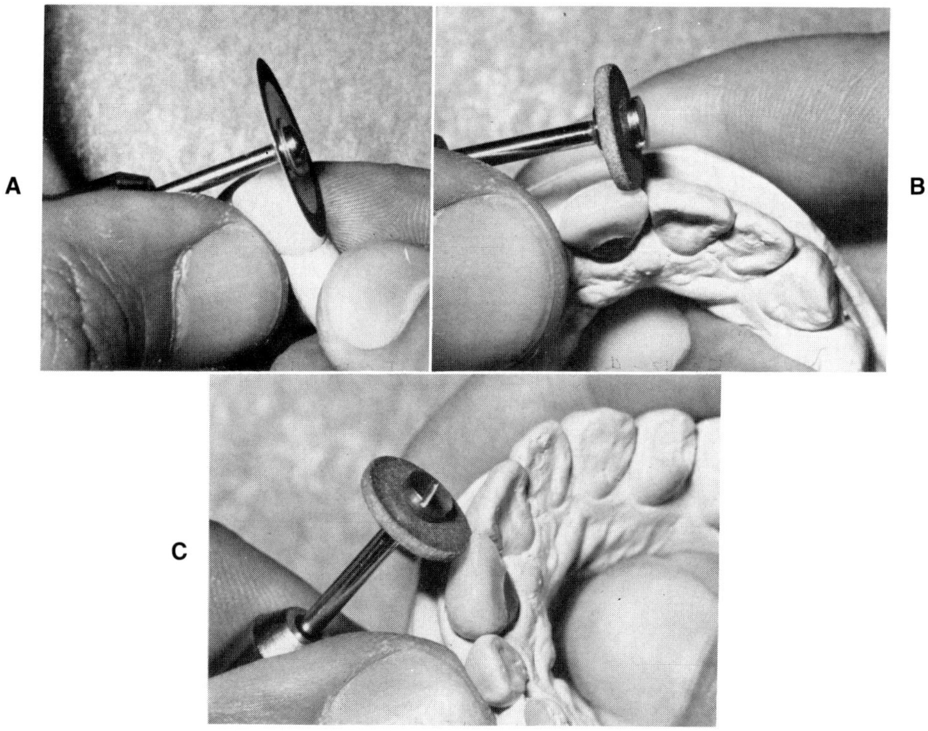

Fig. 11-26. A, Contouring porcelain margin. **B** and **C,** Bulk grind-in of form.

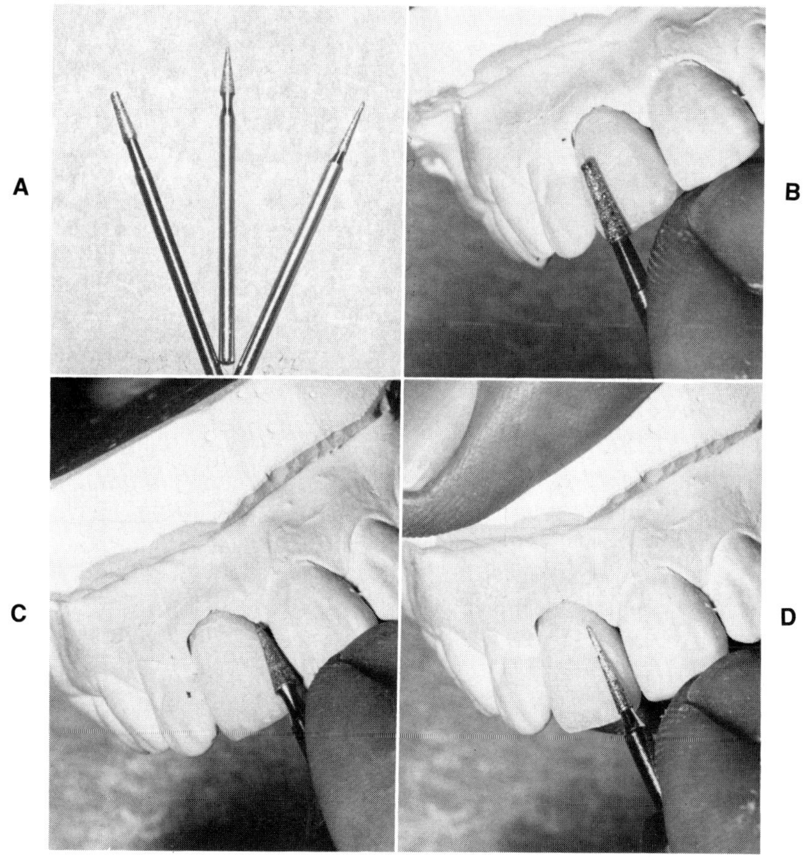

Fig. 11-27. A, Diamond points for final contouring. **B,** Barrel diamond point for facial contouring and texturing. **C,** Short taper diamond point for interproximal contouring. **D,** Long thin diamond point for finishing contour and texture.

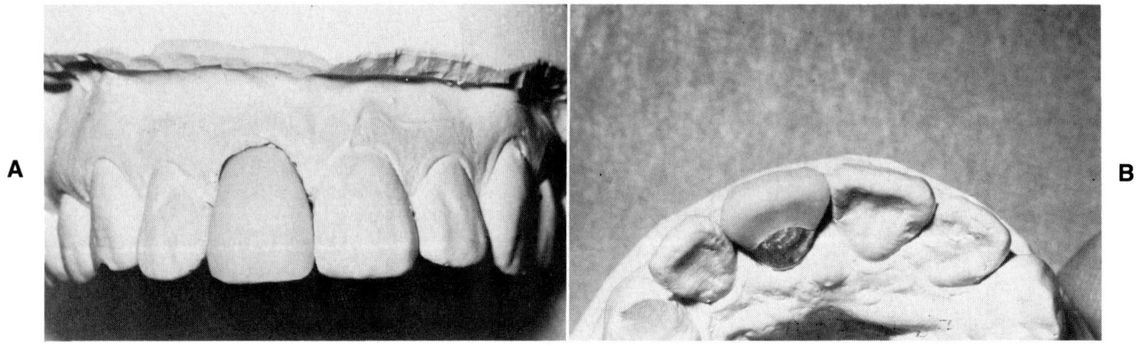

Fig. 11-28. A, Compare texture of adjacent teeth. **B,** Look down incisal aspect to compare developmental lobes of natural tooth.

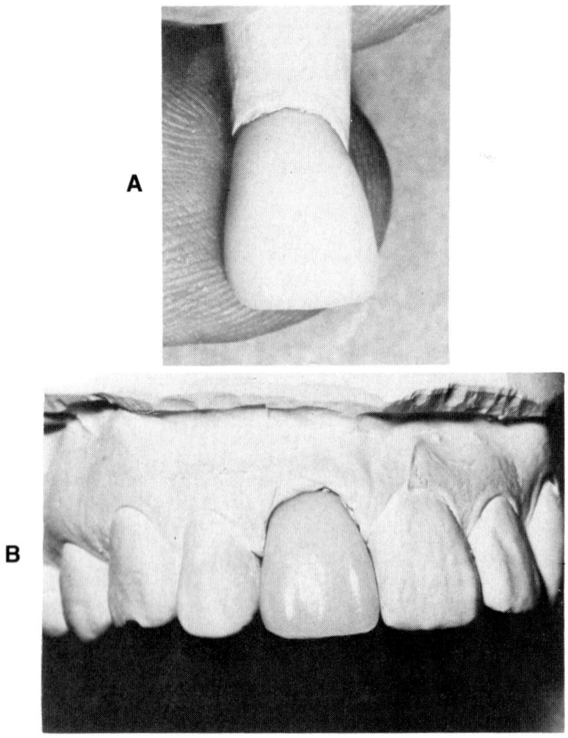

Fig. 11-29. A, Check margin on single die. **B,** Check contacts.

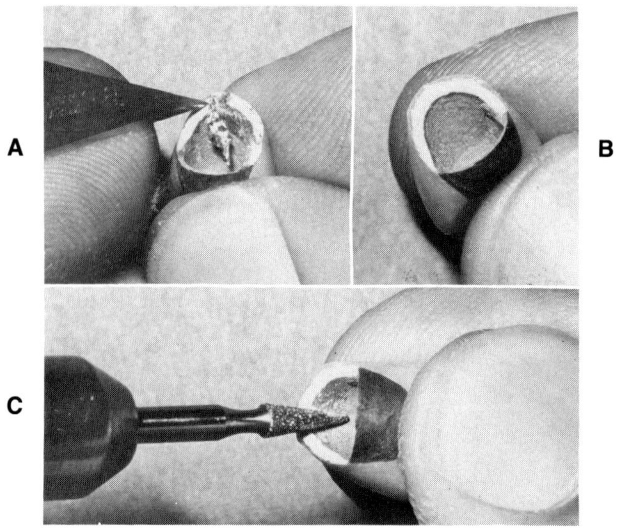

Fig. 11-30. A, Remove platinum. **B,** Check for flaws at margin. **C,** Adjust opaque and metal juncture.

the mouth. The technician can simulate closely by studying the adjacent teeth (Fig. 11-28, *A*). It is also important to study the crown and adjacent teeth by looking down the tooth from the incisal edge for developmental lobes and how they are formed (Fig. 11-28, *B*).

GLAZING

PROCEDURE

1. Before glazing the restoration should be checked in the mouth for final contouring and texturing. Compare the shade carefully, and adjust as is necessary.

2. Remove and clean the crown. If staining is necessary, restain and glaze the crown. A low-fusing overglaze on restorations may reflect light in such a way as to look false. The time and temperature glaze, done properly, comes much closer to nature and also increases the vitality of the porcelain.

3. After glazing, check, the crown on the die, and verify the facial margin (Fig. 11-29, *A*).

4. Place the crown on the cast and check the contacts (Fig. 11-29, *B*).

5. Remove the platinum carefully with a sharp blade, and inspect it for any flaws (Fig. 11-30, *A* and *B*).

6. Using a diamond point at slow speed, smooth out the opaque-gold juncture in the area relieved on the die (Fig. 11-30, *C*).

7. Seat the crown on the die to check the porcelain margin (Fig. 11-31). The crown in now ready for cementation.

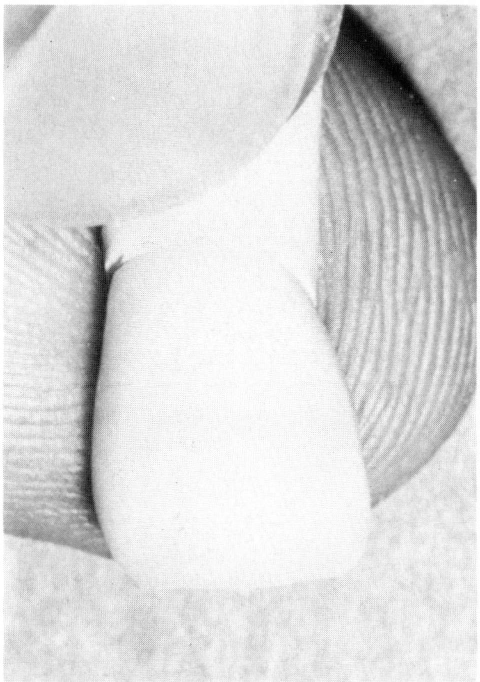

Fig. 11-31. Verify on single die before cementing.

PART TWO

Aluminous porcelain jacket crown

The aluminous porcelain jacket crown has been selected to illustrate the technical procedures involved in the fabrication of porcelain jacket crowns. Although an additional step is involved in fabrication of the reinforcing aluminous core, other steps illustrated are identical to those involved in conventional porcelain jacket construction.

Aluminous porcelain is considered to be the strongest porcelain jacket material and offers the best esthetics in anterior restorations. Due to its fine grain size and self-glazing qualities it is well accepted by the tissue.

PREPARATION DESIGN

The key to successful construction and placement of an esthetic and durable porcelain jacket crown lies in proper evaluation of the clinical condition (occlusion and spatial relationships) and proper preparation design. Reduction of all axial tooth surfaces should be at least 1.0 mm or more, with approximately 2.0 to 3.0 mm reduction of the cervicoincisal length of the crown. Exposed points and line angles should be rounded. This amount of tooth reduction is necessary for proper shade reproduction in the porcelain. Adequate preparation for use of Vita Dur-S* porcelain is illustrated in Fig. 11-32.

A solid working cast and single dies are necessary to fabricate all restorations in the laboratory. This technique allows control over contour by leaving tissue landmarks while fabricating the restoration. It also gives the technician accurate control of contacts.

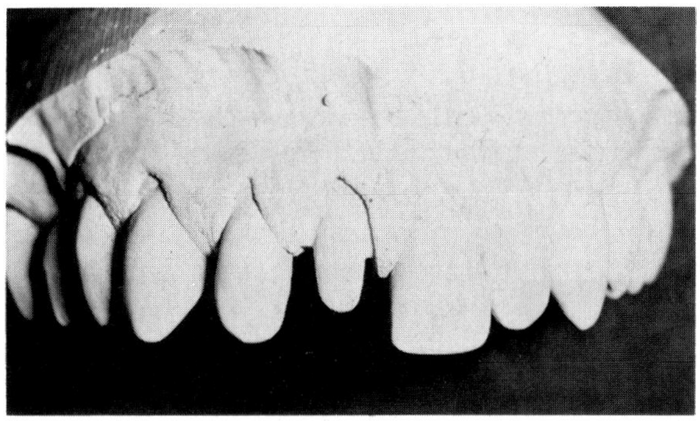

Fig. 11-32. Proper preparation design.

Trimming the die

PROCEDURE

1. There should be no undercut areas below the margin of the die. Trim the die without ditching or placing any undercut areas; any naturally occurring undercut areas should be eliminated with undercut wax or modeling compound. This will allow better matrix adaptation and prevent distortion upon removal of the apron beyond the margin.

2. Apply a thin coat of cyanoacrylate cement to the die using a cotton swab (Fig. 11-33, *A*). Immediately

*Unitek Corp., Monrovia, Calif.

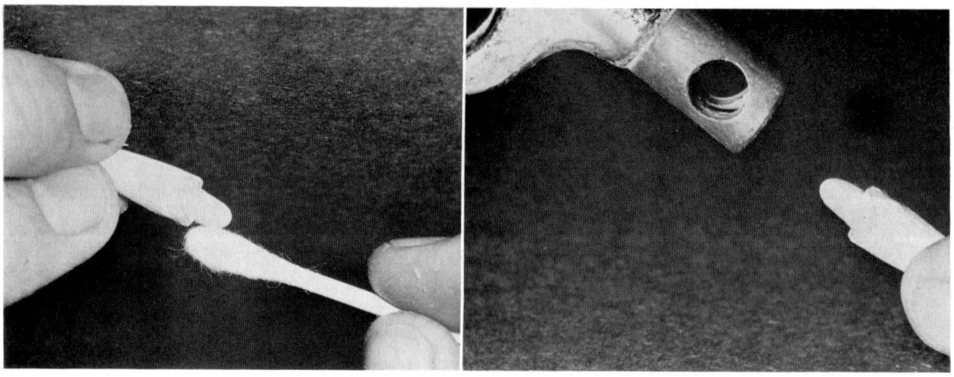

Fig. 11-33. A, Application of cyanoacrylate cement. **B,** Application of air pressure to dry cyanoacrylate cement.

apply air pressure to force the cement into the stone die (Fig. 11-33, *B*). This procedure will give the stone die adequate strength to absorb burnishing of the platinum matrix without eroding the die. If a copperplated or silver-plated die is being used this step can be eliminated.

The basic tools for forming the platinum foil matrix are shown in Fig. 11-34: 0.001-inch thick dead-soft platinum foil, a pair of specially designed tweezers, a pair of sharp scissors, and an orangewood stick shaped with a point at one end and a flat chisel at the other. A plastic matrix former is helpful.

3. Place the matrix former over the platinum foil, using a sharp instrument to cut out as outlined in Fig. 11-35, *A*.

4. Using finger pressure, adapt platinum to the die, being careful to line up the two ends at either the mesial or distal interproximal side (Fig. 11-35, *B*). Mold firmly with finger pressure around the die, and press the free ends firmly together with the tweezers at the proximal and incisal area (Fig. 11-36, *A*).

5. Now cut the excess platinum parallel to the die on the proximal and incisal surfaces, leaving 2 mm excess in each position (Fig. 11-36, *B*).

6. Carefully remove the platinum from the die, and with scissors shorten one side of the proximal and incisal excess by about 1 mm. Trim the marginal apron to form a 1-mm apron all the way around the tooth.

7. Replace the matrix on the die, and re-form the edges on the proximal and incisal surfaces with the tweezers. Lap the longer edge over the shorter edge at both the incisal and proximal surfaces. Using tweezers, firmly crimp the platinum matrix together making a so-called tinner's joint. Next cut an angled section on the incisal on both the mesial and distal sides (Fig. 11-36, *C*).

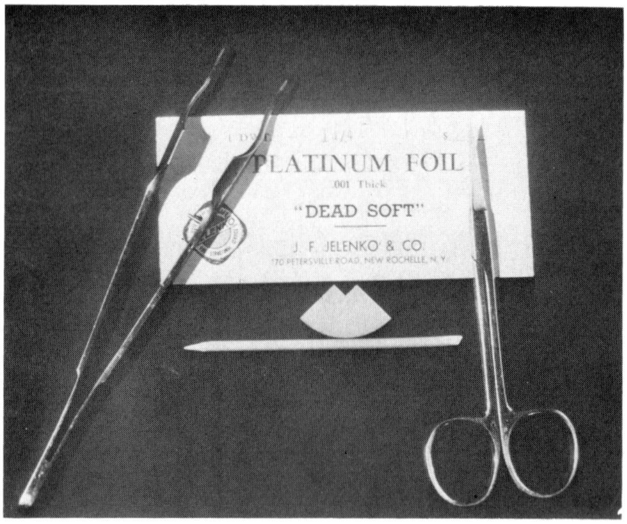

Fig. 11-34. Tools and materials needed to form platinum matrix.

8. Fold the lapped ends of the platinum foil over the die with finger pressure. Adapt the platinum matrix closely to the die by burnishing from the incisal side toward the shoulder with the orangewood stick. The matrix should fit firmly on the die with as few wrinkles in the platinum matrix as possible (Fig. 11-37).

9. Anneal the platinum in the furnace or with a gas flame. This will remove any foreign matter and enable accurate adaptation of the matrix to the die. At this point avoid touching the matrix with the fingers.

10. Now begin applying the opaque or core buildup. It is important to remember that the strength of the aluminous jacket lies with the core buildup. Apply the core material nearly to full contour on the lingual

A 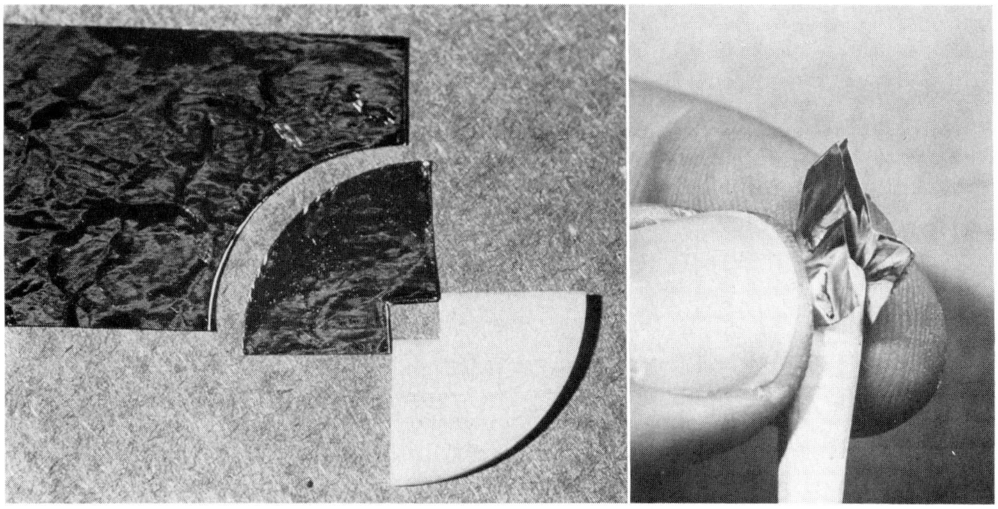 B

Fig. 11-35. A, Cutout of platinum for matrix. **B,** Wrap matrix around die with finger pressure.

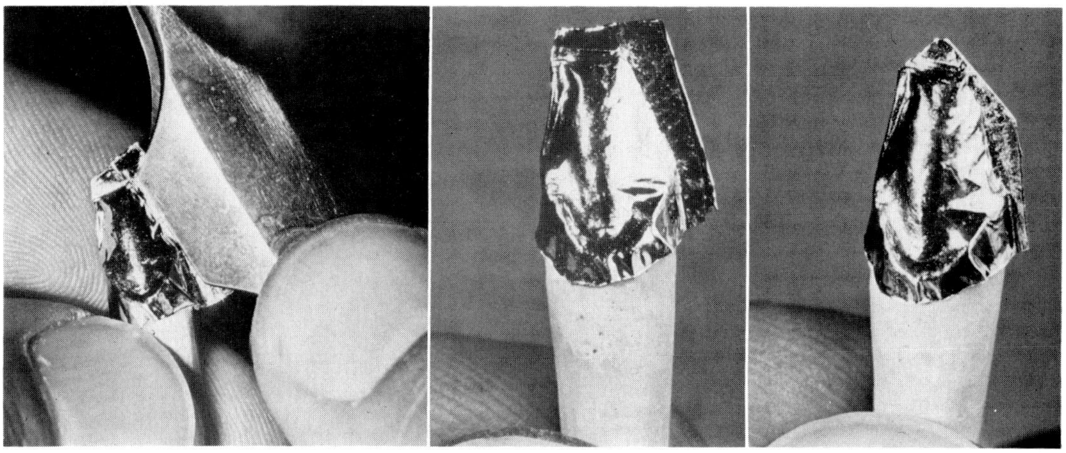

A B C

Fig. 11-36. A, Crimp top and proximal ends together. **B,** Cut top and proximal edges of platinum evenly. **C,** Bevel mesial and distal incisal edges.

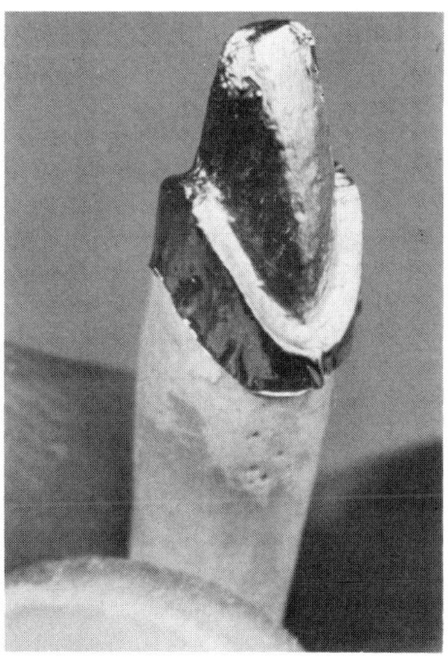

Fig. 11-37. Platinum matrix adapted properly with orangewood stick.

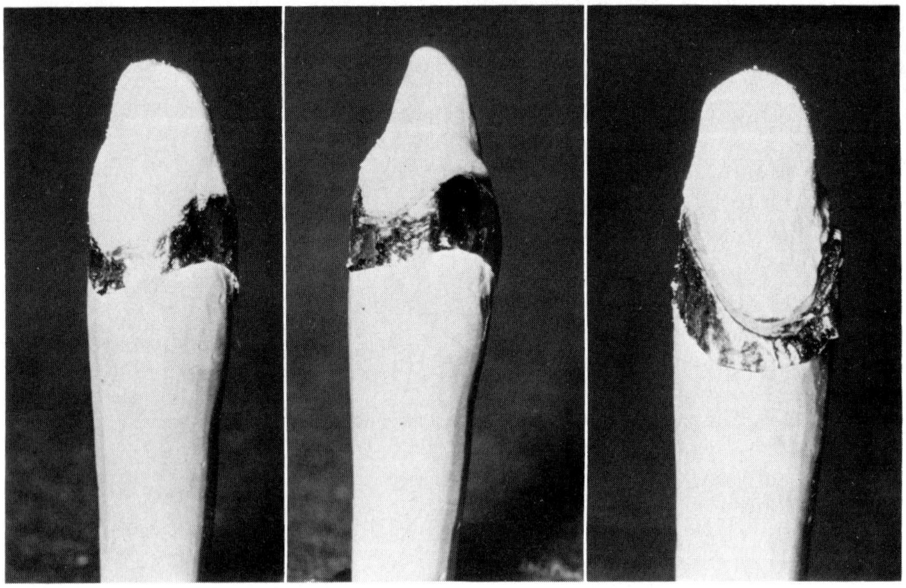

A B C

Fig. 11-38. A, First application of core material. **B,** Ditch around entire margin before first bake. **C,** Place matrix on die, and readapt platinum around margin.

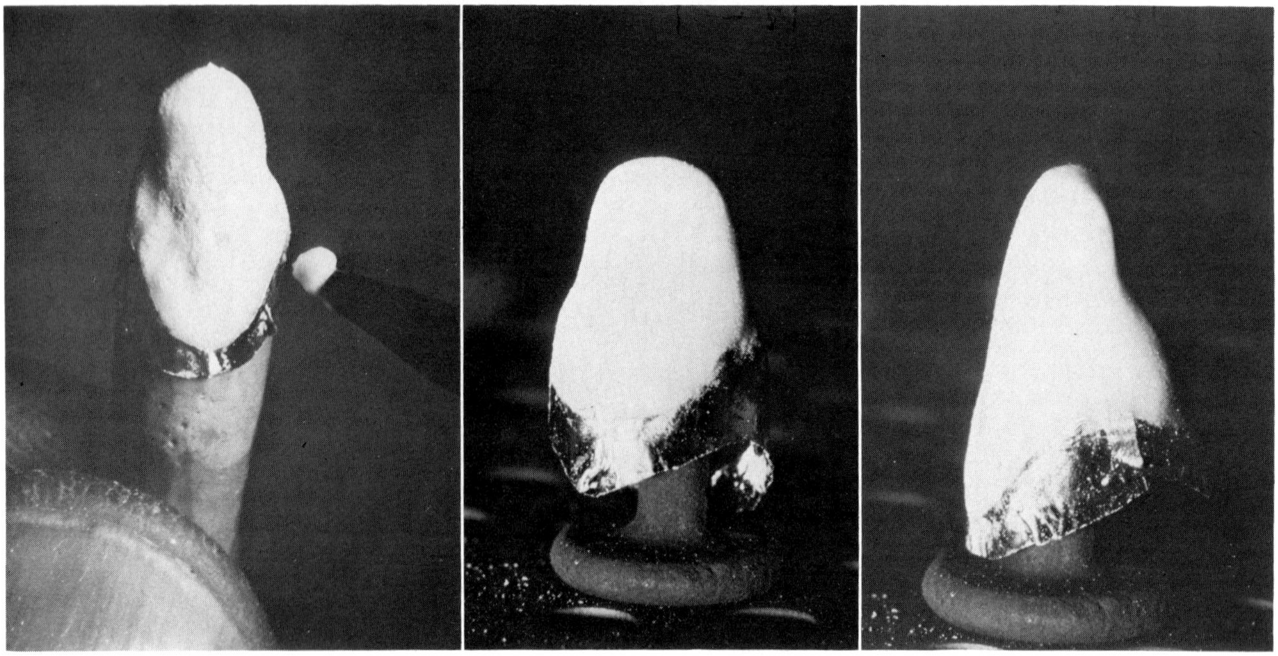

A B C

Fig. 11-39. A, Add core material around margin prior to second bake. **B,** Core buildup before second bake. **C,** Check core for additional bakes.

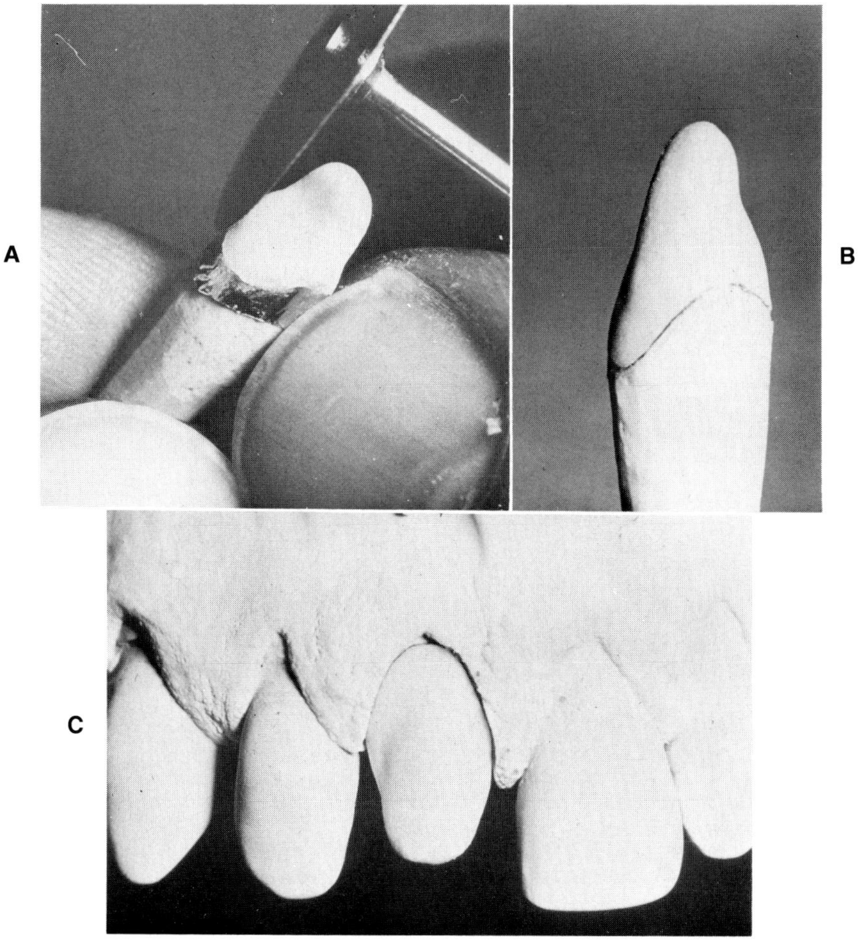

Fig. 11-40. A, Trim core margin, and remove platinum apron with diamond disk. **B,** Verify marginal adaptation. **C,** Check for incisal and lingual clearance.

and proximal areas for strength. Allow about 0.3 mm for dentin or body porcelain and more at the inciso-proximal areas for esthetics (Fig. 11-38, *A*). The facial surface should have only a thin layer to allow adequate thickness for dentin, enamel, and effect powders.

11. After condensing the core material, use either a brush or a finger to adapt the opaque core material over the margin.

12. Before the first opaque firing, make a small ditch completely around the shoulder at the margin (Fig. 11-38, *B*) using a fine metal carver.

13. Fire the first opaque at the manufacturer's recommended temperatures. After cooling, place the matrix back on the die, and readapt the platinum at the margins (Fig. 11-38, *C*).

14. Add opaque at the margins where shrinkage has occurred (Fig. 11-39, *A*), condense with a brush, and bake (Fig. 11-39, *B*).

15. After cooling, replace the crown on the die and check for any defects or deficiencies in contour. Make a corrective bake as necessary (Fig. 11-39, *C*). Carefully trim the excess platinum foil at the margin (apron) with a diamond disc (Fig. 11-40, *A*). At this time verify marginal adaptation of the matrix (Fig. 11-40, *B*).

16. Place the jacket on the working cast, and check for lingual clearance with opposing occlusion and facial and incisal clearance (Fig. 11-40, *C*), and adjust as necessary.

Body and incisal application

PROCEDURE

1. Apply a thin wet layer of body procelain over the entire core, and dry with a tissue. Build up the entire tooth with body porcelain. Be sure to allow for shrinkage, especially at the incisal edge (Fig. 11-41, *A*). Follow the buildup procedure outlined for the porcelain facial margin.

2. Using a brush or tools, shape the body buildup to resemble the final contour (Fig. 11-41, *B*).

A B C

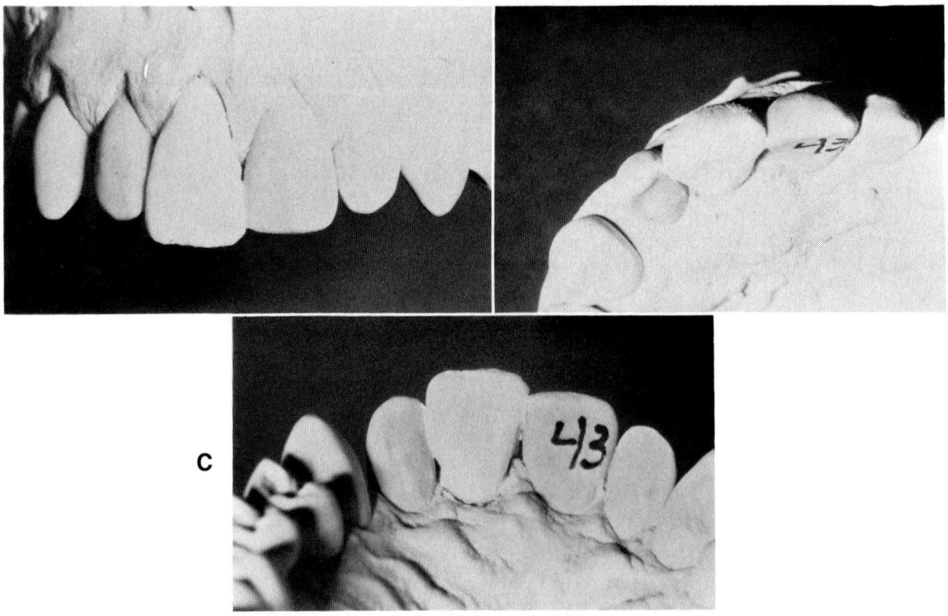

Fig. 11-41. A, Buildup with dentin porcelain. **B,** Model dentin porcelain with brush or tools to ideal tooth form. **C,** Adjust lingual surface to opposing occlusion.

A B C D

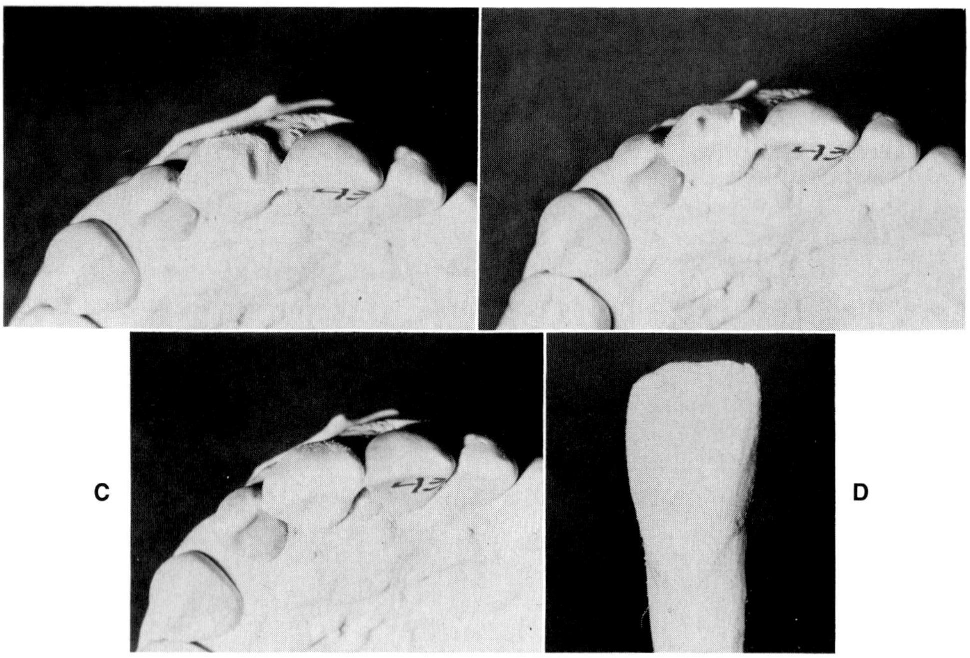

Fig. 11-42. A, Bevel dentin porcelain to allow for enamel overlay. **B,** Addition of translucent rods and color modifiers. **C,** Final contour after enamel application. **D,** Add contacts and margin on single die.

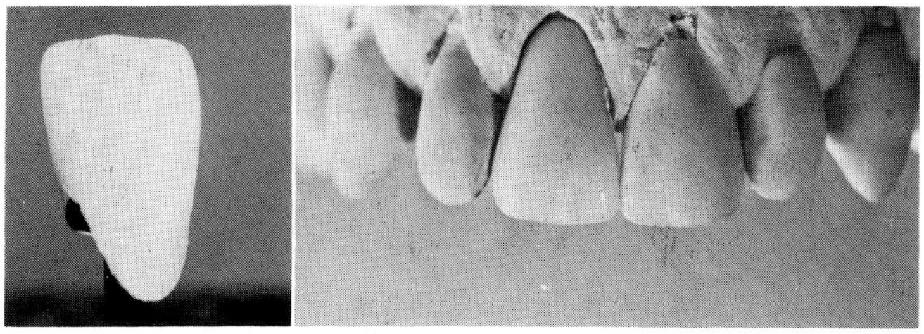

Fig. 11-43. A, Check for add-ons after first bake. **B,** Final contour with diamond points and glaze.

Incisal application

PROCEDURE

1. Using a sharp-bladed instrument bevel the body porcelain to allow room for the enamel overlay, taking care to not expose the core material. Cut V shaped grooves (Fig. 11-42, *A*) for translucent rods at the incisal edge, and add any wet staining or other color modifiers, if needed, at this time. It is important to moisten the porcelain slightly before adding the clear rods and stains.

2. Build the translucent rods out to the final facial contour (Fig. 11-42, *B*).

3. Use a sharp blade to narrow the contour to the desired width.

4. Moisten the porcelain surface, and apply the incisal porcelain on each side of the rods first to keep them from changing position. Fill in the rest of the enamel, and shape to contour (Fig. 11-42, *C*).

5. Remove the crown from the working model, fill in the contacts and margins, and shape them lightly with a soft artist's brush (Fig. 11-42, *D*).

6. Bake according to the porcelain manufacturer's directions. After cooling (Fig. 11-43, *A*), check for deficiencies of contour at contact areas or margins. Make a corrective bake as necessary.

7. Contour with diamond points and glaze (Fig. 11-43, *B*).

PROBLEM AREAS

During the fabrication of the porcelain jacket crown some problems are frequently observed; their probable causes and suggested solutions are listed in Table 11-1. At the time the porcelain jacket crown is verified in the mouth the following problems may be noticed:

1. The gingival margin is open. The porcelain jacket crown technique is frequently criticized for poor margin fit, criticism that is not justified if proper precautions are observed. The platinum foil must be properly adapted to the die. Before the first bake, ditch the core material at the margin. This allows the addition of new porcelain. Do not fail to readapt the platinum foil to the margin after the first bake.

2. Open interproximal contacts are another frequent source of frustration. A solid working cast is recommended. Technicians who use removable dies should constantly guard against excessive movement of the pinned die. The adjacent tooth contacts should be relieved 0.25 mm and then protected with cyanoacrylate cement.

3. Porcelain chipping or fracture during try-in is usually due to improper tooth preparation (undercut), or the die has been abraded. The tooth preparation should have a 1-mm shoulder finish line for adequate bulk of porcelain, and the instrumentation of the shoulder can cause critically parallel or undercut axial walls. The internal surface of the labial and lingual walls on the porcelain jacket crown should be relieved with a diamond instrument if a critical preparation is suspected. The technician should, if a stone die is used, protect it with cyanoacrylate cement. For any technique that requires burnishing platinum foil to the margins, an amalgam die, or metal-plated die is recommended.

4. The restoration may be too short at the incisal edge. A removable die may not be completely seated, or the gingival area has not been properly relieved on a solid working cast. In other words, use care that the crown is completely seated on the working cast before final contouring. The crown should be slightly longer incisally, just as it is best to have interproximal contacts on the tight side. The adjustments to the length and width of the crown take only a few minutes.

PROBLEM AREAS

Several problems can arise with the porcelain facial margin technique. The problems, their probable causes, and solutions are listed in Table 11-2.

1. A metal die is recommended for any technical procedure that requires the adaptation of platinum foil to the shoulder margin; however, if a stone die is used, it should be coated with cyanoacrylate cement.

2. The platinum foil can be securely attached to the metal framework (coping) by spot welding. This procedure is much simpler than soldering. For a proper weld, the platinum foil should extend 2 mm inside the

Table 11-1. Aluminous porcelain jacket crown

Problem	Probable cause	Solution
Jacket fractures at try-in	Erosion of die due to handling	Protect die with cyanoacrylate cement before handling
	Preparation design	Design preparation without sharp edges; have 1-mm shoulder all around
Open contacts	Movement of pinned die	Use solid working cast
	Distorted model	New impression is necessary
Incorrect shade	Insufficient tooth reduction	Vitadue-S crown requires 1 mm or more tooth reduction
	Failure to select proper shade	Learn terms used in determining shades and seeing color in its three dimensions (hue, chroma, and value)
	Overbuilding core material on facial margin	Allow at least 0.5 to 0.8 mm for dentin and incisal porcelain
Open margin	Platinum adaptation	Do not ditch undercut at margin when trimming die
	Failure to ditch core before first bake	Ditch core material around margin before firing
	Failure to readapt platinum around margin after first bake	Use glass rod or orangewood stick to readapt platinum around margin
	Distorted die	Take new impressions
Crown high	Too much core and body buildup on lingual side	Check core on solid model before proceeding to body buildup and adjust
Crown length short at incisal edge after first bake	No allowance for shrinkage	Allow 1 to 1.5 mm extension of incisal edge to compensate for shrinkage
Lamination of porcelain between body and incisal porcelain	Failure to moisten body porcelain before applying to incisal edge	Moisten body porcelain before adding incisal overlay
	Drying with tissue from facial surface	Hold tissue on lingual side when adding incisal porcelain
Cracks in porcelain after first bake	Not enough drying time	Allow at least 5½ minutes drying before inserting in muffle; follow manufacturer's instructions
	Too rapid firing cycle	Check manufacturer's suggestions for rate of temperature climb
	Drying outside layer of porcelain without removing moisture from within	Always hold tissue in opposite area of add-on; remove moisture as crown is built up
Crown displays milky appearance	Failure to apply vacuum	Apply vacuum
	Applied vacuum too late	Apply vacuum at correct temperature
	Oven out of calibration	Recalibrate oven
Loss of crown form after glaze	Too high temperature	Check manufacturer's suggestion for glazing temperature
	Held in oven too long	Check time and temperature rate of climb for oven
	Furnace calibration	Calibrate furnace

coping, and the metal surface must be clean at the weld area.

3. The coping with the platinum apron must seat completely on the master cast before building the porcelain in order to develop proper incisal length and interproximal contact areas. The seating of the coping is verified after opaquing. The die is slightly relieved on the axial surface in the weld area, and the platinum apron is trimmed with a diamond disk so there is no possible seating interference.

4. The porcelain can separate from the coping after the first bake, if the opaqued surface was dry. The opaque should be moistened with a thin slurry mix of dentin porcelain before the buildup of porcelain is started. An open margin after the first bake can usually be traced to the failure to ditch the porcelain at the shoulder before the first bake.

5. Before the crown is seated on the prepared tooth, sharp incisal angles should be rounded, and the inside of the facial and lingual wall should be relieved. If the

Table 11-2. Porcelain labial margin

Problem	Probable cause	Solution
Margin breaks during try-in	Eroded margin on die	Coat die with cyanoacrylate cement to harden
	Tooth reduction	Preparation must have minimum 1-mm shoulder from proximal-to-proximal contact
	Casting did not seat properly with foil	Relieve die in area where platinum is under metal coping
Finished crown has opaque show-through	Inadequate tooth reduction	Wax to full contour before cutting back and investing
	Metal coping too thick on facial margin	Metal should allow for 0.08 mm of body, enamel, and effect colors
	Opaque too thick	Control opaque buildup by putting on several thin layers
Porcelain bubbles when fired	Contaminated bur(s) used for metal shaping	Use only bur(s) and stones recommended by metal manufacturer
	Trapped debris in fold of metal	Shape metal in one direction; bake one opaque layer, and strip in acid before proceeding
Porcelain crazes during firing	Metal design	Check that there are no sharp points, corners, or angles on porcelain-bearing surface
	Too rapid firing cycle	Check manufacturer's firing schedule
Platinum fails to weld to metal coping	Not enough platinum inside coping	Allow at least 2 mm of platinum to extend inside coping
	Failure to remove opaque in area on coping to be welded	Remove opaque from coping in area around margin before firing
	Not enough amperage set on welder	Increase amperage
Opaque lifts margin after firing	Opaque too thick	Apply thin layers of opaque
	Failure to adapt platinum properly	Adapt platinum carefully with tool before opaquing; remove from die carefully
Crown does not seat on solid model after opaquing	Opaque inside casting	Check and remove any opaque before firing
	Failure to remove platinum apron	Trim platinum apron off with diamond disk
Porcelain lifts at metal juncture after baking	Failure to wet surface with thin slurry mix	Wet opaque with thin slurry mix of dentin before building up crown
Enamel fails to fuse to dentin porcelain	Failure to moisten dentin porcelain before application of enamel porcelain	Always moisten porcelain before adding to buildup
	Failure to extract moisture from opposite side of buildup	Hold tissue away from area of porcelain additions
Margin opens after first body bake	Failure to ditch around margin before firing	Ditch margin before first bake
Incisogingival length too short after first bake	Failure to allow for porcelain shrinkage	Overbuild incisal length 0.5 to 1 mm
Shade too bright after insertion	Failure to select appropriate value	Select appropriate value, as well as chroma and hue value with true complimentary color
	Porcelain too thin over opaque	Use complimentary opaque modifiers; try texturizing facial surface to reduce value
Shade too gray when inserted in mouth	Too much incisal overlay	Reduce depth of cut and bevel into body porcelain
	Selected wrong shade	Select proper shade
	Too much surface texture	Smooth out facial surface

labial wall of the coping is stressed, the porcelain can craze or fracture. Also, the porcelain shoulder should be carefully inspected for minute excess porcelain at the margin. Again during seating chipping of porcelain could occur.

SUMMARY

In this chapter the technical procedures and potential problem areas for the fabrication of a metalceramic crown with a porcelain facial margin and an aluminous porcelain jacket crown have been described.

Plastic veneering materials will continue to be developed to give the dentist a treatment alternative to metalceramic restorations. These plastic materials are highly technique sensitive, and the manufacturer's instructions must be observed.

The aluminous porcelain jacket crown was selected to illustrate the technical procedures involved in the fabrication of porcelain jacket crowns. Special emphasis was given to the technique of the porcelain buildup for the jacket crown and ceramometal crown.

A porcelain facial margin is technically the most demanding feature of the metal-ceramic crown. For this reason, the fabrication of a porcelain facial margin crown was described to represent metal-ceramic restorations in this chapter.

BIBLIOGRAPHY

Brecker, S.C.: The porcelain jacket crown, St. Louis, 1951, The C.V. Mosby Co.

Foote, H.: Personal communication, 1954.

Ingraham, R., Bassett, R.W., and Koser, J.R.: An atlas of cast gold procedures, ed. 2, Buena Park, Calif., 1969, Uni-Tro College Press.

Johnston, J.F., Mumford, G., and Dykema, R.W.: Porcelain veneers bonded to metal castings, Practical Dental Mongraphs, March, 1963.

Koper, A., and Gordon, D.C.: Esthetics in oral restorations (course), San Francisco, Dec. 3, 1971, University of California.

Kornfeld, M.: Mouth rehabilitation: clinical and laboratory procedures, St. Louis, 1974, The C. V. Mosby Co.

McLean, J.W.: The alumina reinforced porcelain jacket crown, J.A.D.A. **65**:621, 1967.

McLean, J.W.: The science and art of dental ceramics, New Orleans, 1974, Louisiana State University.

Mumford, G.: The porcelain fused to metal restoration, Dent. Clin. North Am. **9**:241-249, 1965.

Sheu, J.S., and Nielsen, J.P.: Study of the bond between gold alloys and porcelain, J. Dent. Res. **41**:847-851, 1962.

Shillingburg, H.T., Hobo, S., and Whitsett, L.D.: Fundamentals of fixed prosthodontics, Berlin, 1976, Die Quintessence.

Shooshan, E.D.: The reverse pin porcelain facing, J. Prosthet. Dent. **9**:284-301, 1959.

Stein, R.S.: Ceramo-metal and aluminous porcelain restorations (course), Charleston, S.C., Dec. 11-12, 1971, University of South Carolina College of Dental Medicine.

Tanner, H.M.: Personal communication, 1965.

CHAPTER 12

THE DICOR CASTABLE CERAMIC CROWN

KENNETH A. MALAMENT

The Dicor* castable ceramic material has been developed jointly by Corning Glass Works† and Dentsply International. Laboratory and clinical techniques have been in the process of development since 1978 under the direction of Peter J. Adair. An extensive research program, including physical and biologic testing, has resulted in a viable alternative, along with conventional dental porcelain and metal-ceramic systems, for esthetic and cosmetic restoration of individual teeth.

The Dicor castable ceramic material is one of the Pyroceram ceramics manufactured by Corning Glass Works. It is comprised of oxides from silicone oxide, potassium oxide, and magnesium oxide. It also contains fluoride from magnesium fluoride, minor amounts of aluminum oxide and zirconium oxide incorporated for durability, and a fluorescing agent added for esthetic purposes. These components are readily available chemical compounds obtainable in high purity. The material is manufactured in large quantities with stringent quality control that ensures batch-to-batch standardization.

The Dicor castable ceramic has several advantageous features (Fig. 12-1):

1. It is compatible with dental clinical and laboratory procedures most commonly used.
2. It can reproduce conventionally formed wax patterns precisely by using a simple casting system, which allows the generation of detailed occlusal anatomy to meet the requirements of any occlusal scheme.
3. It affords excellent marginal accuracy and strength.
4. It is a smooth, nonporous material that is biocompatible to gingival tissue.
5. The natural translucence eliminates the problem of opacity inherent in metal-ceramic systems and permits development of selective in-depth color.

A detailed discussion of the technical and clinical procedures developed for this castable ceramic material is necessary for complete understanding and successful use of this unique modality.

TOOTH PREPARATION

Tooth preparation, in all instances when the teeth are to be restored with porcelain or ceramic materials, must incorporate sufficient removal of tooth structure to allow an adequate thickness of porcelain for strength and color saturation. When castable ceramic materials are to be employed, tooth reduction of all surfaces must be no less than 1.2 mm to ensure adequate strength. It is recommended that incisal or occlusal reduction be from 1.5 to 2.0 mm and that facial and lingual reduction be from 1.0 to 1.5 mm. Proximal reduction will vary according to individual tooth morphology. It is necessary that the gingival margin design be either a chamfer with a rounded cavosurface junction of 135 degrees or

*Dentsply/York Division, Dentsply International York, Pa. 17405

†Corning Glass Works, Research and Development, Corning, N.Y. 14831

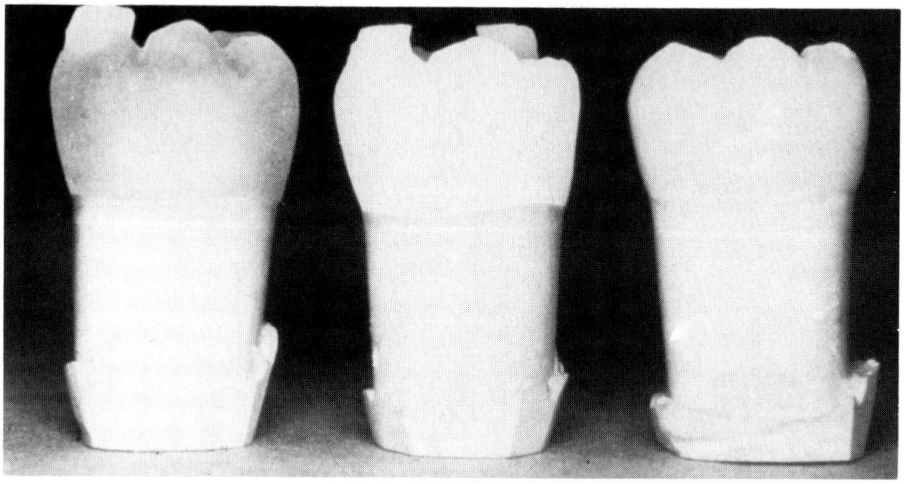

Fig. 12-1. The Dicor castable ceramic exhibits uncomplicated fabrication from full wax-up to casting, ceramming, and coloring procedures.

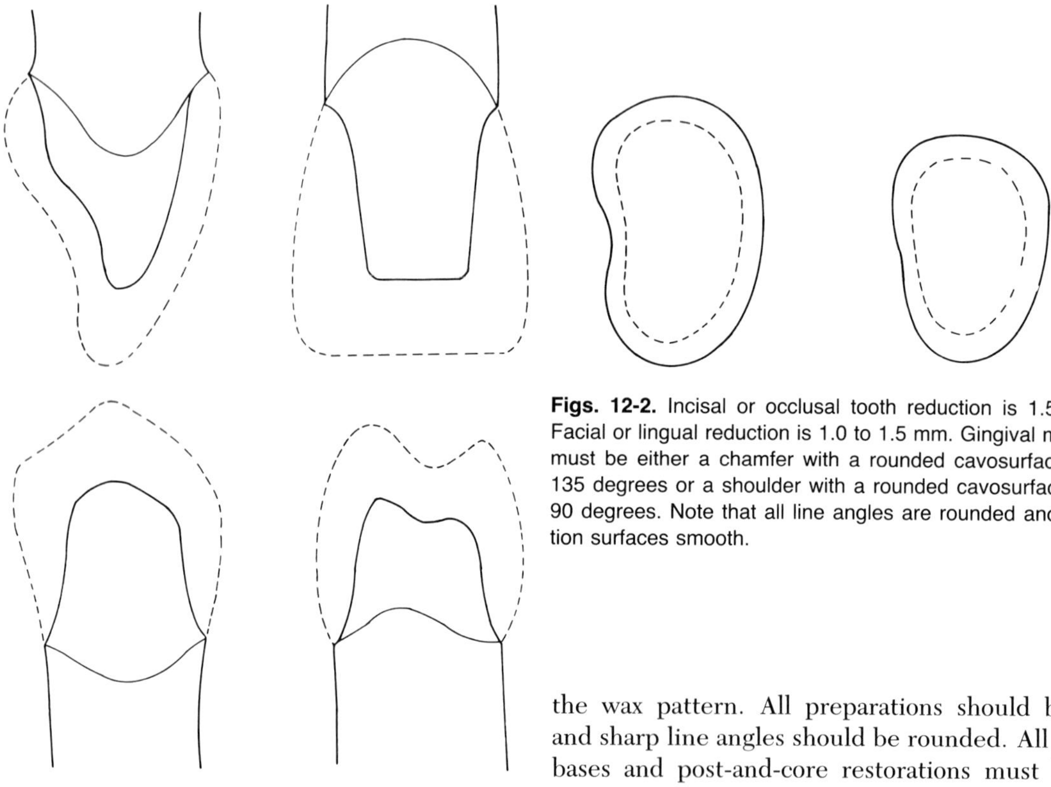

Figs. 12-2. Incisal or occlusal tooth reduction is 1.5 to 2.0 mm. Facial or lingual reduction is 1.0 to 1.5 mm. Gingival margin design must be either a chamfer with a rounded cavosurface junction of 135 degrees or a shoulder with a rounded cavosurface junction of 90 degrees. Note that all line angles are rounded and all preparation surfaces smooth.

a rounded shoulder with a cavosurface junction of 90 degrees (Fig. 12-2). Beveled margins, knife-edged margins, feather-edged margins, slice preparations, and light chamfer margins should not be used, because inherently weak margins will be created in the ceramic material. A 6- to 8-degree taper is recommended for axial surfaces, consistent with the path of withdrawal for the wax pattern. All preparations should be smooth, and sharp line angles should be rounded. All foundation bases and post-and-core restorations must be of adequate strength. Gold post-and-core or silver amalgam foundation bases are strongly recommended.

CAST SELECTION AND DIE PREPARATION

Standard impression techniques can be employed. Use of an improved die stone is preferred because of its ease of manipulation, hardness, and wear resistance. Although epoxy die materials can be used, careful attention to their physical properties and dimensional accuracy must be stressed.

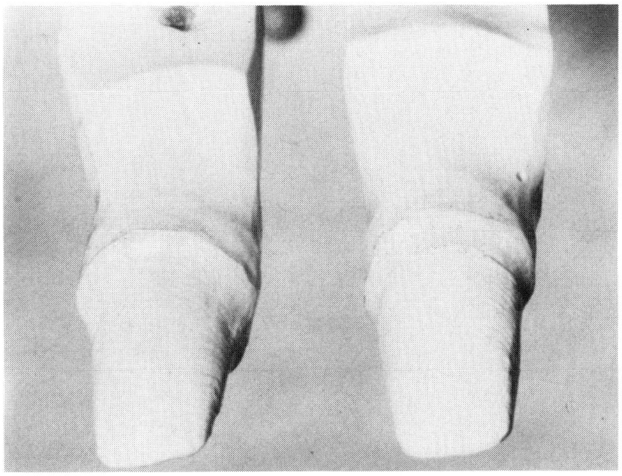

Fig. 12-3. Die preparation involves proper margin definition. A die sealer and a tooth colored die spacer are placed onto prepared die. Note that left die has only sealer placed, while right die has both sealer and colored spacer.

All casts should be free of occlusal artifacts, bubbles, or other inaccuracies. Dies should have an adequate indexing system to prevent rotation and to ensure stability in the base portion of the cast. The dies should be sectioned, trimmed, and refined, taking care that the marginal areas are not damaged. Any existing undercut areas should be blocked out to ensure wax pattern removal without distortion. A die sealer should be used. It is recommended that a tooth-shaded die spacer be employed to aid in determining wax thickness during the waxing process and to facilitate subsequent fitting of the casting. The tooth-shaded die spacer is also valuable in the coloring procedures that follow.

A series of colored die spacers* corresponding to a shade chart is available for use with the technique. A die spacer of appropriate shade, as determined from the shading chart, should be applied evenly to the die to within 1 mm of the margin (Fig. 12-3). One or two coats of the spacing material usually provides adequate thickness for relief of the casting. During the coloring procedure, the die spacing layer, transmitting through the translucent ceramic material, simulates the effect of the natural tooth and aids in proper application of colorants to produce the desired effect.

WAXING

Die lubricant should be applied directly over the die spacer to prevent adherence of the wax to the die. The wax pattern is developed in a manner identical to that employed in the fabrication of a cast gold crown.

All contours of the wax crown should have a minimum thickness of at least 1 mm to ensure adequate strength of the cast ceramic crown. Calipers are valuable in verifying adequate thickness of wax.

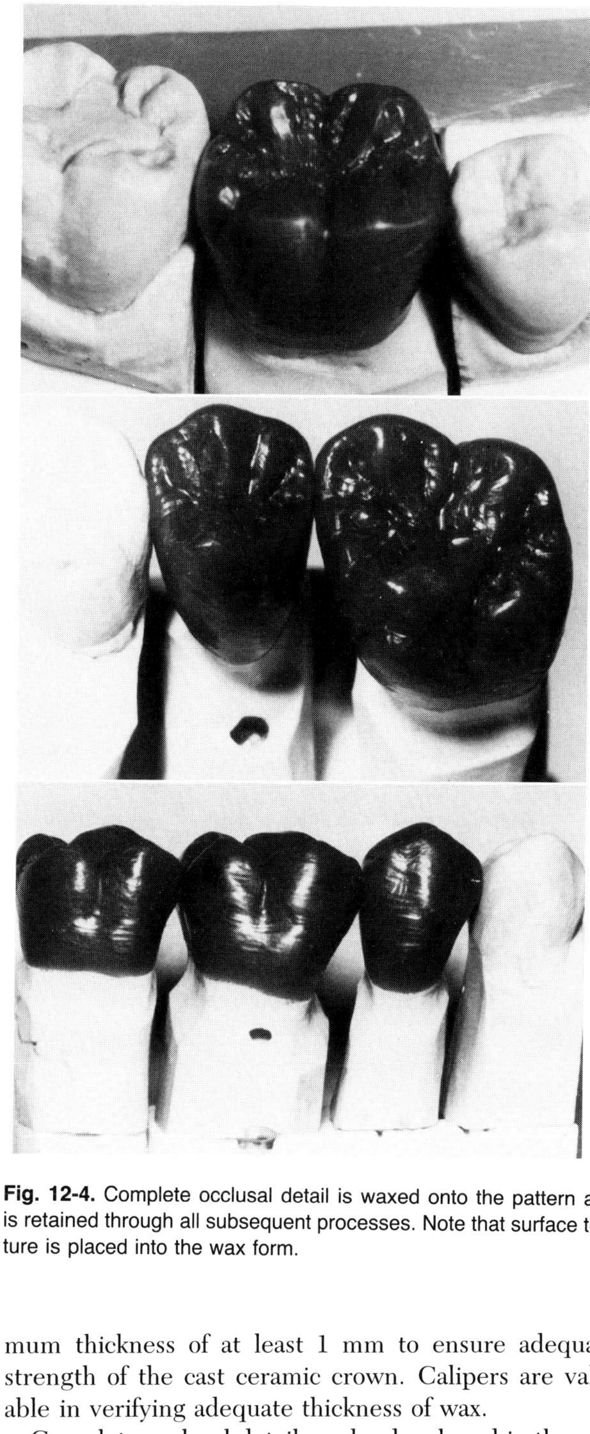

Fig. 12-4. Complete occlusal detail is waxed onto the pattern and is retained through all subsequent processes. Note that surface texture is placed into the wax form.

Complete occlusal detail can be developed in the wax pattern and will be retained through all subsequent processes (Fig. 12-4). The casting and ceramming processes will result in accurate castings that preclude the need for overbuilding of axial and occlusal contours.

The use of an electric wax spatula will aid materially in producing consistent results (Fig. 12-5). A smooth and completely formed internal surface of the waxed crown is necessary. Remelting and refining of margin

*Dentsply International, York, Pa.

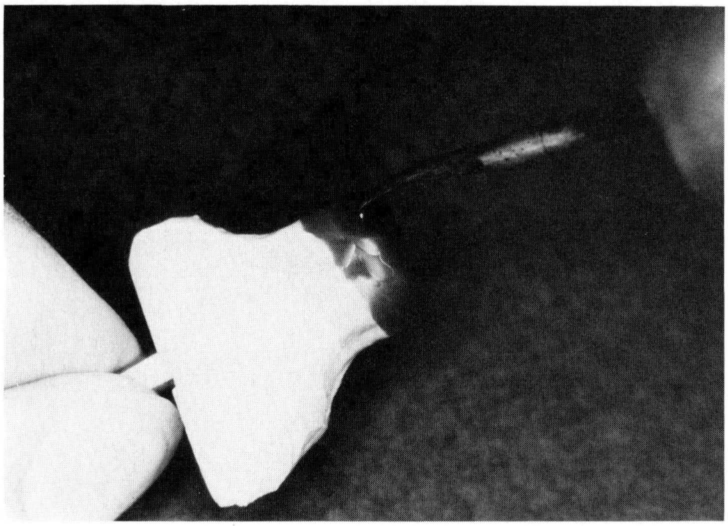

Fig. 12-5. An electric wax spatula will aid in producing fine wax patterns.

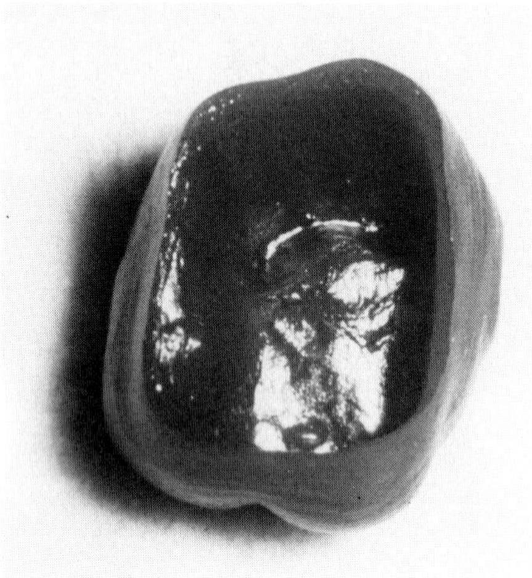

Fig. 12-6. Wax margin areas must be smooth, displaying no wrinkles or creases.

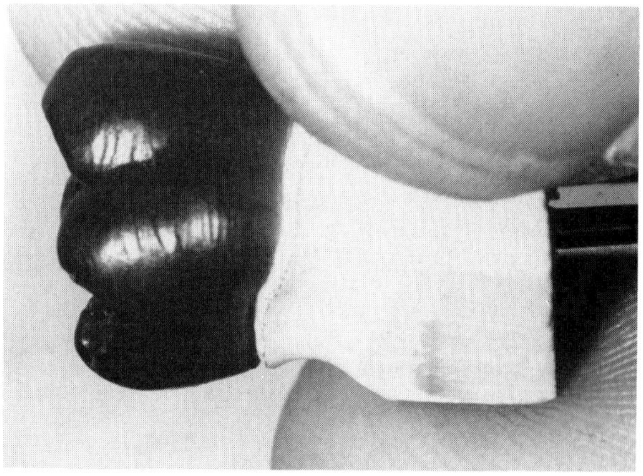

Fig. 12-7. Wax margins should have no overextensions.

areas should not produce internal wrinkles or creases but should be well blended and have adequate thickness (Fig. 12-6). Care should be exercised that waxed margin areas have no overextensions (Fig. 12-7). If thin overextensions remain and are cast, chipping of the glass ceramic can result during the fitting or try-in procedures. Final wax patterns should be examined carefully under magnification, preferably 10 to 30X, to determine marginal integrity (Fig. 12-8).

SPRUING

Several different sprue designs have produced successful castings. One 8- or 10-gauge wax sprue, attached to the incisal surface of anterior patterns, provides an adequate gate for ingress of the ceramic material (Fig. 12-9). Patterns for posterior teeth usually require two 10-gauge wax sprues attached to the facial and lingual cusp tips. Sprue placement on molar patterns should be diagonally opposed for more uniform flow of the fluid ceramic (Fig. 12-10). A sprue design incorporating a perpendicular reservoir has also produced adequate castings (Fig. 12-11).

Wax sprue length should be approximately 3.0 to 4.0 mm. The pattern should be located so that its most distal point is approximately ¼ inch (6 to 7 mm) from the open end of the casting flask (ring) to allow adequate diffusion of mold gasses through the investment.

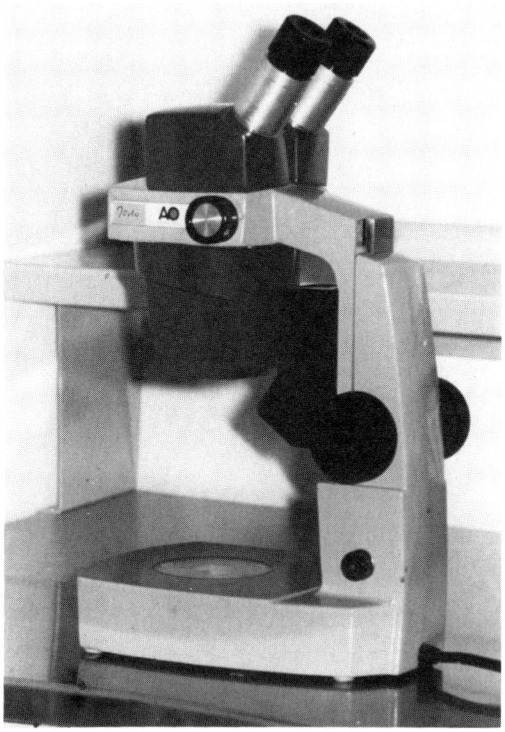

Fig. 12-8. Close examination of wax pattern margins under magnification with a dissecting microscope is highly recommended.

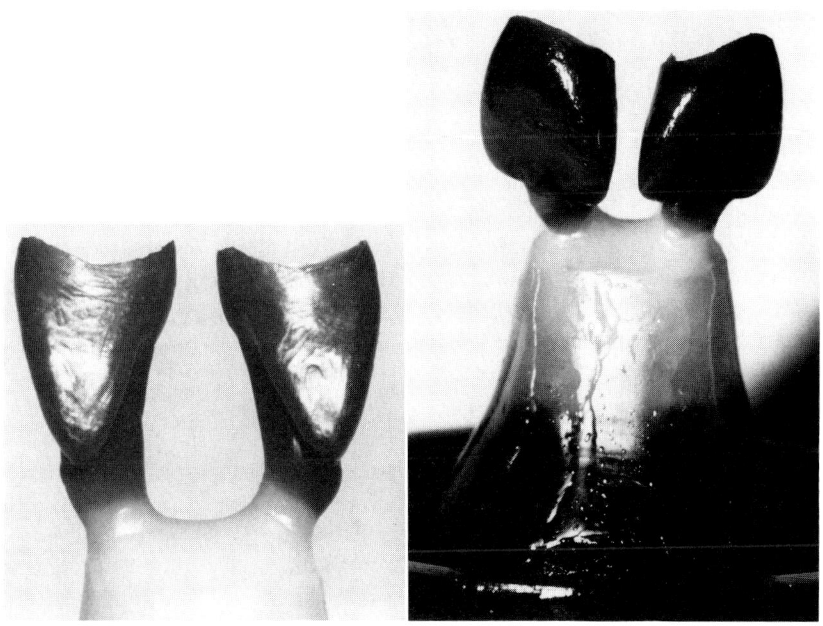

Fig. 12-9. Anterior patterns are sprued by using one 8 or 10 gauge wax sprue attached to incisal edge.

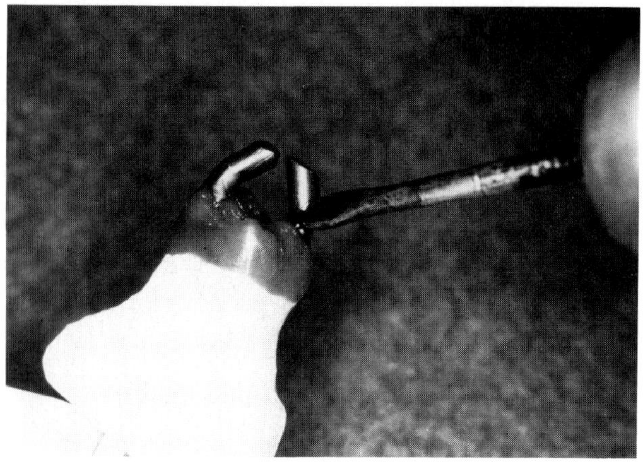

Fig. 12-10. Posterior teeth are sprued by using two 10 gauge sprues attached to facial and lingual cusp tips diagonally opposing each other on molar.

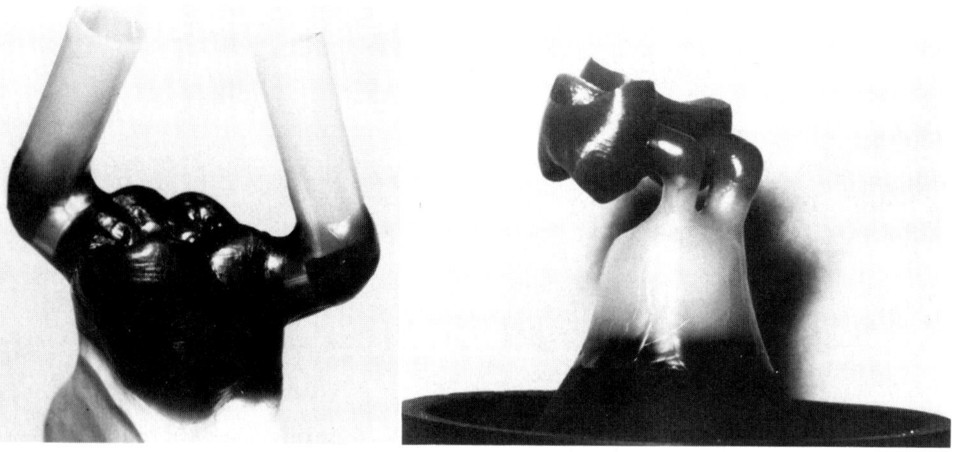

Fig. 12-11. Posterior teeth are sprued using a perpendicular reservoir design.

INVESTING

A conventional wax pattern cleaner should be used to clean the sprued pattern. Any excess should be removed with a gentle application of compressed air. Non-corroding casting flasks (rings) that are resistant to oxidation at high temperatures should be used. Prepare the casting flask by using two layers of Kaoliner* lining material (an asbestos line substitute) suitable for high heat mold conditioning (Fig. 12-12). The liner should be placed with its flat side outward toward the flask. Two layers of lining material should be sufficient to permit the required expansion of the investment material. Saturate the lining material by placing in water for approximately 10 seconds before seating the flask on the crucible former.

A specially formulated phosphate-bonded investment* is used for this casting process. It exhibits virtually no setting expansion but produces approximately 1.5% thermal expansion at temperature.

Measurements of liquid and powder are critical: 8 ml of distilled or deionized water should be mixed with 60 gm of the Dicor castable ceramic investment for 30 seconds under vacuum with power spatulation (Whip-Mix combination mixer).* After spatulation additional vibration under vacuum should be continued for an additional 20 to 30 seconds. The mixed investment should be carefully applied to the pattern with a small sable or camel's hair brush. Extreme care should be exercised to avoid entrapment of air bubbles against the pattern (Fig. 12-13).

After the pattern is carefully filled and coated, the remaining investment material should be vibrated into the flask allowing an excess to remain above the open end of the flask (Fig. 12-14). After bench setting for 1

*Dentsply International, York, Pa.

*Whip-Mix Corporation, Louisville, Ky.

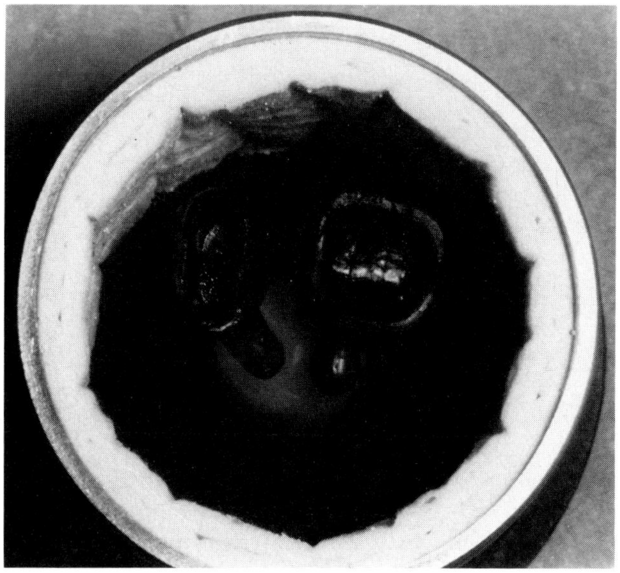

Fig. 12-12. Prepare casting flask (ring) by using two layers of Kaoliner investment ring liner.

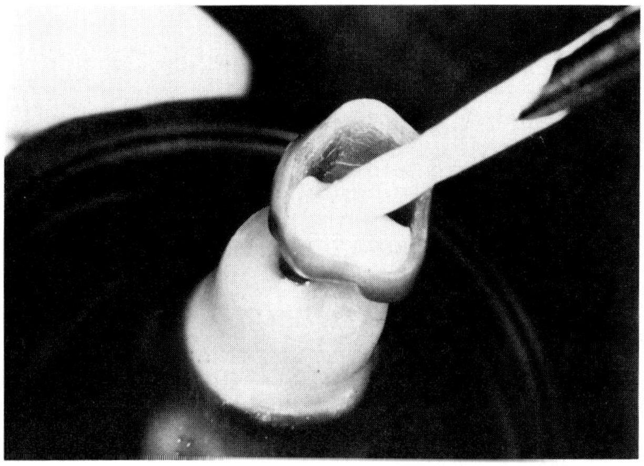

Fig. 12-13. Dicor investment is carefully adapted to all surfaces of the wax pattern using a fine soft brush and vibration.

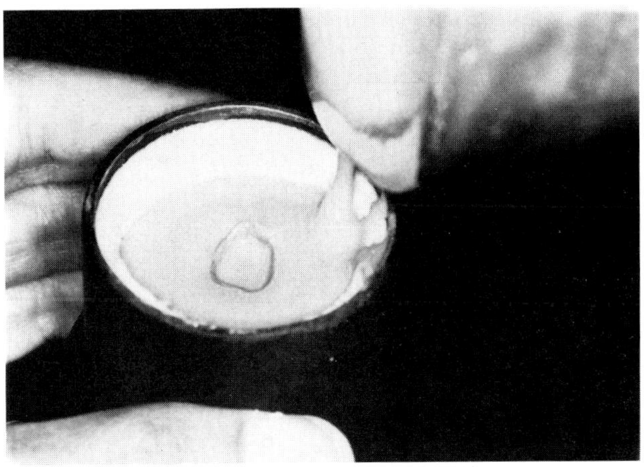

Fig. 12-14. When the pattern is filled, vibrate investment into ring and allow excess to remain.

hour, the excess investment should be trimmed even with the top of the casting flask.

MOLD CONDITIONING

A two-stage mold conditioning should be employed. The invested pattern should be placed in a cold furnace and the temperature raised to 480° F (249° C). This temperature should be maintained (heat soak) for 30 minutes; 10 minutes of additional time should be added for each additional flask if more than three flasks are being processed at one time. The temperature should be raised to 1650° F (899° C) and that temperature maintained (heat soaked) for 2 hours. Similarly, 10 minutes of additional time should be allowed for each additional flask in the furnace.

CASTING

A 4-gm ingot of the Dicor castable ceramic material* is loaded into the ceramic crucible* (Fig. 12-15). It is necessary to determine the amount of ceramic material that will be needed to make a satisfactory casting. When multiplied by a conversion factor of 2.6, the weight of the wax pattern, sprues, and button should not exceed 4 gm to ensure that there will be sufficient Dicor glass to produce a complete casting. As a general rule, two patterns can be cast in one flask. At least 1.5 gm should always be allowed for the weight of the cast glass button.

The Dentsply Dicor casting machine* features a platinum, electric resistance–type muffle mounted on an electrically driven straight centrifugal casting arm (Fig. 12-16). The machine is fitted with a special receptacle to hold the Dicor crucible. This casting machine requires a separate 30 ampere, 230 volt AC, 60 hertz power source. There are specific operating instructions for the equipment.

*Dentsply/York, Dentsply International, York, Pa.

PROCEDURE

1. Maintain an idle temperature of 2010° F (1100° C) for 10 minutes to stabilize the muffle.
2. Open the rear muffle door and insert the crucible containing the glass ingot. A specially marked tool is used to position the crucible at the proper depth inside the muffle for melting the glass.
3. Close the rear door and adjust the melt temperature to 2475° F (1360° C). Turn on the melt switch.
4. When the muffle temperature has reached 2475° F (1360° C), an indicator tone will sound and the temperature will be maintained for 6 minutes.
5. Open the rear muffle door. Remove the casting flask from the burnout furnace and place it in the cradle with the crucible and gate facing the muffle.

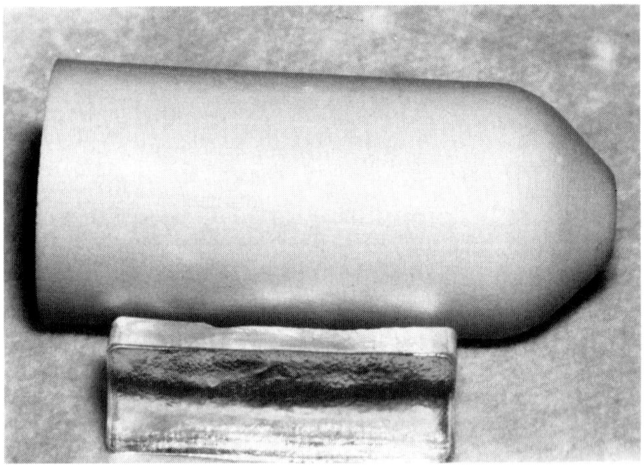

Fig. 12-15. Dicor castable ceramic crucible and 4 gm ingot.

A

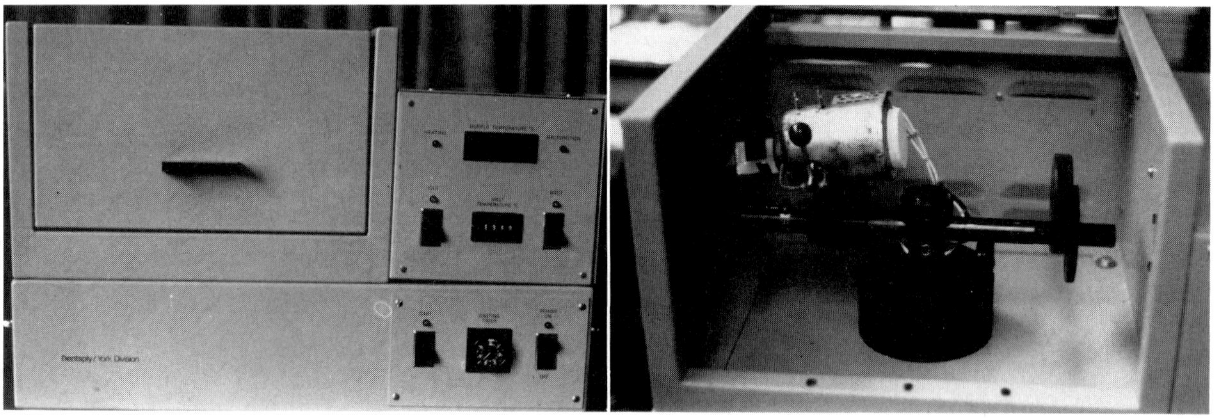

B

Fig. 12-16. Dentsply Dicor casting machine. **A,** Exterior; **B,** interior.

6. Open the front muffle door and slide the muffle assembly forward toward the casting flask until it is seated.

7. Close the casting machine cover and turn on the "cast" switch. The casting arm will now spin automatically for 4½ minutes and then stop. The casting will cool during the spin cycle.

8. Remove the casting flask from the machine and allow it to cool (bench cool) for 45 minutes before deflasking.

DIVESTING

After cooling, the investment is removed from around the edges of the casting flask to a depth of approximately ¼ inch (6 to 8 mm). The investment mass can be forced out of the retaining flask by pushing with the fingers. The bulk of the investment material can be broken away from the casting with finger pressure. Caution should be exercised to avoid sharp glass edges, which may be present on margins or button (Fig. 12-17). The remaining investment should be removed with an air abrasive tool using 25 μm aluminum oxide at 40 p.s.i. (Fig. 12-18). The margin areas should be protected by covering with the finger to prevent possible chipping.

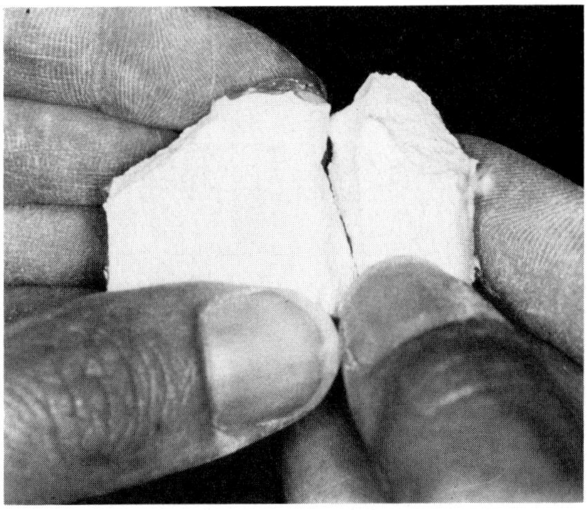

Fig. 12-17. Use finger pressure to break off bulk of investment.

SPRUE REMOVAL

The cast crown is slowly cut off at the junction of the sprue and button using a suitable single- or double-sided diamond disk. The sprue is cut near the glass button to avoid chipping. The casting, at this stage, is composed of noncrystalline glass (Fig. 12-19). The casting should be examined under magnification for unacceptable inclusions, porosity, or voids. The remaining button must be discarded and cannot be reused because the glass is altered during melting cycle.

EMBEDDING

The acceptable casting is next embedded in the castable ceramic embedment material,* so that the ceramming process can take place. It is during this ceramming procedure that the glass in the casting is converted to a 55% crystalline form.

The glass casting is embedded in a mixture of 18 ml distilled water and 50 gm of embedment powder. Hand mixing is sufficient to incorporate the water and embedment powder. The inside of the crown is carefully filled with the embedment mix and is then placed

*Dentsply/York, Dentsply International, York, Pa.

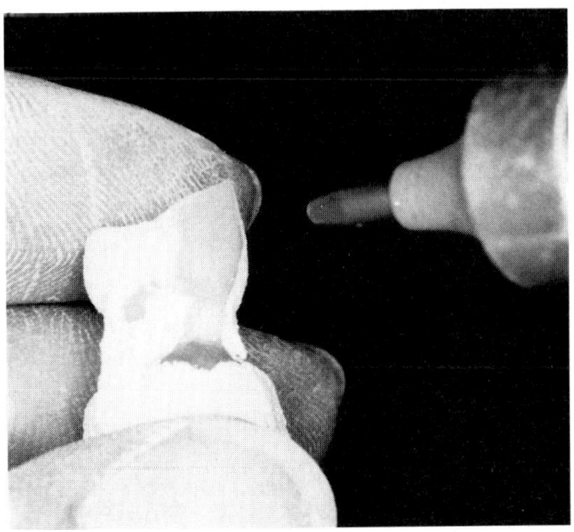

Fig. 12-18. Remove remaining investment with air abrasive tool using 25 μm aluminum oxide at 40 p.s.i.

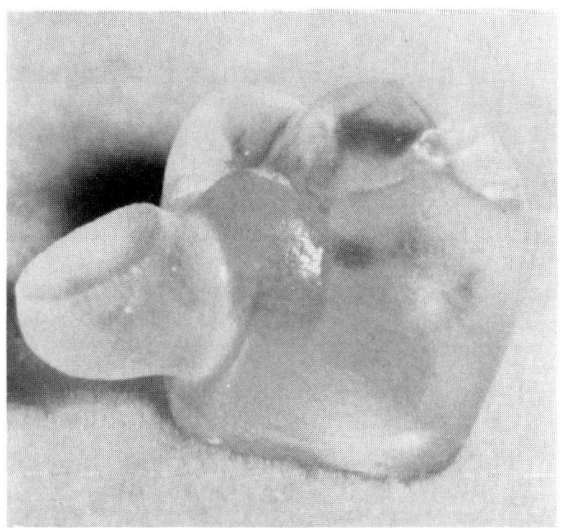

Fig. 12-19. The parent glass casting is in a noncrystalline form. The casting should be examined under magnification for unacceptable inclusion bodies, porosities, and voids.

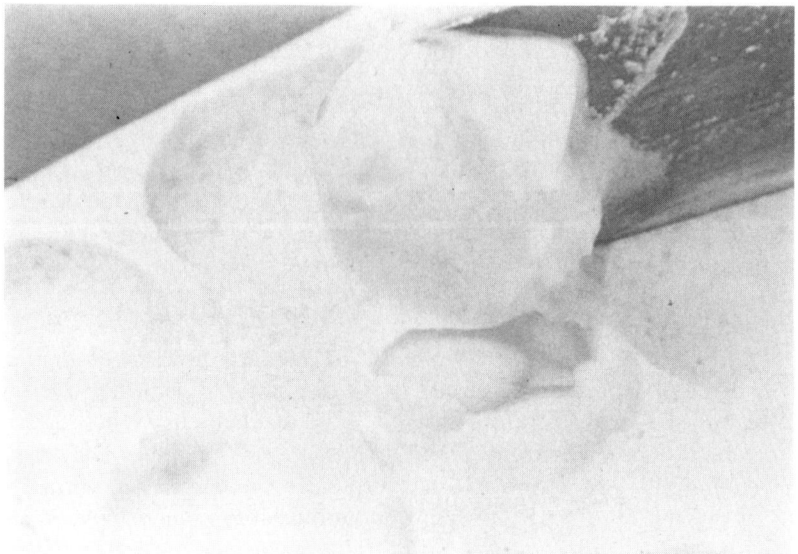

Fig. 12-20. The noncrystalline casting is placed into mixed embedment and covered with additional embedment.

A

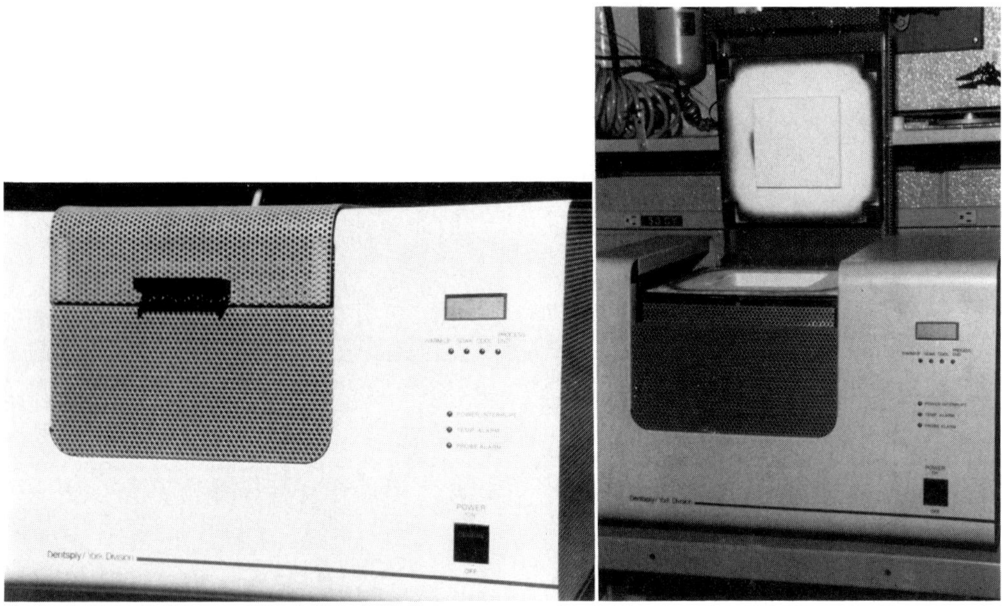

B

Fig. 12-21. Dentsply ceramming furnace. **A,** Exterior; **B,** Interior.

on a tray* with a concave receptacle in which additional embedment material is placed. Additional embedment is used to completely cover and protect the glass crown (Fig. 12-20). The material should be allowed to set for 45 to 60 minutes.

*Dentsply/York, Dentsply International, York, Pa.

CERAMMING

The ceramming process is accomplished in a precisely controlled ceramming furnace* (Fig. 12-21). The furnace temperature is gradually increased to 1960° F (1075° C) for 3.6 hours. This temperature should be maintained automatically for 6 hours. The furnace is cooled to a temperature of 392° F (200° C) and the embedment tray removed. The proper ceram cycle is verified by the use of a pyrometric cone* (Fig. 12-22, A). The characteristic droop will provide verification that proper time and temperature has allowed the de-

*Dentsply/York, Dentsply International, York, Pa.

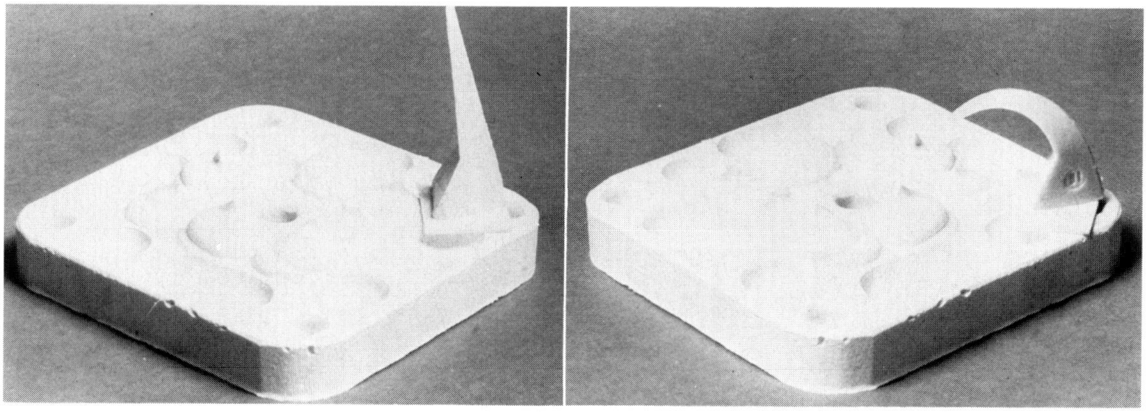

Fig. 12-22. A, A pyrometric cone placed on embedment tray will confirm that ceramming has occurred at the proper temperature and time periods. **B,** Characteristic droop limit of the pyrometric cone indicates proper ceramming.

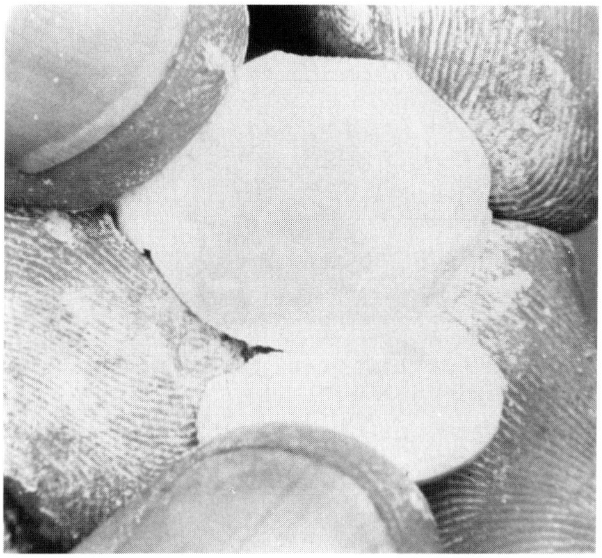

Fig. 12-23. Use finger pressure to break embedment apart.

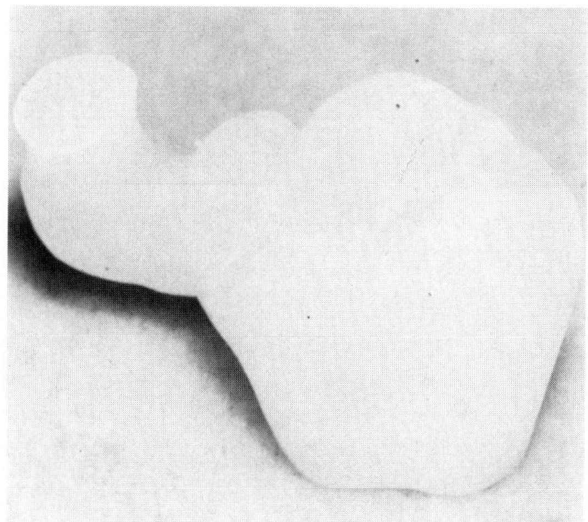

Fig. 12-24. Inspect crystalline glass ceramic crown for internal nodules or irregularities.

velopment of the desired crystalline properties in the casting (Fig. 12-22, *B*).

POSTCERAM DIVESTING

The tray is allowed to cool to room temperature. The embedment is broken away from the casting with finger pressure (Fig. 12-23). The crown is cleaned by air-blasting with 25 μm aluminum oxide at 40 psi at a distance of approximately 6 inches. The margin areas of the crown should be protected with the pad of the finger during the blasting process.

CROWN FINISHING

Before finishing, the crystalline glass ceramic crown should be inspected for internal nodules or irregularities, which may interfere with seating of the casting on the die (Fig. 12-24). Irregularities can be removed with extrafine diamond points (Fig. 12-25). The crown is carefully seated onto the die and examined for marginal overextensions (Fig. 12-26). Irregularities and overextensions must be removed with a fine white point or rubber wheel rotating at slow speed to prevent chipping when the crown is completely seated on the die or tooth. The remaining sprue stub is removed with a double-sided diamond disc rotating at slow speed (Fig. 12-27).

The fine opaque-white "skin" that covers the crown surface must be removed. The sprue area is finished and the "skin" is lightly removed with a fine (Dentsply Fascut no. 2) rubber abrasive wheel.* After removal of

*Dentsply/York, Dentsply International, York, Pa.

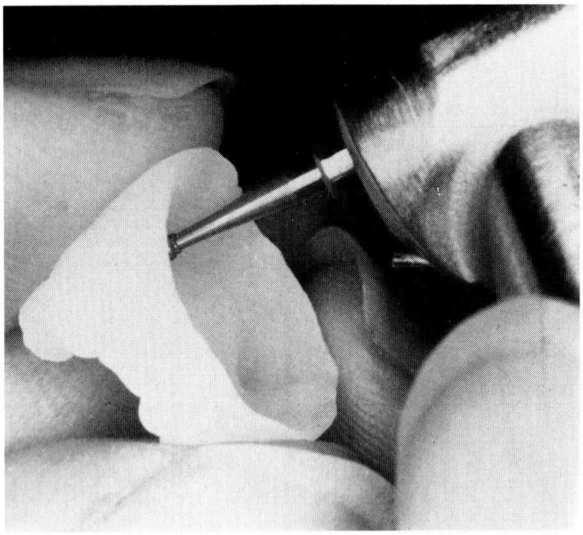

Fig. 12-25. Remove irregularities that may interfere with seating crown on die by using extra fine diamond points.

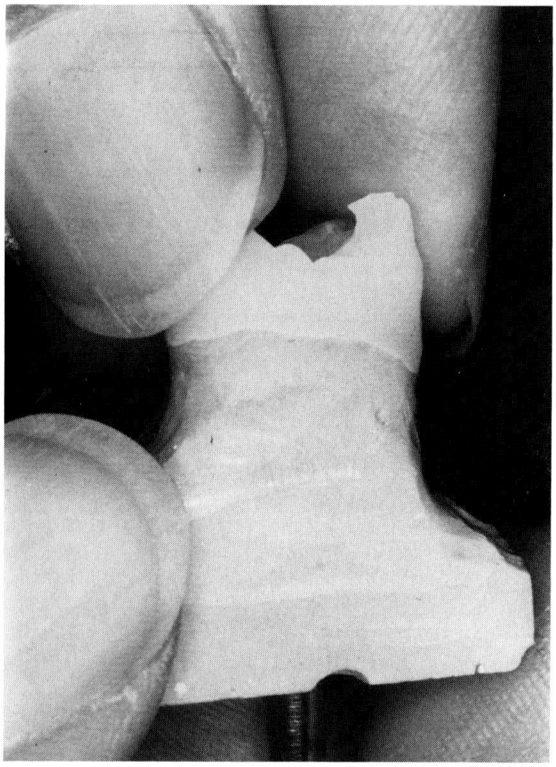

Fig. 12-26. Seat crown onto die and examine for marginal overextensions.

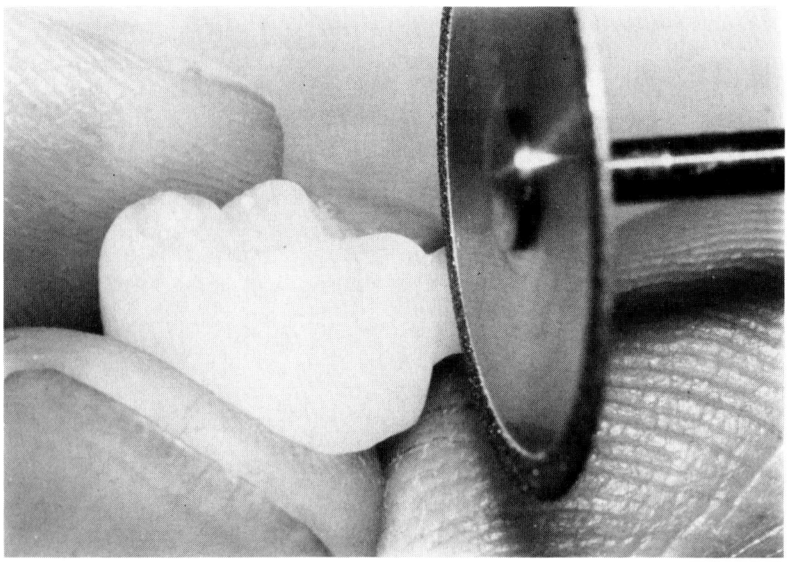

Fig. 12-27. Remove sprue with double-sided diamond disk at low speed.

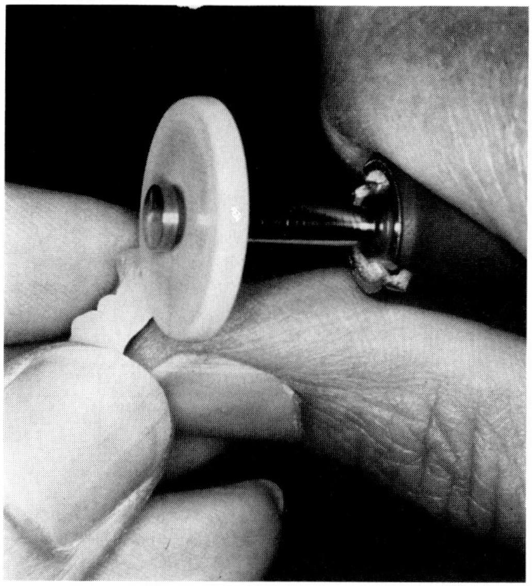

Fig. 12-28. Use a Dentsply Faskut no. 2 rubber abrasive wheel and lightly abrade the glass ceramic surface to remove the "skin" layer. Note the margin area is dressed with a rubber wheel.

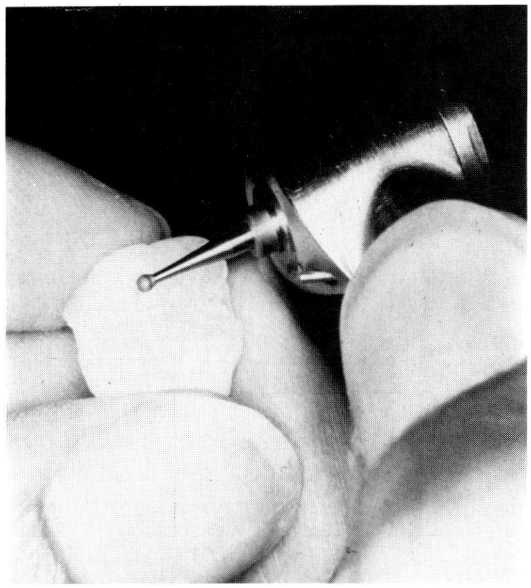

Fig. 12-29. Occlusal surfaces are adjusted for centric occlusion and excursive movements with a fine diamond point.

the "skin," the crown is lightly air-blasted with 25 μm aluminum oxide at 40 psi. The margin area is dressed with a suitable rubber abrasive wheel (Fig. 12-28). Axial surface texture and characterization to produce a natural-appearing surface should be placed, using fine diamond points. Occlusal surfaces can be adjusted when centric occlusion and excursive movements are refined, using fine diamond points (Fig. 12-29). Primary and secondary occlusal anatomy may be defined with suitable small round and inverted cone tungsten carbide burs (Fig. 12-30). Small chips or voids can be corrected with add-on correction material.* Defects in the glass ceramic may be repaired by light grinding of the area and correction made by placing and condensing a thick slurry of the add-on material over the affected area. The casting is dried in front of the open muffle at a temperature of 1100° F (593° C), and then introduced into the muffle and fired under vacuum to a temperature of 1775° F (968° C). The vacuum is released and the temperature maintained for 1 minute. The added porcelain can be shaped and adjusted to the desired contour.

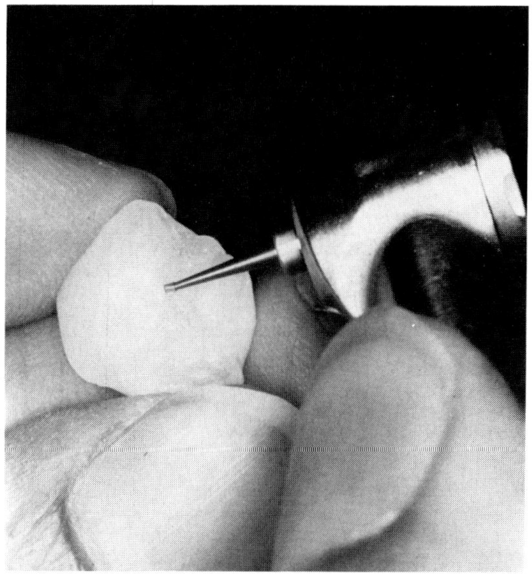

Fig. 12-30. Occlusal anatomy is detailed with suitable small round or inverted cone tungsten carbide burs.

COLORING

The application of colorants onto the translucent castable ceramic and the ability to develop the proper degree of color saturation by application of successive layers of colorant affords a flexibility and control of hue and chroma heretofore unattainable. Other ceramic systems require the building of colors into the crown mass at the time of fabrication and allow only minor modification of value, hue, and chroma in the finishing stages.

There is no opaque substructure to affect natural translucency and color brightness (value) of the Dicor-crown. Metal-ceramic systems historically have been plagued by high value levels caused by the shining

*Dicor Add-on Correcting Porcelain, Dentsply/York, Dentsply International, York, Pa.

through of the underlying opaque layer of porcelain. In such instances it is difficult to maintain proper value while attempting to modify chroma levels. Castable ceramics present a distinct improvement by diffracting and scattering light in a manner similar to natural tooth enamel.

The Dicor shading porcelain* has been developed to complement the castable ceramic translucency. After the ceramming process has been completed, the ceramic is achromatic (Fig. 12-31). The desired hue is determined by addition of the shading porcelain (Fig. 12-32). Additional applications of shading porcelain control the degree of saturation of that hue. If a low chroma is required, only one or two applications of colorant may be necessary. Higher chroma may require three or more layers. Blending of hues may at times be necessary to simulate varying colors within the tooth. Value may be adjusted by the selection of enamel shading porcelain of the desired brightness. Individual characterization may be fired into the crown, and further application of colorant may be placed over those areas, creating an in-depth color.

The blending of enamel and body colors must occur while they are wet. The crown with the applied shading porcelain should be dried by holding the crown near the open furnace door at a temperature of 1292° F (700° C). The glazing temperature should be maintained for approximately 12 seconds. Several applications of shading porcelain are usually required to complete the coloring and characterization process (Fig. 12-33). The first and second applications of the colorant should be fired at a slightly lower temperature to prevent overglazing

*Dentsply/York, Dentsply International, York, Pa.

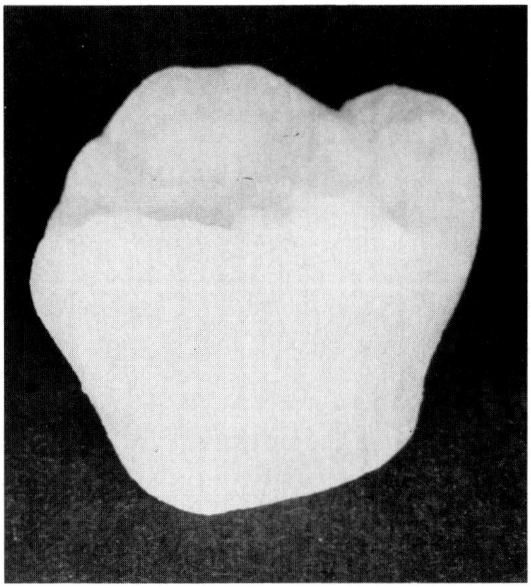

Fig. 12-31. The crystalline castable ceramic crown is achromatic.

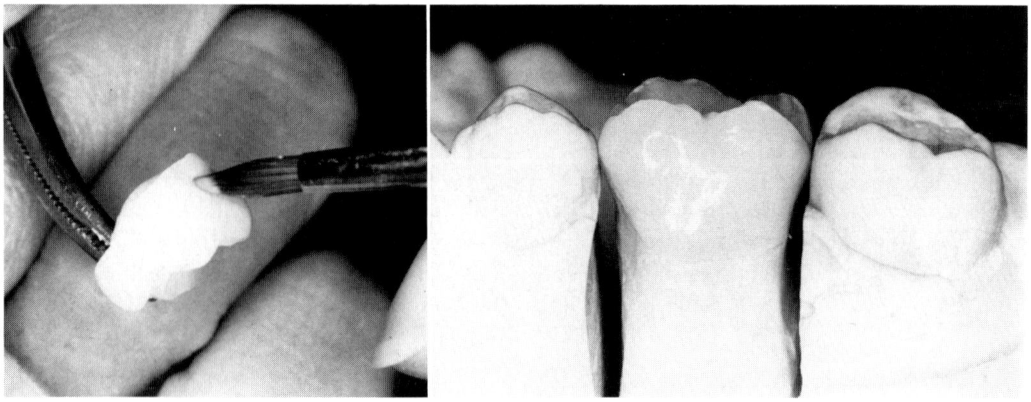

Fig. 12-32. Externally applied shading porcelain determines the desired hue, chroma, and value.

and glassy appearance of the final restoration. Castable ceramics may be fired repeatedly in a conventional glazing oven without affecting the physical properties or marginal integrity of the material. The ability of the dentist or technician to achieve the desired color depends primarily upon color perception, artistry, and patience. The constraints against repeated firings associated with conventional porcelain systems is not a limitation with this cast ceramic system. An overglazed appearance may be retextured with diamond points running at slow speed and refired to produce the desired effect. It is also possible to introduce surface texture into the viscous porcelain colorants with porcelain carving instruments before firing.

FITTING OF THE CROWN

Adjustments of contact areas or the occlusion of a crown may be necessary before cementation. The crown is lightly placed onto the tooth preparation, as marginal chipping may occur if the crown is forced into a tight contact area. Adjustment of contact areas may be made with superfine diamond points. After correction, contact areas should be polished with abrasive rubber wheels. Deficient contact areas can be corrected by removal of colorants from the area, adding additional corrective porcelain, and refiring. Internal adjustments can be made by using superfine diamond points. Occlusal adjustments can be made using superfine diamond points, followed by polishing with abrasive rubber wheels.

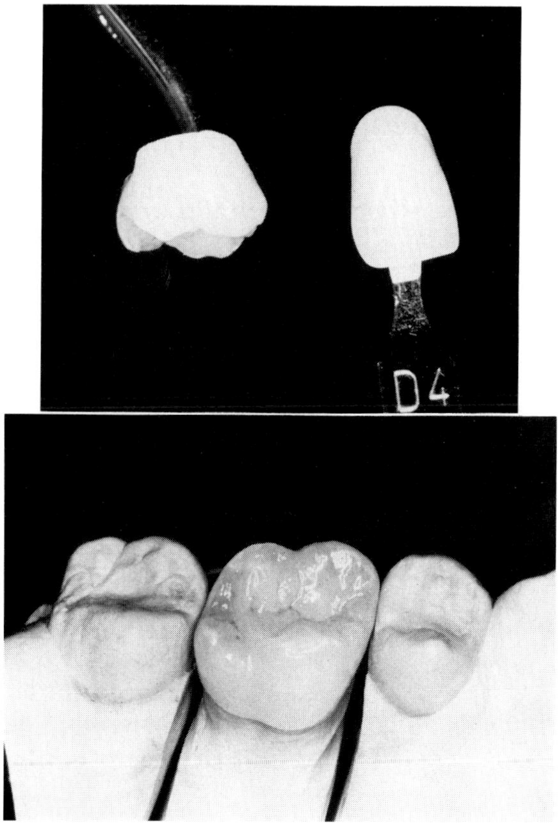

Fig. 12-33. Several applications of shading porcelain may be required to complete the coloring and characterization process.

CEMENTATION

The color value of the cast ceramic may be modified by a series of Dentsply shaded cements.* The greatest effect will be noticeable in the gingival third of the crown. These cements are color-coordinated with the die spacers that were used earlier in the technique and are extremely convenient for minor shade modification. If a natural-colored tooth preparation exists, a translucent glass ionomer cement may be indicated. In those cases in which discolored tooth structure or a metal core is present, the use of properly colored cement can be of inestimable value.

During the cementation process, controlled, positive finger pressure should be used to seat the crown onto the prepared tooth. Excess cement should be completely removed after setting is complete.

SUMMARY

The cast ceramic system is a different approach to esthetic restoration in both anterior and posterior teeth. Clinical testing and clinical application up to the present time indicate that very durable cosmetic restorations can be placed using crowns fabricated with the technique. Failure caused by fracture of the crystalline ceramic after cementation has been rare.

The technique demands excellence at every step of the procedure, from proper initial preparation of the teeth to final cementation, in order to achieve optimum results.

*Dentsply/York, Dentsply International, York, Pa.

BIBLIOGRAPHY

Adair, P.J., Bell, B.H., and Pameijer, C.H.: Casting technique of machinable glass ceramics, J. Dent. Res. **59**:475, 1980.

Adair, P.J., and Grossman, D.G.: The castable ceramic crown, Int. J. Periodont. Restor. Dent. **4**:33-45, 1984.

Adair, P.J., and Grossman, D.G.: Esthetic properties of lost tooth structure compared with ceramic restorations, J. Dent. Res. **61**:292, 1982.

Adair, P.J., and Hoekstra, K.E.: Fit evaluation of a castable ceramic, J. Dent. Res. **61**:345, 1982.

Adair, P.J., Sackett, B.P., and Cammarato, V.T.: Preliminary clinical evaluation of cast ceramic full crown restorations, J. Dent. Res. **61**:292, 1982.

American National Standards Institute/American Dental Association: Addendum to recommended standard practices for biological evaluation of dental materials, January 4, 1982.

Celenza, F.V.: Occlusal morphology, Chicago, 1980, Quintessence Publishing.

Grossman, D.G., Adair, P.J., and Pameijer, C.H.: Evaluation of the color of a cast ceramic restorative material, J. Dent. Res. **59**:542, 1980.

Internal measurements, Physical Properties Department, Corning Glass Works, Corning, N.Y., 1984.

Pameijer, C.H., Grossman, D.G., and Adair, P.J.: Physical properties of a castable ceramic dental restorative material, J. Dent. Res. **59**:474, 1980.

Preston, J.D., and Bergen, S.F.: Color science and dental art, St. Louis, 1980, The C. V. Mosby Co.

Schillingburg, H.T., Hobo, S., and Whitsett, L.D.: Fundamentals of fixed prosthodontics, Chicago, 1976, Quintessence Publishing.

CHAPTER 13

ATTACHMENTS AND SEMIRIGID CONNECTORS

MERRILL C. MENSOR

Attachments are mechanical devices for the fixation and stabilization of a dental prosthesis and include frictional, internal, intracoronal, extracoronal, key and keyway, parallel, precision, and slotted types (Boucher, 1976).

Steiger and Boitel (1959) write that a precision attachment in dentistry is a means of bodily junction for a removable bridge or partial denture. The word precision refers to a procedure that is held to low tolerance in manufacture, whereas semiprecision can refer to any attachments that have a lesser degree of tolerance than the precision unit.

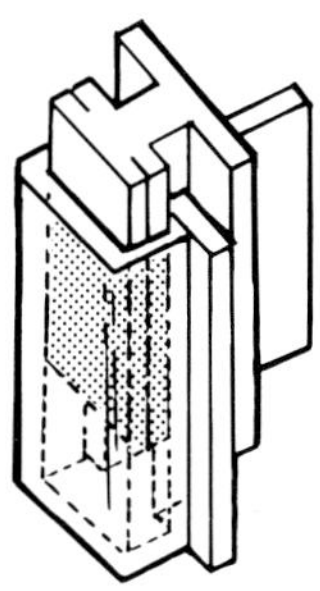

Fig. 13-1. I I-type frictional attachment. Double split in male part provides frictional retention when activated.

PRECISION ATTACHMENTS

precision attachments Precision attachments, as used in dentistry, refer to prefabricated devices used to join a prosthesis with its fixed or removable component.

intracoronal attachments Attachments that usually consist of a two-part unit: one part is a flange generally of a straight or tapered T or I beam, which is joined to the prosthesis, and a negative of the flange, which is incorporated in a retainer with the outside surface slotted to receive the flange.

Preiskel (1979) subclassifies these intracoronal attachments according to those whose retention is entirely frictional (group I) (Fig. 13-1) and augmented by a mechanical lock (group II) (Fig. 13-2).

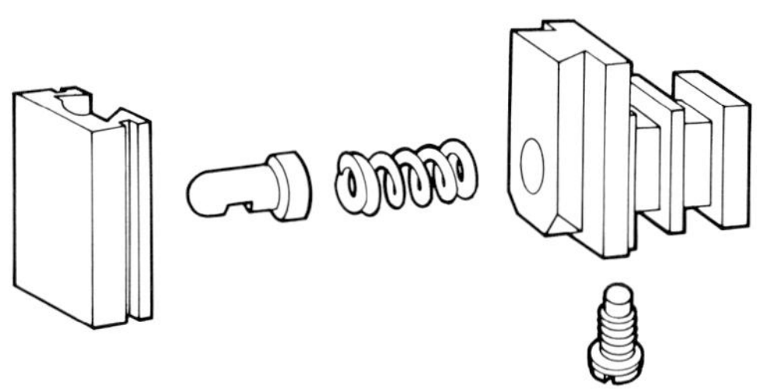

Fig. 13-2. Schatzmann represents pawl-type spring-loaded mechanical lock attachments. Bolt of connector is retained by screw from gingival side. Detent on female aids insertion. Retention flanges provide fixation in resin base.

extracoronal attachments Attachments that consist of two or more parts and are used to join a prosthesis to a retainer. Part or all of their mechanisms is outside the contour of the retainer.

A

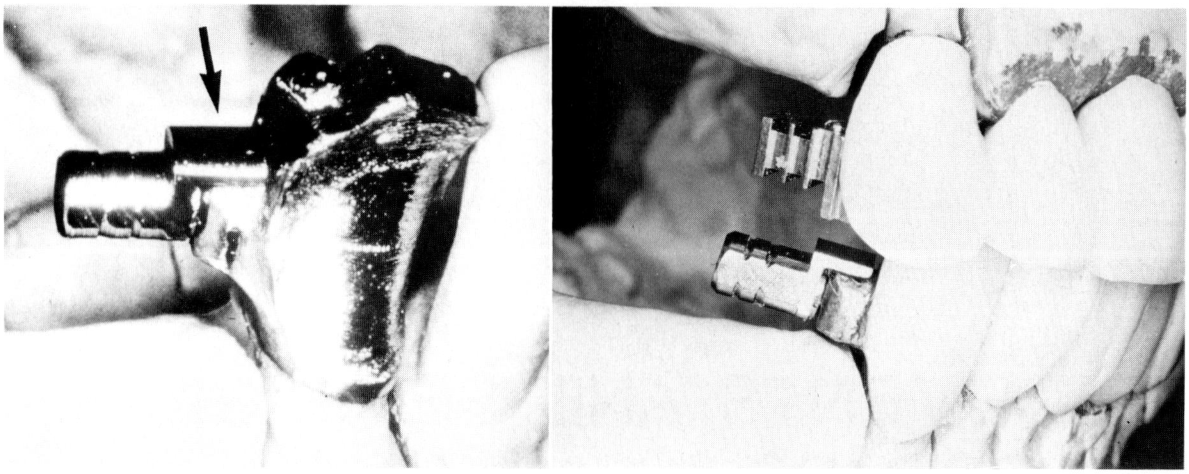

B

Fig. 13-3. A, ASC-52 attachments are spring-loaded universal joint stress directors. Miniature indirect retainer of protect configuration *(arrow)* prevents lift (mandibular) or drop (maxillary) of saddle. **B,** ASC-52 opposing Schatzmann.

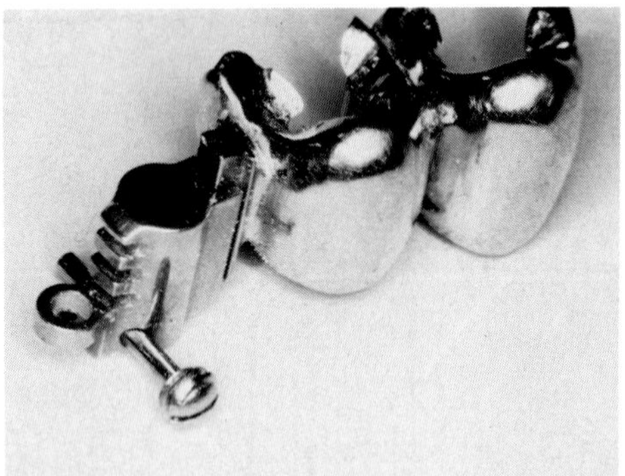

Fig. 13-4. Dalbo-Fix provides separable hinge action for telescope crowns, clasps, or milled retainers. Threaded pin secures attachment components; internal spring provides vertical resilience.

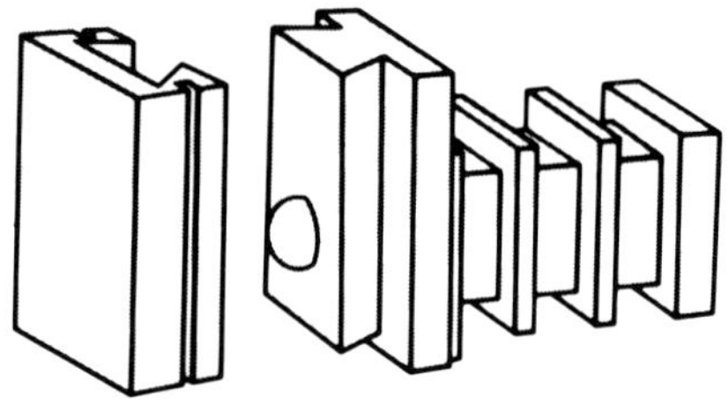

Fig. 13-5. Schatzmann attachment (assembled male, intracoronal female) classified as combined intracoronal-extracoronal attachment.

Preiskel (1979) states that their main application concerns the distal extension partial dentures, although bounded spaces may be restored with them. Preiskel further subclassifies extracoronal attachments into (1) projection units, such as the ASC-52 (Fig. 13-3); (2) connecting units, such as the Dalbo-Fix used between a clasp or telescope crown and the partial denture (Fig. 13-4); and (3) combined attachments, such as the Schatzmann (Fig. 13-5), consisting of an intracoronal section with a projection.

stress directors The term stress director is preferable to "stress breaker" and refers to the potential directional movement of a resilient attachment. Stress cannot be "broken"; it can only be selected, altered, or blocked.

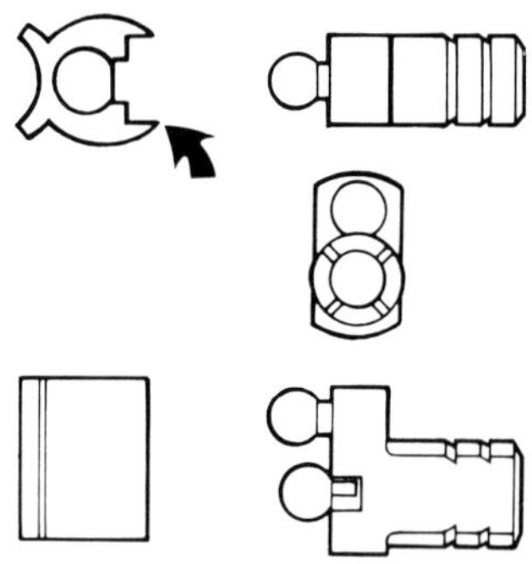

Fig. 13-6. Bival attachments are hybrid ASC-52s with dual fixation rigid or hinge action. Extensions on female *(arrow)* provide lateral stability.

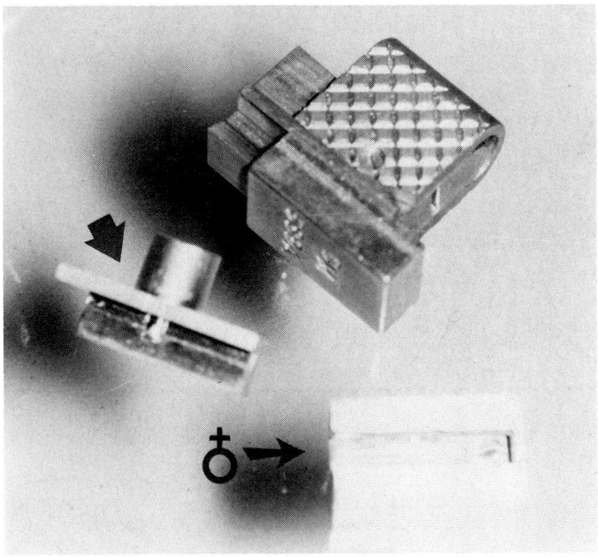

Fig. 13-7. Crismani resilient joint (partially assembled) and rigid Crismani connector *(arrow)* use common female *(lower arrow)*.

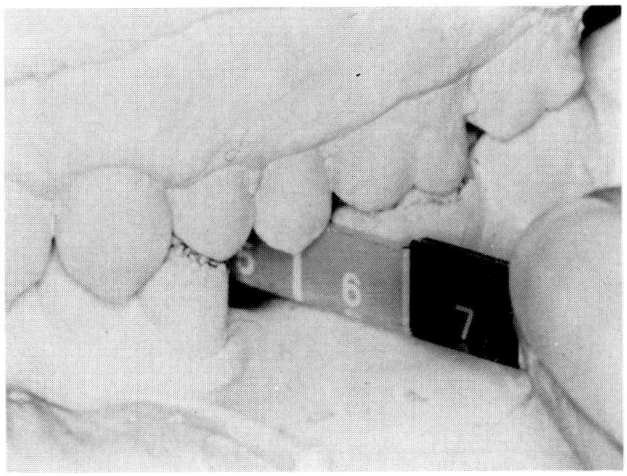

Fig. 13-8. Place EM gauge next to occluded abutment. Use color-coded numerical readout with EM Attachment Selector to choose attachments.

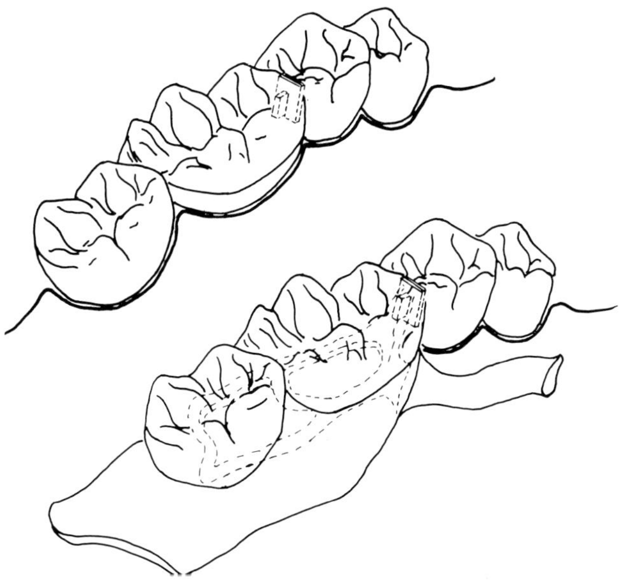

Fig. 13-9. Future planning. Bounded partial dentures *(top)* may be converted to free-end partial dentures *(bottom)* using same attachment.

Stress-director attachments usually consist of the extracoronal attachments with resilience, such as the Bival (Fig. 13-6), or the combined extracoronal-intracoronal attachment, such as the Crismani (Fig. 13-7).

Requirements

The retentive design or mechanical-retentive design of both intracoronal and extracoronal attachments of group I and II (Mensor, 1973) limits their application to clinical crowns that are no shorter than 3 mm occlusogingivally. Many attachments can be shortened occlusogingivally from the size provided by the manufacturer as noted on the EM Attachment Selector,* and this will determine attachment selection. No attachment should be selected without consulting the measurement of the occlusogingival space available from occluded casts (Fig. 13-8). An intracoronal attachment requires axial reduction of the coronal preparation by the dentist to provide space for the female housing, or the retainer will be overcontoured.

Most intracoronal attachments can be converted to extracoronal attachments by reversing their orientation. The occlusal side of the attachment becomes the tissue side, and the male flange is attached to the retainer while the female becomes a part of the prosthesis.

Any rigid system or limited resilient system carrying a free-end partial denture should incorporate multiabutment fixation on the mandibular design and should consider multiabutment fixation for torque reduction on the maxillary arch if palatal support is minimal. Future planning with attachments can allow conversion from a fixed bounded unit to a free-end partial denture without changing the primary attachments (Fig. 13-9).

Universal joint systems, such as the ASC-52 and the Crismani, carrying a free-end partial denture, may be used with single abutment anchorage if there is sufficient osseous support of the abutment tooth. Attachment-retainer retention will be enhanced if auxiliary retention grooves are developed in the retainer preparation (Fig. 13-10).

*EM Attachment Selector, Bell International, Inc., Burlingame, Calif.

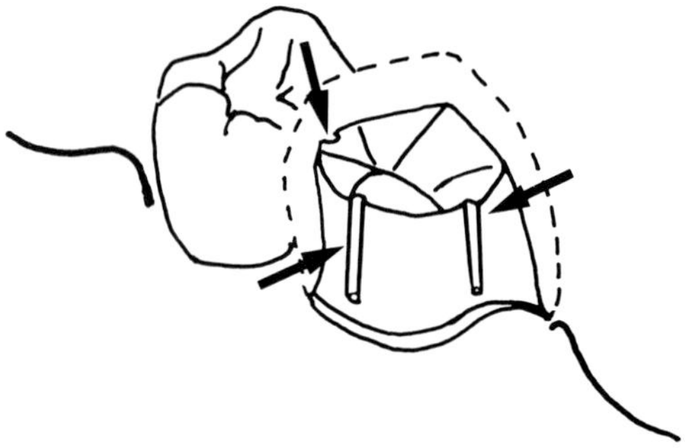

Fig. 13-10. Principle attachment retainer preparation must have parallel retention grooves *(arrows)* to prevent rotation or dislodgment of casting.

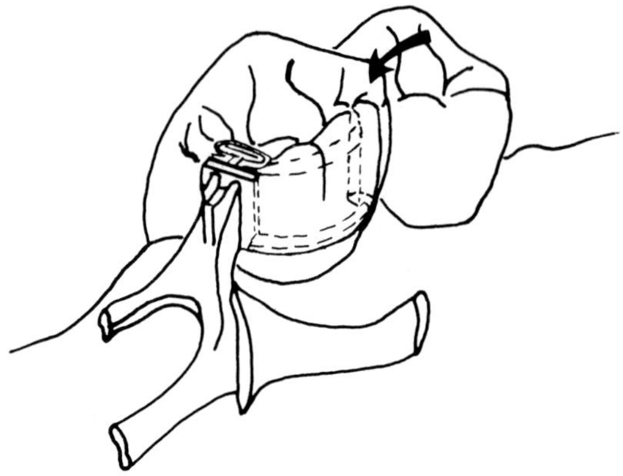

Fig. 13-11. Milled lingual retentive arms require retentive inset *(arrow)* opposite attachments.

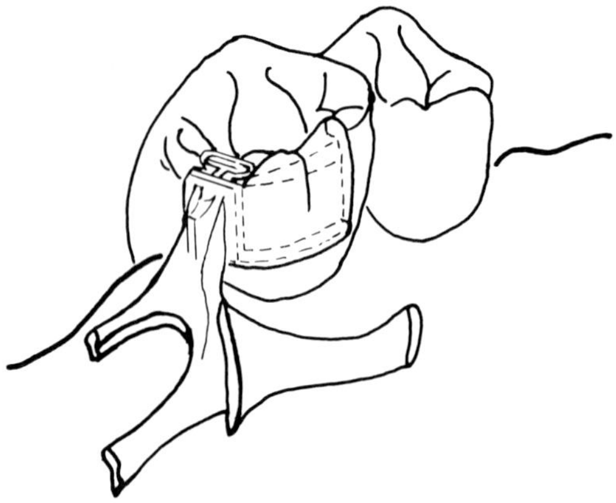

Fig. 13-12. Milled lingual bracing arms have only passive retentive function. Used primarily with rigid attachment systems.

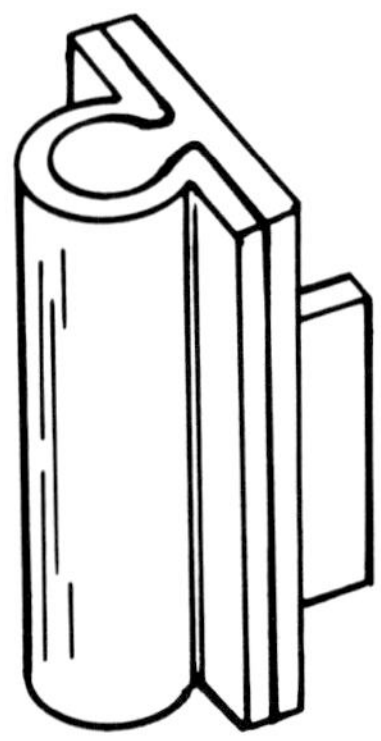

Fig. 13-13. Interlocks are nonfrictional T-type attachments used for splinting and nonparallel abutments.

Milled lingual retentive arms

Milled lingual retentive arms are required for any nonretentive attachment that has little or no adjustment capability (Fig. 13-11). The lingual retentive arm may also be used with the combined extracoronal attachment, whether it is resilient or nonresilient. The shorter the attachment, the greater the need for the lingual arm retention.

Milled lingual retentive arms may be converted to bracing arms (Fig. 13-12) if the attachment retention is fully adjustable and retentive. The arm may be eliminated where the retention is adequate or where either the attachment or extension component is resilient.

Attachments, such as the Interlock (Fig. 13-13) are used in fixed partial dentures for "mechanical soldering" of ceramometal sections. Many attachments are used to allow placement of fixed bridge units with divergent abutments (Fig. 13-14). Attachments are used in periodontal prosthodontics for fixed-removable elements in unilateral and bilateral bounded units (Fig. 13-15).

Framework design

MANDIBULAR PARTIAL DENTURES

The elimination of clasps from the partial denture removes any orientation of the framework to the master cast unless lingual bracing-retentive arms have been milled into the design. As such, two temporary indirect retainers (minor connectors) are waxed up as part of the framework (Fig. 13-16) and provide a means of proper orientation for either picking up the attachments in the mouth or off the master cast. Failure to use these minor connectors will eliminate the orientation of the lingual bar to the relief area and cause lingual tissue impingement in the mouth. In the case of the resilient attach-

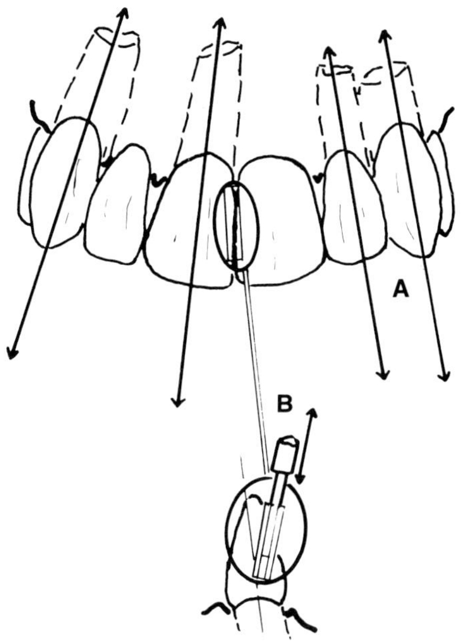

Fig. 13-14. Determine placement path of main retainer *(A)* to establish attachment orientation *(B)*.

A 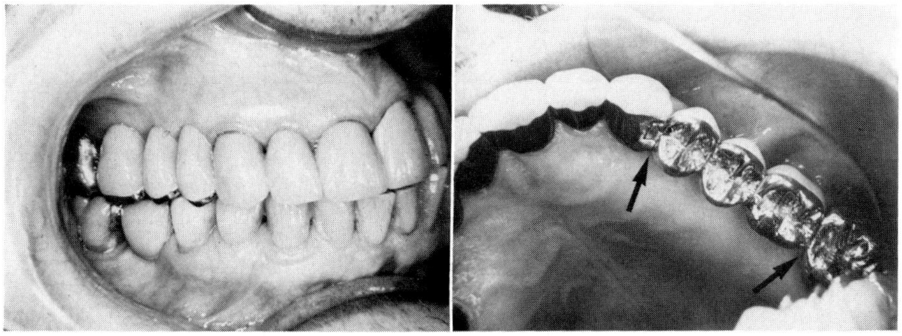 B

Fig. 13-15. A, Facial view of fixed removable pontics replacing Nos. 3 to 5. Attachment females in Nos. 2 and 6. **B,** Unilateral attachment units *(arrows)* must be parallel with each other and opposite side for conversion to bilateral bounded units with crossarch splinting.

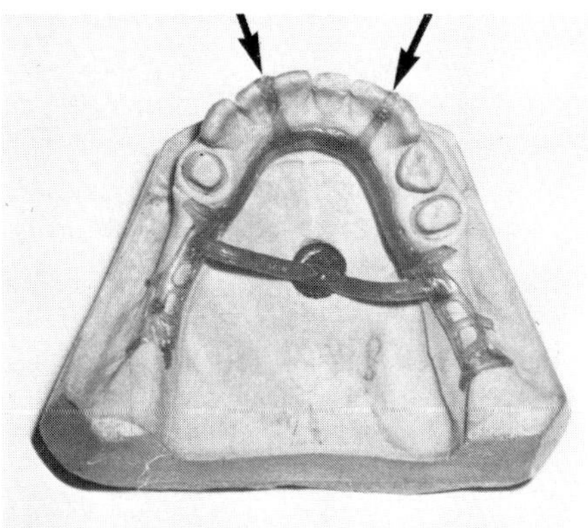

Fig. 13-16. Wax two temporary indirect retainers *(arrows)* in embrasures for frame orientation.

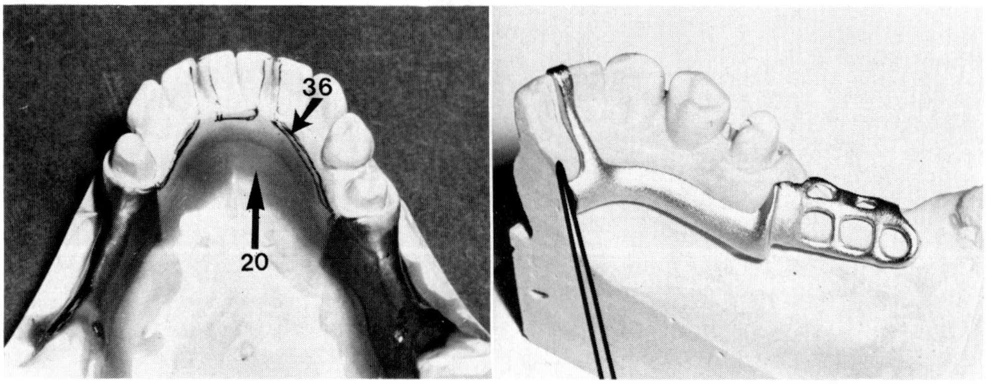

Fig. 13-17. A, Wax out 36-gauge relief occlusally and 20-gauge relief gingivally, and cast in refractory investment. **B,** Relief provides space for vertical and angular displacement.

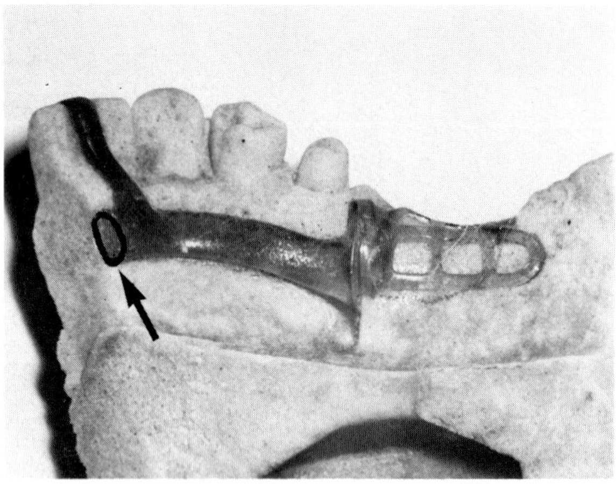

Fig. 13-18. Egg contour *(arrow)* on refractory cast prevents tissue impingement.

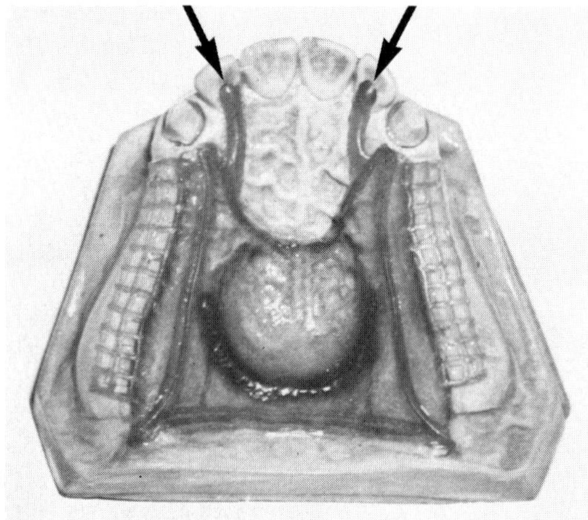

Fig. 13-19. Wax maxillary framework with two temporary indirect retainers either in embrasures or on cingula *(arrows)*. This position can be determined from contact of opposing teeth.

ment, the lingual bar will impinge upon the lingual tissue and make the appliance useless.

The indirect retainer further allows the repositioning or resin pickup of attachments, when necessary, before final delivery of the prosthesis. At that time the minor connectors are removed from the framework.

Relief for nonresilient partial dentures is developed on the master cast before duplication to provide for normal jaw flexion. This is in the order of 30-gauge wax relief with finish lines and saddle stops.

Relief for resilient partial dentures must provide for both vertical and angular displacement; therefore the relief starts at 36 gauge occlusally and increases as a wedge to 20 gauge gingivally (Fig. 13-17). After duplication the lingual bar is waxed with a definite egg contour toward the floor of the mouth (Fig. 13-18).

MAXILLARY PARTIAL DENTURES

The maxillary framework also requires temporary minor connectors for the orientation and testing of the framework, as well as the resin pickup of attachments in the mouth (Fig. 13-19). Under no circumstances should a horseshoe palate design be used, since maximum stability is achieved with broad palatal coverage of the skeletal support bone of the palate. Double beading will ensure palatal seal, but this should be done in concurrence with the dentist's digital palpation of the palate. The bead is usually 2 mm in from the posterior border of the impression on the master cast and to the depth of a No. 2 round bur; the second bead, parallel to the first, is 2 mm further in. Palatal relief is provided over thin areas when indicated. A postpalatal seal, as is normally used in complete maxillary dentures, may also be employed.

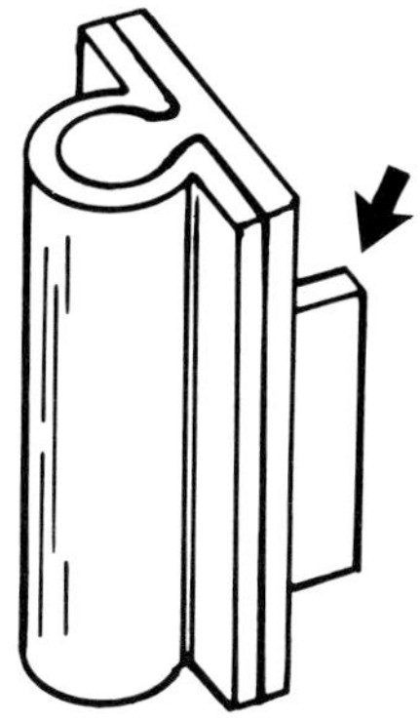

Fig. 13-20. Interlocks or Omega attachments are available in metal-ceramic, precious metal, and resin pattern forms. Two parts are female boxing and corresponding male with extension *(arrow)* for ease of assembly.

Intracoronal attachments

Three representative attachments will be used to illustrate standard techniques for laboratory assembly of the intracoronal section.

Interlock attachment

The Interlock* (Fig. 13-20) is one of the most popular attachments for long-span sectional bridgework and is ideal for anterior nonparallel abutments. It is virtually undetectable because of its buccal-lingual width of 1.5 mm. The length of 6 mm, at times, provides two attachments, and the metal flanges prevent rotation of the components. The flange may also be tapered to match the incisal contour without reducing the effectiveness of the unit. The attachment is provided in ceramometal for direct fusion with the precious alloys. Under no circumstances should precious metal attachments be cast to nonprecious alloys. Such a procedure may result in recrystallization of the attachment and for an incomplete casting of the crown (Moffa, 1976). The Ney M-S† attachment provides the resin form of this system to use with nonprecious metals as well as precious metals.

PROCEDURE

1. Prepare the master cast from the impression, and mount it on an articulator with the opposing cast.
2. Trim and seal the dies, and determine the path of retainer insertion with a surveyor from that of the preparations (Fig. 13-21).
3. Place the Interlock female by means of a parallelometer mandrel in the wax-up, and invest it in a phosphate bond investment.

*APM-Sterngold, Stamford, Conn.
†The J. M. Ney Co., Bloomfield, Conn.

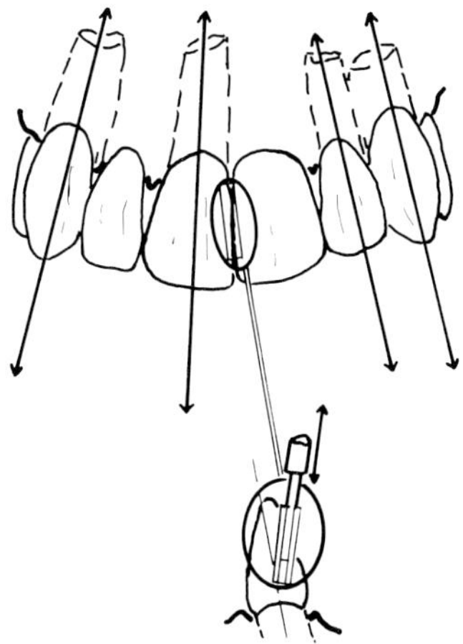

Fig. 13-21. Insertion path must be parallel to shed of bridge unit to be cemented.

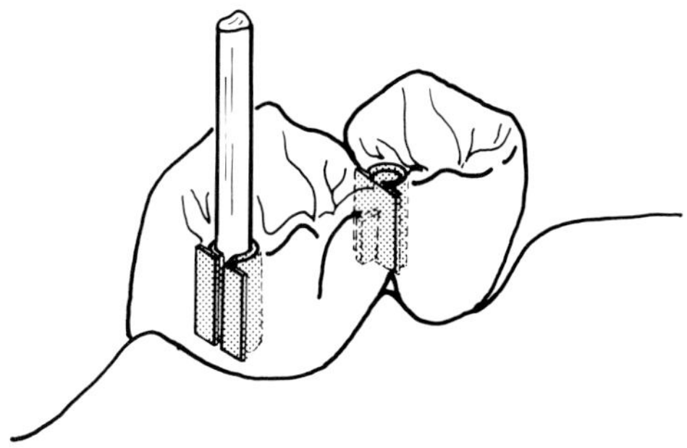

Fig. 13-22. Place second interlock parallel with first when splinting.

4. Heat the mold temperature to 1350° F (737° C) in 1 hour, and make the casting at this mold temperature to ensure metallurgical bonding.
5. Cool a normal crown and bridge alloy or self-annealing alloy with attachments from 850° to 450° F (455° to 235° C) ½ hour and then quench it in water to reharden the metal. (In the case of metal-ceramic restorations the heat treatment of the attachment and metal is automatic in firing the porcelain.)
6. Rough finish the attachment crown, and place the male interlock in the female.
7. Begin the second wax-up with the next abutment as previously described (Fig. 13-22). As an alternate procedure, the male portion of the attachment may be incorporated in the wax-up of the pontic framework (Fig. 13-23).

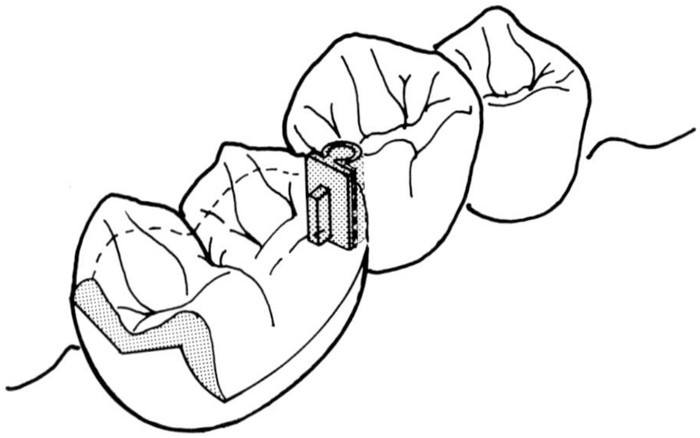

Fig. 13-23. Assemble interlock. Incorporate male with pontic wax-up.

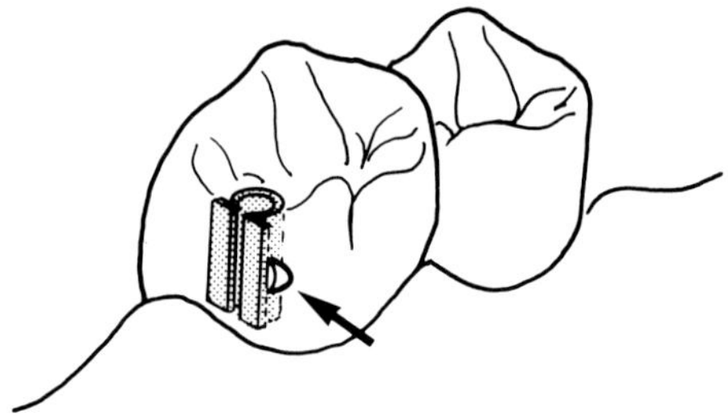

Fig. 13-24. Provide trough *(arrow)* to flow solder to interlock and retainer.

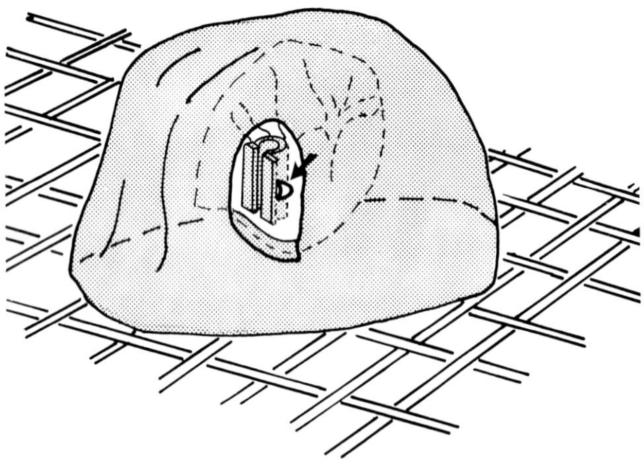

Fig. 13-25. Provide clearance in solder investment *(arrow)* for heat transfer about attachment.

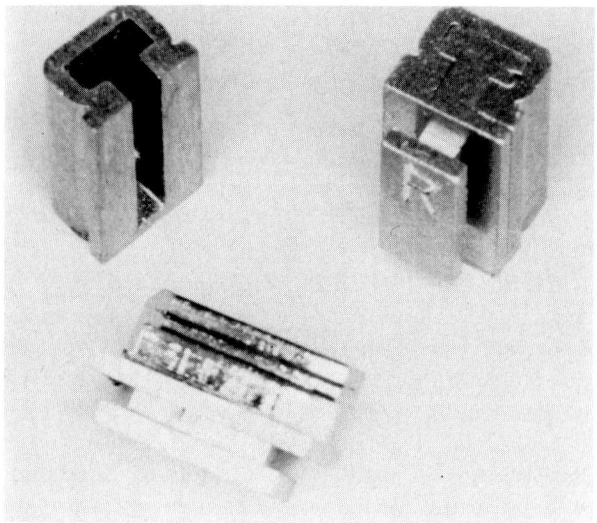

Fig. 13-26. McCollum attachments are H-type with right or left vertical split. Activated split provides frictional retention.

ALTERNATE PROCEDURE

1. Follow steps 1 and 2. Wax the attachments to the crown and then remove them.
2. Invest, cast, and rough finish the crown, and open the lingual area (Fig. 13-24, arrow).
3. Position the attachment in the crown with sticky wax, invest, and solder (Fig. 13-25). NOTE: This was the method prior to the advent of the metal-ceramic attachments and is still the required technique for some attachments.
4. Follow steps 5 to 7. NOTE: If the attachments are too snug, fine-grain graphite with glycerin placed about the attachment will ease the coupling.

McCollum attachment

The McCollum* attachment (Fig. 13-26) is classic and is representative for laboratory procedures of the majority of intracoronal precious metal attachments.

The basic design is that of an I beam with a corresponding female housing. One part of the beam consists of an adjustable flange, which engages the female, and the other is a solid plate that contacts the like member outer plate of the female to provide rigidity of the components. The attachment is available in platinum and gold for soldering or a high-fusing, platinum-gold alloy for direct casting, the latter being the most common form. The attachment is provided with a right and left configuration for ease of adjustment when combined with a lingual bracing arm and is provided with a taper at the gingival part of the female for ease of insertion.

There are two sizes; the small size is 5 mm in length by 2.8 mm in width, and the large size is 6.4 mm in length by 3.4 mm in width, and both have a 2-mm thickness. Each size is provided with a parallelometer

*APM-Sterngold, Stamford, Conn.

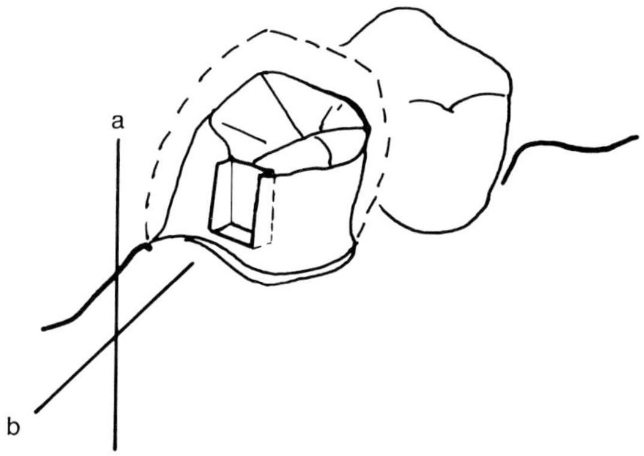

Fig. 13-27. Make diagnostic preparation with axis *a* parallel to long axis of tooth and perpendicular to ridge crest *b.* Axis must also parallel intended path of insertion for partial denture. Box preparation should be 1 mm above gingival margin.

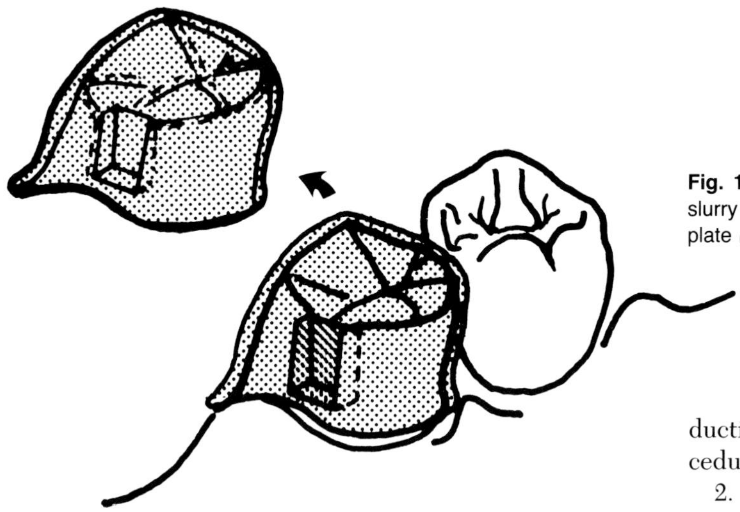

Fig. 13-28. Cast impression of preliminary retainer preparation in slurry stone. Prepare boxing, and make Omnivac or DuraLay template *(arrow).*

mandrel. The vertical clearance may be reduced to 3 mm, but some form of lingual bracing arm should be used with free-end partial dentures.

The McCollum attachment is used as a connector for bounded or free-end partial dentures and as a connector for posterior fixed and fixed removable bridgework.

PROCEDURE

1. The retainer preparations must provide space and positional orientation for the intracoronal attachment, or the castings will be overcontoured. To accomplish this, occlude the diagnostic cast on an articulator to check for vertical orientation of the attachments, and make diagnostic preparations on the study cast to locate the parallel box preparations for the attachments (Fig. 13-27). Sometimes a boxing preparation coping is made as a casting from a preliminary preparation model or a DuraLay* pattern (Fig. 13-28). This step provides an exact orientation of the attachments without overreduction of the teeth and is a chargeable laboratory procedure.

2. Cast the working model from the master impression, mount on an articulator with the opposing cast, and trim the dies.

3. Complete the wax-up of the abutments in the usual manner and prepare for spruing. Lingual bracing arms are recommended for increased stability, reduction of wear, and ease of insertion and removal (p. 334).

4. Determine the attachment position, and remove some wax in the box area until the attachment will almost fit in the hand.

5. Use the parallelometer mandrel to position the attachments at least 1 mm above the gingival margin of the preparations. This is done by warming the attachment with a heated spatula and moving the attachment into the wax-up (Fig. 13-29).

6. Finish the wax-up, invest it in a phosphate bond investment, and ready it for casting.

7. Increase the mold temperature to 1350° F (737° C) in 1 hour. The casting is made at this mold temperature to ensure metallurgical bonding.

8. Clean the castings with an abrasive blaster and an ultrasonic cleaner. Avoid stripping the casting or electrolytic polishing because surface metal removal will reduce the precision of the attachments.

*Reliance Dental Manufacturing Co., Chicago, Ill., or equivalent.

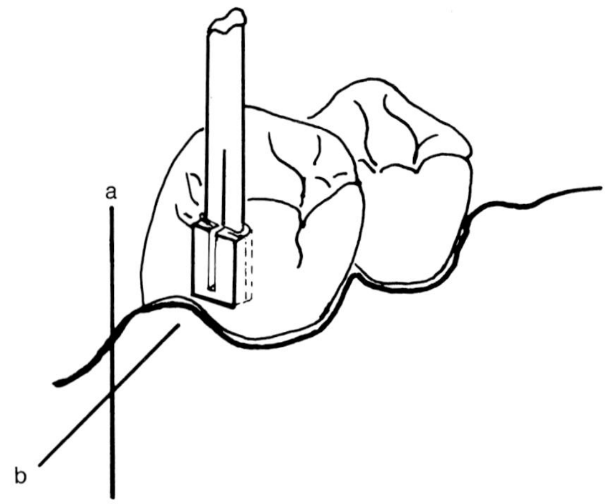

Fig. 13-29. Use mandrel to place attachment in wax-up. Warm attachment with hot spatula and move into wax-up.

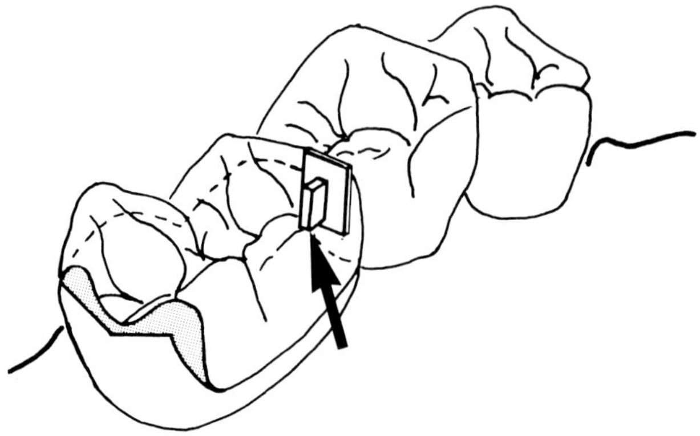

Fig. 13-30. Wax pontic about male extension *(arrow).*

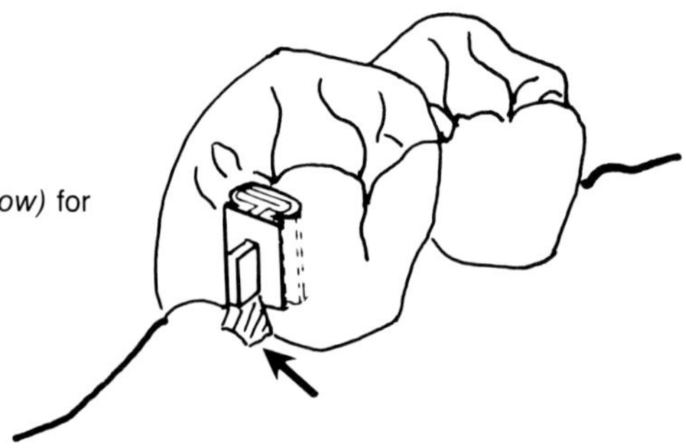

Fig. 13-31. Block out male extension with undercut wax *(arrow)* for removable partial denture duplication.

9. Rough finish the castings, and fit the male to the female on the master cast. (If the attachments are too tight, a graphite powder with glycerin will ease the insertion.)

The procedures indicated for the Interlock attachment can be used for an alternate method of preparing the McCollum attachment.

PROCEDURE FOR FIXED REMOVABLE PARTIAL DENTURES

1. Assemble the attachments on the master cast. Reduce the occlusal extensions of the attachments to occlude with the opposing cast, and include the male extension in the wax-up of the pontics (Fig. 13-30).
2. Invest and cast the pontic section according to steps 6 to 9 described previously.
3. Heat treat any attachment component by heating the castings to 850° F (455° C) and oven cooling to 450° F (235° C) for ½ hour followed by quenching in water. (Heat treating the attachment casting is automatically a part of the procedure for ceramometals when porcelain is fired.)
4. Finish the attachment bridge for delivery to the dentist. The tight fit is normal to attachment bridges, and this may be reduced by using a graphite-glycerin lubricant in the attachments.

An alternate procedure for fixed removable partial dentures is to wax the pontic and cast it separately. It is then soldered to the male attachment and heat treated.

PROCEDURE FOR REMOVABLE PARTIAL DENTURES

1. Fit the male to the female on the master cast and block out the area between the attachment and the ridge crest with undercut wax.*
2. Duplicate the master cast, and wax up the partial denture framework about the attachment section (Fig. 13-31).
3. Elevate the crown on the die with a 12-μm strip of plastic† to provide for cement elevation of the crown. (An alternate method is to seal the die with a cyanoacrylate cement, lubricate the die, and temporarily cement the crown with a mixture of ProTem‡ and a small

---

*The J.M. Ney Co., Bloomfield, Conn., or equivalent.
†Leader Tape, 3M Co., Minneapolis, Minn., or equivalent.
‡ProTem, Professional Products Co., San Diego, Calif., or equivalent.

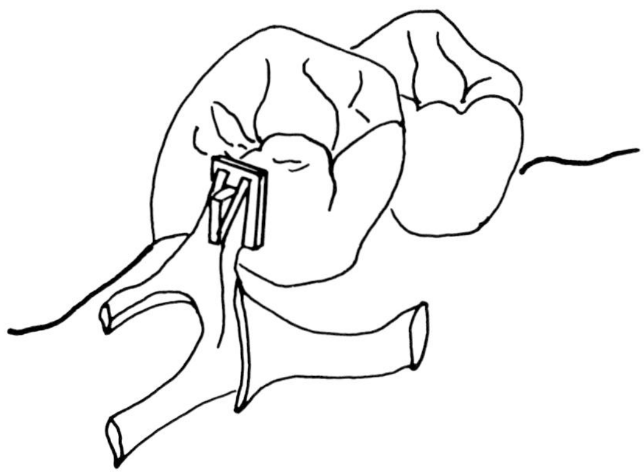

Fig. 13-32. Fit framework to male of attachment, sticky wax, invest, and solder.

amount of the crown and bridge cement powder used by the dentist.)

4. Fit the framework to the attachment, sticky wax it in place, and invest it for soldering (Fig. 13-32). Craig (1976) recommends the use of .585 solder with fluoride flux for austenitic metals and .650 solder with borax flux for precious metals.

5. After soldering, heat treat the framework and attachment male.

6. Complete and finish the partial denture in the usual manner.

7. Retention is *not* activated by the laboratory. This is usually done by the dentist some time after placement of the removable partial denture.

PROBLEM AREAS

Several problems can arise with the intracoronal attachment. Most of them are related to laboratory procedures. The problems, their probable causes, and solutions are presented in Table 13.

1. Metallurgical bond failure is a common error in the direct casting technique due to the mold temperature being held well below 1350° F (737° C) prior to casting and this can be best achieved by casting at the mold temperature or doing an oven soldering to correct the problem.

2. The attachment will sag or melt during porcelain placement if a gold-platinum alloy is used instead of an alloy that is specifically designed for ceramometal procedures.

3. Porosity about the attachment-crown interface is a result of using too high a temperature for soldering with a borax flux. The glass formation blocks the solder flow. The use of a Ney digital furnace* with a clear-view muffle for oven soldering and a temperature range of 1485° to 1515° F (807° to 825° C) is recommended.

4. Porosity about the crown and fracture of the attachment when cast to nonprecious metals is due to the recrystallization of the attachment metal because of the intense heat. Precious metal precision attachments should only be soldered to nonprecious metals with a .585 solder, using a fluoride flux to prevent discoloration.

5. The male will not engage the female for several reasons. The attachments may have oxides or exhibit distortion and require careful fitting with a graphite lubricant. Any burs or high spots should be reduced with a mounted rubber point. Sometimes the occlusal entrance is rolled in from grinding and can be corrected by flaring the entry and beveling the gingival margin of the female if it is not already so manufactured. One very obvious problem of nonentry is the result of the retention having been activated. Under no circumstances should an attachment retention be activated before final placement of the prosthesis.

6. The attachment face will spread or open if it is subjected to a load and the attachment has not been heat treated. Heat treatment in an oven at 850° F (455° C) reduced to 450° F (235° C) in ½ hour, followed by quenching in water will restore 90% of the metallurgical qualities and significantly reduce attachment wear.

7. Loose attachments with adjustable retention may be tightened by simply activating the retention component.

8. Attachments will not seat for several reasons. One of the most obvious is that the insertion pathway is unidirectional, and the ridge undercuts were not blocked out. This is best handled by surveying the master cast, blocking out the undercuts, and processing it on a duplicate cast made from the controlled master cast. The second reason will be either debris in the female, or that the patient has dropped or distorted the partial denture by forcing the appliance. The debris problem is a simple matter, whereas the dropped or forced partial denture may be salvageable only by removing the prosthesis. The distorted section should be identified and corrected if possible before stripping the frame. Preventive maintenance requires thorough instruction to the patient on proper care, insertion, and removal.†

9. Occasionally the prosthesis and crown only fit

*Mark IV digital furnace, J.M. Ney Co., Bloomfield, Conn., or equivalent.

†Patient Information Pamphlet: Your new restoration, APM-Sterngold, Stamford, Conn.

when they are in the saliva and exhibit hyperocclusion of both the retainer and the prosthesis, with no tissue contact because no provision was made for cement elevation of the retainer crown. This is a common problem for technicians accustomed to working with a nonattachment clasp-type partial denture.

Some provision must be made for the cement elevation before the partial denture is constructed, and this may be done in two ways. One system assumes maximum seating of the casting so that a 12-μm plastic film is placed between the casting and the die; the occlusion is established and the partial denture is developed in this relation. The second procedure uses a lubricated cyanoacrylate sealed die with a crown retainer cemented with a mixture of ProTem and some of the powder of the crown and bridge cement to be used, the grain size of the powder establishing the elevation. The entire procedure ensures the same relationship in the mouth as on the articulator and reduces any potential torque load on the abutment teeth.

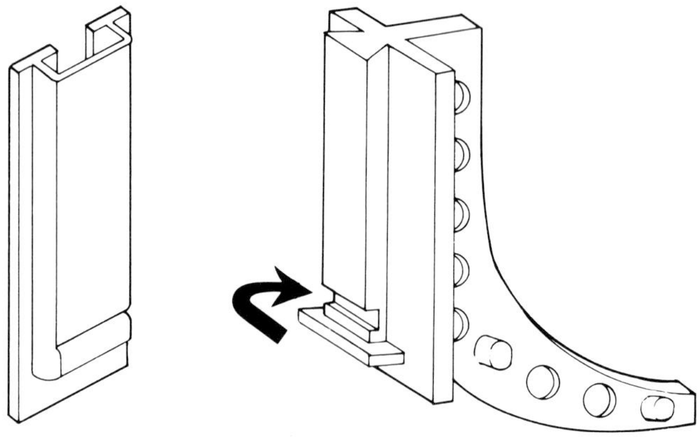

Fig. 13-33. Stern JMS male (right) is redesigned to accept nylon retention jackets (Fig. 13-34). Female (left) is standard .070 G/L series. Notch in male *(arrow)* provides positive snap retention of nylon jackets.

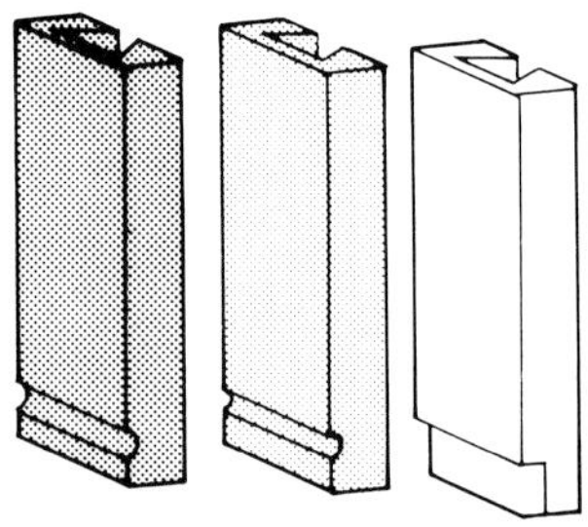

Fig. 13-34. Nylon retention jackets snap on JMS male. Order of retention from right to left: yellow, friction only; red, friction with weak latch; black, friction with strong latch; gray in polycarbonate (not shown), same retention as black.

STERN JMS*

The Stern JMS attachment (Fig. 13-33) represents a total redesign of the intracronal Stern G/L system. The matrix or female is exactly the same as the G/L female described by Baker and Goodkind (1981) and still permits the use of the metal ESI male (part No. 802411) in short bite cases. Stated another way, the JMS male (part No. 802410) may be retrofitted to existing Stern .070 G/L fixed removable or removable partial dentures when retention failure has existed.

The designation "JMS"† stands for Jacket Maintenance System, wherein there are no moving parts or adjustment flanges. The metal patrix or male caries a selection of three precision formed nylon jackets (Fig. 13-34) or a gray polycarbonate jacket, which creates a snug cushioned connection with selective degrees of retention. The nylon or polycarbonate jackets eliminate internal metal contact of the attachment components, so wear and/or loss of retention is only on the replaceable resin parts.

The female JMS housing at its greatest width is 3.5 mm and requires a boxing preparation of greater than 2.3 mm faciolingually and a depth of 1.5 mm to incorporate it within the normal crown contour. The vertical length is 8 mm, including the 1 mm gingival flange extension, which may be reduced to blend with the gingival contour of the retainer. The vertical height of the female may be reduced to conform with the intraocclusal space, but at no time should this reduction exceed 3.5 mm of final height. The female JMS is the same product as the conventional Stern .070 G/L and is available in IP (20% iridium platinum, melting range 2900° to 3000° F) and TF (Thermofit, melting range 2400° to 2500° F). APM-Sterngold states that the IP form can be cast against with virtually any precious or nonprecious alloy.

The male JMS is fabricated from a stellite alloy with a melting temperature of 2465° F. It is machined with a bichanneled vertical extension off the proximal plate and a gingival stop designed to receive the nylon and polycarbonate retention jackets. The male has an extension tail with retention elements (see Fig. 13-33) that allows it to be retained in the removable section by resin, soldering, or cast-to techniques.

The retention shapes of the jackets (Fig. 13-35) provide a snug cushioned connection and prevent wear of the attachment proper. There are four color-coded jackets:

*All copyright illustrations in this section courtesy of APM-Sterngold, Stamford, Conn.

†Personal communication from Joseph M. Sulc, 1983.

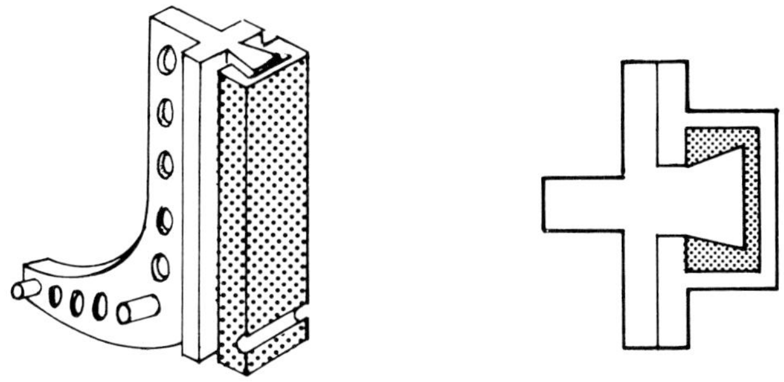

Fig. 13-35. Nylon jackets snap on JMS male, *(left)* and provide snug cushioned fit in female, *(right).*

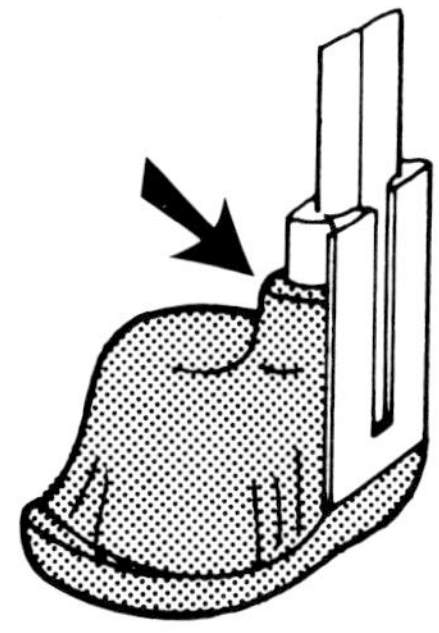

Fig. 13-36. Thin layer of alloy about occlusal portion of attachment *(arrow)* supports female and prevents distortion of attachment or crazing of porcelain.

1. Yellow jacket—nylon jacket for fabrication and initial delivery to the patient. This jacket provides snug frictional fit without snap retention at the gingival.
2. Red jacket—nylon jacket for patients requiring more retention than provided by the yellow jacket. Same frictional fit but with snap retention at the gingival.
3. Black jacket—nylon jacket for patients requiring maximum retention. Same frictional fit with greater snap retention at the gingival.
4. Gray jacket—polycarbonate jacket for patients who keep dislodging or losing the nylon jackets. Requires a cyanoacrylite adhesive.* Same frictional retention and snap as black nylon jacket.

The paralleling mandrel used for the JMS attachment is the same for all Stern .070 females.

The JMS attachment is used as a connector for bounded or free-end partial dentures and as a connector for posterior fixed and fixed-removable bridgework, specifically Kennedy Class I through Class IV.

PROCEDURE

1. Mounted diagnostic casts, as discussed with the McCollum procedure (see Fig. 13-27), should be used to ensure space and positional orientation for the attachments before preparation or the retainer will be overcontoured. Interocclusal space, using the EM gauge (see Fig. 13-8) should not be less than 4 mm (the gingival flange extension may be reduced 0.5 mm and the entire attachment can be reduced 3.5 mm if needed). The faciolingual space should be no less than 2.3 mm and the mesiodistal reduction should be 1.5 to 2 mm.

2. Cast the working model from the master impression, mount on an articulator with the opposing cast, and trim the dies.

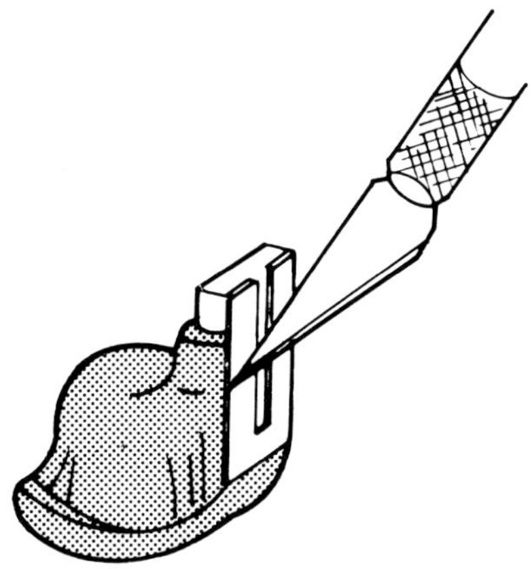

Fig. 13-37. Keep wax off face plate by grooving wax around face plate to prevent metal from flashing into female.

3. Survey the working model and establish a common path of insertion and complete the wax-up in the usual manner. Lingual bracing or retentive arms are recommended for increased stability and ease of insertion and removal (p. 334).

4. Determine the attachment position and remove some wax in the box area until the attachment will almost fit hand-held.

5. Metal occlusal: Use the parallelometer with the Stern .070 mandrel and position the females at least 1 mm above the gingival margin of the preparations by warming the attachment with a heated spatula and moving the attachment into the wax-up (see Fig. 13-29); complete to final contour.

6. Porcelain occlusal: Follow the steps outlined in procedure 5. Full-coverage porcelain requires the attachment to have a thin layer of alloy supporting the attachment above the occlusal portion of the coping. This will prevent distortion of the female or porcelain from contacting the attachment (Fig. 13-36), and will ensure against checking of the porcelain.

7. Use a sharp Bard-Parker knife (Fig. 13-37) and

*JMS Adhesive, APM-Sterngold, Stamford, Conn.

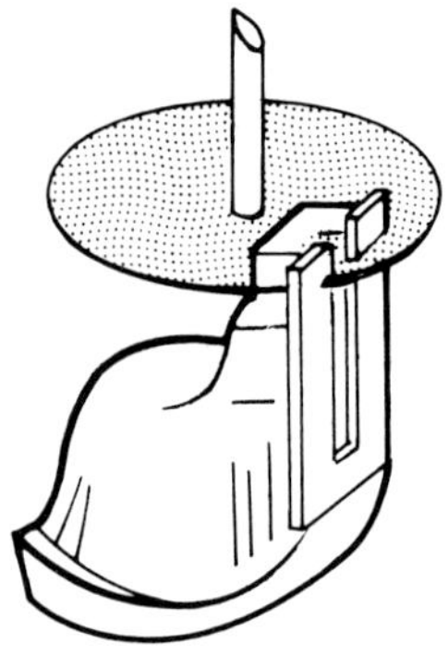

Fig. 13-38. Use thin separating disk for height reduction and remove any metal "folds" with sharp knife.

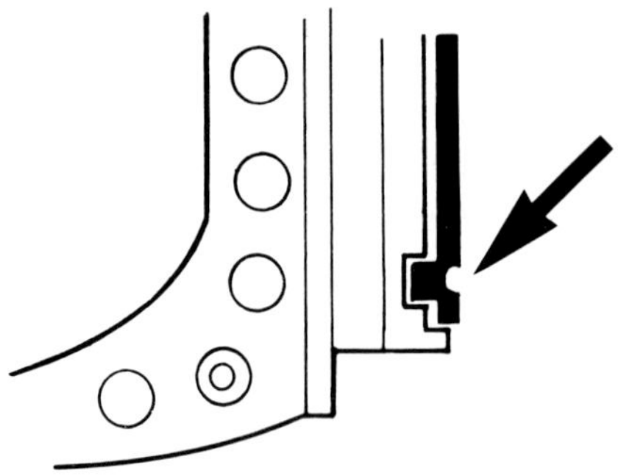

Fig. 13-39. Grooved end of the yellow nylon jacket *(arrow)* must be placed toward gingival of metal core.

scribe the wax about the faceplate of the attachment; this will prevent alloy from flashing over the faceplate and inside the attachment.

8. Sprue the wax patterns so that the alloy will not flow directly to the attachment, and mount on the sprue former to allow direct access to the attachments.

9. Use a phosphate bonded investment* and paint the investment into the attachments. Complete the investment procedure in the usual manner.

10. Increase the mold temperature to 1350° F (737° C) in 1 hour. The casting is made at this mold temperature to ensure metallurgic bonding.

11. Divest and protect the attachment with your finger. Carefully debride the investment from the casting with an air eraser. Use a fiberglass brush† to clean the attachment. Complete the debridement by ultrasonic cleaning.

12. Place the individual attachment retainers on their respective dies and reduce the occlusal extension of the attachments to the desired height with a thin separating disk (Fig. 13-38).

13. Correct any edge fold of the attachment with a sharp knife and insert an ESI male (part No. 802411)† into the attachment several times to ensure that there are no sharp edges or burs. Follow this by polishing the occlusal entry of the attachment with a rubber point. This will protect the nylon or polycarbonate jackets from being "shaved" during misaligned insertion attempts and during the following assembly procedures.

14. Place the yellow nylon jacket on the metal male by aligning the grooved end toward the gingival of the metal core (Fig. 13-39) and snap the sleeve down against the metal bottom plate (the snap-lock can be felt engaging the male recess).

*Ceramco II, Whip-Mix Corp., Louisville, Ky.
†APM-Sterngold, Stamford, Conn.

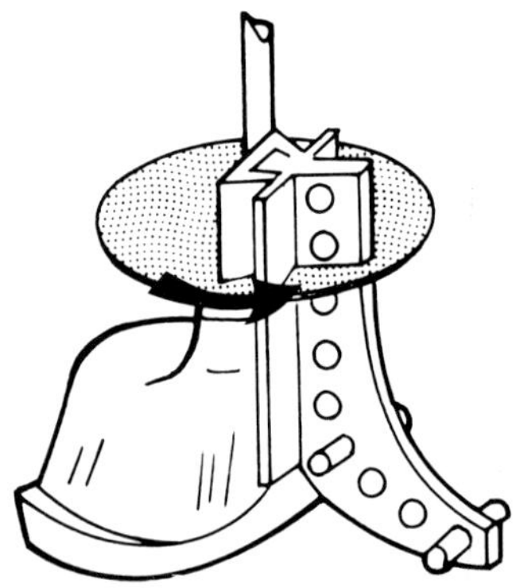

Fig. 13-40. Male with yellow nylon jacket is assembled to female and reduced to occlusal height with thin separating disk. Jacket must be cut toward metal to avoid distortion.

15. Insert the assembled male into the female, making sure that it is fully seated. Use a thin separating disk to cut the nylon toward the metal male, thereby reducing the male to the height of the female (Fig. 13-40).

16. Fixed or fixed-removable bridge male placement: Duplicate the master cast or transfer the retainers from a try-in master impression and begin final assembly. (NOTE: to compensate for final cement elevation, use crown-and-bridge cement powder with glycerine when placing the castings on the working dies or at try-in with the castings before making the new transfer impression.)

17. Use a separating disk and remove a portion of the male's retention tail necessary for pontic construction (leave enough for a mechanical as well as a metallurgic bond; melting point of this stellite alloy is 2465° F).

18. Complete the wax-up of the pontics, remove the yellow nylon jackets (Fig. 13-41), invest and cast the

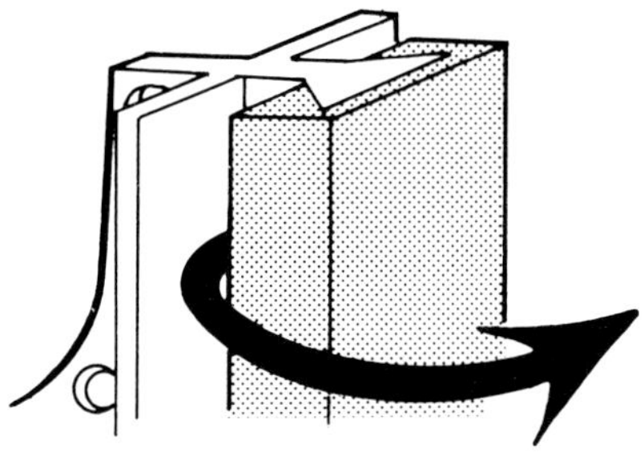

Fig. 13-41. Nylon jackets are removed by peeling off either side, as illustrated by arrow.

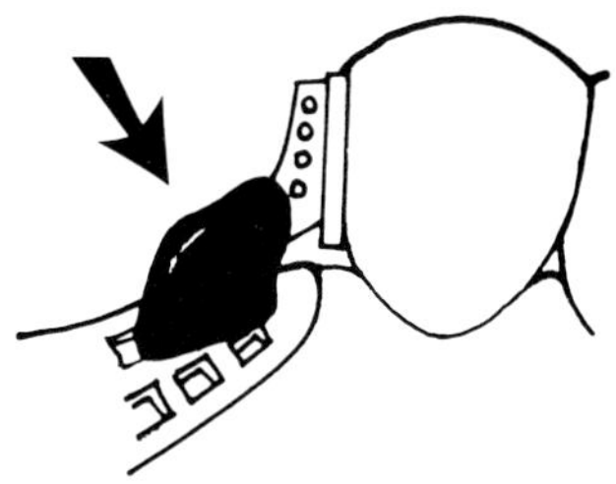

Fig. 13-42. Male attachment is fitted with yellow nylon jacket and related to retainer/partial denture framework with autopolymerizing resin *(arrow).*

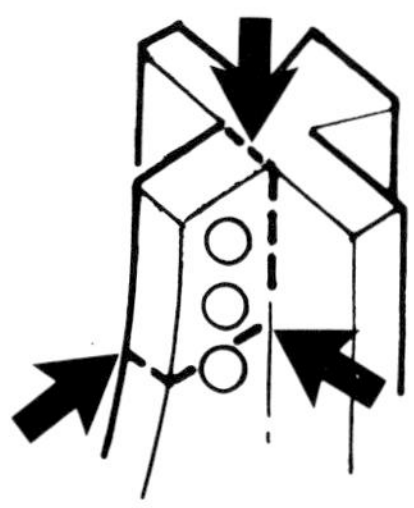

Fig. 13-43. Male retention should always be reduced to provide space for denture tooth or cast metal occlusal *(arrows).*

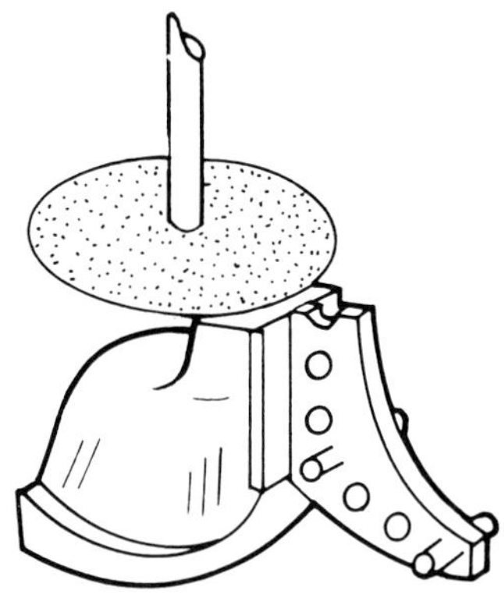

Fig. 13-44. Fit all jackets to individual attachments by (1) reduction with separating disk running toward male JMS then (2) smoothing with sandpaper disk.

pontic section in the usual manner, finish, and assemble by replacing the nylon jackets.

19. Removable partial denture male placement: Duplicate the master cast or transfer the retainers from a try-in master impression and begin final assembly. (NOTE procedure 16.)

20. Fabricate the removable partial denture framework (see Figs. 13-16 through Fig. 13-19). The usual technique assumes resin pickup (Fig. 13-42); however, the retention tails may be waxed up and become a direct part of the framework, as discussed with the pontics in procedure 18.

21. Use a separating disk (Fig. 13-43) and remove a portion of the male retention from the occlusal to allow placement of the first denture tooth against the faceplate without reduction (provides space for cast metal occlusals).

22. Prepare the saddle areas for an altered cast procedure by the dentist.

23. Remount the altered cast with the new occlusal records, complete the wax-up of the removable partial denture, invest, process, and finish in the usual manner.

24. Place new yellow nylon jackets on the males of the fixed-removable partial dentures. Reduce the jackets first with a separating disk (a knife blade will distort the nylon). Follow by final reduction with a sandpaper disk (Fig. 13-44).

25. Prepare extra nylon jackets and package them labled for the side to be replaced.

26. Deliver the appliances. Instruct the patient relative to cleaning the jackets so they will not be dislodged accidently.

27. If dislodgement is a problem, the polycarbonate jacket may be used instead of the nylon jacket. The polycarbonate jacket may be secured with a drop of JMS cyanoacrlate cement.*

*APM-Sterngold, Stamford, Conn.

Table 13-1. Intracoronal attachments

Problem	Probable cause	Solution
Metallurgic bond failure	Mold temperature too low at casting	Use silicophosphate investment and keep mold temperature above 1350° F (737° C)
Attachment sags or melts during placement of porcelain	Gold-platinum alloy attachment used instead of metal-ceramic attachment	Use only high-fusing attachment for metal-ceramic procedures
Porosity about attachment-crown interphase (soldering)	Soldering temperature too high, causing glass formation	Oven solder and use liquid flux*
Porosity about attachment with nonprecious crown	Metal temperature too high at cast	Solder precious metal to nonprecious with .585 solder and fluoride flux
Failure of attachment nonprecious crown	See above; also causes recrystallization of attachment and fracture	See above
Dark discoloration of metal about solder area nonprecious crown	Borax flux and .650 solder	See above
Male will not engage female	Oxidation or casting distortion	Use graphite lubricant and work in; remove burs with rubber point
	Occlusal entrance flared in from grinding or hyperfunction	Bevel gingival margin of male or place slight bevel on occlusal margin of female boxing
	Attachment retention activated before fitting	Do not activate attachment retention until needed
Attachment face spreading open	Not heat treated to restore metallurgic properties	Remake crown or remove; repair it; and heat treat; always heat treat in oven 850° F (455° C) and drop to 450° F (235° C) in ½ hour, quench in water
Attachment wearing	See above	See above
	Part of attachment heat treated, part of it not	See above
	Attachments not parallel	Use parallelometer with mandrel for attachment placement
Attachment loose	Retention not activated	Activate attachment
Nylon jacket distorted, disengaged	Acrylic overextended about first denture tooth	Remove nylon jacket, check for contact of metal faceplates: reassemble
Nylon jackets abraded and dislodged	Burs in female housing or occlusal entry bent	Check insertion with ESI‡ metal male and bevel entry
Retention minimal	Requires more retention	Replace yellow nylon jacket with red or black nylon jacket
Nylon jackets dislodged	Patient may dislodge by insertion or cleaning	Replace nylon jackets with polycarbonate and acrylic cement fixation
Attachment prosthesis will not seat	Undercuts not blocked out prior to processing	Use PIP† for interference and relief; block out all undercuts and process on duplicate casts
	Debris in female	Check and clean
	Patient forced prosthesis to place or dropped	Adjust or possibly remake; instruct patient to never force appliance in or out
Prosthesis in hyperocclusion; base not touching tissue	Crown was not elevated with plastic strip to compensate for cement elevation and partial was related to crown with resultant loss of contact	Always elevate crown with strip of film

*T-Flux, Degussa, Inc., Placentia, Calif., or equivalent.
†Pressure Indicator Paste, Mizzy, Inc., Clifton Forge, Va.
‡ESI Metal Male, APM-Sterngold, Stamford, Conn.

PROBLEM AREAS

The problems discussed on pp. 341-342 and in Table 13-1 are also valid for the Stern JMS with the following additions:

1. The nylon jacket will distort and disengage if the acrylic around the first denture tooth is overextended (Fig. 13-45). Make sure the faceplates of the male and female are in positive contact before placing the nylon jackets.
2. The nylon jackets will abrade if the female housing is not checked for burs and if the occlusal entry is not given a slight bevel. Check insertion and removal path with an ESI metal male (part No. 802411)* before assembly of nylon jackets.
3. Retention reduction may be controlled by substituting the red and black nylon jackets.
4. Frequent dislodgement of the nylon jackets by the patient can be controlled by replacing the nylon jackets with the polycarbonate jackets, as discussed in procedure 27.

Lingual bracing and retentive arms

lingual retentive arms Lingual retentive arms are cast extensions of the partial denture framework that complete the lingual contour of the retainer fitting a milled vertical wall space that is parallel to the path of attachment insertion and has a gingival shoulder. The retentive component is a milled proximal half-cylinder groove parallel to the milled wall and path of insertion. It is both bracing and retentive (Fig. 13-46). Retentive arms are used with both retentive and nonretentive rigid attachment systems.

lingual bracing arms Lingual bracing arms are the same as lingual retentive arms minus the retentive component. These provide bracing only and are used where the attachment retention is fully controllable (Schatzmann and Bival attachments).

Attachments wear and most wear occurs over a period of time from insertion and removal or from functional flexion in the prosthesis. Any binding insertion or removal increases the wear factor. Lingual bracing and retentive arms help reduce this type of wear, assist the patient in finding the correct path of insertion, assist in removal, and reduce lateral surface wear of the attachments.

PROCEDURE

1. Prepare the diagnostic cast reduction to provide normal contour for the bracing arm. This will require axial reduction of the lingual component to a depth of 1.8 to 2 mm (Fig. 13-47) and the gingival margin to a shoulder preparation above the chamfer finish area.
2. The milling procedures are best done on a metal die; however, a stone die may be used by either waxing

*APM-Sterngold, Stamford, Conn.

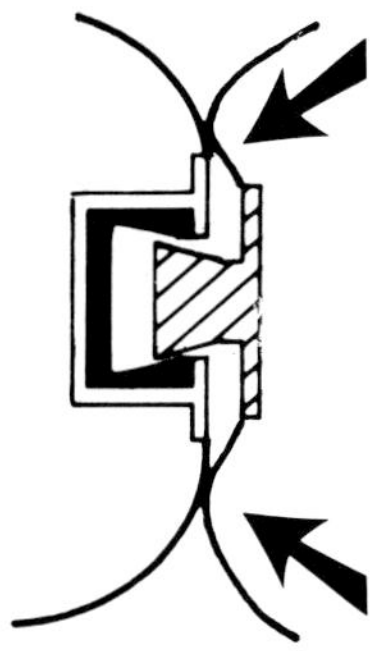

Fig 13-45. Interference *(arrows)* by overcontouring or overextension of resin base distorts nylon jacket and binds attachment.

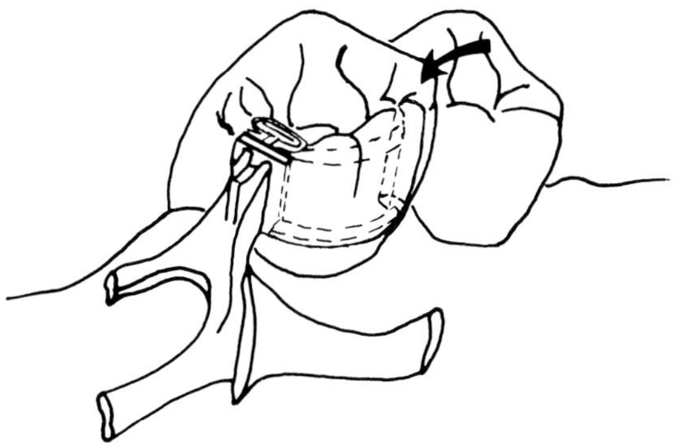

Fig. 13-46. Mill retentive section as half-cylinder groove for maximum retention. Place groove *(arrow)* to parallel and oppose attachment.

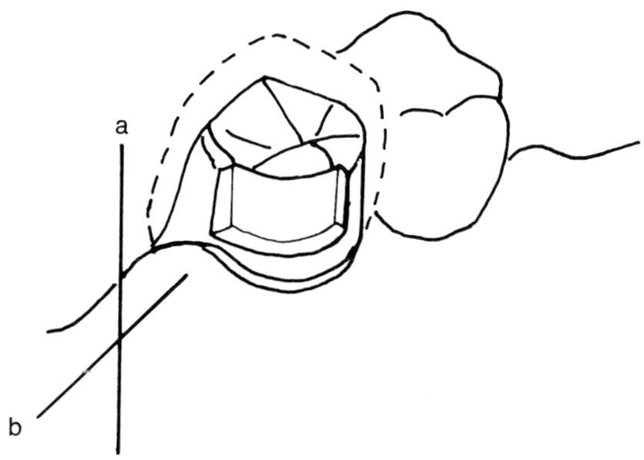

Fig. 13-47. Make diagnostic preparation for milled retainer to avoid overcontouring.

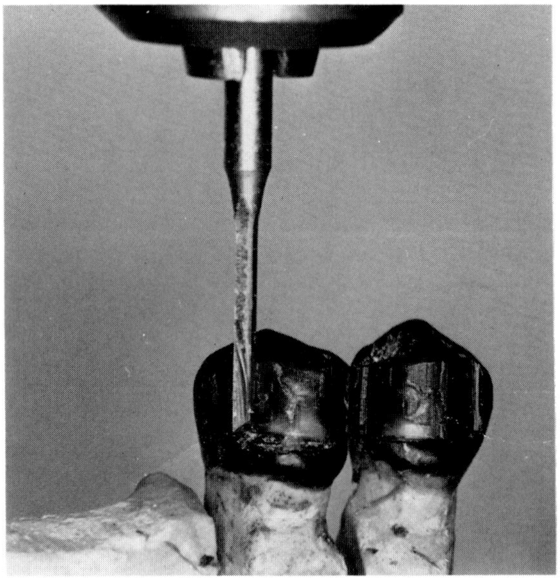

Fig. 13-48. Use end cutting and side cutting wax knife to contour wax-up. Stay at least 2 mm above gingival margin.

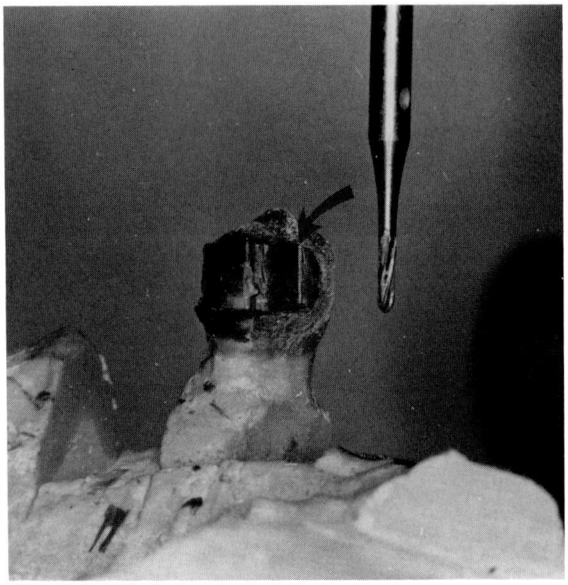

Fig. 13-49. As bracing arm, finish lingual extension as curved surface *(arrow)* with round-end cylinder bur.

against an Omnivac* coping (Fig. 13-48) or using two different color waxes. In the waxing technique, 22-gauge pink sheet casting wax† is adapted to the die, and the wax-up is completed with a contrasting wax such as Whip-Mix* regular blue or green inlay wax.

3. Use a parallel blade wax knife with a parallelometer, such as the Bachmann or similar instruments† (Steiger and Boitel, 1959).

4. Use the pantostat of the Bachmann to reduce the axial wall of the wax-up until the "pink" color just shows through the contrasting wax (cutting through the pink wax will damage the die and violate the seal of the crown).

5. Use the base of the wax knife to establish the gingival seat.

6. *As a bracing arm,* finish the end of the arm as a curved surface (Fig. 13-49).

7. *As a retentive arm,* develop the proximal groove as a half-cylinder depression by rotating a 0.7-mm wax knife in the proximal groove area (Fig. 13-50).

8. Invest the pattern and complete steps 6 to 9 as described for attachment castings in the McCollum procedure.

9. Transfer the individual abutment casting to milling model bases (Fig. 13-51), and mill with Gaerny‡ millers.

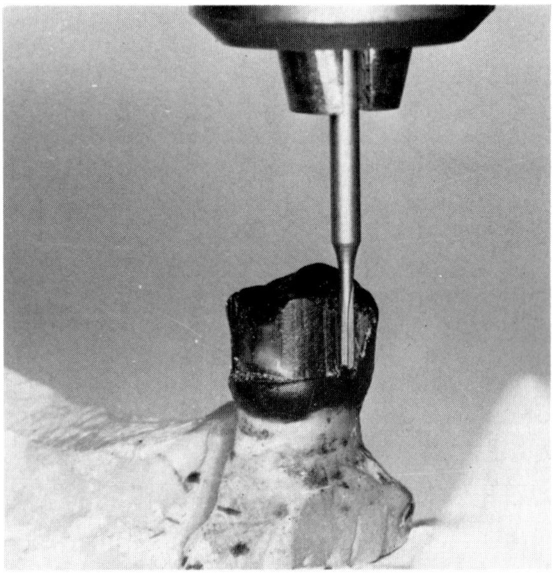

Fig. 13-50. As retentive arm, rotate 0.7-mm wax knife to develop half-cylinder profile.

10. Establish a slight rabbet bevel on the occlusal portion of the parallel wall to provide guidance and bulk (Fig. 13-52, *A*), and place a gingival bevel about the shoulder to provide closure finish of the retaining arm (Fig. 13-52, *B*).

11. Lubricate the milled casting with DuraLay lubricant, and make a customized DuraLay pattern to normal tooth contour about the milled area by the paint-on method (Steiger and Boitel, 1959). Allow the casting

---

*Whip-Mix Corp., Louisville, Ky., or equivalent.
†Kerr Manufacturing Co., Romulus, Mich., or equivalent.
†Parallel drilling and milling instruments, Cendres & Métaux, S.A., Biel, Switzerland; Métaux Précieux, S.A., Neuchâtel, Switzerland, Bell International, Inc., Burlingame, Calif., or equivalent.
‡Gaerny Millers, Brassler USA, Savannah, Ga.

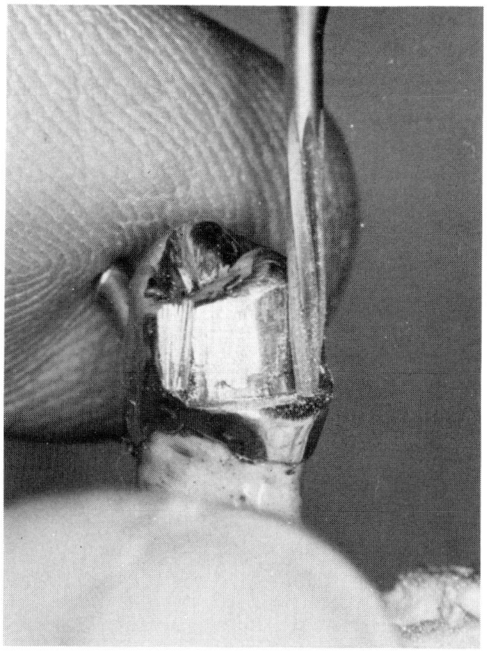

Fig. 13-51. Mill casting with Gaerny cylinder milling bur.

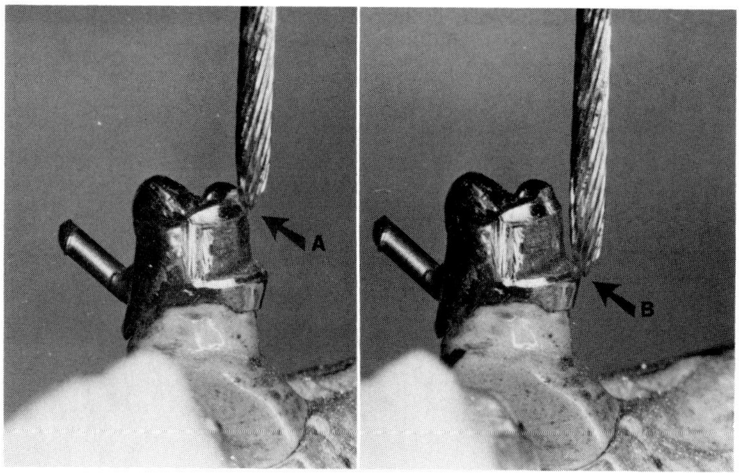

Fig. 13-52. Mill rabbet bevel occlusally *(A)* for occlusal bulk and seal. Mill gingival bevel *(B)* for gingival shoulder and seal.

to set for ½ hour. Then finish the pattern with sandpaper disks, and polish. Fit it to the crown, and remove any undercuts.

12. Either cast the patterns separately and solder them to the framework, or fit them to the duplicate investment cast and make them a part of the framework casting.

13. After casting, rough clean the framework with a shellblaster, and fit the bracing arms to the castings by using a Paasche Air Eraser* to dull the inner surface or Pascal Occlude† to locate the interference points.

*Paasche Air Eraser, Paasche Airbrush Co., Chicago, Ill.
†Occlude, Pascal Co., Inc., Seattle, Wash.

Intracoronal-extracoronal combined attachment (Schatzmann)

The Schatzmann* attachment (Fig. 13-53) is an example of a rigid combined intracoronal-extracoronal class I connector and is unique because of its spring-loaded pawl retention. It is used as a major connector for removable partial dentures, removable bridgework, and particularly distal extension partial dentures. The Schatzmann consists of a female boxing 4.7 mm in length, by 3 mm wide, by 1.6 mm in depth and has

*APM-Sterngold, Stamford, Conn.

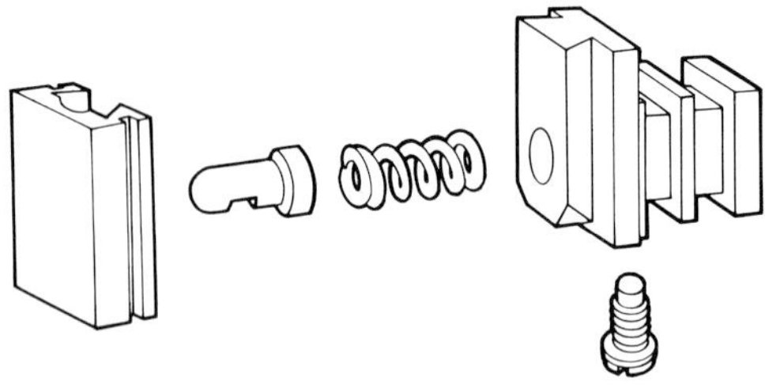

Fig. 13-53. Schatzmann attachments (4.5 mm) are used for maxillary partial dentures and may be used on mandibular partial dentures when opposing maxillay free-end partial dentures or complete maxillary dentures.

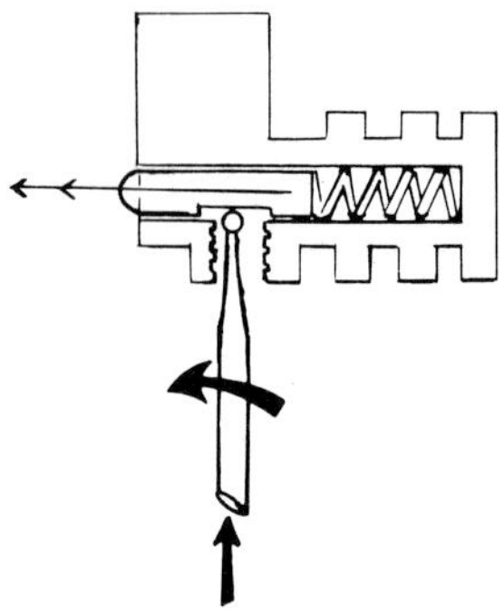

Fig. 13-54. Remove gingival retention screw. Insert No. ½ round bur to remove pawl plunger.

occlusal gingival retention grooves to provide mechanical, as well as metallurgical bonding. The internal design is open at the occlusal surface and face, with an engagement or detent groove at the occlusal surface for the pawl plunger. The internal area is an angular dovetail that forms a contact frictional retention flange with the male. The axial wall 2.5 mm from the base has a hemispheric depression to engage the pawl plunger.

The alloys available are Elitor for use with normal crown and bridge golds and Ceramicor for direct casting with phosphate type investments* for the precious ceramometal techniques.

The male has a corresponding dovetail to engage the female flange and is beveled at the gingival to allow ease of insertion. The axial face of the male has a round opening 2.5 mm from the base to receive the spring and pawl plunger, and the undersurface of the extension housing is threaded to receive the stainless steel locking screw for the plunger. This screw retains and limits the movement of the latter. The housing that is the extension of the male is multiflanged and not only holds the pawl plunger, but is also the connecting unit for the partial denture. Since the plunger and housing are the limiting units of the Schatzmann attachment, the male/female section may be reduced to as low as 3 mm occlusogingivally. All parts are interchangeable and replaceable, and the attachments are provided with a paralleling mandrel and a threaded reline post.

PROCEDURE

1. Fabricate the male of the Schatzmann attachment as described in steps 1 to 9 of the McCollum assembly.†

*Ceramigold Investment, Whip-Mix Corp., Louisville, Ky.

†It is important to keep any attachment at least 0.5 mm away from any area to be covered with porcelain to avoid porcelain stress or fracture.

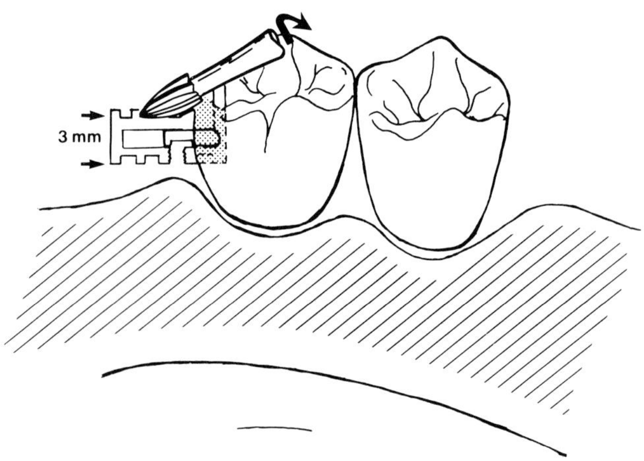

Fig. 13-55. Reduce retention flanges on male (3 mm maximum) to occlude when necessary.

2. Remove the contents of the male housing by first removing the stainless steel locking screw at the base of the housing and then inserting a No. ½ round bur into the hole to contact the plunger, pushing outward until it can be removed digitally or with a pair of cotton pliers. The spring can now be easily extracted (Fig. 13-54).

3. With the contents removed, assemble the male to the female using a few drops of a graphite lubricant, and reduce any excessive occlusal height, including the occlusal portion of the retentive flanges, to 3 mm if necessary to occlude the casts (Fig. 13-55).

4. If the reduction has been done in the previous step, then establish a new detent groove using a No. 7104 flame carbide bur,* and then polish the detent groove with a rubber point of the same dimension (Fig. 13-56).

*No. 7104 flame carbide bur, Brassler, U.S.A., Savannah, GA.

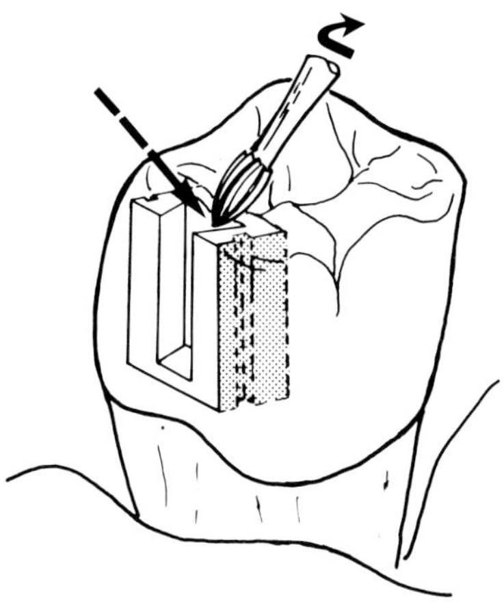

Fig. 13-56. Reestablish detent groove with No. 7104 flame bur after any reduction of attachment.

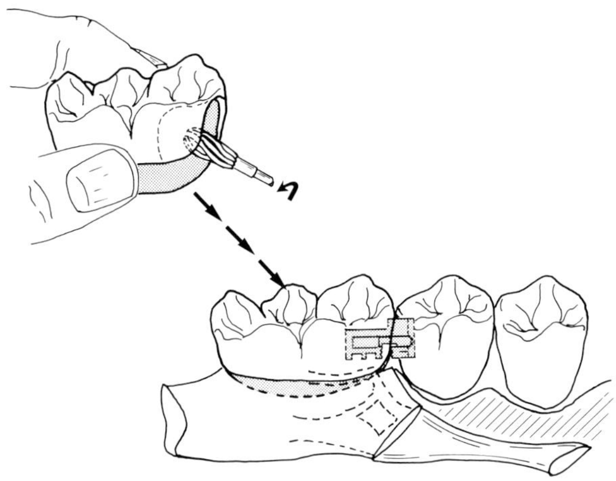

Fig. 13-57. Hollow grind resin tooth to fit about attachment.

5. Elevate the retainer crown on the die with plastic film.* Relate the male to the framework on the master or duplicate processing cast, and join it to the frame by either soldering with a .650 solder for precious metal frame or a .585 solder with a fluoride flux for austenitic metals or with self-curing resin.† (If soldering is done, the casting and attachment must be heat treated by placing them in an oven at 850° F [455° C] and dropping the temperature to 450° F [235° C] in ½ hour, followed by quenching in water.)

6. Fill the space temporarily in the housing with Rubber Sep‡ or Impregum§ and close the base hold with a reline post that is reduced to fit the ridge (this post provides an access hole on the finished prosthesis for placing the stainless steel retentive screw).

7. Hollow grind a resin tooth to fit over the male extension (Fig. 13-57), and seal the inside with a self-curing resin opaque of choice.

8. Complete the wax-up, invest, and complete the work as described in steps 3 to 7 of the McCollum procedure for removable partial dentures.

ALTERNATE PROCEDURE

Temporarily cement the crowns in the mouth, position the framework with the processed base using the indirect retainers or guides, and index the attachments to the frame with self-curing resin. An altered cast technique is used to relate the saddle areas to the retainers followed by steps 6 to 8.

*Refer to step 3 of the procedure for the McCollum attachment, removable partial dentures.

†Resin pickup is the preferred method, since there is no possible change to the metallurgy, and the attachment may be easily replaced or repositioned if needed.

‡APM-Sterngold, Stamford, Conn.

§Premier Dental Products Co., Philadelphia, Pa.

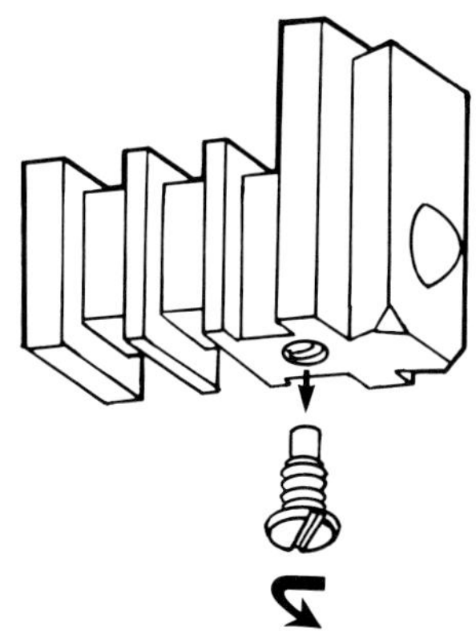

Fig. 13-58. Remove stainless steel retention screw.

DELIVERY OF THE SCHATZMANN APPLIANCE

The Schatzmann appliance is delivered without the retention plunger and spring, but with the stainless steel retention screw.

PROCEDURE FOR ACTIVATING THE ATTACHMENT

After a period of 2 to 12 months, the prosthesis is returned to the laboratory for placement of the pawl retention system.

1. Remove the stainless steel retention screw (Fig. 13-58).

2. Clean the housing and prosthesis in an ultrasonic cleaner, and flush the housing chamber with air and water.

3. Place the helical spring in the facial access hole on

Table 13-2. Intracoronal-extracoronal combined attachment (Schatzmann)

Problem	Probable cause	Solution
Female (Table 13-1)		
Male pawl retension blocks entry, will not depress	Detent removed on occlusal reduction of female	Reestablish detent with No. 7104 carbide bur
Pawl plunger will not hold	Spring is weak	Replace spring
	Pawl plunger is worn	Replace pawl plunger
Pawl plunger too tight	Spring too strong	Cut one turn of spring
Excessive wear of male	Alignment off	Use mandrel in surveyor to set attachments
	In case of soldering to framework, partial denture was not heat treated	Use resin pickup or heat treat if soldered, by placing in oven at 850° F (455° C) and cool to 450° F (235° C) in ½ hour, followed by quenching in water

the male, then place the plunger with the flat end entering first.

4. Place a No. ½ round bur through the base access to locate the recess of the plunger.

5. Place the stainless steel retention screw.

6. If the retention spring is too strong, reduce it by cutting the length of the spring by one turn. (Replace the spring retention on demand or on the average of 6 months to 1 year.)

PROCEDURE FOR REBASING THE SCHATZMANN PROSTHESIS

1. Remove the pawl retention screw.
2. Block the base access hole with impression wax.
3. Correct the denture base with a "wash" impression using the impression material of choice.*
4. Return the "washed" base to the laboratory where the wax plug is removed and the space replaced by the reline screw, which extends beyond the surface of the impression material. Seal the proximal housing with Rubber Sep or silicone.†
5. Pour the cast in the usual manner.
6. Reline the denture base with the material of choice, and reassemble it according to the procedures for activation.

PROBLEM AREAS

The problem areas for the intracoronal-extracoronal combined attachments, such as the Schatzmann, are the same as for the female components (Table 13-1). Additional points are presented in Table 13-2.

1. The male pawl retention will sometimes block the entry into the female. This is usually the result of occlusal reduction of the female and requires reestablishment of the detent using a No. 7104 carbide bur.

2. The pawl plunger will not hold for two reasons. Either it is worn and requires replacement, or the spring is weak and requires replacement.

3. If the retention is too tight, the spring may be reduced in length by one turn.

4. Excessive wear of the male can be the result of improper alignment. A surveyor-mounted mandrel is essential for most attachment procedures. The wear could also be the result of not heat treating the attachment, following soldering to the framework. Most of these attachments are designed to be resin processed in the partial denture, however, if they are soldered, heat treatment will restore 90% of the metallurgical structure to the attachment.

Extracoronal combined attachments

Bival attachment

The Bival* attachment (Fig. 13-59) is an example of a posterior combined rigid-resilient extracoronal class II connector and is a hybrid of the ASC-52.† It is unique because of its adjustable spring-loaded ball-dowel connector and the secondary pivot-retention ball dowel. The Bival consists of a platinum-iridium alloy female housing open at the top and back with matched parallel extensions that embrace the corresponding machined surface of the male. It is 4.5 mm occlusogingivally, by 4.6 mm long, by 4.1 mm wide and has a groove retention flange to facilitate waxing. A special screw mandrel

*Surgident Multiform Impression Paste, Lactona Products Division, Morris Plains, N.J.

†Dow Corning No. 7 Compound, Dow Corning Corp., Midland, Mich.

*Bival, Bell International Inc., Burlingame, Calif.

†Bival, ASC-52, Bell International, Inc., Burlingame, Calif.

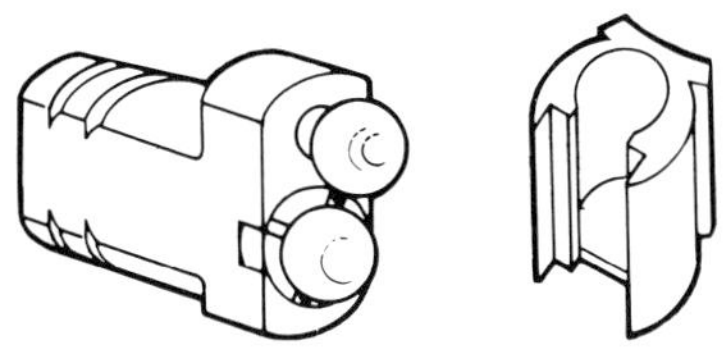

Fig. 13-59. Bival dual-function rigid or resilient attachments (4.5 mm) may be used for maxillary or mandibular partial dentures.

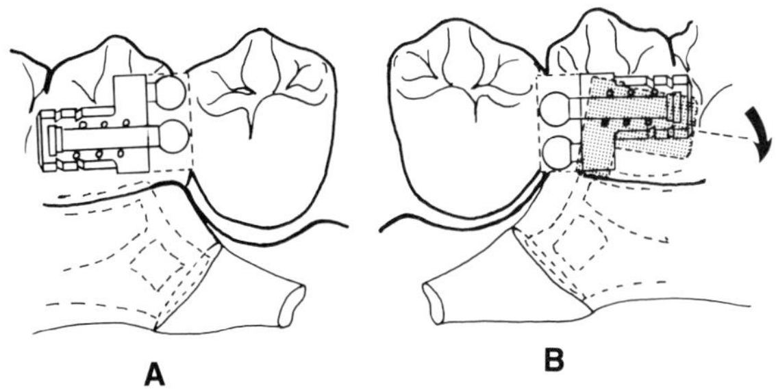

Fig. 13-60. Bival rigid mode **(A)** may be converted to hinge resilience mode **(B)** by rotating male of attachment 180 degrees.

allows easy placement of the female part of the attachment.

The male Bival consists of stainless steel housing with retention grooves and an outside diameter of 3.5 mm; the front 3 mm is machined to engage the female and has a vertical extension of 1 mm that carries a rigid ball dowel, which engages the female sleeve. The main ball dowel is an extension of the housing and is locked in with a female and carries an internal stainless steel helical coil spring that is fixed to the ball dowel by the small collar.

The Bival is a dual function attachment; in the resilient mode (Fig. 13-60, *B*) it pivots as a hinge off the solid ball; in the fixed mode (Fig. 13-60, *A*) it is held rigid by the solid ball and braced laterally by the machined female extensions. It may be used like the Schatzmann attachment in both bounded and free-end saddle partial dentures with any full coverage retainer design and usually double abutment fixation. It should have some form of cross arch stabilization.

PROCEDURE

1. Pour the master cast from the impression, trim and seal the dies, and begin the wax-up of the crowns.
2. As a rigid unit, the attachments may be parallel to each other or divergent if more than one is used. Either way they should lie over the crest of the alveolar ridge.
3. As a resilient attachment, the Bival must be parallel to its like member if the design is a bilateral free-end application, because the Bival is a unidirectional hinge.
4. Determine the path of insertion (Fig. 13-61), and hold the female in position with the mandrel until it is waxed into place.
5. Close the mandrel by turning the screw (Fig. 13-62) and release it from the attachment.
6. Invest the attachment retainers in a phosphate bonded investment, and cast as described for the McCollum attachment, steps 5 to 9.
7. Fit the male to the female, and then relate them to the framework as for the Schatzmann assembly, steps 5 to 8. (Fill the resilient housing with silicone grease* to keep any resin from entering the housing during processing.)
8. The gingival contact of the female housing with the crown should have a V-shaped opening to provide an embrasure for protection of the gingival cuff about the tooth.

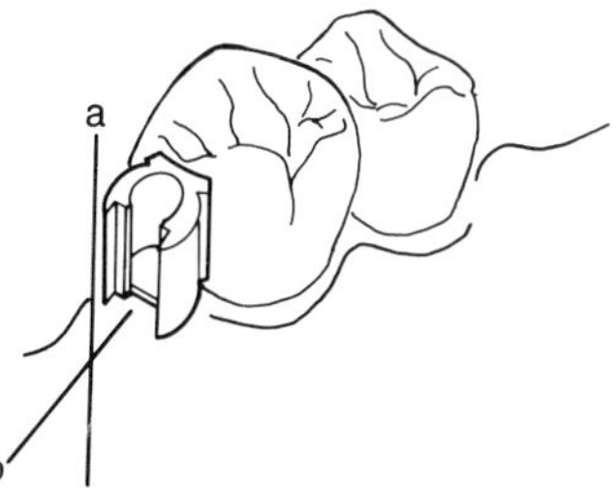

Fig. 13-61. Determine attachment position parallel to partial denture path of insertion and crest of ridge. If hinge action mode is used, make attachments parallel to each other.

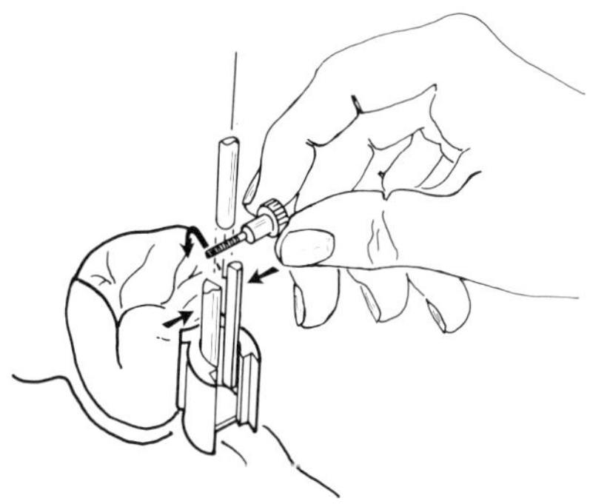

Fig. 13-62. Lute Bival attachment to wax-up, and release mandrel by turning screw.

DELIVERY AND SERVICE

The Bival attachment is delivered with the retention removed until the patient learns the path of insertion

*Dow Corning No. 7, Dow Corning Corp., Midland, Mich.

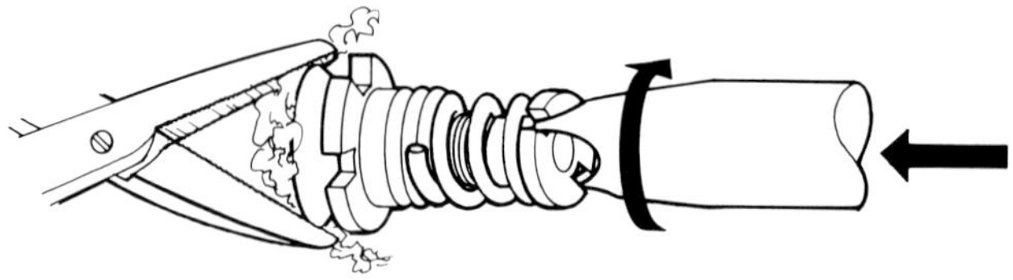

Fig. 13-63. Adjust spring retention by holding ball dowel and turning small collar.

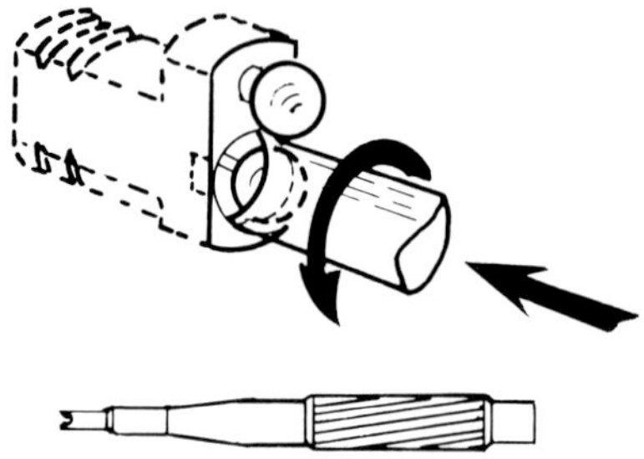

Fig. 13-64. Open male with screwdriver, and remove contents.

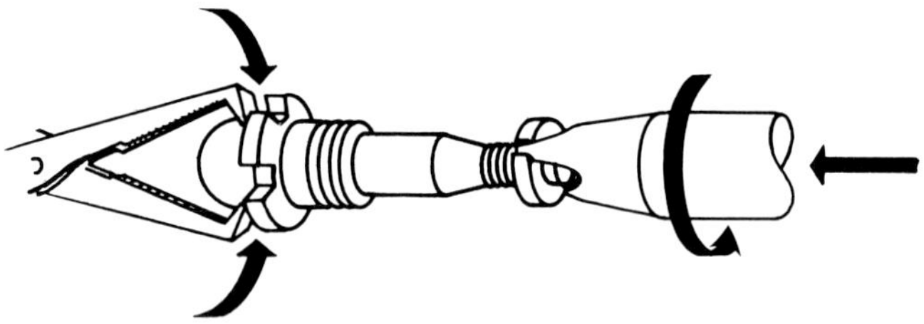

Fig. 13-65. Hold ball dowel with rat tooth pliers, and unscrew small collar.

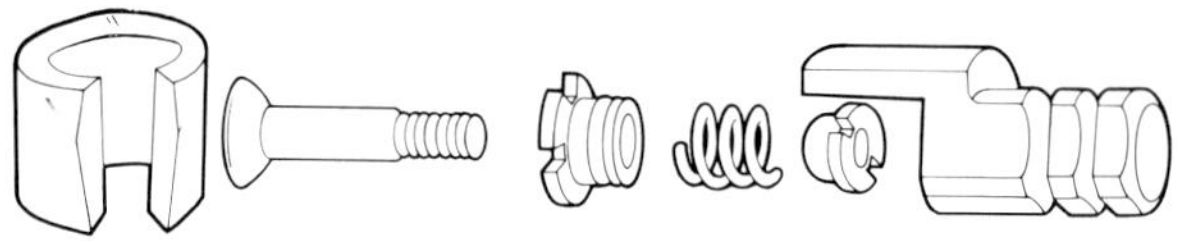

Fig. 13-66. ASC-52 attachments (2.8 to 3.5 mm) are universal joint units that may be used for all resilient free-end partial dentures, but not opposing each other. From left to right, platinum iridium female, ball dowel, ferrule, spring, small collar, protect housing.

and removal. The retention spring may be increased or decreased by adjusting the small collar (Fig. 13-63). The retention spring should be replaced on demand or every 6 to 12 months.

PROCEDURE FOR REPLACING THE SPRING

1. Open the male attachment with a screwdriver (Fig. 13-64).
2. Hold the ball with a special pliers, and unscrew the small collar (Fig 13-65).
3. Remove and replace the spring.
4. Reassemble in reverse order.

ASC-52 attachment

The ASC-52* (Fig. 13-66) is a group II universal joint resilient extracoronal attachment. It consists of a female housing that is open at the top and bottom as well as the face. The face has a dual bevel that assists in the retention with the spring-loaded ball inside and the ferrule outside. There are two types of females for both the spherical and hemispherical configurations. One is flat occlusally and has stops to limit the ball dowel travel gingivally, and the other is curved occlusally with no stops and depends on the protect flange for an occlusal stop. This description applies to the platinum-iridium, gold and stainless steel models. The plastic pattern configurations for nonprecious alloys are all curved with vertical travel stops.

The female housings range from 3.5 mm high, by 4 mm wide, by 3 mm long and may be reduced to match the housing height on the nonprotective configurations.

The standard male attachment ASC-52 consists of a stainless steel housing with a ball or hemispherical dowel, a ferrule, a helical coil spring, and a small collar with a housing diameter of 2.8 to 3.5 mm. The spring action of the dowel provides a "disk brake" retention to the female portion and a universal joint action to the male segment.

The protect male segment ASC-52 is the same as the standard with the addition of the protect flange, which engages the occlusal surface of the female attachment and rotates about it. The protect is the most popular configuration of this system and also provides an occlusal stop for the opposing stamp cusp. The attachments are provided with processing/reline/heating plugs, special screwdrivers, and adjustable screw parallelometer mandrels all in a special laboratory assembly kit.

This attachment system is unique because as a universal joint it does not require parallelism, it does not torque the abutment teeth, and it can be used with a

*ASC-52, Bell International, Inc., Burlingame, Calif.

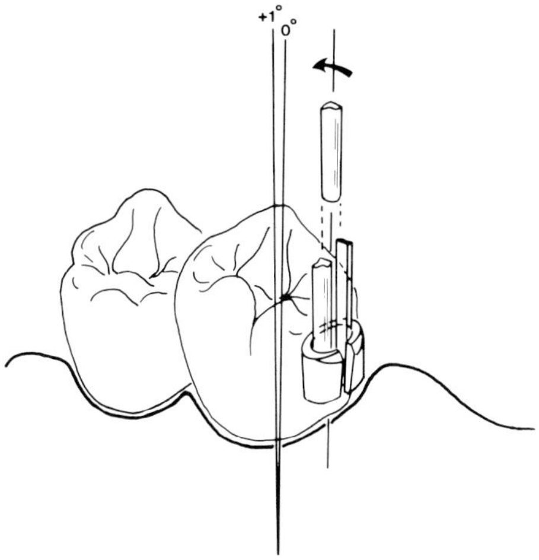

Fig. 13-67. Align attachment in harmony with partial denture path of insertion 0 degrees, and tilt +1 degree for tracking effect *(arrow)*. Ridge orientation all cases attachment over crest of ridge opposing opposite stamp cusp.

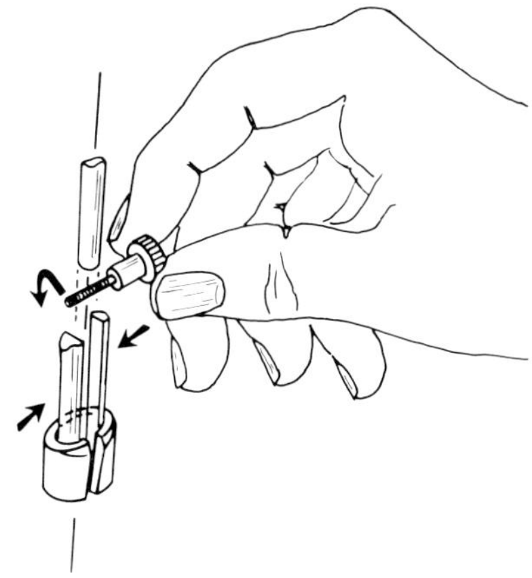

Fig. 13-68. Release mandrel by closing mandrel jaws.

single abutment support when it has a cross arch stabilizer.

PROCEDURE

1. Pour the master cast from the impression, trim and seal the dies, and fabricate the wax patterns of the crowns.
2. Mark the crest of the ridge,* and mark the opposing stamp cusp position (setting the attachment opposite the opposing stamp cusp will give the attachment the maximum functional potential available, and the path of closure of the jaw and insertion path of the partial denture is established) (Fig. 13-67).
3. Wax the platinum-irridium attachments to the crown, at least 1 mm above the gingival margin, using the special mandrel with controllable jaws that are adjusted to fit the female housing. Turn the screw clockwise to close, and counterclockwise to open.
4. Release the mandrel from the attachment by turning the screw clockwise (Fig. 13-68).

Invest the attachments and retainer in a phosphate bonded investment and cast as for the McCollum attachment, steps 5 to 9.

ALTERNATE PROCEDURE USING GOLD

1. Wax the gold-platinum alloy attachments as for steps 1 and 2 above and then separate them from the wax-up.

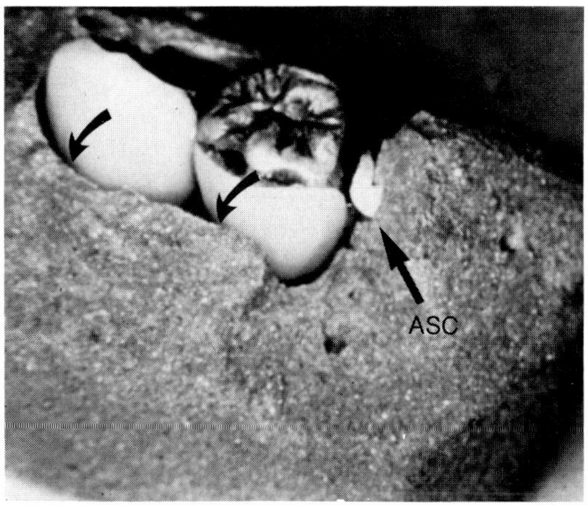

Fig. 13-69. Postsoldering of attachment. Wax out ceramic area *(curved arrows)* before placement in soldering investment. Note investment cleared about ASC-52 female *(straight arrow)*.

2. Invest the casting, cast and finish it, and then sticky wax the attachment to the casting.
3. Invest the casting with the attachment, and oven solder with a .650 solder (Fig. 13-69).
4. Clean the casting, and heat treat by placing it in an oven at 850° F (455° C) and lowering the temperature to 450° F (235° C) ½ hour before quenching in water.
5. The attachment is now readied to receive the male counterpart.

*Universal joint attachments do not have to be parallel when used in bilateral free-end partial denture constructions.

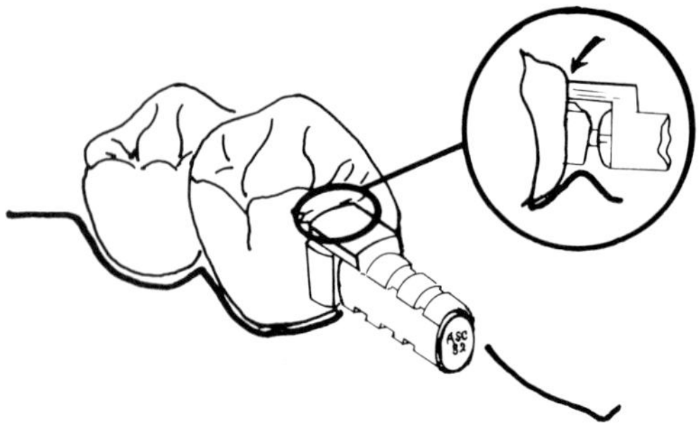

Fig. 13-70. Overwax axial wall between marginal ridge and attachment female *(inset)* to ensure positive contact of protect flange *(circle).*

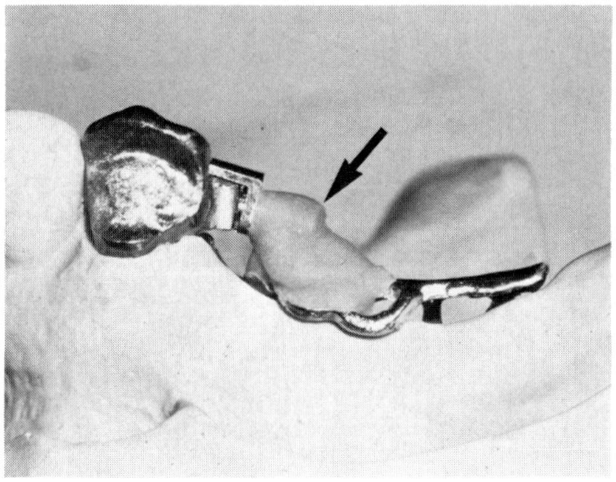

Fig. 13-71. Relate attachment to framework with Getz Minit-Weld *(arrow).*

ALTERNATE PROCEDURE USING STAINLESS STEEL

This method* is used with nonprecious metals.

1. Repeat steps 1 to 3 for gold except that the stainless steel is oven soldered with a .585 solder and a fluoride flux.
2. Spot weld the attachment to the crown and solder it.
3. The attachment may be laser welded.

ALTERNATE PROCEDURE USING A RESIN PATTERN

Resin is used for nonprecious metal alloys only.

1. Repeat steps 1 to 3 of the standard procedure except that the resin pattern is waxed up to the retainer, invested, and cast in the nonprecious alloy of choice.

PROTECT CONFIGURATIONS. Attachments of the protect configuration require overwaxing the area between the marginal ridge and the occlusal surface of the attachment to provide a positive contact of the protect blade (Fig. 13-70). The positive contact prevents a lifting or dropping of the partial denture. The area is overwaxed and cast. The male attachment is fitted to the female housing, and the overcontoured area is reduced until positive orientation is obtained.

PROCEDURE FOR MALE AND FRAMEWORK ASSEMBLY

1. Fit the male segment to the female counterpart, and relate the entire unit to the framework as for the Schatzmann assembly, steps 5 to 8 (Fig. 13-71).
2. Use the master cast or duplicate processing cast, and replace the abutment retainers with the female attachments, as well as the contents of the male housing, with a processing plug (Fig. 13-72).

*Too high a heat will destroy the stainless steel properties and cause corrosion in the mouth.

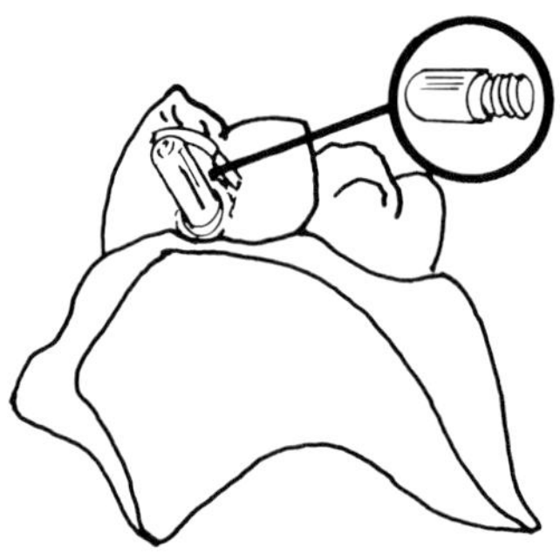

Fig. 13-72. Remove contents of male and replace with processing plug.

3. After processing return the assembled male retention to the housing, and fit the prosthesis to the retainer casting.
4. The spring retention, control, and replacement are the same as for the Bival delivery, servicing, and replacement.

An alternate procedure is to orient the attachment in the mouth using autopolymerizing acrylic resin for attachment directly to a temporary indirect retainer and processed resin base. An altered cast technique is used to relate the castings to the partial denture.

PROCEDURE FOR REPOSITIONING THE MALE

1. Remove the contents of the male housing.
2. Place the processing/heating rod in the housing.
3. Use an electric soldering iron to transfer heat to the attachment (Fig. 13-73).
4. When the resin is softened, remove the attachment (Fig. 13-74).
5. Open the area lingual to the attachment, and enlarge the housing space.
6. Assemble and test the prosthesis for clearance.

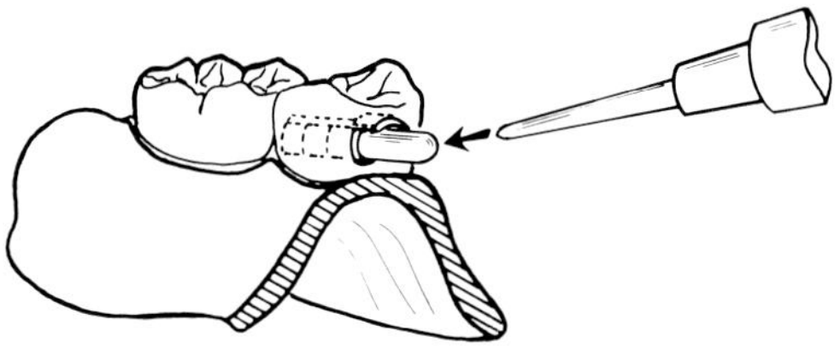

Fig. 13-73. Transfer heat to attachment *(arrow)* with soldering iron until attachment moves.

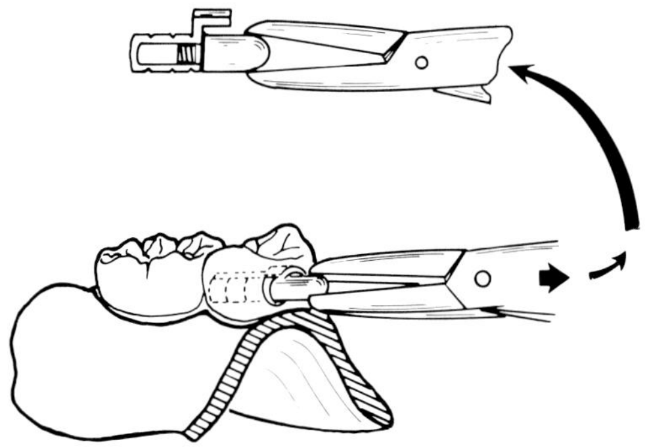

Fig. 13-74. Use pliers to remove attachment from base.

7. Flow self-curing resin about the attachment (this is done either at the bench or in the mouth) (Fig. 13-75).

8. Add more resin according to standard procedures for denture repair, and reassemble the male portion.

Dalbo attachment

The Dalbo* (Fig. 13-76) is the best known extracoronal vertically resilient hinge attachment of group II. It consists of a T-shaped male beam with a ball-shaped appendix based on Roach's design of a channel conjuctor (Nally, 1961). The female portion consists of a housing closed at one end, open at the other, and the face with two retentive spring lamellae and two extensions to engage the T beam. It contains a helical coil spring that functions over the ball extension of the T beam. The regular series has pin retention for processing† only in the U.S. market, whereas the Mini has no spring or processing pin.

The manufacturer‡ of the Dalbo attachment has recently introduced the Sholder-Dalbo or Dalbo-S, which has a step on the T shaped beam designed to block any vertical travel of the female housing in vertical translation exceeding 0.4 mm. The concept is primarily mechanical as an attempt to reduce failure of the resilient spring. Application and laboratory assembly procedures are exactly the same for all Dalbo attachments. The step design is poor and must be slightly rounded to achieve a pure hinge movement in maximum translation.

The alloys available are Ceramicor and Ellitor for the male and Ellitor only for the female. There is a special

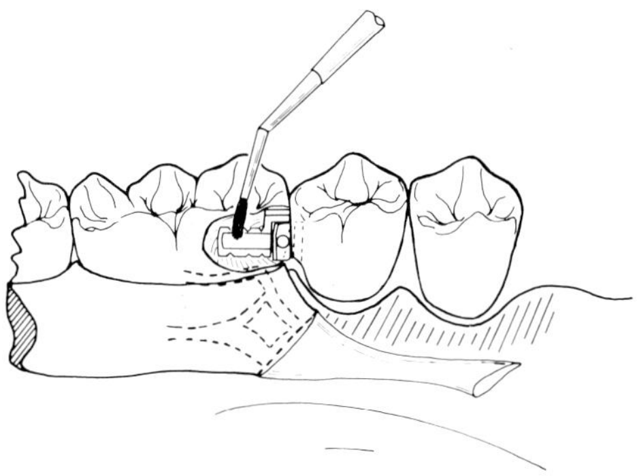

Fig. 13-75. Reposition framework. Hollow out attachment area providing lingual window. Paint in self-curing resin to set. Remove and finish.

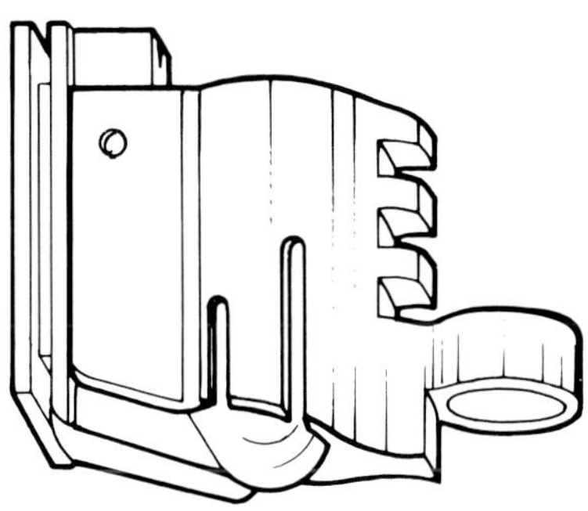

Fig. 13-76. Dalbo resilient joints (4.5 and 5.5 mm) consist of T-shaped beam with ball appendix and spring-loaded frictional retained housing. Dalbo joints are used for maxillary and mandibular partial dentures.

*APM-Sterngold, Stamford, Conn.

†P.G. Larson, President, APM-Sterngold, Burlingame, Calif., personal communication, Mensor Design, 1965.

‡Cendres & Metaux SA, Biel-Bienne, Switzerland.

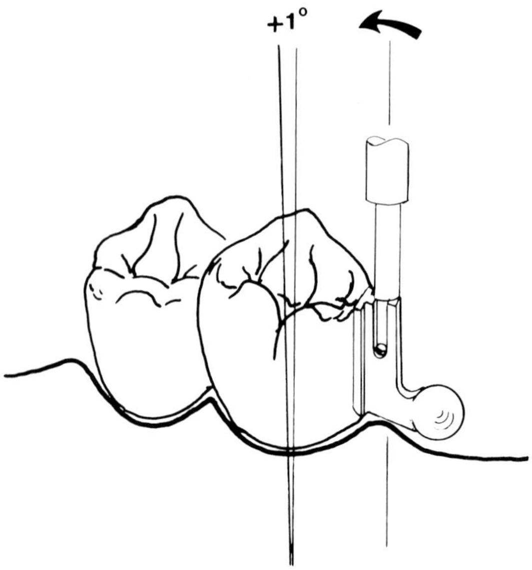

Fig. 13-77. Align male Dalbo +1 degree to path of insertion for tracking *(arrow)*. On bilateral application make both attachments parallel to each other.

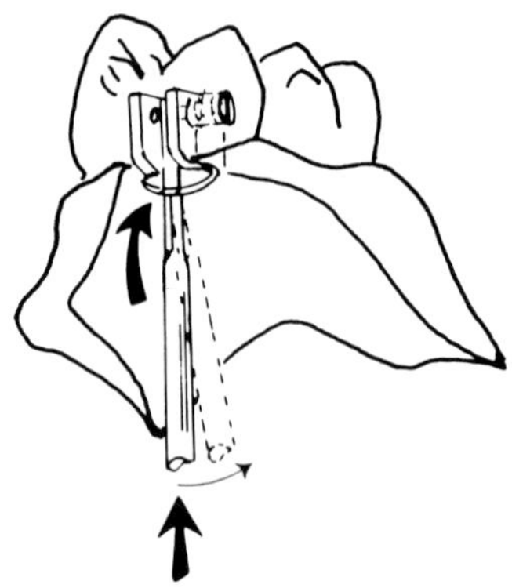

Fig. 13-78. Place hot spatula between lamellae and resin. Activate as shown by arrows.

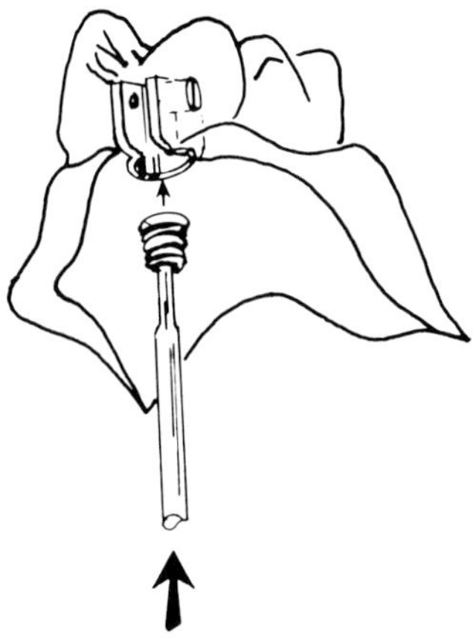

Fig. 13-79. Insert spring with large end first *(small arrow)*.

mandrel for the Dalbo series, which is available as a unilateral and bilateral attachment in large, small, and miniature configurations.

The Dalbo attachment has been used as a connector for both free-end and bounded partial dentures and can have its vertical resilience eliminated by substituting resin for the spring.

PROCEDURE

The attachment orientation follows exactly the procedure of the Bival attachment, steps 1 to 6, and the McCollum attachment, steps 5 to 9, with the following exceptions:

1. Orient the male segment to have a slight plus inclination (Fig. 13-77) occlusogingivally to allow the female portion to track the male and positive seat in function. (A negative orientation would tend to unseat the attachment.)
2. Use the pin for the assembly through the entire processing phase.
3. Use double abutment fixation because the functional attachment will torque the abutments with any load outside the area of function of the attachment.
4. Block out the area between the attachment and the ridge before processing with Rubber Sep or dental stone to provide space for insertion and removal of the prosthesis.
5. After processing, remove the pin, and clear the attachment female of investment. Clear the spring lamellae to function by placing a hot spatula between the outside of the lamellae and the resin of the saddle (Fig. 13-78).
6. Insert the helical coil spring with the large end seating (Fig. 13-79) and further seat it by compression with a laboratory male.
7. If the spring is to be replaced by resin, remove it, and place self-curing resin in the housing with a laboratory male "pinned" in the female to establish the resin limits.
8. Clear the occlusal surface about the T beam to allow for the vertical movement of the prosthesis, and cut an embrasure V at the gingival contact of the male to the retainer to protect the gingival tissue cuff.

PROCEDURE FOR REPLACEMENT OF FEMALE HOUSING

1. Remove the old attachment using a heated ball burnisher that fits inside the housing.
2. Open the attachment area from the lingual side, and clear it for a new female attachment.
3. Assemble the new female segment with the pin,

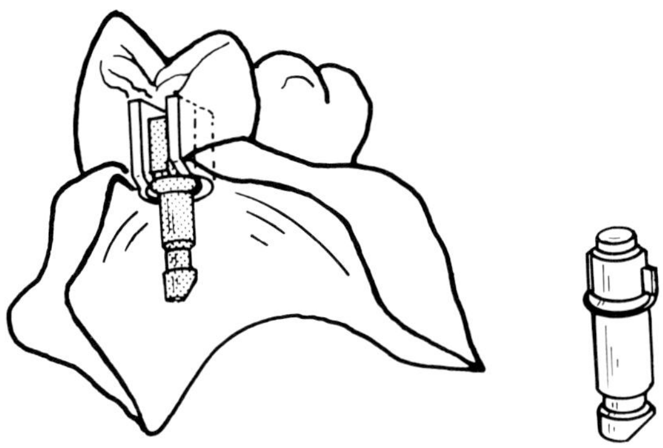

Fig. 13-80. Remove spring and insert reline plug for rebasing.

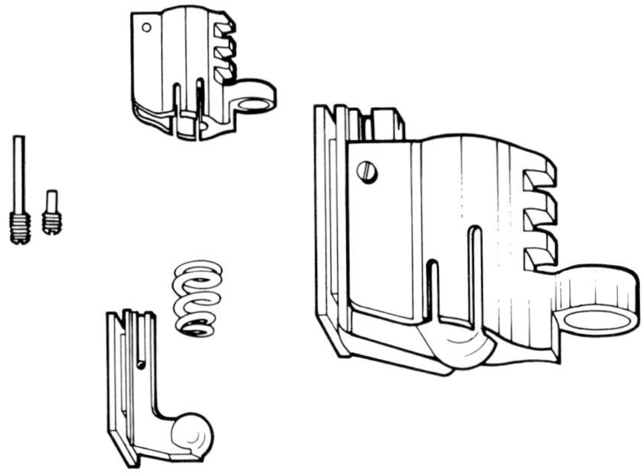

Fig. 13-81. Dalbo-M configuration uses unilateral male. Addition of screw and groove converts Dalbo joint into trifunctional attachment. Screw in female is coincident with base of male groove at rest.

and join the prosthesis to the attachment with resin. Complete the process at the bench following normal repair procedures. (It is important to advise the dentist to block out the space between the male attachment and tissue with an elastomeric impression material during this phase to avoid locking the prosthesis in the mouth.)

PROCEDURE FOR REBASING

1. Remove the spring, and replace it with a metal reline plug (Fig. 13-80).
2. "Wash" the base with the material of choice, and return it to the laboratory.
3. Replace the reline plug with the processing plug and process as for normal rebasing.
4. Replace the spring and clear the spring lamellae according to step 5 for assembly. NOTE: Mini-Dalbos require bending in of extension flanges to ensure proper relationship of male to female for resin pickup of the attachment in the mouth as well as standard laboratory procedures.

MODIFICATIONS OF THE DALBO SYSTEM

A screw and groove configuration of both the male and female components has produced a new trifunctional attachment known as the Dalbo-M attachment* (Fig. 13-81), which has been described thoroughly by Kornfeld (1974).

The basic description is the same as the Dalbo except that the male has a bilateral channel open at the top with a hole at the base of the channel halfway down the T beam. The channel engages a small screw whose diameter is coincident with the channel width. A longer second screw with a longer threaded head locks the attachment together for processing and establishes the thread in the denture base for the functional smaller screw. The attachment has three functions, one with a locked mode and two in the release mode.

In the *locked mode* the screw engages the channel and provides a rigid system like the Schatzmann. It also provides a positive reline position to the opposing occlusion, a fixed platform for functionally generated path procedures and a fixed unit for gnathologic procedures and equilibration. In the *release mode* the attachment can have a combined vertical resilient function, or it can be a hinge only if the spring is replaced by resin.

Outside the United States the Dalbo-M is available in precious metal as unilateral, standard, and miniature attachments.* An M configuration is available in the United States as both a standard unilateral and miniature unilateral attachment for the nonprecious market† in the form of a channeled resin pattern for casting the male and as a special elastic 18-8 stainless steel alloy for the female. The sides of the T beam have been further modified to have retention notches to facilitate wax-up and the male pattern has an extension dowel, which is a built-in parallelometer mandrel (Fig. 13-82).

PROCEDURE

The procedure is the same as for the Dalbo and the Bival attachments, with the exception that after the attachment pattern is placed, the mandrel is removed by passing a hot spatula through the middle of the thin section. A carbon rod obturator is placed in the screw hole, and an extra burnout time of 1 hour is required to ensure complete elimination of the wax and plastic.

---

*Mensor, M.C.: U.S. Patent No. 3,448,521, 1965, San Mateo, Calif.

*Dalbo-M, No. 63.05.2/63.05.5, Cendres & Métaux, S.A., Biel, Switzerland.

†Ultra-M, Ultratek Attachments and Technology, Inc., Concord, Calif.

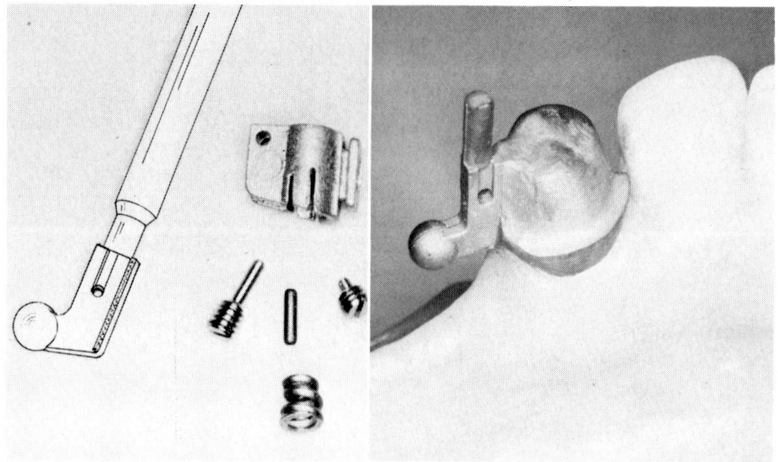

Fig. 13-82. A, Ultra-M is for nonprecious metal only. Male is resin pattern form. **B,** Typical casting in nonprecious alloy.

After casting, the excess of the mandrel is removed to occlusion.

Caution: Under no circumstances should the patterns be used to cast precious metal male attachments, because the resultant casting will not be precise and will have excess wear and possible porosity. Under no circumstances use the nonprecious metal female with the precious metal male attachment. They will retrofit, but they will cause excessive wear of the male and failure of retention.

The nonprecious metal female housing is materially matched to the cast nonprecious metal male. A precious metal female will wear if used with a nonprecious metal male because of the filelike action of the nonprecious metal to the precious metal. Highly finishing the male will eliminate the precision fit, and oxidation during porcelain firing will again produce the file effect wear potential for a precious metal female.

PROBLEM AREAS

The problem areas for the extracoronal combined attachments such as the Bival, ASC-52, and Dalbo are the same as problem areas given in Table 13-1 for metallurgy, wear, discoloration, fracture, porosity, and melt. Additional problems, their probable causes, and solutions are presented in Table 13-3.

1. Stainless steel failure with nonprecious metals occurs as an incomplete bond because of oxide formation. The surfaces should be clean, and using a high-frequency casting machine with an argon gas atmosphere will reduce this problem.

2. Stainless steel corrosion will occur in the mouth if too high a heat is used, since the stainless steel properties will be destroyed. The problem may be solved by spot welding and post soldering with a .585 solder and fluoride flux (a nonpetroleum jelly base).

3. Resin patterns can produce an oversize casting of the investment if casting techniques are not followed precisely for the alloy used, including proper venting and spruing to eliminate porosity.

4. The ball retention of the Bival or ASC-52 will not enter the female if the occlusal surface of the female has been reduced, and the bevel has been removed. The solution is simply the matter of rebeveling the female (Fig. 13-83).

5. The hemisphere of the ASC-52 will enter the female only if the occlusal surface was flared. Reducing the spring tension will increase the movement and will also allow entry of the attachment.

6. If the ASC-52 or Bival attachment is too loose, either the spring is broken or fatigued. The problem is solved by tightening the spring or replacing it.

7. If the ASC-52 prosthesis drops or lifts, the space between the marginal ridge and the attachment was not overwaxed to engage the protect flange (Fig. 13-84). The problem is in assembly, but can be corrected by a resin extension to contact the adjacent prosthesis tooth or contact with a cast metal occlusal.

8. The Dalbo female will show excessive wear if it is retrofitted to a nonprecious metal cast male because of the file effect of the unfinished metal due to the oxides from a porcelain application. If the cast male is highly polished it will not have the precision fit that the machined units exhibit. The solution is to use only nonprecious metal females with nonprecious metal males.

9. The Dalbo attachment has many negative factors in retention. If the ball shows wear and the retention is loose, tighten the spring lamellae. If the balls are flat

Table 13-3. Extracoronal combined attachments (Bival, ASC-52, Dalbo)

Problem	Probable cause	Solution
See application section, Table 13-1; same as female for attachment wear, discoloration, fracture porosity, metallurgical bond, and melting		
Stainless steel failure to join nonprecious metal crown	Oxide surface	Clean surface; use flux and high-frequency casting with argon gas
Stainless steel corrosion	Too high heat destroys stainless properties	Use .585 solder with fluoride flux; spot weld and post solder as above
Resin pattern female and crown oversized (nonprecious metal)	Too much expansion	Check investment and casting technique
Resin pattern female oversized (nonprecious metal)	See above	See above
Porosity in casting and resin pattern attachment (nonprecious metal)	Contamination of metal	Use only new alloy
	Improper spruing and venting	Sprue as recommended by manufacturer
Ball retention will not enter female (ASC-52, Bival)	Nonprotect occlusal surface has been reduced and bevel removed	Rebevel nonprotect spherical female
Hemisphere will not enter female (ASC-52)	Occlusal of female was flared	Do not flare female; spring tension may be reduced to allow entry; refer to assembly instruction
Attachment is too loose (ASC-52, Bival)	Spring is broken or fatigued	Tighten spring or replace spring
Prosthesis lifts or drops in protect configuration (ASC-52)	Crown was not overcontoured to engage protect flange	Assembly technique must be followed exactly: extend resin tooth to contact distal side of abutment or cast metal occlusal to do same
Excessive wear of female (Dalbo)	Precious metal used with nonprecious metal male "file" effect*	Never use precious with nonprecious metals; replace with nonprecious metals
Retention inadequate (Dalbo)	Ball wearing	Tighten spring lamellae
Ball worn flat on side (Dalbo)	Metallurgical problem	Replace attachment
Ball flat or grooved on top hinge limited (Dalbo)	Spring cutting into ball	Smooth off and replace with resin; see instructions
Angular side movement (Dalbo)	Housing extension spreading because of misalignment and jaw flexion	Align resilient Dalbo attachments parallel to each other; bend lamellae extensions inward
Abutment tooth loose (Dalbo, Bival)	Attachments torque single abutments in function	Use double abutment fixation or universal type (ASC-52); use cross arch stabilization
Prosthesis in infraocclusion (Dalbo)	Spring is broken or missing, ridge has resorbed	Replace spring, reset occlusion, and rebase; replace spring with resin
Prosthesis infraocclusion (Dalbo reline)	Overdisplacement from hinge opening	Use Dalbo-M attachment in locked mode; repeat procedure, guiding patient into terminal hinge closure (dentist procedure)

*Dalla Bona, H.: Personal communication, 1965.

on the sides with no retention, it is a metallurgical problem and the attachment must be replaced. If the ball is grooved and flattened, the top of the spring is cutting into the ball, reducing the hinge action with infraocclusion. Replace the spring with resin. (See assembly procedures.)

10. The Dalbo attachment has excessive angular side movement due to a spreading of the housing extensions. This is the result of nonparallel alignment and jaw flexion. Bend the extension inward as a temporary procedure.

11. The abutment teeth are sometimes loose with the Dalbo and Bival attachments, particularly on the mandibular application. These attachments can torque single abutments in function and require either double abutment fixation with some form of cross arch stabili-

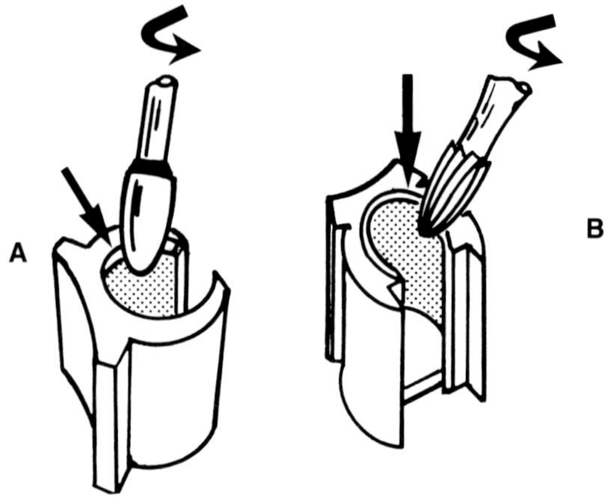

Fig. 13-83. A, Bevel ASC-52 *(straight arrows)* spherical female. **B,** Bevel Bival female.

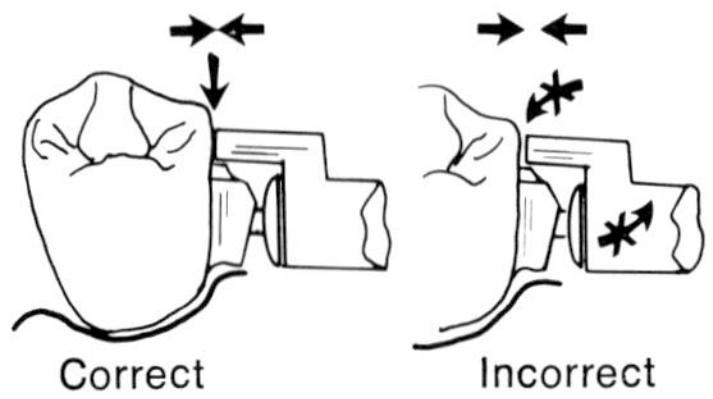

Fig. 13-84. Always overcontour retainer to have correct contact of flange.

zation or replacement of the unit with a universal joint attachment (ASC-52).

12. The Dalbo prosthesis can be in infraocclusion if the spring is broken or missing and will accelerate ridge loss. This can be controlled by frequent spring replacement, substitution of a resin plug for the spring, and rebasing of the prosthesis. The Dalbo attachment can also be in infraocclusion following rebasing due to a hinge over displacement. The problem may be solved by guiding the patient to terminal hinge closure in the reline or by using the Dalbo-M attachment in the locked mode.

SEMIPRECISION ATTACHMENTS

The semiprecision attachments consist of a number of systems that use resin pattern forms or wax or ceramic cores to form the attachments. The best known of these resin systems are the Ney* series (Fig. 13-85), such as the M-S (minimal space), Mortice-Rest, and Mini-Rest, and the P.D. attachment of Natomah,† which is an industry standard available in two sizes and used extensively in several teaching programs and commercial laboratories. The Straus wax‡ and ceramic core and the Howmedica§ ceramic core are representative of other semiprecision attachments used for precious and nonprecious metals.

Indications and application

The Mini-Rest and the P.D. attachments are used as major connectors in combination with the Thompson-Dowel technique or with milled lingual retentive arms.

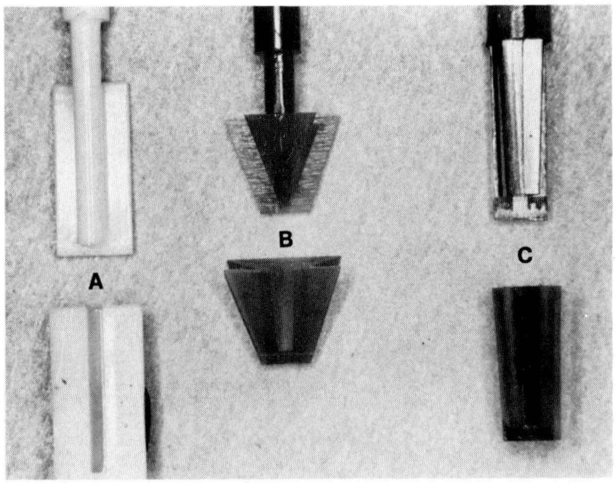

Fig. 13-85. Ney resin pattern interlocks and rests. *A,* M-S. *B,* Mortice Rest. *C,* Mini-Rest.

They are also used as internal rests for splinting, sectional contruction, and as connectors for nonparallel abutment teeth (Shillingburg, Hobo, and Whitsett, 1976).* The nonrigid connector provides a fulcrumfree broken-stress mechanical union of the retainer and pontic on multiple abutment bridges. A characteristic of most of the resin pattern semiprecision attachments is that they have a molded mandrel as an integral part of the male unit. (The keyway should generally be in the distal end of the anterior abutment, and the key should be on the mesial end of the adjacent abutment or pontic.) One of the chief indications for using any of these semiprecision attachments is to compensate for the po-

*The J.M. Ney Co., Bloomfield, Conn.
†Dentalloy, Dental Products, Inc., Stanton, Calif.
‡APM-Sterngold, Stamford, Conn.
§Howmedica, Inc., Chicago, Ill.

*One of the best sources on design and application of the keyway attachment system.

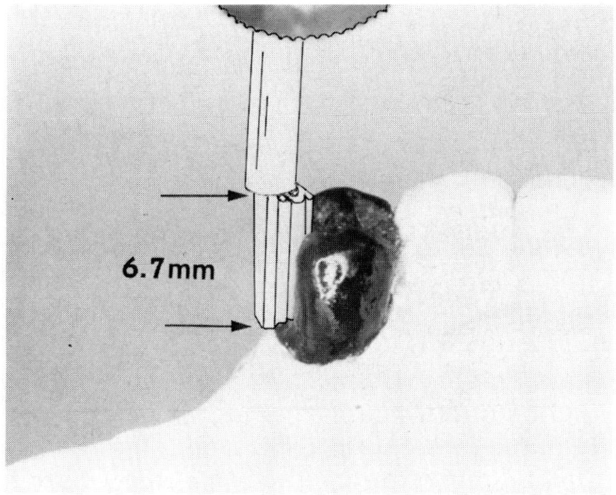

Fig. 13-86. P.D. attachments are used as interlocks or rests in fixed partial denture construction. The 6.7-mm height of female is reduced after casting.

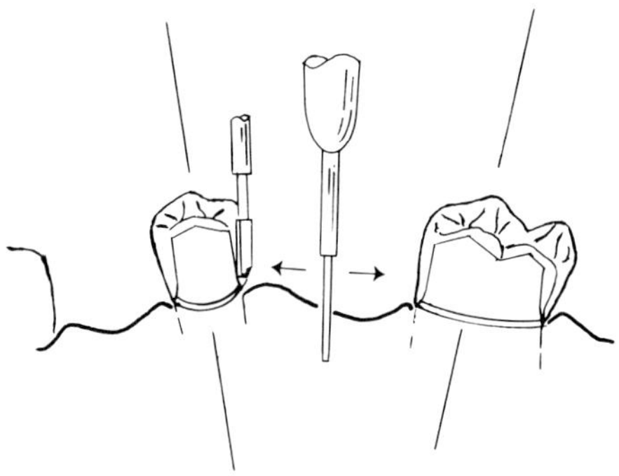

Fig. 13-87. Align attachment parallel with primary retainer shed (molar).

tential peridontal damage or the separation of a retainer from an abutment due to bending of the mandible under function.

P.D. attachments

The P.D.* attachments (Fig. 13-86) are representative of all resin pattern semiprecision attachments for laboratory assembly. They belong to auxiliary group V,† E Interlocks, and G Rests, depending on their use. The P.D. attachment is a tapered, angular dovetail resin pattern, in an "H," design, and the isthmus is short, generally to provide a positive seat in the female. A mandrel is molded as an extension of the occlusal surface of the male. The female boxing is also a resin pattern that is a negative of the male with a flat contact plate that engages the contact plate of the male. The dimensions of large P.D. attachments are 6.7 mm high, by 3.6 mm wide at the top, by 2.5 mm at the bottom. The thickness of the female is 0.5 mm, and the dimensions of the smaller male are 6.7 mm high, by 2.5 mm wide at the top, by 2 mm wide at the bottom.

PROCEDURE

The P.D. attachments, like the Ney Mini-Rest and Mortice-Rest attachments, are dimensionally small and do not require special crown preparation to compensate for possible overcontour.

1. Pour the master cast from the impression, trim and seal the dies, and survey the cast for the most favorable path of insertion (Fig. 13-87). (The fixed unit of a divergent abutment bridge determines the path of insertion, whereas the preparation shed determines the sectional construction position. When used as a major connector partial denture, the path of insertion must correspond to the ridge survey as well.)
2. Complete the wax-up in the usual manner, and create the recess in the pattern, using the assembled pattern/mandrel mounted on the surveyor (Fig. 13-88, *A*).
3. Trim the female, if necessary, and finally seal it into the wax pattern (Fig. 13-88, *B*).
4. Incorporate the male into the female pontic pattern by removing sufficient proximal wax to provide the required space, and then seal it to the pattern (Fig. 13-89). (This step may be done after casting the female and is the technique for partial dentures.)
5. Check the waxed units for proper seating on their dies and the male to its position in the female. Remove the plastic mandrel by passing a hot spatula through the mandrel above the attachment.
6. Sprue, invest, and cast the patterns.* Care must be taken to prevent air entrapment during investing and a partial paint-on; the vacuum investment technique is recommended. The patterns are of a nonresidue resin, but extra burnout time of 1 hour should be allowed to ensure complete elimination of the wax and plastic.
7. Finish the crowns in the normal manner, but use care to avoid abrasives on the attachments.
8. Finish the female proximal plate by placing waterproof silicon carbide paper† on a flat surface and stroking the plate lightly to produce a flat, smooth surface.
9. Lightly brush the male with a wire brush, and check it for nodules and fins. Remove any roughness

*Dentalloy Dental Products, Inc., Stanton, Calif.
†EM Attachment Selector, Bell International, Inc., Burlingame, Calif.

*A type III alloy should be used to reduce attachment wear.
†3M Co., Minneapolis, Minn.

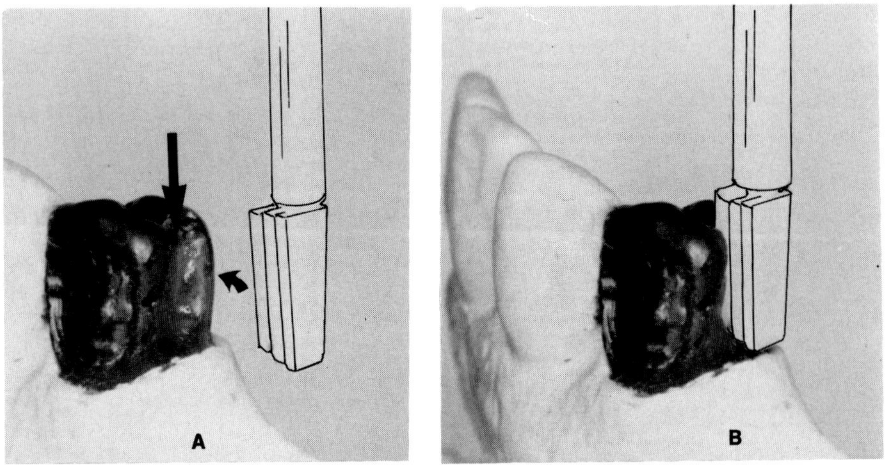

Fig. 13-88. *A,* Remove wax to make room for resin pattern. *B,* Place attachment and complete wax-up.

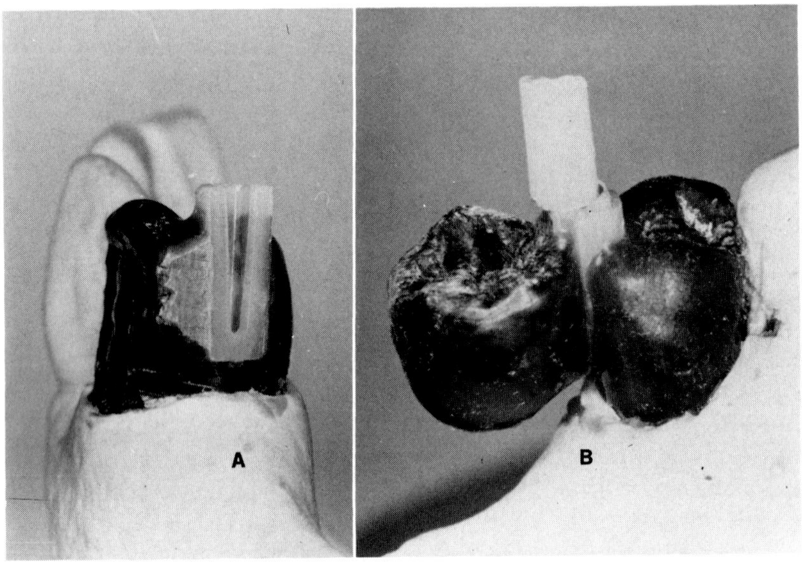

Fig. 13-89. *A,* Remove male and finish contour. *B,* Wax-up pontic with male.

with a rubber point, and fit the attachments with the aid of a graphite lubricant until seated. (An oxidized male will highlight interferences or use Pascal Occlude.)

10. Heat treat the castings at 850° F (455° C) and cool them to 450° F (235° C) in ½ hour before quenching in cold water.

11. Complete final polishing before delivery.

ALTERNATE PROCEDURE FOR FIXED REMOVABLE PARTIAL DENTURES

1. Carry out steps 1 to 4. Wax a P.D. tube into the crown carrying the female opposite the side of the housing, either from the facial or lingual aspects (Fig. 13-90).

2. Carry out procedures 5 to 11.

3. Place the P.D. drill in the sleeve, and tap it into the assembled attachment to establish a hemispherical lock depression.

4. Use the P.D. tap to establish the screw thread.

5. Place the P.D. screw, and shorten it to conform with the crown contour (Fig. 13-90).

6. Establish a screw head, and the unit is ready for delivery.

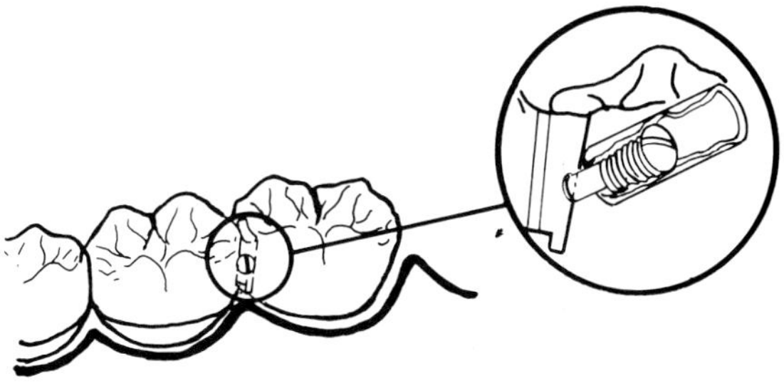

Fig. 13-90. Modify P.D. attachment as screw lock bridge. Wax P.D. tube at angle to occlusal. Cast and fit screw to attachment *(circle)*.

Table 13-4. Semiprecision attachments

Problem	Probable cause	Solution
Attachments will not fit	Different expansion factors, different techniques	Invest and cast together or follow same technique each time
Attachments too tight	Casting too precise	Use powdered graphite lubricant to work attachments and wirebrush male to reduce interference
Female attachment obstructed	Investment procedure did not remove air bubbles and investment did not enter attachment	Use paint-on and vacuum investing technique
Male attachment with fins	Mold temperature too high, investment cracked	Use high-heat investment for high temperature
Attachments wearing	Castings not heat treated Too soft alloy was used	Heat treat all castings to get maximum hardness Use type III alloy

ALTERNATE PROCEDURE FOR REMOVABLE PARTIAL DENTURES

1. Carry out steps 1 to 3.
2. If lingual retentive bracing arms or milled bracing arm minor connectors are used, then complete the procedure on the wax-up before investing.
3. Carry out procedures 6 to 8.
4. Complete the machining of the crown as part of step 7 in the discussion of milled lingual bracing arms.
5. Seat the crowns on their dies with a 12-μm plastic film elevation. Place the male plastic patterns in the females, and remove the mandrel section.
6. Develop the bracing arm section in DuraLay, and join it at the attachment male, or wax it on the investment cast.
7. Block out undercuts with a special blockout wax* and use pressure sensitive wax† following the procedure for resilient mandibular partial dentures.
8. Cast the duplicate impression in the investment stone of choice.
9. Carry out the wax-up in the usual manner to include the plastic parts.
10. An extra burnout time of 1 hour is required over the recommended time to ensure complete burnout of the plastic.
11. Complete steps 9 to 11 of the basic procedure.
12. Set up, invest, process, and finish the partial denture in the usual manner.*

*The J.M. Ney Co., Bloomfield, Conn., or equivalent.
†Kindt Collins Co., Cleveland, Ohio, or equivalent.

PROBLEM AREAS

Several problems can arise with semiprecision attachments, but the problems are unique in themselves compared to the prefabricated units. The problems, their probable causes, and solutions are presented in Table 13-4.

1. The attachments will not fit only because of different expansion factors and casting techniques. The solu-

*The technique for Thompson-Dowel is reported by Koper (1973) and is available as a syllabus from The University of Southern California School of Dentistry, Los Angeles, Calif. The technique for ceramic core attachments varies only in that they require dissolving the porcelain with hydrochloric acid to establish the female space.

tion is to invest and cast together if possible; otherwise, follow the same technique.

2. The attachments fit, but are too tight, the result of too precise a casting. Use powdered graphite lubricant to work the attachments after the male has been burnished with a wire wheel brush to reduce interferences.

3. The female attachments may be obstructed or incompletely defined because the investment procedure did not remove air bubbles, nor did the investment enter the attachment. A paint-on vacuum investing technique will eliminate this problem.

4. If the male attachment has fins, the mold temperature was too high, and the investment cracked. A high-heat investment should be used for high temperature castings.

5. Wear in semiprecision attachments indicates two things: (1) the castings were not heat treated and (2) too soft an alloy was used. The solution to wear reduction is to heat treat all castings and use a hard type III alloy.

SUMMARY

This chapter on attachments in fixed and fixed-removable prosthodontics introduces the technical aspects of a representative selection of attachments used in the fabrication of the bounded and free-end prosthesis. Only the clinical phases that are directly related to the laboratory techniques have been presented. The procedures represent techniques common to all attachments of each design group. The tables for each group of attachments represents a cross section of clinical and laboratory failures and how to solve them. There has been no attempt to include cross arch stabilizers, since they are auxillary to the unilateral free-end partial denture. The footnotes for attachment manufacturers provide a source and related technical information.

REFERENCES

Baker, J.L., and Goodkind, R.J.: Theory and practice of precision attachment removable partial dentures, St. Louis, 1981, The C.V. Mosby Co.

Craig, R.G., editor: Restorative dental materials, ed., St. Louis, 1985, The C.V. Mosby Co.

Koper, A.: An intracoronal semi-precision retainer for removable partial dentures—the Thompson dowel, J. Prosthet. Dent. **30**(5):759-768, 1973.

Kornfeld, M.: Mouth rehabilitation: clinical and laboratory procedures, ed. 2, vol. 2, St. Louis, 1974, The C.V. Mosby Co.

Mensor, M.C.: Classification and selection of attachments, J. Prosthet. Dent. **29**(5):494-467, 1973.

Moffa, J.P.: Personal communication, 1976.

Nally, J.N.: The use of prefabricated precision attachments, Int. Dent. J. **11**:192-216, 1961.

Preiskel, H.W.: Precision attachments in dentistry, ed. 3, London, 1979, Henry Kimpton, Publishers.

Shillingburg, H.T., Hobo, S., and Whitsett, L.D.: Fundamentals of fixed prosthodontics, Berlin, 1976, Die Quintessence.

Steiger, A.A., and Boitel, R.H.: Precision work for partial dentures, Zürich, 1959, Berichthaus.

Zwemer, T.J., editor: Boucher's clinical dental terminology, St. Louis, 1982, The C.V. Mosby Co.

CHAPTER 14

FIXED-REMOVABLE PARTIAL DENTURES

JOHN E. RHOADS

The replacement of missing teeth and restoration of lost alveolar contour has always presented a problem in treatment of those patients who have suffered traumatic injury, congenital defects, or other deformity that has resulted in the loss of anterior dentition. Many of these injuries are of moderate severity and, except for excessive loss of or damage to the residual ridge, would be candidates for restoration with a fixed partial denture.

The loss of contour and size of the residual ridge, however, precludes or makes extremely difficult an esthetic and hygienic restoration with a conventional fixed prosthesis (Fig. 14-1). The pontic must have a passive, minimal contact with the residual soft tissues. If loss of the facial bony plate of the alveolar ridge has occurred from either trauma or natural resorption, the replacement teeth in the pontic area cannot be placed in the most esthetic arrangement, compensate for soft tissue loss, and still maintain the proper contact relationship with the edentulous ridge area.

It remains, then, for the replacement to be predicated on the use of a removable prosthesis to supply the missing contour and provide a means of positioning the replacement teeth in their natural relationships. The use of a conventional removable partial denture must incorporate coverage of soft tissues by major connectors and other necessary elements of the prosthesis and involve several of the teeth as suitable abutments for stabilization.

A number of approaches to the treatment of such problems have been conceived whereby a removable pontic section could be supported directly by adjacent abutment teeth in a manner similar to that of a fixed prosthesis (Fig. 14-2). Such an appliance would have a number of advantages: (1) it could cover a minimum of soft tissue, (2) it could afford a means of replacement of teeth with optimum esthetic arrangement, (3) it could compensate for soft tissue defects, and (4) it could be removed for easy day-to-day hygiene (Fig. 14-3 and 14-4).

BACKGROUND INFORMATION

The concept of removable pontic sections supported by abutment teeth certainly is not new. Evidence of attempts to develop and employ such a modality has been presented in textbooks and periodical literature dating back at least to the early 1900s.

An approach by Fossume using a round bar attached to abutment crowns that supported a suprastructure appears to be one of the first attempts to construct a fixed-removable partial denture (Fig. 14-5). Undoubtedly further perusal of the literature would disclose even earlier attempts at this modality. Other variations that employed the "bar and clip" concept for retention and that relied on extended tissue coverage for rotational stability were presented by Dolder (Steiger and Boitel, 1951), and more recently by Baker and Hader (Fig. 14-6) and by Andrews (Fig. 14-7).

The first use of a precision or semiprecision "bar and sleeve" assembly that provided for rotational stability gained directly through the substructure bar and the

A 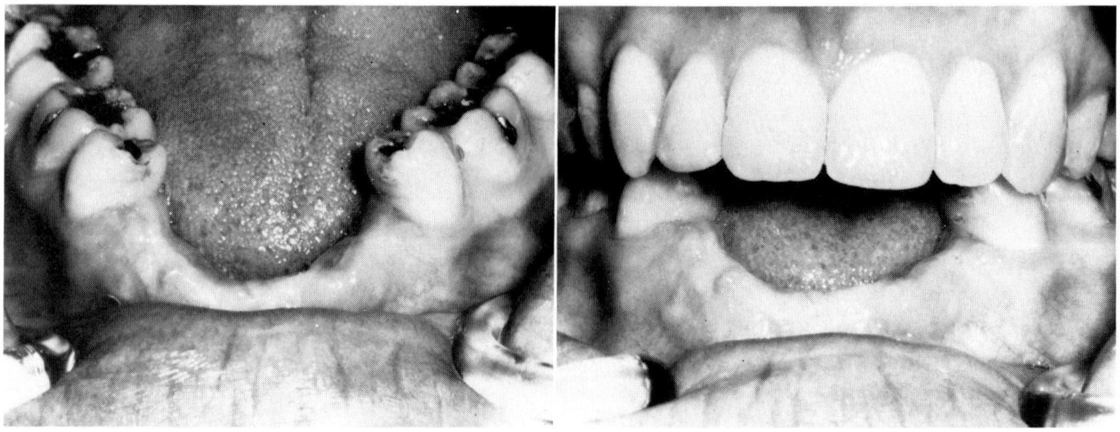 B

Fig. 14-1. A, Excessive loss of alveolar bone or damage to the residual ridge makes esthetic and hygienic restoration difficult. Because of constraints of fixed pontics in relation to the residual ridge, use of a fixed partial denture is contraindicated. **B,** degree of loss of alveolar process resulting from traumatic injury is evident when posterior teeth are in occlusion.

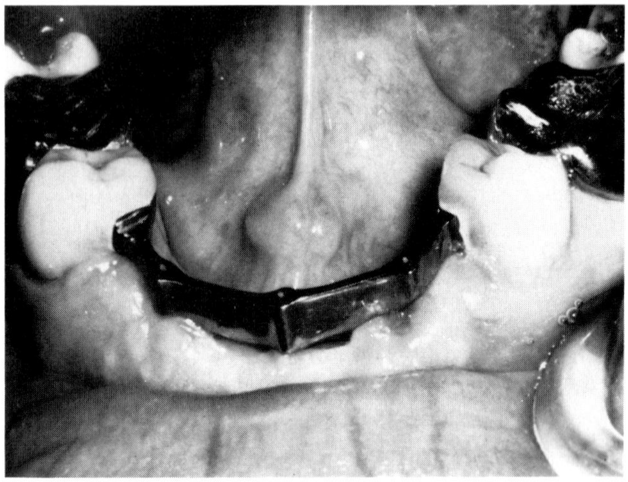

Fig. 14-2. Fixed substructure bar attached to abutment teeth provides support and stabilization for removable suprastructure. Arcuate design of substructure bar required by loss of teeth and osseous structure dictated use of multiple abutment retainers.

A 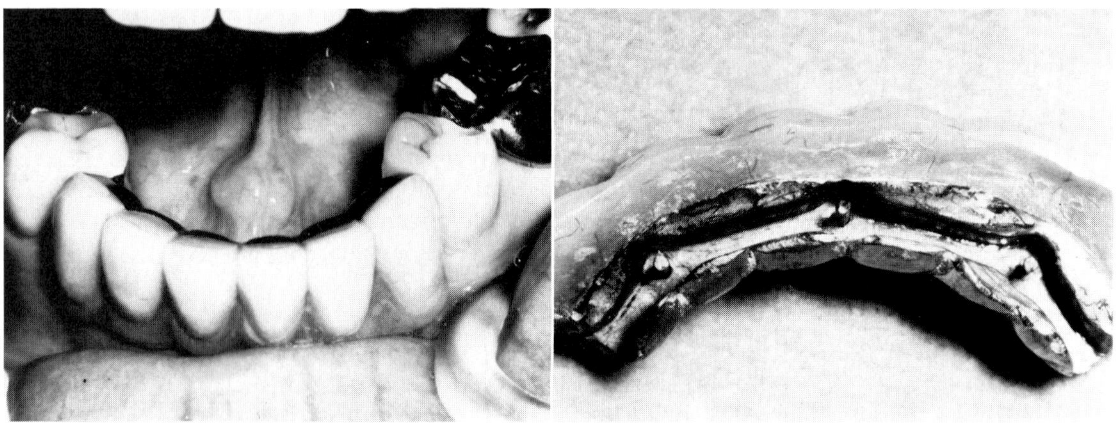 B

Fig. 14-3. A, Removable suprastructure mated to substructure provides support for replacement teeth. **B,** Underside of suprastructure shows broad frictional surfaces and retentive pins that mate to corresponding contours of substructure.

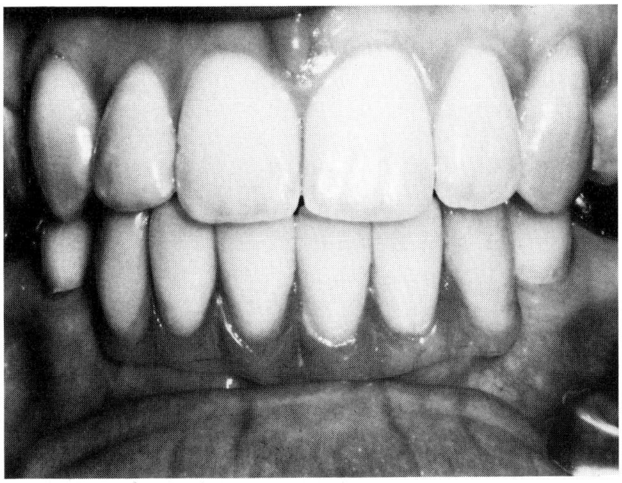

Fig. 14-4. Replacement teeth are placed for optimum function and esthetics, and missing contours are restored with acrylic resin denture material.

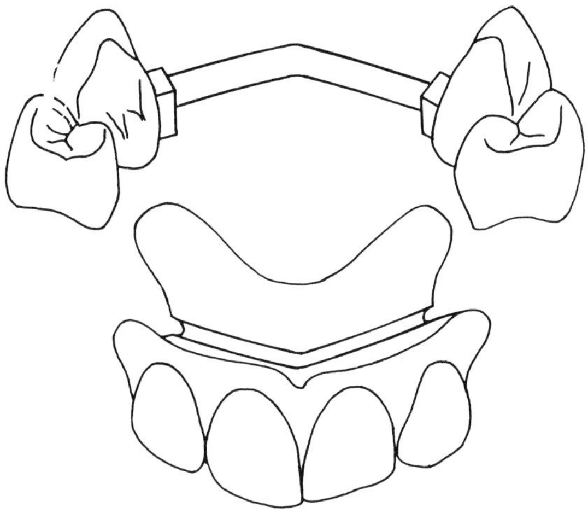

Fig. 14-5. An early attempt in development of fixed removable concept was presented by Fossume. Device employed a round bar attached to abutment crowns that supported suprastructure. Rotational stability was provided by flanges covering soft tissues.

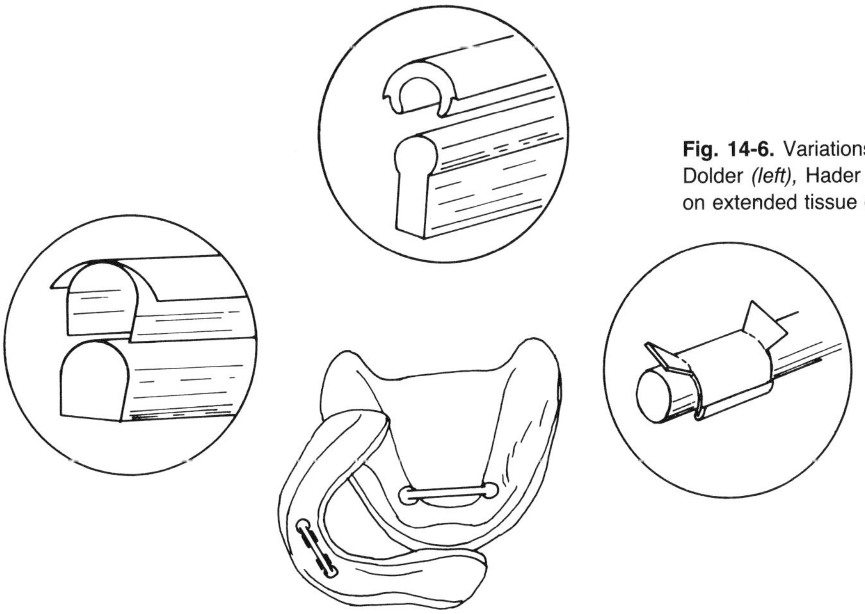

Fig. 14-6. Variations in "bar and clip" concept were developed by Dolder *(left),* Hader *(top),* and Baker *(right).* These concepts relied on extended tissue coverage for rotational stability.

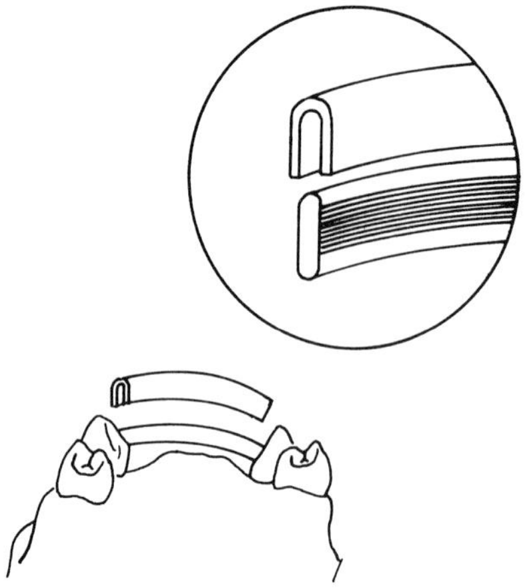

Fig. 14-7. Development by Andrews consisted of a prefabricated arch bar and matching sleeve to which replacement teeth and other suprastructure elements were attached.

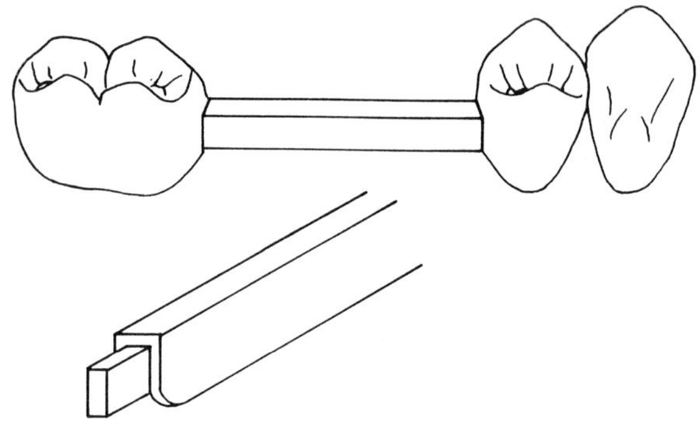

Fig. 14-8. Bennet Blade appears to be first attempt to use a precision or semiprecision bar and sleeve assembly that provided for rotational stability to be gained directly through substructure and abutment teeth.

A

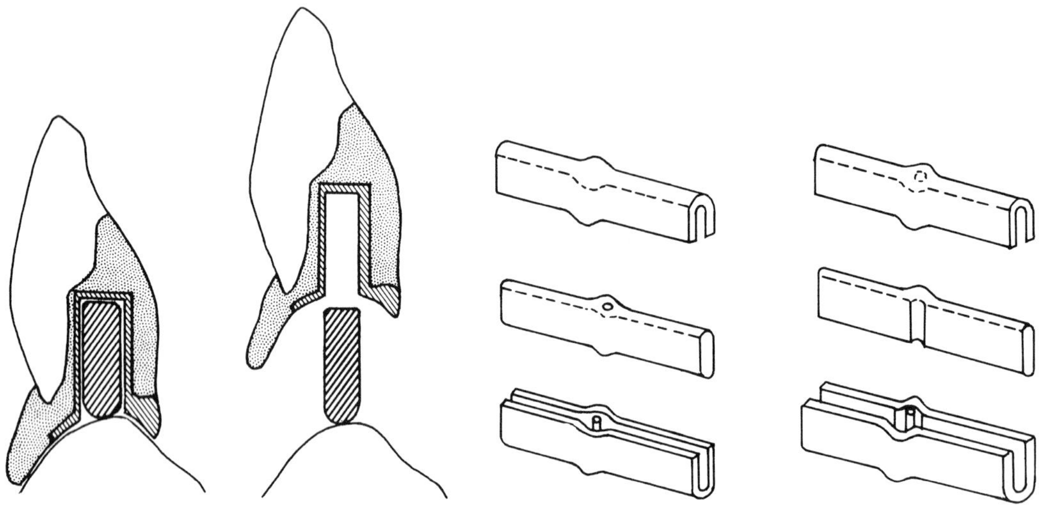

B

Fig. 14-9. A, Refined approach to blade concept has been presented by Steiger and Boitel. Substructure bar is rigidly attached to abutment teeth. Suprastructure, which mates precisely with substructure bar, serves for mounting of replacement teeth and restoration of lost tissue contour. **B,** Variations of bar and sleeve assembly as presented by Steiger and Boitel in 1959 illustrate great variation in design possible with this modality.

abutment teeth thus far discovered was the approach by Bennett—the so-called Bennett Blade (Fig. 14-8). Although precise information has not been found, the modality was probably developed between 1915 and 1920. It appears to be the ancestor of the technique to be described.

In recent years many variations of this concept have been developed by the laboratory craft and precious metal manufacturers. Such information does not necessarily appear in the dental literature. Introduction has been primarily through advertisement in the trade literature. Although some have been illustrated by Schwartz (1948) the origin and history of many of these techniques are difficult to trace.

The Bennett blade is illustrated by Steiger and Boitel, who describe a refined modification of the modality applicable to a variety of situations (Fig. 14-9).

The particular approach described herein was brought to the attention of American Dentistry about 1950 by Downs.* The technique is a versatile one and

*Downs, B.H.: Personal communication, 1955.

A 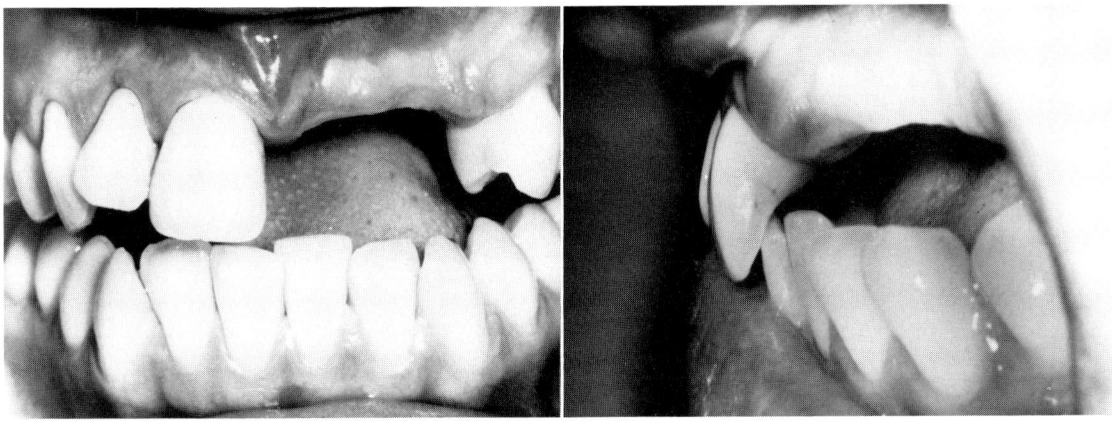 B

Fig. 14-10. A, Preoperative condition of patient. Loss of facial plate of alveolar process in edentulous area, a result of trauma, precludes restoration by means of a conventional fixed partial denture. Undamaged condition of abutment teeth dictates use of conservative abutment retainer preparations. **B,** Lataral view of preoperative condition showing vertical and horizontal overlap of remaining anterior teeth in occlusion. Note space between residual ridge and opposing teeth, which must be restored by prosthesis.

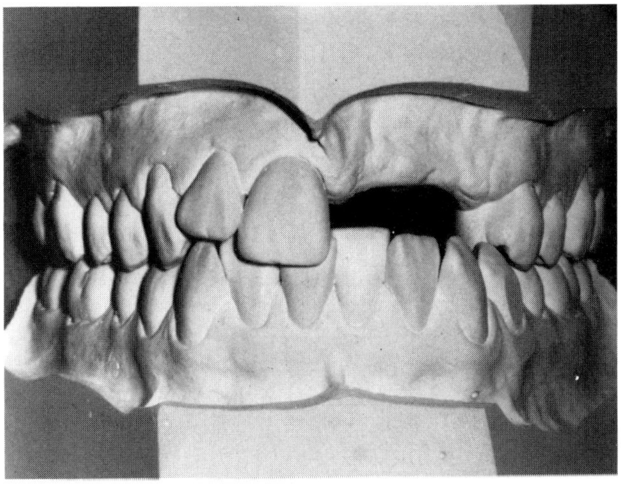

Fig. 14-11. Preoperative diagnostic cast demonstrating occlusal relationships of remaining teeth and contour of edentulous area. Note displacement of labial frenum toward edentulous area, which can create a problem with esthetics of prosthesis.

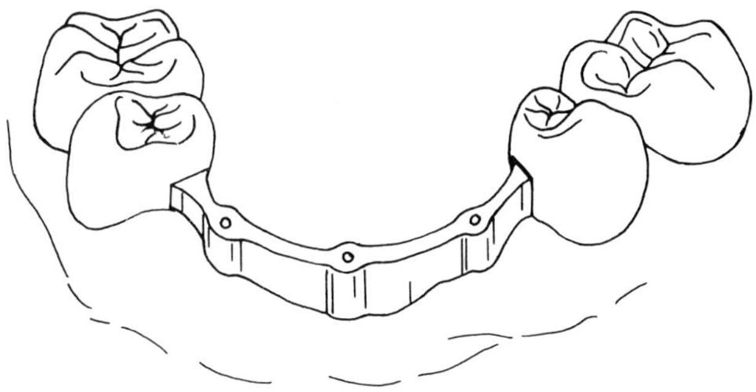

Fig. 14-12. Supporting structure for prosthesis is milled substructure bar (designed for specific contours of problem being treated) that is rigidly attached to abutment castings.

is sufficiently adaptable to varied conditions that little modification of the technical procedure has been made during many years of application (Fig. 14-10).

Although the concept of the fixed-removable partial denture is sufficiently flexible to allow adaptation to both anterior and posterior replacements, the basic principles involved in the technique will be illustrated with step-by-step procedures for fabrication of a prosthesis to restore defects in the anterior part of the mouth (Fig. 14-11).

DESCRIPTION

The fixed removable prosthesis consists of a milled substructure bar (designed for the specific contours of the problem being treated) that is rigidly attached to abutment castings (Fig. 14-12). The bar is specifically designed and fabricated to the contours of the residual ridge. A matching suprastructure, to which the replacement teeth are attached, is fabricated and fitted accurately to the substructure (Fig. 14-13). The irregularly arcuate contour provides exceptional retention and resistance to rotational forces for the suprastructure. Positive retention to minimize vertical displacement is achieved through the use of precious metal spring wire pins, attached to the suprastructure, which traverse parallel mating channels or holes in the substructure (Fig. 14-14).

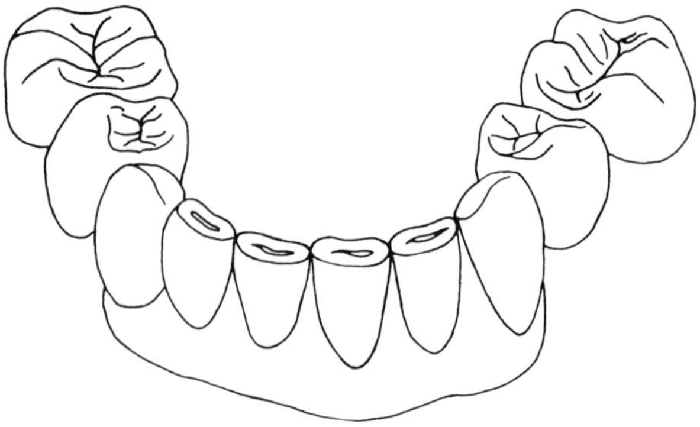

Fig. 14-13. Matching suprastructure to which replacement teeth are attached is fabricated and fitted to substructure.

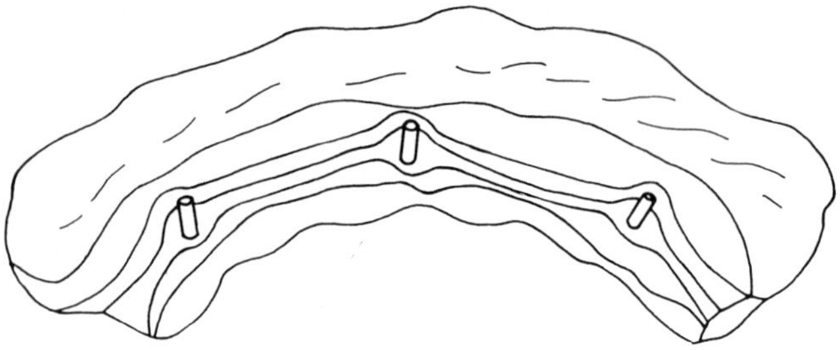

Fig. 14-14. Positive retention to minimize vertical displacement is achieved through use of precious metal spring pins, attached to suprastructure, which traverse parallel mating channels or holes in the substructure.

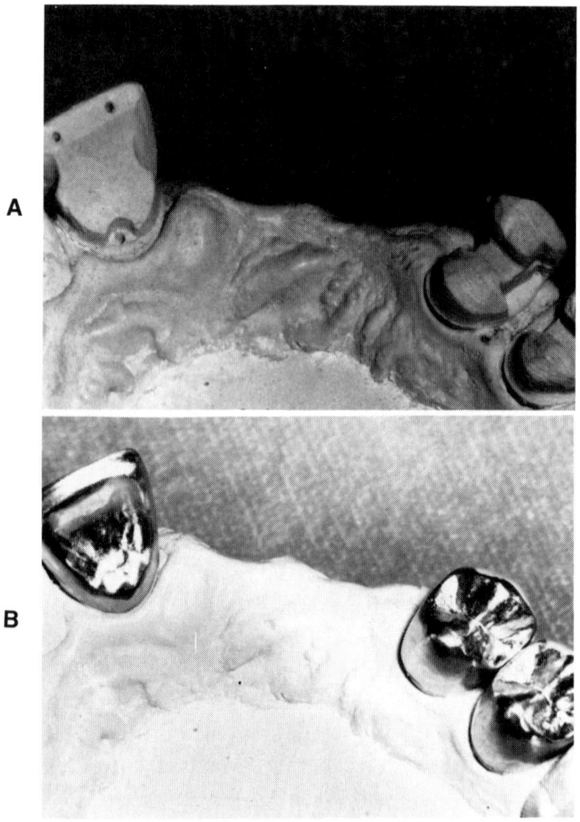

Fig. 14-15. A, Master cast of maxillary arch with abutment teeth prepared to receive partial veneer crowns. Properly engineered preparation design provides adequate retention form, minimal proximal extension to achieve an esthetic result, and minimal reduction of tooth structure. **B,** Completed abutment castings after fitting to the teeth, adjustment of occlusion, and verifying marginal integrity.

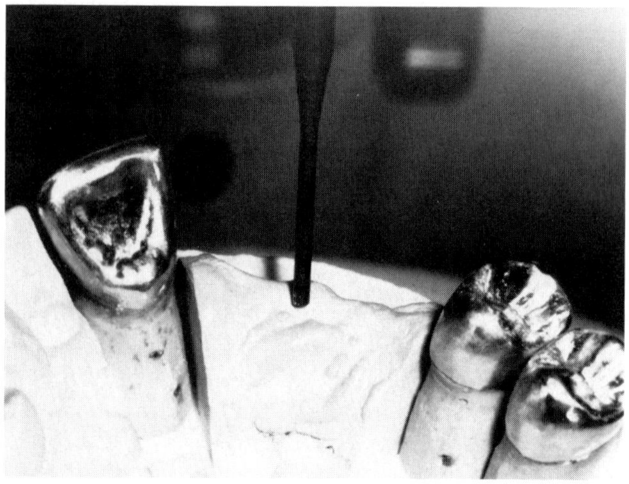

Fig. 14-16. Path of placement of suprastructure, while essentially vertical in direction, should provide for insertion from a facial direction toward lingual to allow minimizing of embrasures between abutment teeth and replacement teeth.

FABRICATION OF THE SUBSTRUCTURE BAR

Determination of path of placement

The path of placement, although essentially vertical in direction, should allow the suprastructure to be placed from the facial aspect toward the lingual to minimize the embrasures between the abutment teeth and the replacement teeth (Figs. 14-15 and 14-16).

The replacement teeth should be selected and fitted to the edentulous area of the diagnostic cast before any definitive treatment is commenced. This will allow the esthetic result to be determined beforehand and can do much to eliminate time-consuming modifications later in the procedure. These teeth will also provide an important guide in the subsequent placement of the substructure bar.

In many instances exact reproduction of the natural teeth will not be available from commercial sources. It

A 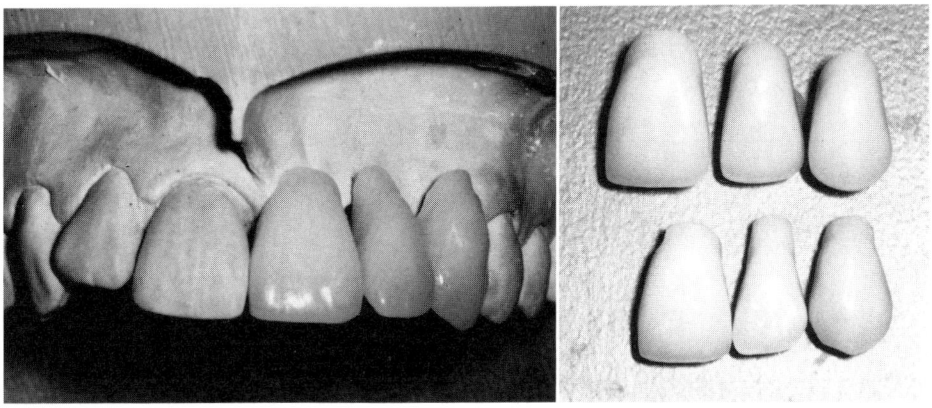 B

Fig. 14-17. A, Replacement teeth have been recontoured and fitted to edentulous area, achieving optimum esthetic arrangement. Prearrangement of these teeth aids in determining optimum position for substructure bar. **B,** Stock denture teeth before and after recontouring and customizing to imitate contours of patient's remaining teeth. Acrylic resin denture teeth can be recontoured and repolished easily. Porcelain denture teeth, after recontouring, must be reglazed using appropriate stains and glazes in a porcelain glazing oven.

may be necessary to reshape the artificial teeth by recontouring, modifying proximal surfaces, or changing the surface contour and texture (Fig. 14-17). Such modification is most easily accomplished using resin teeth, which can be polished by conventional agents. Porcelain denture teeth can also be modified and refinished using porcelain stains and glazes. In most instances, because of the degree of loss of soft tissue, the optimum arrangement of the replacement teeth will not allow contact with the residual ridge. This area is brought to full contour with wax that is later replaced with denture base resin.

The working cast should be mounted on a suitable platform that will allow easy removal and replacement on the milling apparatus without loss of the plane of orientation (Fig. 14-18).

Positioning the substructure bar

The position of the substructure bar is determined largely by the position of the replacement teeth. It should be placed immediately lingual to these teeth so that excessive bulk in the lingual contour of the suprastructure can be avoided or minimized.

Positioning of the retentive pins

The position of the retentive pins should be determined after the replacement teeth have been oriented and stabilized with a removable plaster core (Fig. 14-19). The most advantageous pin placement is opposite the interproximal spaces of the adjacent replacement teeth. Such placement allows increased thickness of metal in the substructure bar that is necessary for reinforcement around the retention holes.

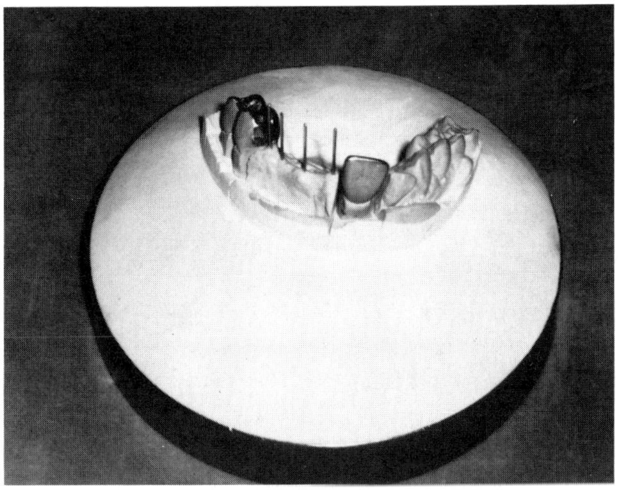

Fig. 14-18. Master cast is mounted securely on a milling platform so that subsequent milling procedures will produce lateral surfaces that are exactly parallel with retentive pins.

After pin positions have been selected, holes of a size comparable to the pins (0.7 mm) are drilled parallel into the respective ridge areas of the working cast to a depth of approximately 2 mm. These holes will accept and stabilize stainless steel pins in a parallel relationship during the subsequent fabrication of the substructure bar (Fig. 14-20).

Fabrication of the substructure bar

The substructure bar is developed in wax around the prepositioned stainless steel pins (Fig. 14-21). The bar is carved to approximate dimension to minimize the

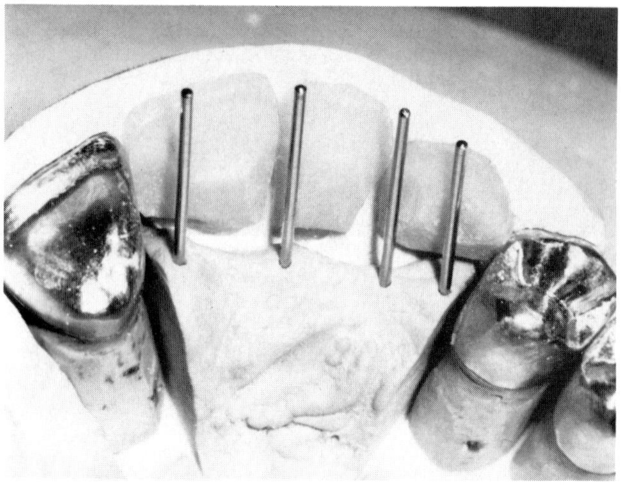

Fig. 14-19. Retentive pin position is determined after replacement teeth have been positioned and stabilized with removable plaster core. Most advantageous position is in interproximal spacing.

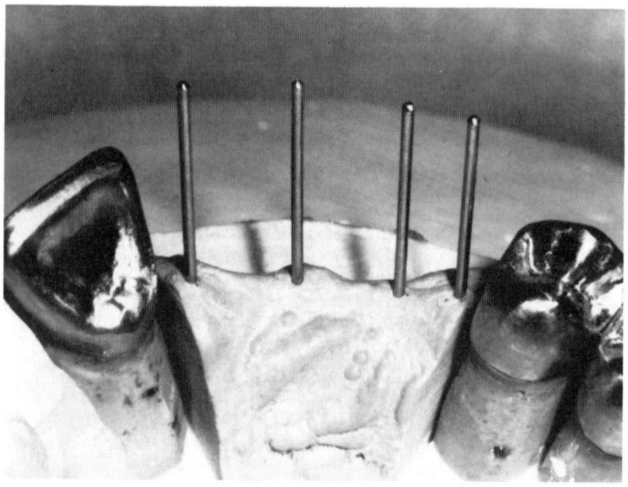

Fig. 14-20. Stainless steel pins that will form retentive holes in substructure bar are positioned by drilling holes of appropriate size into cast to a depth of approximately 2 mm.

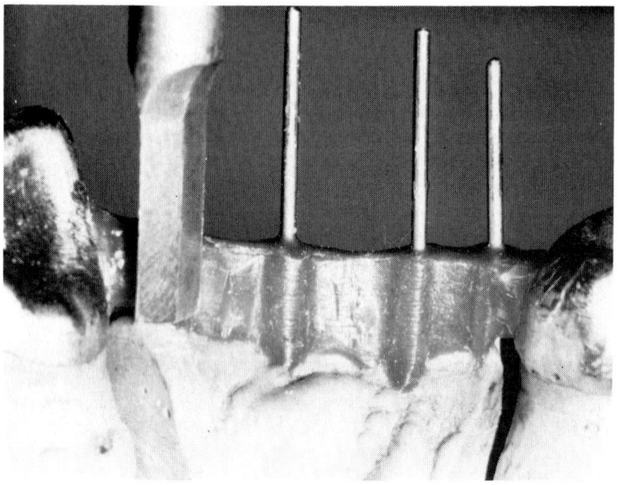

Fig. 14-21. Substructure bar is developed in wax around prepositioned stainless steel pins. It is carved to approximate dimension to minimize subsequent milling procedures.

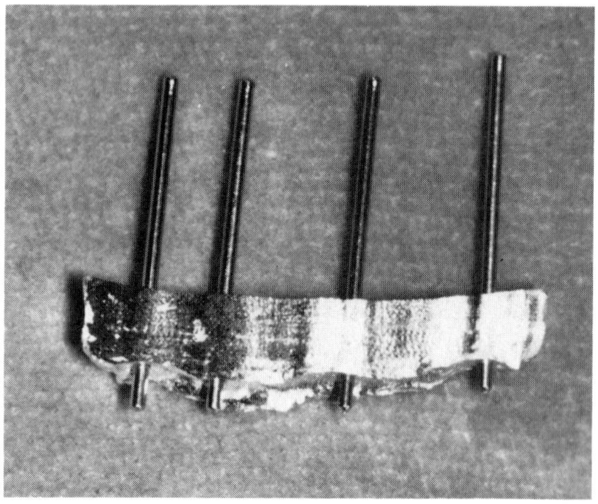

Fig. 14-22. Waxed substructure is invested and cast in Type IV partial denture gold alloy. Stainless steel pins are maintained in wax pattern as it is invested and are removed from casting later in fabrication procedure.

milling of metal in the subsequent steps. The sides of the wax substructure bar should be carved parallel to each other with a suitable blade mandrel affixed to the surveyor spindle or modelling arm of the milling apparatus.

The wax bar is removed from the cast, invested, and cast in type IV partial denture gold alloy. The parallel pins are maintained in the wax pattern to be removed from the casting at a later point in the procedure (Fig. 14-22).

After casting, the bar is reoriented into alignment with the path of insertion and joined to the abutment castings by soldering. When the abutments are to be metal-ceramic crowns, assembly of the substructure bar to the abutments can be accomplished using a post soldering technique (see section on assembly of dental castings, p. 244).

After assembly of the bar to the abutments, the parallel pins are removed from the casting by tapping to loosen them and drawing them out with pliers. The holes are cleaned and reamed with spiral drills or jeweler's broaches of appropriate size. Carbon rods (0.7 mm diameter*) may be used in place of stainless steel

*Scripto "Cassette" 0.7 mm pencil.

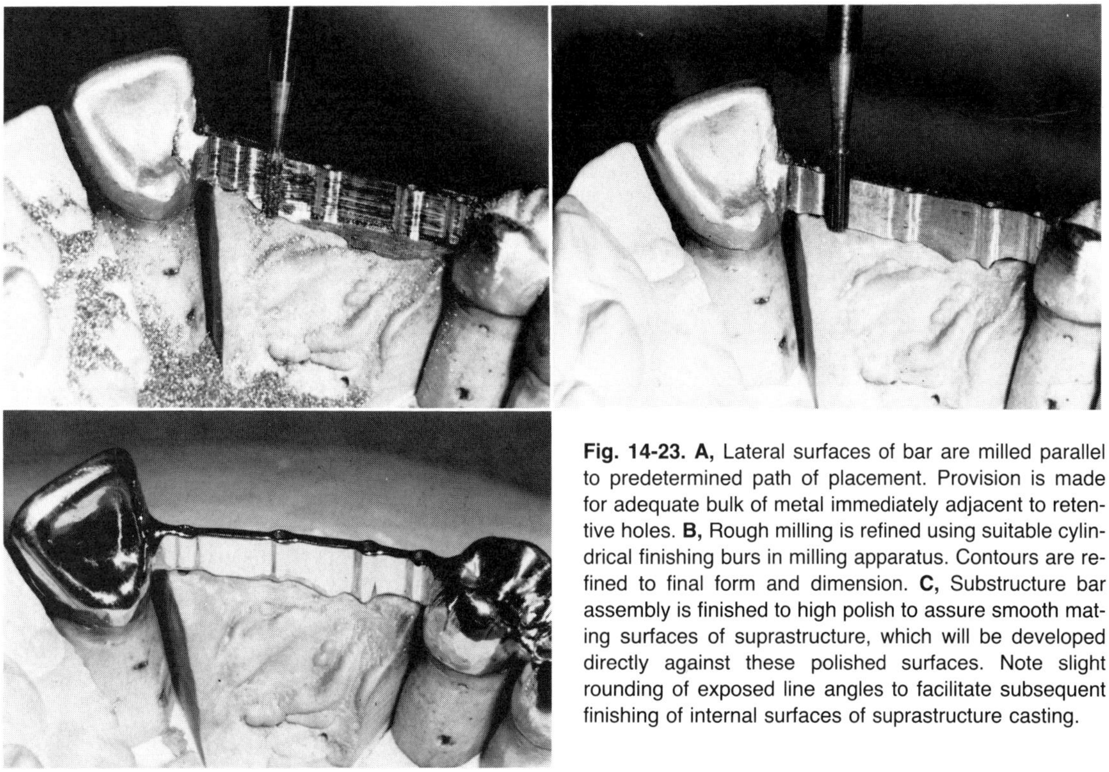

Fig. 14-23. A, Lateral surfaces of bar are milled parallel to predetermined path of placement. Provision is made for adequate bulk of metal immediately adjacent to retentive holes. **B,** Rough milling is refined using suitable cylindrical finishing burs in milling apparatus. Contours are refined to final form and dimension. **C,** Substructure bar assembly is finished to high polish to assure smooth mating surfaces of suprastructure, which will be developed directly against these polished surfaces. Note slight rounding of exposed line angles to facilitate subsequent finishing of internal surfaces of suprastructure casting.

pins if difficulty is experienced in obtaining metal pins of appropriate dimension.

The assembled substructure is returned to the working cast and placed on the milling apparatus for refining of the lateral surfaces (Fig. 14-23). The surfaces are milled parallel to each other, with provision being made for adequate bulk of metal in the immediate area of the retentive holes. The parallel milled surfaces are smoothed with cylindric milling and finishing burs and then polished to a fine finish (Fig. 14-24). After completion of the *suprastructure*, the tissue surface of the substructure bar is rounded and polished to minimize contact with the residual ridge and to facilitate hygiene.

FABRICATION OF THE SUPRASTRUCTURE

New stainless steel pins are inserted into the retentive holes in the substructure bar (the pins should have a light frictional fit). The plaster core supporting the replacement teeth is repositioned, and pattern resin* is applied in small increments to the lubricated substructure bar. After the initial veneer layer of pattern resin has been applied to the bar, the remainder of the suprastructure is built to the desired contour with additional pattern resin or with inlay wax (Fig. 14-25).

A thin even coating of petroleum jelly has proved to

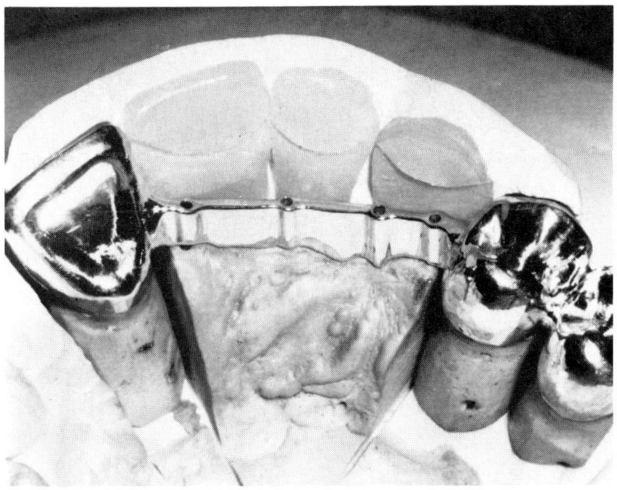

Fig. 14-24. Finished substructure bar with replacement teeth, in their plaster matrix, in position. Note finish lines to enable production of a close adaptation of suprastructure metal to replacement teeth.

*Duralay, Reliance Dental Mfg. Co., Worth, Ill.

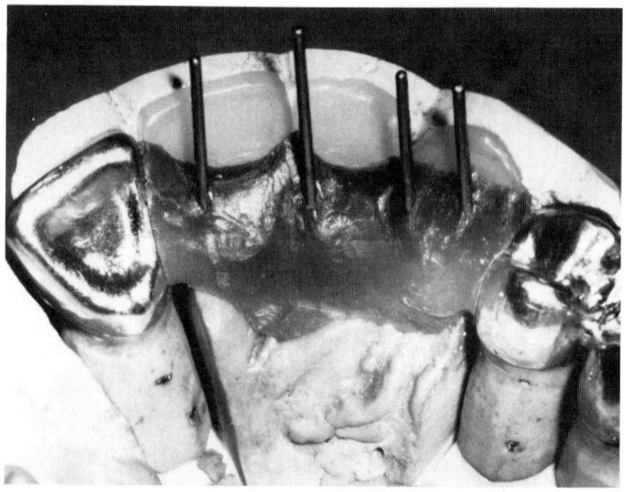

Fig. 14-25. Initial layer of pattern resin is applied in increments to lubricated substructure bar to assure uniform adaptation. Remainder of suprastructure is built to desired contour with additional pattern resin or with inlay wax. Natural contour of lingual surfaces of teeth being replaced is simulated to minimize excessive bulk of finished prosthesis. New metal pins have been placed in holes of substructure bar and will be withdrawn with suprastructure pattern.

A

B

C

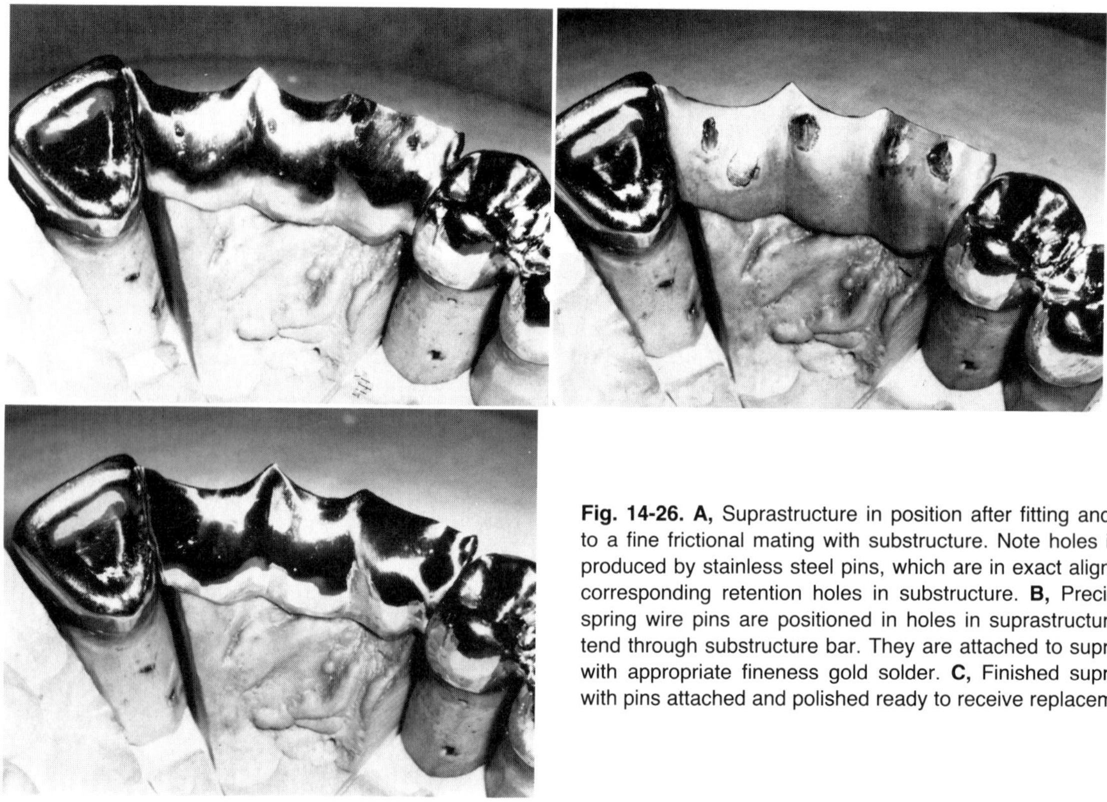

Fig. 14-26. A, Suprastructure in position after fitting and polishing to a fine frictional mating with substructure. Note holes in casting, produced by stainless steel pins, which are in exact alignment with corresponding retention holes in substructure. **B,** Precious metal spring wire pins are positioned in holes in suprastructure and extend through substructure bar. They are attached to suprastructure with appropriate fineness gold solder. **C,** Finished suprastructure with pins attached and polished ready to receive replacement teeth.

be an excellent release agent (lubricating or separating material), which will facilitate removal of the completed pattern from the substructure bar. Care should be exercised to employ as thin a layer of separator as is practical so that accuracy of the pattern mating surfaces is maintained.

Retentive elements in the form of loops, buttons, bars, or other surface irregularities should be placed upon the facial aspect of the suprastructure pattern to provide adequate retention for the resin that will be used to attach the replacement teeth.

The suprastructure pattern is removed from the substructure, examined for completeness, invested, and cast in an appropriate gold alloy (type IV).

After casting, the stainless steel pins are removed and the inner surface of the casting is carefully finished with cylindrical finishing burs to produce an accurate frictional fit on the substructure. After the internal por-

A B C

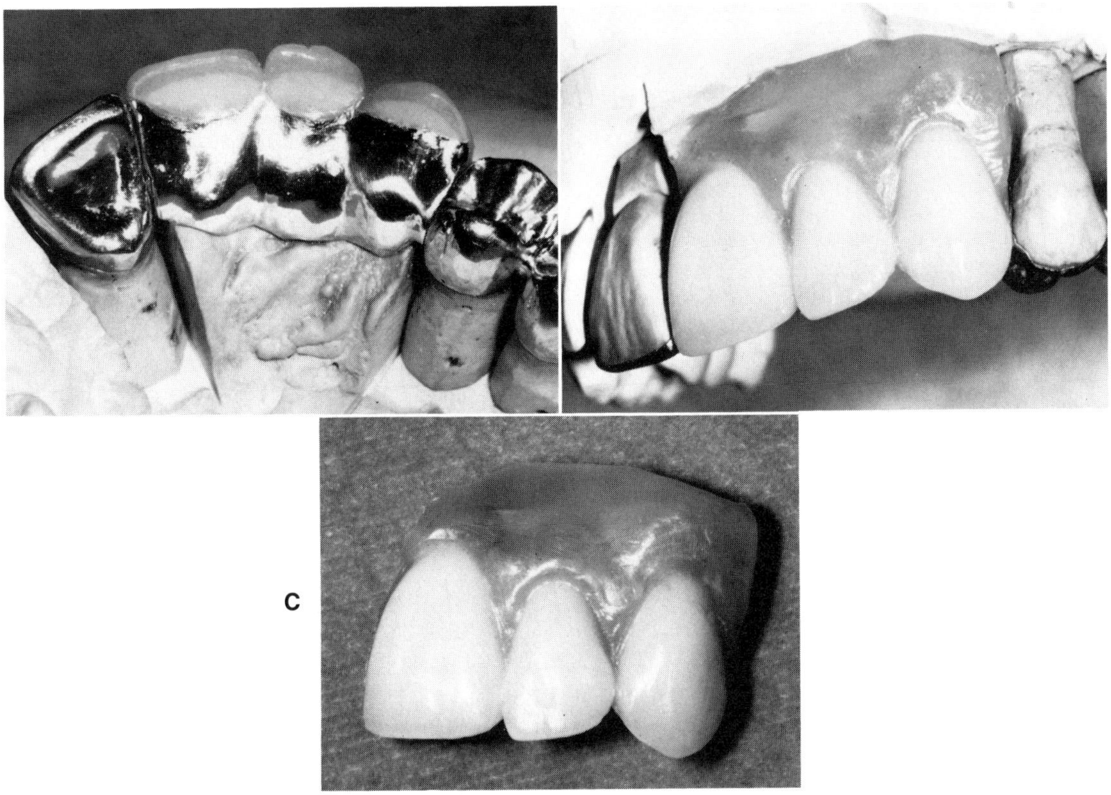

Fig. 14-27. A, Replacement teeth properly positioned to suprastructure. Note close adaptation of metal to finish lines prepared in replacement teeth. **B,** Replacement teeth are arranged on suprastructure and simulated gingival tissues have been developed. **C,** Replacement teeth are attached to suprastructure and wax contour developed and finished, ready for processing.

tion of the suprastructure is finished and polished the final precious metal retentive pins* are oriented and affixed by soldering (Fig. 14-26). The precious metal spring wire pins of appropriate diameter are fitted through the suprastructure and attached with sticky wax. The suprastructure is carefully withdrawn, soldering investment introduced around the pins inside the retentive slot, and the pins soldered to the suprastructure with appropriate fineness gold solder.

After final wax-up the replacement teeth are attached to the suprastructure with suitable denture base acrylic resin formed to the desired facial contour (Fig. 14-27).

EVALUATION OF THE MODALITY

Advantages

Flexibility of design

The basic elements of the system lend themselves to a variety of applications to meet the requirements of many different situations. Being custom made to the contours and alignment of each individual condition, the substructure affords opportunity for wide variation in design, placement, contour, and retentive capability (Figs. 14-28 to 14-30).

Oral hygiene

The fixed substructure's narrowness in its contact with the underlying tissue permits optimum hygiene of abutment teeth and adjacent tissue. The removal of the suprastructure permits easy cleaning of the underlying tissues, an inherent problem associated with conventional fixed partial dentures.

Minimal tissue coverage

Being greater only where loss of contour of the residual ridge has occurred, the tissue contact and coverage can approximate that of the fixed partial denture. By comparison, it is unnecessary to cover extensive areas of palatal or lingual tissue with the prosthesis (major connectors) and to involve a number of teeth with clasp retainers, which are necessary elements of a conventional removable partial denture.

The bulk of the prosthesis that essentially replaces the contour of missing dental structures (and only that) affords greater acceptance by the patient.

*Orthoclasp wire (Baker); Elasitcor wire (Metaux).

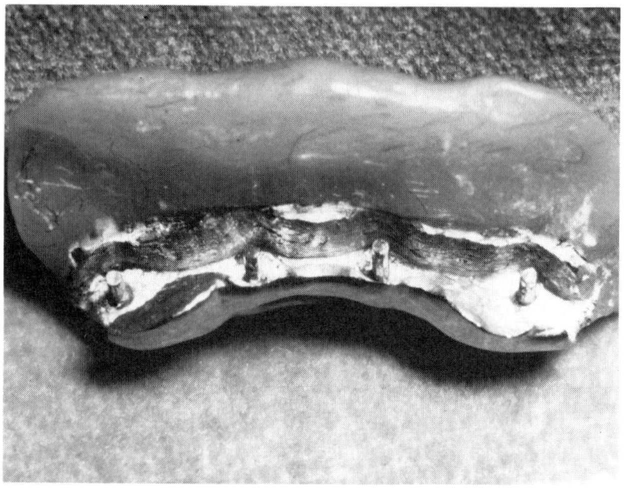

Fig. 14-28. Tissue surface of acrylic and channel in suprastructure mate with corresponding contours of substructure. These irregularly arcuate surfaces produce great resistance to rotational dislodgement of suprastructure. Note parallel retentive pins that fit into corresponding holes in substructure.

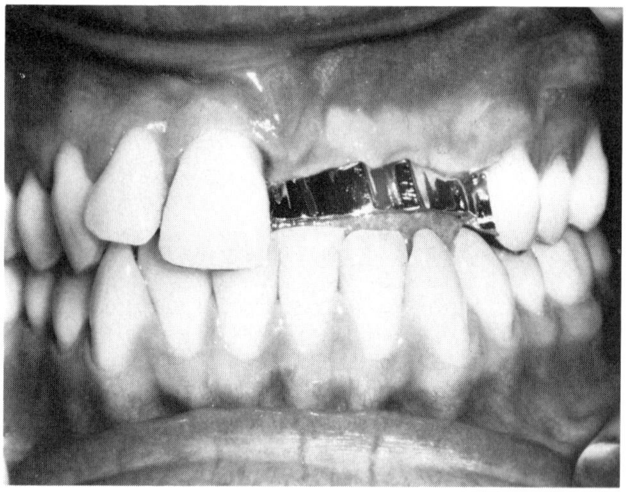

Fig. 14-29. Substructure bar in position. Tissue surface of bar has been rounded and polished (after fabrication of suprastructure) to afford minimal contact with tissue and to facilitate cleansing.

A

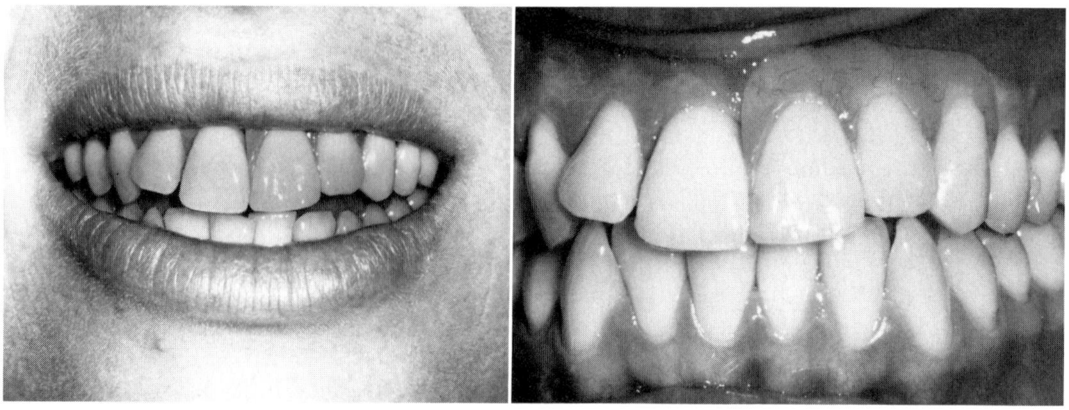

B

Fig. 14-30. A, Suprastructure is in position and replaces missing teeth and alveolar process lost as a result of an automobile accident. **B,** Suprastructure in position. Unsightly triangular embrasure between central incisor teeth has been minimized by favorable path of insertion of suprastructure. Note almost nonexistent display of metal, which can be achieved by properly executed retainer preparation.

Durability

Experience has shown this approach to be most durable and to have presented few maintenance problems. Breakage and major repair have been found to be infrequent.

Esthetic results

The wide selection of replacement teeth and restorative materials that can be used allows optimum esthetic results to be attained even for patients presenting considerable deformity.

Ease of adjustment

The broad frictional areas presented by the lateral surfaces of the mating parts enable an inherently stable prosthesis to be developed. The wear of the frictional surfaces, which occurs with time, is distributed over a large surface with relatively little effect on the retentive character of the suprastructure. The retentive pins that traverse the corresponding holes in the substructure can be adjusted easily to provide adequate frictional retention as the necessity arises.

Limitations

In general, the limitations associated with use of the fixed removable prostheses are similar to those encountered in conventional fixed partial dentures.

Abutment requirements

The abutment requirements for the fixed removable partial denture are identical to those of the fixed partial denture. Both modalities derive their entire support from the abutment teeth, none from the residual ridge or teeth in other areas of the arch.

Common path of insertion

All abutment teeth are tied or splinted together through the rigid connection to the substructure bar, a condition comparable to that in the fixed partial denture when the abutments are affixed to one another through the interposed pontic section. Accordingly, the path of placement and removal of the retentive elements of the abutment preparations must be in directional harmony with each other. Long axes of the teeth that are to serve as abutments must be sufficiently harmonious so that the preparation of the teeth may present the required degree of parallelism and occlusogingival length to provide adequate retention and stability. An even more critical relationship exists in those instances wherein multiple abutments are used. The feasibility of placing a fixed or fixed removable prosthesis can be severely compromised if serious misalignment of the abutment teeth is encountered.

Crown to root ratio

The bony support of the abutment teeth as influenced by root morphology and length, amount and character of supporting bone, and ratio of root length embedded in bone to tooth length coronal to the alveolar crest is vital to the success and longevity of any fixed prosthesis. With due consideration to the reported results of recent investigations on periodontal-prosthetic rehabilitation, the prosthodontist is limited in the planning of treatment by the condition of the abutment teeth and their alveolar support (Nyman, 1981; Polson, 1978).

Rotational forces

The axiom of geometry stating that the "shortest distance between two points is a straight line" can be applied to fixed prosthodontics when the relationships of abutments and pontic area are considered. The forces of occlusion applied to the pontic are best resisted by the abutments when members are in comparative alignment (Tylman and Malone, 1978). The more arcuate the pontic in its configuration, the greater the rotational moment that is reflected to and must be resisted by the abutment teeth and the attached prosthesis. The length of span and curvature of the pontic from axial alignment of the abutment teeth are limiting factors to the use of the modality (Schillingburg et al., 1978).

Interocclusal space requirements

A minimum occlusogingival height of 3 to 4 mm is necessary for proper function of the prosthesis. Accordingly, the interocclusal space available between the residual ridge and opposing teeth is a determining factor in the decision to use the fixed removable concept. From a practical standpoint, however, there is usually more than adequate occlusogingival space available since most patients under consideration present damaged ridges and lost alveolar process.

Disadvantages

Gingival response to fixed substructure

When a fixed part of a prosthesis is in continuous contact with soft tissue, patient hygiene of the region becomes a potential problem. This is true with fixed partial dentures and also with the substructure of the fixed removable partial denture.

Being of narrow dimension (1.5 to 2 mm in width) and rounded faciolingually where tissue contact is made, the fixed substructure presents a minimum contact area that can be cleaned easily by the patient with toothbrush and dental floss. Although a distinct possibility, tissue proliferation in the region of contact of bar and ridge has been infrequent.

Precise technical procedures

A limiting factor in the decision to use the fixed removable partial denture as a treatment modality is the availability of personnel familiar with and trained in the technique. Although the technique is not extremely difficult to carry through, a certain degree of fine craftsmanship is necessary. Technicians trained in the use of precision attachments, milled crowns, and other precision and semiprecision elements should experience little difficulty in fabrication. The technique is more time consuming than either a removable partial denture or conventional fixed partial denture.

DISCUSSION

The concept of the fixed removable partial denture provides a combination of some of the best attributes of both fixed and removable partial dentures. It minimizes many of the shortcomings of each modality.

It has proved to be a useful method of restoring moderate-sized defects in the anterior region of both jaws. It has proved to be a comparatively trouble-free treatment modality with a service expectancy of many years. Repairs of the suprastructure can be made with ease. Failure of the substructure assembly has been found to be infrequent. When such failure has occurred, however, it has required major modifications similar to those experienced with corresponding failure of a conventional fixed partial denture.

The concept is one that lends itself to a variety of treatment variations. It can be a most useful part of a dentist's armamentarium for treatment of defects in the anterior region of the mouth.

REFERENCES

Nyman, S.: Prosthetic treatment of patients with advanced periodontal disease. Presented before the American Academy of Restorative Dentistry, 1981.

Polson, A.: Prosthetic rehabilitation of patients with advanced periodontal disease. Presented before the Academy of Denture Prosthetics, 1978.

Schillingburg, H.T., Hobo, S., and Whitsett, L.D.: Fundamentals of fixed prosthodontics, Chicago, 1978, Quintessence Publishing Co.

Schwartz, J.R.: Modern methods of tooth replacement, Dent. Items Interest, 1948, p. 240.

Steiger, A.A., and Boitel, R.H.: Precision work for partial dentures, Zurich, 1951, Buchdruckerei Berichthaus.

Tylman, S.D., and Malone, W.F.P.: Tylman's theory and practice of fixed prosthodontics, ed 7. St. Louis, 1978, The C.V. Mosby Co.

CHAPTER 15

PROVISIONAL CROWNS, SPLINTS, AND FIXED PARTIAL DENTURES

WAYNE V. CAMPAGNI and C. WAYNE CASWELL

provisional restoration A dental prosthesis worn for varying periods of time which maintains esthetics, provides masticating surfaces, and protects the hard and soft tissues.

The provisional restoration is frequently the patient's first impression of the final prosthesis. It should be representative of the final esthetic result, but even more importantly, it must replace the missing tooth structure and maintain a healthy environment for the adjacent soft tissues (Fig. 15-1).

A provisional restoration should satisfy the following criteria:

1. It should afford protection and stability for the prepared teeth.
2. It should provide masticatory function and its contours should provide a basis for proper phonetics.
3. It should provide an esthetic replacement of missing tooth structure and should provide the patient a preview of the cosmetic possibilities of the final result.
4. It should provide a stable and functional occlusion in the anterior as well as the posterior region of the mouth.
5. It should promote good oral hygiene and prevent irritation of the gingival tissues.
6. It should exhibit strength and wear resistance and be color stable.

Provisional restorations are placed to protect the abutment teeth from the insults of function and extreme temperatures so that the patient may remain comfortable until the prescribed restoration is placed. They must be contoured to allow adequate plaque control using routine methods of oral hygiene so that optimum tissue health may be maintained during this phase of treatment (Fig. 15-2).

The provisional restoration should be fabricated to resemble the final restoration as closely as can be envisioned. It is at this stage of the treatment sequence that modifications of occlusion and alteration of tooth contour for appearance and hygiene can be made quickly and easily. Cosmetic modification should be made with input from the patient and used as a guide for the fabrication of the final prosthetic treatment.

Skurow and Lytle (1971) have stated, "Probably the most predictable way to establish an adequate and healthy embrasure zone is with the provisional restoration, moving to the final restoration by changing materials only." The provisional restoration should incorporate the highest standards of physiologic form in regard to occlusion, axial contours, proximal embrasures, pontic form, and marginal integrity that the material used for its fabrication will allow.

Many materials have been used for the fabrication of provisional restorations. For single posterior crowns, a well-adapted aluminum crown may suffice. In those instances where a number of teeth are involved and cosmetic provisional restorations are required, one of the tooth-colored resin materials should be employed.

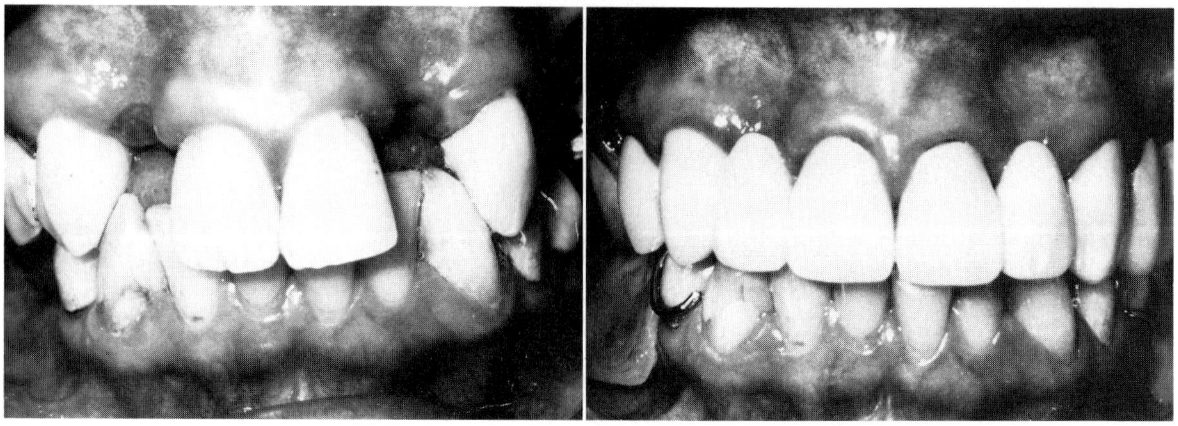

Fig. 15-1. A, Poor esthetics from missing and damaged teeth. **B,** Provisional restorations restore esthetics and maintain good tissue health. Note open gingival embrasures, which allow proper hygiene and improve tissue health.

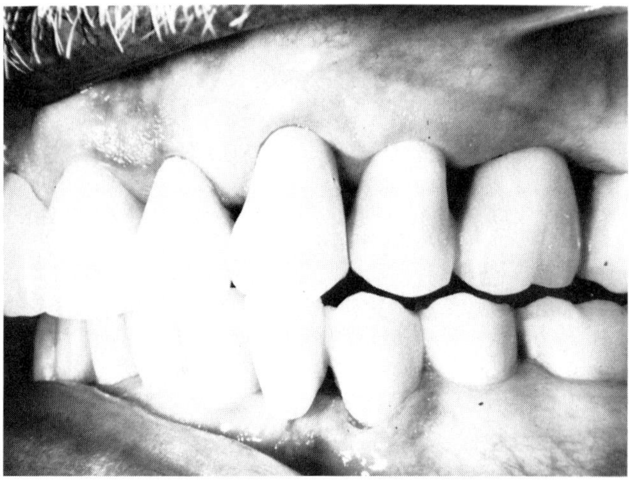

Fig. 15-2. Provisional restoration with proper axial contour, marginal integrity, and embrasure form to allow optimum oral hygiene. (Photograph courtesy Dr. Han Ook Scuble.)

USE OF PROVISIONAL RESTORATIONS AS DIAGNOSTIC AIDS

Provisional restorations can be very useful in diagnosis for the following factors:

1. Establishment of occlusal plane
2. Replacement of missing teeth
3. Determining path of insertion
4. Evaluation of pontic design
5. Evaluation of patient's esthetic demands
6. Establishment of proper tooth contour and form

Diagnostic waxing may be developed to evaluate and reestablish the occlusal plane. At the same time pontic contours may be developed, the completed waxup duplicated with irreversible hydrocolloid (alginate impression material), and a durable cast made for fabrication of matrices (templates) to be used in the fabrication of provisional restorations (Fig. 15-3).

TYPES OF PROVISIONAL RESTORATIONS

Preformed crowns

Various types of preformed crowns have been and are readily available from several different manufacturers. Such products find greatest use for protection of individual teeth that are being restored and need protection for only a short period of time. Thin metal crown forms of aluminum or tin-silver can be adapted to the occlusion, contact with adjacent teeth, and trimmed to the contour of the marginal gingivae (Fig. 15-4).

Provisional coverage of individual anterior teeth can be made quickly with crown forms of clear celluloid (Fig. 15-5) or tooth-colored shells of polycarbonate (Fig. 15-6, *A* and *B*). These crown forms can be trimmed to conform to the gingival contour and filled with autopolymerizing resin. After setting of the resin the excess can be trimmed and polished and the crowns seated

A B C D E

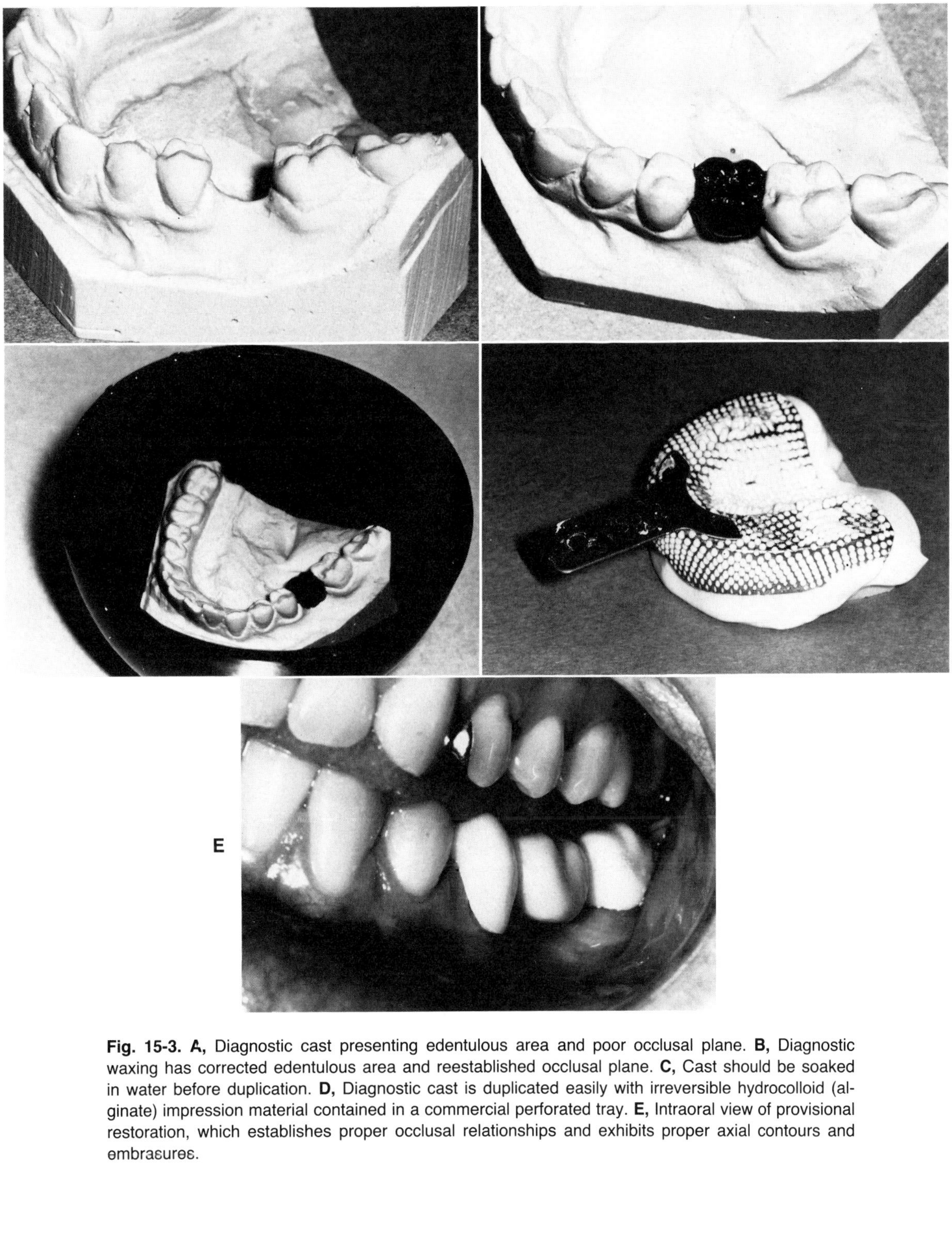

Fig. 15-3. A, Diagnostic cast presenting edentulous area and poor occlusal plane. **B,** Diagnostic waxing has corrected edentulous area and reestablished occlusal plane. **C,** Cast should be soaked in water before duplication. **D,** Diagnostic cast is duplicated easily with irreversible hydrocolloid (alginate) impression material contained in a commercial perforated tray. **E,** Intraoral view of provisional restoration, which establishes proper occlusal relationships and exhibits proper axial contours and embrasures.

A

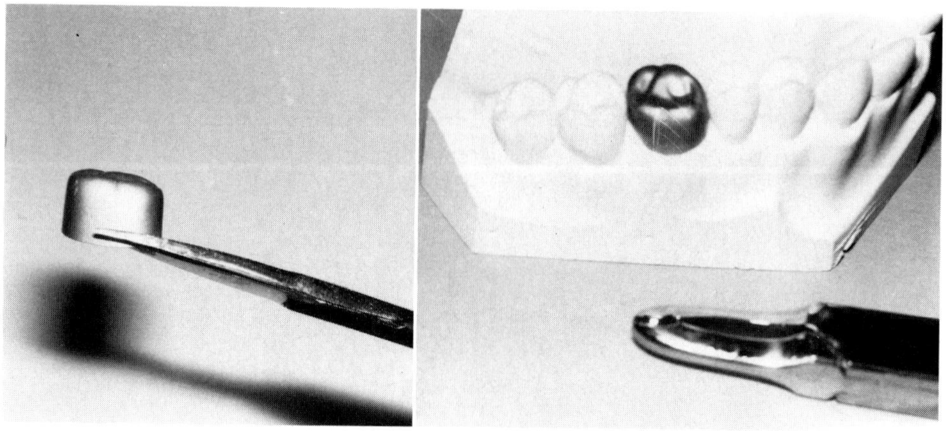

B

Fig. 15-4. A, Aluminum shell crown can be trimmed to approximate gingival contour and adapted to serve as a provisional crown for a short period of time. **B,** Thin metal shell crowns properly contoured with contouring pliers.

A

B

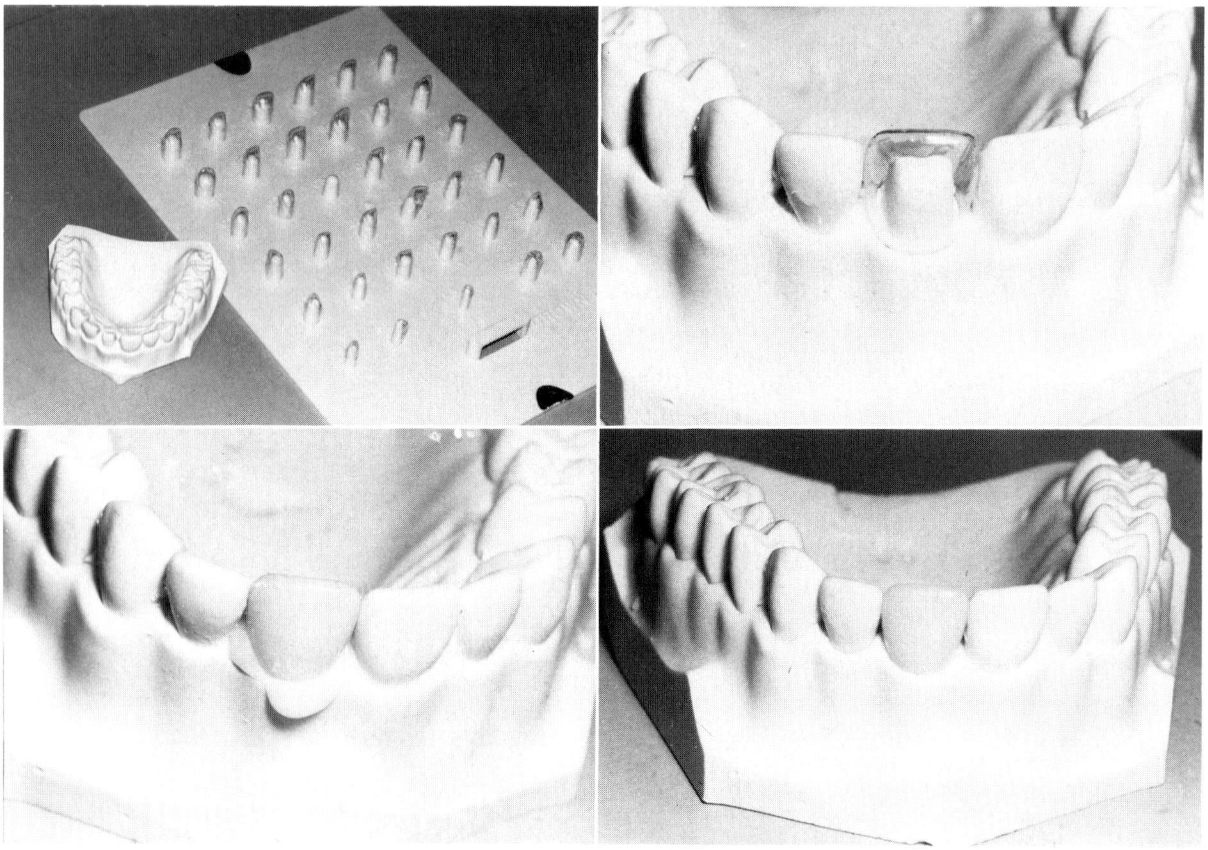

C

D

Fig. 15-5. A, Celluloid crown forms may be used as a matrix to fabricate esthetic resin provisional crowns. **B,** Proper-size celluloid crown form adapted to contour of gingival margin. **C,** Acrylic resin is adapted to prepared tooth in a celluloid crown form. **D,** Well-adapted and contoured acrylic resin provisional crown fabricated with a celluloid crown.

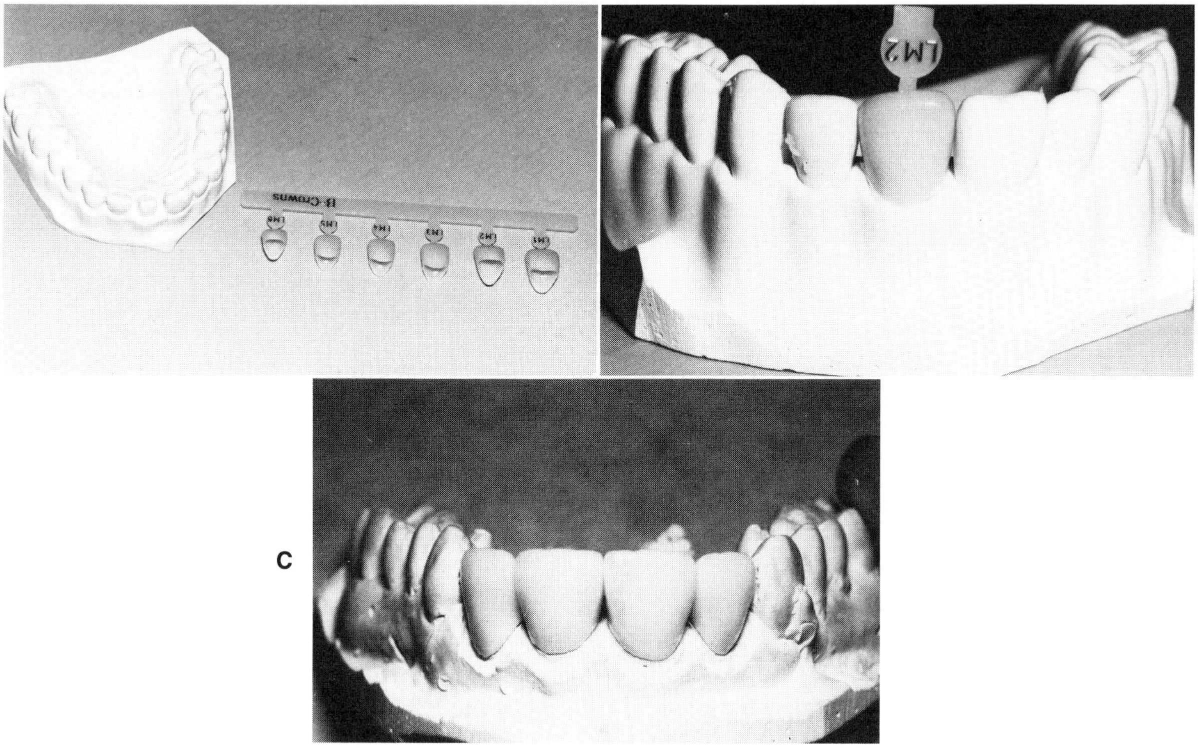

Fig. 15-6. A, Polycarbonate shell mold guide for selection of proper sized crown form. **B,** Adapted and contoured polycarbonate crown. **C,** Multiple polycarbonate crowns.

with a provisional cement (preferably one not containing eugenol) (Fig. 15-6, *C*).

MATERIALS FOR PROVISIONAL RESTORATIONS

Several different types of autopolymerizing resins are currently available and are suitable for the fabrication of provisional restorations: (1) polymethyl methacrylates, (2) polyethyl methacrylates, (3) epimines, and (4) hybrids. Table 15-1 lists these materials with their advantages and disadvantages. Table 15-2 is a list of several of the commercial products available in each classification.

Polymethyl methacrylates

Polymethyl methacrylate is the acrylic resin most often used in dentistry. These materials resemble those used for complete dentures, except that they are tinted with tooth-colored pigments rather than varying shades of pink. They possess the best physical properties of the acrylic resins available for provisional restorations. They have the disadvantage of a high heat of polymerization (165°F, 71°C) and the monomer is irritating to the pulpal and gingival tissues. In addition they have a high volumetric shrinkage. When they are fabricated correctly, however, they provide restorations that are durable enough to last from several months to a year.

Color stability is good, they are capable of a high polish, and they can be finished to a fine margin. Crowns and splints made with these resins are acceptable biologically and may serve as a long-term interim protection in more extensive prosthetic or periodontal-prosthetic treatment.

The material is supplied in two parts: a monomer (methyl methacrylate) and a powder (polymethyl methacrylate). The polymer contains pigments, an activator (benzoyl peroxide) to start polymerization, inhibitors to increase shelf life, and cross-linking agents to prevent crazing.

Polymerization of polymethyl methacrylate and other resins can occur in two different ways: first, a chemical activation of the benzoyl peroxide by a tertiary amine such as dimethyl-*p*-toluidine. This is contained in the monomer. When the monomer and polymer are mixed, polymerization occurs at room temperature. This is called self-curing, cold curing, or autopolymerization. Second, benzoyl peroxide can be activated by heat. When the mixture of monomer and polymer is heated to 165°F (74°C), the benzoyl peroxide is activated and polymerization occurs.

Table 15-1. Classification of resins for provisionals

Material	Advantages	Disadvantages	Indications
Polymethyl methacrylates (PMM)	Best abrasion resistance Best color stability Good polishability Good marginal finish	High heat of polymerization (165°F) High shrinkage Monomer irritating to pulp Eugenol deteriorates resin	Indirect techniques Long-term provisionals
Polyethyl methacrylates (PEM)	Low shrinkage Rubber stage to set Lower heat of polymerization (125°F) Longer working time	Poor hardness Poor abrasion resistance Poor color stability Poor finishability Eugenol deteriorates resin	Short-term provisionals (1 to 3 weeks) Direct technique
Epimine	Lowest shrinkage Negligible heat of polymerization Lowest pulpal irritability Eugenol does not affect resin	High cost/unit Air bubbles Poorest in color stability, hardness, abrasion resistance Cannot be corrected by additions	Most biologically compatible when used in direct technique
Hybrids	See text	See text	Require further clinical testing to establish efficacy

Table 15-2. Partial list of resins for provisionals according to type

Material	Product	Manufacturer
Polymethyl methacrylate (PMM)	Jet Acrylic Durlay Temporary C & B Kit Temporary Bridge Resin	Lang Dental Mfg. Co., Chicago, Ill. Reliance Dental Mfg. Co., Worth, Ill. L. D. Caulk Co., Milford, Del.
Polyethyl methacrylate (PEM)	Splint line Trim Snap Aristocrat HTC	Lang Dental Mfg. Co., Chicago, Ill. H. J. Bosworth Co., Skokie, Ill. Parkell Biomaterials Division, Farmingdale, N.Y. Healthco Dental Supply, Boston, Mass.
Epimine	Scutan	Premier Dental Products Co., Norristown, Pa.
Hybrids	Kind (PEM + Bis GMA) Kind Radiopaque (barium glass added) Dentalon (PMM + isobutyl methacrylate monomer) Protemp (Bis Acrylic composite)	Den-Mat Corp., Santa Maria, Calif. Kulzer Inc., Irvine, Calif. ESPE-Premier Sales Corp., Norristown, Pa.

Polyethyl methacrylates

The polyethyl methacrylates do not possess the hardness and abrasion resistance of the polymethyl methacrylates. In addition, they are not capable of as fine marginal adaptation and polish as are the harder materials. Their advantage lies in a lower heat of polymerization (125°F, 51.5°C). They also pass through a rubbery stage in the setting reaction which allows ease of removal from the teeth with miminal distoration. They exhibit a long working time. These properties, paired with their lower shrinkage values, make them especially well suited for use in direct provisional techniques. The low abrasion resistance, hardness, and relatively poor color stability should limit their application to short-span restorations that require a short period of service.

Epimines

Only one epimine resin (Scutan*) is currently available for use by the profession for the fabrication of provisional restorations. The material exhibits a very low polymerization temperature (102°F, 39°C) and has a low residual monomer content (4% after polymerization). One of its greatest advantages is its very low shrinkage upon polymerization. Its accuracy makes it particularly well suited for "direct" techniques.

Hybrids

Several new hybrid products are available to the profession. They are a combination of two or more types of materials. One (Pro-temp*) is a bis-acrylic composite resin and should possess high strength. It can be corrected by addition. It is intended for use in long-span restorations. Limited clinical experience with this material has found it to be brittle in service. Repairs and additions are difficult. Mixing is more difficult than with the other resins and bubbles are easily incorporated into the mass.

Another new hybrid material (Kind†) is a polyethyl methylacrylate filled with a bis-acrylic resin. It exhibits a very high heat of polymerization. It is also available with barium glass as a filler to make it radiopaque. This radiopaque material, however, does not flow as readily as do some of the other materials.

A third material (Dentalon) is a polymethyl methacrylate meshed with an isobutyl methacrylate monomer. It has physical and handling properties that place it between the polymethyl methacrylates and the polyethyl methacrylates. At this time only limited clinical testing has been done with this hybrid material, and its long-term advantage still must be determined.

MATRICES FOR PROVISIONAL RESTORATIONS

Many different materials have been employed to serve as matrices for forming the autopolymerizing resin used to fabricate provisional restorations. The matrix or overimpression can be made of wax (softened and placed in a suitable carrier), irreversible hydrocolloid (alginate), or silicone putty material. Matrices of this type may be made directly upon the teeth before they have been prepared or upon a cast of the teeth that has had the edentulous spaced blocked out and undercut areas eliminated (Figs. 15-7 and 15-8). The silicone putty and wax (after chilling) provide a more positive seat against the teeth and adjacent tissues than does the alginate matrix and are generally preferred.

*Premier Dental Products Co., Norristown, Pa.
†Den-Mat Corp., Santa Maria, Calif.

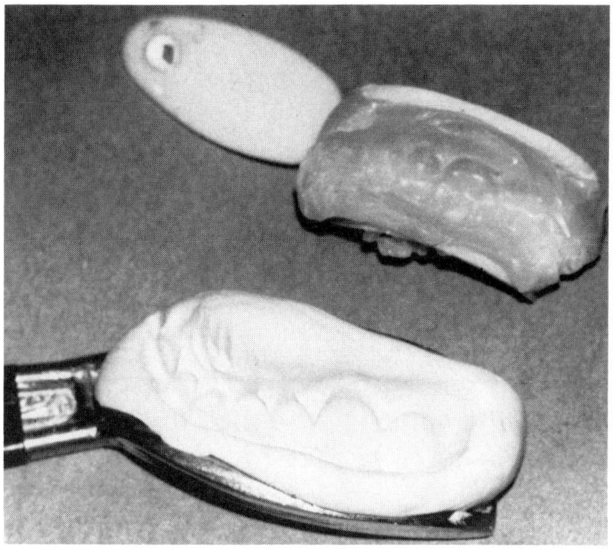

Fig. 15-7. Overimpressions of wax and silicone putty made directly from teeth for fabrication of a provisional restoration.

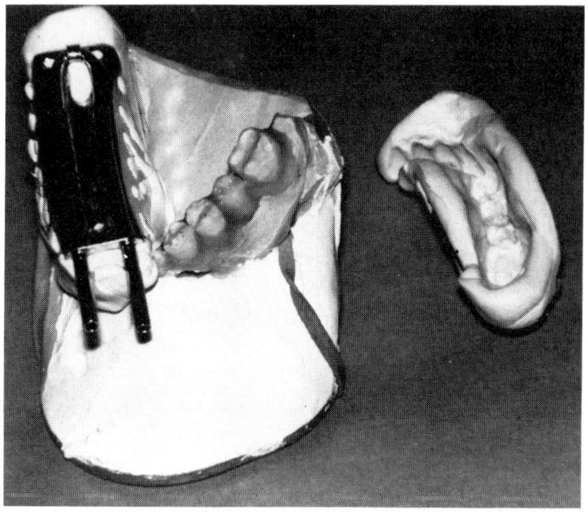

Fig. 15-8. Diagnostic cast with a denture tooth positioned in edentulous space and gingival undercut areas filled to provide additional bulk of resin during fabrication of the provisional restoration. Silicone putty impression will serve as a matrix for making provisional restoration.

Silicone putty matrix

Silicone putty, when properly adapted, produces a very accurate negative reproduction of the cast. The matrix should extend at least one tooth on either side beyond the teeth to be prepared (Fig. 15-9). In those instances where the last tooth in the arch is to be covered with a provisional restoration, the matrix material should be extended onto the adjacent residual ridge. The most efficient and versatile matrices, however, are

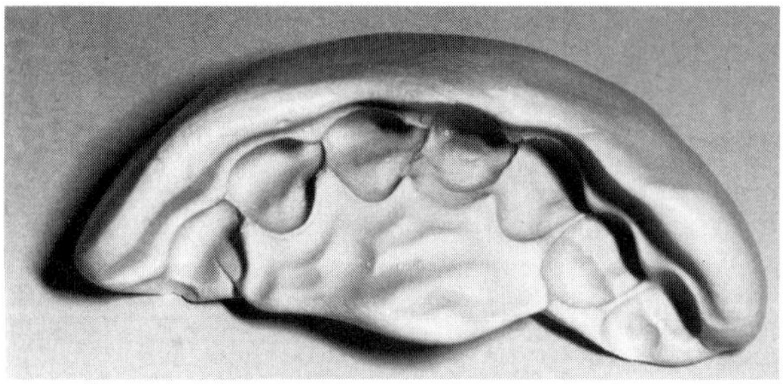

Fig. 15-9. A silicone putty matrix of anterior teeth showing details that can be copied.

those made of thin polypropylene, polyvinyl, or acetate sheet. The softened sheet plastic is adapted to a cast of the patient's dental arch either by vacuum forming or by compression molding with a counter die system.

These thin plastic matrices have many other uses in addition to fabricating provisional restorations. Krug (1973) and Preston (1976) have described other uses for the plastic matrices:

1. Use as preparation guide to determine adequate tooth reduction.
2. Fabricate provisional restorations directly or indirectly.
3. Develop full contour waxing.
4. Aid in cutback design and metal frame design for metal ceramic restorations.

Fabrication of polypropylene, polyvinyl, or acetate sheet matrices

Vacuum/pressure method

Vacuum-forming apparatus (Fig. 15-10, *A*) has an important position in the dental laboratory. The equipment has found many uses. Fabrication of resilient mouth guards, occusal splints, record bases, custom impression trays, templates, and matrices are only a few of the numerous applications of which this versatile apparatus is capable.

PROCEDURE FOR THIN PLASTIC MATRICES

1. The diagnostic cast to be replicated is placed on the vacuum grid (Fig. 15-10, *B*).

2. A sheet of polypropylene or polyvinyl resin 0.020 inch in thickness is mounted below the heating element and heated until it softens and sags approximately 1½ to 2 inches.

3. The vacuum is turned on and the holder that retains the plastic sheet is dropped to form a seal on the vacuum plate (Fig. 15-10, *C*).

4. As the air is evacuated around the cast, the softened plastic sheet will be adapted closely to the contours of the cast (Fig. 15-10, *D* and *E*).

5. The adapted matrix is removed from the cast and trimmed to proper extensions.

In those instances where the cast is large or where small matrices are desired, the cast may be sectioned and individual matrices may be formed for each segment (Fig. 15-10, *F* and *G*).

Compression forming method

A stone cast is used as a base for the matrix, which will be closely adapted by pressing the soft sheet plastic against it. After cooling, the matrix is trimmed to the desired dimensions. The necessary items for this technique are:

1. A bunsen burner
2. A wire frame to support the plastic sheet while it is heated
3. Silicone spray mold release agent to prevent adherance of the softened plastic to the cast
4. Silicone putty with which to adapt the matrix material to the cast (Fig. 15-11, *A*)

PROCEDURE

1. The plastic sheet (0.020 inch polypropylene or polyvinyl) is placed in the wire holder and sprayed with silicone mold release agent (Fig. 15-11, *B*). The cast to be replicated is also sprayed with the mold release agent to prevent adherence of the plastic (Fig. 15-11, *C*).

2. The plastic is heated over a bunsen burner slowly and evenly until it is completely softened, clear, and sagging. Heating should take place around the edges or periphery first, gradually moving the heat toward the center of the plastic (Fig. 15-11, *D*).

3. The soft plastic sheet is placed over the cast and the silicone putty pressed firmly against it to adapt it to the critical areas of the cast. The plastic should be allowed to cool before separation from the cast is attempted (Fig. 15-11, *E* and *F*).

4. The closely adapted resin matrix can be removed from the cast and excess material trimmed with scissors (Fig. 15-11, *G*).

At times it may be necessary to reproduce contours developed in a diagnostic waxup of casts, either from modification of occlusal plane and occlusal relation-

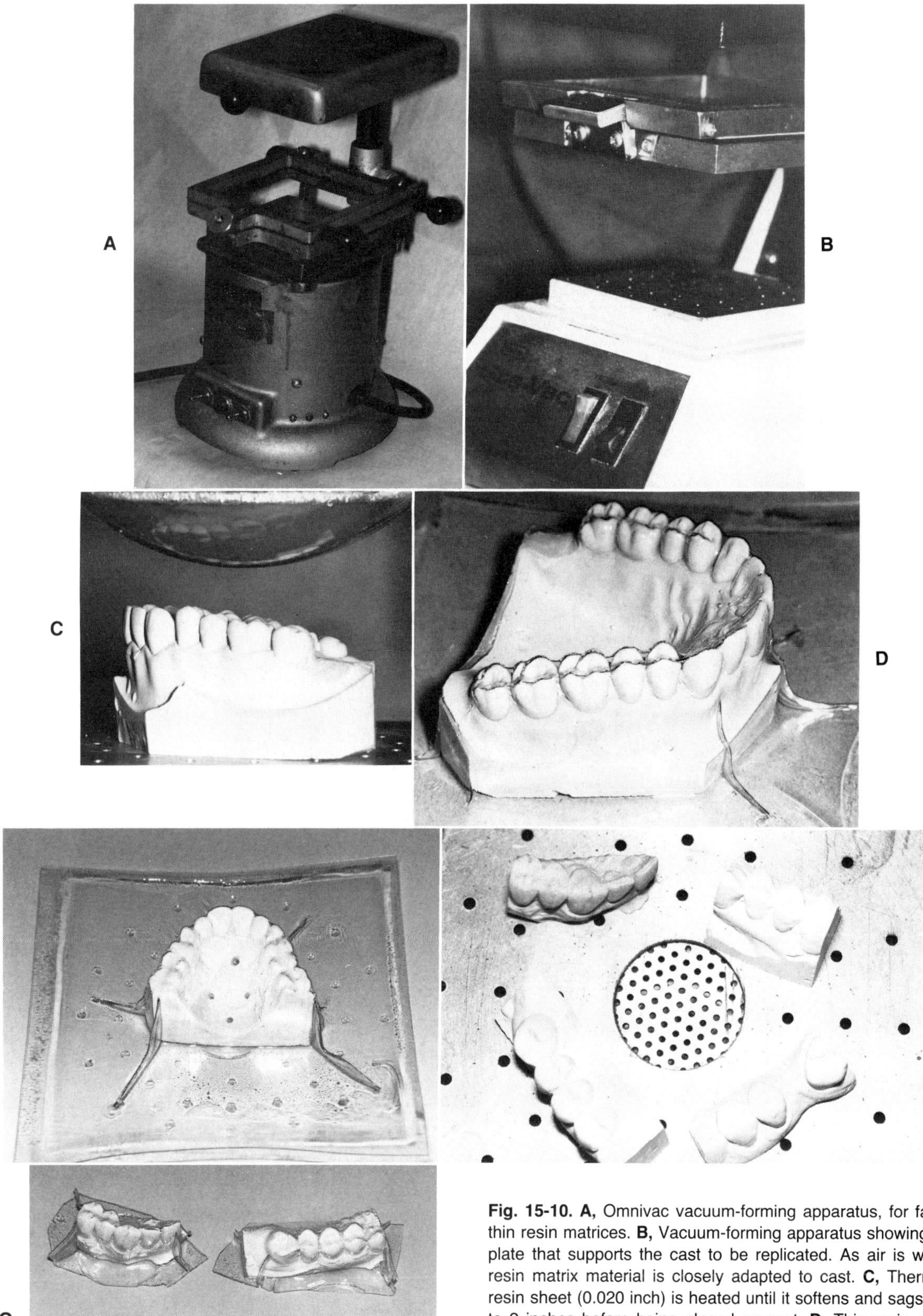

Fig. 15-10. A, Omnivac vacuum-forming apparatus, for fabricating thin resin matrices. **B,** Vacuum-forming apparatus showing vacuum plate that supports the cast to be replicated. As air is withdrawn, resin matrix material is closely adapted to cast. **C,** Thermoplastic resin sheet (0.020 inch) is heated until it softens and sags from 1½ to 2 inches before being placed on cast. **D,** Thin resin sheet has been closely adapted to contours of teeth on cast. **E,** Holes placed in center of cast aid in withdrawal of air during vacuum-forming adaptation. **F,** Multiple matrices may be formed simultaneously with the vacuum-forming procedure. **G,** Small casts that have had matrices adapted simultaneously.

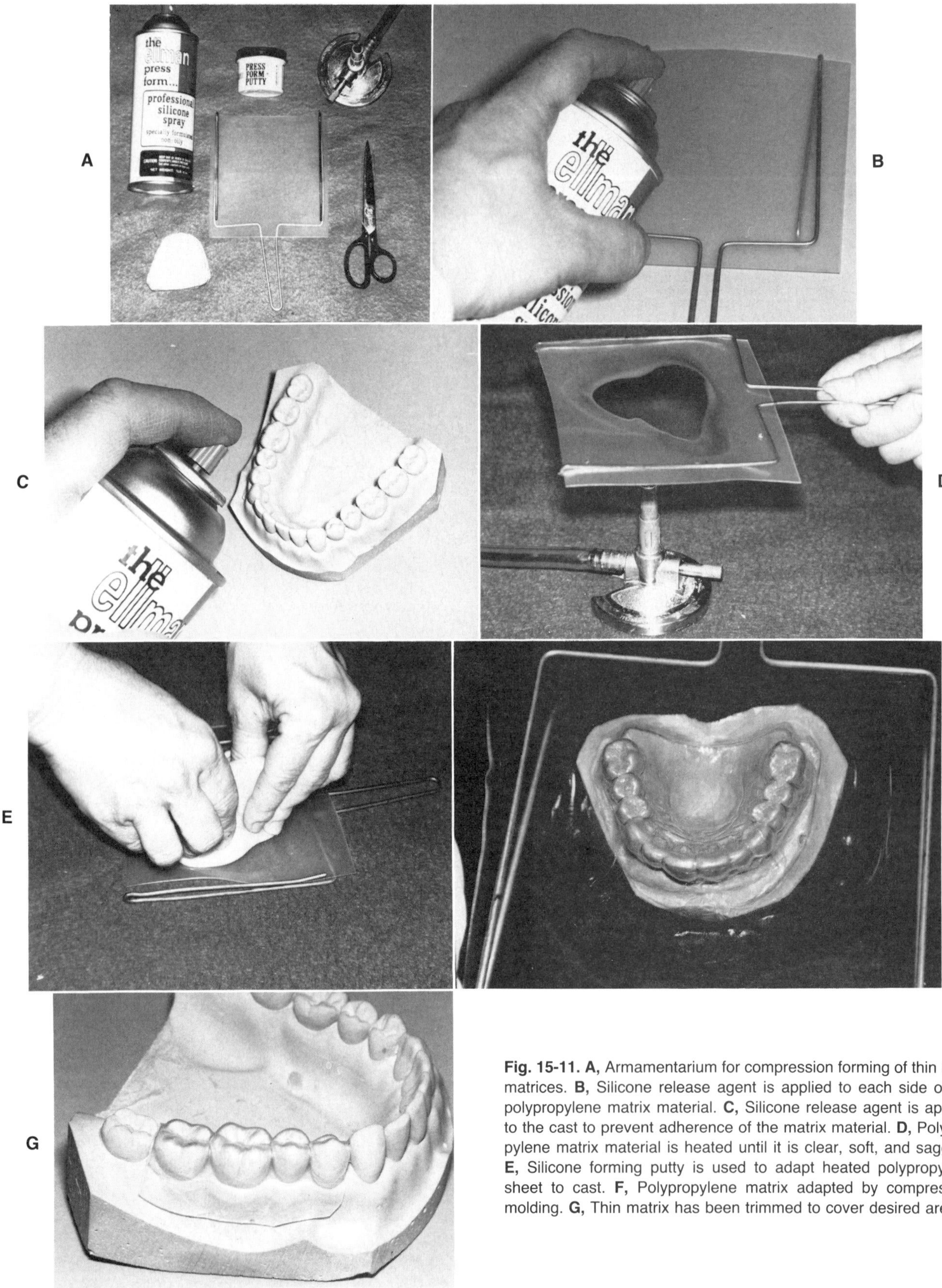

Fig. 15-11. A, Armamentarium for compression forming of thin resin matrices. **B,** Silicone release agent is applied to each side of the polypropylene matrix material. **C,** Silicone release agent is applied to the cast to prevent adherence of the matrix material. **D,** Polypropylene matrix material is heated until it is clear, soft, and sagging. **E,** Silicone forming putty is used to adapt heated polypropylene sheet to cast. **F,** Polypropylene matrix adapted by compression molding. **G,** Thin matrix has been trimmed to cover desired area.

A

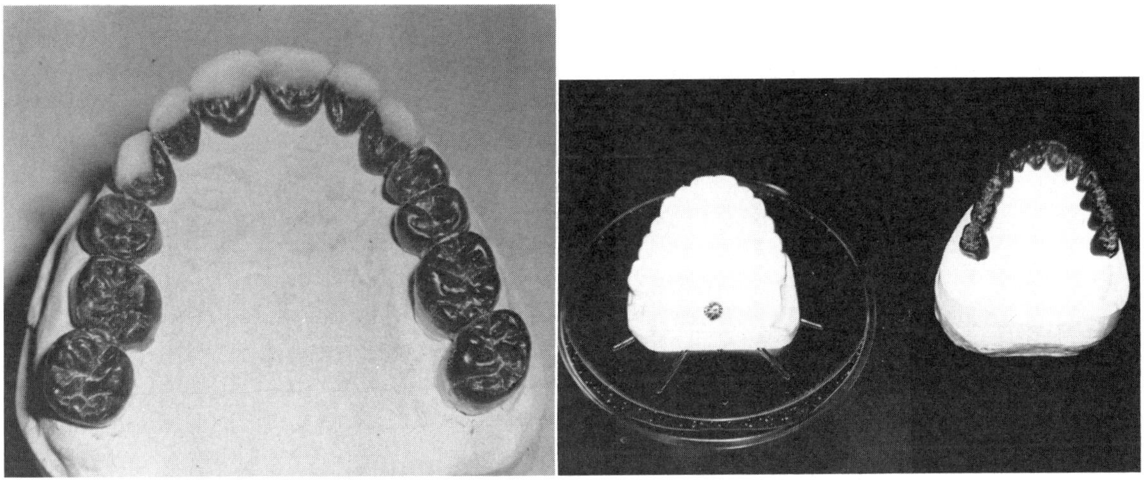

B

Fig. 15-12. A, Diagnostic cast has been modified extensively. **B,** Diagnostic waxup and duplicate cast made from an irreversible hydrocolloid impression.

ships, or where cosmetic realignment of the teeth has been made (Fig. 15-12, *A*). Wax contours cannot be replicated directly because of wax distortion in contact with the hot plastic. The diagnostic waxup is duplicated with irreversible hydrocolloid (alginate) and the resultant cast used to form the thin plastic matrix (Fig. 15-12, *B*).

Techniques for provisional restorations

The three techniques for provisional restorations are (1) direct, (2) indirect, and (3) indirect direct reline (eggshell). All techniques require that a preimpression or matrix be made to serve as a form or mold for the restoration. This mold or form is filled with an autopolymerizing resin and carried to position directly over the prepared teeth or onto a cast of the teeth after they have been prepared.

Custom-made restorations

There are several methods by which custom-made provisional restorations may be fabricated. The particular method employed will be determined, in part, by the extent and complexity of the coverage required and by the length of time it is anticipated that the appliance will be needed.

DIRECT TECHNIQUE

The direct technique entails fabrication of a provisional restoration with autopolymerizing resin directly upon the prepared teeth.

PROCEDURE

1. The diagnostic cast of the arch to be treated is modified as necessary by diagnostic waxing, an impression made with irreversible hydrocolloid (alginate), and a cast produced (Fig. 15-13).

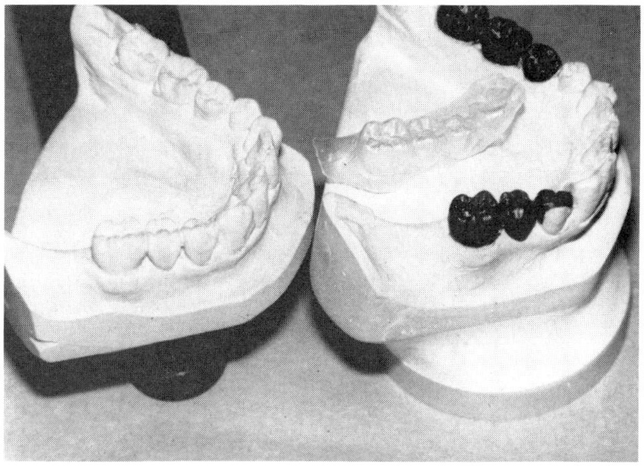

Fig. 15-13. Diagnostic cast modified by waxing duplicate cast.

2. A thin plastic shell or matrix of polypropylene or polyvinyl, 0.020 inch in thickness, is formed and trimmed as illustrated in Fig. 15-13.

3. After the teeth are prepared, and the soft tissue displaced from the subgingival margins, silicone grease is applied to the prepared tooth surfaces for protection against the irritating effects of the monomer.

4. Autopolymerizing resin is placed in the matrix, which is seated over the prepared teeth. One advantage of the plastic matrix is that the thinness allows the patient to close his teeth, thereby allowing occlusion to be developed more accurately (Fig. 15-14). Cool water should be played over the matrix to minimize the heat developed during polymerization. The setting of the

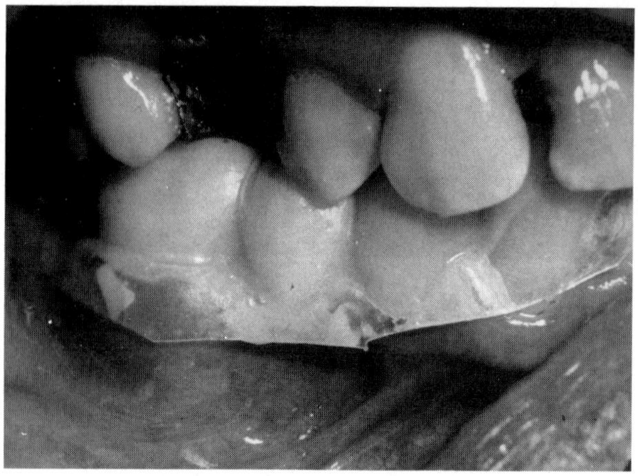

Fig. 15-14. Thin resin matrix filled with autopolymerizing resin being used to fabricate a provisional restoration by direct technique.

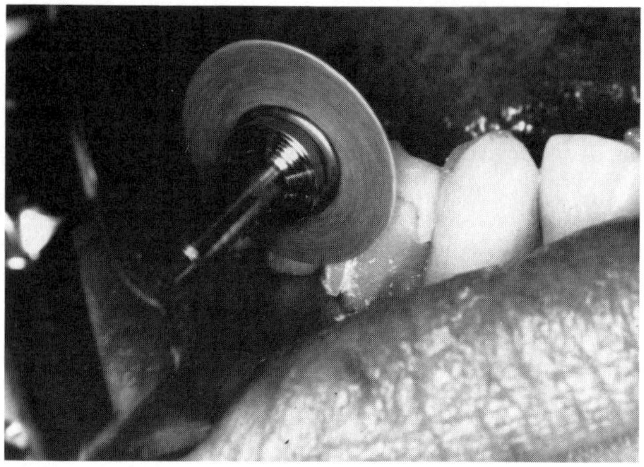

Fig. 15-15. Nonabrasive side of sandpaper disk can be used to remove bulk and refine accessible margins of provisional restoration. Care must be exercised that delicate margins of preparation not be damaged or modified by the disk.

resin should be tested at regular frequent intervals to determine the degree of hardness.

If undercut areas are present, or if there is any misalignment of the prepared teeth, it is appropriate to remove the matrix and the resin mass before it has become completely polymerized. Failure to do so may result in the teeth being subjected to excessive heat of polymerization and the material becoming tightly locked onto the teeth.

5. The provisional restoration that has been cast is removed from the matrix, and excess material over margins trimmed and contours refined.

6. The restoration is refitted to the teeth. Any marginal discrepancies can be corrected by addition of small increments of new resin with a small sable or camel's hair brush.

7. Marginal overhangs may be trimmed with suitable small stones and disks, care being taken not to alter any fine exposed margins of the prepared teeth (Fig. 15-15).

8. Occlusion is refined; the restoration is removed from the teeth, polished, and seated with provisional cement.

INDIRECT TECHNIQUE

The fabrication of provisional restorations by an indirect technique has a number of advantages. Restorations made in this manner are usually stronger, fit the teeth more accurately, and because, of their increased density are more biocompatible. The higher density and strength achieved by polymerization of polymethyl methacrylate under pressure at an elevated temperature permits finer margin finish and higher surface polish. Improved fitting of the crowns is achieved through processing against a cast, which limits polymerization shrinkage. Biocompatibility is a result of higher polish, better margin adaptation, and teeth and tissue not being subjected to irritation from the monomer and heat of polymerization.

PROCEDURE

1. Preparation for actual fabrication of the provisional restoration is similar to that described for direct technique. Any necessary diagnostic waxing is performed on the cast, and a duplicate cast embodying those modifications is obtained. A thin polypropylene (plastic) matrix is formed over the modified cast.

2. The teeth are prepared, and the soft tissues are retracted as necessary (Fig. 15-16).

3. An impression is made of the prepared teeth using either irreversible hydrocolloid or other material (reversible hydrocolloid or elastomeric impression material) (Fig. 15-17).

4. The impression is poured with quick-setting plaster, either impression plaster* or "accelerated" stone made by mixing hydrocal powder with "slurry" water. After setting (5 to 10 minutes) the cast is separated, any artifacts (bubbles, etc.) removed, and the peripheral areas trimmed on a margin trimmer (Fig. 15-18).

5. The matrix is fitted to the cast and its complete seating verified (Fig. 15-19).

6. After the trimming away of the portions of the cast that represent gingivae extending above or obscuring the gingival margins, the cast is generously coated with an alginate foil substitute (Fig. 15-20).

---

*Impression Plaster No. 2, Kerr/Sybron, Romulus, Mich.

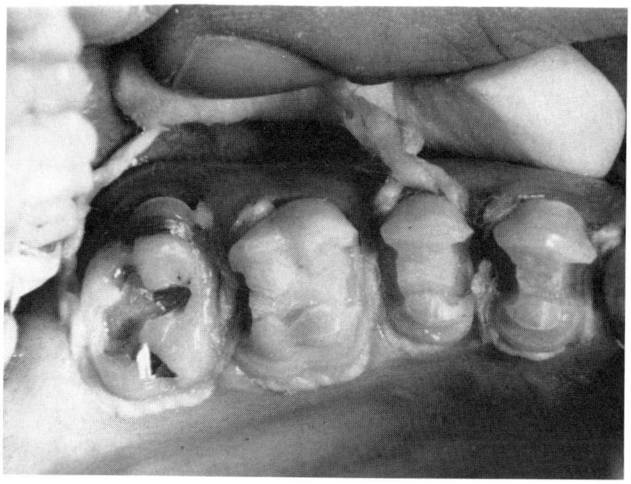

Fig. 15-16. Teeth have been prepared and tissues retracted before fabricating provisional restoration.

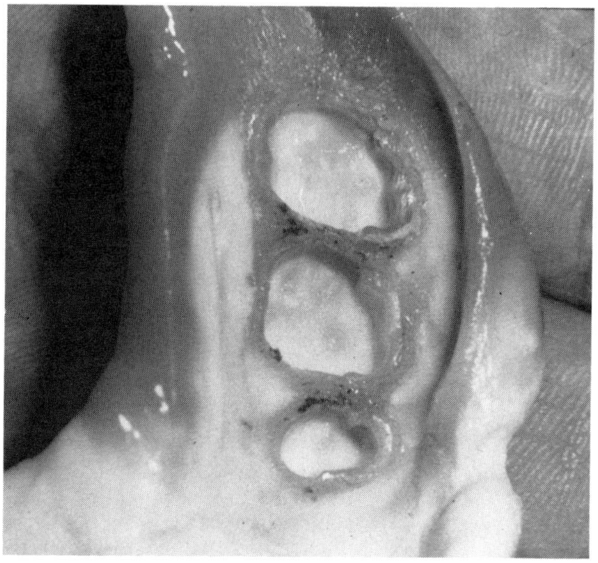

Fig. 15-17. Impression of prepared teeth to be used in fabrication of provisional restoration.

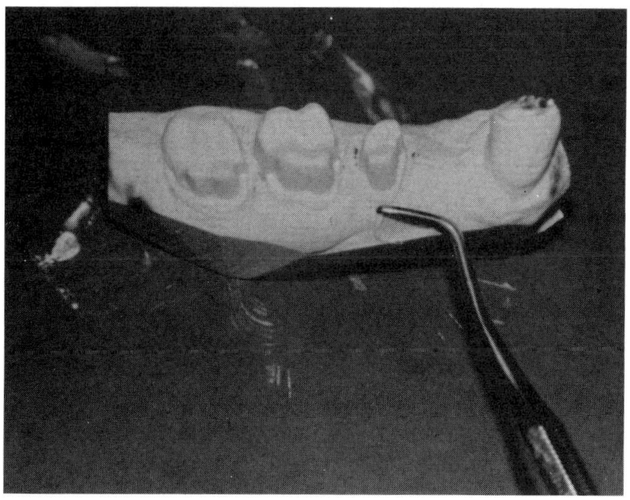

Fig. 15-18. Cast after separation from impression. Artifacts are removed and gingival tissue obscuring subgingival margins is trimmed.

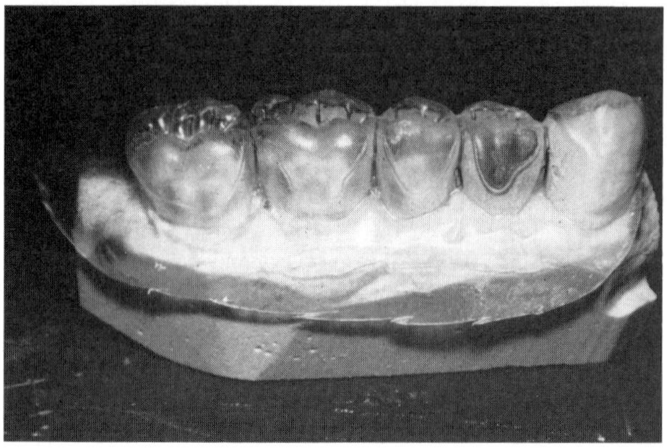

Fig. 15-19. Matrix is placed on trimmed cast to verify seating.

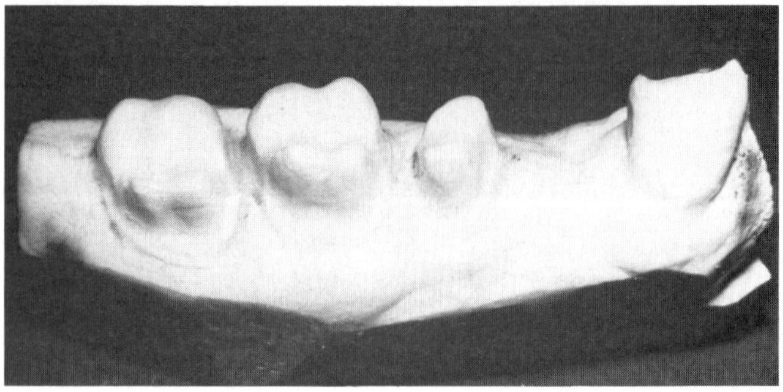

Fig. 15-20. Cast is generously coated with alginate for substitute.

A

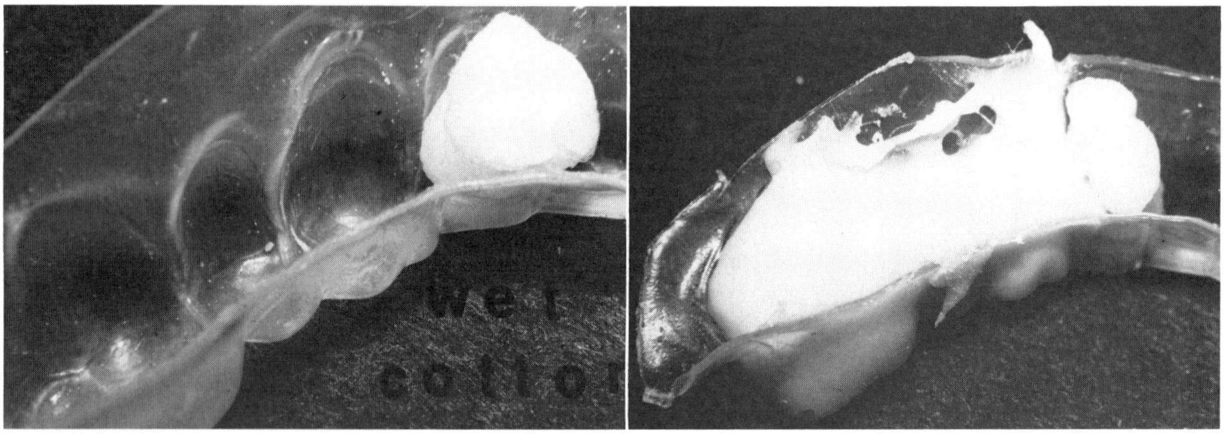

B

Fig. 15-21. A, Areas not to be included in provisional restoration are dammed off with cotton. **B,** matrix is filled with autopolymerizing resin, which is allowed to reach the "frosty" stage.

7. Areas not to be included in the provisional restoration are blocked with wet cotton (Fig. 15-21, *A*).

8. The matrix is filled with a semifluid mix of autopolymerizing acrylic resin of proper shade. When polymerization has progressed to the point that the material has a "frosty" appearance (Fig. 15-21, *B*), the matrix is seated completely on the cast and secured lightly with a rubber band (Fig. 15-22).

9. The cast is placed into a pressure vessel* containing warm water (125° to 130°F, 51° to 54°C) and allowed to complete polymerization under pressure of 20 to 25 p.s.i. for approximately 10 minutes. After removal from the pressure vessel, the matrix is stripped from the polymerized resin, which should be examined for thin areas, voids, or other defects. Before removal from the

*Pronto II Pressure Vessel, Vernon-Benshoff Co., Albany, N.Y.

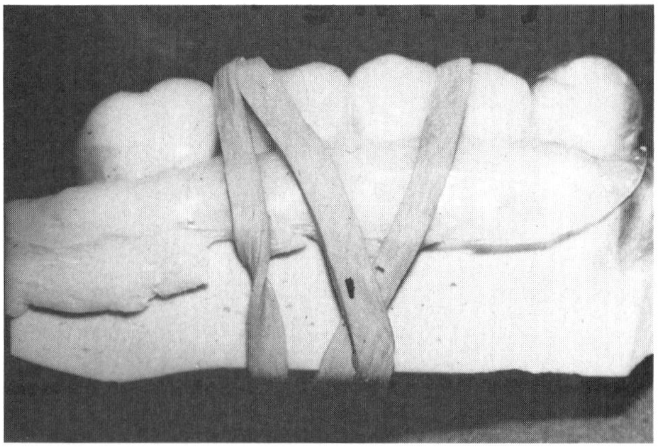

Fig. 15-22. Wet cotton plugs are removed from matrix, which is then completely seated on the cast. Matrix is stabilized lightly with rubber bands and placed in a pressure vessel (125°F at 25 p.s.i.) for polymerization.

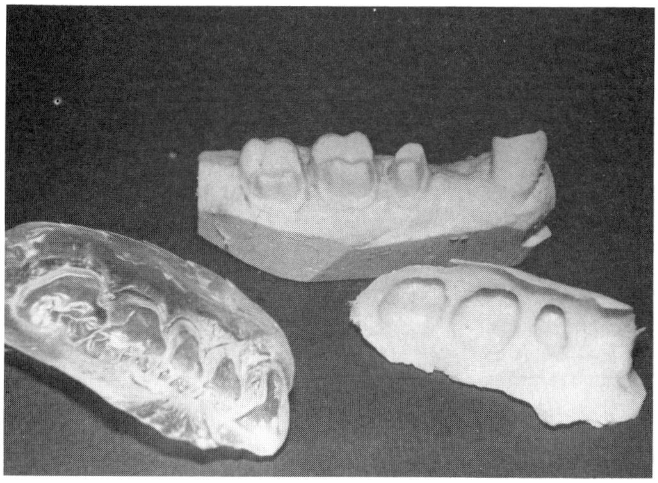

Fig. 15-23. Polymerized provisional restoration separated from the cast and matrix, ready for trimming.

cast any defective areas should be corrected with additional acrylic resin applied with a small sable or camel's hair brush. Any addition should be polymerized under heat and pressure by being returned again to the pressure vessel for several minutes.

10. The rough resin casting of the provisional restoration is removed from the cast (Fig. 15-23). Excess resin is removed with disks and appropriate laboratory burs, and the restoration contoured to the approximate form desired.

11. The restoration is fitted to the teeth; final trimming of gingival margins, gingival embrasures, and axial contours is performed.

12. The occlusion is refined; the restoration is removed, polished, and cemented with appropriate provisional cement.

The indirect-direct reline (eggshell) technique

The indirect-direct technique combines a preexisting "shell" of the provisional restoration with a chairside reline procedure after the teeth have been prepared. The advantage of the technique is that the "shell" can be fabricated as a laboratory procedure prior to the appointment at which the teeth are prepared. A corrective "reline" procedure can be performed easily and quickly after preparation of the teeth. The technique enables fabrication of the provisional restoration, which fits the teeth accurately, which has proper contour, esthetics, and occlusion, and which has been produced with minimum time commitment for the patient.

PROCEDURE

1. The diagnostic cast is modified as necessary by diagnostic waxing, and undercut areas are eliminated with wax to provide for additional bulk of resin later in the procedure (Fig. 15-24).

2. The modified cast is duplicated with irreversible hydrocolloid and a cast is made (Fig. 15-25).

A

B

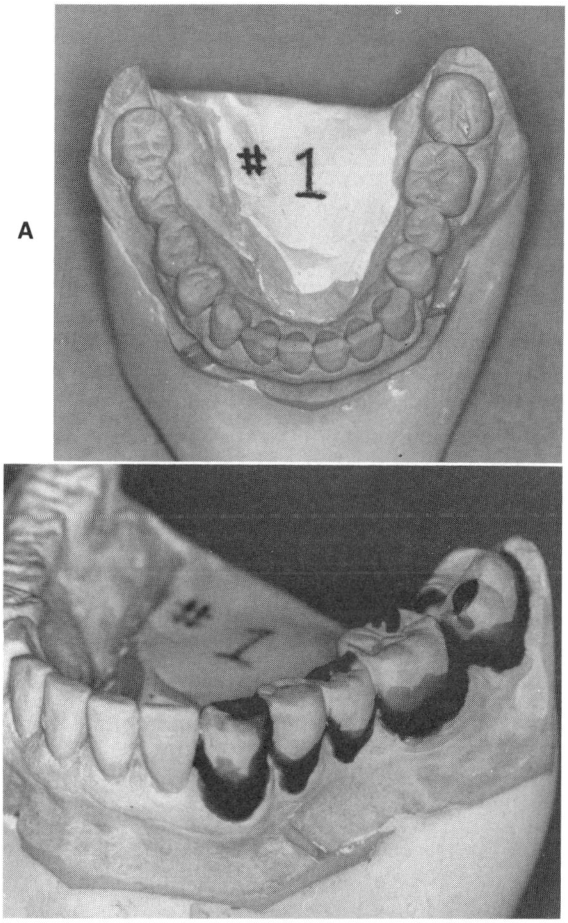

Fig. 15-24. A, Diagnostic cast before modification. **B,** Diagnostic cast after modification of occlusal areas and elimination of undercut areas near gingival margins. Additional bulk of resin will be formed in this area during fabrication to assure adequate thickness for proper trimming of margins.

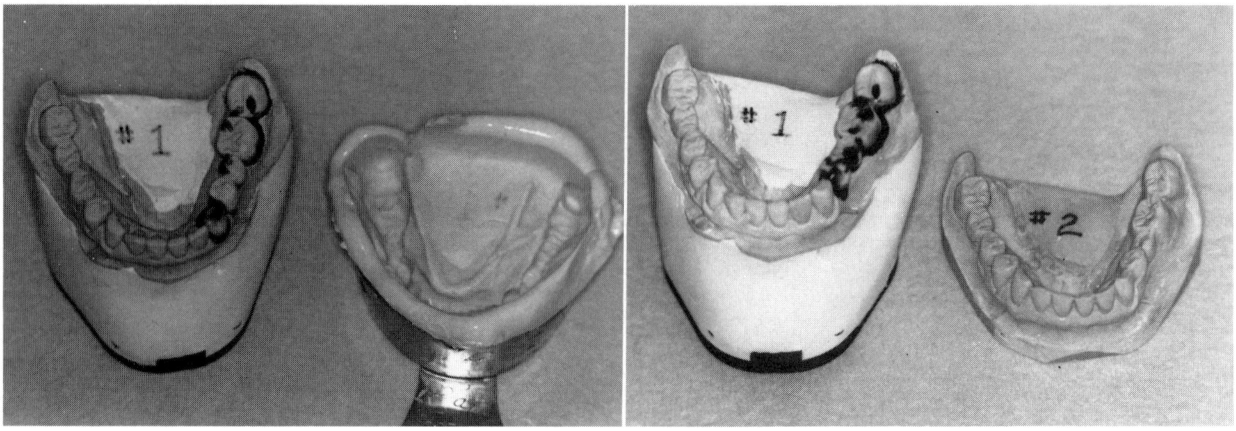

Fig. 15-25. A, Irreversible hydrocolloid after separation from modified diagnostic cast. Maxillary tray has been used so that trimmed area representing the tongue space will be reproduced. **B,** Modified diagnostic cast and duplicate.

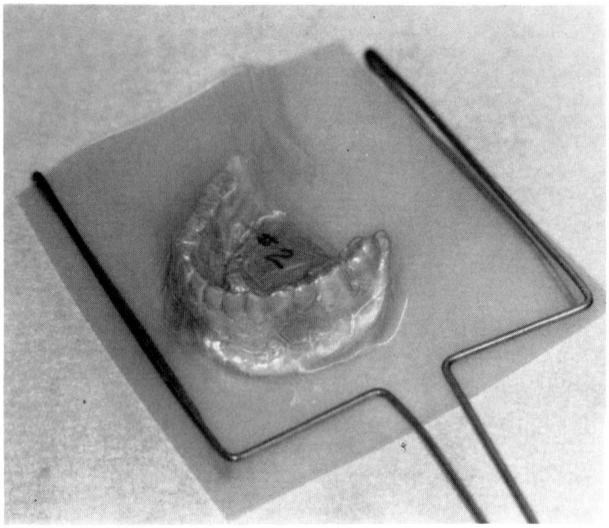

Fig. 15-26. Matrix adapted to duplicate cast.

3. A thin (0.020 inch) matrix of polypropylene or polyvinyl resin is fabricated upon the modified cast (Fig. 15-26).

4. The teeth to be included in the provisional restoration are reduced on the cast to the approximate form anticipated in the actual preparation of the teeth. The preparation of the teeth on the cast should be conservative and reduced less than that planned for the natural teeth so that interference between the preformed shell and the prepared teeth will not occur (Fig. 15-27).

5. The "shell" provisional restoration is fabricated upon the modified cast. A coating of foil substitute is applied to the stone surfaces that will be involved; autopolymerizing polymethyl methacrylate is placed into the matrix, positioned on the cast, and polymerized in a pressure vessel (125°F at 20 p.s.i.). The "shell" provisional restoration casting is removed from the cast, separated from the matrix, and roughly trimmed in preparation for the subsequent reline procedure (Fig. 15-28).

6. At the preparation appointment the teeth are prepared and the soft tissues retracted to expose the subgingival margins. The "shell" is fitted to the teeth. Care should be exercised that no interference is present between the internal surface of the shell and the prepared teeth. The shell should fit freely and completely over the teeth (Fig. 15-29).

7. The "shell" is filled with autopolymerizing resin (either polymethyl methyacrylate or polyethyl methacrylate) that is allowed to undergo partial polymerization (Fig. 15-30) and positioned on the teeth, which have been lubricated with silicone jelly. The patient is instructed to close into normal occlusion to completely seat the reline "shell." During the polymerization period the restoration is released and reseated several times to free the resin from adhering to the teeth. The relined shell should be removed from the teeth immediately before final hardening occurs to prevent possible locking of the resin to the teeth and to avoid subjecting the teeth to the rapid temperature rise which occurs upon final polymerization (Fig. 15-31).

8. The provisional restoration is trimmed, shaped, adjusted for occlusion, polished, and cemented as described in the section on finishing techniques (Fig. 15-32).

A 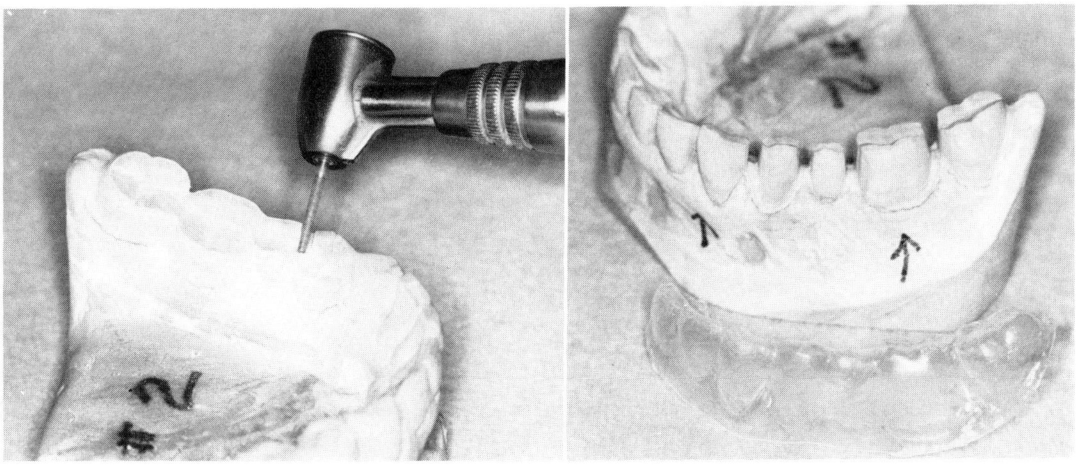 B

Fig. 15-27. A, Teeth on duplicate cast are prepared to approximate preparations planned for the teeth. **B,** Teeth on cast are reduced slightly less than planned reduction of teeth. Conservative reduction or underreduction will prevent interference between prepared natural teeth and inner surface of "shell" provisional restoration, which is to be relined.

A 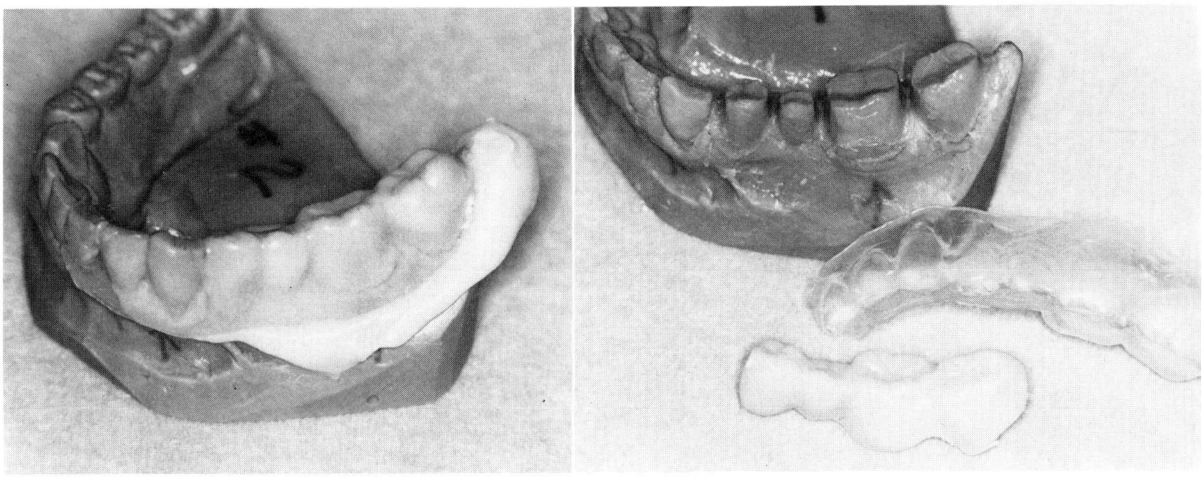 B

Fig. 15-28. A, Matrix filled with autopolymerizing resin seated on duplicate diagnostic cast, which has had "approximate" preparations prepared on stone teeth. **B,** Provisional "shell" removed from cast and matrix before trimming.

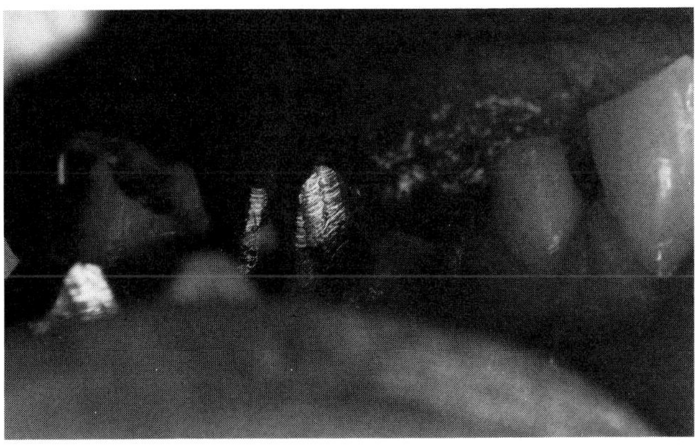

Fig. 15-29. Teeth have been prepared and tissue retracted, ready for reline procedure.

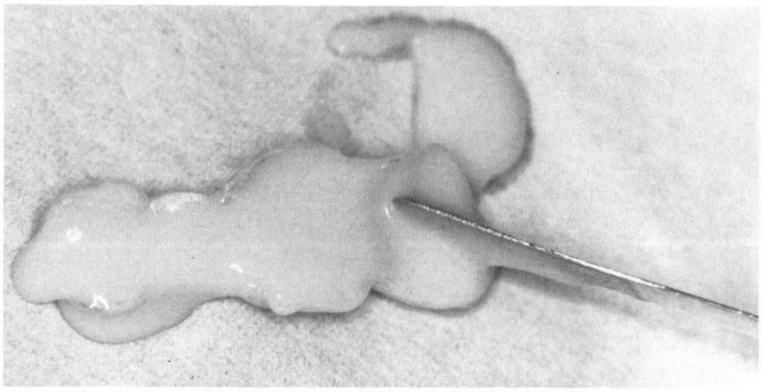

Fig. 15-30. Fluid autopolymerizing resin is placed in "shell" in preparation for reline procedure.

Fig. 15-31. "Shell" with autopolymerizing resin filler seated upon teeth. Patient has closed teeth into occlusion to assure complete seating of "shell."

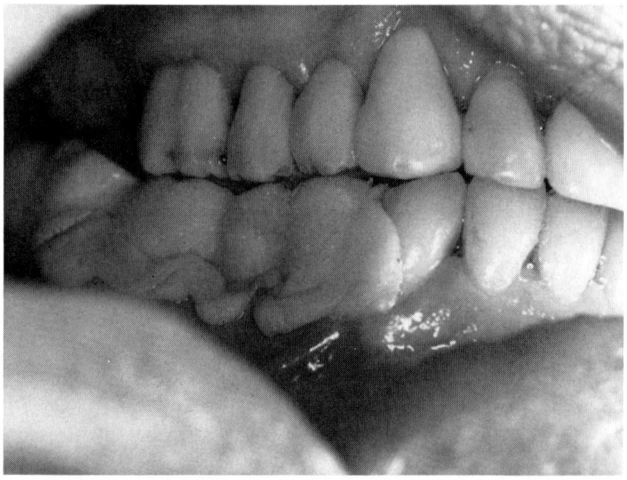

Fig. 15-32. Relined provisional restoration after trimming and polishing. Note close adaptation of margins and axial contours to allow proper hygiene.

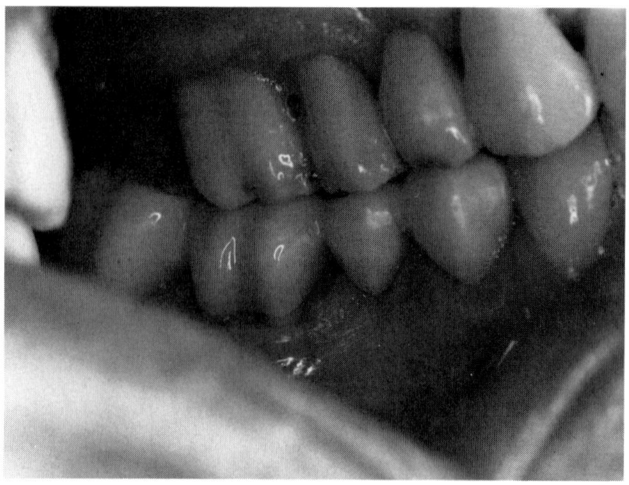

HEAT-CURED PROVISIONAL RESTORATIONS

When very strong, long-lasting provisional restorations are necessary, a conventional heat-cured acrylic resin should be used. Such techniques are more time consuming in the laboratory but produce a restoration that is superior in both appearance and durability. Several tooth-colored acrylic resin products* are available that provide a wide range of shades. So that the resin may be properly processed, it is necessary that the wax buildup of the provisional restoration be invested in a suitable processing flask.

PROCEDURE

1. A thin plastic matrix is formed over a duplicate diagnostic cast. The teeth to be involved in the provisional restoration are prepared on the cast to the approximate form of the actual preparations. Care should be taken that slightly less reduction is made on the cast than is anticipated for the reduction of the teeth themselves (Fig. 15-33).

2. Ivory-colored wax is melted (Fig. 15-34, *A*); the matrix is filled with fluid wax (Fig. 15-34, *B*).

3. The wax-filled matrix is guided into position upon the cast, which has been lubricated with a suitable wax release agent (Fig. 15-35). The matrix is stripped from the wax and the contours refined to the desired bulk and contour (Fig. 15-36).

4. The waxed-up restorations are invested in a separable flask in a manner similar to that used for complete dentures. In most instances the prepared cast, with the waxup in place, is invested. This supplies an accurate form for the inner surfaces of the provisional restoration (Fig. 15-37).

An alternate method, to supply the core for the resin to be processed against, is that of introducing die stone into the inner surfaces of the waxed crowns. This produces a die of the internal surfaces, which can be used for processing the acrylic resin (Fig. 15-38).

5. The wax is eliminated with very hot water and then cooled, and the stone surfaces are coated with a foil substitute (Fig. 15-39).

*Vita, K & B; Biolon, Dentsply/York, Dentsply International, York, Pa.; Jet, Lang Dental Mfg. Co., Inc., Chicago, Ill.

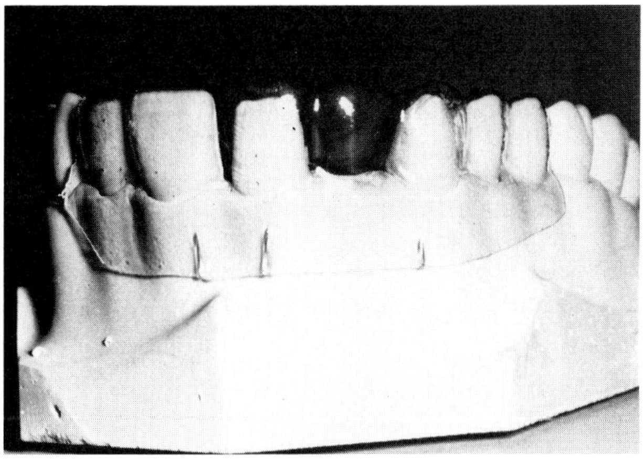

Fig. 15-33. Resin matrix over diagnostic cast that has had teeth prepared in preparation for waxing of a heat-cured provisional restoration.

A

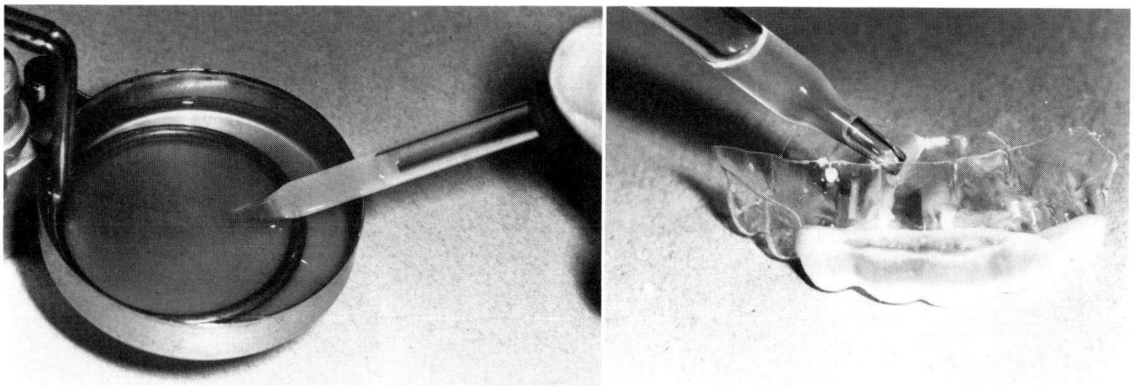

B

Fig. 15-34. A, Ivory colored inlay wax is melted and drawn into medicine dropper for transfer to matrix. **B,** Lubricated resin matrix is filled with melted wax.

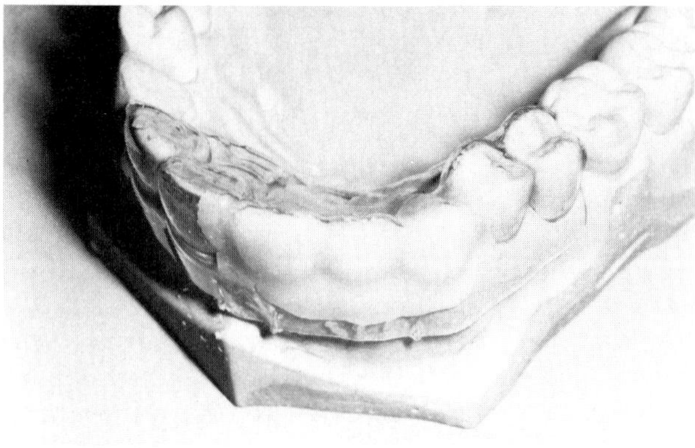

Fig. 15-35. Wax-filled matrix is seated on "prepared" diagnostic cast.

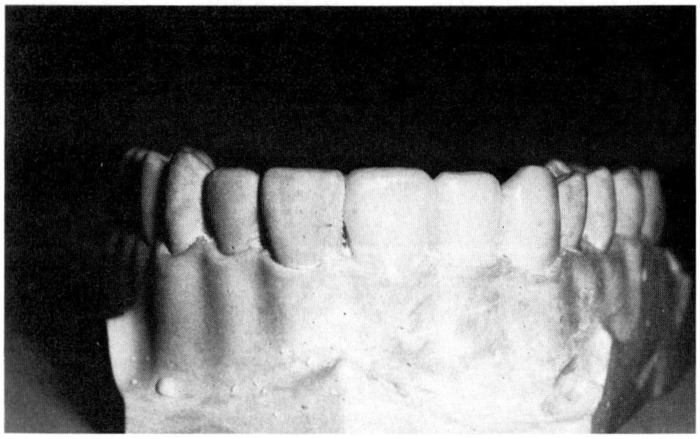

Fig. 15-36. Resin matrix is stripped from wax, excess wax removed, and contours refined.

Fig. 15-37. Invested provisional restoration has been "boiled-out" and stone cast coated with alginate foil substitute.

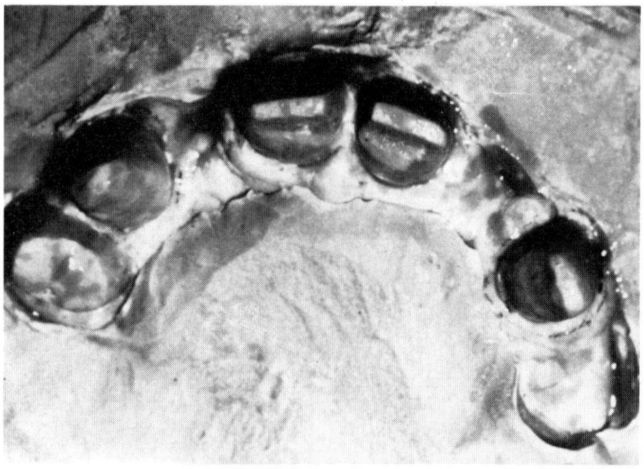

A

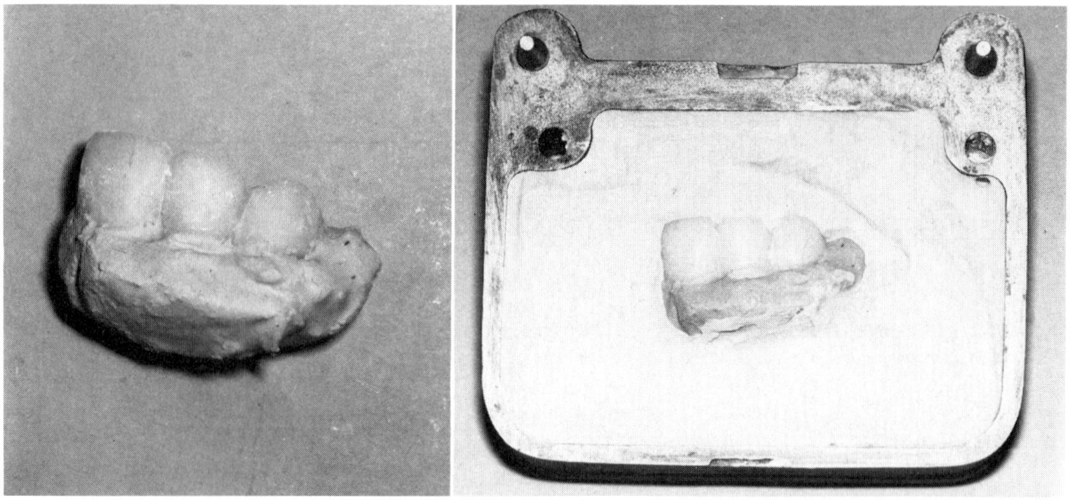

B

Fig. 15-38. A, Alternate procedure: waxed provisional pattern is removed from cast and dental stone introduced into wax crowns. After setting, cast is invested and used for processing of "heat-cure" acrylic resin. **B,** Waxed provisional restoration on stone processing cast embedded in cast.

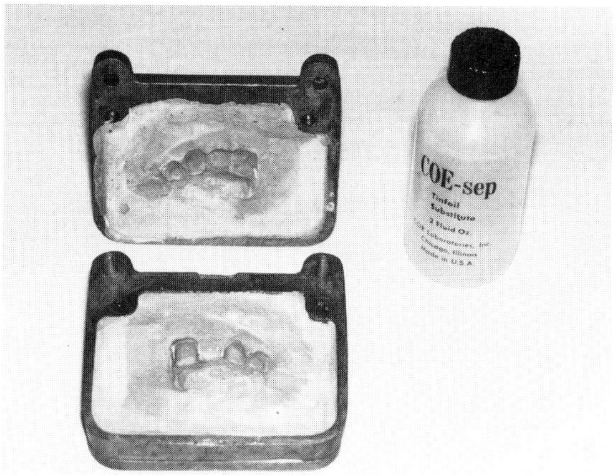

Fig. 15-39. Separated flask with wax eliminated, foil substitute placed, ready for resin placement.

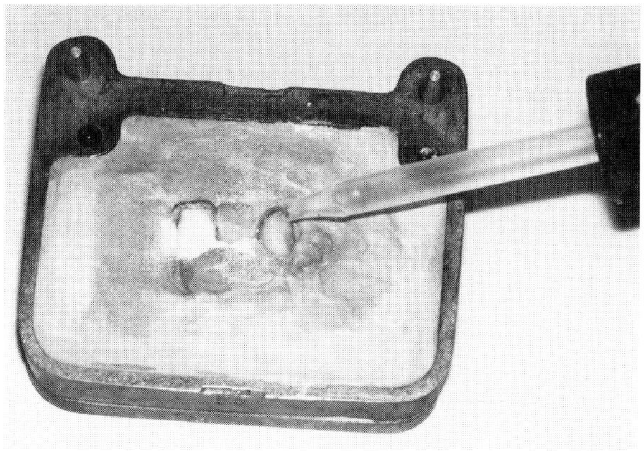

Fig. 15-40. Resin polymer of appropriate color is sprinkled into mold and moistened with monomer. Process is repeated until mold has been overfilled.

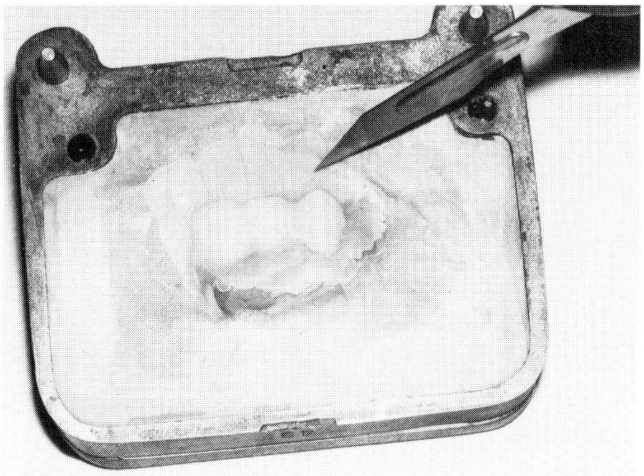

Fig. 15-41. After trial packing flask is opened and excess "flash" is trimmed.

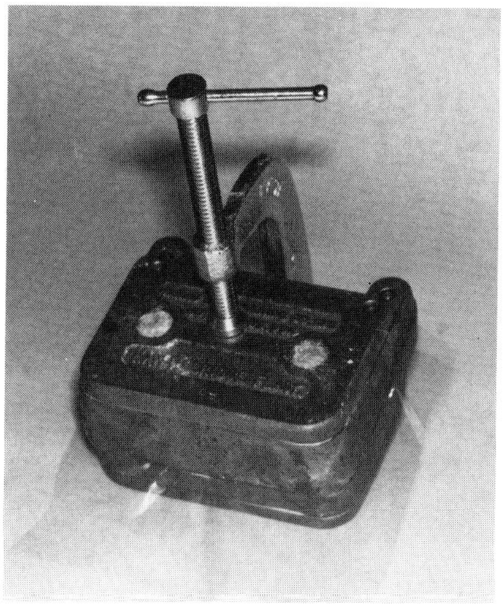

Fig. 15-42. Flask is closed, placed in clamp, and resin polymerized.

6. Acrylic polymer powder is sprinkled into the areas to be cast and moistened with acrylic monomer. The procedure is repeated until the contours have been overbuilt. Incisal, body, and gingival colors can be developed on the facial surfaces by careful application of each colored acrylic powder into its particular area. The graduation of color can be established easily if one area is allowed to dry slightly before the next color is applied (Fig. 15-40).

7. The flask is closed in an appropriate press with a sheet of cellophane or trial pack separating film. The flask is separated and excess flash is removed. Packing under pressure ensures dense resin in the cured provisional restoration (Fig. 15-41).

8. The flask is closed with a sheet of separating film over the facial surface of the molded restoration and held tightly together with a suitable clamp or press (Fig. 15-42).

9. The resin is polymerized by immersing in water at 212°F (100°C) for 30 to 60 minutes.

TRIMMING AND POLISHING

Finishing techniques are the same regardless of the method used to fabricate the provisional restoration.

Smooth, polished surfaces on correctly contoured restorations that provide good marginal adaptation are necessary to maintain optimum health.

PROCEDURE

1. Gross trimming of the resin is accomplished with large burs and disks. Care should be taken that overheating of the resin does not occur, in order to avoid distortion (Fig. 15-43).
2. Contouring is refined with small laboratory burs to trim marginal areas and blend facial and lingual contours into the interproximal embrasures (Fig. 15-44).
3. Separating disks and sandpaper disks should be used to develop properly shaped embrasures (Fig. 15-45). Gingival embrasures should be opened to provide adequate space to accommodate the interdental papilla and to allow access for proper hygiene. Embrasures adjacent to pontic areas should allow ready access for dental floss or small pointed periodontal brushes.
4. The occlusion should be adjusted to provide positive uniform but minimal contact areas in maximal in-

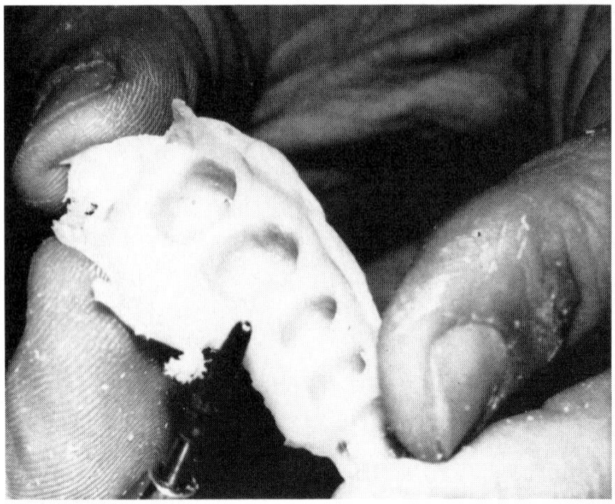

Fig. 15-43. Polymerized resin is roughly shaped with large laboratory burs.

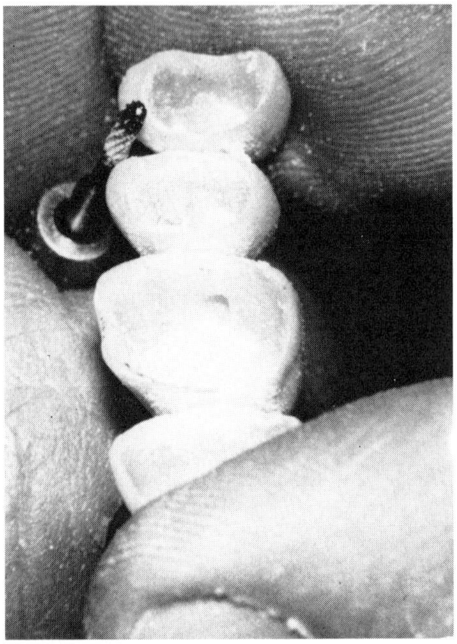

Fig. 15-44. Contours are refined with smaller burs to blend axial contours with interproximal embrasures.

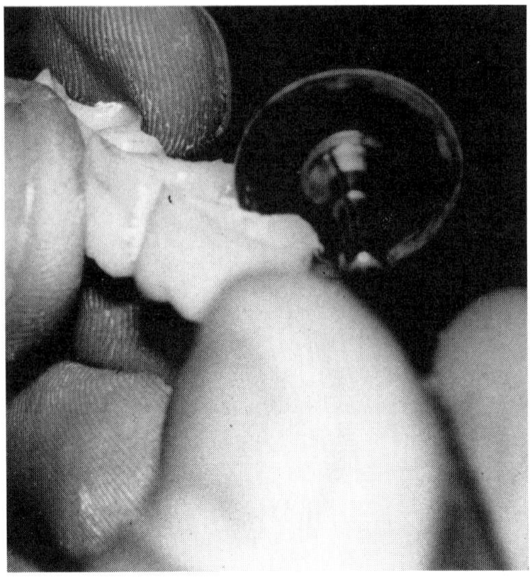

Fig. 15-45. Interproximal embrasures are refined with sandpaper disks.

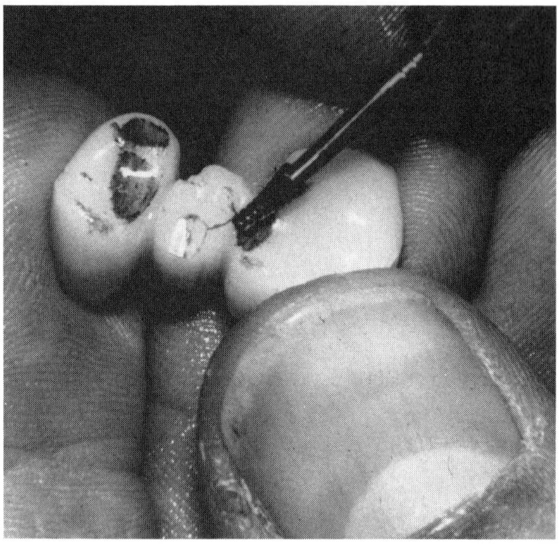

Fig. 15-46. Occlusion is adjusted to centric contact and eccentric excursions. After centric contacts have been identified supplementary grooves and sulci may be developed.

tercuspal position. Contact in lateral excursions should be eliminated if possible in the posterior regions and provide proper, even contact in the anterior. Occlusal tooth form (grooves and sluiceways) can be developed after centric occlusal stops have been identified (Fig. 15-46).

5. Marginal areas should be examined with the provisional restoration seated upon the teeth to assure smooth blending of the surfaces of the teeth with the contours of the resin. Any overhanging margins, which will cause gingival irritation, should be removed.

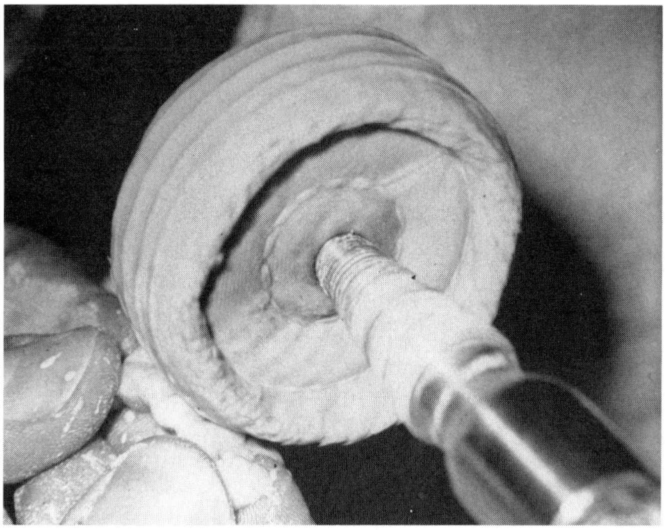

Fig. 15-47. Smooth surfaces are polished with fine pumice and rag wheel at low speed. Margins should be protected during polishing to prevent damage.

6. Polishing of the smooth axial surfaces of the restorations should be performed with fine pumice and a large ragwheel running at slow speed. Fine margins should be protected by covering with the ball of the finger (Fig. 15-47).

7. Interproximal areas should be polished with a flexible rubber cup and fine pumice (Fig. 15-48). The satin finish produced by fine pumice and ragwheel is usually sufficient to simulate the surface smoothness of natural enamel. Higher polish may be achieved through the use of fine soft bristle brushes* and fine polishing agents (Fig. 15-49).

CEMENTATION

Cementation of provisional restorations should be carried out with the same degree of care exercised in the rest of the fabrication procedure. Provisional cement, like permanent luting agents, can be very irritating if not removed from the gingival sulcus. The following steps will aid in the complete removal of provisional cement from the adjacent tissues after placement of the provisional restoration.

PROCEDURE

1. A small syringe (normally used for the placement of composite restorations) that accepts fine disposable

*Abbott-Robinson Bristle Brushes, #11 soft, Buffalo Dental Mfg. Co., Inc. Brooklyn, N.Y.

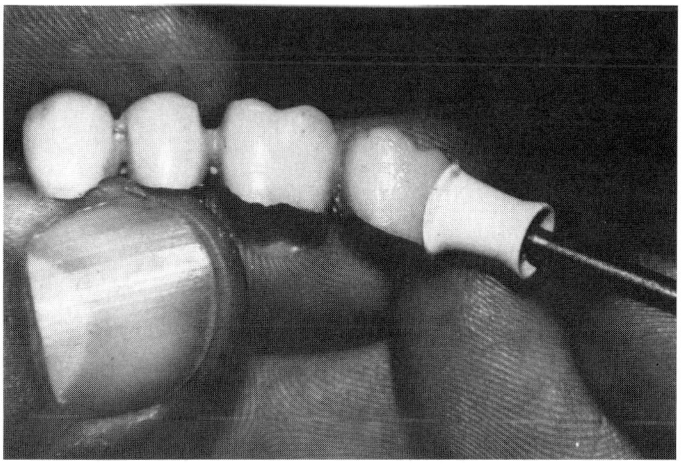

Fig. 15-48. Interproximal areas are polished with fine pumice and flexible rubber cup.

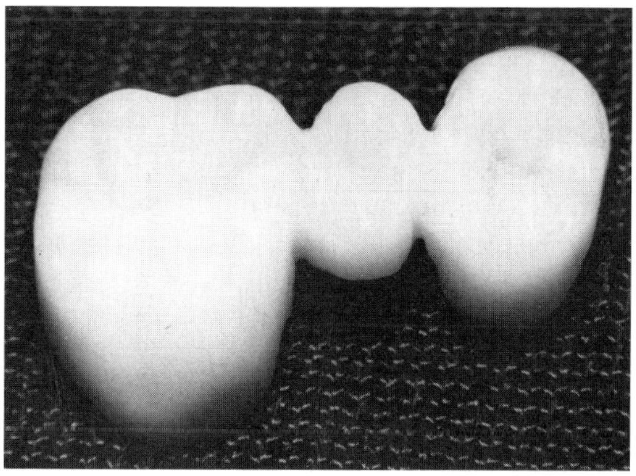

Fig. 15-49. Provisional restoration ready for cementation.

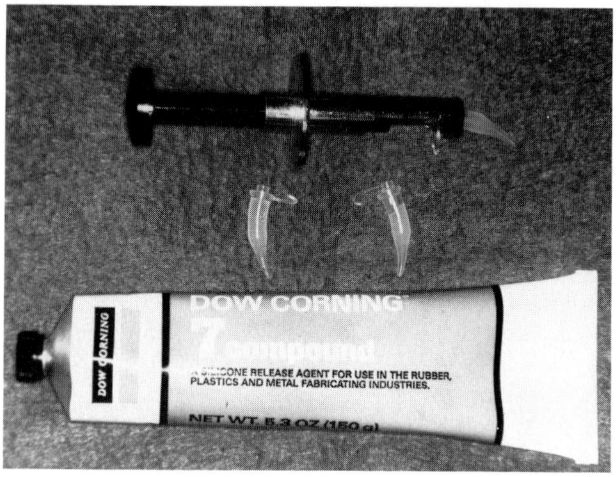

Fig. 15-50. Small "composite" syringe with disposable tips filled with silicone grease.

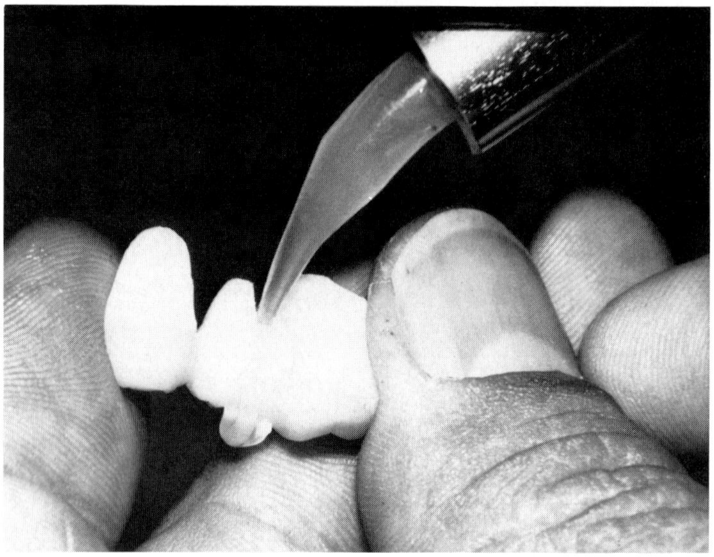

Fig. 15-51. Silicone grease is applied to interproximal embrasures, tissue surfaces of pontics, and smooth surfaces near the margins, to prevent adherence of provisional cement to resin. Careful application will prevent material from coating inside of crowns.

tips should be used to place silicone grease on critical external surfaces of the restoration to prevent adherence of the cement (Fig. 15-50).

2. Interproximal embrasures, tissue surfaces of pontics, and other critical areas should be filled or coated with a protective layer of silicone grease. Care must be exercised that the material does not coat the inner surfaces of the crowns, especially at the marginal areas (Fig. 15-51). It has been found that eugenol-containing cements cause deterioration and softening of acrylic resin crowns.

3. Provisional cement (preferably one containing no eugenol) should be placed as a small band about 2 mm wide around the inner surface of the crowns adjacent to the margins. As the provisional restoration is seated on the teeth, the preplaced cement will be forced between the prepared tooth and the closely adapted resin. The small amount of cement used will limit the excess cement, which is forced out of the crown and into the gingival sulcus. The removal of excess cement after setting and debridement will be greatly facilitated by this simple procedure. It will be found upon subsequent removal of the restoration that the provisional cement had been forced up inside the crown, completely sealing the space between the tooth and the closely adapted resin restoration.

4. All provisional cement should be cleaned carefully from the gingival sulcus and embrasures. The silicone grease that was applied to the crowns before cementation prevents the cement from adhering to the resin

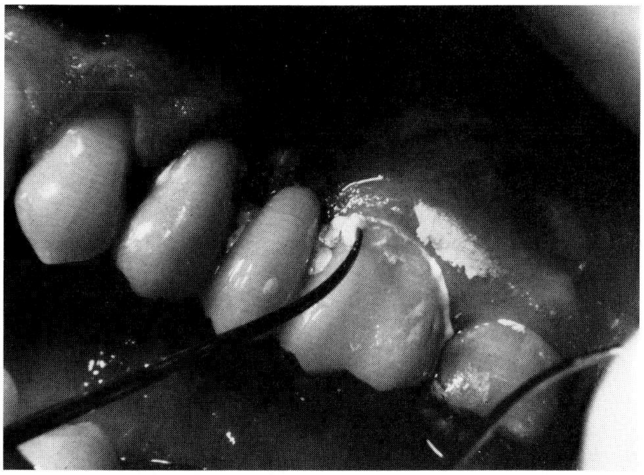

Fig. 15-52. Cement is removed carefully from interproximal areas and gingival sulcus. Incomplete removal will cause irritation of gingival tissues.

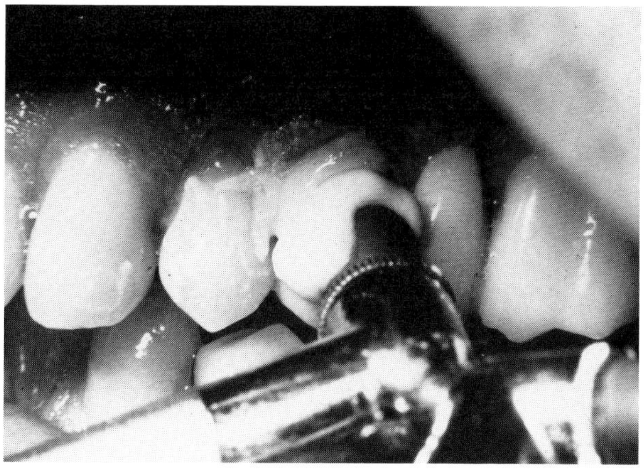

Fig. 15-53. Surfaces of provisional restoration are cleaned with fine pumice and rubber cup in prophylaxis handpiece.

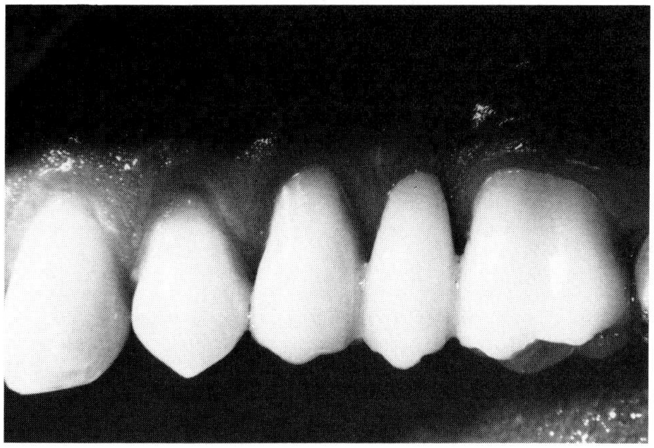

Fig. 15-54. Provisional restoration after cementation. All cement has been removed from interproximal areas and gingival sulcus. Contours of restoration promote good hygiene and tissue health.

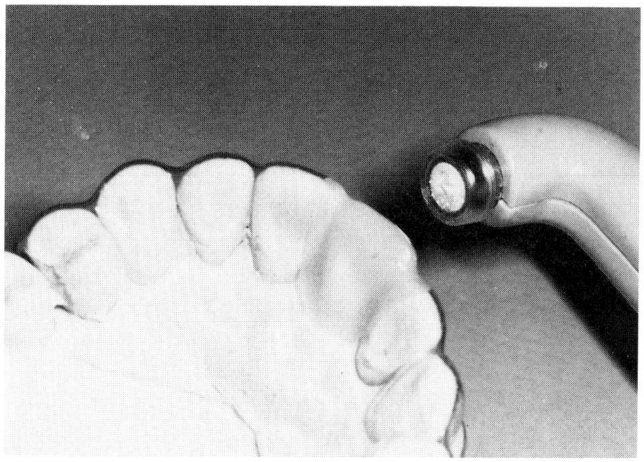

Fig. 15-55. Visible light source is used to cure provisional restoration fabricated with light-curing resin.

and allows it to be removed quickly and easily (Fig. 15-52).

5. The gingival sulcus and embrasure areas should be carefully inspected to assure that no small pieces of cement remain. The surfaces of the teeth, margins, and subgingival areas should be cleaned with fine pumice and rubber cup in a prophylaxis handpiece (Fig. 15-53). Carefully constructed provisional restorations that are properly placed will contribute to the health of the soft tissues (Fig. 15-54).

LIGHT-CURED RESIN

Improvements in and availability of resins that can be polymerized by exposure to light make possible their use in the fabrication of provisional restorations. A celluloid or clear plastic matrix can be used as a carrier to position the material over the cast, which has been coated with an alginate foil substitute. A visible light source applied at close range (2 mm) to all surfaces of the clear matrix for 40 to 60 seconds will produce complete curing of the material (Fig. 15-55).

The material can also be built up in successive layers to enable close control of shading and characterization of the restorations.

After curing of the material, the restoration can be removed from the cast, trimmed, contoured, and polished in a manner similar to that of the heat-cured materials (Fig. 15-56).

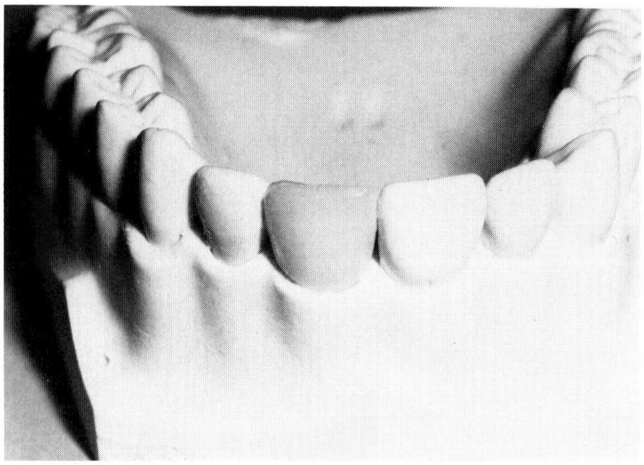

Fig. 15-56. Provisional restoration fabricated with light-curing resin.

SHADE MODIFICATION AND CHARACTERIZATION

Proper shading and characterization of provisional restorations, especially those which must serve in the anterior region, has become an essential consideration in their fabrication. Provisional restorations that are to serve for only a few days or weeks are usually fabricated from only one shade of polymer. Those that are more extensive, must serve for a longer period of time, or are to be placed for patients with higher esthetic demands, can be characterized, and have basic shadings modified to meet the more stingent cosmetic requirements. In some instances the modifications can be subtle; in others intense or dramatic characterizations are necessary.

Intrinsic characterization

The addition of color modifiers within the mass of the restorative material tends to lend depth and naturalness to the appearance of the restoration. Other modifications can be made by application of surface colorants either to the exterior surface of the restoration or to the internal surface where the color is reflected through the resin material.

Colorants applied to the inner surface crowns

The shading of crowns can be modified by coating the inner surfaces of crowns with varying colors of fast-curing liquid plastic stains.* These stains have been developed for shade modification of resin crowns. Several different shades are available. When placed on the inner surfaces of resin crowns, a marked modification of shading can be made as the color is transmitted through the resin of the restoration. This procedure is not particularly effective for pontic areas because of the increased thickness of the resin (Fig. 15-57).

*Minute Stain, George Taub Products, Jersey City, N.J.

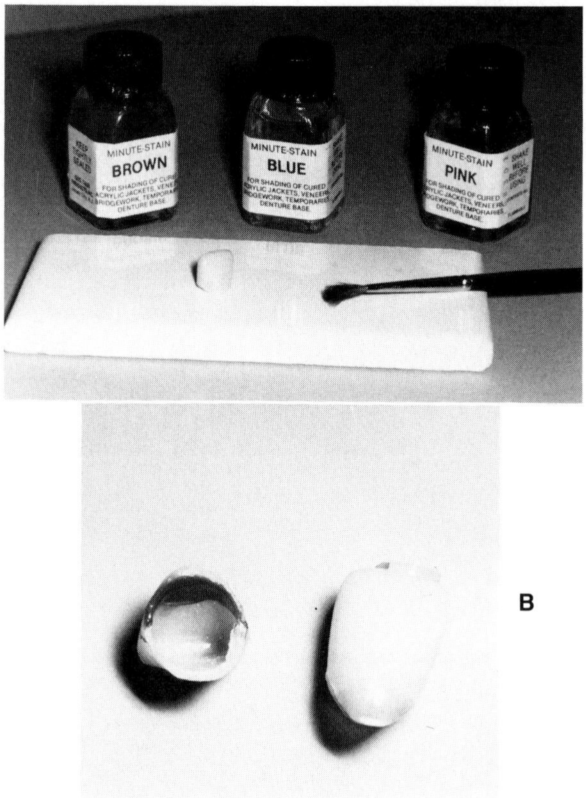

A

B

Fig. 15-57. A, Acrylic surface stains used for shade modification. **B,** Shade modification placed on inner surface of a polycarbonate crown.

Addition of color modifiers to polymer powders before mixing

The shade and appearance of resin powders (polymer) can be modified by addition of pigments. Filings from colored chalks* can be mixed with the polymer powder to produce the desired modification of shade. At the present time such modifications must be made carefully and by "trial and error" to determine the proper proportions that will produce the desired result. Additive pigments are very intense and should be added carefully in small amounts until the desired effect is produced. Knowledge gained through experimentation with these materials will enable the development of individualized restorations (Fig. 15-58).

Premixed acrylic polymer shades that correspond to the shade guide colors are available for fabrication of heat-cured provisional restorations (Fig. 15-59, *A* and *B*). These polymer powders are applied in successive layers, each being wetted by monomer before the next layer is applied. The technique permits individualized color variations to be developed within the restoration (Fig. 15-59, *C*).

*Colored Chalk, Binney and Smith, Inc., Easton, Pa.

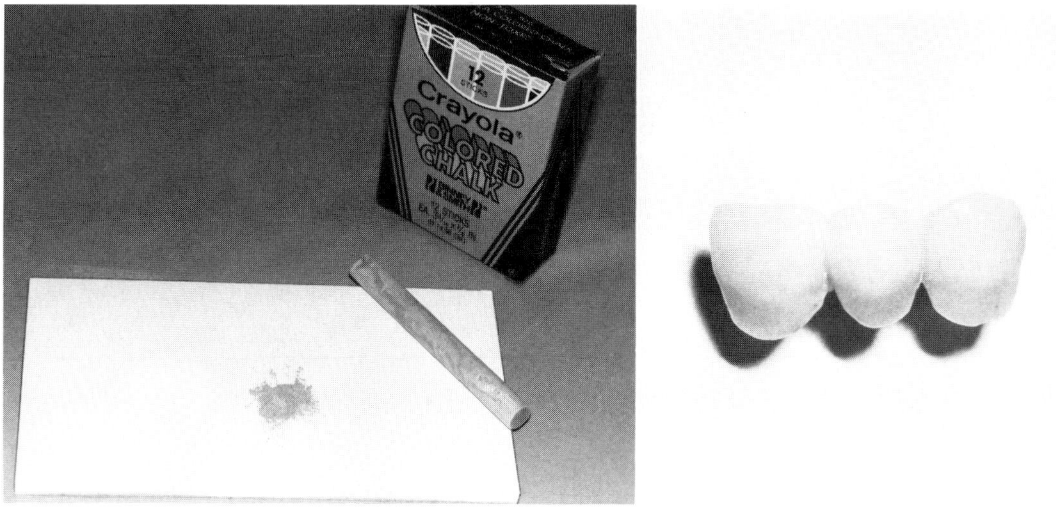

Fig. 15-58. A, Chalk filings can be mixed with acrylic polymer powder to modify basic shades. Pigments are intense and must be employed carefully for desired effect. **B,** Provisional restoration with gingival and body colors modified with pigments.

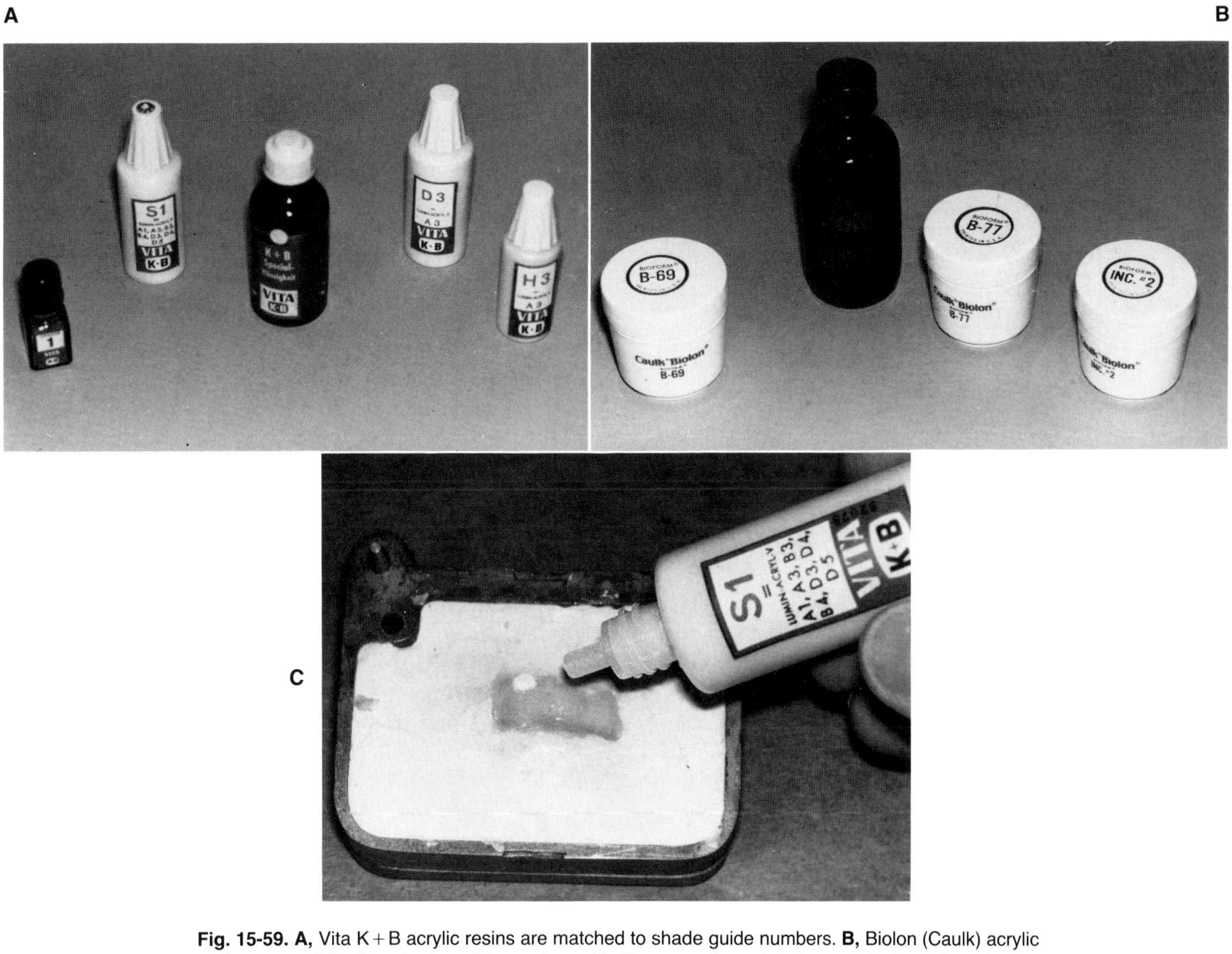

Fig. 15-59. A, Vita K + B acrylic resins are matched to shade guide numbers. **B,** Biolon (Caulk) acrylic resins are matched to shade guide numbers. **C,** Proper and careful placement of acrylic polymers into mold can create natural tooth shades.

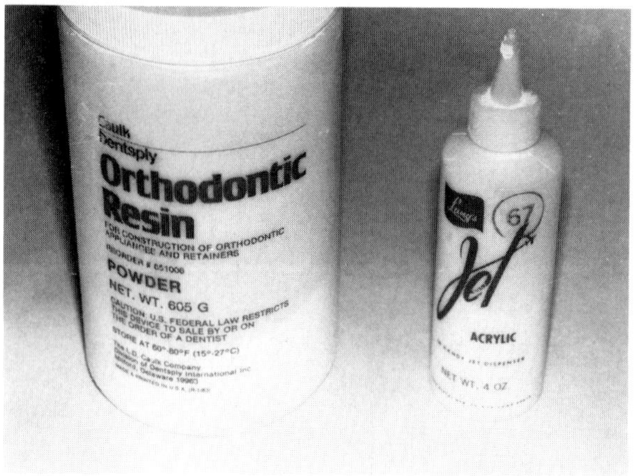

Fig. 15-60. Clear orthodontic acrylic polymer can be used as a dilutant and modifier to increase translucence in incisal area of provisional crowns.

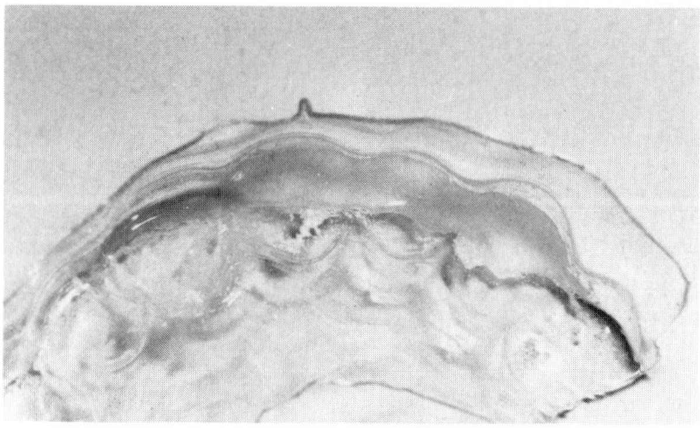

Fig. 15-61. Clear resin can be used as a thin layer or blended with incisal and body shades. Careful use will avoid demarcation lines.

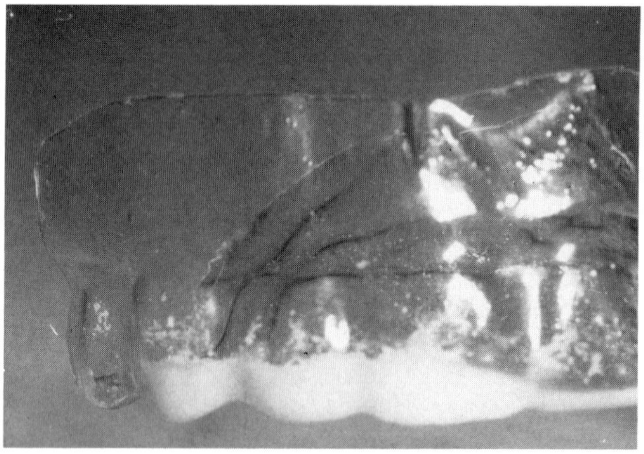

Fig. 15-62. Incisal shade modified with clear acrylic is built up within matrix.

Translucence or incisal area

The incisal third of any restoration is a very important part of its esthetic or cosmetic makeup. Aside from the contour, thickness, and surface characteristics, the value and degree of translucence of adjacent teeth must be carefully simulated. This is a vital part of the final restoration. It is also an important consideration in the development of an esthetic provisional restoration.

The value, color, and translucence of the incisal portion of acrylic provisional restorations can be modified by addition of clear polymer powder* to the incisal or body shades that are available (Fig. 15-60). Clear acrylic can be added as a thin veneer or used as a dilutant to increase the translucence of other polymer powders. The clear resin should not exceed 30% to 40% of the total amount of powder. Excessive proportions of the clear material will result in an incisal area that is too translucent (Fig. 15-61).

If the restoration is built up in increments in a processing flask, the incisal area is the last portion to be added before trial packing. If, on the other hand, the restoration is to be built within a matrix, the incisal portion is added first and blended with the selected body shades to avoid sharp demarcation areas (Fig. 15-62).

Extrinsic characterization

Extrinsic characterization of provisional restorations allows the placement of colorants and modifiers in specific areas. Lowering of value, increasing of intensity of a color, modification of color, placing of specific details of characterization, and simulation and accenting of interproximal areas are a few of the applications of external modifiers.

Several products are available that lend themselves to surface modification of resin restorations (Fig. 15-63). The minute stain* is applied to the surface with a fine brush, using even strokes. The material cures very quickly. Streaking of the colorant may occur if the material is applied thinly or too slowly. Properly employed, the material is effective for surface detailing and for shade or value modification (Fig. 15-64, *A*).

The Rembrandt† material is a new light-cured resin

*Orthodontic Resin, Clear, L.D. Caulk Co., Dentsply International, Inc., Milford, Del.

*Minute-Stain, Taub Products, Inc., Jersey City, N.J.
†Rembrandt Surface Pigments Den-Mat, Santa Maria, Calif.

A

B

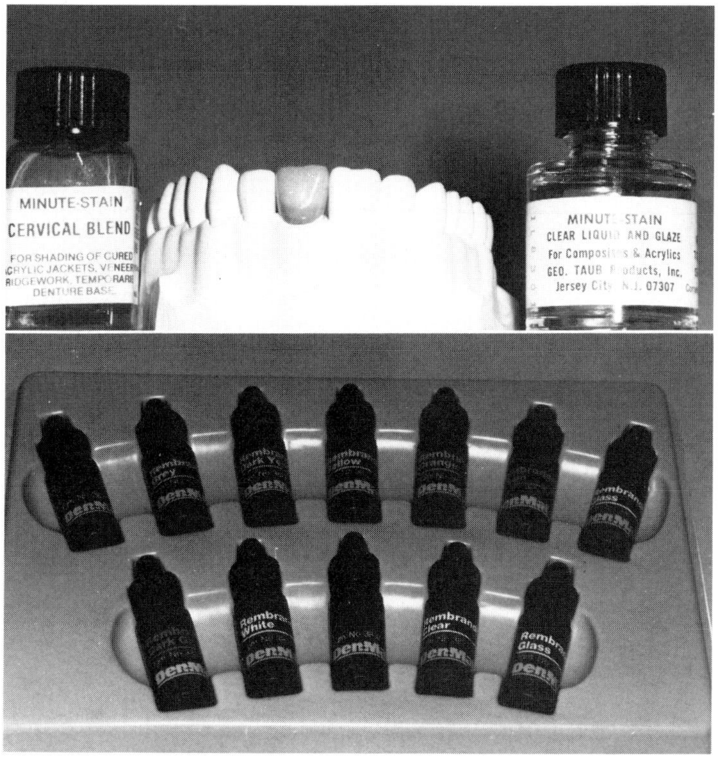

Fig. 15-63. A, Acrylic stains applied to surface can modify basic shades. Value can be lowered, hue changed, and chroma increased. **B,** Light-curing color pigments for characterization and shade modification.

A

B

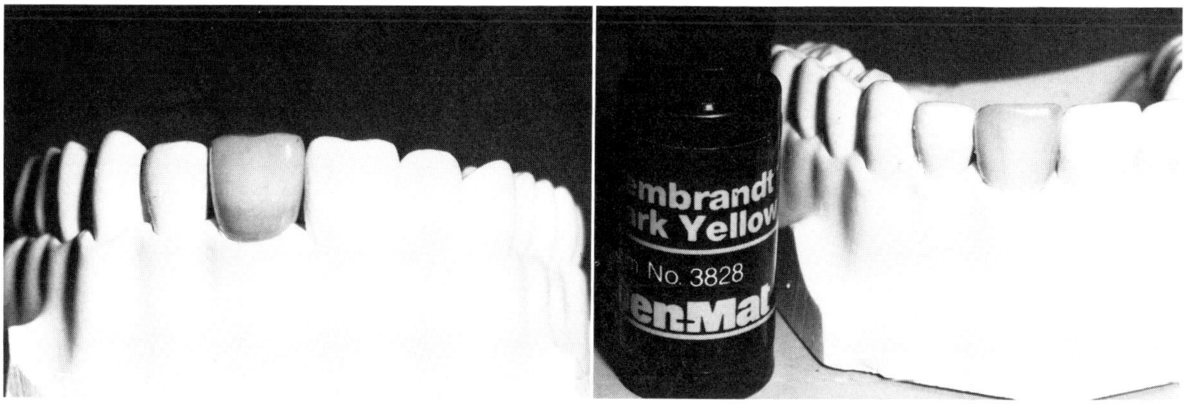

Fig. 15-64. A, Subtle characterization of anterior provisional restoration. **B,** Characterization and modification can be developed carefully with "Rembrandt" colorants. When desired effect is produced material is polymerized with visible light source. Clear glaze can be applied as protective layer over colorants.

in the field of surface characterization. The colors are more subtle than other surface pigments. Increased working time is possible for the development of the desired effect, as setting is activated by exposure to the light source. A clear "glaze" can be applied to serve as a protective layer for the pigments (Fig. 15-64, *B*).

REFERENCES

Krug, R.S.: Multiple uses of plastic templates in fixed prosthodontics, Dent. Clin. North Am. **19**:313, 1973.

Preston, J.D.: A systematic approach to the control of esthetic form, J. Prosthet. Dent. **35**:393, 1976.

Schmidt, J.B., Dill, G.C., and King, C.J.: Anterior temporary coverage, So. Carolina Dent. J. **27**:5-8, 1969.

Shillingburg, H.T., Hobo, S., and Whitsett, L.D.: Fundamentals of fixed prosthodontics, ed. 2, Chicago, 1981, Quintessence Publishing Co.

Skurow, H.W., and Lytle, J.D.: The interproximal embrasure, Dent. Clin. North Am. **15**:3:641, 1971.

Stein, J.: Pontic-residual ridge relationship: a research report, J. Prosthet. Dent. **16**:252-285, 1966.

Talkov, L.: Temporary acrylic fixed bridgework and splints, J. Prosthet. Dent. **2**:693-702, 1952.

Tonn, J.H., and Cook, J.A.: Esthetic temporary crowns from plastic denture teeth, J. Michigan Dent. Assoc. **53**:118-120, 1971.

Tylman, S.D., and Malone W.F.P.: Tylman's theory and practice of fixed prosthodontics. ed. 7, St. Louis, 1978, The C.V. Mosby Co.

Wood, M., Halpern, B.G., and Lamb, M.F.: Visible light cured composite resins: an alternative for anterior provisional restorations, J. Prosthet. Dent. **51**:192-194, 1984.

CHAPTER 16

REPAIR TECHNIQUES

RYLE A. RADKE

Repair of any existing restoration should be made only after careful evaluation to determine the ability to meet the biologic and clinical requirements necessary to serve as a clinically acceptable restoration. If these requirements cannot be met, then provisions for a remake must be instituted, or the appliance should be removed and the teeth given proper temporary protection until a more expedient time for remake presents itself.

The types of repairs presented represent the most common clinical problems encountered in a fixed prosthodontic practice. The procedures are meant to be modified as varied clinical problems are encountered. Space does not permit presenting every possible variation of repair. Repairing parts of pontics, for example, with quick-cure acrylic or composites has been left out because of the poor clinical results attained with this method. The repairs described take considerable time and are usually indicated where a large multiple splint or an extensive bridge makes the time expenditure reasonable.

The reason for failure of the appliance is in many instances due to a flaw in its original design or construction. A repair will often be followed by another failure and subsequent loss of patient confidence, so a careful analysis of the faulty appliance is imperative before treatment. Pontic repairs usually fall into the following categories: (1) ceramometal repair using an overcasting; (2) ceramometal repair using parallel pins; and (3) pin pontics and Tru-pontics using a split-cast technique.

PONTIC REPAIR

Metal-ceramic repair using an overcasting

First, the extent of the pontic fracture is evaluated. If the gingival adaptation of the porcelain is adequate, this will simplify procedures.

PROCEDURE

1. Prepare the framework and facial surfaces of the fractured pontic with a medium-grit tapered diamond. Establish finish lines on the proximal surfaces of the adjacent teeth, making an incisal path of insertion for the restoration (Fig. 16-1).

2. Remove sufficient bulk of material for esthetics, and make the reduction with the retentive principles of a full-crown restoration. The proximal connector walls are short because of the solder connector, so place a facial groove to augment retention and increase parallelism (Fig. 16-1, *B*, arrows).

3. Establish finish lines on the remaining gingival porcelain. Use care to gain sufficient length and reduction of the lingual surface of the framework for occlusion and retention.

4. Make an elastic impression after preparation, and construct a working cast with a removable die. Then construct a thin overcasting from the cast. Bake porcelain on this thin ceramometal overcasting, and shape carefully to be well adapted to the interproximal finish lines while still allowing ease of withdrawal from the working model (Fig. 16-1, *A*).

5. Carefully adjust the restoration to eliminate occlusal interferences, and then cement it into place (Fig. 16-1, *D*).

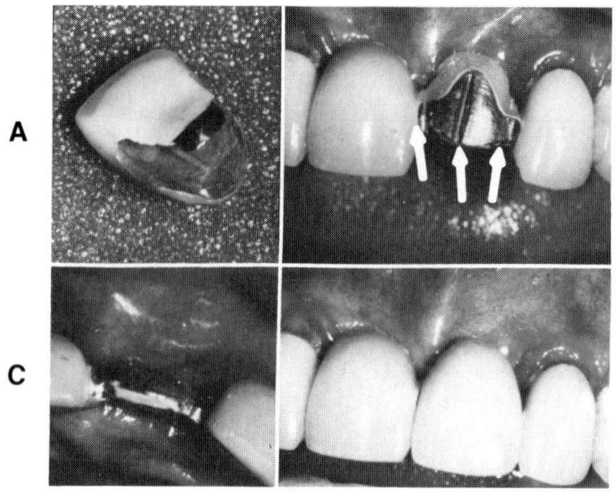

Fig. 16-1. A, Finished casting, showing short interproximal walls. **B,** Labial view of preparation, showing facial grooves and interproximal finish lines *(arrows)*. **C,** Incisal view of preparation, showing relationship of finish lines on adjacent teeth. **D,** Finished repair.

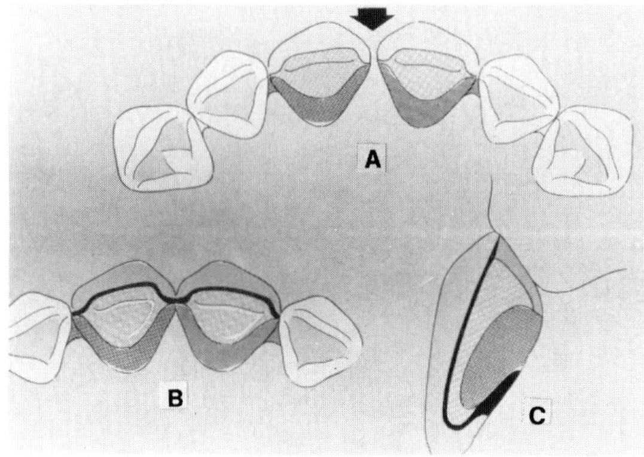

Fig. 16-2. *A,* Anterior bridge with fractured solder joint between central incisors prepared for overcastings. *B,* Overcastings in place. *C,* Faciolingual view, showing relationship of overcasting to substructure.

This method of repair can be used in the event of connector failure in an extensive bridge or splint (Fig. 16-2, *A*). Preparations are made on the pontics adjacent to the failure as described previously. Facial grooves will greatly enhance retention. An elastic impression is made, then a double overlay (Fig. 16-2, *B* and *C*). The porcelain is baked and carefully adjusted to the interproximal spaces. The appliance is tried in the mouth, and all occlusal interferences are carefully removed before it is cemented into place. Repairs made in this manner are durable, esthetic, and capable of providing excellent service for the patient.

Metal-ceramic repair using parallel pins

Fractured anterior pontics in cases with deep anterior overbite or insufficient clearance on the lingual surface, precluding the overcast procedure, can be repaired with a facially withdrawing casting. This procedure can also be used where the gingival adaptation of the pontic is lost, and a new pontic tip must be reconstructed and readapted to the tissue.

PROCEDURE

1. Remove the porcelain from the facial aspect with a medium-grit diamond, and place the parallel pins (Fig. 16-3). Prepare the incisal edge in the path of withdrawal of the pins, and prepare the interproximal porcelain of the adjacent teeth with finish lines.

2. Place the pins with an Auto-Klutch drive,* using a .027 drill. The pinholes should be a minimum of 2 mm deep, oriented gingivally for added length. If convenient, the pinholes should extend completely through the framework.

3. Lubricate the drill with petroleum jelly, or wax to minimize binding.

4. Place size .026 plastic pins in the pinholes, and make an impression with rubber-base impression material in a facially withdrawing tray. Pour the impression, and make a thin casting to which porcelain is baked.

5. Carefully adjust the finished restoration in the patient's mouth to remove all occlusal interferences, and then cement it (Fig. 16-4).

In the case of a pontic needing a new porcelain tip adapted to the tissue, the procedure previously described can be modified as follows:

1. The preparation must withdraw gingivally and incisally, as well as with the pins (Fig. 16-3, *C*, arrows). Make the impression with a facially withdrawing tray, and place a lingual stent of compound to control the flow of impression material in the pontic area.

2. Make a split cast to facilitate adaptation of the gingival porcelain of the pontic.

These procedures are readily adaptable and provide excellent long-lasting and esthetic repairs. It is again emphasized that these repairs are used in long-span bridges and extensive splints where the repair time is warranted.

Pin pontics and Tru-Pontics using split-cast technique

Sheets (1966) describes a split-cast procedure for replacing Harmony pin pontics by an indirect method. This procedure is adequate for porcelain or acrylic replacement. The split cast can also be applied to the repair of ceramometal pontics where the gingival porcelain has been fractured or new gingival adaptation is needed.

*Whaledent, Inc., New York, N.Y.

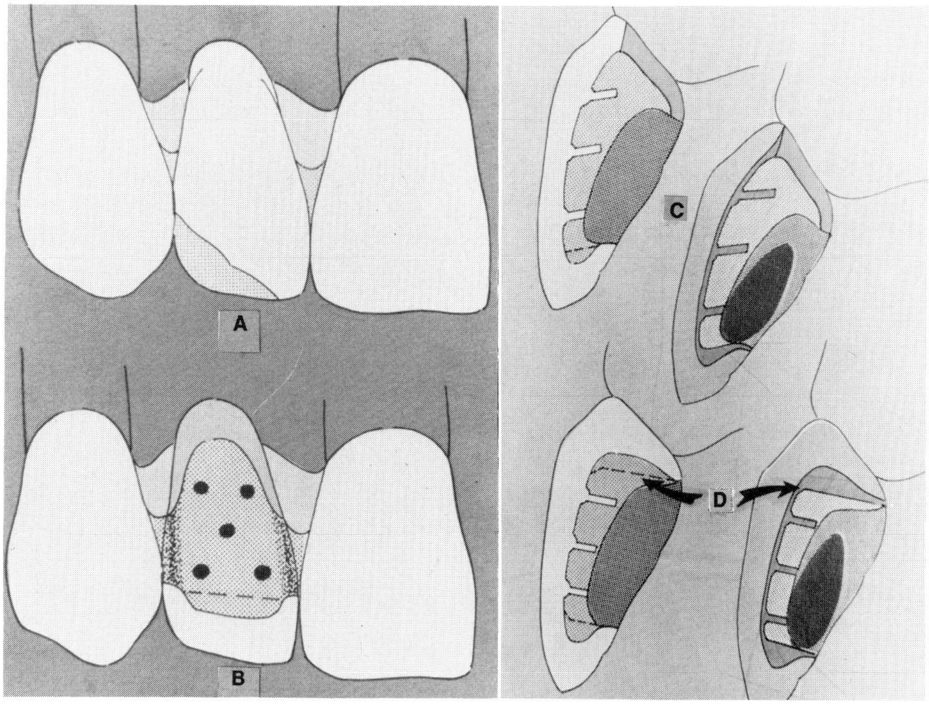

Fig. 16-3. *A,* Facial view of fracture. *B,* Facial view of preparation. *C,* Faciolingual view of preparation when gingival porcelain is intact *(arrows). D,* Faciolingual view of preparation, showing replacement when gingival porcelain is fractured. Dotted lines show outline of preparation. Relationship of casting in gingival portion is shown by arrow.

A

B

C

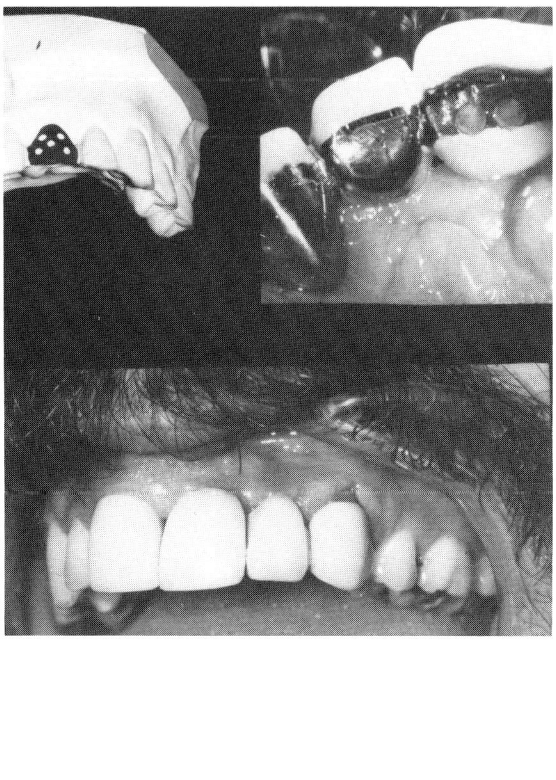

Fig. 16-4. A, Facial view of working model of preparation. **B,** Lingual view of cemented facing, showing pins extending through casting. **C,** Facial view of complete repair.

PROCEDURE

1. Make an alginate impression of the bridge, and pour a cast. From this cast, make a lingual template of compound to restrict the flow of the elastic impression material.

2. Trim the compound so that the impression material is not blocked from critical areas of the backing.

3. On the facial aspect, make a plastic tray that extends at least one tooth either side of the pontic and covers enough of the gingival area to permit readaptation of the pontic. This tray should have some relief to allow for thickness of the impression material. The tray should extend slightly over the occlusal surfaces of the bridge to provide a definite stop for aligning the tray in the mouth (Figs. 16-5 and 16-6).

4. Place a preformed metal pin in the pontic backing, and make and trim a rubber-base impression.

5. Place the impression on a flat piece of carding wax, occlusal surface down, in preparation for boxing and pouring in stone (Fig. 16-7).

6. Check the pins for alignment, and pour the impression until the cervical margins of the teeth are covered (Fig. 16-8).

7. Allow the stone to set, and cut positioning grooves into the stone.

8. Lightly lubricate the stone with petroleum jelly, and make a second pour.

After setting, we have a split cast (Fig. 16-9) that will allow adaptation of the pontic to the original backing. The gingival portion is then ground in, using the base of the split cast. The new pontic should show excellent tissue adaptation (Fig. 16-10).

The identical procedure can be used for repair of the

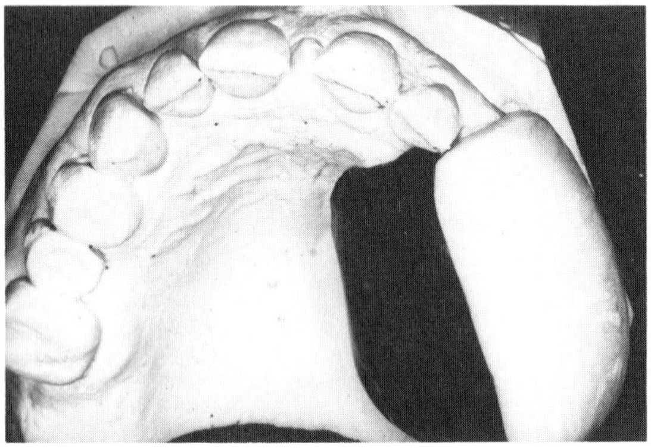

Fig. 16-5. Study cast with facial plastic tray and compound lingual stint.

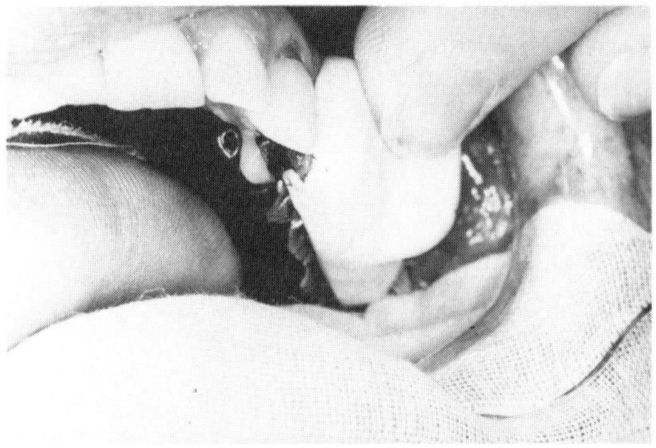

Fig. 16-6. Tray and stent in place in mouth.

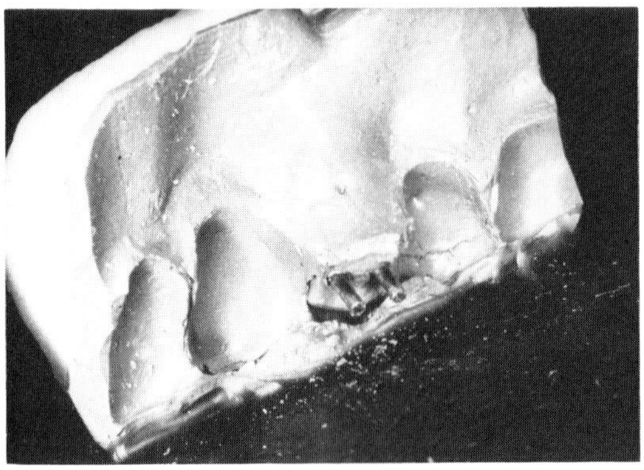

Fig. 16-7. Rubber-base impression with metal pins in place and boxed with utility wax in preparation for pouring.

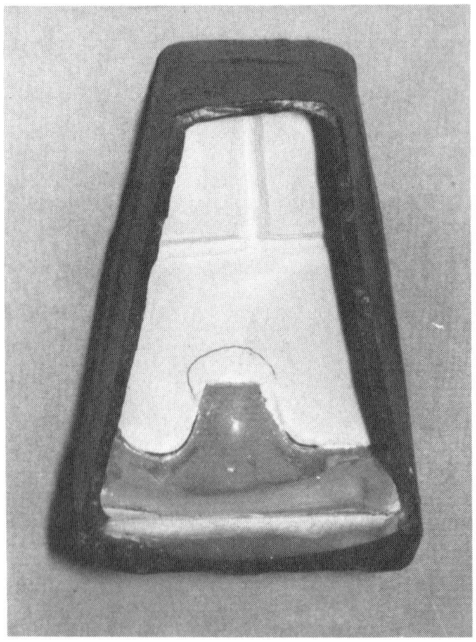

Fig. 16-8. First pouring is completed up to necks of teeth and backing. After setting, stone is scored and lubricated in preparation for second pour.

Steele's Tru-Pontics. Preformed plastic or metal tracks* are placed in the impression of the backing, and the impression is double poured in the same way. The pontic is adapted to the backing and then to the removable ridge area.

Clinical experience shows that the porcelain facing usually fails due to flexing of the backing from insufficient rigidity. Repairs with heat-processed acrylic are usually indicated in these cases, since a porcelain repair will almost always fail again.

*The Columbia Manufacturing Co., New York, N.Y.

REPAIR OF FRACTURED ABUTMENT FACINGS
Use of an overcasting

Fractured facings present a more difficult challenge than pontics due to the lack of faciolingual space and limitations as to pin placement. In many instances, the crown must be removed and reconstructed. The repair procedure is lengthy and time consuming and is not recommended except in conjunction with multiple splints and extensive bridges. The chair time involved in the repair can exceed a remake of the old bridge. The overcast procedure can be used if there is sufficient room for a metal substructure and for porcelain buildup (Fig. 16-11).

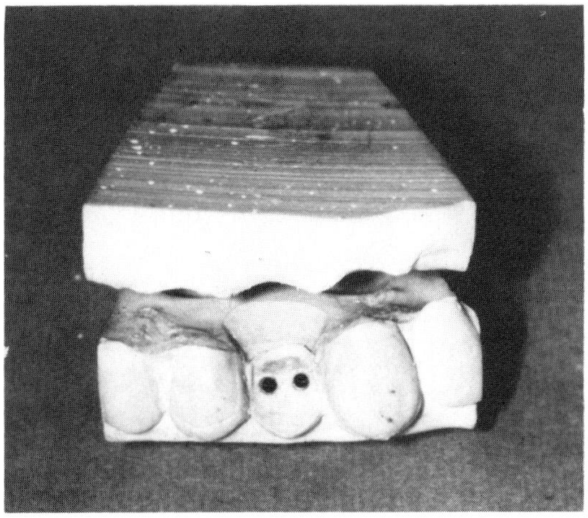

Fig. 16-9. Complete cast with pins removed, showing separation. Pontic can now be fitted to backing and then adapted to gingival portion in two stages.

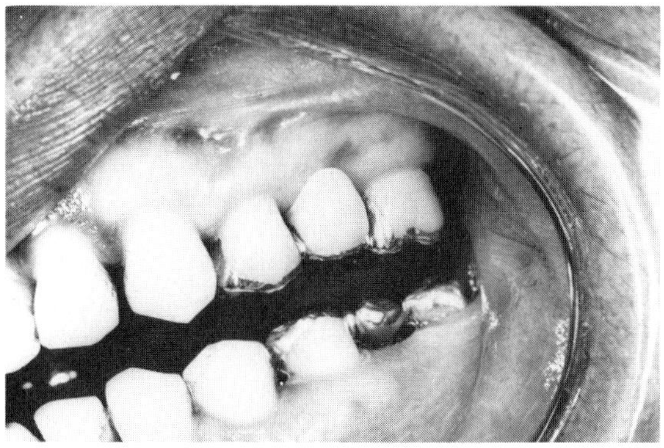

Fig. 16-10. Completed repair.

A

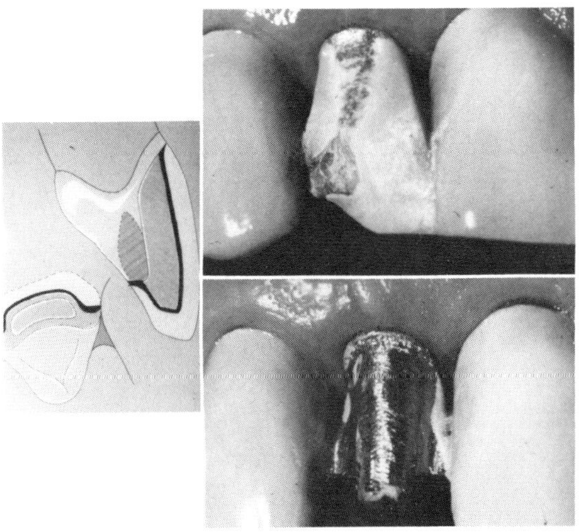

B

C

Fig. 16-11. A, Cross section of overcasting and incisal view, showing relation of overcasting *(dark line)* to preparation and to porcelain. **B,** Fractured abutment in ten-unit splint. **C,** Preparation of metal and porcelain interproximal walls.

PROCEDURE

1. Remove the porcelain, and establish proximal finish lines as described. The most difficult challenge is to gain sufficient length of the lingual wall to get adequate retention.
2. After the preparation is complete, make an elastic impression and make two casts on which the overcast is constructed (Fig. 16-12).
3. Start the wax pattern on the solid cast, and finalize it on the removable die.
4. Fabricate the finished restoration, check it carefully for occlusal prematurities, and then cement it.
5. If an adequate lingual wall cannot be established, then construct a facially withdrawing pin-retained casting, or incorporate a new casting into the splint with semiprecision attachments.

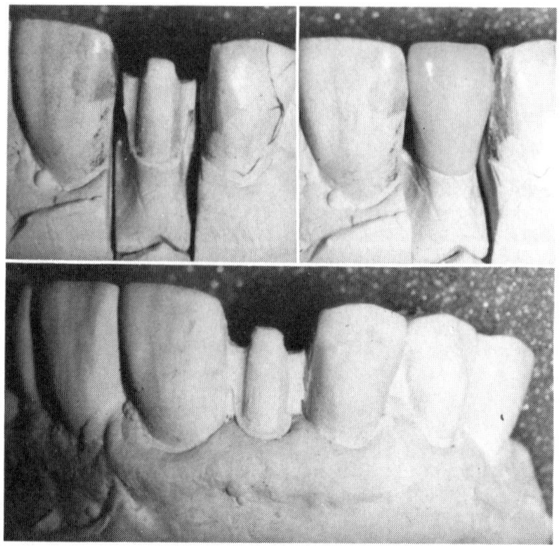

Fig. 16-12. A, Working model with removable die. **B,** Finished restoration. **C,** Solid working cast for start of wax-up.

Parallel pins

A pin procedure can be used for repairing a facing. The only variation of the previously described pontic repair is that the pins must be placed interproximally, and as a rule only two pins can be placed.

Retainer replacement and incorporation in splint or bridge with semiprecision attachment

In the case of a multiple splint with a fractured facing or loose abutment, one procedure is to remove the casting and prepare the metal of the interproximal connecting areas as male semiprecision attachments (Fig. 16-13). This repair can be used in the middle of a multiple splint or as a terminal abutment. The resistance to lateral displacement is excellent.

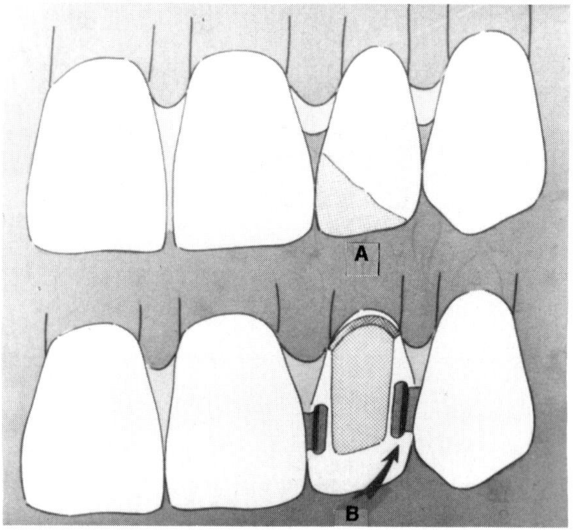

Fig. 16-13. *A,* Fractured facing in splint. *B,* Prepared male attachment *(arrow)* formed from connector.

PROCEDURE

1. Cut the casting, and carefully remove it in sections, leaving the interproximal connectors intact.
2. Carefully shape the interproximal connectors into male attachments (Fig. 16-14), and, with care, form them to make a most retentive key that will provide excellent stability. The male attachment is best formed with a small medium-grit diamond, and the isthmus is refined with a No. 169L carbide bur.
3. Make an elastic impression, and make a working cast (Fig. 16-14), using a two-impression procedure.

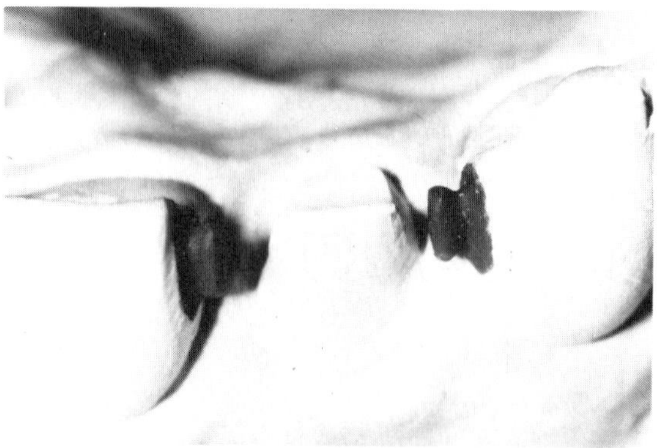

Fig. 16-14. Working model; male connectors show dark.

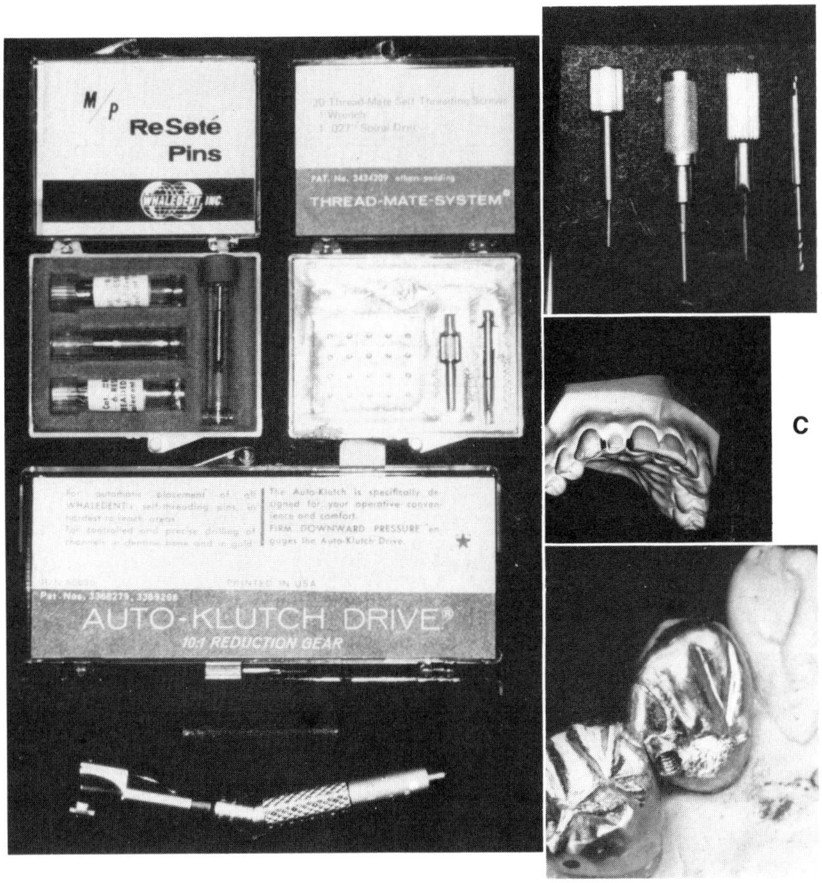

Fig. 16-15. A, ReSeté pin set and Auto-Klutch Drive. **B,** T.M.S. pin, .027; ReSeté pin, .027; tap, .027; drill, .027. **C,** Facial view of working model. **D,** Threaded pinholes from lingual aspect.

4. Form the wax pattern on a solid master cast, and refine the margins on a separate die after the pattern is adapted to the attachments and the preparation.
5. Make a casting, carefully adjust it on the master cast, and bake on the porcelain.
6. Equilibrate the restoration in the patient's mouth, and cement it. This restoration gives excellent resistance to lateral forces in the splint.

If resistance to vertical displacement is necessary, the Auto-Klutch drive and a drill and tap set for the ReSeté pin system (Fig. 16-15) can be used from the lingual side of the attachment. Drilling all the way through the keyway is not necessary. All that is required is an indentation, and when the ReSeté is screwed into place and tightened, the castings are effectively immobilized (Lum, 1977).

Direct and indirect plastic repairs

In the case of an extensive splint or bridge where, for mechanical or esthetic reasons, the previously described metal-ceramic repairs are not applicable, the plastic repairs can be used.

PROCEDURE

1. Make a preliminary impression (alginate), and construct a plastic facially withdrawing tray. It must extend at least one tooth on either side of the repair site and have sufficient occlusogingival width to encompass the entire outline of the repair area.
2. Make an impression (elastomeric) of the fracture site (Fig. 16-16, *A* and *B*), which has been prepared with undercuts to provide retention.
3. Construct a working cast, and fabricate a facing with heat-cured acrylic resin.
4. Cement the new facing with an autopolymerizing crown and bridge resin of the proper shade.
5. If retention is insufficient due to the framework design, tap .027 pinholes, and place pins in the metal backing.
6. Note the location of the pins, and relieve the interior of the facing relieved; cement the new facing with autopolymerizing crown and bridge resin of the proper shade. Judgment must be exercised in placing the pins and correcting their length for esthetics.

A useful modification of this procedure is to hollow

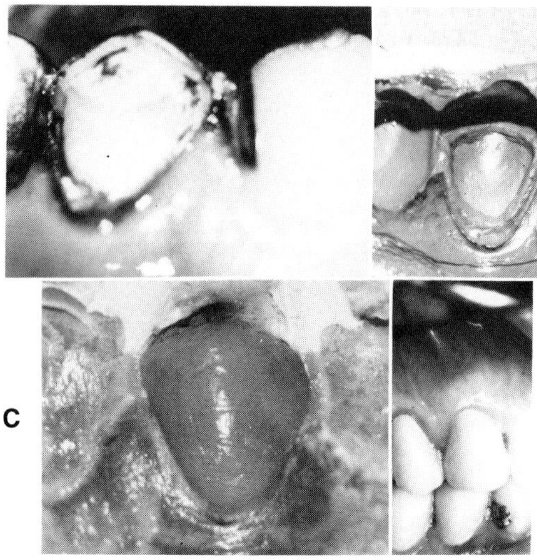

Fig. 16-16. A, Damaged facing. **B,** Impression of prepared facing. **C,** Heat-cured replacement. **D,** Final restoration.

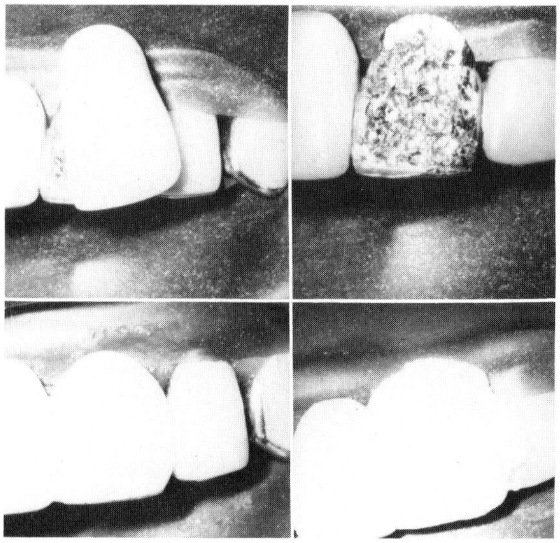

Fig. 16-17. A, Plastic denture tooth of proper mold and shade. **B,** Prepared backing. **C,** Facing fitted. **D,** Facing cemented with autopolymerizing crown and bridge cement.

grind a plastic denture tooth (Portnoy, 1973) of the proper mold and shade for the site (Fig. 16-17, *A*). Prepare the backing with undercuts (Fig. 16-17, *B*) and, if necessary, use pins in the metal to gain added retention. After careful adaptation, cement the facing with autopolymerizing crown and bridge resin of the proper shade (Fig. 16-17, *C* and *D*). Hard-setting crown and bridge acrylics such as Neopar are preferred. After the plastic has set, careful trimming and polishing make a most esthetic and long-lasting repair. This same procedure can be done by the indirect technique on a cast, saving chair time.

REPAIR OF ABUTMENTS IN MULTIPLE SPLINTS OR LARGE BRIDGES

A loose abutment can be detected by pulling occlusally on the splint or bridge, then drying the gingival margins and pressing the appliance into place. If saliva comes out, the abutment is loose. Another clinical sign is a foul odor about which the patient complains or which the operator detects in an otherwise clean mouth.

Repairing a splint with a loose abutment is one of the more exasperating problems facing the dentist. A quick solution is essential because rapid breakdown of the abutment by caries is assured. In one clinical case, a canine of a multiple abutment bridge with no lesions was reduced to a soft mass to the gingival margin in less than 6 months after insertion.

Removal of the bridge and recementation

This procedure involves a potential risk of crown or root fracture. It does not solve the basic problem of why the appliance has become loose, and is not recommended.

Parallel or nonparallel pins used to repair bridge with fractured solder joint or abutment failure

PROCEDURE USING PARALLEL PINS

1. Prepare the area to be joined with dovetails in the pontic area (Fig. 16-18, *A*) and pinhole preparations.
2. Make an impression (elastomeric) of the prepared site and a casting (Fig. 16-18, *B*) that is retained in the dovetails. The metal thickness of the dovetail should be at least 2 mm deep.
3. Cement the casting in place (Fig. 16-18, *C*).

PROCEDURE USING NONPARALLEL PINS

The nonparallel pin procedure (Grunwald, 1974) can be used for correcting posterior abutment failure.

1. If a sufficient bulk of gold is present, prepare the dovetails in the pontic.
2. Impress the area and construct a new abutment with the male attachment.
3. Place this casting in the repair site, and drill, tap, and retain with .027 nonparallel pinholes and .027 threaded screws from the buccal and lingual aspects.

The nonparallel pin procedure is more advantageous than the parallel pin procedure because the pins can be oriented to the optimum thickness of gold in the pontic. A variation of this procedure is illustrated in Fig. 16-19, where thickness of gold is inadequate, or a pontic with a porcelain occlusal surface is present. A male attachment is prepared in the connector area, using medium-grit diamonds (½DTL and 169L or 170L fissure burs). Two impressions of this area are required, one

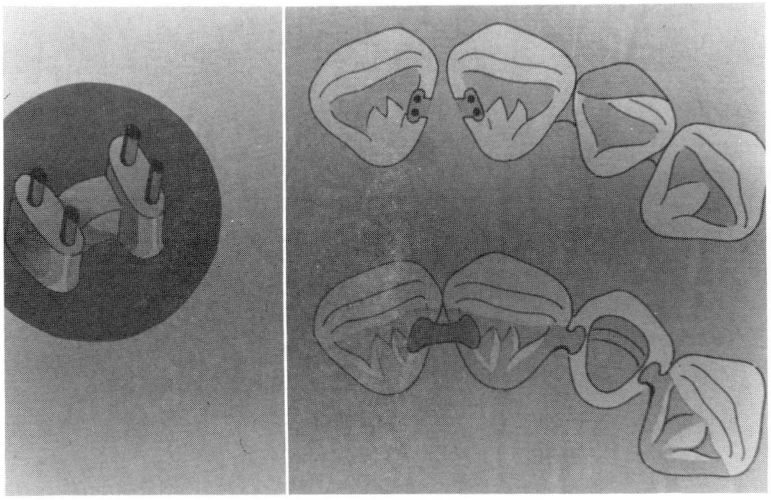

Fig. 16-18. A, Dovetail preparations. **B,** Casting. **C,** Casting in place with dovetails.

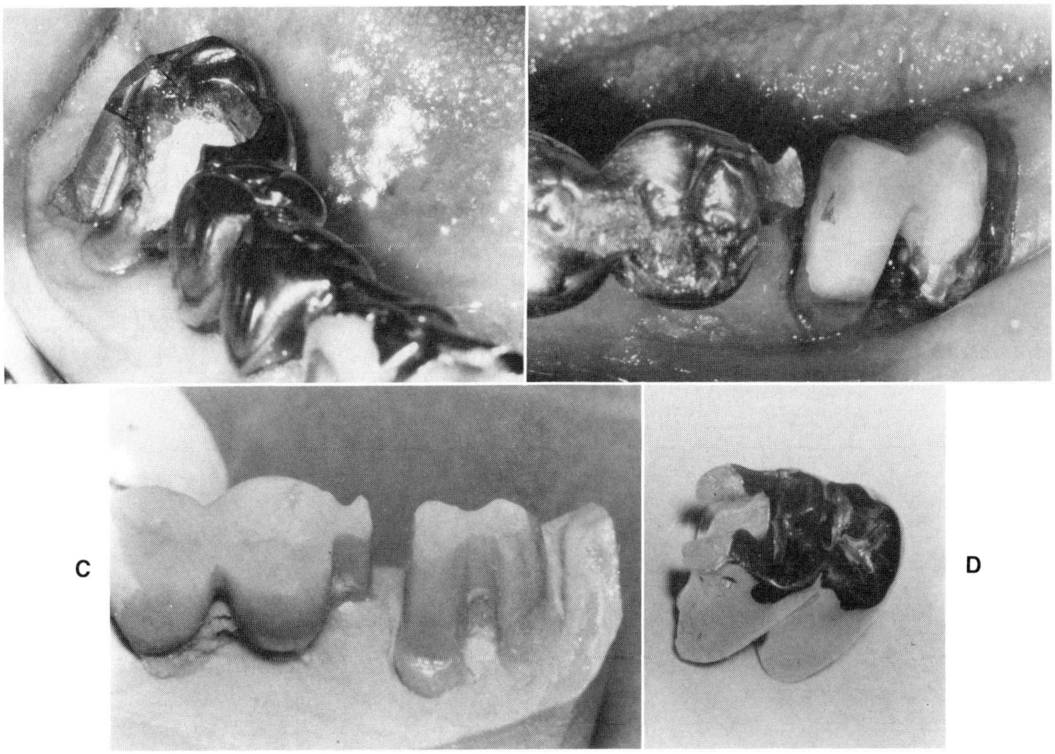

Fig. 16-19. A, Sectioning of old crown to preserve connector area. **B,** Prepared male attachment. **C,** Solid working cast. **D,** Finished casting.

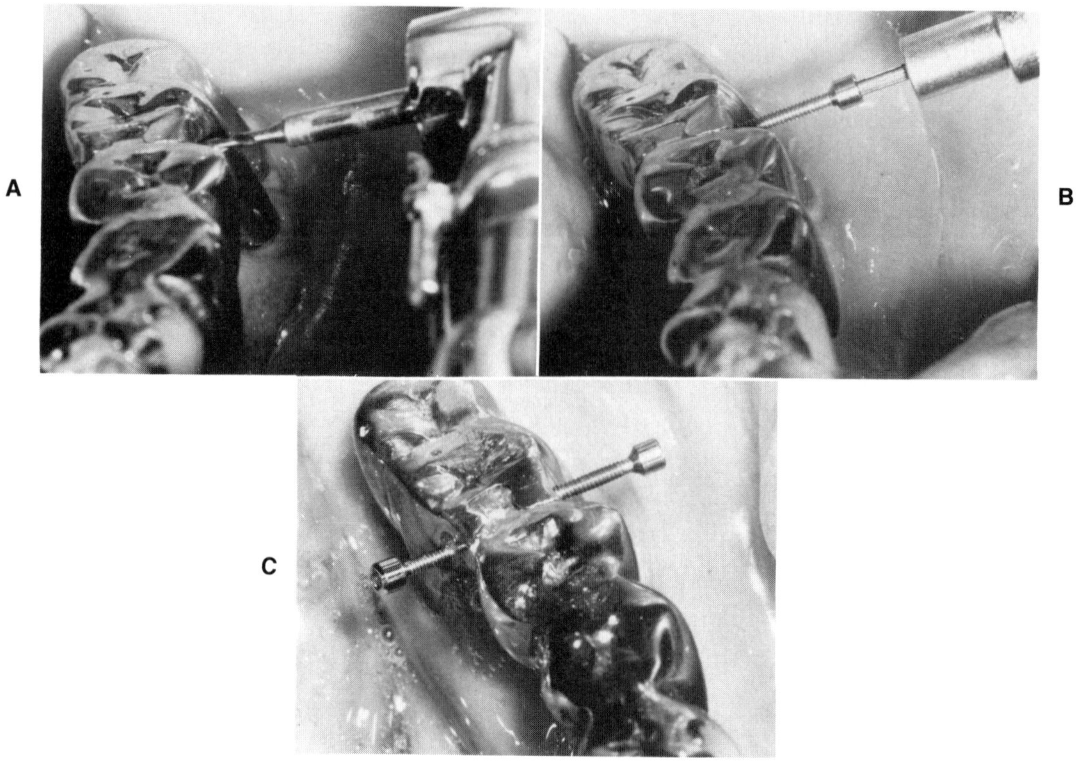

Fig. 16-20. A, Casting in place and .027 drill hole being placed. **B,** Tap (.027) in use. **C,** ReSeté pin being placed faciolingually.

for the die and one for the working model. The wax-up is built on the working model, and marginal adaptation is completed on the die. A casting is made and cemented in place. The connector area is drilled and tapped, and .027 Reseté pins placed buccolingually lock the casting in a solid unit (Fig. 16-20).

Chairside repairs

With certain periodontal splints, one of the teeth must be removed. The splint can be kept in place by sectioning the root(s) and removing it. The remaining clinical crown with root is smoothed and polished into the shape of a conical pontic. An amalgam or composite restoration is placed to obturate the remaining root canal and pulp chamber.

A temporary chairside repair of a loose retainer can be made using the free-flowing properties of the carboxylate cements. A hole is placed on the lingual surface of the casting. The preparation is debrided with sodium hypochlorite, using the lingual access hole. Carboxylate cement is placed in a Jiffy Tube with the tip cut to fit tightly into the lingual access hole. The assistant pulls down on the loose casting with a loop of dental tape through the solder joint, and the carboxylate cement is squeezed into the preparation until it comes out of the gingival margins.

This does not solve the basic problem of the retainer springing loose from the abutment in the first place. Careful equilibration might make this repair fairly long lasting, but it should be carefully monitored, and the operator should plan for a more definitive restoration.

REPAIRS OF HOLES IN CROWNS, ABUTMENTS WITH RECURRENT CARIES, AND DEFICIENT GINGIVAL MARGINS

Amalgam

Amalgam repairs of holes in crowns and abutments with recurrent caries have been successful clinically. The advantages of amalgam are its ease of manipulation and excellent sealing properties that help prevent caries from recurring. In repairing gingival margins, the amalgam is well tolerated by the tissue and is easily polished for better patient acceptance.

A disadvantage is that there will be corrosion between the gold and alloy in contact (Arvidson, 1975). Clinically this does not appear to endanger the integrity of the restoration. I have been able to observe repairs of this nature for periods of more than 10 years. A good amalgam technique that incorporates the minimum amount of mercury, plus careful polishing of the restoration after a 24-hour set, results in a smooth restoration acceptable to the patient.

Resin

Repairs with composite resins are essential in the anterior area where esthetics is of prime importance (Ribbons, 1973; Chan, 1972). The composites are also useful for the repair of holes on the occlusal surfaces, but will wear away from the margins rather quickly when put into an area of high stress or abrasion. A rubber dam is essential for proper placement of composites.

Gold foil

Repair with gold foil is the most permanent and esthetically acceptable restoration. It is indicated where access is readily available. Use of the rubber dam is necessary for this procedure to assure a long-lasting seal.

CONSTRUCTING A CROWN UNDER AN EXISTING PARTIAL DENTURE

A direct-indirect procedure (Thurgood, 1973; Staffanou, 1978) or an indirect procedure can be used to construct a crown under an existing partial denture. This repair should be used only when the framework can be definitely seated, with all saddle areas and clasps properly aligned.

DIRECT-INDIRECT PROCEDURE

1. Prepare the tooth, and make an impression for a die.
2. Construct a thin plastic coping over the die (Fig. 16-21). At the next appointment, flow wax on the coping, and seat the partial denture on the soft wax to get imprints of the clasps and rest seat.
3. Lute the pattern to the partial framework with DuraLay (Fig. 16-22). Fit a large alginate tray, and take an alginate impression, being careful not to displace the partial framework.
4. Remove the impression with the partial framework and the plastic coping attached to the framework.
5. Replace the original die in the plastic coping, lubricate the die, and pour the working model after blocking out undercuts in the saddle areas (Fig. 16-23).

This provides a very accurate relationship between the partial framework and the die, allowing for precise placement of rests and retentive areas for the clasps in the finished restoration (Fig. 16-24).

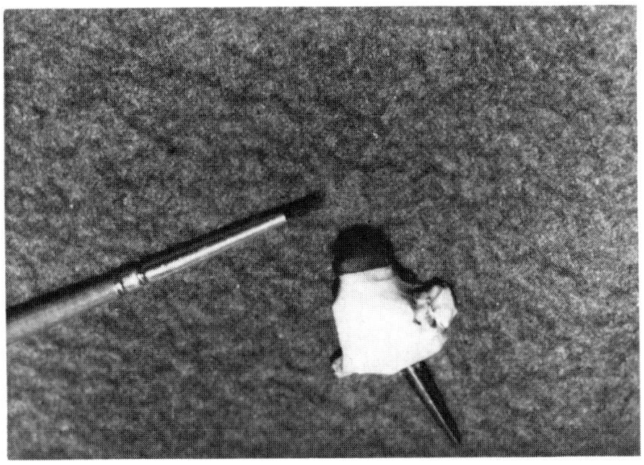

Fig. 16-21. Duralay coping on die.

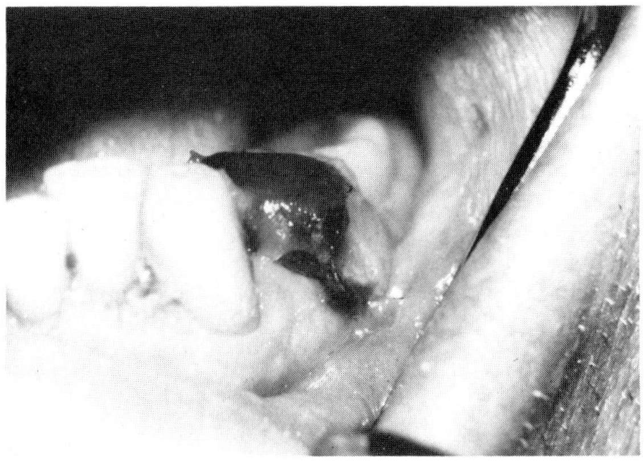

Fig. 16-22. Coping in place on abutment tooth, rests and clasp ir dents placed and luted to framework with Duralay.

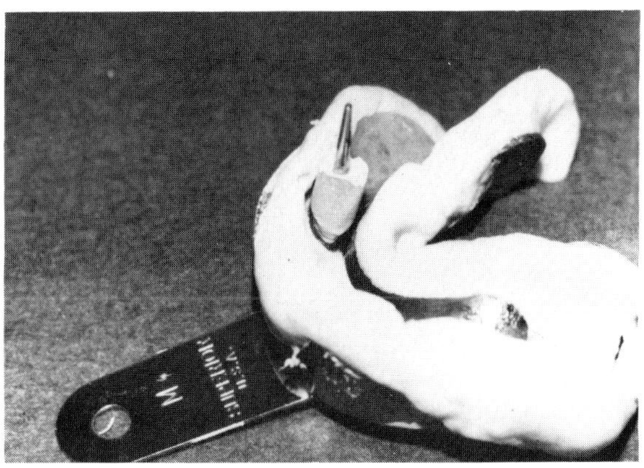

Fig. 16-23. Die replaced in coping.

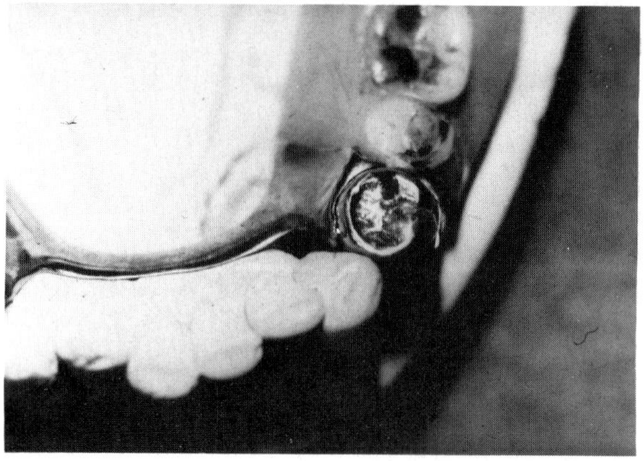

Fig. 16-24. Finished restoration.

INDIRECT PROCEDURE

1. Make a preliminary impression, and construct a quick-cure tray extending at least two teeth on either side of the abutment; the two teeth are to include the partial denture teeth.
2. Prepare the tooth, making sure adequate bulk is available for a minimum of 2 mm from all clasps and rest-seat areas to be incorporated in the gold restoration. If porcelain is to be used, a 2.5- to 3-mm clearance is required.
3. Retract the tissue, and make an impression (elastomeric). Seat the partial denture, assuring that the remaining clasps and indirect retainers are positively seated. Place the loaded tray over the preparation, and stabilize the appliance and tray. Remove the partial denture and impression.
4. Block out undercuts in the acrylic saddle, and pour the impression.
5. Make a separate impression for the die. Develop the wax pattern on the working cast, and transfer it to the die for completion of the margins.

READAPTATION OF CAST CROWN THAT HAS SEPARATED FROM TOOTH

Occasionally a crown will be constructed when the dentinal support is minimal or, more commonly, a crown is placed on an endodontically treated tooth that has not been properly reinforced with a post and core. These castings frequently result in a fracture of the remaining dentinal support. However, the cast crown that has separated from the tooth can be readapted to the damaged tooth by the use of a post and core technique, thus prolonging the clinical life of the casting.

The damage to the tooth structure falls into two categories: (1) fractures where the marginal integrity of the restoration remains intact, and (2) fractures that necessitate readaptation of the margin. In the first type, where the marginal integrity is intact, the tooth must be endodontically treated, if necessary, before the restoration is begun and the canal prepared for a dowel space. A preformed plastic form of the proper size is used to facilitate the construction of the casting, for example, Starlite Endowel or Parkell C.I. Kit (Fig. 16-25, *A*). Notch and shape the pattern so the casting appears as in Fig. 16-25, *B*. At this stage the casting should seat fully on the tooth and the crown should precisely fit the margin of the tooth. Carefully lubricate the interior of the crown with Duralay lubricant. Flow Duralay into the interior of the casting and firmly seat on the lubricated tooth. Place firm pressure on the crown until the Duralay reaches a doughy consistency. Remove the casting, trim away the excess Duralay, and firmly reseat on the tooth. Repeat these steps if necessary to be sure that the marginal adaptation is proper (Fig. 16-25, *C* and *D*). The relationship of the Duralay to the crown and the core is shown by the arrow in Fig. 16-26, *A*. Allow the Duralay to cure and remove the crown. The result is a plastic pattern that has reestablished the integrity of the lost tooth structure.

Remove this direct pattern and carefully place the sprue (Fig. 16-26, *B*). Attach the sprue where it can be cut off easily without affecting the internal adaptation. Invest the pattern with a phosphate-bonded investment and adjust the liquid/powder ratio to minimize expansion of the casting. Burn out the pattern at 1100° F for at least 1 hour, to assure that the post pattern is brought up to full mold temperature. When casting, be sure that the gold is very fluid before releasing the casting machine. Remove the casting, carefully remove the sprue, and check the fit of the cast core inside the crown with gold rouge and chloroform (Fig. 16-26, *C*). Note that the new gold is retained mechanically by the notches in the pattern. The casting is now ready for clinical verification. However, it is prudent to place a cement escape channel on the post to prevent splitting of the root or incomplete seating from hydraulic pressure at cementation.

Although it is possible to make a post and core casting from a direct pattern in one step to readapt a casting to a damaged tooth, it is advisable to use the described technique because of the difficulty in precisely fitting this type of casting and obtaining proper adaptation of the crown.

In the second type of fractures the marginal integrity of the crown is lost, thus creating a more difficult technical correction (Fig. 16-27, *A*). Prepare the tooth with a new finish line and provide a proper ferrule effect of 2 mm. When the preparation of the post space and margins are complete, make an impression of the prepared tooth, and make a die (Fig. 16-27, *B*).

Make a wax pattern of the post and wax up the core

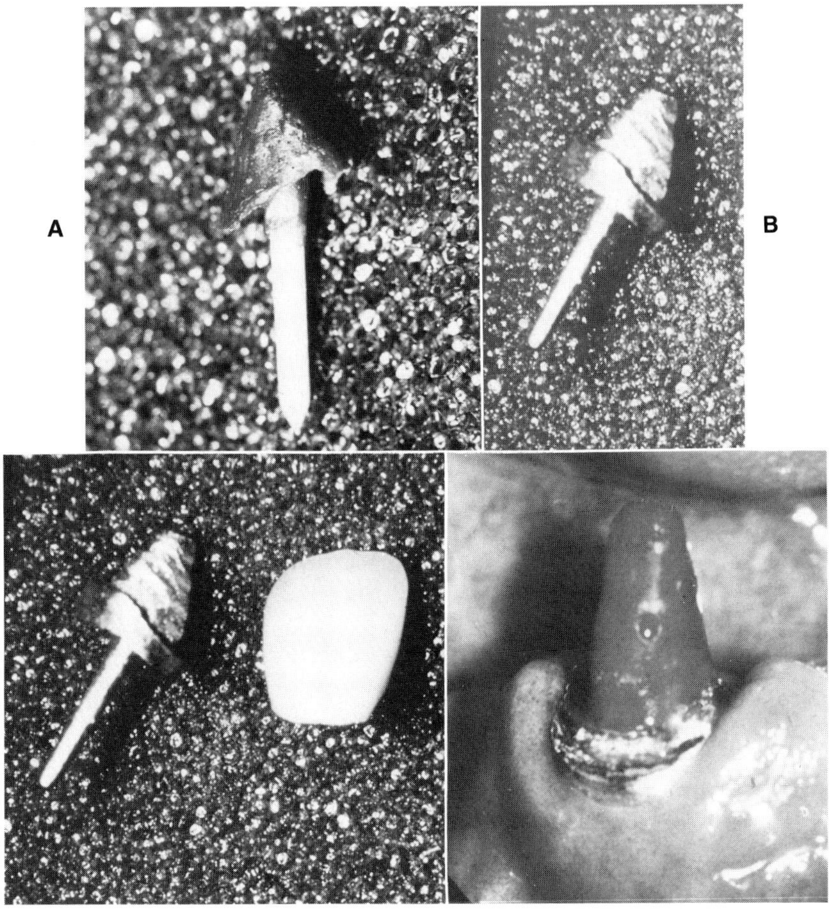

A B C D

Fig. 16-25. A, Post and core pattern using Starlite Endowel and Duralay. **B,** Cast pattern with undersized core. **C,** Core is adjusted so that crown does not touch. **D,** Crown is seated with Duralay to correct fit.

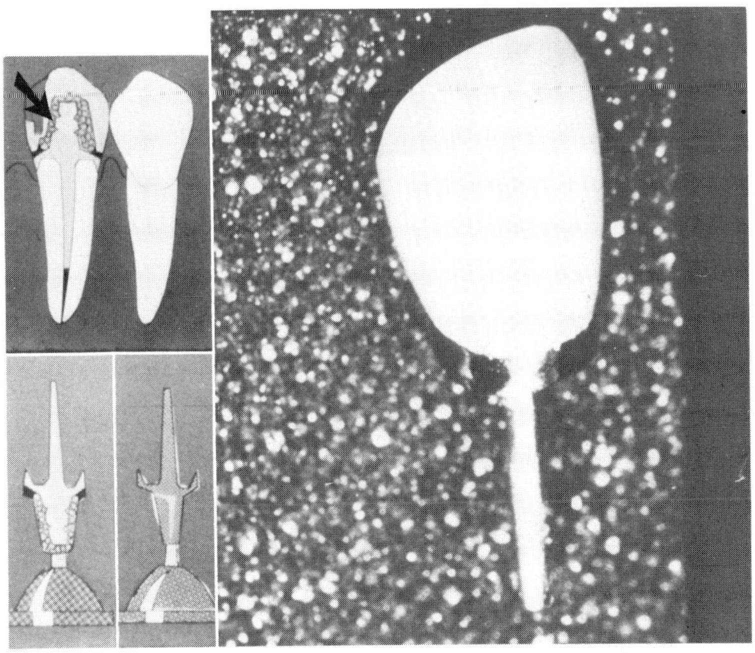

A B C

Fig. 16-26. A, Cutaway showing relationship of core, Duralay, and crown. Arrow shows Duralay correction. **B,** Investing for casting; Duralay correction. **C,** Assembled castings ready for try-in.

A 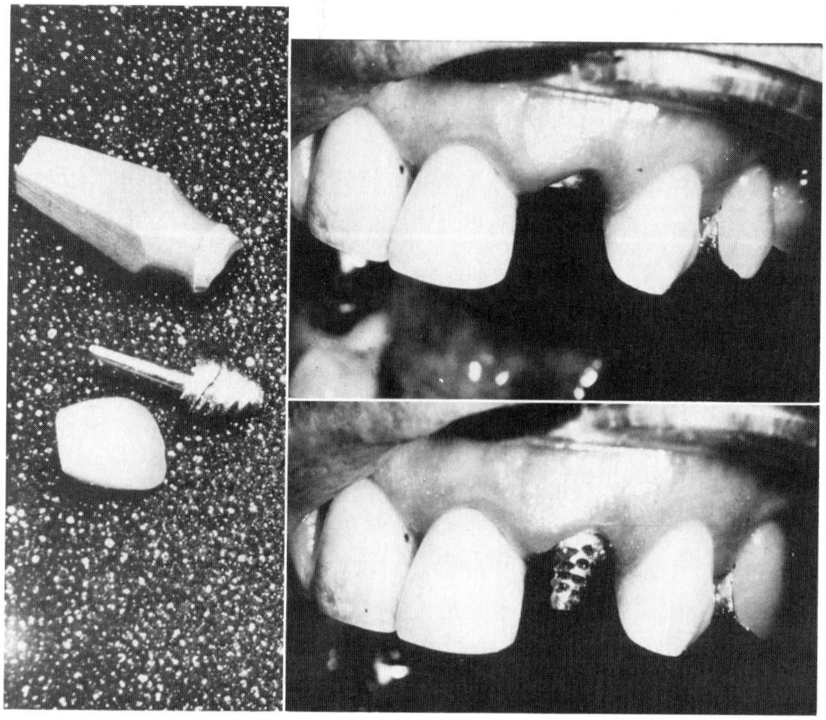 B C

Fig. 16-27. A, Marginal integrity of crown lost. **B,** Die of reprepared tooth; post and core fits new margins. **C,** Casting with undersized core verified on tooth.

A 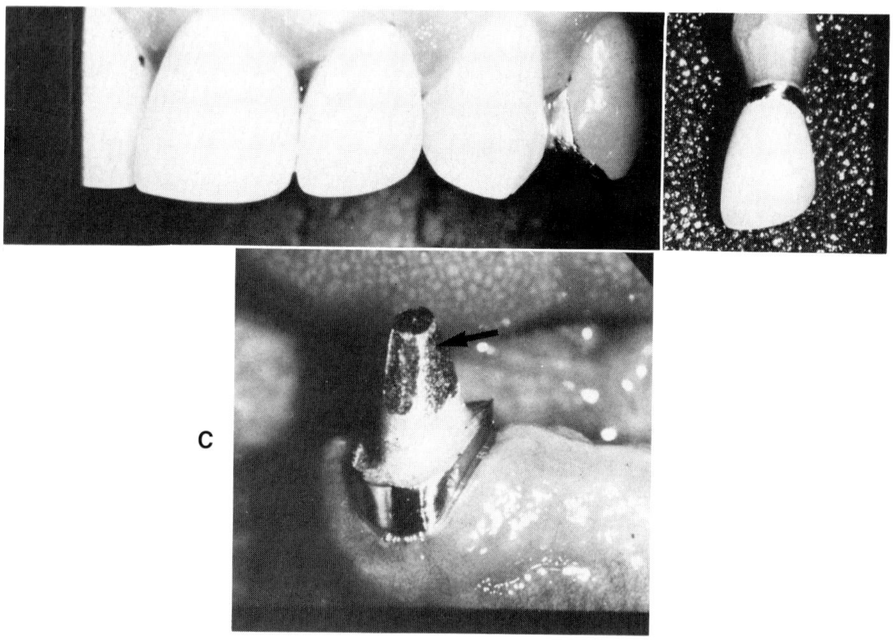 B C

Fig. 16-28. A, Crown adapted with Duralay. Position and occlusion verified. **B,** Assembled post and core with crown in place to verify fit. **C,** Corrected casting in mouth. Arrow shows new casting to original undersized core.

with the margins of the preparation incorporated in the pattern. The core is deliberately undersized (Fig. 16-27, *C*). As in the technique described for other fractures, verify the post and core on the tooth and position the crown in relation to the adjacent teeth. Verify the occlusion to ascertain any interferences between the crown and the undersized core (Fig. 16-28, *A*). Make a mix of Duralay. Place the casting and hold it in proper relation until the Duralay reaches a doughy stage. Remove the casting and reseat it. Take care to maintain proper position of the casting (Fig. 16-28, *B*). After the Duralay is cured, invest the pattern and cast as previously described. In Fig. 16-28, *C*, the arrow shows the newly cast gold.

This repair can be very useful in prolonging the life of a partial denture when one of the abutment crowns fails. The same procedures are used for the build-up of the tooth. After the casting with the undersized core is fitted, the crown is rerelated in the mouth with the partial denture in place (Fig. 16-29). These repairs are also very useful in maintaining the continuity of anterior restorations when a failure of the dentinal support occurs.

PROBLEM AREAS

Common problems in repair techniques, their probable causes, and solutions are identified in Table 16-1. The overcasting and pin-retained casting repairs are predicated on precise casting techniques carried out on solid working casts. Bubbles in a casting or faulty working casts magnify the errors to a point where the repair is not feasible. Attention to detail in the preparation of the framework with the principles of preparation design incorporating resistance and retention form are necessary. Pin placement and length have to be planned. A pin less than 2 mm in length is marginal in its retentive capability.

1. In the repairs of all pontics, rigidity of the framework has to be analyzed. A framework that is worn to the point that it flexes is incapable of holding a porcelain repair and any repair will have to be plastic, and will in all probability be very limited in longevity.

2. Repairs using semiprecision attachments are predicated on careful preparation of the male or female attachment. The use of diamond points to initiate the shape of the attachments is helpful. A finishing bur can be used to finalize the shapes of the attachment.

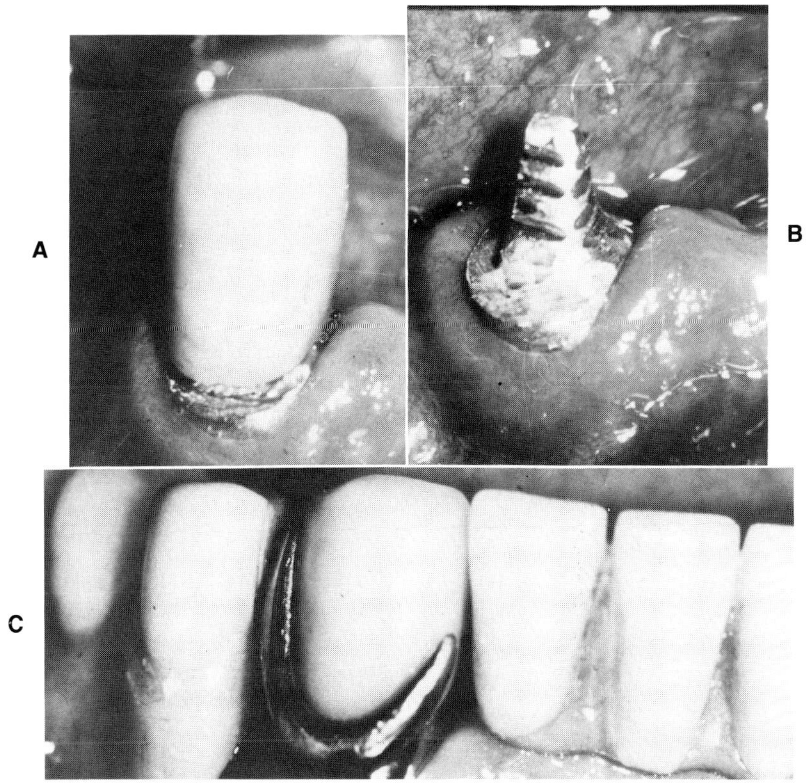

Fig. 16-29. A, Undersized core seated on fractured tooth. In this case margins are to be reestablished in post and core casting. **B,** Crown tried in to ascertain there is no interference to core. **C,** Lubricated crown seated with Duralay on post and core. Partial denture in place to reposition accurately.

Table 16-1. Repair techniques

Problem	Probable cause	Solution
Overcasting repair not seating	Excess porcelain on proximal surfaces	Adjust proximal contacts with Busch-Silent stone after marking interference with articulating paper or occlusal indicator spray
	Distorted impressions	Block out area under connector with wax to minimize distortion of impression
Overcasting repair not retained due to lack of retention	Facial groove not placed on facial surface	Use all retentive principles of parallelism as well as auxillary grooves to enhance retention (Fig. 16-1, *B*)
Insufficient room for overcasting repair	Anterior overbite or excessive vertical overlap	Use facially withdrawing pin casting
Pin casting not seating	Excess porcelain in interproximal space	Adjust interproximal porcelain with Busch-Silent stone after marking interferences with occlusal indicator spray or articulating paper
	Pin not parallel	Bevel pinholes with No. 6 round bur, and straighten pins if necessary
	Distorted impression	Nylon bristles used during impression technique touched tray; place appropriate stops on tray to allow relief of the tray
	Bristles pulling out of impression	Place "nail head" on bristle to retain it in impression material
Pin casting not retained	Pins too short	Pins should be at least 2 mm long or completely penetrate the backing; burnish with green stone at cementation
Pin pontic or Tru-Pontic repair refracturing	Framework flexing or worn out	Use heat-cured plastic pontic
Shaping male attachment	Burs chattering and lack of control	Use medium-grit diamond
Semiprecision attachment repair not seating	Distorted impression	Use hydrocolloid or block out under attachment with wax if silicone or rubber impressions are made
	Attempted repair with removable die	Use solid working model and transfer wax pattern to separate die
Twist-drill binding	Insufficient lubricant	Use wax for lubricant and proceed slowly; if drill binds, reverse handpiece, and relubricate drill before proceeding again
Insufficient retention for plastic-facing repair	Thin gold backing	Drill and place pins in gold backing for retention
Post and core not seating	Overexpansion of casting or defects on casting	Use careful investing technique; do not use liner in ring and increase liquid 1 ml over normal when investing
Second casting not fully forming	Mold temperature not high enough; gold not fluid enough	Increase mold temperature and get gold very fluid before casting; use extra wind on casting machine
Crown not fitting or seating	Check for proper sprue removal	Use chloroform and gold rouge, or sandblast the casting for detection of interferences

3. Impression making is critical, and hydrocolloid seems to be an excellent choice for this technique. Cross-pin stabilization for this procedure is easily accomplished with the Thread Mate System drills and pins available. Binding of the drills is a problem, but careful reversing of the handpieces and use of wax for a lubricant overcomes this problem. The pinholes can be tapped. Self-tapping pins can also be used for pin placement.

4. Crown placement under an existing partial denture is an extremely critical procedure. The partial framework has to be carefully related to the working cast. The technique using the Duralay coping has the best clinical results of the techniques that have been used.

SUMMARY

Techniques for repairs have been described that have been used successfully on large splints and bridges in which a remake would be a great physical and financial burden for the patient. It is important that the basic design of the appliance be biologically acceptable before the repair is undertaken.

REFERENCES

Arvidson, K.: Corrosion studies of a dental gold alloy in contact with amalgam under different conditions, Sven. Tandlak. Tidskr. **68**(4): 135-139, 1975.

Chan, K.C., Nareander, H., Soni, P., and Khowassah, M.A.F.: Tissue reactions to two composite resins, J. Prosthet. Dent. **27**:176-180, 1972.

Grunwald, D.C.: A simplified partial denture, J. Acad. Gen. Dent. **22**:20-21, 1974.

Lum, L.: Personal communications, 1977.

Portnoy, L.L.: Repairing a bridge using threaded non-parallel pins, J. Calif. Dent. Assoc. **41**:471-474, 1973.

Ribbons, J.W., and Pearson, G.J.: A composite filling material: a two-year clinical assessment, Br. Dent. J. **134**:389-391, 1973.

Sheets, C.E.: A split cast procedure for the replacement of pontics, J. Prosthet. Dent. **16**:948-954, 1966.

Staffanou, R.S.: Personal communications, 1978.

Thurgood, B.W., Thayer, K.E., and Lee, R.E.: Complete crowns constructed for an existing partial denture, J. Prosthet. Dent. **29**:507-512, 1973.

CHAPTER 17

DIAGNOSTIC AND TREATMENT APPLIANCES

CHARLES McNEILL III

Occlusal therapy in the form of removable and fixed appliances or splints is an important adjunct to prosthodontic procedures. Pathologic manifestations of the masticatory system require reversible diagnostic and intermediate treatment measures before finalization of any prosthodontic treatment. Temporomandibular joint disorders, bruxism, instability of the maxillomandibular relationship, vertical dimension or other bite alterations, tooth mobility and/or periodontal involvement, extreme tooth wear, and fracture all demand proper sequential management.

The sequence of treatment begins with all proper diagnostic procedures mentioned in previous chapters. Occlusal appliances or splints must be considered when the occlusion is suspected as the cause of the patient's problems, or if the occlusion is to be altered by any discernible magnitude that would change the maxillomandibular relationship. Furthermore, after the diagnostic procedures many prosthodontic patients need reevaluation before the treatment is finalized.

The periodontal, pulpal, and temporomandibular joint health must be evaluated before progressing to the final steps of the case. Once the final treatment plan is determined, an occlusal appliance still may be included in the overall treatment regimen.

There are many types of diagnostic and treatment appliances. They can be fixed or removable. In this chapter only a few representative forms of appliances will be shown and discussed. Diagnostic and treatment appliances can be divided into the following three catagories: (1) diagnostic interocclusal and/or bruxism appliances, (2) orthopedic repositioning appliances, and (3) orthopedic stabilizing appliances.

The purpose of these appliances, as stated by Clark (1984), is to perform one or more of the following: (1) to stabilize and improve the function of the temporomandibular joints, (2) to improve the function of the masticatory motor system and reduce abnormal muscle activity, and (3) to protect teeth from attrition and adverse traumatic loading.

DIAGNOSTIC TEMPOROMANDIBULAR JOINT (TMJ) AND/OR BRUXISM APPLIANCES

Occlusal splints are quite helpful in diagnosing TMJ disorders related to occlusion and articulation problems. The artificial masking of occlusal prematurities or deflective contacts allows for a decrease in muscle fatigue, spasm, and tenderness; joint edema, inflammation, and tenderness, and tooth mobility and sensitivity. Furthermore, the tendency for bruxism is usually diminished or eliminated by an occlusal appliance (Ramfjord, 1961).

Anterior palatal bite plates can be easily fabricated for short-term or intermittent use as a diagnostic appliance (Fig. 17-1). The appliance simply separates or disengages the posterior tooth contacts, allowing for several physiologic changes to occur within the stomatognathic system (Perry, 1969). First, any existing posterior occlusal prematurities are immediately eliminated both in the intercuspal position and during func-

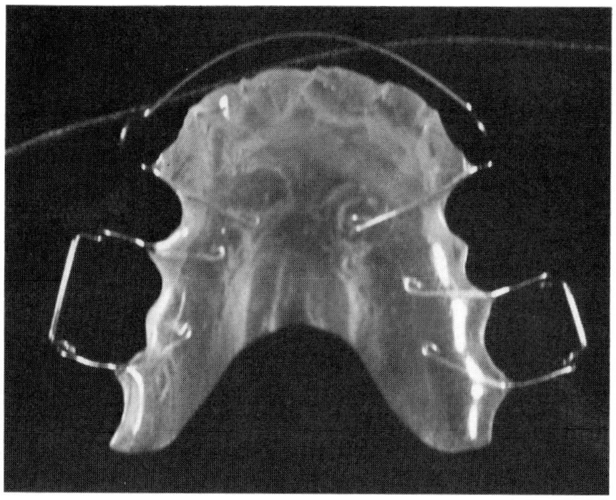

Fig. 17-1. Anterior bite plate.

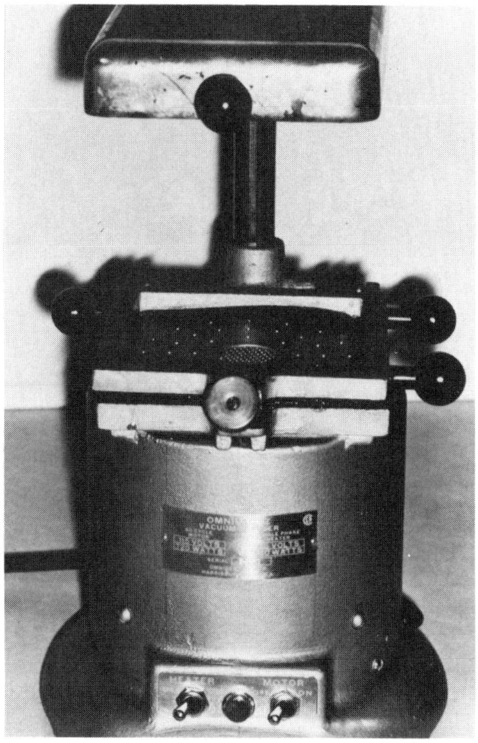

Fig. 17-2. Omnivac vacuum machine.

tional and parafunctional movements of the mandible (Bakke and Moller, 1980; Krough-Poulsen and Olsson, 1966). These premature contacts can act as fulcrums that reflexly increase mandibular muscle activity biomechanically and adversely affect condylar position (Roth, 1973). Second, the fact that there are only anterior contacts on the appliance causes a decrease in elevator activity during lateral jaw movements, as explained by Williamson (1983). An added advantage is that the anterior contacts allow for a rapid repositioning of the mandible without requiring intricate and time-consuming corrections.

"Emergency splints" can be fabricated directly in the mouth with acrylic. The acrylic is moulded only over the maxillary anterior teeth to prevent closure of the mandible into full intercuspation, as described by Langer (1975). These appliances are suggested for short-term use only for patients with muscle trismus and limited mandibular opening ability.

Resilient splints and other temporary or limited-use splints should be used either for short duration of full-time wear or for limited time periods of wear. The reason is that the resilient mouthguard material fatigues easily, and the partial-coverage appliance permits tooth movement, such as overeruption, rotation, and migration. Therefore instead of the splint being a reversible form of treatment or purely a diagnostic aid, it can cause irreversible changes in the occlusion. These changes may, in fact, create an occlusion that is more traumatic than the original one. The advantage of the soft splint and temporary splint is the ease of construction and low cost.

Only the fabrication of the mouthguard resilient bruxism splint and the anterior bite plane splints will be described. It should be pointed out that one retrospective study and clinical assessments claim that resilient appliances have slightly decreased effectiveness when compared to hard acrylic full-arch appliances (Posselt, 1963).

Vacuum-formed TMJ resilient splint

PROCEDURE

1. Pour the maxillary or mandibular impression with dental stone. Do not invert the impression.

2. Prepare the cast for vacuum adaptation. Trim the base flat and as thin as possible. Trim the sides square with the base. Cut a 5-mm hole in the deepest part of palate to provide good palatal adaptation of material.

3. Adapt the mouthguard blank. Place the cast on the vacuum plate of the Omnivac II Precision Vacuum Adapter* (Fig. 17-2), Biostar Universal Pressure Molding Machine† (Fig. 17-3), or vacuum machine of choice. Swing the heating unit to the rear, and turn it on. Raise

*Buffalo Dental Manufacturing Co., Brooklyn, N.Y.
†Great Lakes Orthodontic Products, Inc., Buffalo, N.Y.

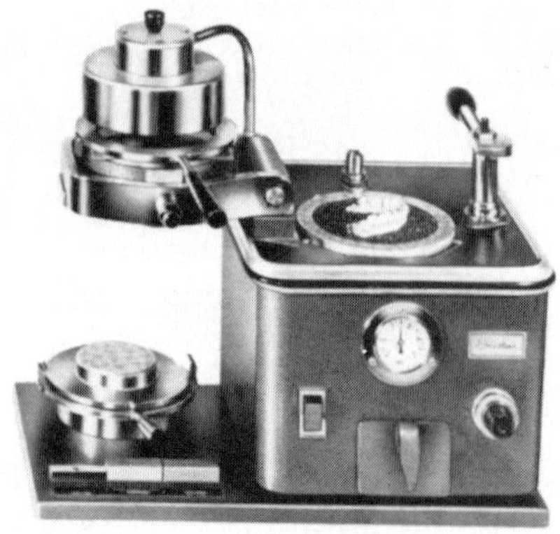

Fig. 17-3. Biostar universal pressure molding machine.

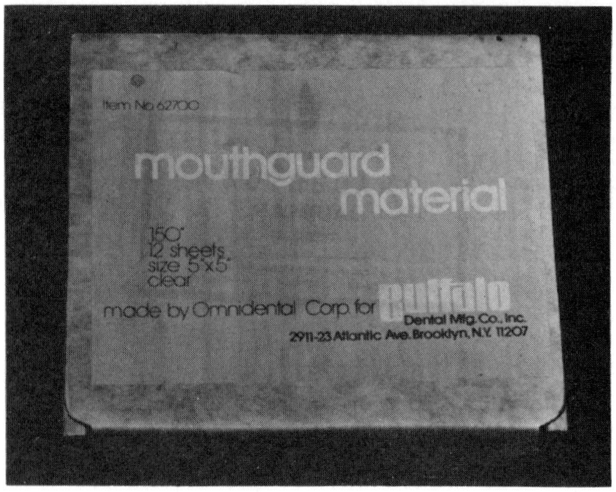

Fig. 17-4. Mouthguard material.

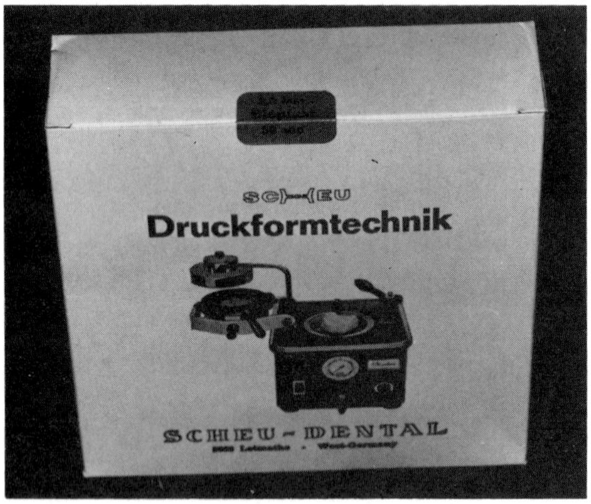

Fig. 17-5. Bioplast resilient material.

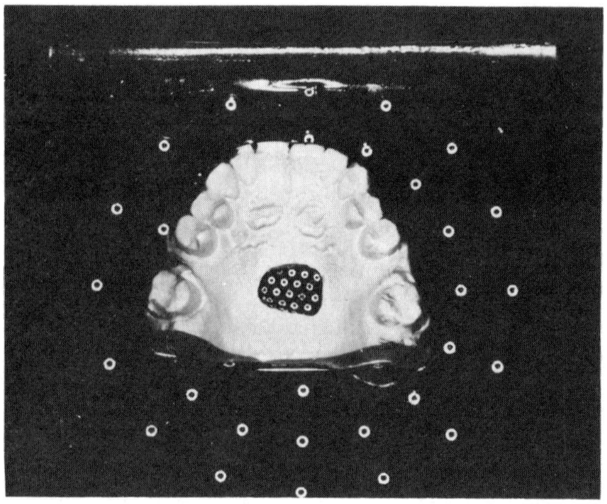

Fig. 17-6. Mouthguard material adapted over cast.

the hinged frame until it clicks into the heating position. Place a 5 × 5-inch (13 × 13-cm) mouthguard material* (Fig. 17-4) or Bioplast† 1.5, 1.0, or 3.0 (Fig. 17-5). Swing the heating unit into position over the resin material. When the material begins to sag, approximately ½ to ¾ inch (13 to 19 mm), turn on the motor switch, and lower the frame over cast. Leave the heating unit in place over the cast until the adaptation process is completed (15 seconds) (Fig. 17-6). Swing the heating unit out of the way, and allow the adaptation to cool for at least 30 seconds, with the motor running.

4. Remove mouthguard material blank. Trim the excess material off the cast with scissors (Fig. 17-7). Continue to trim the splint as depicted with scissors and a large Melite acrylic bur or Parkell Trim Bur No. 514* (Fig. 17-8).

5. Adjust the occlusion of the appliance on an articulator or in the mouth. Use large carbide acrylic burs (No. 84T). Adjust the occlusion until there is 0.5 mm of thickness of material over the first prematurity.

6. Finish the splint. The splint should allow for an even bilateral contact of all mandibular or centric relation. Festoon the soft splint with the same large bur (Fig. 17-9). Smooth the splint with orange solvent, and wash it in cold water (Figs. 17-10 and 17-11). Deliver the splint to the operatory with its retainer box (Fig. 17-12).

*Buffalo Dental Manufacturing Co., Brooklyn, N.Y.
†Great Lakes Orthodontic Products, Inc., Buffalo, N.Y.

*Parkell, Farmingdale, N.Y.

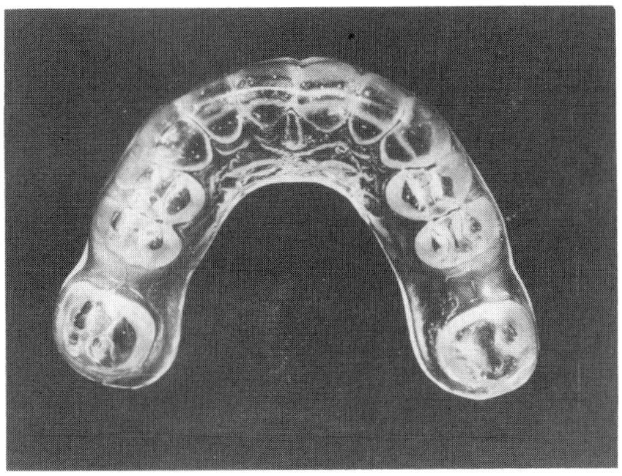

Fig. 17-7. Excess material trimmed.

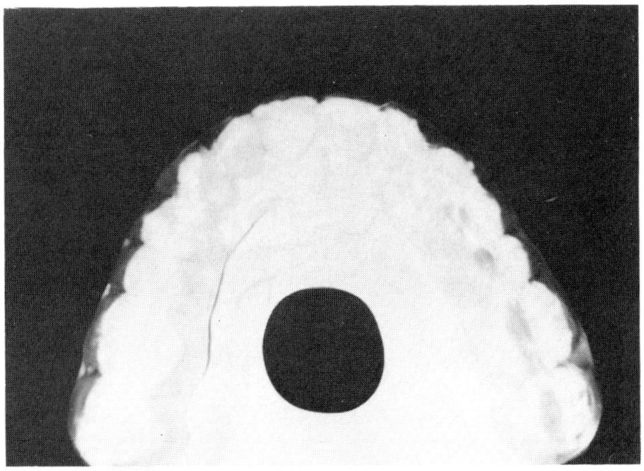

Fig. 17-8. Trimmed splint.

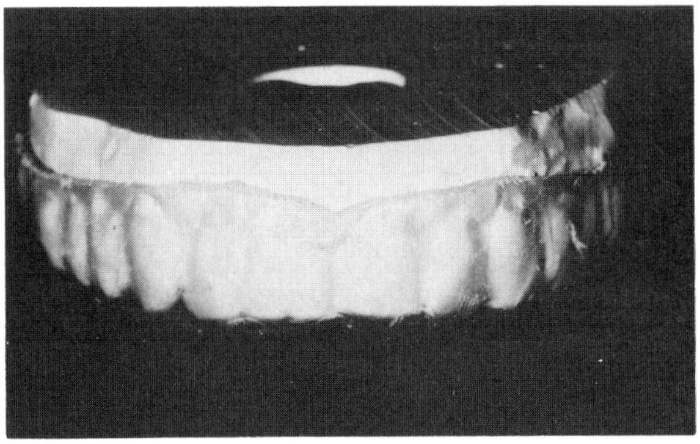

Fig. 17-9. Festooned splint.

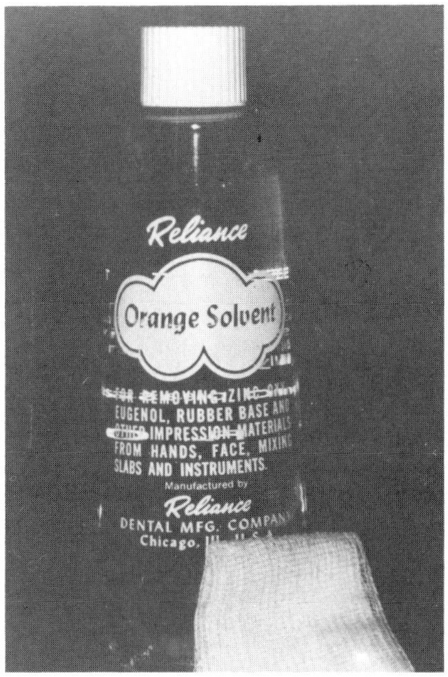

Fig. 17-10. Orange solvent.

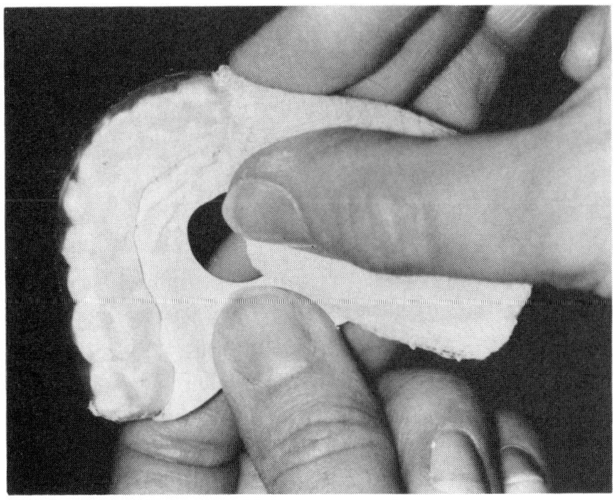

Fig. 17-11. Smoothing and polishing splint with orange solvent on 2 × 2-inch gauze.

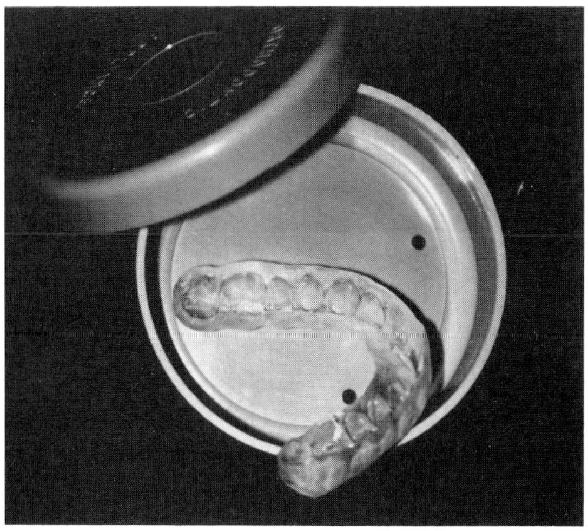

Fig. 17-12. Resilient splint in retainer box.

ORTHOPEDIC APPLIANCES

The concept of utilizing an interocclusal appliance for more complex diagnostic problems and for treatment of craniomandibular (TMJ) disorders is well established (Ramfjord and Ash, 1983). Usually these appliances are fabricated with definitive invasive therapy in the mind of the clinician. The advantage of reversible, noninvasive appliance therapy prior to definitive therapy can be essential. The importance of stabilizing the maxillomandibular relationship before definitive occlusal therapy was discussed by Dyer (1974), by Shore (1967), and others. It is mandatory to establish as much as is clinically possible, a physiologic optimum position of the condyle-disk assembly, "normal" integrated neuromuscular activity, and a stable interocclusal relationship.

There are four prerequisites for proper fabrication of an occlusal appliance that would be used for long-term therapy (over 3 weeks) and/or full-time wear. It should be noted that full-time wear provides for a much more rapid and greater relief of symptoms. The prerequisites are as follows:

1. The splint should be as unobtrusive and comfortable as possible.
2. The splint must cover all teeth in the arch to prevent eruption.
3. All teeth in the arch must be stabilized to prevent migration, rotation, and tipping.
4. The splint must be retentive enough to prevent movement or slipping during mastication.

Orthopedic repositioning appliances

Orthopedic repositioning appliances are the most common form of nonsurgical treatment for internal derangements of the temporomandibular joint. There are many variations in the design of these appliances. Regardless of the design, the main purpose of a repositioning appliance is to biomechanically induce a change in the relationship of the articular structures, thus improving function. There are primarily two types of appliances. One appliance is an anterior repositioning appliance, and the other is a superior repositioning appliance. Both appliances are fabricated using a vacuum and/or positive air pressure forming machine (see Figs. 17-2 and 17-3).

Anterior repositioning appliance

The anterior repositioning appliance is used for internal derangements related to the malrelationship of disk-condyle assembly (Farrar and McCarty, 1982). The appliance is utilized for disk-interference disorders such as disk displacement, chronic distal thrust of the mandible (Ricketts, 1966), and/or locking with and without reduction. Anterior displacement of the disk is usually associated with a posterior-superior positioning of the condyle in the closed jaw position (Weinberg, 1979). Thus, treatment with an anterior repositioning appliance attempts to bring the mandible (condyle) forward and downward (anterior-inferiorly). After disk "recapturing" occurs, a period of "healing and/or adaptation" allows the condyle to be returned to a reasonably normal physiologic position by making subsequent adjustments on the appliance. As this repositioning of the disk-condyle assembly occurs into the fossa, the symptoms may or may not return. If they do return, then other modalities may be necessary, including surgery. An anterior repositioning appliance may also be beneficial in cases of disk perforation and localized degenerative joint disease. In these cases the degenerative tissues can cause a posterior and superior positioning of the condyle. As in disk displacement, these conditions can also benefit from a biomechanical approach that postures the mandible downward and forward.

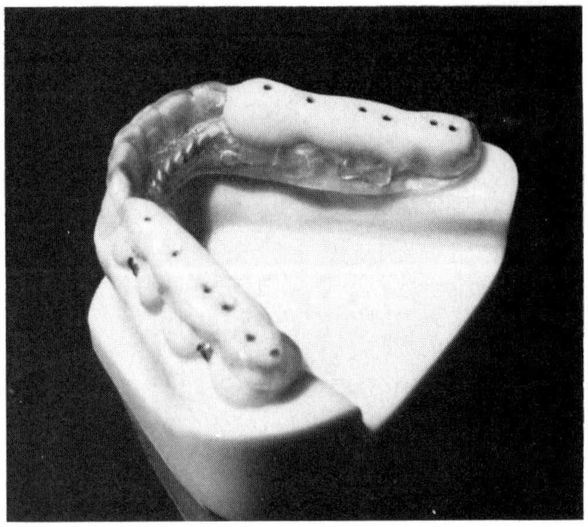

Fig. 17-13. Autopolymerizing acrylic on occlusal surface of mandibular appliance.

An appliance that is used to reposition the disk-condyle assembly must be worn 24 hours a day to be effective. They can be made on either arch, but the lower arch is usually preferred. A lower appliance is most often more esthetic; thus, patients are more willing to wear the appliance full time (Gelb, 1977). If an upper appliance is used, many times a ramp must be developed on the lingual aspect of the anterior part of the appliance in order to keep the mandible forward. This results in a large amount of visible acrylic.

The occlusal contacts on the appliance are placed in such a manner that the condyles are maintained in a downward and forward position on closure. The occlusal stops or contacts can be fabricated on mounted casts or added directly in the mouth with autopolymerizing acrylic (Fig. 17-13). The position that determines the exact location of the occlusal contacts is the mandibular

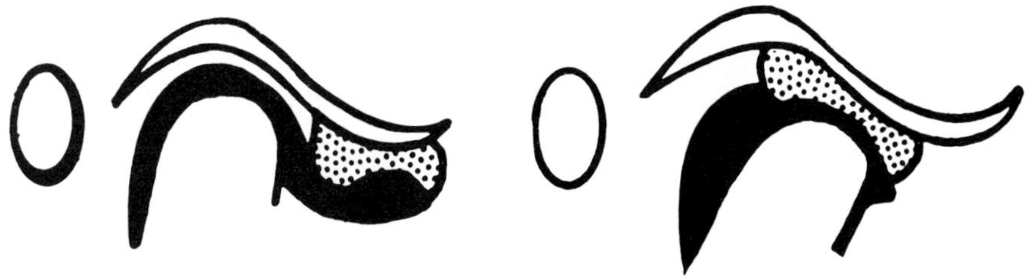

Fig. 17-14. Early reciprocal click. Second position with proper condyle-disk relationship ("recaptured disk").

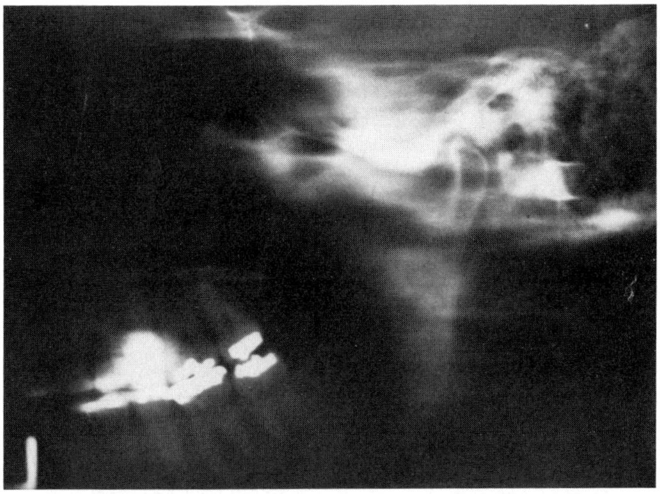

Fig. 17-15. Tomogram of left condyle in posterior position in articular fossa due to anteriorly displaced disk.

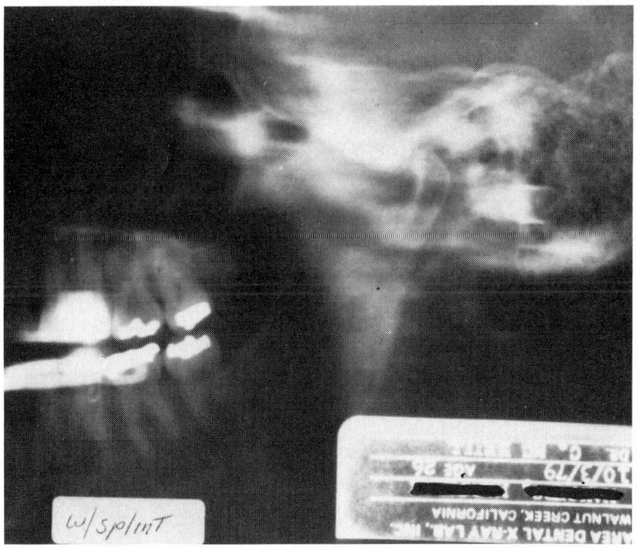

Fig. 17-16. Tomogram of same condyle with proper disk/condyle relationship with anterior repositioning appliance in place.

position immediately before the closing click (Fig. 17-14).

The appliance must be worn for a minimum of 6 weeks, and possibly as long as 6 months. During this time an attempt is made by repeated occlusal adjustments to reposture the corrected disk-condyle assembly into its physiologic position in the fossa. At that time an evaluation must be made whether the appliance can be utilized as an ongoing stabilizing appliance or if further therapy is necessary (Figs. 17-15 and 17-16).

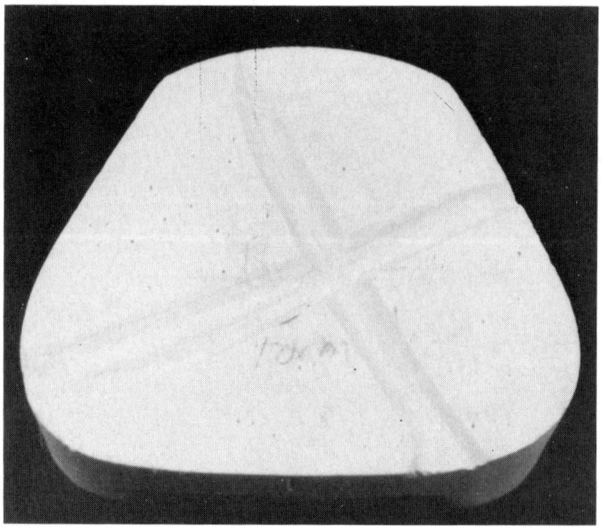

Fig. 17-17. Base of working cast coated with separating medium.

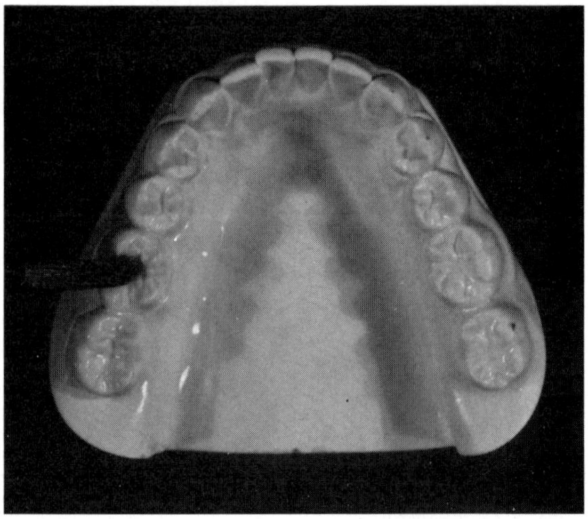

Fig. 17-18. Separating medium being applied to occlusal surface.

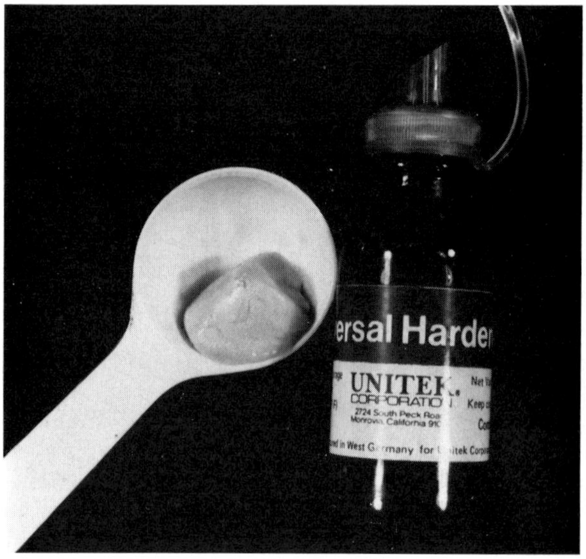

Fig. 17-19. Optosil blockout material, Type I, with Universal hardener.

PROCEDURE FOR VACUUM-FORMED ANTERIOR REPOSITIONING APPLIANCE

1. Take impression of mandibular arch in either alginate or hydrocolloid impression material.
2. Pour impression in hard white dental stone.
3. Trim cast with a flat base and score base with an X for an index for taking cast with appliance back to articulator. Coat undersurface with separator* (Fig. 17-17).
4. Mount cast with intraocclusal record on semiadjustable articulator.
5. Remove cast from mounting and apply separator to teeth surfaces of cast (Fig. 17-18).
6. Block out undercuts on cast with Optosil,‡ using ¼ scoop of Optosil and 6 to 8 drops of Universal Hardener§ (Fig. 17-19).
7. Bend four .032 ball clasps* for retention on the right and left between bicuspids and between first and second molars (Figs. 17-20 and 17-21).
8. Place sticky wax clasps in the four buccal embrasure areas.
9. Bend gold supporting wire* to fit lingual area from cuspid to cuspid, 3 to 4 mm below gingival sulcus of six anteriors. Place sticky wax wire (Figs. 17-22 and 17-23).
10. Add autopolymerizing acrylic* to attach supporting wire to the bicuspid clasps (Fig. 17-24).
11. Allow acrylic to polymerize in hot water in curing unit for 3 to 5 minutes (Fig. 17-25).
12. Remove supporting wire and bicuspid clasp unit from cast in order to clean sticky wax from underneath tissue side of supporting wire and from cast.

---

†Great Lakes Orthodontic Products Inc., Buffalo, N.Y.
‡Optosil Hard, Type I, Unitek Corporation, Monrovia, Calif.
§Unitek Corporation, Monrovia, Calif.

*Great Lakes Orthodontic Products, Inc., Buffalo, N.Y.

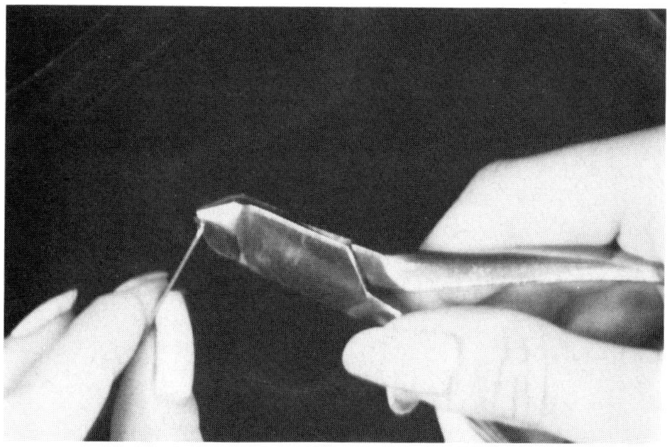

Fig. 17-20. Bending 0.032 ball clasp material with bird beak pliers.

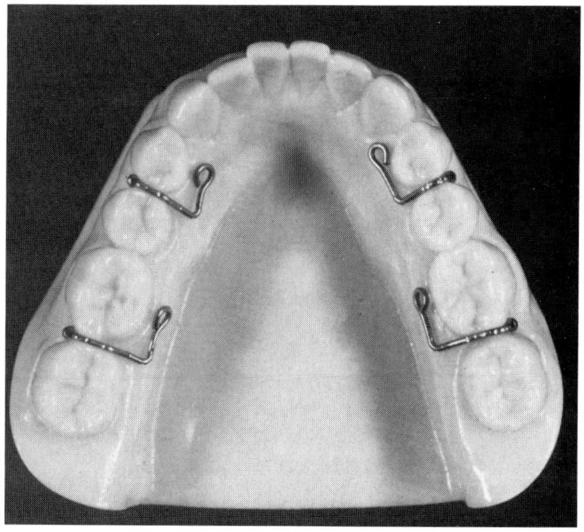

Fig. 17-21. Ball clasps in position ready to be sticky waxed to cast.

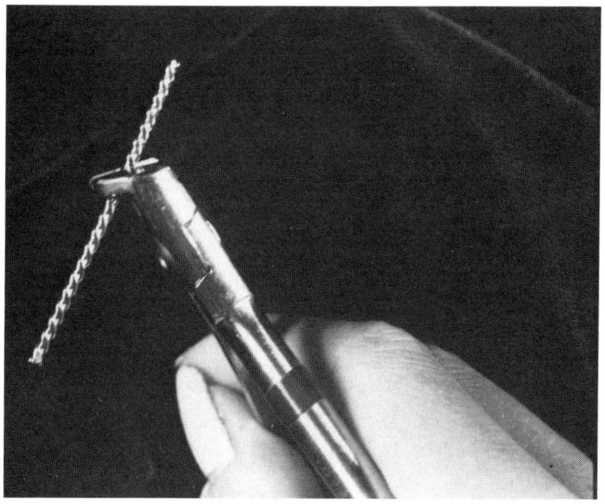

Fig. 17-22. Bending gold-plated, lingual support wire.

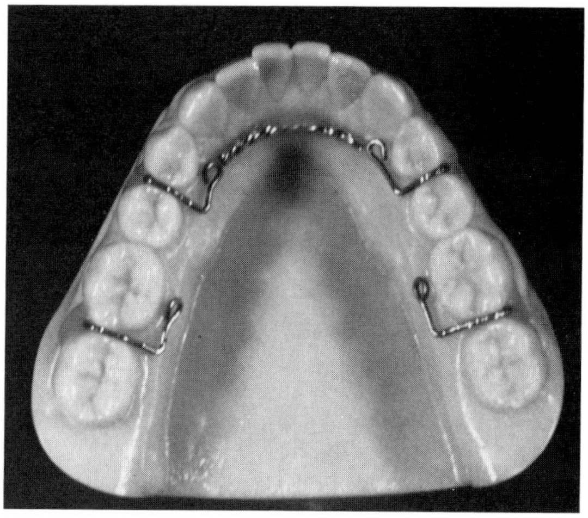

Fig. 17-23. Support wire placed in cast from cuspid to cuspid area.

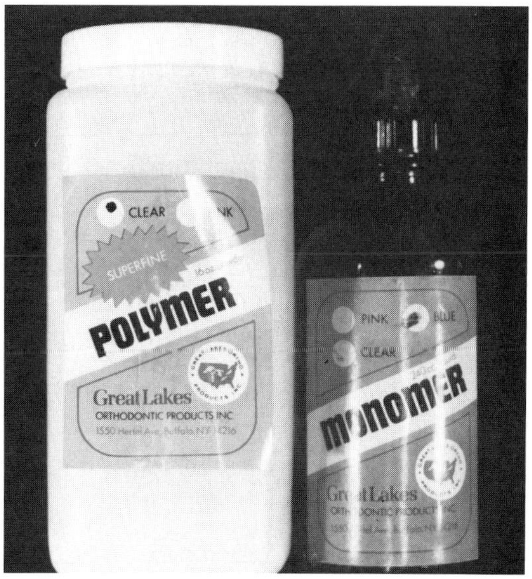

Fig. 17-24. Autopolymerizing acrylic for attachment of clasps and support wire.

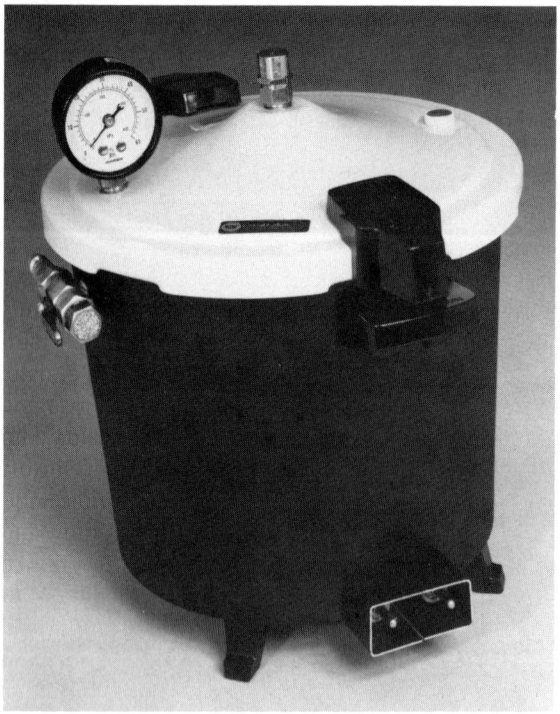

Fig. 17-25. Electric pressure pot for dense polymerization of acrylic.

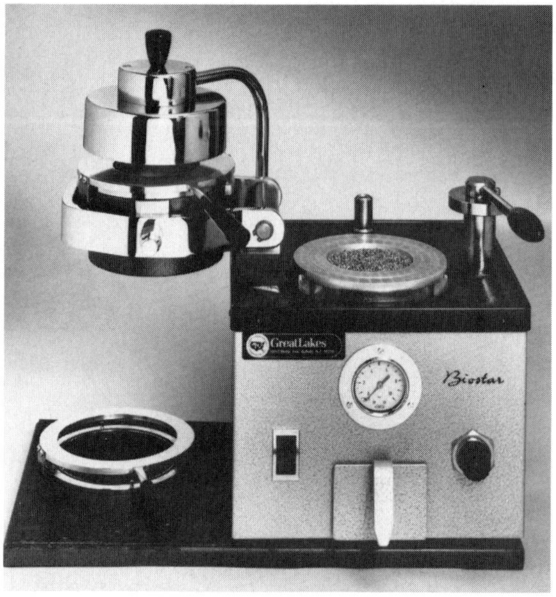

Fig. 17-26. Positive air pressure adaptation instrument for forming Biocryl II disks to working casts.

13. Turn on Biostar* unit to allow infrared heating element to heat for 5 minutes prior to forming Biocryl‡ (Fig. 17-26).

14. Place 2 mm thick Biocryl in holding frame ring of Biostar with corresponding spacer adapter (Fig. 17-27).

15. Submerge appliance design cast in lead pellets, in Biostar, to block out undercuts in nonsplint facial areas.

16. Place heating element over Biocryl material to begin softening.

17. Mix the autopolymerizing acrylic again and add to all clasps and supporting wire to aid in embedding same in appliance material.

18. Quickly place Biostar in position over cast and lock in place with locking handle.

19. Allow cast to remain under pressure for 3 minutes.

20. Activate pressure release button and remove cast from Biostar unit (Fig. 17-28).

21. Using a No. 265 cutting bur,* remove excess Biocryl II from cast (Figs. 17-29 and 17-30).

22. Cut excess acrylic to the approximate periphery of the appliance with double-sided sintered diamond disk.*

23. Return cast to mounting and glue in place with MDS adhesive.†

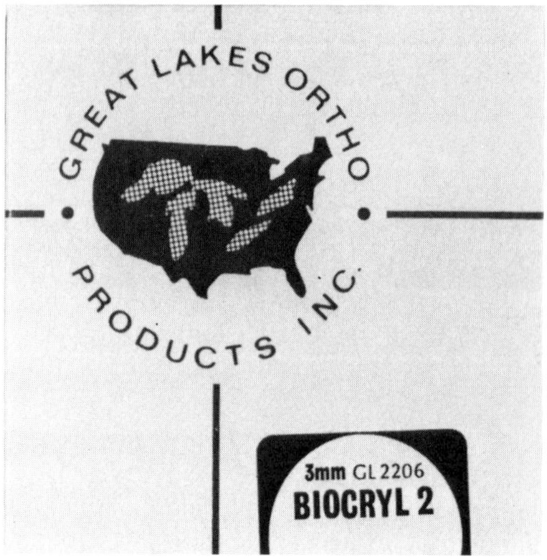

Fig. 17-27. Biocryl II disks, 3 mm in thickness, for lower appliance.

*Great Lakes Orthodontic Products, Inc., Buffalo, N.Y.

*Diamond disc, #7941, 4 mm thickness, Brasseler USA, Inc., Savannah, Ga.

†MDS Adhesive, QX-4, MDS Products, Inc., Anaheim, Calif.

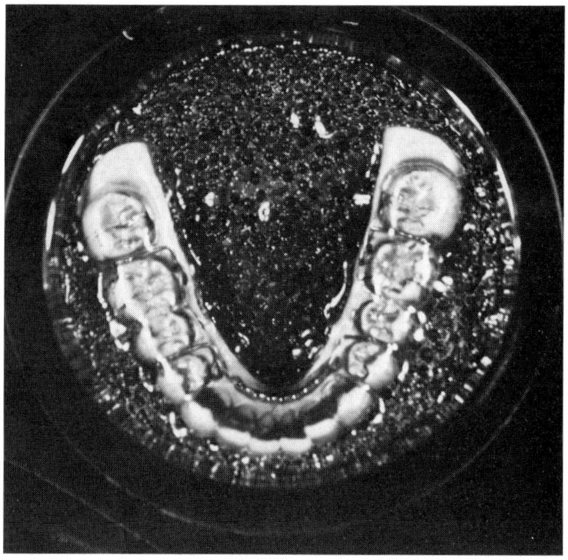

Fig. 17-28. Biocryl II disk formed to mandibular cast.

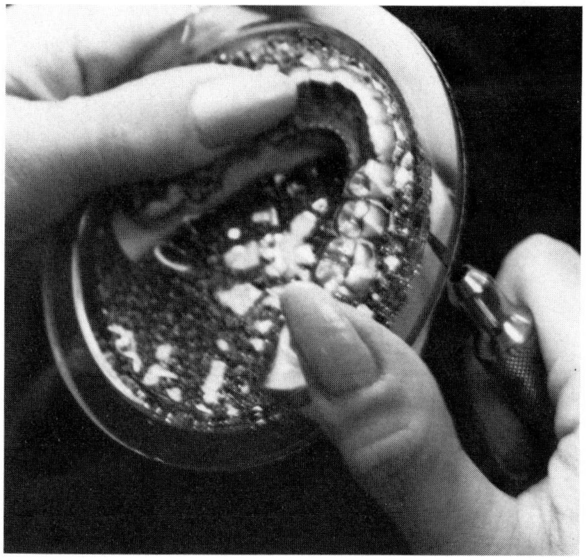

Fig. 17-29. Initial cutting for removal of biocryl II disk.

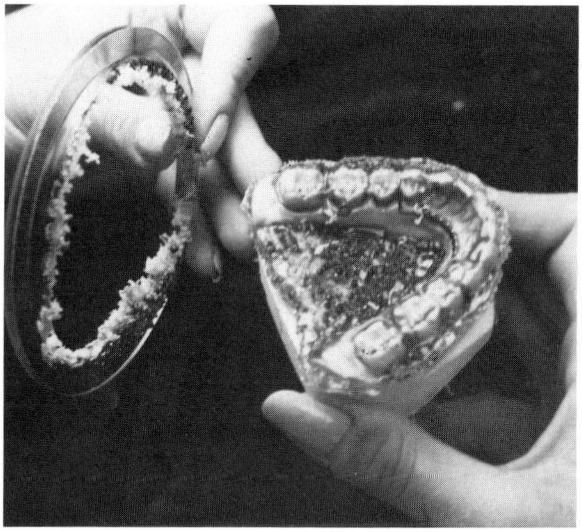

Fig. 17-30. Excess material separated from cast.

24. Return mounted cast to articulator and proceed with adjusting occlusion using Arti-Fol Plastic* and a No. H251EF acrylic bur† (Fig. 17-31).

25. Continue to establish contact for each upper posterior lingual cusp, developing the final bilateral even occlusion with a No. H261EF bur.† Develop 2 mm deep fossae on appliance. NOTE: This step can be accomplished in the laboratory or directly in the mouth (Fig. 17-32).

26. Remove appliance from cast with laboratory knife and cut out lingual acrylic to periphery with cutting bur.

*Bausch Dental KG, West Germany
†Brasseler USA, Inc., Savannah, Ga.

27. Contour and finish all borders and surfaces of appliance with No. H251EF bur, contouring lingual to provide as much space as possible for the tongue but leaving enough acrylic for strength (Fig. 17-33).

28. Using Bard-Parker blade No. 25, remove any flash of the autopolymerizing acrylic from around all clasps and anywhere on periphery.

29. Polish on lathe and wet ragwheel with No. 2 medium coarse pumice.*

30. Final polish appliance with dry ragwheel and Fabulustre Polish† (Fig. 17-34).

*Kerr Dental Products, Emeryville, Ca.
†Great Lakes Orthodontic Products, Inc., Buffalo, N.Y.

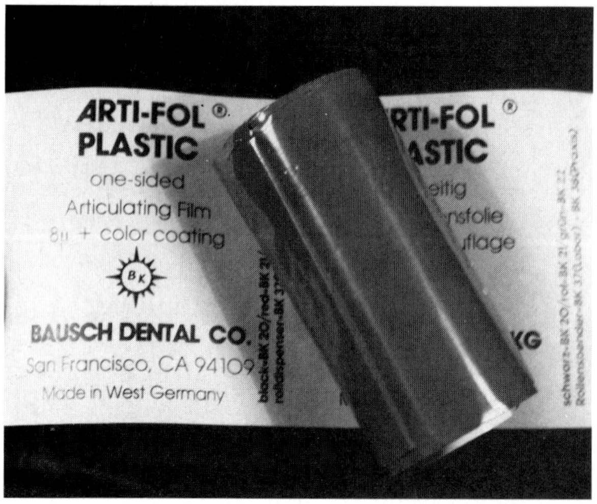

Fig. 17-31. Ultrathin, extremely accurate articulating foil.

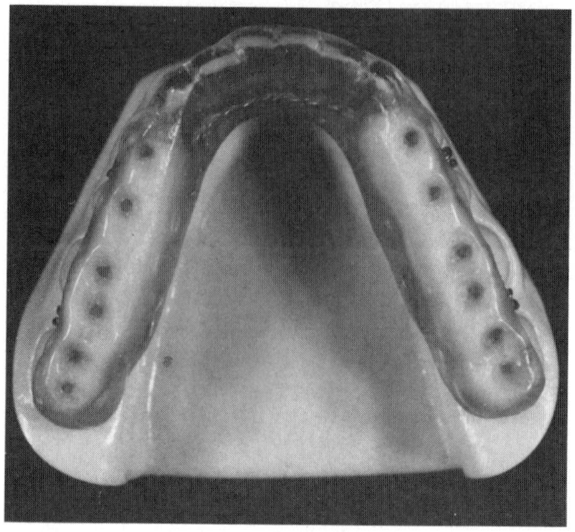

Fig. 17-32. Bilaterally even fossae, 2 mm in depth, for maxillary lingual cusps. Acrylic may also have to be added to anterior part of splint for anterior contact with maxillary teeth.

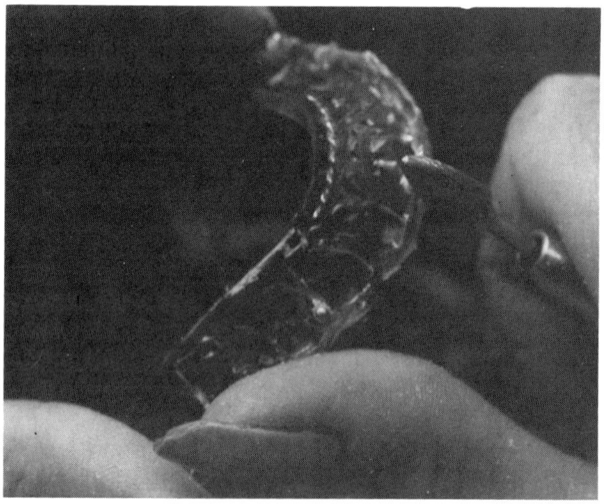

Fig. 17-33. Final contouring and smoothing with acrylic bur.

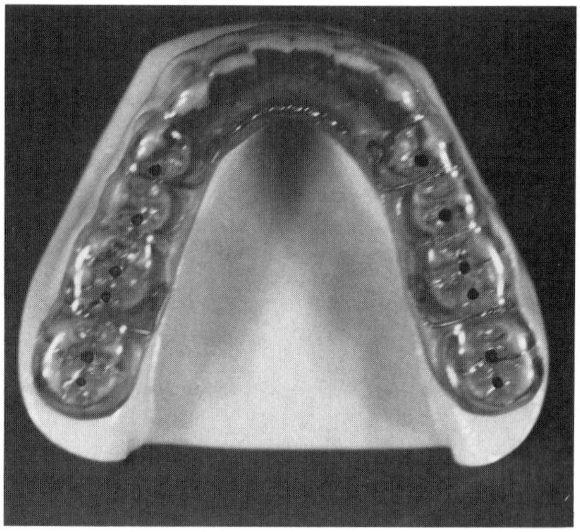

Fig. 17-34. Polished anterior repositioning appliance. Note occlusal contacts were established in laboratory on this appliance, whereas occlusion was established in mouth on appliance in Fig. 16-32.

31. Remove polish with Orange Solvent. Be sure to rinse off Orange Solvent thoroughly; if left on, it will make appliance gummy.

Superior repositioning appliance

The superior repositioning appliance is the one of choice when the condyle is displaced posteriorly and inferiorly rather than posteriorly and superiorly; thus there is a distraction of the articular structures rather than a compression. The cause of this specific articular disturbance is a posterior premature occlusal contact or fulcrum creating a distraction of the condyle away from eminent contact with the disk and posterior slope of the eminence. In order to properly seat or position the condyle against the disk and eminence, a superior repositioning appliance is used (Roth, 1973; Williamson, 1981) (Figs. 17-35 and 17-36).

The biomechanical advantage of an anterior bite plane is used initially in an attempt to allow the condyles to physiologically seat in the fossa (Shore, 1967). The anterior bite plane acts like an anterior jig (Lucia, 1978) or leaf-gauge (Long, 1973; Williamson, 1980). Anterior contact only on the bite plane prevents posterior occlusal fulcrum and corresponding distraction of the

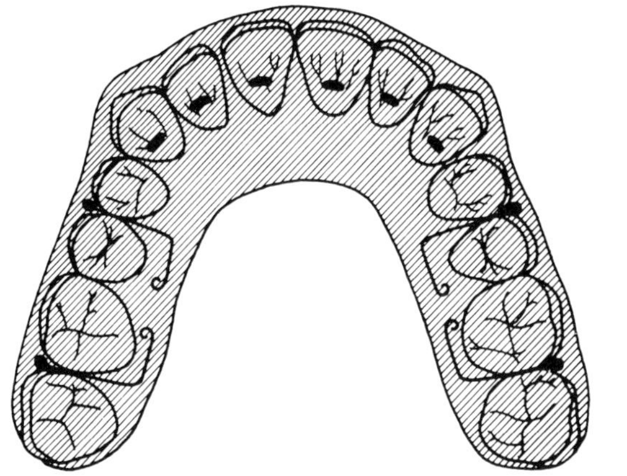

Fig. 17-35. Anterior contacts only in area of cuspid to cuspid creating anterior bite plate or jig effect, allowing condyles to establish physiologic seating.

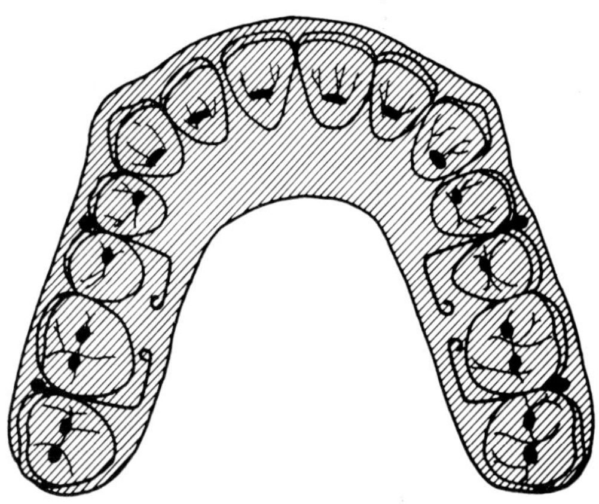

Fig. 17-36. After 1 week posterior occlusal stops are added to maxillary appliance in order to prevent extrusion of lower posterior teeth.

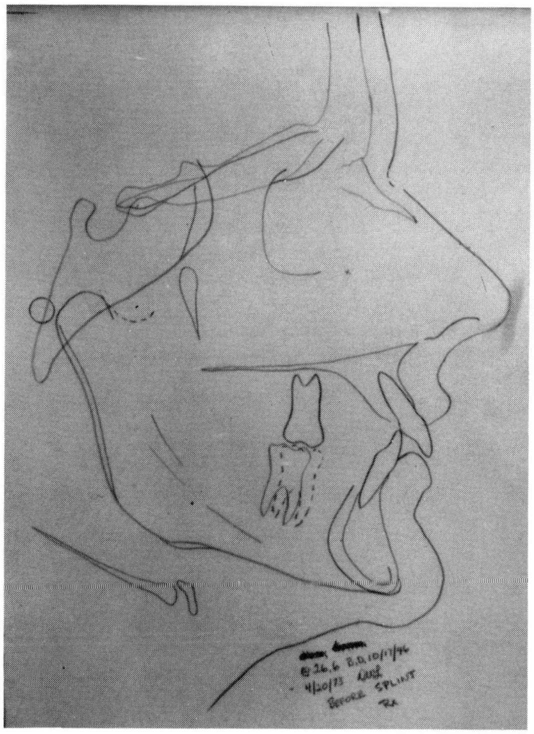

Fig. 17-37. Symptomatic unstable centric relation of patient before TMJ therapy.

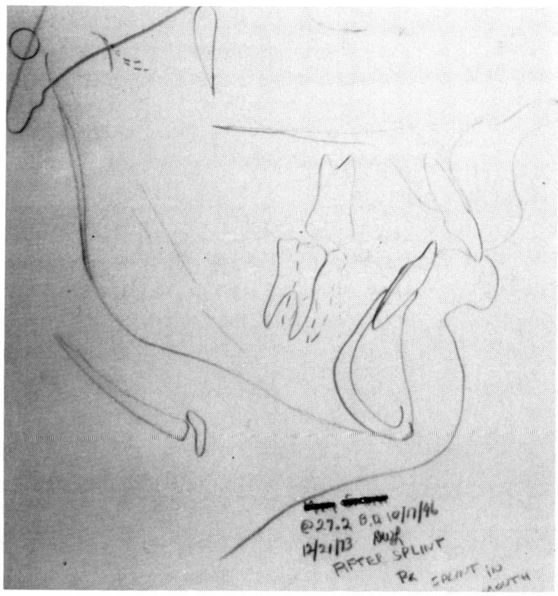

Fig. 17-38. Symptom-free, stable centric relation of patient following TMJ therapy.

condyle. The mandible can now act as a class III lever system, with the joint being the fulcrum rather than the posterior premature contact. This appliance can be used only for 1 to 2 weeks, at which time *posterior occlusal contacts must be established.* Otherwise, eruption of the opposing posterior teeth can occur. Thus, the appliance is changed over to a stabilizing appliance very early in the treatment. Subsequent occlusal adjustments of the appliance over a 3- to 6-month period allow for the final repositioning and stabilization of the jaw relationship (Figs. 17-37 and 17-38).

The biomechanical approach to superiorly repositioning the condyles can be provided by either an upper or lower appliance. Usually the upper arch is preferred since better control of the anterior occlusal contacts can be provided. If a lower appliance is used, it would be more difficult to provide an anterior stop. Furthermore, in an attempt to establish therapeutic criteria of a treat-

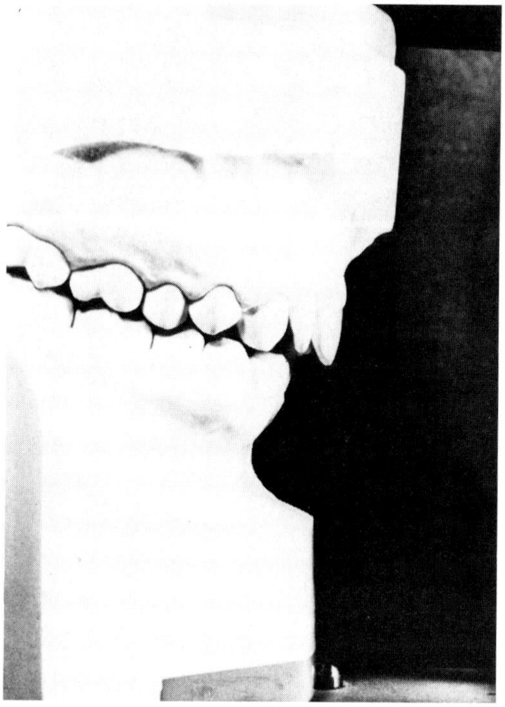

Fig. 17-39. Incorrect jaw relationship caused by increased muscle activity and posterior occlusal fulcrums or interferences.

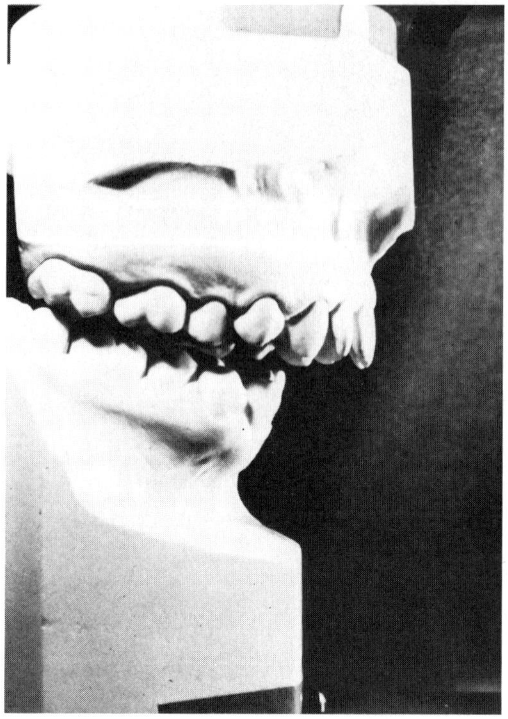

Fig. 17-40. Stabilized maxillomandibular relationship following therapy.

ment occlusion, anterior or cuspid guidance is easier to establish on an upper appliance.

The appliance is best fabricated on mounted casts in the retruded, contact position. An appliance can be fabricated in autopolymerizing acrylic, in heat-cured acrylic, or from a vacuum or positive-air–formed appliance to which autopolymerizing acrylic is added. Anterior contacts on the appliance are established in the laboratory such that there is a 1 to 1.5 mm clearance between the posterior occlusal surface of the appliance and the opposing teeth. After 1 to 2 weeks of wear the posterior occlusal contacts must be added with autopolymerizing acrylic directly in the mouth in the new, more superiorly seated condylar position. Again articulation treatments or adjustments are performed on the appliance to keep pace with the continuous changes in maxillomandibular relationship. These must be continued until the relationship becomes stabilized (Figs. 17-39 and 17-40).

PROCEDURE FOR VACUUM-FORMED SUPERIOR REPOSITIONING APPLIANCE

1. Make impression of maxillary arch with either alginate or hydrocolloid impression material.
2. Pour impression in hard white dental stone.
3. Trim cast with a flat base and score base with an X for an index for taking cast with appliance back to articulator. Coat undersurface with separator.*
4. Mount cast with intraocclusal record on semiadjustable articulator.
5. Remove cast from mounting and apply separator to teeth surfaces of cast.
6. Block out undercuts on cast with Optosil,* using ¼ scoop of Optosil and 6 to 8 drops of Universal Hardener† (Fig. 17-41).
7. Bend four .032 ball clasps† for retention on the right and left between bicuspids and between first and second molars (Fig. 17-42).
8. Place sticky wax clasps in the four buccal embrasure areas.
9. Turn on Biostar* unit to allow infrared heating element to heat for 5 minutes before forming Biocryl.*
10. Place 2 mm thick Biocryl in holding frame ring of Biostar with corresponding spacer adapter (Fig. 17-43).
11. Submerge appliance design cast in lead pellets, in Biostar, to block out undercuts in nonsplint facial areas.
12. Place heating element over Biocryl material to begin softening.

*Great Lakes Orthodontic Products, Inc. Buffalo, N.Y.
†Unitek Corporation, Monrovia, Calif.

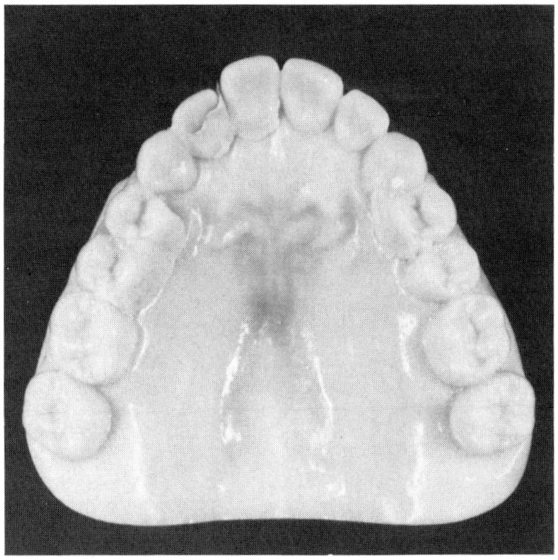

Fig. 17-41. Blockout material added to lingual of bicuspid areas and right lateral and central incisors.

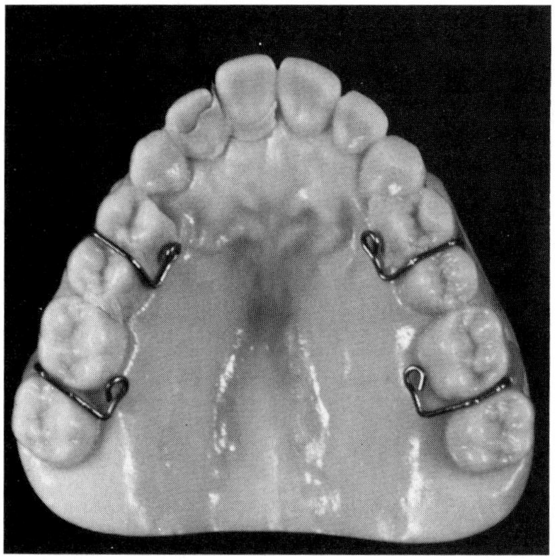

Fig. 17-42. Ball clasps formed and placed on working cast.

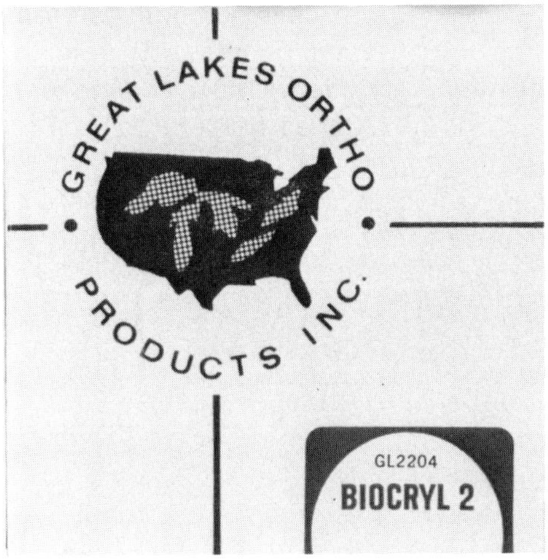

Fig. 17-43. Biocryl II material, 2 mm thick, for maxillary appliances.

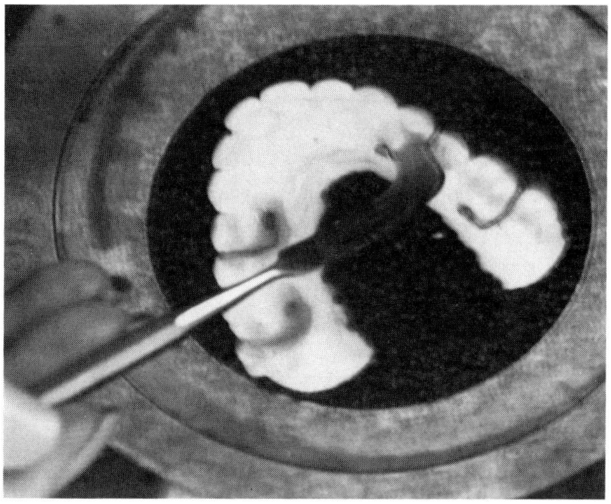

Fig. 17-44. Addition of autopolymerizing acrylic around clasps for retention in Biocryl II disk during adaptation.

13. Mix small amount of autopolymerizing acrylic* and add to all clasps to aid in embedding same in appliance material (Fig. 17-44).
14. Quickly place Biostar in position over cast and lock in place with locking handle.
15. Allow cast to remain under pressure for 3 minutes.
16. Activate pressure release button and remove cast from Biostar unit.
17. Using a No. 265 cutting bur,* remove excess Biocryl II from cast.
18. Cut excess acrylic to the approximate periphery of the appliance with double-sided sintered diamond disk.*
19. Return cast to mounting and glue in place with MDS adhesive.†
20. Return mounted cast to articulator and proceed with adjusting occlusion using Arti-Fol Plastic‡ and a No. H251EF acrylic bur.§
21. Continue to establish full contact with a No. H261EF bur,§ adding autopolymerizing acrylic

*Great Lakes Orthodontic Products, Inc.,

*Diamond disk, No. 7941, 4mm thickness, Brasseler USA, Inc., Savannah, Ga.

†MDS Adhesive, QX-4, MDS Products Inc., Anaheim, Ca.

‡Bausch Dental KG, West Germany.

§Brasseler USA, Inc., Savannah, Ga.

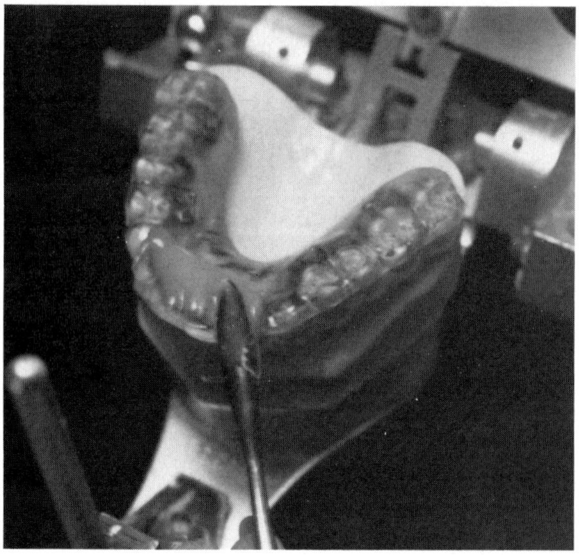

Fig. 17-45. Addition of autopolymerizing acrylic to anterior of appliance in order to establish anterior bite plate.

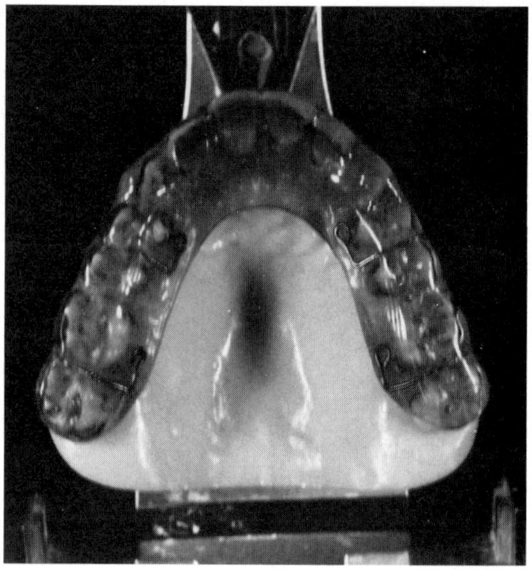

Fig. 17-46. Appliance contoured with acrylic bur.

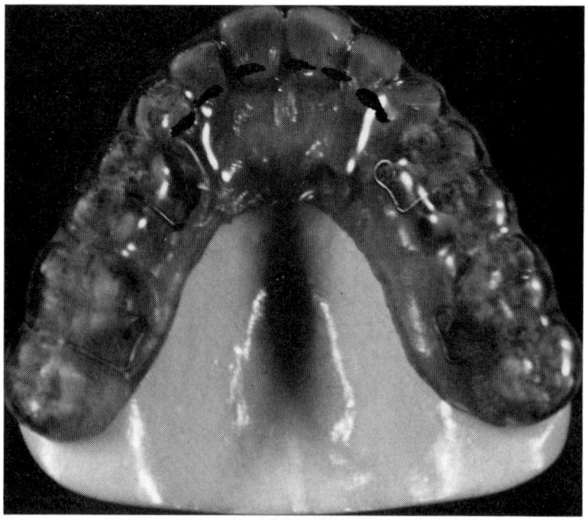

Fig. 17-47. Anterior stops for lower six anterior teeth established in laboratory on mounted casts.

plane on anterior if necessary to establish full contact, cuspid guidance, and a 1 mm deep fossa (Fig. 17-45).

22. Remove appliance from cast with laboratory knife and cut out lingual acrylic to periphery with cutting bur.

23. Contour and finish all borders and surfaces of appliance with No. H251EF bur, contouring lingual to provide as much space as possible for the tongue, but leaving enough acrylic for strength (Fig. 17-46).

24. Using Bard-Parker blade No. 25, remove any flash of the autopolymerizing acrylic from around all clasps and anywhere on periphery.

25. Polish on lathe and wet ragwheel with No. 2 medium coarse pumice.*

26. Final polish appliance with dry ragwheel and Fabulustre Polish† (Fig. 17-47).

27. Remove polish with Orange Solvent. Be sure to rinse off Orange Solvent thoroughly; if left on, it will make appliance gummy.

Observe the occlusal contacts. Lower buccal cusps

*Kerr Dental Products, Emeryville, Ca.

†Great Lakes Orthodontic Products Inc., Buffalo, N.Y.

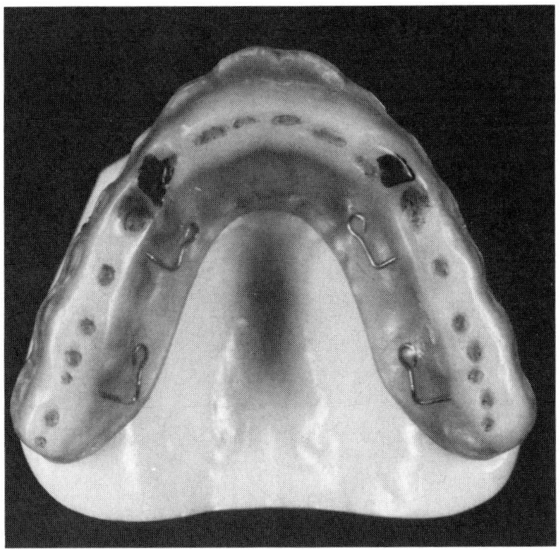

Fig. 17-48. Anterior guidance and posterior occlusal stops established in mouth with temporary autopolymerizing acrylic.

and lower incisal edges of the anteriors in terminal hinge centric relation should have even contact. There should be no mesial slide from the terminal hinge relation of the teeth to their occlusal, fully intercuspated position. Protrusive contact should be evenly available on the mesial slopes of the buccal cusps of the lower first premolars engaging the distal side of the upper canine areas of the appliance. A continuation of the protrusive excursion will separate the contacts of all posterior teeth. In the working side excursion, the lower canine contacts the lingual plane of the upper appliance, resulting in a separation of all possible contact of the posterior teeth (Fig. 17-48).

Orthopedic stabilization can be accomplished by (1) mandibular orthopedic stabilizing appliances, (2) occlusal adjustment, (3) restorative therapy, (4) prosthodontic therapy, (5) orthodontic therapy, (6) surgery, or (7) any combination of these. The decision to provide these treatments is based upon the belief that long-term stability of the occlusion in relation to the temporomandibular joints is a necessity for a particular patient (Okeson, 1983).

Orthopedic stabilization

Invasive, nonreversible forms of tooth structure modification procedures should be deferred until after the acute symptoms have been controlled and the jaw relationship stabilized. Otherwise, intracapsular edema, disk displacement, and muscle splinting can all cause a malposition of the condyle within the fossa. Injudicious alteration of the occlusion at this time could result in further complications, more complex treatment, and additional cost to the patient. Furthermore, it is important to note that it is not always necessary to alter the occlusion after the acute condition has been controlled, providing the occlusal relationships return to an acceptable state.

Because of the complexity of some of these forms of treatment, the decision may be made to continue the use of a mandibular orthopedic stabilizing appliance indefinitely. They are usually fabricated in heat-cured acrylic with cast clasps in an effort to provide a more durable and retentive appliance. The appliance is waxed on hinge-axis mounted casts (Dyer, 1974). It is usually constructed on the upper arch for two reasons: (1) it provides better control or stabilization of the upper and lower anterior teeth; and (2) anterior or cuspid guidance in both the lateral and protrusive ranges is easier to achieve.

Instructions for the care of the appliance by the patient should routinely be given for all types of appliances. Often the patient's recovery can progress to the point that night-time use of the appliance is sufficient to prevent recurrence of symptoms. This is especially true if the patient has learned to control or modify parafunctional habits during the day.

Instructions for care of craniomandibular orthopedic appliance

1. The plastic device in your mouth is a SPECIAL ORTHOPEDIC APPLIANCE. Other terms for this device include "occlusal night guard," "occlusal splint," and "orthotic." It protects your teeth from the damaging effects of clenching, grinding, and other occlusal habits. It will also help your jaw joint (TMJ or temporomandibular joint) to heal and become more what stable and comfortable.

2. **Wear it all the time.** To be effective, the appliance must be worn 24 hours each day. Take it out only to clean it.

3. **Insert and remove carefully.** Use pressure on the cheek side of your back teeth to remove the appliance for cleaning. The appliance fits snugly to prevent movement. You may have to experiment to find the easiest way to insert and remove the appliance.

4. **Keep it clean.** Clean the appliance daily in a denture soak solution. This is the only time you should remove the appliance.

5. **Speech will be affected.** Your ability to make certain sounds, such as the "s" and the "th" sounds, will be temporarily affected. With some practice you can quickly overcome this minor inconvenience.

6. **Avoid vigorous chewing.** The appliance makes it possible to close your jaws together without straining the joint. Therefore, eat only soft or prepared foods that do not require vigorous chewing. Remember, the objective of the splint is to relieve bite stresses.

7. **Your jaw joint will change as it heals.** You may then notice that your lower teeth no longer fit properly against the appliance. When this occurs, healing stops and symptoms may recur. Periodic adjustments assure the greatest possible comfort and most rapid healing.

8. **The appliance can be a diagnostic aid.** If you have permanent damage or habitually clench or grind your teeth, some or all of the symptoms may remain. When the damage is reversible, the signs and symptoms will disappear.

9. **Three months without changes generally indicates stability of the jaw joint,** which means that the muscles and bone have adapted and stabilized in their proper, healthy positions. Then an analysis can reveal exactly what will be required to establish a healthy bite relationship between the upper and lower teeth.

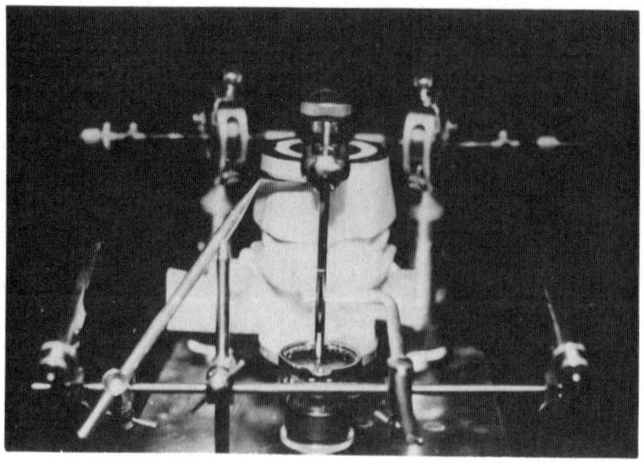

Fig. 17-49. Mounting maxillary cast on semiadjustable articulator.

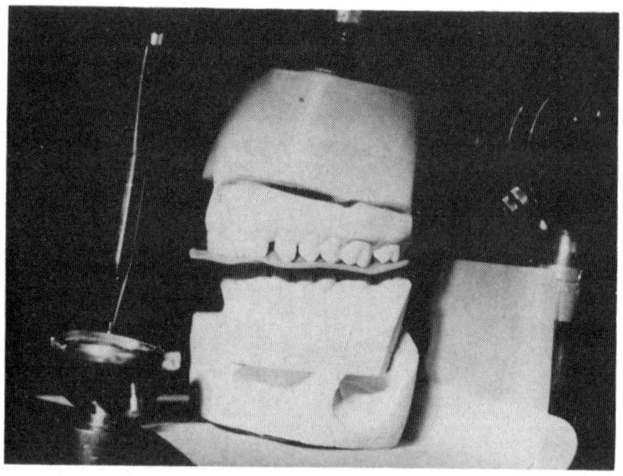

Fig. 17-50. Mounting mandibular cast with interocclusal record.

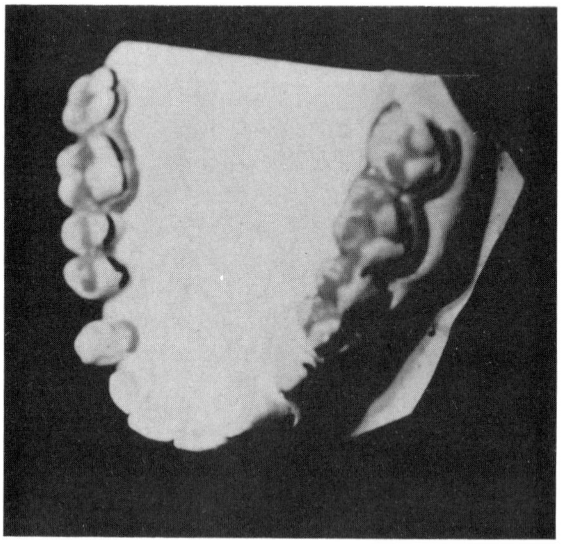

Fig. 17-51. Working cast that has been surveyed and undercuts blocked out.

Maxillary orthopedic stabilizing (processed-acrylic) appliance

PROCEDURE

1. Mount the maxillary cast on the articulator. Use a face-bow adjusted to an arbitrary terminal hinge as located by condyle palpation (Fig. 17-49).

2. Mount the mandibular cast on the articulator. Use a terminal hinge maxillomandibular (interocclusal) record (Fig. 17-50).

3. Bead the palate of the upper master cast in a U-shaped outline at the desired palatal periphery for the appliance with a No. 6 round bur.

4. Duplicate the master cast in stone (working cast). This cast is for the final wax-up and processing of the plastic.

5. Survey the cast for clasps, and block out undesirable undercuts, including occlusal fissures (Fig. 17-51).

6. Duplicate the working cast in investment material (refractory cast) for casting clasps (Figs. 17-52 and 17-53).

7. Wax and cast the clasps (Figs. 17-54 and 17-55). Usually double molar clasps (buccal and lingual) and double premolar and canine clasps are indicated. NOTE: More recently, rather than the molar clasp being brought over the marginal ridges of the molars, it has been wrapped around the distal side of the second molar, like a circumferential clasp. This minimizes breakage of the splint in the molar area.

8. Mount the working cast on the articulator. Make plastic terminal hinge records from the original mounting, and use them to mount the upper duplicate cast (Fig. 17-56). Set incisal pin to permit a 1 mm thickness

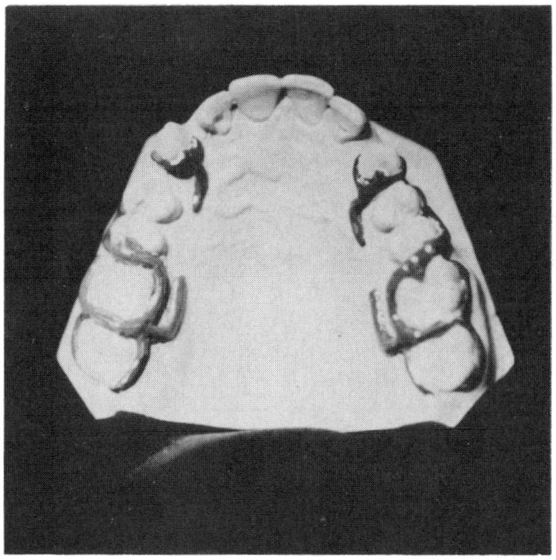

Fig. 17-52. Refractory cast with waxed clasps.

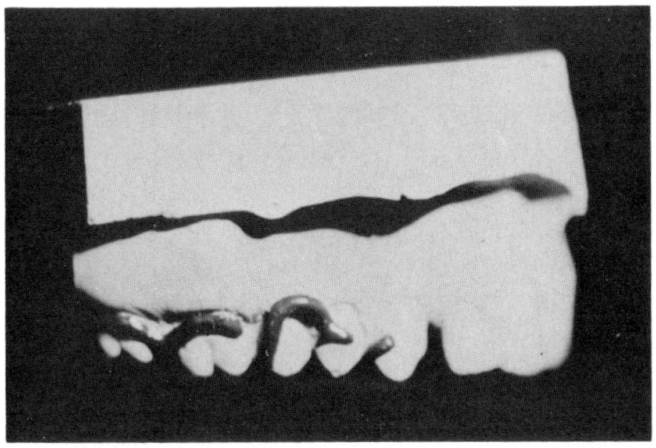

Fig. 17-53. Refractory cast with waxed clasps.

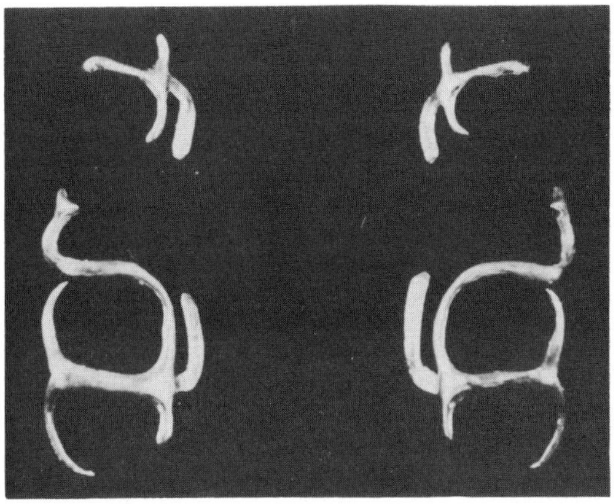

Fig. 17-54. Separate cast clasps.

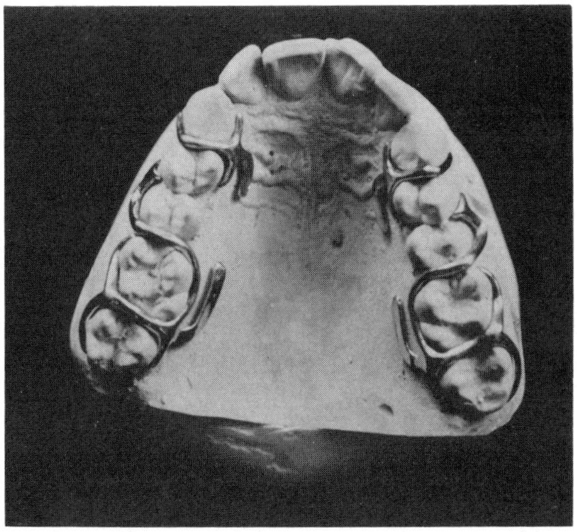

Fig. 17-55. Cast clasps placed on working cast.

Fig. 17-56. Mounting maxillary working cast to mandibular master cast.

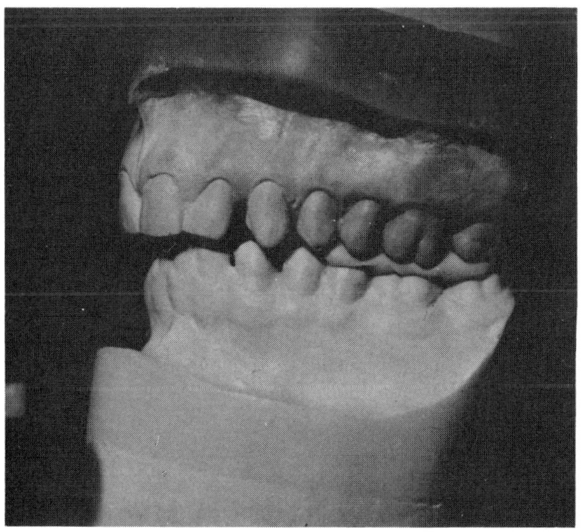

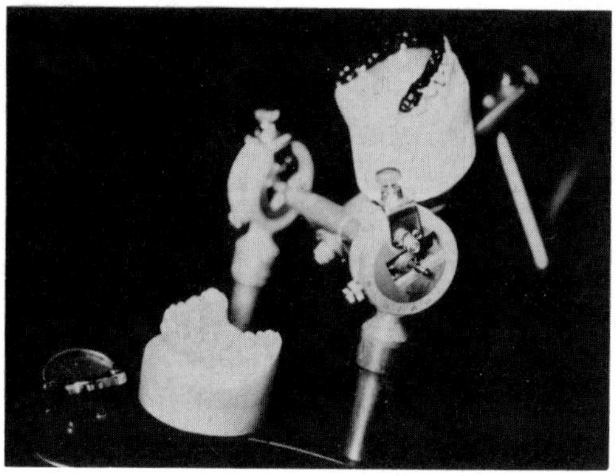

Fig. 17-57. Waxed maxillary orthopedic appliance.

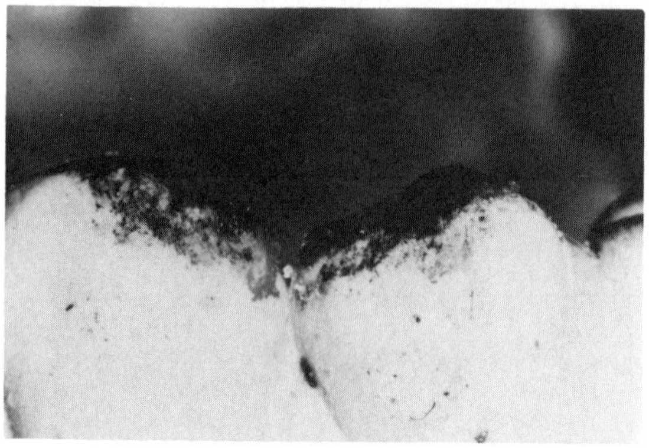

Fig. 17-58. Articulator ribbon markings on distal side of lower canine and mesial side of first premolar.

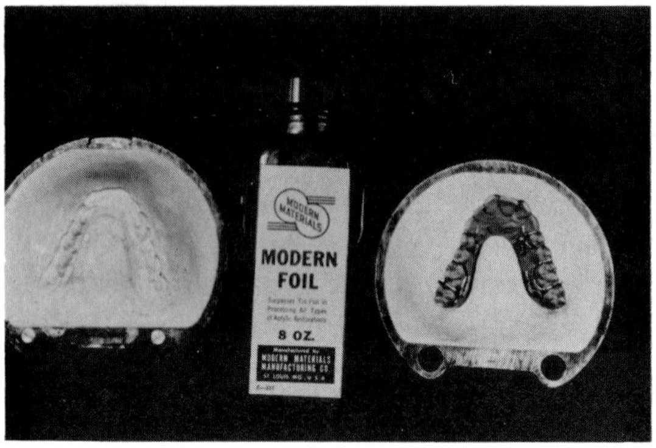

Fig. 17-59. Boiled-out flask in preparation for packing heat-cured acrylic.

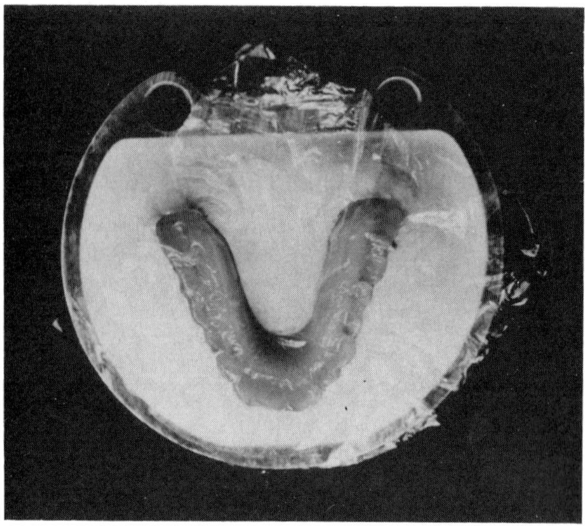

Fig. 17-60. Packing acrylic.

of wax at the first prematurity. Position the clasps on the working cast. Proceed with the wax-up. Establish the cusp-fossa relation in inlay wax (Fig. 17-57). Establish the anterior guidance through correctly placed canine protection. Note the articulator ribbon markings for working contact on the distal side of the canine and for protrusion contact on the mesial side of the lower first premolar, just as occlusion was determined for the previous appliance (Fig. 17-58). Add one thickness of baseplate wax to complete outline of appliance. Process the appliance on the working cast (Figs. 17-59 and 17-60).

9. Fit the processed appliance on the master stone cast (Fig. 17-61).

10. Adjust the appliance on the articulator, following the basic rules for equilibration (Figs. 17-62 and 17-63).

11. Retain the original casts to serve as a base of rebuilding the appliance if treatment procedures eventually make this necessary (Fig. 17-64).

NOTE: If this appliance is to be constructed without the clasps, then omit steps 5 to 7. However, if clasps are not used, then have wax cover most of the facial surface of posterior teeth, depending on the undercut relationship of the facial surface (the facial undercuts

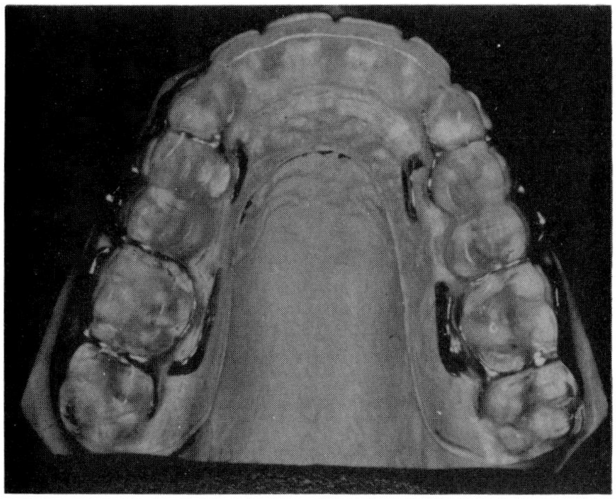

Fig. 17-61. Processed appliance on master cast.

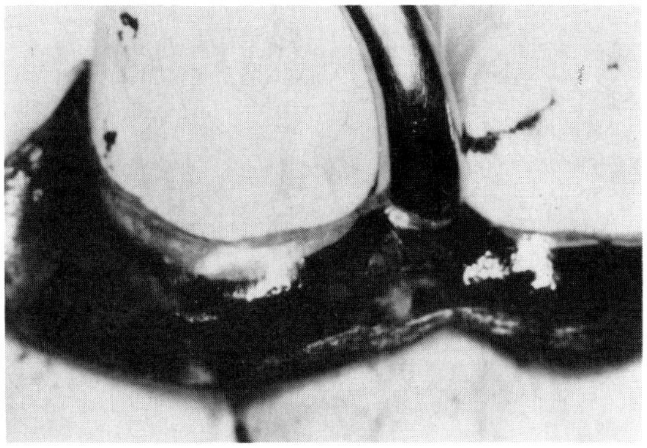

Fig. 17-62. Appliance in centric relation in canine region.

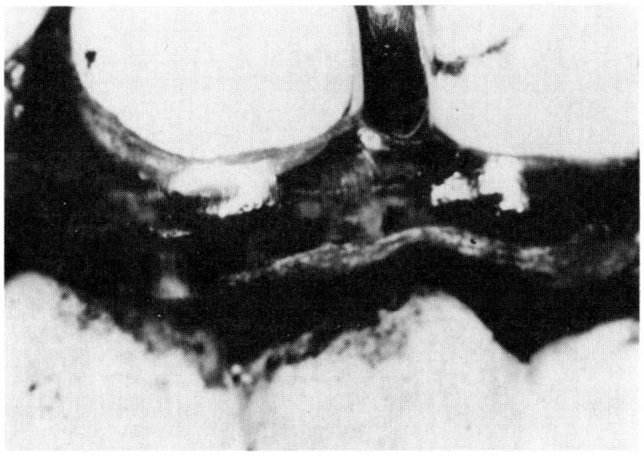

Fig. 17-63. Canine rise in working excursion, separating posterior teeth from splint on both working and balancing sides.

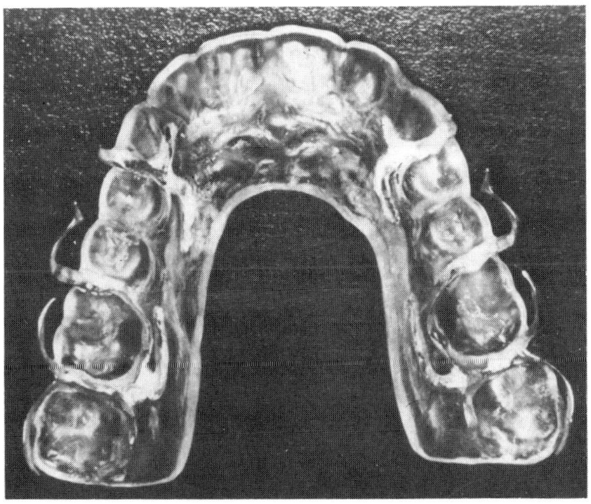

Fig. 17-64. Finished appliance ready for delivery.

Table 17-1. Vacuum-formed autopolymerizing-acrylic repositioning appliance

Problem	Probable cause	Solution
Incomplete adaption of resin blank to cast	Insufficient heating of blank, or lack of opening in palatal area	Allow more heating time with vacuum machine; be sure to add palatal opening
Uneven thickness to adapted resin blank	Too thick base on cast	Trim base of cast as thin as possible
Extreme difficulty in removing adapted resin blank from cast	Undercuts not properly blocked out	Use blockout material around pontics and other severe undercuts
Loose-fitting splint	Lack of proper cooling of resin blank before removing from cast	Allow vacuum-formed blank to cool before removing from cast

Table 17-2. Processed acrylic stabilizing appliance

Problem	Probable cause	Solution
Incomplete seating of processed splint back on working cast	Undercuts not properly blocked out	Be sure to survey master cast and block out undercuts *and* deep occlusal grooves on fissures
Occlusion on working cast remounted to lower master cast severely off	Distorted occlusal records used for mounting of working cast and/or improper flasking of appliance	Use dimensionally stable interocclusal recording medium; use proper flasking and processing techniques for each denture fabrication step to save time in long run
Porous splint	Improper packing, flasking, and processing	Do not use shortcuts in these important steps

will serve for retention of the appliance). Overextend into the buccal and proximal embrasure undercuts initially when processing. It is much easier to reduce this extension later than to try to make up for inadequate retention.

DISCUSSION

1. The use of vacuum-formed or positive pressure-formed resin appliances offers an inexpensive means of fabricating a diagnostic or treatment appliance. However, the material can be easily misused. Incomplete adaptation of resin to the cast, uneven thickness of the adapted resin, or a loose fitting splint are avoided by proper cast preparation; that is, the base of the cast should be trimmed as thin as possible, and the palatal area could have a perforation approximately 5 mm in diameter. Insufficient heating of the resin blank and/or insufficient vacuum pressure will cause incomplete adaptation to the cast. The result is a loose-fitting splint or irregular thickness. Distortion of the splint can also be caused during removal of the resin blank from the cast prior to proper cooling (Table 17-1).

Undercuts in the cast, especially in pontic areas, must be blocked out before a resin blank is adapted. This will facilitate removal and minimize any distortions to the splint.

2. The major problem areas for the processed acrylic appliances are due to incomplete seating of the splint back on the working cast, usually because undercuts and deep occlusal grooves and embrasures have not been blocked out before the cast was duplicated (Table 17-2).

Occlusal discrepancies found when the splint is processed and reseated on the master cast can be prevented by using dimensionally stable interocclusal records and by proper flasking technique. Porosity in the processed acrylic, also, can be traced to improper packing, flasking, and processing.

3. The fabrication of the resilient splint is similar to that of the vacuum-formed autopolymerizing-acrylic splint in that resin blanks are heated and pressure molded to a working cast (Table 17-3). The base of the working cast must be thin and have a palatal opening for optimal vacuum adaptation of the heat-softened resin blank. Only the deepest undercuts on the master cast need to be blocked out when resilient splint material is used.

Table 17-3. Resilient splint

Problem	Probable cause	Solution
Incomplete adaptation of resilient splint material	Insufficient heating of material or lack of opening in palatal area	Allow more heating time with vacuum machine; be sure to add palatal opening
Uneven thickness to adapted resilient splint material	Overheating of material or too thick base on cast	Follow manufacturer's heating instructions; trim cast base as thin as possible
Uneven edges of splint	Lack of proper finishing technique	Use large acrylic bur after scissors to smooth periphery
Splint seems to become ill-fitting after polishing	Too much orange solvent, or solvent not thoroughly washed off splint	Use limited amount of orange solvent on 2 × 2-inch (5 × 5-cm) gauze; wash thoroughly in cold water after using solvent

Table 17-4. Anterior bite plane

Problem	Probable cause	Solution
Extreme difficulty in removing splint material from cast	Undercuts not properly blocked out	Use blockout material around pontic areas and other severe undercut areas
Splint material too loose on cast	Insufficient heating of material	Follow heating instructions closely
Porous areas in autopolymerizing acrylic added to anterior	Some areas allowed to dry when resin applied to splint material	Keep area moist with monomer to prevent drying when applying resin; be sure to cover with lubricant and use curing unit
Autopolymerizing acrylic does not adhere to splint material	Acrylic too dry when applied, or splint material not compatible for addition of autopolymerizing acrylic	Keep acrylic moist, and be sure that acrylic will adhere to particular splint material; many materials do not allow adhering of acrylic

4. Autopolymerizing acrylic is effectively used for fabricating an anterior bite plane or when corrective additions are needed to a processed acrylic appliance (Table 17-4). Any addition of resin to resin requires a roughened surface of the previously processed resin and that the surface is moistened with monomer. If the resin is applied by the sprinkle-on technique, excess monomer should be present to prevent porosity when autopolymerizing.

SUMMARY

This chapter discusses various diagnostic and treatment appliances used for patients with temporomandibular joint disorders, bruxism, unstable maxillomandibular relationships, vertical dimension alterations, and periodontally compromised dentitions. The procedures for the fabrication of temporomandibular joint, bruxism, and orthopedic appliances were discussed.

In dental practice today, the treatment of temporomandibular joint disturbances has become commonplace. The technician should be familiar with the procedures for fabricating various treatment appliances needed.

REFERENCES

Bakke, M., and Møller, E.: Distortion of maximal elevator activity by unilateral premature tooth contact, Scand. J. Dent. Res. **88**:67, 1980.

Celenza, F.V., and Nasedkin, J.N.: Occlusion, the state of the art (Lucia, V.O.: Position paper), Chicago, 1978, Quintessence Publication Company.

Clark, G.T.: A critical evaluation of orthopedic interocclusal appliance therapy: design, theory, and overall effectiveness, J. Am. Dent. Assoc. **108**:359, 1984.

Dyer, E.H.: Importance of a stable maxillomandibular relation, J. Prosthet. Dent. **30**:246, 1974.

Farrar, W.B., and McCarty, W.L., Jr.: A clinical outline of temporomandibular joint diagnosis and treatment, Montgomery, 1982, Normandie Publications.

Gelb, H.: Clinical management of head, neck, and TMJ pain and dysfunction, Philadelphia, 1977, W.B. Saunders Co.

Krough-Poulsen, W.G., and Olsson, A.: Occlusal disharmonies and dysfunction of the stomatognathic system, Dent. Clin. North. Am. Nov., 1966, p. 627.

Langer, B.: The immediate palatal plate, J. Prosthet. Dent. **34**:422, 1975.

Long, J.H.: Locating centric relation with a leaf gauge, J. Prosthet. Dent. **29**:608, 1973.

Okeson, J.P., et al.: Evaluation of occlusal splint therapy and relaxation procedures in patients with temporomandibular disorders, J. Am. Dent. Assoc. **107**:420, 1983.

Perry, H.T.: Relation of occlusion to temporomandibular joint dysfunction: the orthodontic viewpoint, J. Am. Dent. Assoc. **79**:137, 1969.

Posselt, U.: Treatment of bruxism by bite guards and bite plates, J. Canad. Dent. Assoc. **12**:773, 1963.

Ramfjord, S.P.: Bruxism, a clinical and electromyographic study, J. Am. Dent. Assoc. **62**:21, 1961.

Ramfjord, S.P., and Ash, M.M.: Occlusion, ed 3. Philadelphia, 1983, W.B. Saunders Co.

Ricketts, R.M.: Clinical implications of the temporomandibular joint, Am. J. Orthodont. **52**:416, 1966.

Roth, R.H.: Temporomandibular pain—dysfunction and occlusal relationships, Angle Orthod. **2**:136, 1973.

Shore, N.A.: A mandibular autorepositioning appliance, J. Am. Dent. Assoc. **75**:908, 1967.

Weinberg, L.A.: An evaluation of occlusal factors in TMJ dysfunction-pain syndrome, J. Prosthet. Dent. **4l**:198, 1979.

Williamson, E.H.: Occlusion and TMJ pain and dysfunction, J. Clin. Orthod. **15**:333, 1981.

Williamson, E.H., and Lunquist, D.P.: Anterior guidance: its effect on electromyographic activity of the temporal and masseter muscles, J. Prosthet. Dent. **6**:816, 1983.

Williamson, E.H., et al.: Centric relation—a comparison of muscle determined position and operator guidance, Am. J. Orthodont. **77**:133, 1980.

CHAPTER 18

DENTAL LABORATORY EQUIPMENT

JOHN E. RHOADS

Much of the equipment used routinely in the dental laboratory has become standard and for some time has changed relatively little in design or construction. Other equipment changes, however, have reflected modification, improvement, or development of new technology.

Certain techniques have required the development of new apparatus or modification of existing equipment to fulfill the requirements of laboratory processes. High-fusing base metal and palladium alloys for metal ceramic restorations have made more control over the mold conditioning process necessary, and new multiple-stage burnout furnaces have been developed. Metal-ceramic systems and new porcelain formulations demand porcelain furnaces with programmable microprocessor controls that allow more precise firing of porcelains.

Technology associated with resin-bonded metal-ceramic restorations and fixed partial dentures has demanded that appropriate air-blasting equipment and electrochemical etching apparatus be developed.

Greater understanding of occlusion, gnathologic concepts, and jaw (and joint) function has prompted development of more sophisticated articulators and recording equipment.

Major items of equipment currently in use in dental laboratories will be described in this chapter. While it is not possible for all equipment from all manufacturers to be described, representative examples of major items will be illustrated.

ABRASIVE BLASTING EQUIPMENT

The development of efficient abrasive blasting equipment followed the development of metal-ceramic systems and techniques for production of base metal frames for both fixed and removable partial dentures. The actual utility of miniaturized air-blasting was demonstrated in the devesting of hard high-heat (silicate and phosphate bonded) investments and removal of small collections of fired porcelain from the inside of metal-ceramic crowns. Early attempts at air-blasting in dentistry followed the design of equipment used in basic industries for removal of large areas of paint, rust, scale, and other contaminants from walls, metal surfaces, ships' bottoms during drydock procedures, and other similar applications. Such equipment was large, powerful, and designed for the cleaning of large surfaces.

Miniaturization of the concept for use in dentistry was necessary for treatment of smaller, more intricate surfaces with much finer abrasive agents. The problem of recontamination of blasted surfaces by the abrasive was solved by using a system that did not recycle or recirculate the abrasive from a collection chamber. Fresh abrasive was continually introduced into the lines, and spent abrasive was collected by a suction exhaust system. Abrasive particle size was reduced from fine sand to extremely fine aluminium oxide or tiny glass beads 25 to 50 μm in diameter.

Tight, well-lighted cabinets with hand ports incorporating abrasive restricting cuffs to fit around the wrists were developed to confine the blasting process. Miniaturization of fine blasting tips mounted in convenient "pencils" have been developed to allow precise control of areas being subjected to the blasting. Many different manufacturers offer relatively sophisticated equipment of this type.

Dental abrasive blasting units incorporate several important features, which have become standard on most units offered.

1. A small, light, easily manipulated "pencil," which provides a precise continuous stream of extremely fine abrasive blasting material on demand and under control of the operator.
2. An abrasive-tight compartment within which the blasting process can be confined. The apparatus should provide a large viewing window and a good internal light source for visibility. The blasting compartment should incorporate restricting cuffs to fit around the wrists, when the hands are inserted, to prevent escape of abrasive into the air of the laboratory.
3. An adequate suction device to withdraw the spent abrasive from the blasting compartment. Some units incorporate specially designed filters to prevent fine abrasive particles from entering the bearings of the electric motor and causing early failure. Other mechanisms incorporate an air system to generate the necessary suction.

Many products are currently available that are well designed and available for use in the dental laboratory. A few representative examples are described and illustrated.

The Airbrush Workstation (Fig. 18-1), which is available from Oxy Dental Products, has been efficiently designed to use a minimum of bench space. The well-lighted work chamber is designed to reduce etching of the viewing window and incorporates restrictive cuffs to fit the wrists of the user to minimize escape of abrasive from the cabinet. The unit incorporates a self-contained suction and dust collection system.

The Heraeus Dental Gold Company Combilador CL-FSG abrasive blasting unit allows several different abrasive media to be instantly available through a built-in switching system. The model illustrated in Fig. 18-2 is one of several available from this source. Air pressure as well as selection of abrasive can be varied from the control panel on the face of the cabinet.

The Ney Blastmate Non-Recycling Abrasive Blasting Unit (Fig. 18-3) has a large viewing window and access

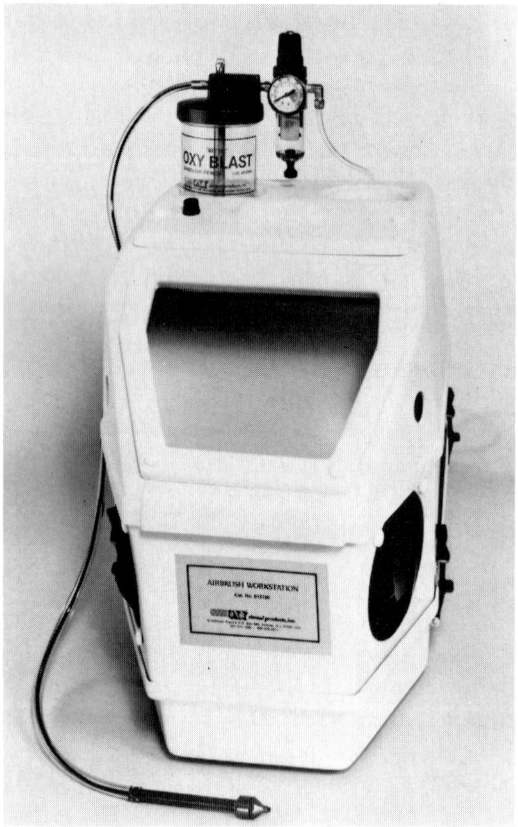

Fig. 18-1. Airbrush Workstation (Oxy) is an efficiently designed unit that occupies a minimum of bench space. Well-lighted cabinet is designed to reduce etching of large viewing window.

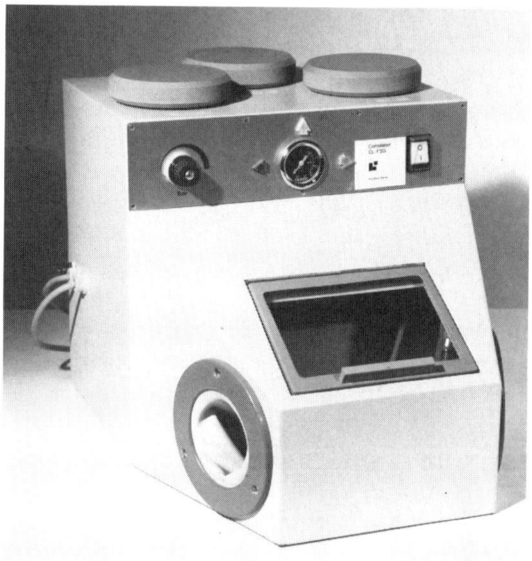

Fig. 18-2. Combilador CL-FSG abrasive blasting unit (Heraeus Dental Gold Co.) allows several different abrasive media to be instantly available through a built-in switching system. Air pressure as well as selection of abrasive can be varied from control panel on face of cabinet.

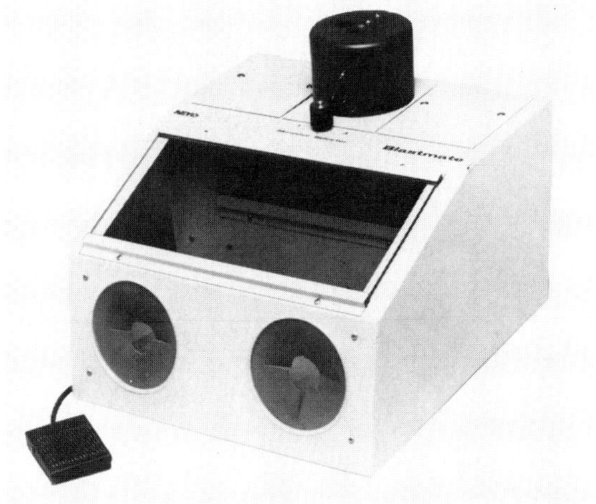

Fig. 18-3. Blastmate Non-Recycling Abrasive Blaster (Ney) has large viewing window and hand access from front of cabinet. Abrasive stream is controlled by foot-control valve.

from the front of the cabinet. Activation of the abrasive stream is controlled by a foot control valve.

The Micro Pencil Air Abrasive Unit (Fig. 18-4) from Sterngold is a high-pressure nonrecycling abrasive blasting apparatus designed for devesting of castings and preparation of metal surfaces to receive porcelain. The unit features a built-in vacuum system powered by compressed air. The system is reported to have extended life because there are no electric motor bearings exposed to fine abrasive dust.

The Mini Max Blaster (Fig. 18-5) from Belle de St. Claire combines features of two other abrasive blasting models produced by Belle de St. Claire. Its compact size allows maximum versatility in a minimum of bench space. Two large abrasive chambers have adequate capacity for production work. Each abrasive chamber is connected to a separate handpiece operated by a conveniently placed push button. The unit assures nonrecirculating, contamination-free abrasive. A separate dust collector system can be attached to the back of the apparatus.

ELECTRONIC BALANCES

The use of precious metals in dentistry has of necessity involved the weighing of alloys consumed in casting. Determination of the amount of metal to be used in making a casting can be determined by assessing the weight of the wax pattern, including the sprue tree, and

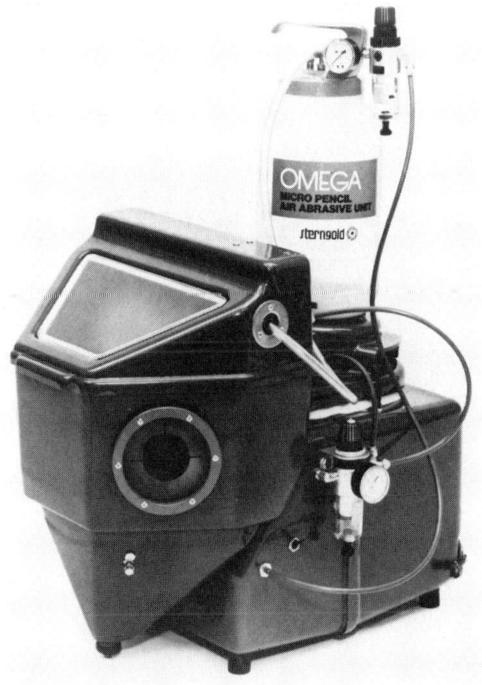

Fig. 18-4. Micropencil Air Abrasive Unit (APM/Sterngold) is a high-pressure nonrecycling abrasive blasting unit that features a built-in vacuum system powered by compressed air.

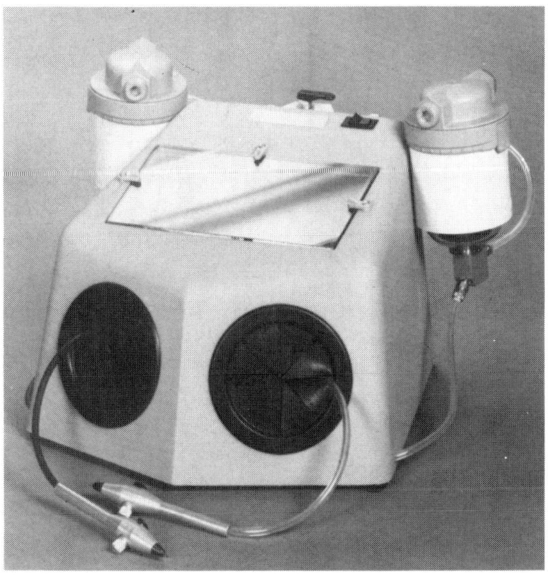

Fig. 18-5. Mini-Max Blaster (Belle de St. Claire) is compact in size and has two large abrasive chambers. Each chamber is connected to separate handpiece operated by push button. System is nonrecirculating and employs a separate dust collector system.

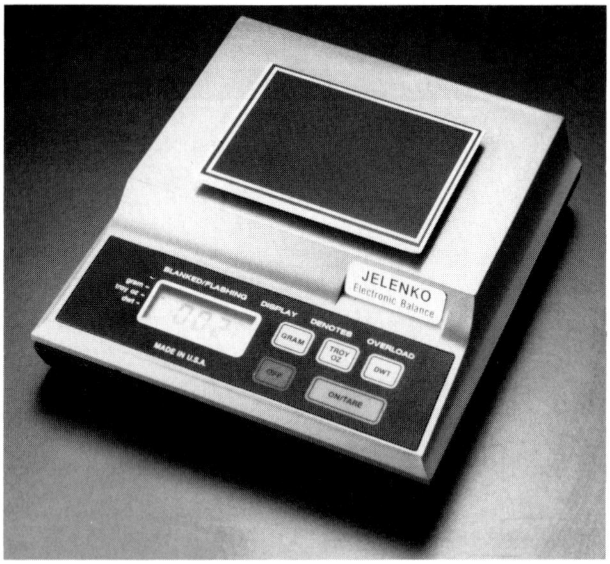

Fig. 18-6. Electronic Balance (Jelenko) provides rapid weighing of wax patterns and casting alloys. Apparatus has capability of weighing in three modes: troy ounces, grams, and pennyweights.

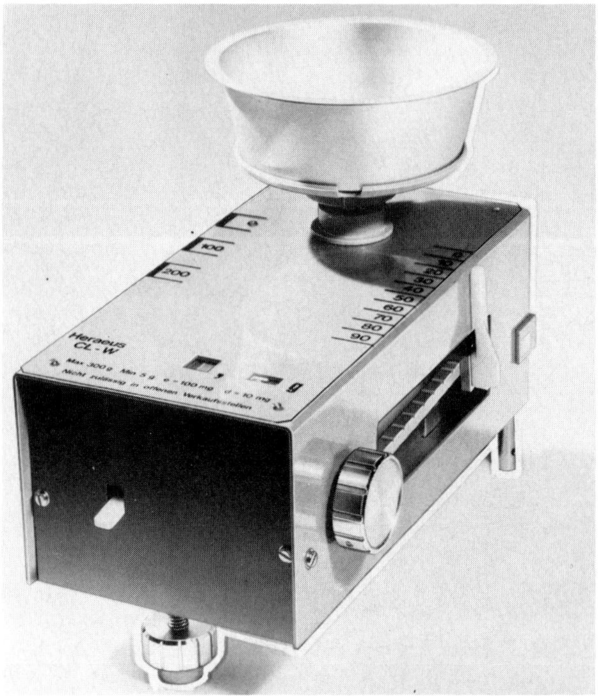

Fig. 18-7. Precision Scale CL-W (Heraeus) uses a series of sliding weights to achieve balance with materials being weighed. Scale is accurate to 0.0005 gm.

multiplying by a factor appropriate to the specific gravity of the alloy.

Traditionally fine weights have been determined by a delicate balance using precise counterweights to determine the exact weight of the sample. In recent years very sensitive electronic balances have been developed and are currently available for use in dentistry, the jewelry industry, and other scientific endeavors.

The electronic balance offered by the J.F. Jelenko Company (Fig. 18-6) provides rapid accurate weighing of wax patterns and alloys. The apparatus has the capability of weighing in three modes: troy ounces, grams, and pennyweights. Readout of weights is on an LED screen.

The precision scale from Heraeus Dental Gold Corporation (Fig. 18-7) employs a series of sliding weights to produce a balance with materials being weighed. The scale is accurate to 0.0005 gm and has a capacity of 300 gm.

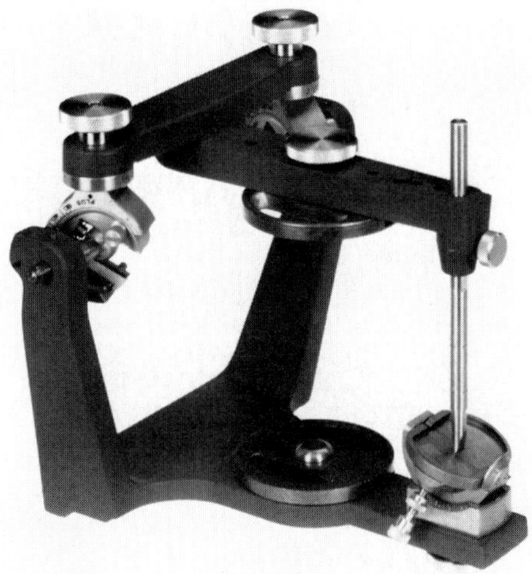

Fig. 18-8. Wide-Vue–184-1 (Hanau) is a semiadjustable arcon-type articulator of enclosed track design, with fixed average intercondylar distance.

ARTICULATORS

The large number of different articulators currently available is an indication of the tremendous need for and use of apparatus that can simulate jaw movement. Such equipment must be able to faithfully simulate varying degrees of jaw movement from simple opening and closure to complicated movements that reflect movement within the temporomandibular joint itself.

Varying concepts of occlusion and jaw function are reflected in the design and construction of these instruments. Apparatus with varying degrees of complexity and sophistication have been developed to meet the needs of various aspects of prosthetic dentistry. In cer-

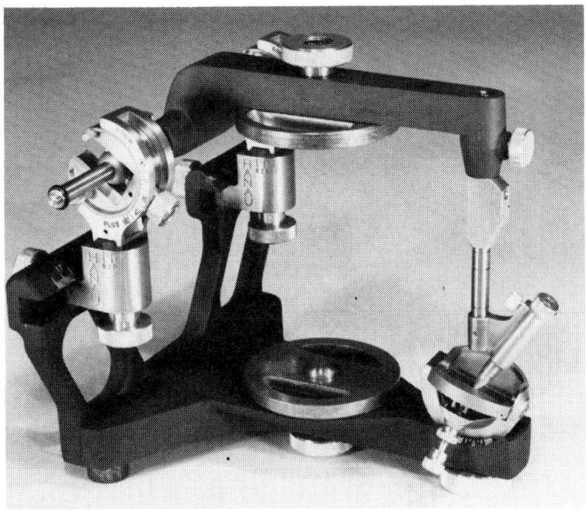

Fig. 18-9. University–130-22 (Hanau) is a semiadjustable, axle-type articulator of enclosed track design. Adjustments and condylar track are affixed to lower member of instrument.

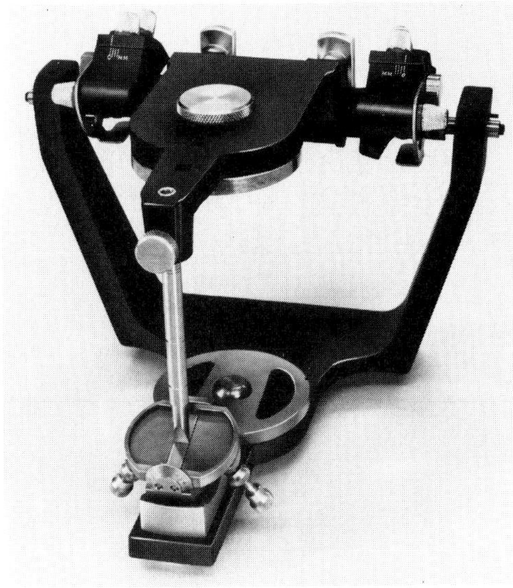

Fig. 18-10. Radial Shift–166-1 (Hanau), an arcon-type articulator, incorporates adjustable side shift from 0 to 3 mm. Curved (¾ inch) superior guiding surface may be inclined from 0 to 60 degrees and progressive side shift from 0 to 30 degrees.

tain cases only a simple closure of the casts into occlusal contact is necessary, while in other instances, where complete occlusal rehabilitation is to be produced, an instrument capable of complete and sophisticated adjustment may be required.

Depending upon the concept, design, and mechanical elements included, articulators are generally classed as simple, semiadjustable, or completely adjustable. Major manufacturers supply a range of models, varying in complexity and capability to meet the needs of varying clinical situations.

The Hanau Wide-Vue No. 184-1 (Fig. 18-8) is a semiadjustable arcon-type articulator of enclosed track design. The instrument incorporates a fixed average intercondylar distance. Release of a centric lock allows the condyle balls, which are attached to the lower member of the articulator, to track adjustable angulations from 0 to 70 degrees. Lateral tracking for progressive side shift is capable from 0 to 30 degrees. It is supplied with an adjustable mechanical incisal table or with a flat anterior table capable of accepting customized acrylic anterior guidance.

The Hanau University Model 130-22 (Fig. 18-9) is a semiadjustable, axle-type articulator of enclosed track design. Adjustments and condylar track are affixed to the lower member of the instrument. Positive centric locks can be released to allow condyle tracking from 0 to 70 degrees. Lateral tracking adjustment to represent progressive side shift from 0 to 30 degrees is possible. The upper member of the instrument can be removed from the lower.

An adjustable incisal pin acts as the anterior stop and prevents alteration of the vertical dimension during adjustment of the adjustable mechanical incisal table.

The Hanau Radial Shift Model 166-1 (Fig. 18-10) is an arcon type instrument incorporating an adjustable side shift from 0 to 3 mm. A ¾ inch curved superior guiding surface may be inclined from 0 to 60 degrees and the progressive side shift from 0 to 30 degrees.

The removable upper member may be returned to exact centric position by engaging centric latches. Anterior guidance is provided by an adjustable mechanical guide table or by a flat plastic table that can be modified and customized with autopolymerizing resin. The instrument requires no wrenches. All adjustments can be made with thumbscrews. Lingual view of casts from the posterior is reported to be excellent.

The Hanau-Mate No. 165-1 (Fig. 18-11) is an average value instrument with condylar inclinations of 30 degrees, progressive side shift of 15 degrees, and fixed anterior guidance of 10 degrees for both protrusion and lateral inclination. It is capable of accepting both earpiece and facia bow mountings. A spring centric return may be released to allow removal of the upper member for waxing. The instrument does not use separable mounting plates. The stone mounting is held in tapered wells by tapered stainless steel pins, which can be removed easily.

The Hanau LTD No. 147-3 (Fig. 18-12) is a simple average value relator with values of 20 degrees protrusion and 15 degrees lateral. A spring returns the casts to centric relationship. A bearing screw posterior to the

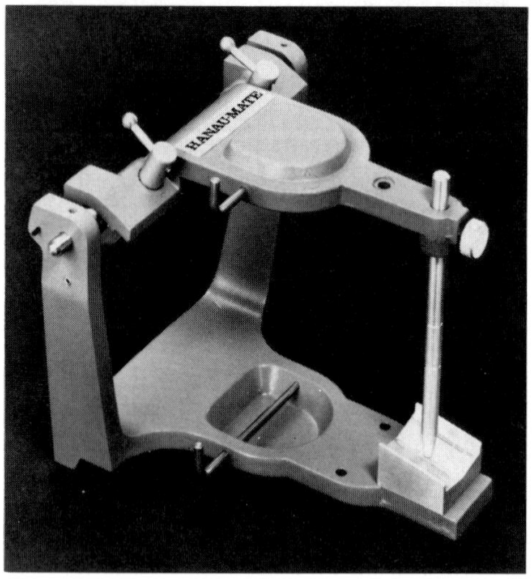

Fig. 18-11. Hanau-Mate–165-1 (Hanau) is an average value instrument with condylar inclination of 30 degrees, progressive side shift of 15 degrees, and fixed anterior guidance of 10 degrees for both protrusive and lateral inclination. It is capable of accepting ear- and face-bow mountings.

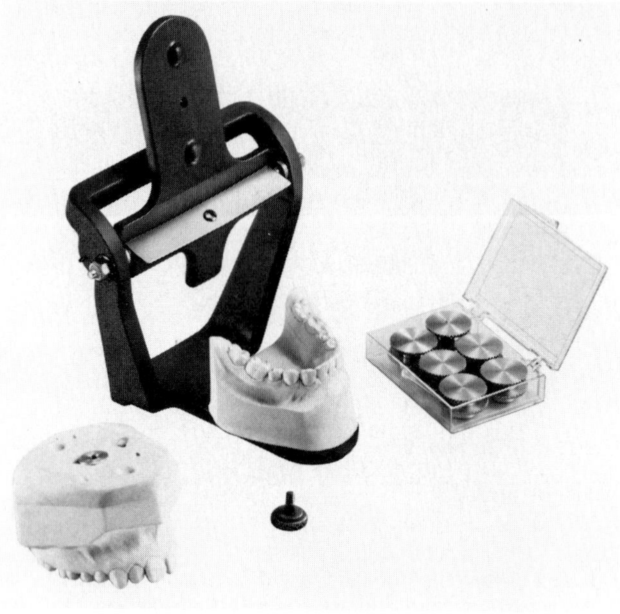

Fig. 18-12. LTD–147-3 (Hanau) is a simple average value relator with values of 20 degrees protrusion and 15 degrees lateral. A bearing screw posterior to the articulator axis maintains vertical relationship. Ear- and face-bow mountings can be accepted.

articulator axis maintains vertical relationship between the upper and the lower members. There is no anterior stop or guidance. The casts mount with disposable inserts and key to circular bosses on the upper and lower members. Ear and facia bow mountings can be accepted.

The Hanau Twin Stage Occluder No. 131-1 (Fig. 18-13) will accommodate functionally generated path techniques. The prepared cast is mounted on the lower member. The opposing cast is mounted in maximum intercuspation on one of the arms and the functional positive core on the other.

The anatomic opposing cast is used to develop esthetics and positional relationships while the positive core establishes ridge and groove direction for functional waxing. No lateral excursions are involved.

The Hanau Condyle Repositioner No. 181-101 (Fig. 18-14) resembles an articulator in appearance. Guidances are adjustable permitting the condyles to be moved upward, downward, forward, or back with accuracy within a range of 3 mm from centric position. The instrument is used for fabrication of splints for temporomandibular joint dysfunction. It is reported that it can be used in conjunction with evaluation of transcranial radiographs of the condyle.

The Dentatus ARH Articulator (Fig. 18-15) is a semi-adjustable axle-type instrument with condyle tracks, which are adjustable to 60 degrees, attached to the

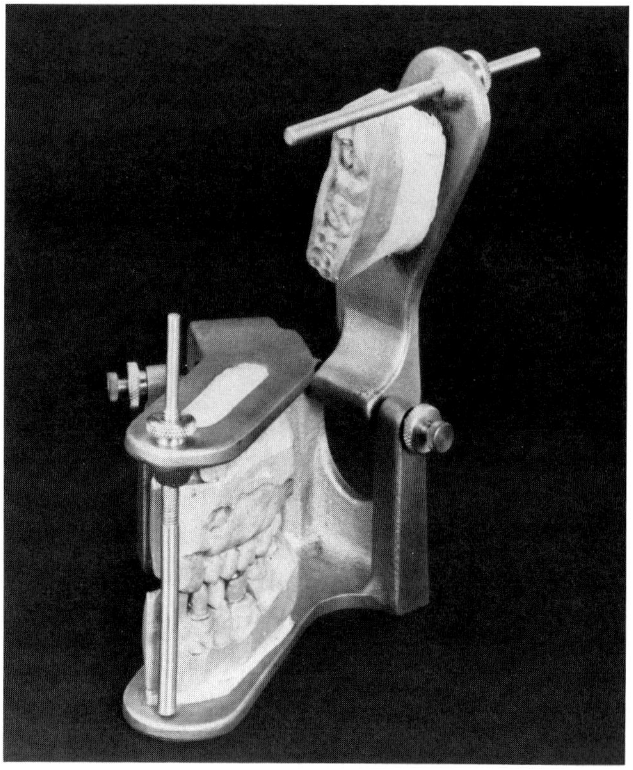

Fig. 18-13. Twin Stage Occluder–131-1 (Hanau) will accommodate functionally generated path techniques. Prepared cast is mounted on lower member. Opposing cast is mounted in maximum intercuspation on one arm and functional positive core on the other.

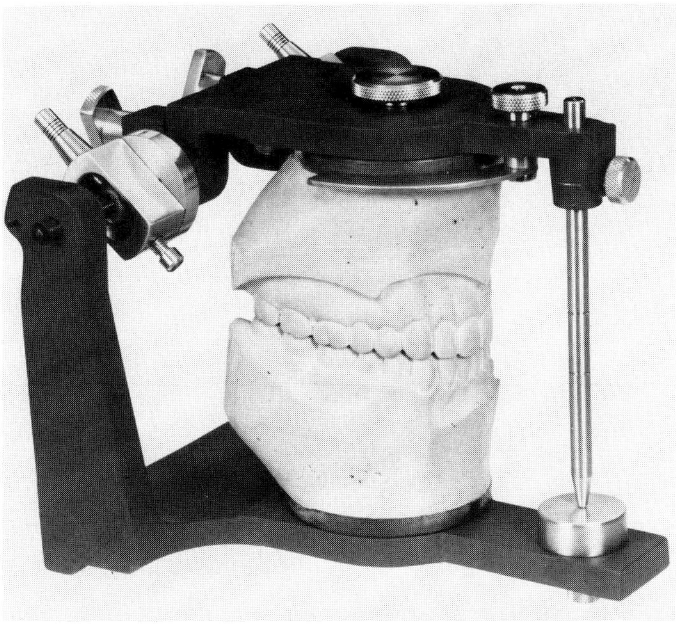

Fig. 18-14. Condyle Repositioner–181-101 (Hanau) resembles an articulator in appearance. Guidance is adjustable, permitting condyles to be moved upward, downward, forward, or back within 3 mm from centric position. It is used for fabrication of splints for temporomandibular joint therapy.

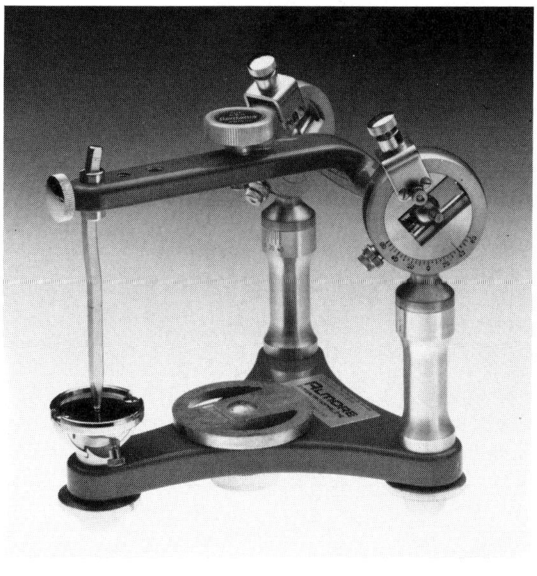

Fig. 18-15. ARH Articulator (Dentatus) is a semiadjustable axle-type instrument. Condyle tracks, attached to the lower member of the articulator, are adjustable to 60 degrees. Transverse axis has extendible calibrated axis pins for orienting face-bow pointers. Curved incisal pin allows constant position on incisal table during opening and closing of vertical dimension.

lower member of the instrument. The condylar transverse axis has extendible calibrated axis pins with centered indentations for orienting face-bow pointers. The curved incisal pin maintains the same position on the incisal table during opening and closing of the upper member of the articulator. A detachable incisal table, which can be tilted anteroposteriorly in the horizontal plane, is standard. The instrument will accept a customized acrylic incisal table.

The Dentatus ARA Articulator (Fig. 18-16) is an arcon-type instrument with an enclosed condyle track design. Spherical balls representing the condyles are supported by a centrally placed column attached to the lower member. Condylar tracks can be adjusted from 0 to 90 degrees and progressive side shift can be adjusted from 0 to 40 degrees.

The curved incisal pin permits the pin to remain in the same position in relation to the incisal table during increasing or decreasing of vertical dimension.

Mounting procedures are assisted by extendible calibrated axis pins with central indentations and an orbital axis indicator to properly orient the face-bow.

The Whip Mix Articulator Model 8500 (Fig. 18-17) is a semiadjustable instrument of arcon design. Condylar inclination and progressive side shift are adjustable. Intercondylar distance can be adjusted to three settings: narrow, average, and wide. The instrument will accept face-bow mountings. Adjustment possibilities have been kept to the necessary minimum. The instrument

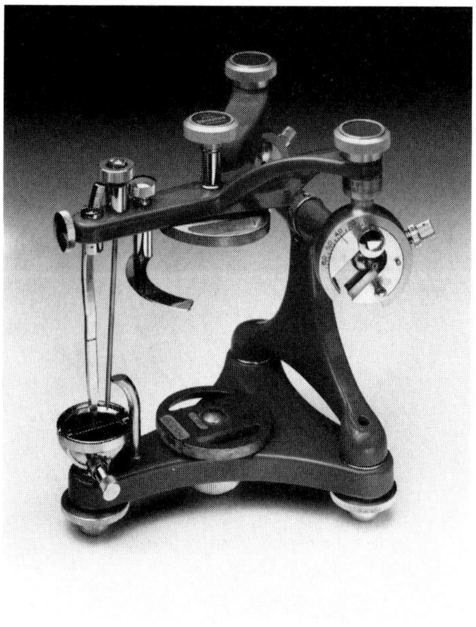

Fig. 18-16. ARA Articulator (Dentatus), an arcon-type instrument with enclosed track design. Spherical balls representing condyles are supported by a centrally placed column attached to lower member.

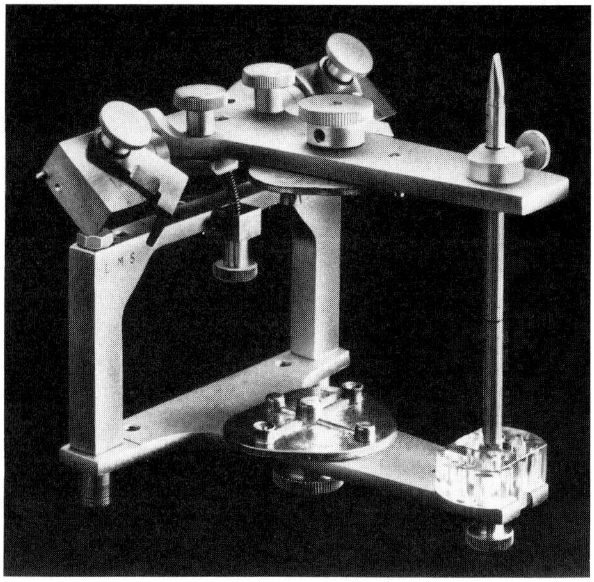

Fig. 18-17. 8500 Articulator (Whip Mix), a semiadjustable articulator of arcon design. Condylar inclination and progressive side shift are adjustable. Intercondylar distance can be adjusted to three settings: narrow, average, or wide. The instrument will accept face-bow mountings. Adjustment possibilities have been kept to a necessary minimum.

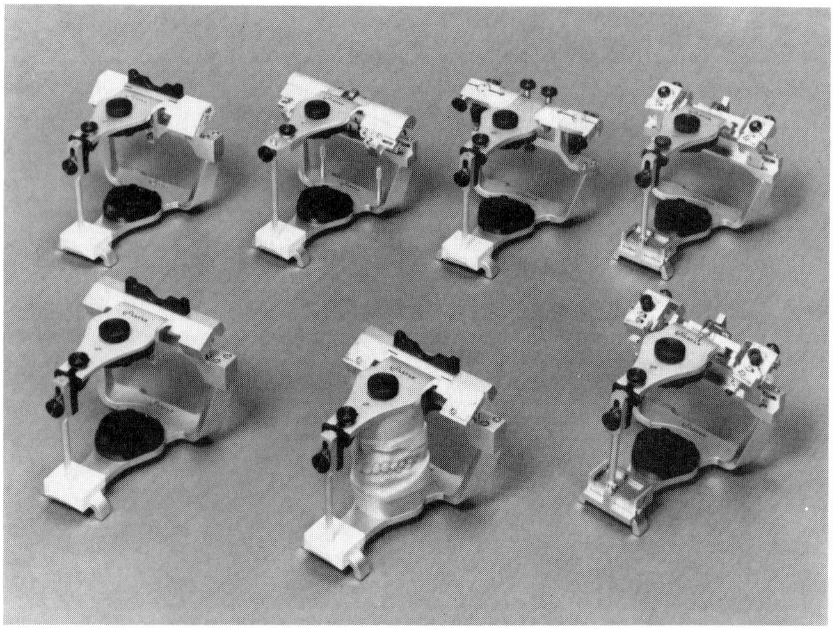

Fig. 18-18. Denar Corporation Articulators. *Lower left,* Automark Articulator, a nonadjustable instrument suitable for static observation of related casts, simple treatment, or transferring casts between office and laboratory. *Lower center,* Mark II Articulator, a simple semiadjustable instrument providing the minimum required adjustment for clinical application. *Upper second right,* Track II Articulator, a semiadjustable articulator with permanently secured upper and lower member, suitable for removable prosthetic procedures. It provides for immediate side shift and has capability for adjustment of centric relation/centric occlusion. *Upper second left,* Gnathomatic Articulator has adjustement capabilities that can simulate condylar paths of clinical significance. Instrument has setting for variable intercondylar distance. *Upper left,* D5A Articulator, a fully adjustable articulator capable of accepting and adjusting to all movements required by interocclusal records and pantographic recordings. Optional fossa inserts (nylon or acrylic) are available. *Lower right,* SE Articulator, a fully adjustable articulator similar to the D5A, provides easy access to medial and superior fossa walls for custom modification. Inserts may be accessed without wrenches.

offers ease in teaching and clinical and laboratory use.

The Denar Corporation offers a complete family of articulators from nonadjustable relators to instruments with fully adjustable capabilities. The differences between models are formulated to complement various theories and techniques of occlusal rehabilitation. All Denar Articulators are designed upon the arcon principle. The upper member is removed easily by disengaging a centric latch to facilitate waxing procedures. Both mechanical and custom incisal tables are available.

The Denar Automark (Fig. 18-18, lower left) is a nonadjustable instrument suitable for static observation of related casts, for simple treatment, or for transferring casts between office and laboratory. The Denar Mark II (Fig. 18-18, lower center) is a simple semiadjustable instrument providing the minimum required adjustment for clinical application. It provides adjustment for immediate and progressive side-shift and eminence (protrusive) inclination.

The Denar Track II (Fig. 18-18, upper row, second right) has permanently secured upper and lower bows, which make it well suited for removable prosthetic procedures. The instrument provides for immediate side shift and has a centric relation/centric occlusion adjustment capability. In addition to complete denture work the articulator can be used in fabrication of removable partial dentures and simple fixed partial dentures.

The Denar Gnathomatic articulator (Fig. 18-18, back row, second left) has adjustment capabilities that can simulate condylar movement paths, which have clinical significance. The instrument is also capable of adjustment for variations in intercondylar distance.

The Denar D5A Articulator (Fig. 18-18, top, left) is fully adjustable and capable of accepting and adjusting to all movements required by interocclusal records or pantographic recordings. Adjustment capabilities include superior fossa wall, rear fossa wall, protrusive inclination, immediate and progressive side shift, and intercondylar distance. Optional fossa inserts (nylon or acrylic) of varying anatomic curvatures are available for medial and superior wall fossae.

The Denar SE Articulator (Fig. 18-18, lower right) is a fully adjustable instrument similar to the D5A, but it provides easy access to medial and superior fossae walls for custom modification for gnathologic evaluation and treatment. The manufacturer states that fossa inserts can be removed and replaced for customizing without wrenches while the pantograph is assembled.

The Denar Omni, semiadjustable articulator (Fig. 18-19) has been designed to fit the needs of both fixed and removable prosthodontics. The instrument allows interchangeability of fossae. Closed (tracking) fossae may be used when the articulator is to be used for removable (complete) prosthodontics. Open fossae used in conjunction with a positive centric latch convert the instrument for use for fixed prosthodontics. The design permits excellent visibility of lingual areas and ready access from the posterior.

The design permits compatibility with other Denar equipment such as face-bows, ear-bows, mounting

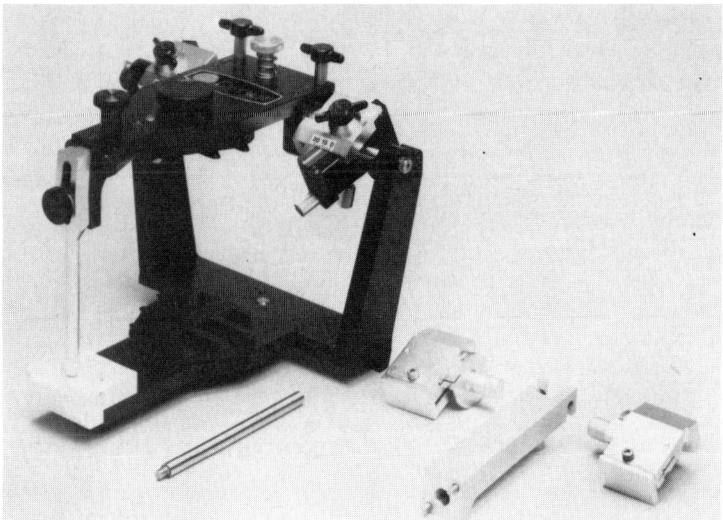

Fig. 18-19. Omni Articulator (Denar), a semiadjustable articulator designed to fit needs of both fixed and removable prosthodontics. It allows interchangeability of articular fossae and permits excellent visibility of lingual areas and ready access from the posterior. It is compatible with other instrumentation of manufacturer.

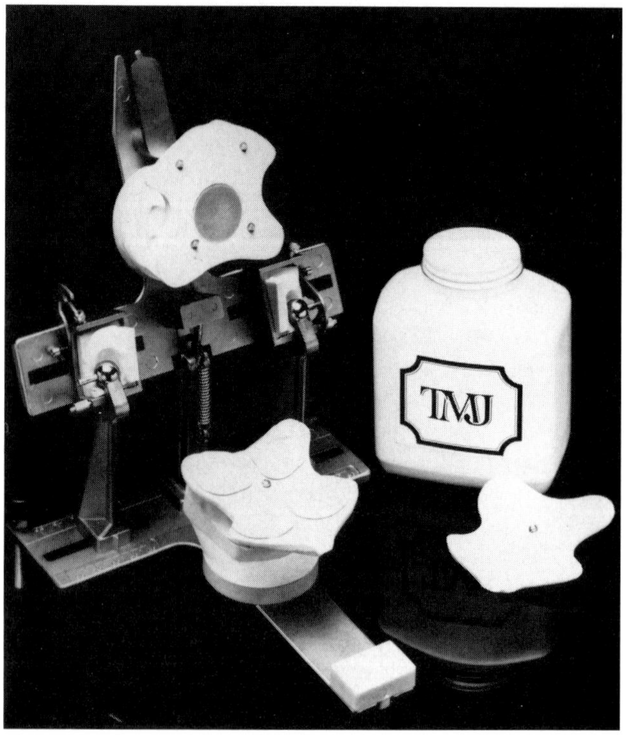

Fig. 18-20. Deluxe Articulator (TMJ), a fully adjustable articulator that can be used with intraoral stereographic recordings to program the instrument. Articulator movements created by following recordings are used to create five-walled fossa analogs.

plates, and custom or mechanical incisal pins and tables.

The TMJ Instrument Company offers a fully adjustable articulator with articular fossa elements that reproduce an analog of mandibular movement. The system incorporates intraoral stereographic recordings and custom-molded fossa analogs. The articulator is so devised that it can also be used as a simple semiadjustable or fixed average path system.

The TMJ Deluxe Articulator can be used as a fully adjustable, semiadjustable, or simple hinge articulator. It incorporates an adjustable intercondylar distance from 80 to 160 mm, a positive centric lock that locks the upper member in terminal hinge position, interchangeable condylar guidance, and a curved incisal pin so that pin position in relation to the incisal table is maintained constant when the vertical dimension is changed.

When employed as a fully adjustable instrument, the articulator is used in conjunction with intraoral stereographic recordings (Fig. 18-20), which are used to program the instrument. The articulator movements created by following these recordings are used to create five walled fossa analogs (Fig. 18-21). This procedure is used in place of pantographic tracings.

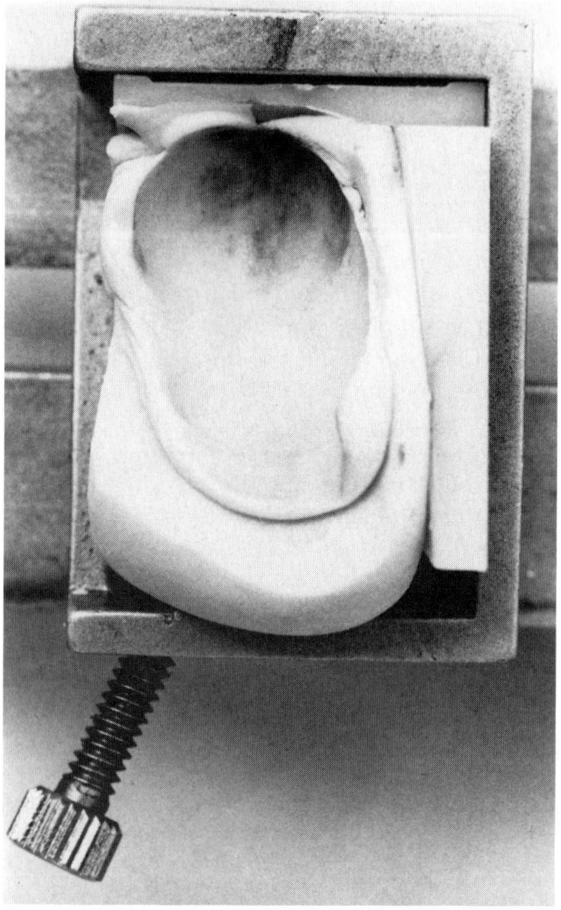

Fig. 18-21. Five-walled fossa analog created in autopolymerizing resin by following intraoral stereographic recordings. Procedure is used in place of pantographic tracings.

The instrument can also be used as a semiadjustable articulator by using preformed analog fossae, which can be quickly inserted in place of the custom-made analog fossae. The articulator can also be fitted with mechanical fossae, which allow adjustable condylar inclination and side shift movements.

The TMJ Mini Articulator (Fig. 18-22) is a somewhat simplified version of the Deluxe Articulator. Major differences are limitation of intercondylar distance setting and a simplified incisal pin. General dimensions of the two instruments are similar.

FACE-BOWS AND MANDIBULAR RECORDING EQUIPMENT

If prostheses are to be fabricated in the laboratory away from the clinical treatment area, some means is necessary to transfer craniomaxillary relationship to the laboratory simulator. Various methods have been devised to measure and record positions and dimensions of the patients' jaws and skeletal structures and to

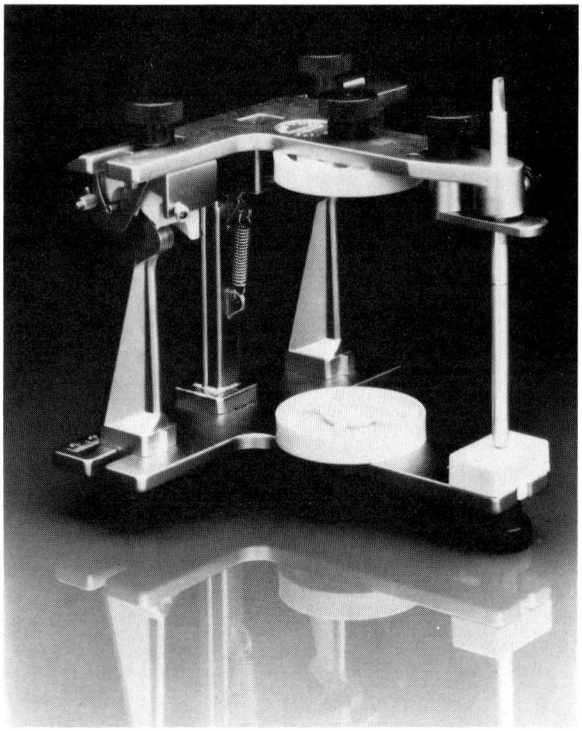

Fig. 18-22. Mini Articulator (TMJ), a simplified version of Deluxe Articulator. Major differences are limitation of intercondylar distance setting and a simplified incisal pin.

transfer that data to laboratory apparatus. Numerous types of face-bows, mandibular movement recorders, and mounting jigs have been fashioned for this purpose. When properly used in conjunction with accurate interocclusal records, reliably mounted working casts can be obtained.

The Hanau Twirl-Bow No. 164-2 (Fig. 18-23, *A*) is an earpiece-type face-bow. Both earpieces traverse equally and parallel to the transverse axis. They are adjusted by turning a single thumb wheel—hence the name "Twirl-bow." An orbital pointer serves as the anterior reference of the Frankfort plane as an aid for orientation of the assembly on the articulator. In the transfer of an anatomic mounting to an articulator (Fig. 18-23, *B*), a mounting guide positions the occlusal index at the same relative position on the articulator to that occupied when the apparatus is adjusted to the patient's landmark points.

The Hanau No. 153-16 (Fig. 18-24) is also an earpiece-type face-bow. Calibrated rods are adjusted equally to suspend the earpieces in each meatus of the patient. A "triad" of meatus/occlusal plane is obtained when an occlusal index is clamped to the body of the face-bow. The assembly is oriented on the articulator, which is equipped with pins that simulate the patient's auditory meatus. These pins are 12 mm posterior to and on the same horizontal plane as the center of the condyle.

The Hanau No. 132-2SM (Fig. 18-25) is a more conventional facia-type bow with calibrated rods for equal adjustment to the palpated area of the condyle or predetermined hinge axis. Two clamps are attached to the body of the apparatus: one for attachment of a bite fork, the other to fix a pointer to a third point of reference.

Whip Mix "Quick Mount" Face-bow No. 8600 (Fig. 18-26) is an ear-bow compatible with all Whip Mix articulators. It can be reset to transfer an approximate relationship from patient to articulator with a minimum of time and instrumentation. The design incorporates a self-centering caliper and plastic earpieces from which interpolation of the patient's hinge axis can be made. The bridge of the nose is used as a third reference point for orientation.

The Denar Corporation offers several types of face-bows and ear-bows. The Slidematic Face-bow allows approximate transfer of positional relationships from the patient to the articulator. It is especially useful in the mounting of diagnostic casts and simple prosthodontic treatment.

The Denar D31AB Face-bow/Ear-bow is used for transfer and mounting of master casts and where extensive rehabilitative procedures are to be undertaken. While the apparatus is usually oriented relative to hinge axis determination, it may also be employed as an ear-bow for approximation to the opening axis.

A 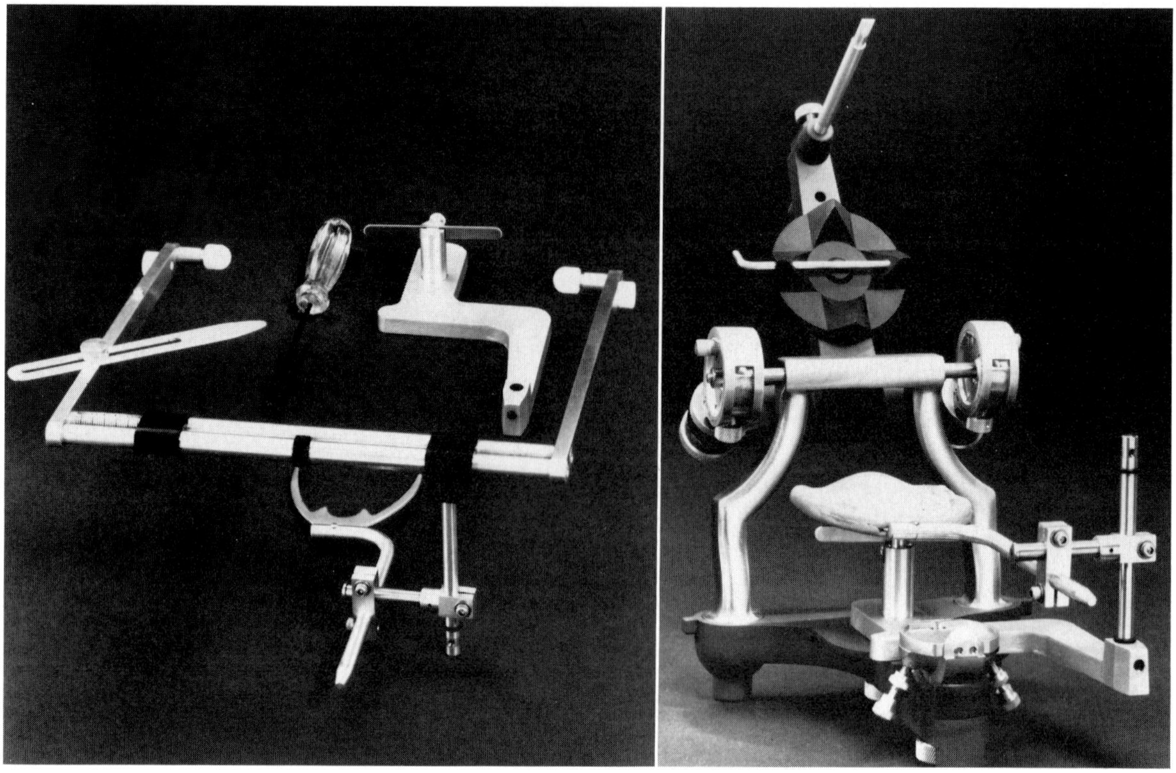 B

Fig. 18-23. A, Twirl Bow–164-2 (Hanau), an earpiece-type face-bow. Earpieces, which traverse equally and parallel to the transverse axis, are adjusted by turning a single thumb wheel. Orbital pointer serves as third point of reference of Frankfort plane. **B,** Face-bow transferred to articulator. Mounting guide positions occlusal index at same relative position to that occupied when adjusted to patient's landmark points.

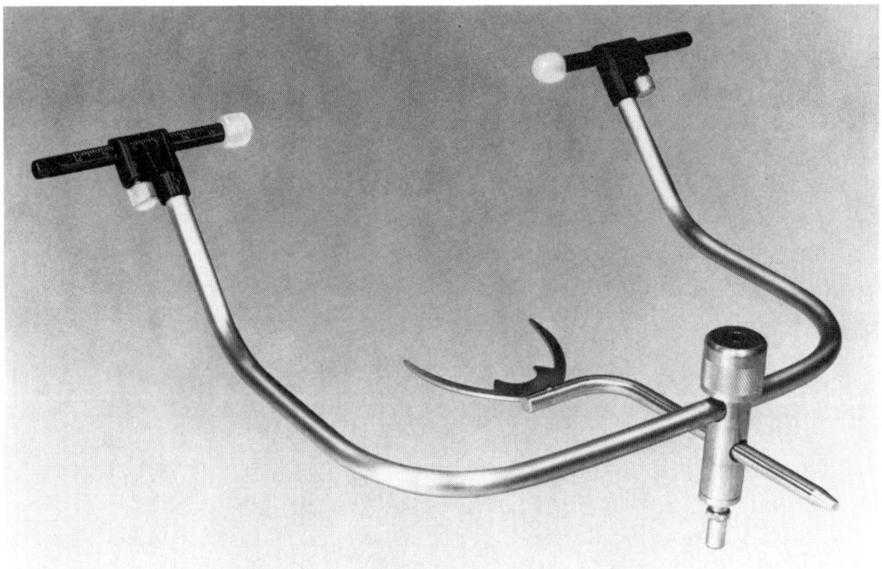

Fig. 18-24. Earpiece face-bow–153-16 (Hanau) Calibrated rods are adjusted equally to suspend earpieces in each meatus of patient. Articulator is equipped with pins 12 mm posterior to and on same horizontal plane as center of condyle.

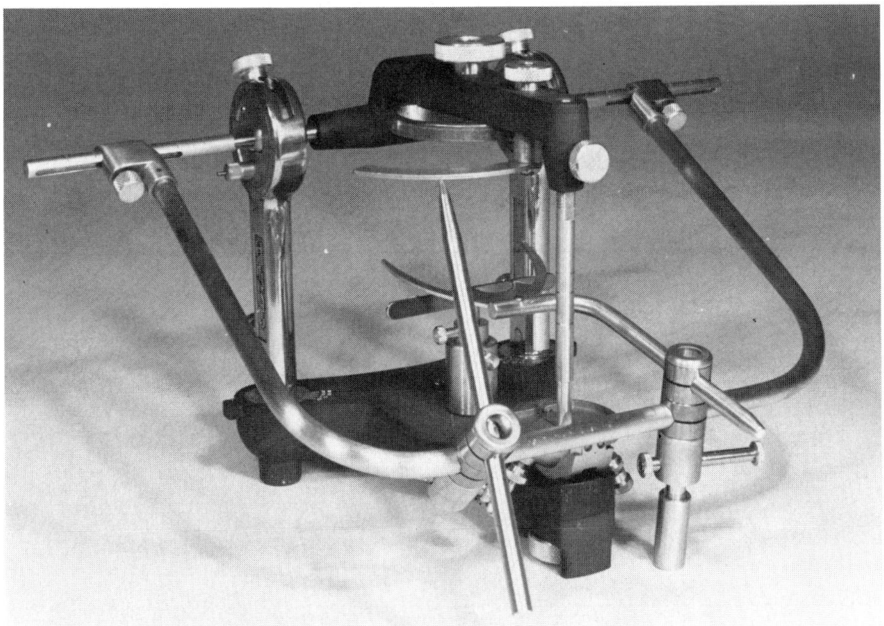

Fig. 18-25. Facia Bow–132-2SM (Hanau), a conventional facia-type bow with calibrated rods for equal adjustment to palpated areas of condyle or predetermined hinge axis. Clamps are attached to body of apparatus for fixation of bite-fork and orbital pointer.

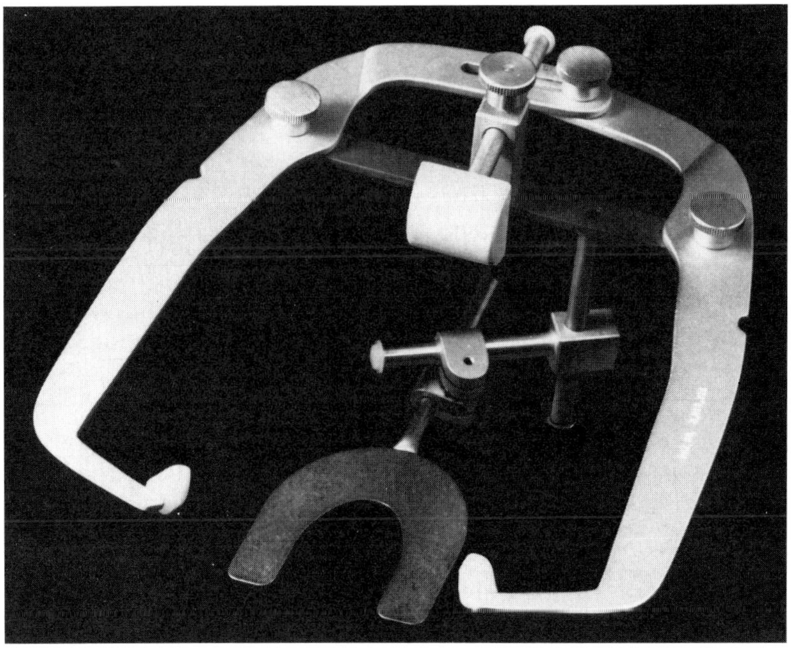

Fig. 18-26. "Quick Mount" Face-bow–8600 (Whip Mix), an ear-bow compatible with all Whip Mix articulators. Design incorporates self-centering caliper and plastic earpieces from which interpolation of opening axis position can be made.

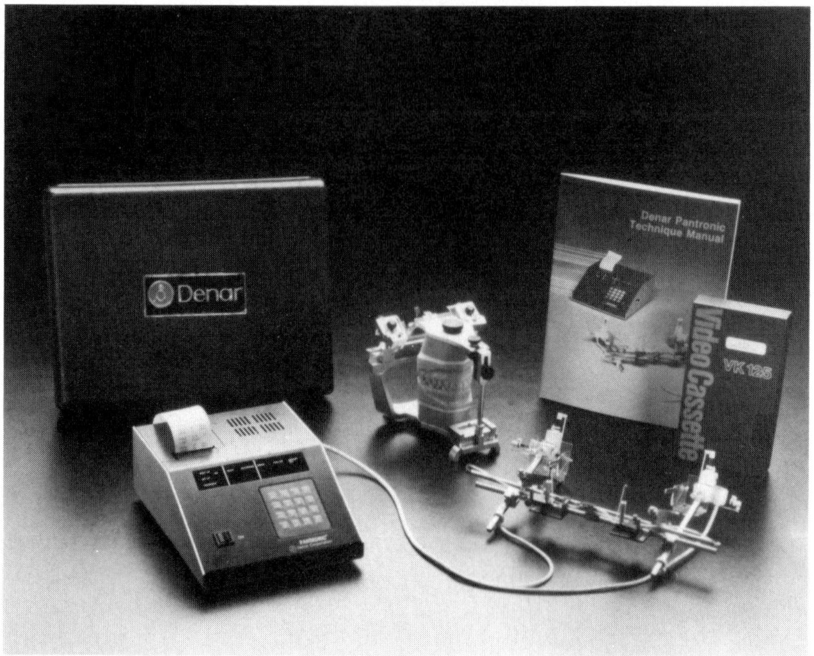

Fig. 18-27. Pantronic Recording System (Denar) employs "state-of-the-art" electronic technology to evaluate temporomandibular joint dysfunction. An outgrowth of manual pantography, it can be used to evaluate muscle coordination through a pantographic reproducibility index (PRI).

A **B**

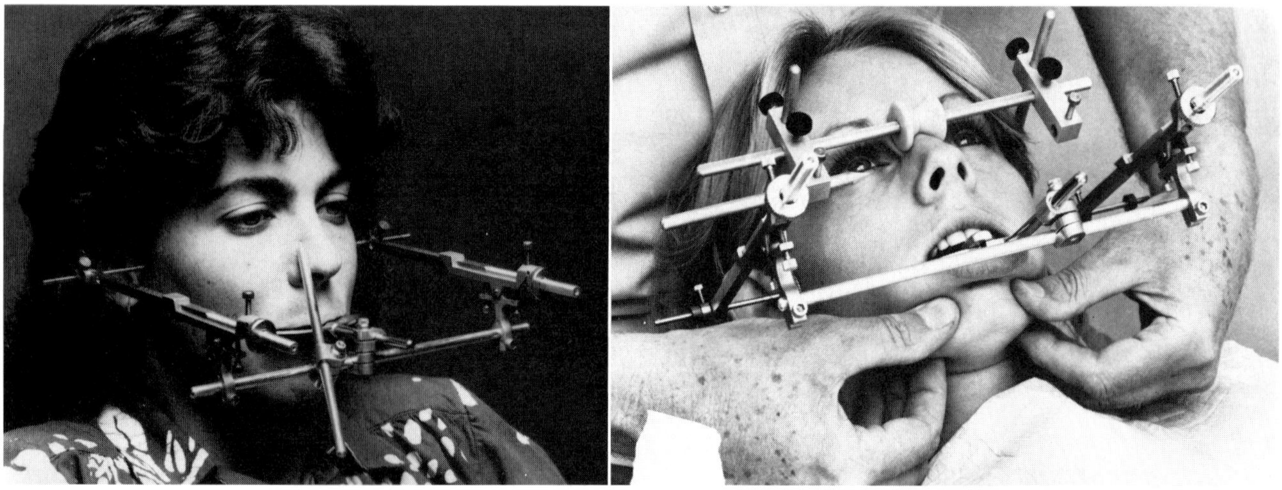

Fig. 18-28. A, Kinematic Face-bow (TMJ) adjustable in all three planes. Face-bow can be used to locate a patient's hinge axis. It can also be used to record arbitrary or approximate axis. With special adapters it can function as an ear-bow. An adjustable orbital pointer provides a third point of reference. **B,** Kinematic Face-bow when used in conjunction with hinge axis "flags" can serve to indicate mandibular movement. Condylar inclination and side-shift measurements can be recorded.

The Denar Mini-Recorder (D3MR) is a mechanical pantographic recording mechanism suitable for tracking border movements of lateral jaw movements. It is extremely useful in the setting and adjusting of fully adjustable articulators for use in occlusal rehabilitation. It is capable of being upgraded to utilize electronic recording systems.

The Denar Pantronic recording system (Fig. 18-27) employs state-of-the-art electronic technology to evaluate temporomandibular joint dysfunction. Originally designed as an outgrowth of manual pantography for the accurate adjustment of articulators for rehabilitative treatment, its capabilities have been enlarged to make it an important diagnostic tool for determination and treatment of temporomandibular joint and muscle dysfunction. The patient's muscle coordination can be measured by employment of a pantographic reproducibility index (PRI). Evidence has been presented that, through the use of such an index, (PRI), measurements can be used to evaluate the condition of the temporomandibular joint.

The TMJ Kinematic Face-bow (Fig. 18-28, *A*) is adjustable in all three planes, enabling the easy location of the hinge axis of the jaw. It can also be used to record an arbitrary or approximate axis. By use of a special adapter it can be employed as an ear-bow. An adjustable orbital pointer permits orientation of an anterior or third point of reference. When used in conjunction with hinge axis flags, the apparatus can function as mandibular movement indicator (Fig. 18-28, *B*). Condylar indication and side-shift measurements can be recorded and maintained to provide a permanent patient record.

CASTING EQUIPMENT

Nearly all of the metals used for casting in dentistry are sufficiently viscous in their fluid or melted state that they will not flow into a small gate or sprue to fill a small intricate mold. As a result, the casting of these metals is usually accomplished by forcing the alloy into the mold rather than relying upon gravity flow of the fluid metal. This is accomplished by use of a centrifuge or by positive air pressure upon the molten metal. The largest percentage of casting equipment in use in dentistry employs a spinning beam to which the mold is attached, to throw the metal into the mold by centrifugal force.

Typical examples of such apparatus are supplied by Penwalt/Jelenko (Broken Arm Casting Machine [Fig. 18-29]) and the J.M. Ney Company–(Emesco Senior Casting Machine [Fig. 18-30]). Both of these machines incorporate a "broken arm" principle, which allows the melting crucible and mold to be positioned at right angles to the spring-propelled beam of the apparatus. As the beam begins its rotation the melted alloy, by its inertia, is carried directly toward the mold. As centrifugal force is generated by the spinning of the arm (beam) the casting flask and mold swing into alignment and become subjected to the full centrifugal force.

More sophisticated centrifugal equipment is available from Penwalt/Jelenko that provides for melting of the alloy through electronic induction (the Production Caster [Fig. 18-31]). It is capable of melting all alloys used in dentistry, both gold alloys and base metal (cobalt-chrome and chrome-nickel). The equipment has the capability for providing an argon atmosphere for cleaner, oxide-free castings. It is well suited for making

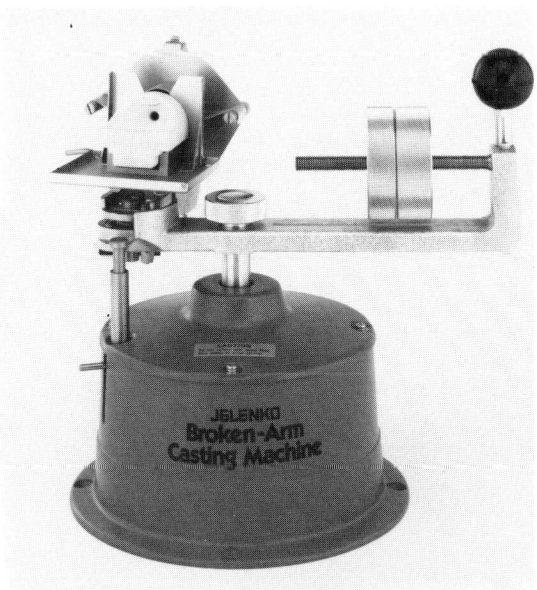

Fig. 18-29. Broken-Arm Casting Machine (Jelenko) incorporates "broken-arm" principle that allows melting crucible and mold to be positioned at right angles to propeller arm of the apparatus. At beginning of rotation melted alloy can flow directly into sprue and mold.

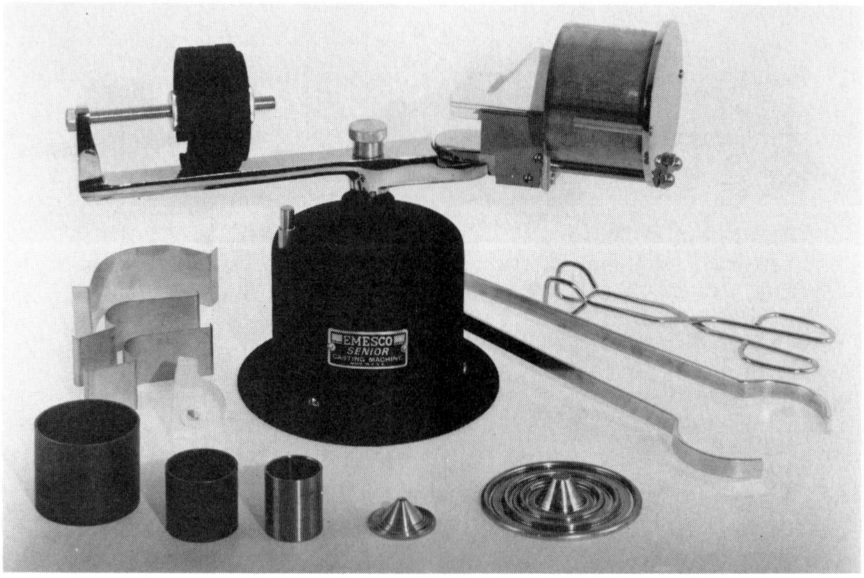

Fig. 18-30. Emesco Senior Casting Machine (Kerr) propellor arm, which has adjustable counterweights, incorporates a swivel joint which allows the crucible and mold to rest at right angles during melting of the metal. Because of its inertia, the molten alloy travels directly from the crucible into mold. As rotation accelerates assembly swings into alignment with arm to provide full effect of centrifugal force on metal being cast.

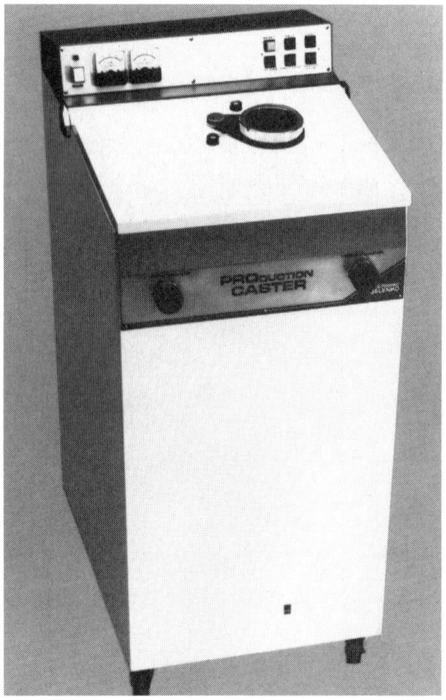

Fig. 18-31. PROduction CASTER (Jelenko) provides for melting of casting alloy through electronic induction. Centrifugal casting machine is capable of casting all metals (precious and base metal) used in dentistry. Equipment provides an argon atmosphere for cleaner, oxide-free castings.

castings for both fixed and removable partial dentures.

A similar unit developed by Unitek—the Autocast Induction Casting Unit (Fig. 18-32)—provides induction heating of the alloy and incorporates an optical pyrometer to determine temperature of the alloy. When the alloy has reached proper temperature, the casting is made by spinning of the centrifugal arm.

Several manufacturers have developed and offer equipment which employs air pressure to force the melted alloy into the mold. Heraeus Dental Gold Corporation offers several different models that employ a combination of melting the metal under vacuum and casting with positive air pressure. The Combilador Vacuum Pressure Casting Apparatus CL-G 2002 (Fig. 18-33) melts the alloy under vacuum in a resistance-type muffle, which surrounds a graphite-lined ceramic crucible. When the alloy reaches casting temperature, the chamber inverts, allowing the metal to enter the mold. Synchronized with the inversion, positive air pressure is applied to force the metal into the mold. The heating and casting cycle is controlled by a programmed microprocessor. Several other models incorporating the same principle are available (Figs. 18-34 and 18-35).

A recent introduction by Heraeus is an apparatus similar to those just described but which incorporates induction heating and temperature sensing with an optical pyrometer (Fig. 18-36). The apparatus provides

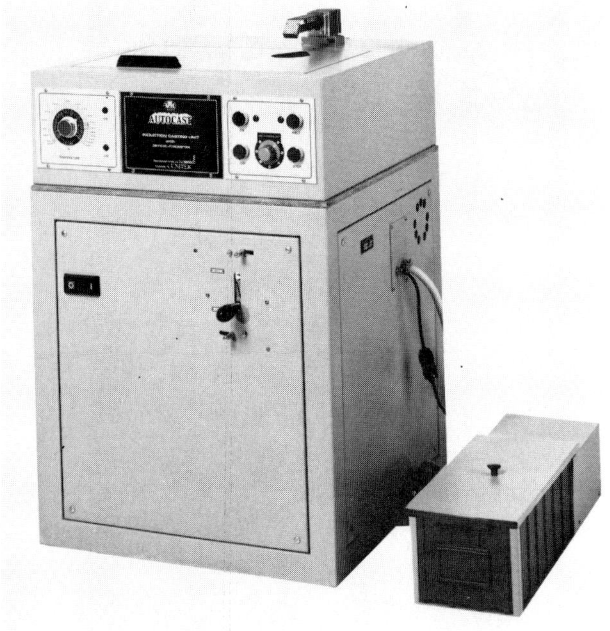

Fig. 18-32. AUTOCAST induction casting unit (Unitek) provides induction heating of metal alloys to be cast and incorporates optical pyrometer to determine temperature of alloy. Casting is accomplished by spinning of centrifugal arm.

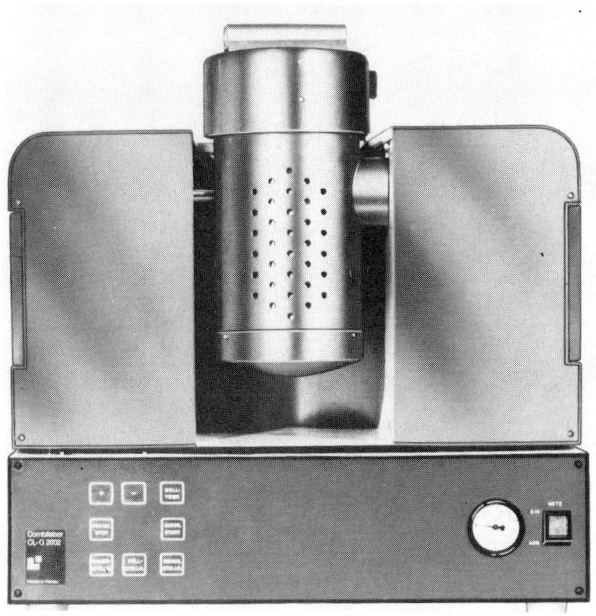

Fig. 18-33. Combilador CL-2 2002 Vacuum pressure casting apparatus (Heraeus). Casting alloy is melted under vacuum in a resistance-type muffle surrounding a graphite-lined ceramic crucible. Casting chamber inverts and positive air pressure is applied to force metal into mold.

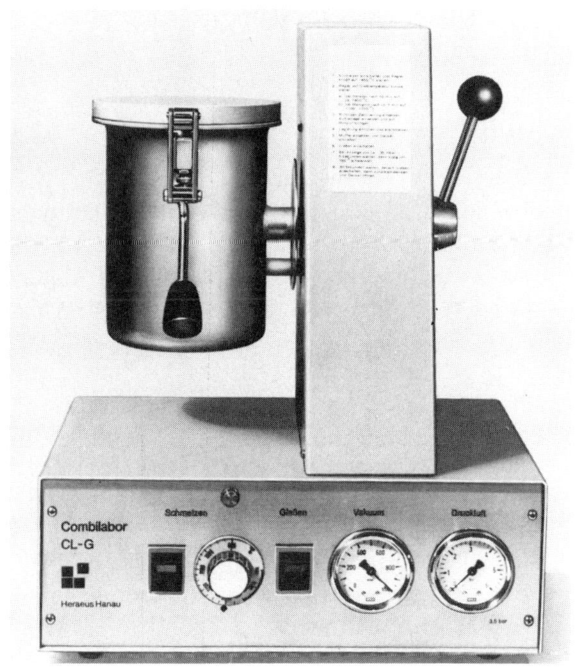

Fig. 18-34. Combilador CL-G Vacuum pressure casting apparatus (Heraeus), a member of the Combilador casting equipment family. This model is inverted by hand.

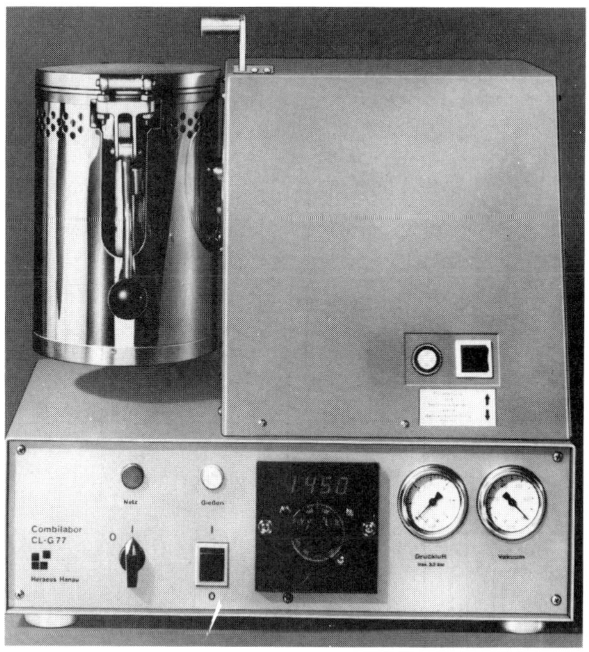

Fig. 18-35. Combilador CL-G77 vacuum pressure casting apparatus (Heraeus). Its design is similar to other Heraeus Combilador casting machines but it includes an electronic readout of metal temperature.

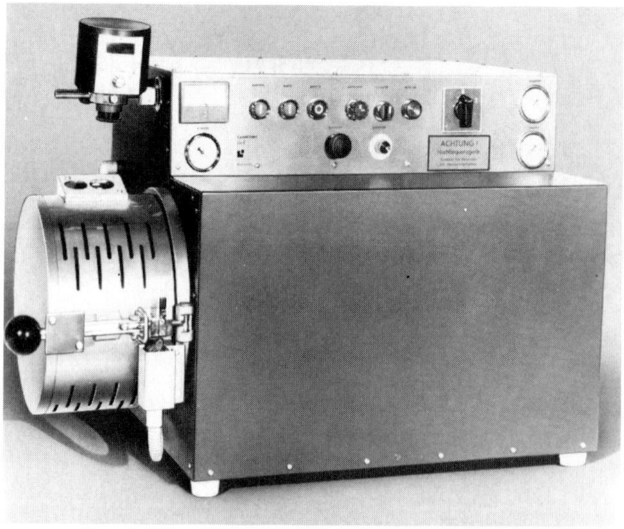

Fig. 18-36. Combilador CL-1 Inductively heated vacuum-pressure casting apparatus (Heraeus). A recent introduction by Heraeus, it incorporates induction heating and temperature sensing with an optical pyrometer. Both precious and base metal alloys can be cast with the equipment. All Heraeus models employ principle of inverting casting chamber to allow metal to flow into mold gate (sprue) at precise time that positive air pressure is applied to force metal into mold.

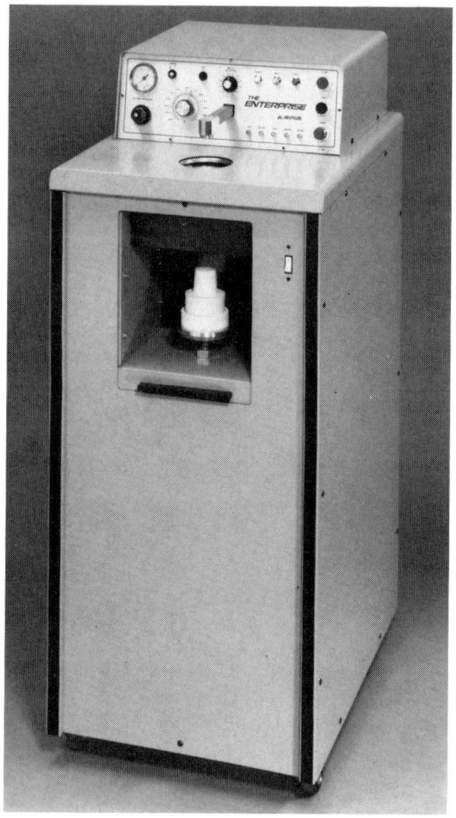

Fig. 18-37. Enterprise Casting Unit (Jelrus Dental Products), a sophisticated air pressure casting machine that incorporates argon atmosphere for melting the metal, an infrared sensor to determine proper casting temperature, and induction heating of all metals used in making dental castings.

the capability for melting and casting of any metal, precious or base, used in dentistry.

All Heraeus models employ the principle of inverting the casting chamber so that the metal alloy is poured from the melting crucible into the mold gate (sprue) at the precise time that positive air pressure is applied to force the metal into the mold.

Another sophisticated casting machine has been developed by Jelrus Dental Products Corporation. The Enterprise Unit (Fig. 18-37) uses a unique method of melting the alloy to be cast by induction heating directly in a preformed crucible area of the casting mold. A small gate or sprue sized to match the surface tension of the melted alloy prevents the metal from prematurely entering the mold. The melting chamber is purged with argon to produce an oxygen-free atmosphere for melting the alloy. Temperature is sensed by an optical pyrometer (infrared sensor). A viewing window allows observation of the melting process by the operator. The casting is made by introduction of positive air pressure (20 to 40 psi) into the sealed casting chamber. One distinct advantage of the method is that virtually all turbulence in the metal is eliminated, as well as effects of centrifugal force upon "leading edge" areas of the casting, as present in centrifugal casting.

DIE PINNING EQUIPMENT

The extensive rehabilitative procedures that have been developed require accurate master casts which provide for removal and replacement of individual dies into their precise positions. Several different methods of producing separable dies have been developed to accomplish this end. The so-called dry pinning technique permits the placement of metal die pins into critical areas of the die base after recovery of the cast from the impression.

The technique involves flattening of the basal surface of the master cast and accurately positioning holes in the base in relation to the teeth which will form the removable dies. In most cases, removal of the palatal area of the maxillary and lingual area of the mandibular cast facilitates separation of the individual dies. Metal pins are cemented into the holes, which have been drilled into the base of the cast. A new base portion is poured against the lubricated and flattened surface of the cast. The cast is sectioned with a fine saw through the interproximal areas. The individual teeth can then

A

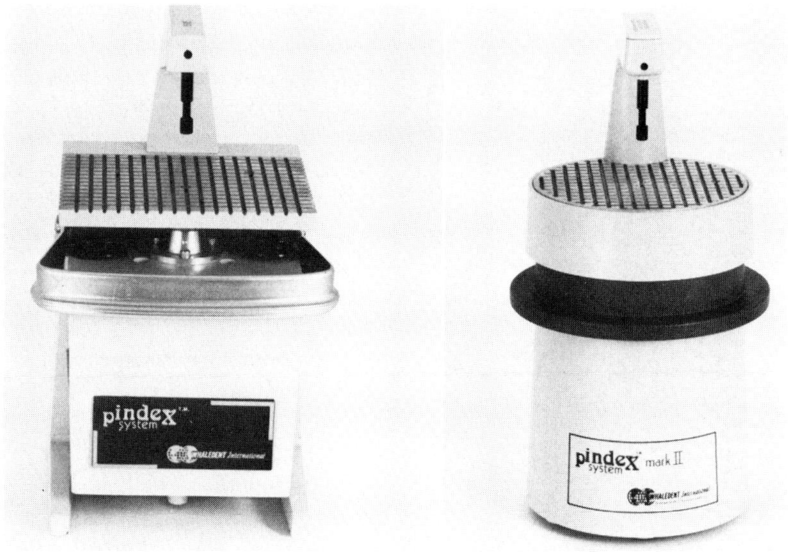

B

Fig. 18-38. A, Pindex System (Whaledent) employs a light beam to orient cast for proper drilling of holes in base of cast. Spring-loaded platform is depressed to allow rotating drill to form precise holes into which metal die pins can be cemented. **B,** Pindex Mark II (Whaledent), a refined version of Pindex System. Apparatus is designed to drill holes in underside of cast in exact alignment with teeth on cast.

be removed and trimmed to serve as removable dies.

The Pindex system (Whaledent International) (Fig. 18-38) employs a light beam to orient the cast for proper drilling of the hole in the base of the cast. As the spring-loaded drilling platform is depressed, the rotating drill is exposed to drill a hole of prescribed depth in the base of the cast and in exact alignment with the light beam. The apparatus is designed to drill holes in the underside of the cast.

A similar apparatus, developed by APM-Sterngold and named the Accudrill (Fig. 18-39), is described as a dowel pin press. The technician places the trimmed "first pour" (of the impression) on the horizontal table and positions the cast so that the pointer, which is in exact alignment with the drill, indicates the position of the desired hole to be placed in the cast base. As the platform is depressed, a hole is drilled in the cast to the predetermined depth. After the appropriate holes are drilled in the base of the cast, brass dowel pins are cemented to place with cyanoacrylate cement. The unit uses standard shank (3⁄32 inch) carbide burs and is compatible with all standard dowel pins as well as the TDI double pin system.

The Oxy Microdrill (Fig. 18-40) has also been developed for the "dry pinning" process. Rather than an overhead indicator, this system employs a mirror beneath the glass drilling table so that the technician can position the drill exactly for drilling the holes in the base of the cast. An adjustable chuck accommodates

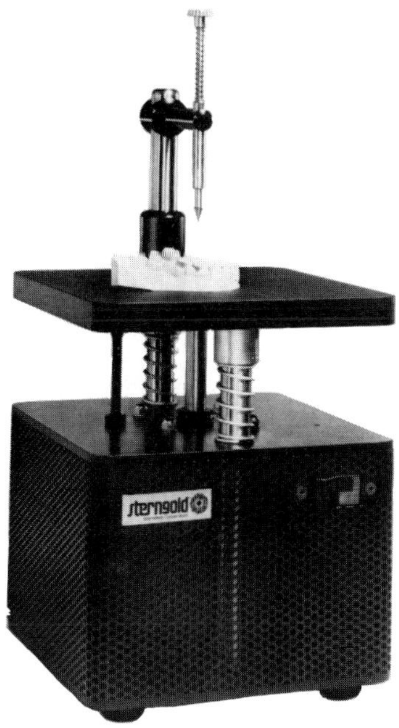

Fig. 18-39. Accudrill (Sterngold), a dowel pin press that orients cast by means of perpendicular spring-loaded pointer or mandrel. Pointer allows exact location of hole position beneath. Depressing platform exposes drill so that precise hole can be formed in base of cast.

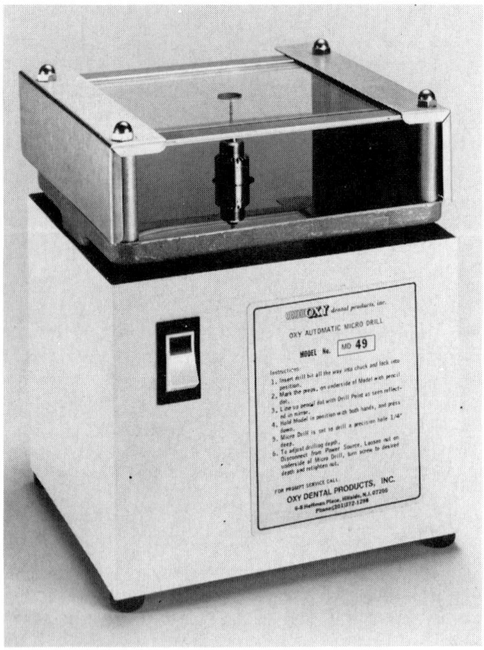

Fig. 18-40. Automatic Micro-Drill (Oxy), which employs a mirror beneath a glass drilling table to allow technician to position drill exactly for drilling holes in base of cast. Adjustable chuck accommodates several different sizes of drills or burs.

drill sizes to 5⁄32 inch. Adjustable drilling depths are possible by adjusting preset stops.

Unitek has developed and offers a router and pin drill set. The Router (Fig. 18-41, *A*) is used to trim away palatal and lingual portions of the cast in preparation for the "dry pinning" process. The "Pin Drill" (Fig. 18-41, *B*) employs an overhead spring-loaded pointer, which is in exact alignment with the drill, to indicate the optimum position of the hole in relation to the working area and base of the die. By depressing the drilling table, the drill produces a precise hole in the cast base. Die pins are subsequently cemented into the holes with appropriate cement.

BURNOUT (MOLD CONDITIONING) FURNACES

Mold conditioning or "burnout" furnaces have become increasingly sophisticated. The first attempts at wax elimination and mold conditioning were gas-fired appliances or other simple arrangements typified by a casting flask (ring) resting upon a wire mesh suspended over a bunsen burner. When the sprue hole appeared "cherry red" it was assumed that the mold was ready to be cast.

Furnaces with electric muffles were developed that permitted adjustment of temperature for high-heat or

A

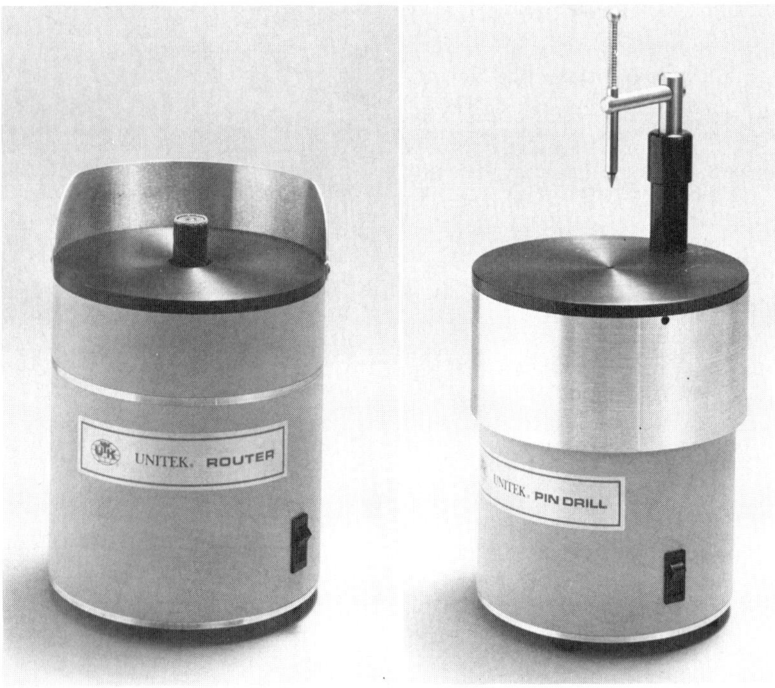

B

Fig. 18-41. A, Router (Unitek) used to trim away palatal and lingual portions of casts in preparation for "dry pinning" process. **B,** Pin Drill (Unitek) employs an overhead spring-loaded pointer that is in exact alignment with drill to indicate optimum position of hole in relation to working areas and base of die.

low-heat casting techniques. Timing devices were added later to signal correct conditioning times. Such improvements greatly facilitated the casting procedure by allowing more precise mold conditioning. Timers also relieved the technician of the responsibility of coordinating burnout time in a busy laboratory.

With the development of high-heat (silicate and phosphate-bonded) investments, the use of multiple stages of burnout temperatures to prevent mold cracking and damage became necessary. At first several different furnaces, each set at a different temperature, were employed, the casting flasks (rings) being transferred from furnace to furnace to suit the appropriate time/temperature requirements.

More recently, furnaces have been developed with controls that allow different temperatures and times within a programmed cycle. Sophisticated electronic timing systems are now incorporated by several manufacturers to allow the programming of a progression of temperatures with proper timing of temperatures (heat soak) to be achieved.

The Neymatic 101 (Fig. 18-42) is a large-capacity furnace that allows for a temperature setting to be selected and set at the press of a button.

Heraeus Dental Gold Company produces several different models with varying degrees of control sophistication. The Combilador CL-VS 2002 (Fig. 18-43) features a microprocessor temperature and time control programmed from a control panel on the face of the apparatus. Time and temperature are displayed by liquid crystal display (LCD). The muffle is protected by new improved insulating material and a built-in extractor flue can be fitted with a postburn catalyzer to control fumes from heated investment and wax during the burnout period.

Oxy Dental Products, Inc., produces several different well-built models of burnout furnaces with three-sided embedded heating elements, and solid state circuitry giving control over both temperature and rate of heat rise. Stainless steel construction makes these units resistant to corrosion. The Midi Model BOD 7S (Fig. 18-44) is moderate in size, with muffle dimensions of 6½ by 5 by 4½ inches.

Unitek supplies several different furnaces designed to fit the needs of different capacity laboratories. The Automatic Dual-Temp Burnout Furnace (Fig. 18-45) allows programming of two different burnout temperatures and holding (heat soak) times.

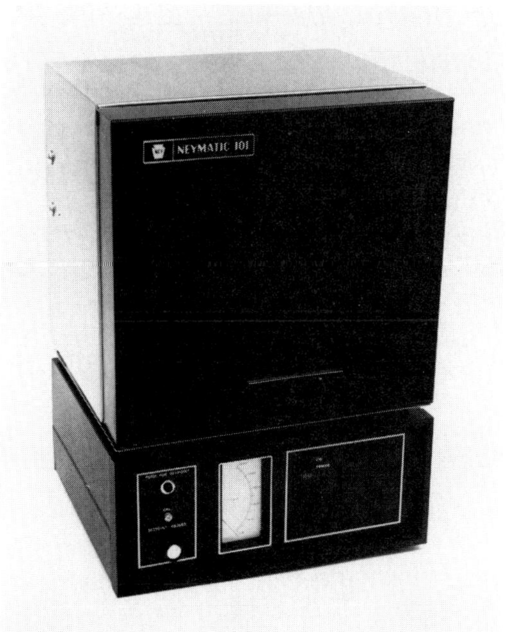

Fig. 18-42. NEYMATIC-101 (Ney), a large-capacity furnace that allows for a temperature setting to be selected and set at the press of a button.

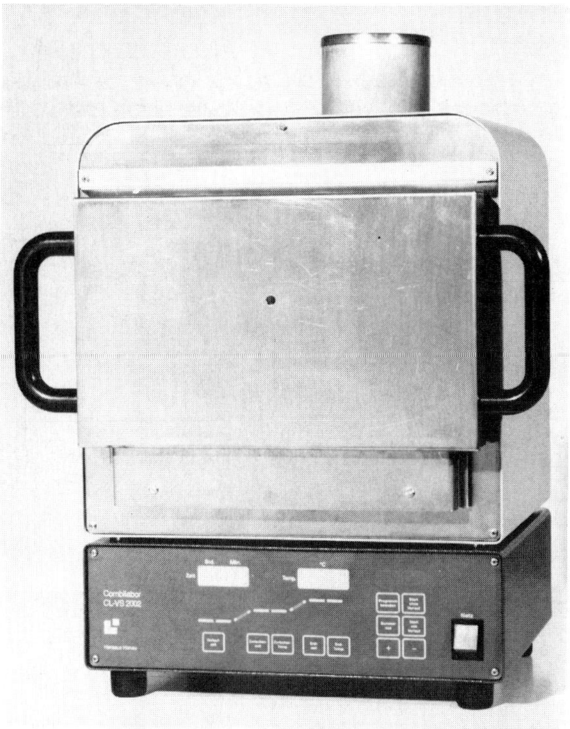

Fig. 18-43. Combilador CL-VS 2002 (Heraeus) features a microprocessor temperature and time control programmed from a control panel on face of apparatus. Time and temperature are displayed on a liquid crystal display (LCD). Furnace can be fitted with postburn catalyzer to control fumes from heated investment and wax during burnout period.

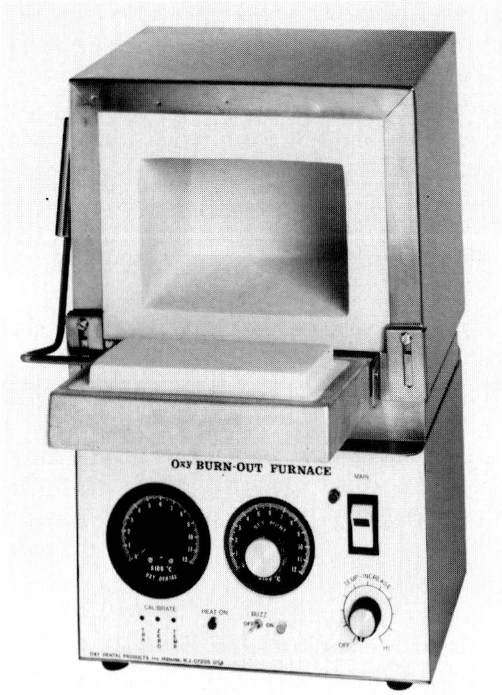

Fig. 18-44. Midi Model BOD 7S Furnace (Oxy Dental Products), a moderate sized furnace with solid state circuitry to control time, temperature, and rate of heat rise. Stainless steel construction provides resistance to corrosion.

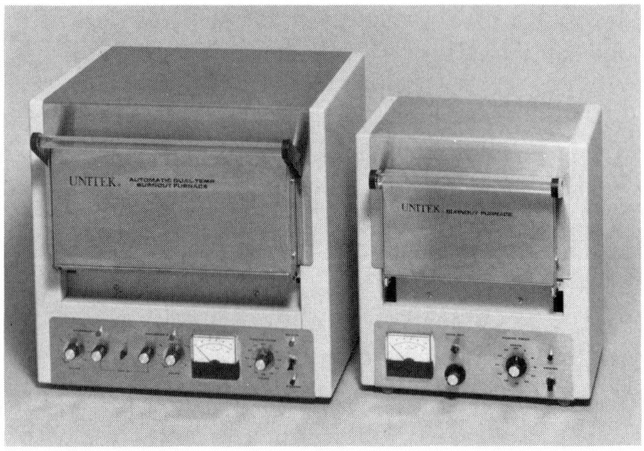

Fig. 18-45. Automatic Dual-Temp Furnace (Unitek) allows programming of two different burnout temperatures and holding (heat soak) times.

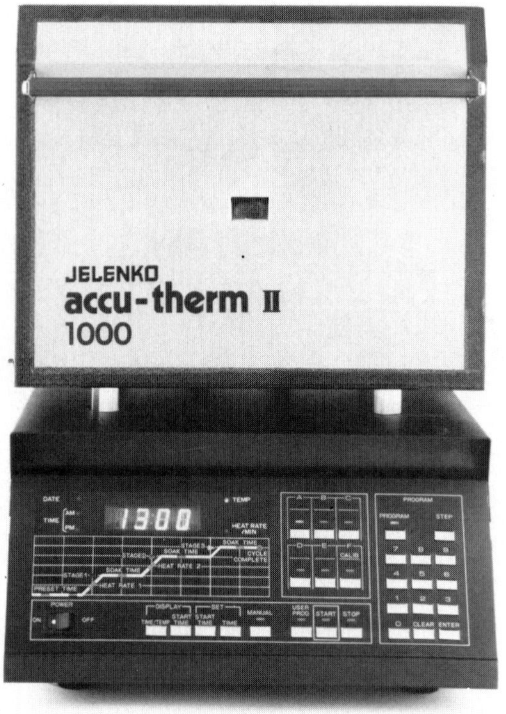

Fig. 18-46. Accu-Therm II 1000 (Jelenko) incorporates three-stage computerized control system. Furnace allows option of elevating temperature in three stages, if desired for uniform mold expansion.

An example of the burnout furnace offered by Jelenko is the Accu-Therm II 1000 (Fig. 18-46). It incorporates a three-stage computerized control and utilizes a graphic heat rate monitoring system. The furnace allows the option of elevating the temperature in three stages, if desired, for uniform expansion. It is stated that the temperature can be reduced after the "heat soak" if necessary to meet the requirements of some Type III gold alloys.

PORCELAIN FURNACES

Furnaces for firing ceramic restorations, like their companion burnout (mold conditioning) furnaces, have undergone marked improvements and have become increasingly sophisticated to meet the demands of different porcelains and ceramic systems.

The Jelenko Flagship furnace (Fig. 18-47) control is very flexible, with 22 different firing cycles and an additional 22 user-programmable firing cycles. It allows much more efficient use of the ceramist's time and is designed to increase the technician's productivity as well as uniformity of porcelain firing. It, along with similar products, represents the current state-of-the-art in furnace design and construction.

Unitek currently produces several porcelain furnaces with varying degrees of sophistication. The Ultra-Mat CDF (Fig. 18-48) represents this manufacturer's contribution to current concepts of design and construction. It includes a programmable computerized control system with a CRT display for temperature and other technical information.

The Oxy Micro-Ten furnace (Fig. 18-49) employs microprocessor circuitry, has a capacity for 30 different programs, displays program status and automatic elec-

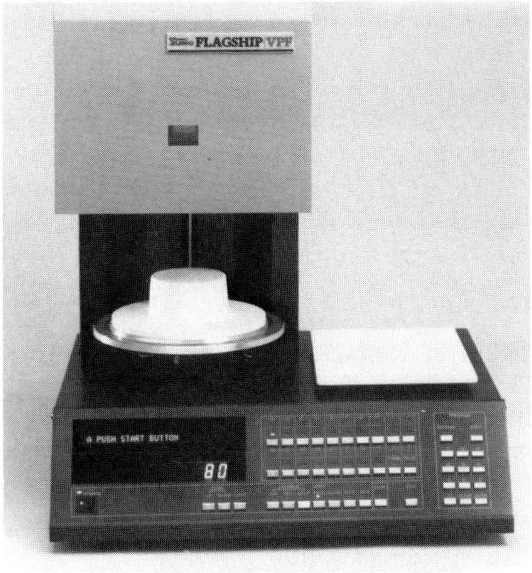

Fig. 18-47. Flagship VPF (Jelenko) computerized control is very flexible, with 22 different firing cycles and an additional 22 user programmable firing cycles. Firing table automatically raises and lowers from firing chamber.

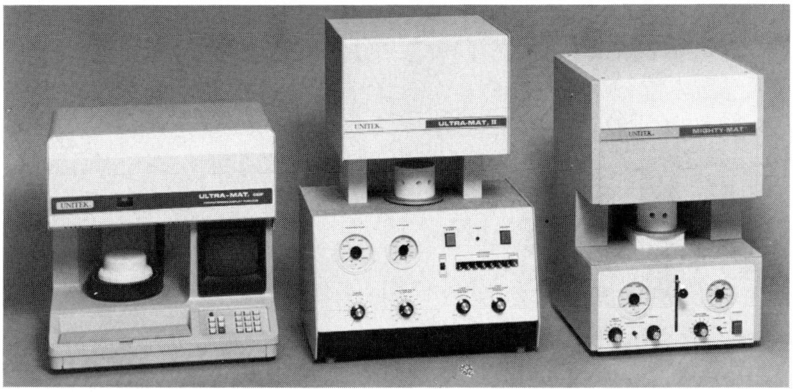

Fig. 18-48. Ultra-mat CDF (Unitek) *(left)* represents Unitek's contribution to current concepts of design and construction. It has a programmable computerized control system with CRT display for temperature and technical information.

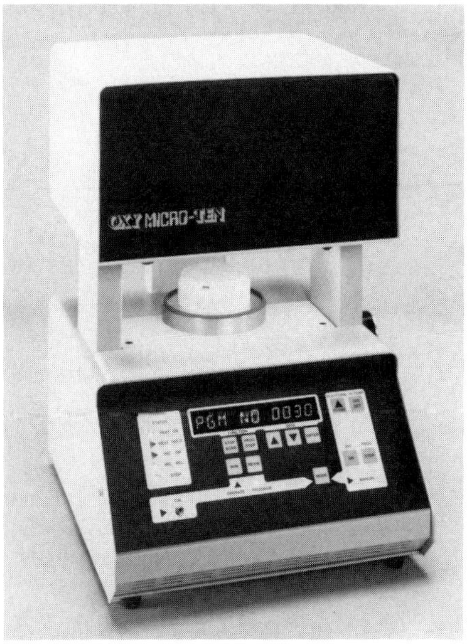

Fig. 18-49. Oxy Micro-Ten (Oxy Dental) employs microprocessor circuitry, has capacity for 30 different programs, displays program status, has automatic electronic calibration, and protects program input with retained program memory in case of power failure.

tronic calibration, and protects program inputs with retained program memory in case of power failure.

LABORATORY HANDPIECES

Electronic and air-driven handpieces are offered by several manufacturers as alternatives to belt-driven handpieces and bench lathes for grinding, trimming, and polishing small items.

The Bell International Laboratory Hand Engine (Fig. 18-50) is capable of operating at 2000 to 35,000 r.p.m. and has a constant torque feature that automatically delivers more power when pressure is exerted on the rotating bur or stone. Noise level is low. The nylon outer casing is of a size and shape that is comfortable to hold and use.

Hanau's Emesco Electric "Micro" motor handpiece (Fig. 18-51) features a foot control to vary rotational speed of the handpiece. Improved air circulation keeps

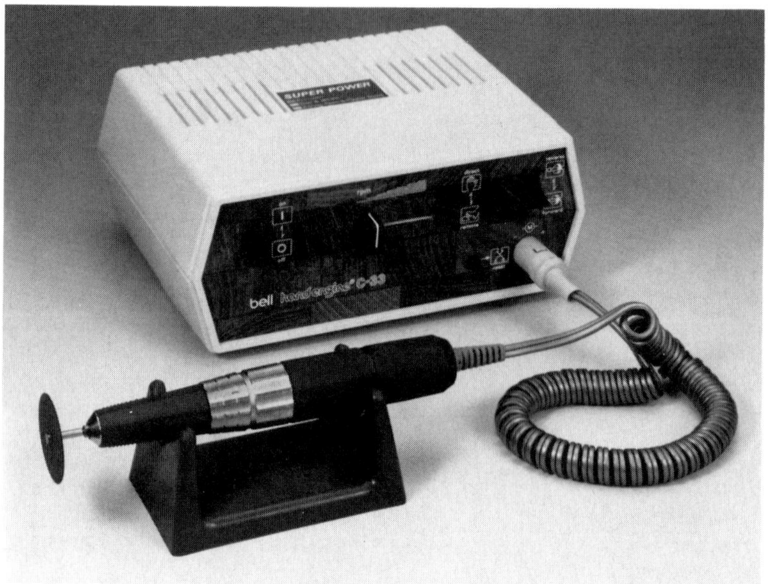

Fig. 18-50. Hand Engine C-33 (Bell International) is capable of operating speeds from 2000 to 35,000 r.p.m. and has a constant torque feature that automatically delivers more power when pressure is exerted on the rotating stone or bur. The nylon outer casing is of a size and shape that is comfortable to hold and use.

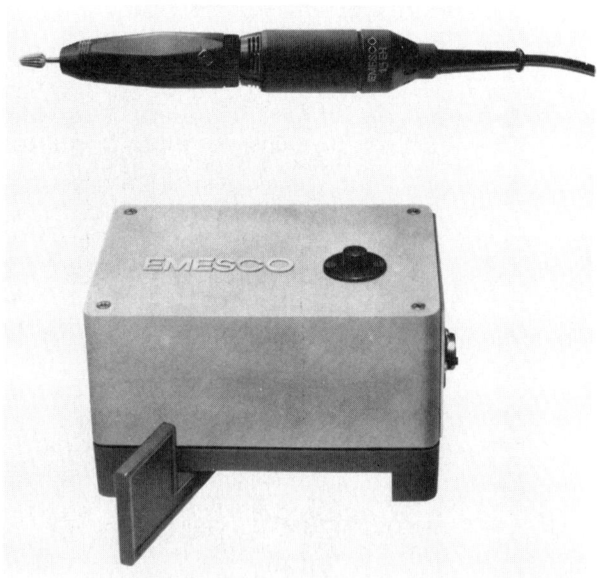

Fig. 18-51. Emesco "Micro" Motor Handpiece (Hanau) features foot control to vary rotational speed of handpiece. Improved air circulation keeps motor from overheating during heavy use. Barrel of handpiece is of a size that is comfortable to hold and minimizes hand fatigue.

the motor from overheating during heavy use. The barrel of the handpiece is of a size that is comfortable to hold and minimizes hand fatigue.

ELECTROCHEMICAL EQUIPMENT

Several manufacturers offer equipment for electroplating impressions with copper or silver to produce metal dies. Hanua is producing an improved version of an electroplating unit which that company has supplied for many years (Fig. 18-52). The unit is capable of electroplating up to 10 individual impressions at one time. Larger sectional impressions may be successfully electroplated by applying a cathode lead to the metallized impression surfaces. Areas not intended to be plated are usually covered with a protective wax coating.

Unitek produces a unique multiplating unit (Fig. 18-53) that has the capability for plating, stripping, or electropolishing. An accessory to the plating unit is a larger vessel for holding electrolyte, which enables simultaneous plating of a number of individual impressions or larger sectional or full-arch impressions. The unit is capable of plating copper, silver, or tin. Unitek also supplies equipment for stripping and electropolishing of partial denture frames and irregular surfaces (Fig. 18-54).

Oxy Dental Products manufactures equipment for etching of metal retainers to be used for resin-bonded prostheses (Fig. 18-55). The unit provides a control timer module, stirring capability for agitation of solutions, holders to support work during the etching pro-

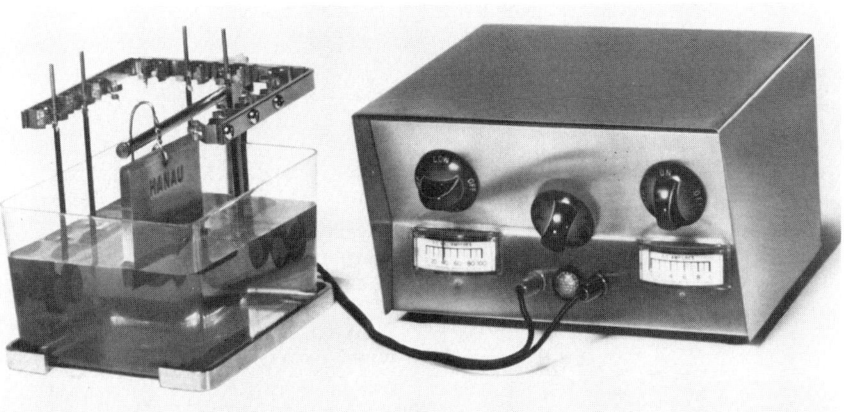

Fig. 18-52. Electroformer 143–1C (Hanau), an improved version of electroplating unit manufacturer has produced for many years. Unit is capable of electroplating as many as 10 individual impression simultaneously.

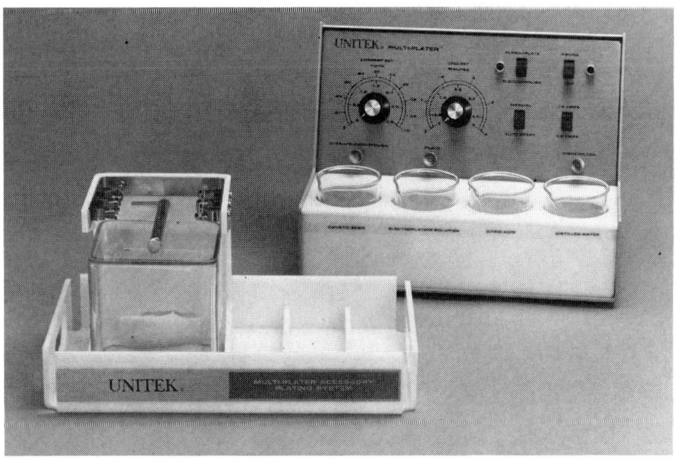

Fig. 18-53. Multi-plater (Unitek), a unique multiplating unit that has capability for plating, stripping, or electropolishing. Accessory vessel allows simultaneous plating of number of individual impressions, larger sectional impressions, or full arch impressions. Unit is capable of plating copper, silver, or tin.

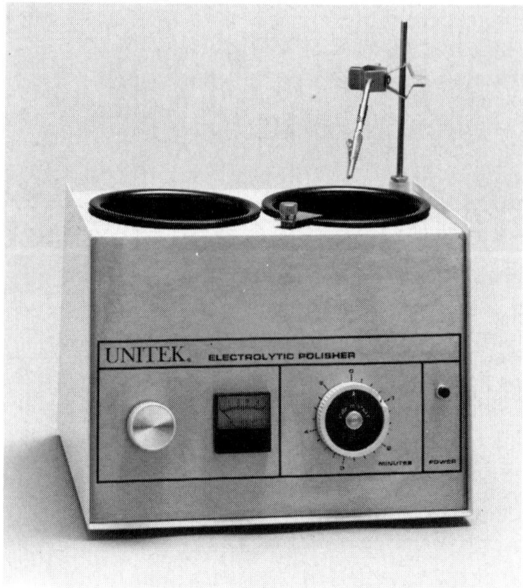

Fig. 18-54. Electrolytic Polisher (Unitek), a deplating unit for stripping and electropolishing of partial denture frames and irregular surfaces.

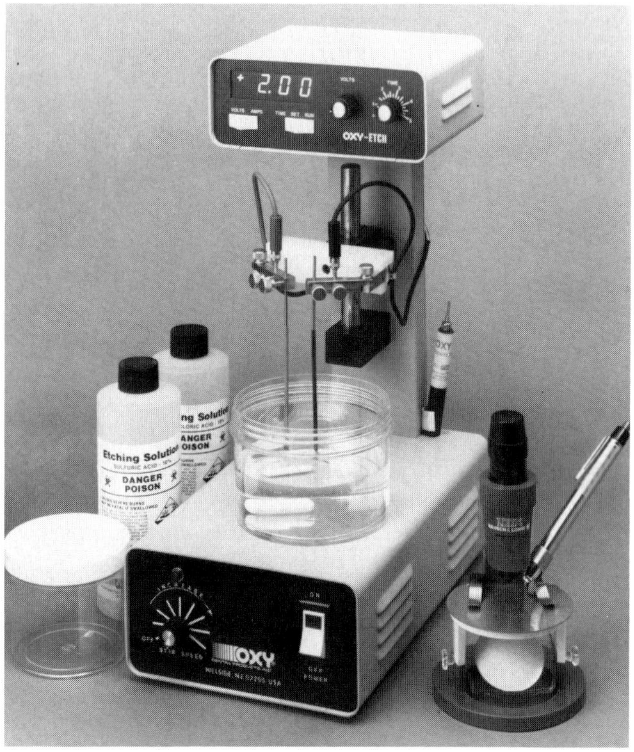

Fig. 18-55. Oxy-Etch (Oxy Dental Products), a unit for etching of metal retainers to be used for resin-bonded prostheses. Proper etching of metal surfaces to be bonded is important for maximum retention of the resin.

cess, and a small microscope for examination of the etched surfaces.

Esmadent Division of Esma Chemicals, Inc., supplies equipment for etching, stripping, and electropolishing of partial denture frames and other small irregular objects. A chemical devesting unit capable of removing all investment and oxide by chemical means has been developed for use in dental laboratories. The unit saves time in abrasive blasting and other preparatory cleaning procedures that are necessary before finishing can be attempted.

MILLING AND PARALLELING EQUIPMENT

The fabrication of milled crowns, telescope crowns, precision and semiprecision attachments, fixed removable partial dentures, and certain types of periodontal splinting would be difficult without the use of paralleling and milling equipment. Most types of equipment

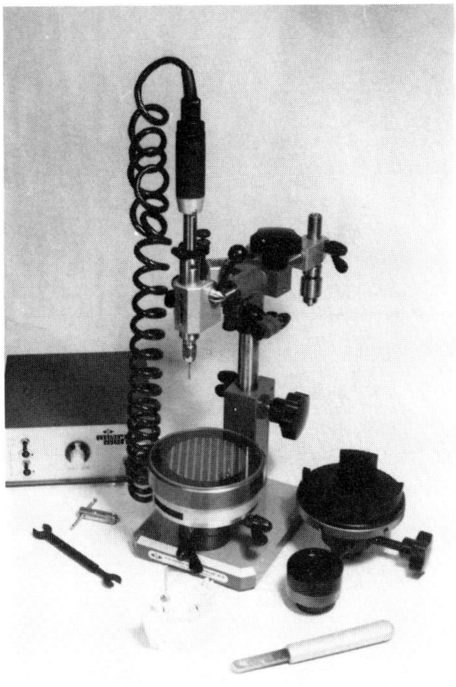

Fig. 18-56. Bachmann Parallelor and Precision Milling Instrument (Sterngold) a precision unit for drilling screw holes and milling crown surfaces, bars with parallel sides, and rests in both wax and metal. Adjustable table permits precise inclination of working cast for surveying and milling operations. Table has magnetic holding device for securing casts in exact alighment.

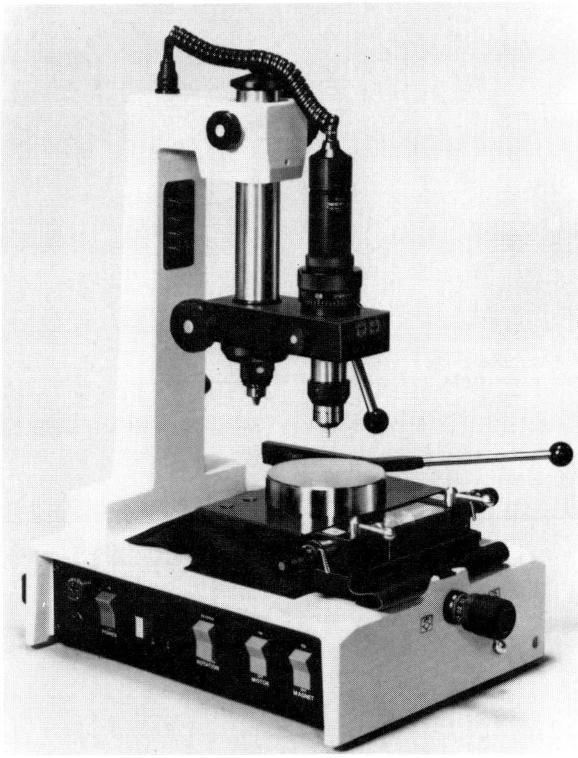

Fig. 18-57. EM Parallellmeter (Bell International), a solid vibration-free apparatus capable of milling in three directions: vertical, horizontal, and circular. Each movement is controlled by micrometer adjustment to 0.01 mm. Precise, quiet, vibration-free milling is accomplished by a specially designed handpiece. Casts are attached by an electromagnetic stage.

made for these purposes are multiuse machines, which include a movable modeling arm for paralleling surfaces in wax and metal, the capacity to serve as a surveying device to determine heights of contour and undercut areas, and a milling head for producing parallel surfaces in crowns, bars, guide planes, and other precise contouring of axial surfaces. Most devices include an adjustable base for mounting of the working cast for surveying and milling procedures.

The Bachmann Parallelor and Precision Milling instrument available from APM-Sterngold (Fig. 18-56) is a precision unit for drilling screw holes and for milling crown surfaces, bars with parallel sides, and rests in both wax and metal. An adjustable mounting table permits precise inclination of the working cast for surveying and milling operations. The table has a magnetic holding device that allows removal and replacement of the mounted cast into exact alignment.

The unit features paralleling/surveying arms for placement of precision attachments, a milling head for precision milling, and an accurate miniature drill press. An optional electric motor drive provides for high-speed milling. Rotational speed of the spindle can be regulated up to 20,000 rpm.

The EM Parallelometer (Fig. 18-57) supplied by Bell International is a solid vibration-free apparatus capable of milling in three directions: vertical, horizontal, and circular. Each movement is controlled by a micrometer adjustment to 0.01 mm. A specially designed hand engine installed on the parallelometer provides precise, quiet milling without vibration. Casts can be attached and removed by an electromagnetic stage. The apparatus can also function as a surveyor.

MODEL TRIMMERS

Model trimmers are essential in any dental laboratory. There are few casts of dental stone made in any laboratory that do not require excess portions of stone removed before use by the technician and dentist.

The Toothmaster Discomat (Fig. 18-58) supplied by Whaledent International is illustrative of the design of nearly all model trimmers. A large flat disk 10 to 14 inches in diameter, driven by a direct drive electric motor and covered in a suitable housing, is supplied

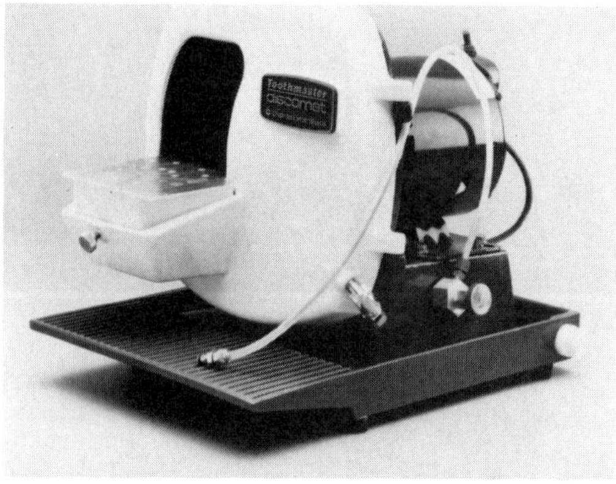

Fig. 18-58. Toothmaster Discomat (Whaledent International). Flat table is used to stabilize and orient casts against flat abrasive disk, which is kept clear of debris by water spray.

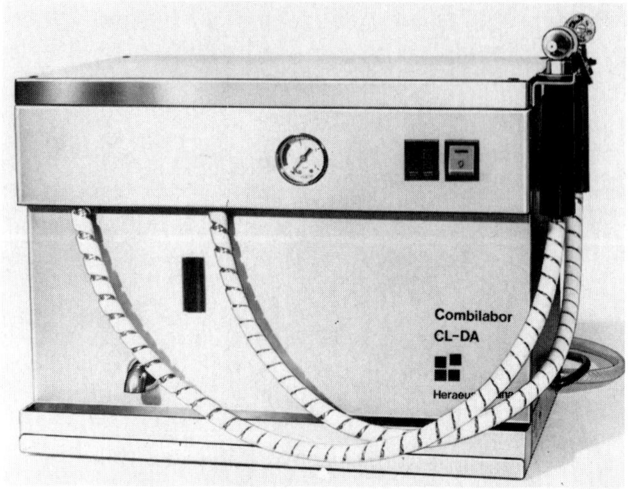

Fig. 18-59. Combilador CL-DA Steam Cleaning Unit (Heraeus) is an efficient, compact, steam cleaning unit that supplies both steam and hot water for removal of grease, wax, and polish from castings, partial denture frames, casts, dies, and procelain.

with a water spray to carry away grindings from the cast. Most are fitted with a flat table to support and orient the cast while it is being trimmed.

STEAM CLEANING EQUIPMENT

Steam cleaners are less glamorous yet essential elements of any complete laboratory operation. Most units have a short heat-up time and supply both steam and hot water. Nozzles attached to flexible insulated hoses allow steam to be directed on the work to be cleaned. The units are extremely valuable for cleaning castings after polish; metal frames to which porcelain is to be applied; wax and polish residues on casts; liquid residues after electroplating, electropolishing, or stripping; and impression trays.

Heraeus Dental Gold Company manufactures an efficient unit, the Combilador CL-DA (Fig. 18-59). The Steam-Klean from Williams Gold Company (Fig. 18-60) is an efficient, ruggedly built, "no-frills" unit. Both products supply hot water or steam as needed for cleaning of metal, porcelain, or casts. The units are simple to operate. Objects being cleaned should be held in suitable tongs or holders to protect hands and fingers from the steam.

ULTRASONIC CLEANERS

Ultrasonic cleaners have become essential in dental laboratory operation; they can be used to clean polish and wax residues from castings, to devest castings, to remove cement from provisional restorations, and to clean porcelain prior to glazing. Equipment is available in many sizes and capacities.

Several major manufacturers offer equipment to fit the needs of dental offices and laboratories. Heraeus Dental Gold Company manufactures the Combilador CL-UI (Fig. 18-61), which uses two sound heads, has automatic adaptation of sound intensity, and has a stainless steel housing.

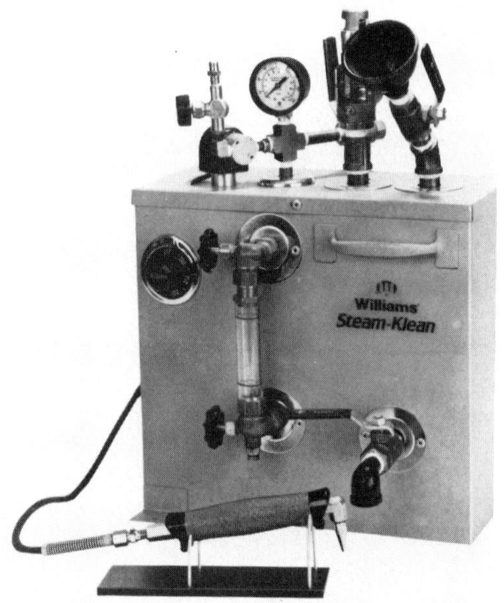

Fig. 18-60. Steam-Klean (Williams), a no-frill utilitarian steam cleaning unit for intensive dental laboratory use, supplies both hot water and steam for degreasing, wax and polish removal, and cleaning of porcelain before glazing.

Unitek supplies several different sizes and capacities of ultrasonic cleaners (Fig. 18-62). The units are well designed, efficient, and easy to maintain.

L and R Manufacturing Company is one of the pioneer manufacturers of ultrasonic cleaners (Fig. 18-63).

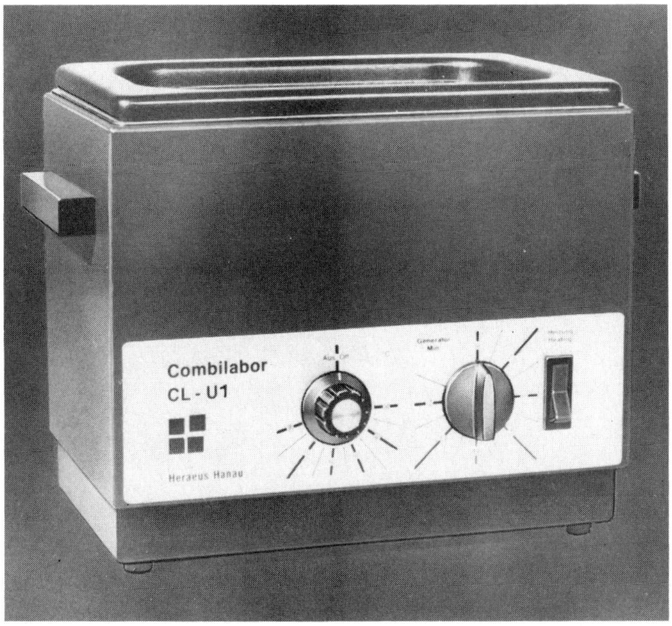

Fig. 18-61. Combilador CL-1 Ultrasonic Cleaner (Heraeus) uses two sound heads and has automatic adaptation of sound intensity. Stainless steel housing makes maintenance of appearance easy.

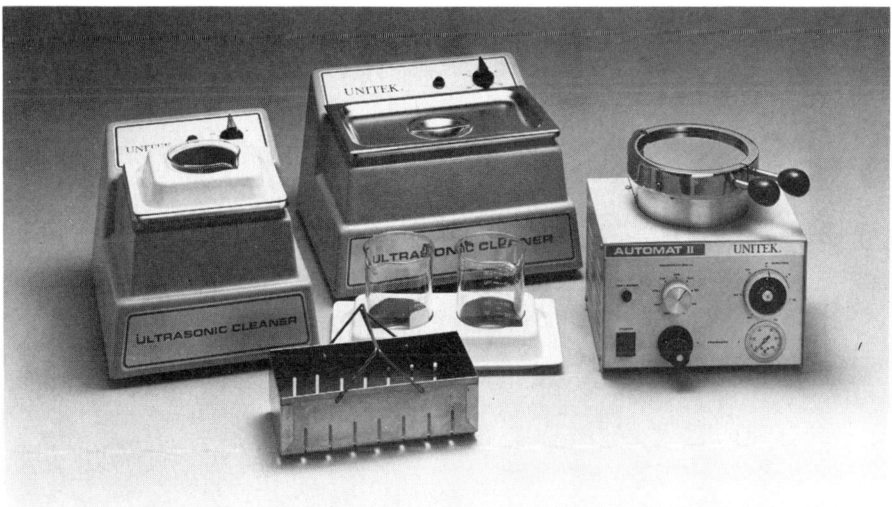

Fig. 18-62. Ultrasonic Cleaner (Unitek). Several different sizes of ultrasonic cleaners are offered by Unitek. The units are well designed, efficient, and easy to maintain.

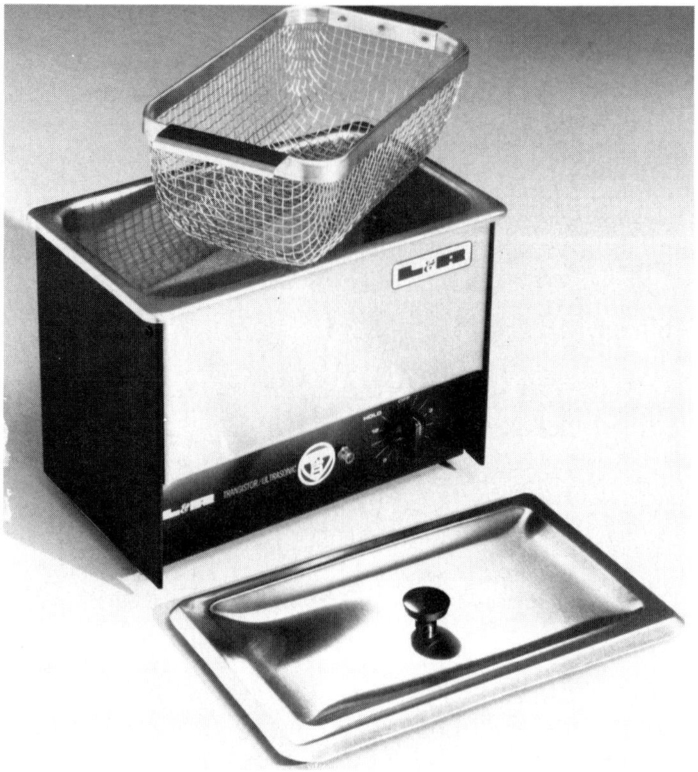

Fig. 18-63. Transistor/Ultrasonic Cleaning Unit (L and R Manfacturing) features solid state electronics and stainless steel holding tanks, are self-tuning, and have high rated cleaning power.

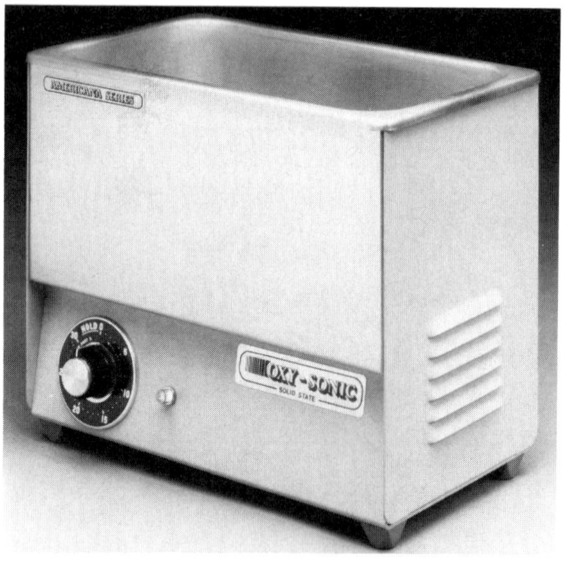

Fig. 18-64. Oxy-Sonic (Americana Series) (Oxy Dental Products). Several models of different size and capacity are available. All have stainless steel tanks and solid state electronics and are self tuning. Infrequent repairs can be made easily with plug-in replacement modules.

Several different models are available, some of which are designed to be used on a bench top, others to be recessed or "flush mounted."

Oxy Dental Products, Inc., supplies ultrasonic cleaners in several sizes and capacities (Fig. 18-64). They are suitable for use by dental laboratories, dental offices, jewelers, manufacturers of precision parts, and other similar operations. They feature solid state electronics and are self tuning. Repairs can be made easily with plug-in replacement modules.

VACUUM INVESTING EQUIPMENT

Mixing equipment for preparation of dental plasters, die stones, and casting investments is necessary in any dental laboratory. The vacuum mixing of investments to eliminate air bubbles from the mix is essential to the production of fine dental castings. Several units are available that provide for both a vacuum source and power spatulation in appropriate carriers or vessels (bowls).

Heraeus Dental Gold Company supplies the Combilador CL-VMR (Fig. 18-65) for the dense, air-free mixing of plasters and investments. The unit can be mounted on either wall or bench top. Mixing vessels are available in three sizes.

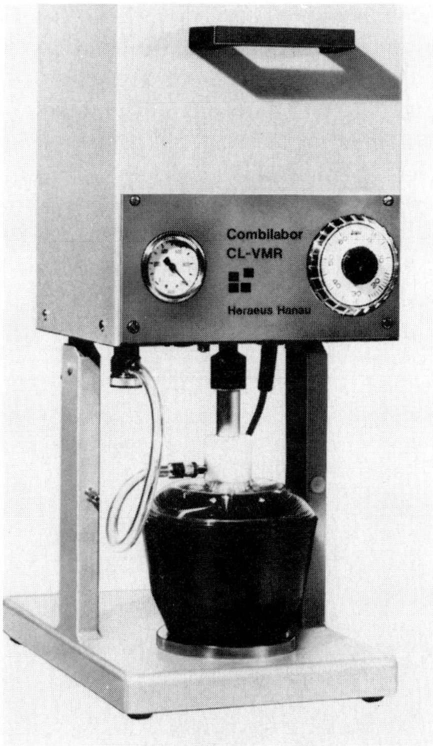

Fig. 18-65. Combilador CL-VMR Mixing Unit (Heraeus) serves as vacuum pump, power mixer, and vibrator. Unit is designed for heavy-duty use. Several sizes of mixing vessels are available.

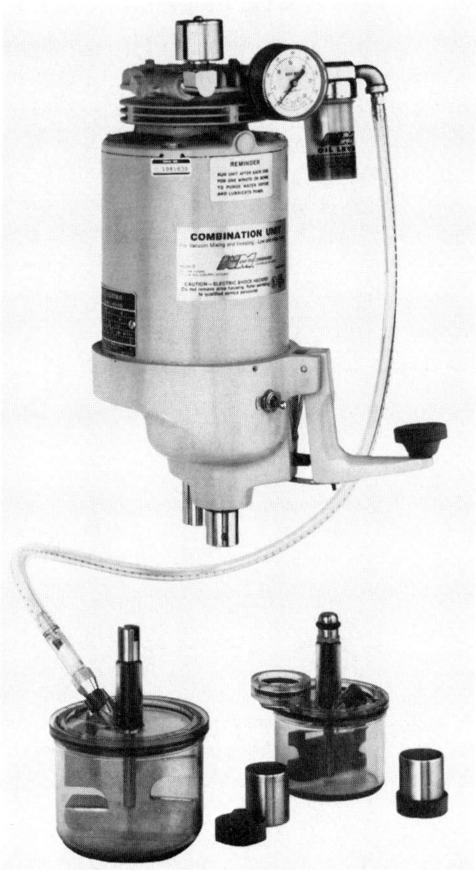

Fig. 18-66. Combination Mixing Unit (Whip Mix) serves as vibrator, power mixer, and vacuum pump. Heavy-duty unit is designed primarily for wall mounting. Different sizes of mixing vessels are available.

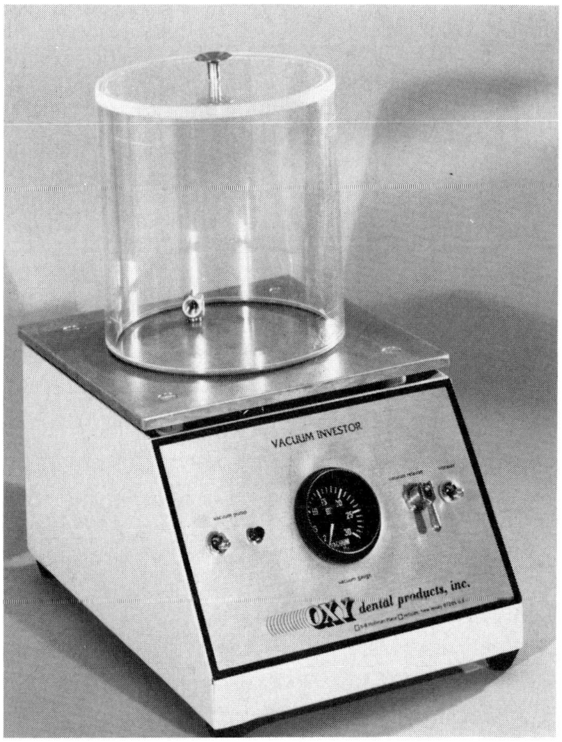

Fig. 18-67. Vacuum Investor (Oxy Dental Products), designed primarily for vacuum investing of wax patterns, is essentially a bell jar for vacuum and vibrator table. Air is withdrawn from mixed investment and vibrated to place within the casting flask (ring).

The Whip Mix Corporation manufactures a combination mixing unit (Fig. 18-66), which serves as a vacuum pump, power mixer, and vibrator. Designed primarily for wall mounting, the unit has several different sizes of mixing vessels for dental stones and investments. The sturdy unit is designed for heavy-duty use.

Oxy Dental Products, Inc., produces a vacuum investor (Fig. 18-67), which is a combination vibrator and vacuum chamber. It is suitable for removing air bubbles from mixed dental stones and investments.

VIBRATORS

Many mixing units provide built-in vibration. The additional use of vibrators for pouring impressions, placing investment around wax patterns in casting flasks (rings), and other similar procedures that do not require the use of vacuum is an integral part of many laboratory procedures. These items are unglamorous workhorses of the laboratory. Most vibrator units offer variation in intensity of vibratory action. Other units offer variation in vibration frequency as well. Most equipment is quite rugged and will provide years of service.

Whaledent International supplies a light duty Toothmaster Investment Vibrator (Fig. 18-68), which is suitable for placement of mixed investment into cast flasks, pouring of sectional impressions, and vibration of other small items. Vibrating intensity of the table can be varied by adjustment of the control knob.

The Combilador CL-R made by Heraeus Dental Gold Company (Fig. 18-69) is a heavy-duty vibrator that offers variation in both intensity and frequency of vibration. The table of the unit is covered by a rubber cushion, which moderates the sharpness of the vibration and facilitates cleaning.

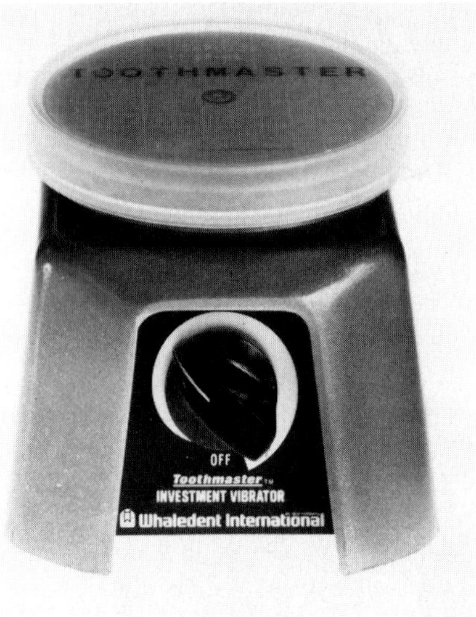

Fig. 18-68. Toothmaster Investment Vibrator (Whaledent International) is designed for light to moderate use. Unit is used primarily for pouring sectional and complete arch impressions and for investing wax patterns. Intensity of vibration can be varied. Vibrating table is covered by a resilient plastic cover that is easily cleaned.

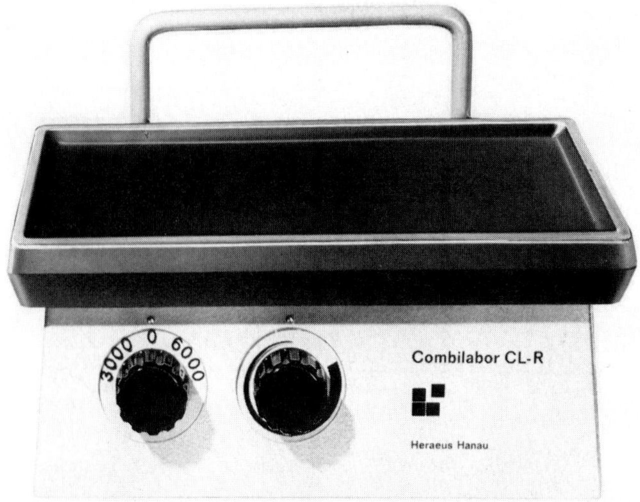

Fig. 18-69. Combilador CL-R Vibrator (Heraeus) is a heavy-duty vibrating unit with a rubber-covered table, to attenuate vibratory shock, that is easily cleaned. Intensity as well as frequency of vibration can be varied by controls on face of apparatus.

ELECTRIC WAX SPATULAS AND WAXING EQUIPMENT

Emphasis on extensive rehabilitation procedures incorporating occlusal reconstruction, on development of occlusion on fully adjustable articulators, and on waxing of frames for ceramic restorations and fixed partial dentures has resulted in the development of equipment to facilitate waxing procedures and techniques. Several manufacturers supply electric wax spatulas and other similar equipment that provides for variation in spatula temperature to match waxes and applications.

Belle de St. Claire provides several items to aid in waxing (Fig. 18-70). The Micromatic waxing unit (upper left) has a wax pen with interchangeable tips and an electric temperature indicator to monitor tip temperature. A larger unit (lower right) provides two wax pens, the individual temperature of which can be varied, and a gas burner in addition. A valuable piece of equipment for waxing of copings for metal-ceramic crowns is a wax dipping pot (upper right) for developing a uniform thickness of wax. Variation in the thickness of the wax can be obtained by increasing or decreasing the temperature of the melted wax. The unit employs a special wax for this purpose.

The Combilador CL-EW electric wax spatula (Fig. 18-71) is made by Heraeus Dental Gold Company. The temperature is controlled by a sliding resistance bar. Interchangeable tips offer a variety of sizes and shapes. The wax tips come to temperature quickly. An integrated electrical circuit in the control protects against overly high temperature and overload.

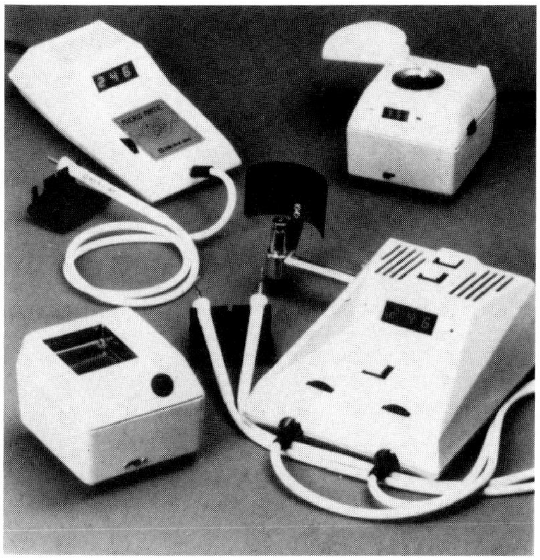

Fig. 18-70. Micro-Matic Waxing Unit (Belle de St. Claire) *(upper left)* has single electric wax spatula with a series of replaceable tips. Tip temperature is shown on LED readout. Temperature can be varied to suit wax and tip size being used. A larger unit *(lower right)* has two wax pens or spatulas individually controlled for temperature. Unit also has provision for gas burner. A wax-pot *(upper right)* is used as dipping pot for waxing of copings for metal ceramic frames. Thickness of wax shell is determined by type and temperature of wax.

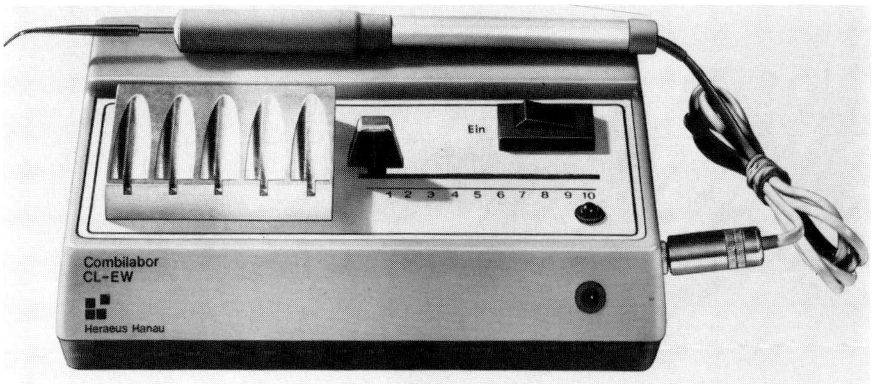

Fig. 18-71. Combilador CL-EW Waxing Unit (Heraeus) has different size and style tips for waxing occlusion and margins of crowns. Temperature of tip can be varied by sliding resistance bar. Novel design of holder for extra tips allows quick and easy change of tips while heated.

ACKNOWLEDGMENTS

The following manufacturers should be thanked for their cooperation and generosity in supplying photographs and descriptions of the equipment illustrated. Without their assistance, the completion of this chapter would have been much more difficult. Sincere thanks are expressed to the following organizations and their dedicated representatives: Almore International, Portland, Ore.; APM-Sterngold, Stamford, Conn.; Belle de St Claire, Van Nuys, Calif.; Bell International, Burlingame, Calif.; Denar Corporation, Anaheim, Calif.; AB Dentatus, Hagerston, Sweden; Esmadent/Esma Chemicals, Inc., Highland Park, IL.; Teledyne/Hanau, Buffalo, N.Y.; Handler Manufacturing Company, Westfield, N.J.; Heraeus Dental Gold Corporation, Queens Village, N.Y.; J.F.Jelenko (Penwalt/Jelenko), Armonk, N.Y.; Jelrus Dental Products Corporation, New Hyde Park, N.Y.; L and R Manufacturing Company, Kearny, N.J.; J.M. Ney Company, Bloomfield, Conn.; Oxy Dental Products Inc., Hillside, N.J.; TMJ Instrument Company, Santa Ana, Calif.; Unitek Corporation, Monrovia, Calif.; Whaledent International, New York, N.Y.; Whip Mix Corporation, Louisville, Ky.; and Williams Gold Company, Buffalo, N.Y.

APPENDIX

MANUFACTURER'S INDEX

Aderer, J. Inc.
21-25 44th Ave.
Long Island City, NY 11101
(212) 392-7272

Almore International
P.O. Box 25214
Portland, OR. 97225
(503) 643-6633
(800) 547-1511)

American Dental Mfg. Co., Inc.
Box 4546
Missoula, MT 59806
(406) 728-7700
(800) 548-9272

American Dental Supply
53 Blenheim Dr.
Easton, PA 18042
(215) 252-1464

American Thermocraft Corp.
60 Franklin St.
East Orange, NJ 070l7
(201) 674-4550

APM-Sterngold
Div. Sterndent
90 Viaduct Rd.
Stamford, CT 06907
(203) 348-5111
(800) 423-9942

Attachments International
328 N. San Mateo Dr.
San Mateo, CA 9440l
(415) 347-5594

Atwood Industries
P.O. Box 655
5501A Reseda Blvd.
Tarzana, CA 91356

Aurium Research Corp.
130 County Courthouse Rd.
Garden City Park, NY 11040
(516) 741-0300
(800) 645-6110

Baldor Electric Co.
5711 S. 7th St.
Ft. Smith, AR 72902
(501) 646-4711
Telex 537425

Bambi Air Compressors
10 Eyre St.
Springhill
Birmingham, B187AA, U.K.

Bausch and Lomb
1400 N. Goodman St.
Rochester, NY 14602
(716) 338-6000

Bell International
1320 Marston Rd.
Burlingame, CA 94010
(415) 348-2055

Belle de St. Claire
16145 Valerio St.
Van Nuys, CA 92406
(213) 988-6644

Harry J. Bosworth, Co.
7227 N. Hamlin Ave.
Skokie, IL 60076
(312) 679-3400

Brasseler U.S.A.
800 King George Blvd.
Savannah, GA 31405
(912) 925-8825
(800) 841-4522

Buffalo Dental Mfg. Co., Inc.
2911 Atlantic Ave.
Brooklyn, NY 11207
(212) 277-5400

Busch and Co.
Postfach 149,5250
Engelskirchen
West Germany 0-22-63/4041

Cadco Products
8890 Regent St.
Los Angeles, CA 90034
(213) 204-1203
(800) 421-0782

Candulor Dental GmbH
7703 Rielasingen-Worblingen 2
Am Riderngraben 4
West Germany 0-77-31/2-29-56

Candulor Dental
Am Wasser 55
8049 Zurich
Switzerland (051) 567773

Carborundum Co.
P.O. Box 156
Niagara Falls, NY 14302

Cast-Rite Tech. Dental Products
Rt.5, Box 240
Murray, KY 42071

L.D. Caulk Co.
Div. Dentsply International, Inc.
P.O. Box 359
Milford, DE 19963
(302) 421-4511
(800) 441-8448

Ceka N.V.
Century Center-de Keyserlei 60, Bus 44
2000 Antwerp, Belgium
(031) 32-06-11
Telex 71147

Cendres and Metaux SA, Ors Dentaire
Rt. de Boujean 122
2501 Biel-Bienne
Switzerland

Ceramco, Inc.
Div. Johnson and Johnson
20 Lake Dr. CN 7065
East Windsor, NJ 08520
(609) 443-3300
(800) 257-9508

Chayes Virginia, Inc.
8233 Baumgart Rd.
Evansville, IN 47711
(812) 867-6451

Clev-Dent
Div., Cavitron Corp.
15400 Commerce Park Dr.
Brook Park, OH 44142
(216) 267-2800

Coe Laboratories, Inc.
3737 W. 127th St.
Chicago, IL 60658
(312) 568-2100

Corning Rubber Co.
578 Gates Ave.
Brooklyn, NY 11221
(212) 574-7557

Cratex Rubberized Abrasives
1600 Rollins Road
Burlingame, CA 94010
(415) 697-1600

Crescent Dental Mfg. Co.
7750 W. 47th St.
Lyons, IL 60534
(312) 447-8050

Cutter Dental
2200 Powell St.
P.O. Box 8817
Emeryville, CA 94608
(415) 420-4203

De Trey A.G.
Nurenberg Str. 19/P.O. Box 566
CH 8037 Zurich
Switzerland

Degussa Dental, Inc.
181 W. Orangethorpe
Placentia, CA 92670
(800) 221-0168 (East)
(800) 323-8124 (Midwest)
(800) 854-3015 (West)

Denar Corp.
901 East Cerritos St.
Anaheim, CA 92805
(714) 776-9000
TWX 910-591-2718

Denram Products
236 W. Maple Ave.
Monrovia, CA 91016
(213) 359-8376

Densco, Teledyne
3840 Forest St.
Denver, CO 80207
(303) 399-0240

Dental Plastics and Products
P.O. Box 894
Kansas City, MO 64141
(913) 782-2112

Dental Technology Systems, Inc.
50 Curtner Ave.
Campbell, CA 95008
(408) 377-4504

Dentsply International
570 W. College Ave.
York, PA 17405
(717) 845-7511

Di-Equi Dental Products
P.O. Box 10165 Church St. Sta.
New York NY 10249
(914) 297-4387

William Dixon Co.
750 Washington Ave.
Carlstadt, NJ 07072
(201) 935-0100
TWX 710-989-0141

Durand-Girard Metaux Precieux
22-23 Rue Junerie
69005 Lyons, France

Duro-Test Corporation
2321 Kennedy Blvd.
North Bergen, NJ 07047
(201) 867-7000

Ellman Dental Mfg. Co.
1135 Railroad Ave.
Hewlett, NY 11557
(516) 569-1482

Emesco, Teledyne
41 Bancker St.
Englewood, NJ 07631
(201) 568-5368

Englehard Industries
700 Blair Rd.
Carteret, NJ 07008
(201) 321-5000
(800) 631-5599

Esmadent
Div. Esma Chemicals
P.O. Box 162
Highland Park, IL 60035
(312) 433-6116

Flexiplast, Inc.
1010 McDonald Ave.
Brooklyn, NY 11230
(212) 438-3270

General Scientific Equipment
Limekiln Pike and Williams Ave.
Philadelphia, PA 19150
(215) 424-1550
(800) 523-0166

Gnathographic Specialties
137 S. Prospect
Tustin, CA 92680
(714) 838-3462

Hammond Dental Mfg. Co.
4496 Industrial St.
Simi Valley, CA 93063
(805) 527-8822

Hanau-Teledyne
80 Sonwill Dr.
Buffalo, NY 14225
(716) 684-0110

Handler Mfg. Co.
612 North Ave.
East Westfield, NJ 07090
(201) 233-7796

Harmony Dental Products
1114 Mission St.
So. Pasadena, CA 91030
(213) 799-0984

Harper Buffing Machine Co.
363 Ellington Rd.
East Hartford, CT 06108
(203) 389-7471

Heat Systems Ultrasonics
38 East Mall
Plainview, NY 11803
(516) 694-9555

Helvoigt "Wax" Torch
1325 Mariners Drive
Newport Beach, CA 92660

Heraeus Dental Gold
222-34 96th Ave.
Queens Village, NY 11429

Higson Industrial Tool
P.O. Box 41274
Los Angeles, CA 90041
(213) 255-5261

Howmedica, Inc.
5101 S. Keeler Ave.
Chicago, IL 60632
(312) 735-0606

Huggins Engineering
2070 Walsh Ave.
Santa Clara, CA 95050
(408) 727-6766

K.H. Huppert Co.
16815 S. State St.
South Holland, IL 60473
(312) 339-2022
Telex Huppert Shnd 25-4276

Hygienic Corp.
1245 Home Ave.
Akron, OH 44310
(216) 633-8460

Injection Specialties
P.O. Box 670
Tuckerton, NJ 08087
(201) 569-4775

International Laser Systems
3404 N. Orange Blossom Trail
Orlando, FL 32804
(305) 843-4731

J.F. Jelenko, and Co.
Div. Pennwalt Corp.
99 Business Park Dr.
Armonk, NY 10504
(800) 431-1785
(914) 273-8600

Jelrus Dental Products Corp.
2020 Jericho Turnpike
New Hyde Park, NY 11040

Jupiter Engineering, Inc.
138 Evernia St.
Jupiter, FL 33458
(305) 746-3984

Justi, H.D. Co.
2233 Stratham Blvd.
Oxnard, CA 93033
(805) 487-9868
(800) 235-4639

Kavo E.W.L.
21-25 44th Ave.
Long Island City, NY 11101

L & R Manufacturing Co.
577 Elm St.
Kearny, NJ 07032
(201) 991 5330

Labline Instruments
Lab-Line Plaza
Melrose Park, IL 60160

Lab-Master Production Tool
4509 Forest Ave.
Kansas City, MO 64110

Lares Manufacturing Co.
1581 Industrial Rd.
San Carlos, CA 94070
(415) 595-5971

Lasco Diamond Products
P.O. Box 33
Chatsworth, CA 91311
(213) 882-2423

MDS Products Co.
1440 S. State College Blvd. 3-14
Anaheim, CA 92806
(714) 991-3606

Microflame, Inc.
3724 Oregon Ave. So.
Minneapolis, MN 55426
(612) 935-3777

Micro-Mega SA
11 Rue des Mouettes
1227 Geneva
Switzerland

Mizzy, Inc.
P.O. Box 632
Clifton Forge, VA 24422
(703) 862-4151

Modern Materials Mfg.
Div. Columbus Dental
1021 So. 10th St.
St. Louis, MO 63104

Motloid Co.
325 W. Huron
Chicago, IL 60610
(312) 944-2448

Moyco Industries, Inc.
21st. and Clearfield Sts.
Philadelphia, PA 19132
(215) 229-0470
(800) 523-3676

Myerson Tooth Corp.
Div. Pfizer Co.
90 Hamilton St.
Cambridge, MA 02174
(617) 876-6501
(800) 225-5774

Mynol Inc.
600 Parkway
Brodnail, PA 19008
(215) 353-6767

J.M. Ney Co.
Ney Industrial Park
Bloomfield, CT 06002
(203) 242-2281
(800) 243-1942

Niranium Corp.
34-37 11th St.
Long Island City, NY 11106
(212) 721-9015
(800) 221-1422

Nobilium/American Gold Co.
Div. of CMP Inustries, Inc.
935 Broadway
Albany, NY 12201
(800) 833-2343
Telex 710-441-8218 VMPINO ALB

Ohaus Scale Corp.
29 Hanover Rd.
Florham Park, NJ 07932

Oxy Dental Products, Inc.
6 Hoffman Place
Hillside, NJ 07205
(201) 372-1298
(800) 526-4911

Paasche Airbrush Co.
1909-1929 W. Diversey Pkwy.
Chicago, IL 60614
(312) 281-6650

Pacific Dental Products/Pacific Alloy
1717 Old Tustin Ave.
Santa Ana, CA 92701
(800) 854-8391
(714) 953-4287

Parkell Products, Inc.
155 Schmitt Blvd.
Farmingdale, NY 11735
(516) 294-1134

Pascal
2929 NE. Northrup Way
Bellevue, WA 98004
(206) 827-4694

Pease and Curren, Inc. (precious metal refiners)
75 Pennsylvania Ave.
Warwick, RI 02888
(401) 739-6350
Telex 952130

Pentron Corp.
125 Plains Industrial Rd.
P.O. Box 771
Wallingford, CT 06492
(203) 265-3886
(800) 243-3100

Pfingst and Co. Inc.
105 Snyder Rd.
S. Plainfield, NJ 07080
(201) 561-6400

Precision Dental Manufacturing Co.
23 S. Wabash
Chicago, IL 60603
(312) 726-9306

Premier Dental Products
1710 Romano Dr.
Norristown, PA 19401
(215) 277-3800

Ransom and Randolph Co., Div. of Dentsply International
P.O. 905
Toledo, OH 4360l
(419) 241-6261

Reliance Dental Mfg. Co.
5805 W. 117th Place
Worth, IL 60482
(312) 597-6694

Rocky Mountain/Ortho
700 W. Colfax
Denver, CO 80217
(303) 292-3570

Rx Jeneric Gold Co.
Div. Jeneric Industries, Inc.
125 N. Plains Industrial Rs.
P.O. Box 724
Wallingford, CT 06429
(203) 265-7397

Sat-Fin Air Brush Co. Inc.
8970 S.W. 87th Ct.
Miami, FL 33176
(305) 271-5322

Shofu Dental Corp.
4025 Bohannon Dr.
Menlo Park, CA 94025
(415) 324-0085

Slaycris Products
1029 S.W. Washington St.
Portland OR 97025

Star Dental Mfg. Co., Inc.
P.O. Box 896
Valley Forge Corporate Center
Valley Forge, PA 19842
(215) 666-9050

AM-Sterngold
Div. Sterndent Corp.
90 Viaduct Rd.
Stamford, CT 06907
(203) 348-5111
(800) 243-9942

Suter Dental Mfg. Co.
P.O. 1329
Chico, CA 95927
(916) 342-1921

Sybron/Kerr
21200 Wick Rd.
Romulus, MI
(313) 946-7800

George Taub Products, Inc.
277 New York Ave.
Jersey City, NJ 07307
(201) 798-5353

Technical Specialties
487 Elliot Ave.
W. Seattle, WA 98119
(206) 282-0997

Tempil Corp.
2901 Hamilton Blvd.
S. Plainfield, NJ 07080

3-M Company
3M Center Bldg. 225-55
St. Paul, MN 55043
(612) 73308018

Ticonium Co.
Div. CMP Industries
413 N. Pearl St.
Albany, NY 12297
(518) 434-3147
Telex 710 441 8218 CMPIND ALB

TMJ Instrument Co., Inc.
3203 W. Pendleton
Santa Ana, CA 92704
(714) 557-4381
Telex 678 401 TABIRIN

Ultratek International, Inc.
1041 Shary Circle
Concord, CA 94518
(415) 939-7434
Telex 335 467 ULTRATEK CNCD

Union Broach Corp.
36-40 37th St.
Long Island City, NY 111-1
(212) 361-9300
(800) 221 1344
Telex 225159 HCEM

Unitek Corp.
2724 S. Peck Rd.
Monrovia, CA 91016
(213) 445-7960

U.S. Borax and Chemical
3075 Wilshire Blvd.
Los Angeles, CA 90010
(213) 381-5311

Vernon-Benshoff Co., Inc.
413 North Pearl St.
Albany, NY 12207
(518) 434-3147
Telex 710 441 8218 CMPIND ALB

Vibrabrush, Inc.
1345 E. 3900 South Ste. 114
Salt Lake City, UT 84117
(801) 272-4239

Wells Extended Pin and Mfg. Co., Inc.
5861 Flynn Creek Rd.
Comptche, CA 95427
(707) 937-0521

Whaledent Intl.
Div. IPCO Hospital Supply Corp.
236 Fifth Ave.
New York, NY 10001
(212) 696-8000

Whip Mix Corp.
P.O. Box 17183
361 Farmington Ave.
Louisville, KY 40217
(502) 637-1415

Wilkinson Co.
31011 Agoura Rd.
Westlake Village, CA 91361
(213) 889-0050
Telex 698213

Williams Gold Refining Co., Inc.
2978 Main St.
Buffalo, NY 14214
(716) 837-1000
(800) 828-1003
Telex 91-224-Will Gold-Buff

Index

Boldface numbers indicate volumes of *Dental Laboratory Procedures* series: **1**, *Complete dentures;* **2**, *Fixed partial dentures;* **3**, *Removable partial dentures.*

B

C

E

F

G

H

O

P

T

U

V